Fundamentals of Surgical Practice

This is the new, expanded and updated edition of the key text currently available for the first stages of the MRCS examination. Mirroring the exam syllabus, it offers the trainee a clear understanding of the core knowledge required for examination success and incorporates new material reflecting recent developments and the new examination. The chapters have been written by acknowledged experts, many of whom are themselves involved in the training and examining of candidates. Designed to achieve maximum efficiency in learning, the content provides ample detail, key points and suggestions for further reading. In addition to a detailed index, each chapter has its own table of contents for ease of use. It will be indispensable for the new trainee and will also provide established surgeons and other healthcare professionals working in the surgical environment with a modern, authoritative overview of the key areas of surgical practice.

Prof. **Andrew N Kingsnorth** is a Consultant Surgeon at Derriford Hospital in Plymouth and Professor of Surgery at Peninsula Medical School, University of Plymouth. He is currently an associate editor of the International Journal of Surgical Investigation and has been an editorial board member for the British Journal of Surgery (1996–1999). Prof. Kingsnorth also spent many years as a Member of the Court of Examiners of the Royal College of Surgeons of England (1994–2000) and has published over 300 articles and invited chapters in 30 books, as well as co-editing 6 books and co-authoring 1 book.

Aljafri A Majid is a Consultant Cardiothoracic Surgeon at University Hospital, Kuala Lumpur and Professor in the Department of Surgery at the Faculty of Medicine, University of Malaya. He is also a member of the Panel of Examiners for the Royal College of Surgeons of Edinburgh.

Fundamentals of
Surgical Practice

Second Edition

Edited by
Andrew N Kingsnorth and Aljafri A Majid

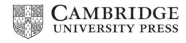

CAMBRIDGE
UNIVERSITY PRESS

CAMBRIDGE UNIVERSITY PRESS
Cambridge, New York, Melbourne, Madrid, Cape Town, Singapore, São Paulo

CAMBRIDGE UNIVERSITY PRESS
The Edinburgh Building, Cambridge CB2 2RU, UK

Published in the United States of America by Cambridge University Press, New York

www.cambridge.org
Information on this title: www.cambridge.org/9780521 677066

First published 1998

Printed in the United Kingdom at the University Press, Cambridge

A record for this book is available from the British Library

Library of Congress in Publication data

ISBN-13   978-0-521-67706-6 paperback
ISBN-10   0-521-67706-8 paperback

Contents

Preface   vii
Contributors   viii

1 Preoperative management   1
F Rosewarne & B Thomson

2 Principles of anaesthesia   16
CMH Gómez & JWW Gothard

3 Postoperative management   39
DM Bowley

4 Nutritional support   50
J Payne-James

**5 Surgical sepsis: prevention
and therapy**   58
QM Nunes, CV Soong & BJ Rowlands

6 Surgical techniques and technology   71
RM Kirk

**7 Trauma: general principles of
management**   89
C Macutkiewicz & ID Anderson

8 Intensive care   111
A Neville & AA Majid

9 Principles of cancer management   149
AP Forrest & MS Duxbury

**10 Ethics, legal aspects and
assessment of effectiveness**   184
SJ Leinster

**11 Haemopoietic and lymphoreticular
systems: anatomy, physiology and
pathology**   199
DC Strauss, AJ Botha & I Taylor

12 Upper gastrointestinal surgery   230
TJ Wheatley

13 Lower gastrointestinal surgery   249
DM Bowley & C Cunningham

14 Hernia management   264
AN Kingsnorth

15 Vascular surgery   286
JR Barwell & ZH Khan

16 Endocrine surgery   304
D Lee & RG Hardy

17 The breast   322
SD Heys

18 Thoracic surgery   351
CP Clarke

19 Genitourinary system   369
N Harris & A Dickinson

20 Head and neck   391
WWK King, JKS Woo & DSC Lam

21 The central nervous system   415
J Palmer

22 Musculoskeletal system   440
SP Frostick & V Sahni

23 Paediatric surgery   493
PKH Tam

Index   525

Preface

One of the first challenges for aspiring surgeons to negotiate is the intercollegiate MRCS examination, which has replaced similar examinations previously run by the four Royal Surgical Colleges. The first edition of Fundamentals of Surgical Practice has become a recommended and standard text for the MRCS examination largely due to the reputation of its contributors. As editors of the second edition we are delighted that the majority of our authors have signed up to a revision and update of their chapters. There are some new contributors and some of our senior authors have revised their chapters with junior colleagues attuned to modern surgical thinking.

Technological aspects of surgery have undergone rapid change in the last two decades. A parallel change has taken place in the educational concepts underpinning transfer of basic knowledge into surgical practice. The knowledge base itself may not have changed a great deal but its method of presentation has. Therefore, we have selected authors with a gift for imparting the enthusiasm of their specialist interest in a straightforward and easily understood way but without missing out on the detail. In this edition the alimentary system has been expanded into two chapters on Upper gastrointestinal and Lower gastrointestinal surgery and a separate chapter on Hernia management has been added to emphasise the importance of surgery of the abdominal wall as an expanding area of specialist interest. The successful format of the previous edition has been retained and we are confident that this book will continue to remain a popular reference source for those beginning their postgraduate training in surgery.

Andrew N Kingsnorth
Aljafri A Majid
February 2005

Contributors

Iain D Anderson
BSc MD FRCS FRCS(Gen)
Consultant Surgeon
Hope Hospital, Manchester
Senior Lecturer in Surgery, University of Manchester
Hillsborough Tutor in Critical Care, The Royal College of
Surgeons of England, Manchester, England

JR Barwell
Consultant Vascular and Renal Transplant Surgeon,
Derriford Hospital, Plymouth, UK

Abraham J Botha
MD FRCS
Department of Upper GI and General Surgery
St Thomas' Hospital, London, UK

Douglas M Bowley
Department of Colorectal Surgery, John Radcliffe Hospital
Headley Way, Headington, Oxford, UK

C Peter Clarke
MBBS(Melb) FRACS FACS FCCP
Senior Thoracic Surgeon
Austin and Repatriation Medical Centre, Heidelberg,
Victoria, Australia
Professorial Associate, Department of Surgery, University of
Melbourne, Victoria, Australia

Christopher Cunningham
Department of Colorectal Surgery, John Radcliffe Hospital
Headley Way, Headington, Oxford, UK

Andrew Dickinson
MD FRCS (Urol)
Derriford Hospital, Plymouth, UK

Mark S Duxbury

Oleg Eremin
MD FRCS(Ed) FRACS
Honorary Consultant Surgeon
Aberdeen Royal Hospitals NHS Trust, Aberdeen
Regius Professor of Surgery, University of Aberdeen, Aberdeen
Examiner in Surgery, Royal College of Surgeons,
Edinburgh, UK

Mark Fordham
FRCS
Consultant Urologist
Royal Liverpool University Hospital
Member, Court of Examiners, Royal College of Surgeons,
England

A Patrick Forrest
FRCS(Ed, Eng, Glasg) MD ChM HonDSc (Wales, Chinese
University of Hong Kong) LLD (Dundee) HonFACS FRACS
FRCS(Can.) FRCR
Professor Emeritus, University of Edinburgh
Senior Lecturer in Surgery, University of Glasgow
Professor of Surgery, Welsh National School of Medicine
Regius Professor of Clinical Surgery,
University of Edinburgh, Member of Council, Royal College
of Surgeons, Edinburgh, UK

Simon P Frostick
MA DM FRCS
Honorary Consultant
Royal Liverpool University Hospital
Professor of Orthopaedics, University of Liverpool,
Liverpool, UK

Carlos MH Gomez
LMS FRCA
Honorary Senior Registrar and Research Fellow
Department of Anaesthesia and Intensive Care, Charing
Cross Hospital, London, UK

John WW Gothard
MBBS Dip(Obst) RCOG FRCA
Consultant Anaesthetist,
Royal Brompton Hospital
Honorary Senior Lecturer, National Heart and Lung
Institute, Imperial College School of Medicine,
London, UK

Roshan Lall Gupta
MS FRCS(Eng) FRCS(Ed) FACS
Emeritus Professor of Surgery
Meerut, India

Robert G Hardy
BSc MB ChB PhD
Department of Endocrinology, Royal Infirmary,
Edinburgh, UK

DR Harper
BSc MD FRCS
Consultant Surgeon
Falkirk and District Royal Infirmary NHS Trust
Honorary Senior Lecturer, Department of Surgery,
University of Edinburgh
Examiner, Royal College of Surgeons,
Edinburgh and Royal College of Physicians and Surgeons,
Glasgow, UK

Neil Harris
MD MRCS(Eng)
Department of Urology,
Derriford Hospital, Plymouth, UK

Steven D Heys
MD PhD FRCS(Glas) FRCS(Ed)
Honorary Consultant Surgeon
Aberdeen Royal Hospitals NHS Trust, Aberdeen
Reader in Surgery, University of Aberdeen, Aberdeen
Examiner in Surgery, Royal College of Surgeons,
Glasgow, UK

Jason Payne-James
19 Speldhurst Road, London, E9 7EH, UK

RV Jeffreys
MChir FRCS(Ed)
Consultant Neurosurgeon
Walton Centre for Neurology and Neurosurgery, Liverpool
Clinical Lecturer in Neurosurgery, University of Liverpool,
Liverpool, UK
Examiner, Royal College of Surgeons, Edinburgh
Member of Specialist Advisory Board in Neurosurgery,
Royal College of Surgeons of Edinburgh
Previously Examiner in Conjoint FRCS (Surgical Neurology),
Edinburgh, UK

ZH Khan
Locum Consultant Vascular Surgeon,
Derriford Hospital, Plymouth, UK

Walter WK King
MD FRCS(Ed) FRCS FACS FCSHK
Chief, Division of Head and Neck – Plastic and
Reconstructive Surgery
Prince of Wales Hospital, Shatin, Hong Kong
Professor of Head and Neck – Plastic and Reconstructive
Surgery, The Chinese University of Hong Kong, Hong Kong,
China

Panel of Examiners (1992–1998), Conjoint Fellowship
Examination of the Royal College of Surgeons of Edinburgh
and the College of Surgeons of Hong Kong
Examiner, Joint Inter Collegiate Higher Specialist
Examination, RCS Edinburgh/CSHK Conjoint Examination
(1996–1998)

Andrew N Kingsnorth
BSc MS FRCS
Consultant Surgeon
Derriford Hospital, Plymouth
Honorary Professor of Surgery, Peninsula Medical School
External Undergraduate Examiner, Oxford, London and
Kuala Lumpur, Malaysia
Member, Court of Examiners, Royal College of Surgeons of
England, UK

RM Kirk
MS FRCS
Honorary Consulting Surgeon
Royal Free Hospital, London, UK

Dennis SC Lam
MBBS DO FRCS FRCOphth
Department of Ophthalmology and Visual Sciences
Prince of Wales Hospital
Associate Professor, Department of Ophthalmology and
Visual Sciences, The Chinese University of Hong Kong,
Hong Kong, China

David Lee
BSc MB ChB FRCS(Ed)
Consultant General and Endocrine Surgeon, Royal
Infirmary, Edinburgh, UK

Sam J Leinster
BSc MD FRCS
Lead Clinician, Breast Cancer Services
Honorary Consultant Surgeon, Royal Liverpool and
Broadgreen Hospitals
Professor of Surgery and Director of Medical Studies,
University of Liverpool
Examiner, Royal College of Surgeons, Edinburgh
Examiner, PLAB, General Medical Council
Member, Training Committee and Examinations
Committee, Royal College of Surgeons, Edinburgh, UK

Roderick Anderson Little
PhD FRCPath FFAEM
Professor of Surgical Science
University of Manchester, Manchester
Head, MRC Trauma Group, Director NWIRC, Member,
Court of Examiners, Royal College of Surgeons, London, UK

C Macutkiewicz
Department of Surgery, Hope Hospital,
University of Manchester, School of Medicine

Aljafri A Majid
MBBS BmedSc(Hons) FRCS(Ed) FRCSEd(CT)
Consultant Cardiothoracic Surgeon
University Hospital, Kuala Lumpur, Malaysia
Professor and Head, Department of Surgery, Faculty of
Medicine, University of Malaya, Malaysia
Member, Panel of Examiners, Royal College of Surgeons,
Edinburgh, UK

Angela Neville
Department of Surgery, University of Southern California,
Los Angeles, USA

QM Nunes
Clinical Fellow in General Surgery, Queen's Medical Centre,
Nottingham, UK

Fred Rosewarne
MBBS FANZLA
Assistant Director
Department of Anaesthesia, Royal Melbourne Hospital
Clinical Instructor, Royal Melbourne and Western Hospital
Clinical School
Supervisor of Training in Anaesthesia, Royal Melbourne
Hospital, Melbourne, Australia

Brian J Rowlands
MD FRCS FACS
Consultant Surgeon
Queen's Medical Centre, University of Nottingham,
Nottingham, UK
Professor of Surgery; Chairman of RCS England Working
Party on Care of the Critically Ill Surgical Patient

RC Smith
MB ChB ChM FRCS(Ed)
Consultant Surgeon
Falkirk and District Royal Infirmary NHS Trust
Honorary Clinical Teacher, University of Edinburgh
Convenor of The Examinations Committee, Royal College of
Surgeons of Edinburgh, Edinburgh, UK

Chee Voon Soong
MB BCH FRCSI
Specialist Registrar in General and Vascular Surgery
Royal Victoria Hospital, Queen's University of Belfast, Belfast
Northern Ireland Postgraduate Surgical Training
Programme, UK

Dirk C Strauss
MBChB, FCS(SA), MMed(Stell)
Department of Upper GI Surgery, St Thomas' Hospital,
London, UK

Paul KH Tam
MBBS(HK) ChM(Liverpool) FRCS(Edin, Glas, Ire) FRCPCH
FHKAM(Surgery) FCSHK
Chief, Division of Paediatric Surgery
Department of Surgery, Queen Mary Hospital
Chair of Paediatric Surgery, Department of Surgery, The
University of Hong Kong Medical Centre
Quandom Fellow, Lincoln College, University of Oxford.
(Formerly, Clinical Reader, Director and Consultant (Hon.)
in Paediatric Surgery, University of Oxford and John
Radcliffe Hospital, Oxford 1990–1996)
Examiner in Fellowship (General Surgery), Royal College of
Surgeons, Edinburgh
Examiner, Intercollegiate Specialty Board in Paediatric
Surgery (UK)
Examiner in Diploma of Child Health, Royal College of
Physicians (UK)
Examiner in Fellowship (General Surgery), College of
Surgeons of Hong Kong, Hong Kong, China

Irving Taylor
MD ChM FRCS
Consultant Surgeon
University College London Hospitals NHS Trust, London
Professor of Surgery and Head of Department of Surgery
University College London, London, UK

Robert JS Thomas
MBBS MS FRACS FRCS
Western Hospital, Victoria, Australia
Department of Surgery, University of Melbourne, Victoria,
Australia

Benjamin Thomson
Department of Surgical Oncology,
Peter MacCallum Cancer Centre

TJ Wheatley
Consultant Upper GI Surgeon, Derriford Hospital,
Plymouth, UK

John Woo
FRCSEd FHKAM (otorhinolaryngology)
Consultant
Department of Surgery, Prince of Wales Hospital, Chinese
University of Hong Kong
Adjunct Associate Professor, Chinese University of Hong
Kong, Hong Kong, China

1

Preoperative Management

Fred Rosewarne[1] and Benjamin Thomson[2]

[1]Department of Anaesthesia, Royal Melbourne Hospital and Western Hospital Clinical School, Melbourne, Victoria, Australia
[2]Department of Surgical Oncology, Peter MacCallum Cancer Centre

CONTENTS

Preoperative assessment	1
Introduction	1
General preparation	2
Preoperative assessment of fitness for anaesthesia and surgery	3
Cardiovascular system	3
Respiratory system	5
Central nervous system	6
Renal system	7
Liver	7
Endocrine system	8
Haematology	9
Lifestyle influences on anaesthetic risk	10
Concurrent drug treatment	11
Prophylaxis of thromboembolic disease	13
Preadmission clinics	14
Routine investigations prior to surgery	14
Further reading	15

goals. A plan for anaesthesia, postoperative care and pain relief can then be constructed and this generally involves:

- informing patient of the proposed procedure;
- obtaining informed consent for proposed procedure, including any risks from not having the procedure;
- assessing pre-existing conditions and estimation of their impact on physiological reserve;
- planning the type of anaesthesia guided by the above information and patient preferences;
- planning postoperative management of any pre-existing conditions;
- planning analgesia.

The American Society of Anesthesiologists' (ASA) classification has found wide acceptance as a broad-based system for classifying the general fitness of patients for surgery and their predicted mortality (Table 1.1).

Factors increasing the operative risk include:
- age >70 years;
- surgery >3 h duration;
- emergency versus elective operation;
- presence of associated illnesses (especially uncontrolled diabetes or heart failure);
- physiological reserve impaired;
- obesity, malnutrition, immunosuppression and cancer;
- radiotherapy, steroid use.

PREOPERATIVE ASSESSMENT

Introduction

The preoperative evaluation of patients is intended to reduce the morbidity and mortality associated with surgery and anaesthesia. The relative benefits of the proposed operation need to be balanced against the possible adverse effects that may result from anaesthesia and surgery. The severity of any underlying medical conditions and their impact on physiological reserve must be assessed. Optimisation of the management of any underlying medical condition is undertaken. It is necessary to take a detailed history, examine the patient and obtain appropriate laboratory investigations to achieve these

Table 1.1. ASA classification of illness.

1	No organic, physiological, biochemical or psychiatric disturbance
2	Mild to moderate systemic disturbance which does not limit normal activities
3	Severe systemic disturbance which limits normal activities but is not incapacitating
4	Severe, life-threatening systemic disorders
5	Moribund with little chance of survival
6	Increasingly ASA 6, is used to designate an organ donor
E	'E' placed after the number, indicates an emergency operation

General preparation

Consent

Consent is a very important process in the preoperative management of patients. It is much more than informing the patient of the risks of the procedure and should include discussion of:

- An explanation of the condition requiring surgery and why that surgical procedure is considered the best option.
- Other treatments that could be considered as well as the expected outcome without treatment.
- A description of what will be done at the time of the procedure (i.e. what will be removed, site of incision and reconstruction).
- The expected anaesthetic management (i.e. general anaesthesia versus regional anaesthesia and sedation).
- What to expect following the anaesthetic (i.e. drain tubes, central venous and urinary catheters, stomas, etc.).
- Expected long-term outcomes and implications of the procedure.
- Confirmation of the side and site of the procedure to avoid 'wrong site or side' procedures.

To aid patient education and consent many surgical colleges and societies produce patient information pamphlets for common procedures.

Discussion of the complications of surgery can be an exhaustive process if all possible problems are discussed. Some patients may require a further consultation for follow-up discussion. Many patients will require the presence of a professional interpreter for the consent process, with family used for translation only when an interpreter is not available. Each patient needs to be individually assessed as some complications may be of greater significance than for other patients, even if very uncommon or rare. The discussion of risk for a procedure should be based on a balance of the benefit of the operation against its complications. In this component of the consent there should be discussion of:

- Common risks of any procedure and plans to avoid them (i.e. the use of heparin to avoid deep venous thrombosis, the importance of postoperative mobilisation in preventing deep venous thrombosis and pulmonary atelectasis);
- Specific risks of the procedure;
- Anaesthetic consent.

The legal interpretation of the consent process often differs to the medical interpretation. The laws regarding the consent process differ in each country. Furthermore, the age a patient is able to give informed consent differs according to the country and social circumstances. Health care providers must acquaint themselves with the particular legal and consent protocols in their locality and health care facility. Some specific situations should be considered in detail:

- *Emergency*: When urgency or the patient's clinical state precludes the obtaining of a valid consent, life-saving treatment may commence. This decision must be documented.
- *Under-age patients*: Parents can consent for their children however the legal situation becomes increasingly complex

Table 1.2. **Effect of age on physiological processes.**

Function	% decline from 20–30 to 60–80 years
Cardiac output	20
Muscle mass	20
Maximal breathing capacity	60
Cortical neurones	50
Hepatic blood flow	25–40

for adolescents over 16 years, with considerable variation between countries and states/provinces. The clinician should be aware of the local practice.

- *Incompetent patients*: Consent should be obtained from the legally appointed guardian or the 'Person Responsible' as defined by the local Guardianship Board or equivalent.
- *Religious and cultural issues*: Restricted consent can be given by patients to allow certain treatments but not for others. A common example is Jehovah's Witnesses who may consent to surgery but not allow blood transfusion. The issues involved with the use of cell-savers and extra-corporeal bypass and specific blood products needs to be discussed in detail with Jehovah's Witnesses because there is some variation in attitudes to ensure there is no misunderstanding. In emergency situations where the patient's wishes are not clearly known, the patient must be treated according to Standard Protocols. In the case of children under 16 where blood transfusion is deemed necessary, application to the appropriate authority will be required if parental consent for transfusion is withheld.

Emergencies

In the emergency situation, estimation of physical status is compromised by the need to manage the presenting illness. A history may need to be taken from relatives during preoperative resuscitation and thorough physical examination may be difficult. Hospital records, if available, are invaluable to exclude systemic illness. Accurate estimation of fluid status is an essential part of successful preoperative management. Knowledge of the time course of the illness is important in guiding this process since previous fluid losses are particularly difficult to assess. Ongoing losses must be documented, bearing in mind that concealed losses are notoriously difficult to estimate. Serum electrolyte concentrations may significantly underestimate fluid losses in the presence of isotonic losses. Correction of problems such as fluid deficit and electrolyte imbalance can proceed while the patient is being prepared for emergency surgery. Preoperative resuscitation can nearly always be performed prior to surgery except in cases of life-threatening haemorrhage.

Age

Increasing age increases perioperative risk because of progressive reduction in functional reserve of organ systems as well as increasing illnesses associated with increasing age. The commonest co-morbidities are arthritis, hypertension, diabetes and cardiac disease (Table 1.2).

PREOPERATIVE ASSESSMENT OF FITNESS FOR ANAESTHESIA AND SURGERY

Cardiovascular system

Cardiac risk factors

Numerous studies have attempted to define the aetiological factors associated with perioperative cardiac complications and several risk assessment indices have been published. Patients may be classified as low risk (<3%), intermediate (3–10%) or high risk (>10%) of major adverse cardiac events.

Major risk factors are:
- myocardial infarction within previous 3 (major risk) or 6 (moderate risk) months;
- unstable angina;
- untreated cardiac failure;
- significant aortic valve stenosis;
- untreated hypertension.

Relative risk factors are:
- prior myocardial infarction;
- jugular vein distension (or S3 gallop);
- non-sinus rhythm;
- ventricular ectopic beats/min;
- age >70 years;
- surgery >3 h duration;
- emergency surgery;
- significant medical impairment: $PaO_2 < 60$ mmHg, $PaCO_2 > 50$ mmHg and $K < 3$ mmol/l;
- chronic liver impairment.

Postoperative cardiac complications result from patients with impaired physiological reserve being unable to cope with the stresses of the perioperative period. Factors impinging on the physiological reserve include:
- myocardial depression from sepsis and anaesthetic agents;
- variable pre- and after-load due to fluid shifts associated with disease, surgery and fluid replacement regimens;
- reduction in oxygen transport secondary to myocardial depression, intrapulmonary shunting, blood loss and pain- or drug-induced hypoventilation;
- miscellaneous factors such as hypotension, acidosis, tachycardia, fluctuating blood levels of therapeutic agents.

Ischaemic heart disease

Recent consensus guidelines from the USA (American Heart Association and American College of Physicians) plus research in Europe has produced algorithms to assist evaluation of at-risk patients prior to non-cardiac surgery (American College of Physicians, 1997; Chassot et al., 2002).

Myocardial infarction

The risk of perioperative myocardial infarction is most strongly correlated with previous infarction history (Table 1.3) or the

Table 1.3. Risk of myocardial infarction.

• No previous infarction	0–5%
• Acute myocardial infarction >6 months previously	6%
• Myocardial infarction 3–6 months ago	10%
• Infarction <3 months ago	30%

Table 1.4. Risk of myocardial infarction.

Class 1	Angina with strenuous exercise
Class 2	Angina with moderate exercise
Class 3	Angina after climbing 1 flight of stairs or walking 1 block
Class 4	Angina at rest

presence of inadequately treated cardiac failure. The mortality rate from perioperative myocardial infarction is high (40–60%). Previously 6 months was considered the minimum time between uncomplicated myocardial infarction and elective surgery, but recent data supports a 3-month minimum period. In the event that surgery cannot be delayed, a full assessment of cardiac function is required and intraoperative monitoring using transoesophageal echo (TOE) or Swan–Ganz catheter may be desirable. Postoperatively, the patient should be cared for on an intensive care unit for the first 24 h because the risk of reinfarction continues in the postoperative period (15% in the first 48 h). In the elective patient, evidence of significant ischaemic changes on stress testing may be followed by coronary angiography and possible percutaneous coronary stents or coronary bypass grafting prior to elective surgery. Prophylactic perioperative beta-blockade has been shown to reduce risk in patients with proven coronary artery disease, although specific protocols are uncommon in clinical practice. A titration of heart rate to ≤65 bpm has been widely supported.

Angina

The clinical assessment of the severity of angina may be based on the grading system devised by the New York Heart Association (Table 1.4). Patients in classes 1 and 2 undergoing low or intermediate risk surgery are at no increased risk with surgery but should have exercise electrocardiograms (ECGs) prior to surgery. Anti-anginal medication should be continued through the preoperative period. Patients in classes 3 and 4, especially those scheduled for intermediate- or high-risk non-cardiac surgery should be considered for coronary angiography and possible revascularisation or coronary stent percutaneous trans luminal coronary angioplasty (PTCA) prior to elective surgery. This is because of the high incidence of myocardial infarction when elective surgery is performed on this group, however to date, no randomised controlled clinical trial has assessed the overall benefit of prophylactic coronary grafting to lower cardiac risk during non-cardiac surgery.

Table 1.5. Classification of hypertension.

Category	Systolic (mmHg)	Diastolic (mmHg)
Normal	<130	<85
High normal	130–139	85–89
Hypertension		
Stage 1 (mild)	140–159	90–99
Stage 2 (moderate)	160–179	100–109
Stage 3 (severe)	180–209	110–119
Stage 4 (very severe)	>210	>120

Investigation

- *Chest Radiograph*: A relatively non-specific test although cardiomegaly and venous congestion associated with cardiac failure can be detected.
- *ECG*: A normal resting ECG does not exclude the presence of ischaemic heart disease. Ambulatory ECG during the 48 h prior to surgery in patients with known coronary artery disease has shown silent ischaemic episodes in 18–40% of patients. However, in the absence of symptoms and signs of coronary disease, there is good correlation between a normal resting ECG and an uneventful preoperative course.
- *Stress ECGs*: A significant correlation with the development of preoperative complications is shown in patients who:
  - show ischaemic changes during exercise;
  - are unable to reach 85% of their predicted maximum heart rate during exercise.
- *Isotopic scanning*: Thallium scanning can determine the ventricular ejection fraction. An ejection fraction of <0.30 correlates with a significantly increased risk of perioperative myocardial infarction.
- *Transthoracic echocardiography (TTE)*: This can detect abnormalities of the ventricular contractility and valve function.
- *Coronary angiography*: This provides definitive evidence of the degree and extent of coronary occlusion and is essential before coronary bypass surgery.

Hypertension

Hypertension is present in approximately 20% of adult patients and the definition of hypertension has changed with greater realisation of the deleterious effects of even modest long-term elevation of blood pressure (BP; Table 1.5).

Mild controlled hypertension in isolation appears to pose no additional operative risk, but uncontrolled hypertension (Stage 3 or 4) has an increased risk of congestive cardiac failure, myocardial ischaemia and unplanned admission to critical care units perioperatively.

Antihypertensive medication should not be discontinued prior to surgery. However, there have been reports of significant induction hypotension in patients treated with angiotensin converting enzyme (ACE) inhibitors. Clinical practice varies, with some authors advocating cessation of ACE inhibitors on the day prior to surgery whilst others continue therapy. Elective surgery should be curtailed if the diastolic BP exceeds 115 mmHg as a diastolic BP >120 mmHg has a well-documented association with perioperative complications. In the emergency situation, intra-arterial monitoring and control of BP using intravenous beta-blockers or glyceryl trinitrate (GTN) should be employed. Management of hypertensive patients during surgery is complicated by their exaggerated responses to noxious stimuli such as pain or endotracheal intubation.

Management principals:
- Assessment and optimisation of BP control.
- Assessment of associated pathology:
  - coronary disease;
  - congestive failure;
  - renal dysfunction;
  - peripheral vascular disease.
- Anaesthetic management (refer to Chapter 2):
  - accurate monitoring of BP;
  - management of intubation hypertension;
  - observation of intraoperative hypertension or signs of ischaemia;
  - avoidance of large swings in BP or periods of prolonged hypotension.
- Postoperative management (refer to Chapter 3):
  - optimal pain control – non-steroid anti-inflammatory drugs (NSAIDs) should be used cautiously, if at all, in patients on angiotensin 2 receptor blockers and diuretics because of a significant risk of development of renal impairment;
  - BP management prior to return of oral medication.

Congestive cardiac failure

Untreated congestive cardiac failure has a high association with postoperative morbidity and is a contraindication to elective surgery. If emergency surgery is necessary in the presence of poorly controlled heart failure, monitoring of left and right ventricular filling pressures will be necessary and consideration should be given to postoperative respiratory support. Patients with treated cardiac failure are at low risk of complications, provided medication is maintained over the preoperative period. The fluid shifts associated with spinal and epidural anaesthesia may precipitate pulmonary oedema in the preoperative period and may be controlled by leg elevation or bandaging, as well as judicious doses of vasoconstrictors such as metaraminol.

Valvular heart disease

Undetected valvular heart disease, especially aortic stenosis, has a high association with postoperative morbidity. In addition to impaired cardiac function, associated organ pathology such as pulmonary, hepatic and renal dysfunction may occur. Clinical assessment is based on history, exercise tolerance and auscultation. The New York Heart Association classification

Table 1.6. New York Heart Association classification of patients with heart disease.

1	Asymptomatic
2	Symptoms with ordinary activity but comfortable at rest
3	Symptoms with minimal activity but comfortable at rest
4	Symptoms at rest

of patients with heart disease is a useful index of functional impairment (Table 1.6).

Assessment requires either TTE, TOE or cardiac catheterisation to determine pressure gradients across the valves. In general, preoperative management of the patient with valve disease involves prophylactic antibiotics, because of the increased risk of bacterial endocarditis, and meticulous attention to fluid management, as well as specific therapy for individual heart problems.

Respiratory system

Risk factors

A list of risk factors which increase the incidence of postoperative pulmonary complications exists in an analogous manner to that for cardiac complications.
- *History*:
  - preoperative symptoms of respiratory disease,
  - preoperative history of chronic obstructive airways disease (COAD),
  - preoperative productive cough,
  - cigarette smoking,
  - poor nutrition,
  - age >60 years.
- *Examination*:
  - obesity,
  - abnormal chest examination,
  - abnormal chest X-ray.
- *Surgery and anaesthesia*:
  - thoracic and upper abdominal surgery,
  - anaesthesia >3 h.

Certain techniques improve preoperative pulmonary performance and reduce the incidence of complications:
- bronchodilator therapy,
- pre- and postoperative chest physiotherapy,
- optimal analgesia,
- cessation of smoking 6–8 weeks prior to major surgery,
- use of the incentive spirometer as an adjunct to physiotherapy,
- early ambulation,
- prophylactic antibiotics if chest infection is present.

Assessment of respiratory function

Clinical history should elicit exercise tolerance, type and productivity of cough and any precipitating factors of respiratory distress, such as lying flat. Examination includes auscultation and percussion of the chest and an assessment of airway patency. Bedside clinical testing of respiratory function provides valuable information, especially in situations where laboratory testing may not be readily available:
- breathlessness on walking a few metres around the ward usually represents decreased cardiopulmonary reserve;
- inability to count beyond 20 at a single inspiration quantifies dyspnoea;
- accompanying the patient during stair climbing verifies the degree of exertional dyspnoea.

Laboratory testing accurately quantifies the degree of impairment as well as recording effects of therapy such as bronchodilator administration. The commonest tests are:
- *Spirometry* which measures the volumes of exhaled gas per unit time. The commonly assessed parameters are:
  - forced vital capacity (FVC);
  - forced expiratory volume (FEV1);
  - FEV/FVC ratio: usually >85%; <50% indicates that postoperative ventilation is more likely;
  - maximum mid-expiratory flow rate (MMEFR);
  - peak expiratory flow rate (PEFR) which measures airflow obstruction at high flow rates.
- Arterial blood gas estimation provides information as to baseline levels of gas transfer and helps guide therapy.

Indicators of *significant risk* of postoperative respiratory failure are:
- respiratory rate >40/min,
- $PaCO_2 > 50$ mmHg,
- $PaO_2 < 60$ mmHg,
- gradient > 300 mmHg on 100% oxygen,
- V_d/V_t ratio 0.6,
- FVC < 15 ml/kg,
- FEV1 < 50% predicted value.

The COAD

The term COAD includes a group of destructive lung diseases generally caused by smoking and characterised by dyspnoea of progressive severity, airflow obstruction and cough. The destructive process leads to hypoxaemia and hypercarbia. Historically, the disease was separated into chronic bronchitis (predominantly obstructive disease) and emphysema (predominantly destructive disease), but they are now generally grouped together, reflecting the fundamentally similar pathophysiology. Intercurrent chest infections are common and right ventricular dysfunction is seen in up to 50% of patients with COAD.

Any increase in quantity or change in appearance of sputum may be indicative of developing infection. Assessment of the severity of COAD requires knowledge of the degree of exercise impairment. The distance a patient can walk on the flat or the number of flights of stairs which can be climbed before developing dyspnoea gives a measure of exercise tolerance. Other conditions such as hip disease or intermittent claudication can limit the value of this clinical test. Some anaesthetists walk up the stairs with patients to verify these facts.

Tests of airflow limitation quantitate the level of impairment. FEV1 is the most commonly used although the MMEFR is more sensitive. The response to β_2 selective agonists such as salbutamol should be ascertained prior to surgery. As with asthma, the patient should take their aerosol with them to the operating room for use prior to surgery. Phosphodiesterase inhibitors (theophyline) are second-line therapy as the narrow therapeutic dose range means toxic symptoms may occur. Ipratropium bromide (atrovent) combined with selective β_2 agonists may give improved and prolonged benefit compared with β_2 agonists alone. Intraoperative arterial blood gas monitoring is advisable in patients with severe COAD and baseline values on room air, prior to surgery and assist planning postoperative care.

Patients with COAD are prone to desaturation during sleep and this has important implications for postoperative care and may contribute to the incidence of myocardial infarction in the early postoperative days. Physiotherapy commencing preoperatively significantly improves the outcome, especially in patients with significant sputum production. Regional anaesthesia, particularly for lower abdominal, limb and vascular surgery, is useful in this group of patients.

Asthma

Asthma is a syndrome of heightened bronchial reactivity to a variety of stimuli, resulting in airflow obstruction of variable severity. The overall incidence in the population is 4% and this is increasing worldwide. Therapy involves the use of bronchodilators alone or in combination with anti-inflammatory agents. Maintenance steroid use is increasing in asthma medication and inhaled steroids cause fewer systemic problems than oral steroids due to their poor absorption from the lungs. Suppression of adrenal function may occur with oral steroid therapy and this may last for up to 3 years after cessation of therapy.

Clinical assessment

In known asthmatics, it is essential to elicit provoking factors, frequency of attacks, length of hospitalisation required and the drug therapy, especially steroid use. Physical examination may be unremarkable between attacks.

Respiratory function test

Spirometry should be performed to assess FVC and FEV1. Spirometry also allows assessment of the response to bronchodilators. Arterial blood gases and chest X-rays are not routinely necessary. Some centres recommend routine full blood testing to detect eosinophilia but this is not universal.

Preoperative preparation requires optimisation of drug therapy and estimation of baseline respiratory function, allowing grading of severity of asthma:

- *Mild asthma* (no hospitalisation): Maintain routine therapy and administer selective β_2-agonist (salbutamol) via aerosol prior to surgery.

- *Moderate asthma* (some functional impairment, routine use of bronchodilators): Maintain routine therapy and administer selective β_2-agonist (salbutamol) via nebuliser prior to surgery.

- *Severe asthma* (significant impairment, current bronchoconstriction): Corticosteroids should be used (e.g. hydrocortisone 1–3 mg/kg) 2 h prior to surgery in addition to inhaled β_2-agonist therapy.

Upper respiratory tract infections

The significance of upper respiratory tract infections (URTIs) on the outcome of surgery has been argued. There is an increase in bronchial reactivity associated with URTI and thus postponement of surgery in asthmatic patients is prudent. In non-asthmatic adults, no effect on outcome has been found. In children, no agreement has been reached on the advisability of postponement of elective surgery during URTIs.

Obstructive sleep apnoea

Patients with obstructive sleep apnoea (OSA) have episodes of upper airways obstruction associated with arterial oxygen desaturation. OSA is defined as the cessation of airflow for longer than 10 s despite continued ventilatory efforts, at least 5 times per hour of sleep. Desaturation during sleep results in bradycardia and ventricular ectopic beats and eventually systemic and pulmonary hypertension develops. The incidence of OSA appears to be increasing with approximately 2–4% of the population affected. It is commoner in males and in the obese ($>60\%$ with OSA are obese). OSA causes episodes of daytime sleepiness and an increase in accidental injuries. At the preoperative interview patients or their partners may volunteer symptoms, but all obese patients should be questioned for occult OSA. Sleep studies should be performed to quantitate the severity of OSA and evaluate therapy prior to surgery. If surgery cannot be delayed, the patient should be assumed to have OSA and managed accordingly. Regional anaesthesia, if practical, is a good option and sedative drugs, particularly benzodiazepines should be avoided. If patients have their own continuous positive airway pressure (CPAP) apparatus this should be brought to hospital with them prior to surgery and postoperative care in a high dependancy unit is advisable.

Central nervous system

Epilepsy

Patients with grand mal epilepsy are at increased risk of fitting in the perioperative period due to:

- inadequate blood levels of anticoaconvulsants because of fasting or impaired absorption due to surgical pathology;
- excitatory effects of some anaesthetic agents or delay in recommencing oral medications.

At the preoperative interview the frequency of attacks, any precipitating circumstances, and current medications should be documented. Anti-epileptic agents should be taken on the morning of surgery and if oral therapy cannot be resumed postoperatively, parenteral anti-epileptic agents should be commenced.

Dementia

The increasing population of elderly patients has increased the number of patients with Alzheimer's dementia and vascular dementia presenting for surgery. The commonest co-morbidities encountered in dementia patients are COAD and atherosclerotic cardiovascular disease. It is common for a deterioration in cognitive function to occur in the perioperative period and this may take weeks to resolve. Neuroleptic drugs appear to increase the incidence of cognitive disorders perioperatively. Patients with chronic brain syndromes pose several problems in preoperative assessment:

- Consent, to be valid, should be signed by the person responsible under the relevant law of the jurisdiction involved or be referred to the local Guardianship Board (or similar).
- Accurate history taking may be impossible and medications may not be remembered. Increased time may be required to allow access to previous medical histories from other hospitals.
- Patient anxiety may lead to extreme agitation and restlessness. Sedative agents injudiciously given may worsen this agitation.
- Underlying pathological processes affecting other organ systems (alcoholism, severe peripheral vascular disease or chronic syphilis) or physical factors (head injury with flexion deformities, bed sores or low-grade urinary tract infections) must be taken into account during surgery and anaesthesia.

Renal system

Chronic renal failure

Patients with chronic renal failure pose many problems for the surgeon and anaesthetist because of the frequency with which surgery is necessary in these patients and the many associated medical problems present in this group:

- *Cardiovascular*:
  - Hypertension and associated complications.
  - Chronic anaemia due to ureamia and reduced erythoropoietin levels. Haemoglobin (Hb) levels of 7–10 g/l are normal in patients with chronic renal failure and injudicious transfusion may precipitate cardiac failure. The patient's weight is a useful guide to the level of hydration in an emergency when dialysis may not be possible prior to surgery.
- *Diabetes*:
  - Associated retinopathy, microvascular disease or autonomic dysfunction should be considered.
- *Acid–base and metabolic*:
  - Metabolic acidosis.
  - *Hyperkalaemia*: Serum potassium >6 mmol/l requires dialysis prior to surgery to prevent further rises during the preoperative period. Factors which may increase serum potassium include the use of suxamethonium,

administration of blood and hypoventilation. In all but dire emergencies, correction of potassium prior to surgery can be accomplished by dialysis, glucose–insulin therapy or Resonium enemas.
  - Hypocalcaemia due to vitamin D deficiency.
  - Hypermagnesaemia.
  - Inability to manage a water load.
- *Immune system*:
  - Concurrent use of immunosuppressants and decreased phagocyte effectiveness combine to increase perioperative risk of sepsis.
- *Coagulation*:
  - Coagulopathy may be present due to reduced platelet adhesiveness. International Normalised Ratio (INR) and antiprothrombin time (APTT) are usually normal.
- *Arteriovenous fistula*:
  - The presence of vascular access fistulas for haemodialysis in the upper limbs limits venous access for non-invasive blood pressure (NIBP) monitoring and drug administration during anaesthesia and recovery. Protection of the function of these fistulas from pressure and periods of hypotension (which may cause clotting of the fistulae) requires continual vigilance until the patient has fully regained consciousness.
- *Miscellaneous*:
  - Delayed gastric emptying (uraemia) and increased gastric acidity increase the risk of reflux and aspiration. Preoperative use of H_2 receptor blockers or proton pump inhibitors is recommended.
- *Medications*:
  - The majority of renal patients have associated hypertension and medication should be continued through the preoperative period. Oral hypoglycaemics should be discontinued the night before surgery and insulin should be managed as discussed in the section on diabetes. Renal failure decreases clearance (but not loading dose) of many drugs. If gentamycin or other aminoglycosides are necessary, blood levels should be monitored perioperatively. Metabolic changes in chronic renal failure affect clearance of NSAID's, pancuronium, pethidine (norpethidine accumulation) and enflurane which should be avoided.
- *Transplanted patients*:
  - Immunosuppressants increase infection risk, steroids increase osteoporosis and risk of pathological fractures. The transplanted kidney is at risk of physical damage during positioning or rejection if immunosuppressants are withheld perioperatively.

Liver

The commonest causes of liver impairment are viral (hepatitis B and C), toxicity (alcohol, paracetamol) and autoimmune disease (primary biliary cirrhosis, autoimmune hepatitis).

Liver failure can be classified by the acuity (i.e. the interval between the onset of jaundice and the development of encephalopathy:
- *Hyperacute*: within 7 days.
- *Acute*: within 7–28 days.
- *Subacute*: within 28 days to 6 months.
- *Chronic*: >6 months.

Pathophysiological features include:
- *Haematological*: coagulation should be checked because many patients will have impaired coagulation due to clotting factor deficiency and impaired platelet function.
- *Respiratory*: pleural effusions or ascites may impair breathing and increase aspiration risk.
- *Cardiovascular*: cardiomyopathy (alcoholic and haemochromatosis) should be excluded.
- *CNS*: encephalopathy is commonest in acute and can be graded:
  - *Grade 0*: alert and orientated.
  - *Grade 1*: drowsy but orientated.
  - *Grade 2*: drowsy and disorientated.
  - *Grade 3*: agitated and aggressive.
  - *Grade 4*: unrousable to deep pain.
- Pharmacological effects include prolongation of muscle relaxants (suxamethonium, mivacurium, vecuronium and rocuronium), as well as accumulation of fentanyl and morphine. Non-steroidal agents should be avoided because of the increased risk of gastrointestinal (GI) bleeding in patients with impaired coagulation.

Assessment of liver function: Serum bilirubin and albumin plus prothrombin time (PT) are markers of global hepatic dysfunction, whilst elevated levels of transaminases can occur with minor liver damage. The Childs–Pugh classification for patients with cirrhosis indicates an increasing chance of hepatic failure.

Endocrine system

Diabetes

Approximately 2.5% of the population have diabetes with the incidence rising in patients >80 years old. The majority (>90%) have non-insulin-dependent diabetes mellitus (NIDDM or Type II diabetes).

Assessment of the diabetic patient undergoing surgery should include:
- *Cardiovascular system*: Microvascular disease is widespread in diabetic patients with between 15% and 60% of insulin-dependent diabetics having ECG changes. This microvascular disease is frequently associated with left ventricular dysfunction.
- *Hypertension*: This is present in over 60% of diabetic patients. Autonomic neuropathy is an uncommon but serious complication of diabetes with impaired cardiovascular responses to exercise and stress. Orthostatic hypotension is a reliable indicator of the presence of autonomic neuropathy.

- *Peripheral vascular disease*: This is frequently present and these patients are at risk of vascular occlusion during periods of hypotension or hypovolaemia.
- *Renal disease*: This is common in diabetic patients with glomerulosclerosis, papillary necrosis and ultimately chronic renal failure.

Preoperative management of blood glucose is necessary to prevent ketosis and acidosis, volume depletion due to osmotic diuresis or complications associated with undetected hypoglycaemia, especially brain cell damage or pulmonary aspiration, whilst unconscious. Blood sugar should be estimated, usually by the finger-prick method, since urine sugar estimations are too unreliable during periods of fluctuating blood sugar and variable urine output.
- For *major* surgery in *insulin-dependent* diabetes patients: insulin–dextrose–potassium infusion is a reliable regimen. Frequent blood sugar monitoring is important to avoid potentially dangerous periods of hypoglycaemia. Follow-up in the perioperative period and consultation between anaesthetist, surgeon and physician is essential.
- For *minor* surgery in *insulin-dependent* diabetes patients: half of the normal morning insulin requirement is given and a 5% dextrose infusion is commenced. If oral feeding does not recommence within 4–6 h, conversion to the regimen as for major surgery should be instituted.
- For *minor* surgery in *NIDDM* patients: withhold oral hypoglycaemic agent on the morning of surgery. Blood sugar should be monitored throughout the preoperative period.
- *Emergency* surgery in diabetics: is frequently undertaken against a background of either infection or acidosis and hyperglycaemia. Meticulous attention to blood glucose control and fluid balance are essential.

Hypothyroidism

Subclinical hypothyroidism affects an estimated 2–8% of the population and this incidence rises to 16% in females over 60 years. Patients with clinical hypothyroidism should be rendered euthyroid prior to elective surgery, because of their increased sensitivity to anaesthetic agents which may cause delayed awakening. L-thyroxine can be given as 50 μg/day initially followed by 150–200 μg/day as a maintenance dose. In elderly patients or those with coronary disease, reduced doses are recommended.

Hyperthyroidism

Medical control of hyperthyroidism using beta-blockers and antithyroid drugs (propylthiouracil or similar) is necessary prior to elective surgery to avoid serious complications such as:
- Thyroid storm, which is an acute episode of profound thyroid hyperactivity associated with tachycardia, pyrexia and cardiac arrhythmias. If untreated, this condition has a high mortality rate.
- Precipitation of angina, myocardial infarction or cardiac failure.

- *Tachyarrhythmias*: episodes of paroxysmal atrial fibrillation (AF) occur in nearly 25% of hyperthyroid patients.

If emergency surgery is indicated in hyperthyroid patients, the following precautions are necessary:
- intravenous administration of antithyroid drugs;
- indwelling arterial monitoring;
- sedating premedication to allay anxiety;
- avoidance of drugs which may provoke tachycardia, such as ketamine, pancuronium, atropine;
- use of beta-blockade to control heart rate during endotracheal intubation and surgical incision;
- adequate depth of anaesthesia to ablate noxious stimuli;
- good postoperative pain control.

Adrenal insufficiency

Two types of adrenal insufficiency exist:
- Primary (Addison's disease) with inadequate levels of glucocorticoids, mineralocorticoids and androgens. Signs include fatigue, anorexia, cutaneous pigmentation and hypotension with hyponatremia and hyperkalaemia.
- Secondary due to inadequate levels of corticotropin-releasing hormone (CRH) or adrenocorticotrophic hormone (ACTH) due to corticosteroid use or hypothalamic or pituitary disease.

Normal cortisol secretion is 25–30 mg/day rising to 75–150 mg with stress such as surgery and peaking at 200–500 mg/day with severe stress. A dose equivalent of prednisolone 20 mg/day for at least 3 weeks in the last year will produce some adrenal suppression. Recommendations for steroid replacement perioperatively vary widely.

A suggested regime is:
- minor surgery IV hydrocortisone 25 mg;
- major surgery:
  - *intraoperatively*: IV hydrocortisone 75–150 mg;
  - *postoperatively*: IV hydrocortisone 50 mg 8 h for 1 day, then 25 mg 8 h for 1 day.

Acute Addisonian crisis is rare and presents with:
- lethargy, weakness;
- severe nausea, vomiting and abdominal pain;
- hypotension with hypovolaemia.

Management involves treatment of cause (if possible), glucocorticoids and fluids. Inotropes are relatively ineffective in Addisonian crisis if steroids are not given.

Phaeochromocytoma

These are catecholamine secreting tumours of chromatin cells. Noradrenaline secretion predominates in most cases, but in 15% of cases adrenaline secretion is predominant. Presenting signs include hypertension either constant or paroxysmal, headache, sweating and palpitations. Catecholamine-induced cardiomyopathy may also be present. Management prior to surgery involves alpha-blockade with phenoxybenzamine or prazocin for between 3 days and 2 weeks. Beta-blockers may be added to alpha-blockade if necessary. Echocardiography to exclude cardiomyopathy is advisable.

Haematology

Anaemia

Chronic anaemia (Hb < 9 g/l) should be corrected prior to elective surgery, because the anaemic patient has reduced oxygen carrying capacity reserve to compensate for intraoperative blood loss. In addition, compensatory mechanisms for the reduced oxygen carrying capacity, such as:
- *Increased cardiac output*:
  - peripheral vasodilation (microvascular control mechanisms);
  - reduced blood viscosity.
- *Increased oxygen extraction*:
  - shift of haemoglobin dissociation curve to the right;
  - local tissue acidosis;

may encroach on cardiac reserve. Correction to Hb 10 g/l is advised using supplemental iron for elective surgery. If transfusion to correct chronic anaemia is necessary when surgery is more urgent, caution is required if >1 unit/day is administered in case pulmonary oedema is precipitated, and packed cells are used in preference to whole blood. Intraoperative blood loss should be promptly replaced and factors increasing postoperative oxygen requirements (especially shivering) should be avoided.

Patients with sickle cell anaemia are at increased risk of sickle cell crises during anaesthesia:
- hypoxic episodes,
- tourniquet use,
- dehydration associated with prolonged fasting of increased fluid losses

Although hydroxyurea has been used to stimulate HbF production which reduces the incidence and severity of sickle cell crises, this work is still in the experimental stages due to concerns regarding mutagenesis and leukemogenesis. Patients from countries with endemic sickle cell disease should be screened prior to surgery.

Coagulation and haemostasis

Coagulation disorders

It is vital to diagnose and appropriately manage patients with these disorders. Some of them are obscure, some of them can be elucidated from the history. A history must be taken of previous operations or spontaneous episodes of bleeding, perhaps from the gums or following trivial injuries. Drug and family history are also essential. Bruising or petechiae may be present on examination. Detection of some conditions will emerge from results of simple routine tests such as PT, partial thromboplastin time (PTT), thrombin time (TT) and platelet count.

In most cases the expert help of a clinical haematologist will be required. In cases that are difficult to interpret, it is better to anticipate and take precautionary measures than to call for help when disaster has struck.

Bleeding disorders may be congenital or acquired:
- *Congenital defects* include clotting factors as in haemophilia and von Willebrand's disease, congenital platelet disorders

and vessel wall defects such as hereditary haemorrhagic telangiectasia.

- *Acquired disorders* include clotting factor disorders resulting from drugs such as anticoagulants, antibiotics and liver disease. Disseminated intravascular coagulopathy (DIC) may complicate sepsis, haemolysis, antibody–antigen complex reactions and advanced neoplasia. Platelet function is notably reduced by aspirin and NSAIDs and in liver, kidney and myeloproliferative disorders. Platelets numbers are reduced in autoimmune thrombocytopaenia, hypersplenism and aplastic anaemia. The integrity of the vessel walls is reduced after taking steroids, in vasculitis and in malnutrition.

Patients on maintenance treatment with anticoagulants who are to undergo operation are at risk from bleeding but if their anticoagulants are stopped they are at risk of thrombosis. Before minor operations it is usual to stop oral warfarin for 2 days preoperatively and to start it immediately afterwards. Those having extensive procedures or with, for example, prosthetic heart valves, should stop warfarin and be maintained on heparin subcutaneously or by intravenous infusion under the supervision of a haematologist. In some cases, an operation may need to be performed as an emergency, or a patient may have bled as a result of taking anticoagulants. In these cases, the anticoagulant effects should be reversed with vitamin K, fresh frozen plasma (FFP) or concentrated clotting factors – again under the guidance of a haematologist.

Patients with coagulation disorders usually need to have blood or blood products available during surgical procedures, such as plasma-reduced cells, platelet transfusions, FFP, cryoprecipitate (which contains fibrinogen, fibronectin and factor VIII) or coagulation factor concentrates. They may, however, have atypical antibodies.

LIFESTYLE INFLUENCES ON ANAESTHETIC RISK

Alcohol
Excessive alcohol ingestion leads to a spectrum of pathology depending on the extent and chronicity of the problem:

- *Increased cellular tolerance* of drugs means that higher than expected doses of anaesthetic agents will be required.
- *Withdrawal symptoms* in the postoperative period require aggressive treatment to prevent the patient from injuring themselves or staff members. Symptoms include: disorientation, hallucinations, tachycardia, hypertension and grand mal convulsions. Management includes thiamine, benzodiazepine sedation and beta-blockers. Mild alcohol withdrawal symptoms occurring within 6–8 h of abstinence require no specific therapy.

Potential perioperative problems include:
- cellular tolerance leading to higher anaesthetic requirements,
- chronic brain syndrome (alcoholic dementia),
- clotting abnormalities,

- increased risk of infection,
- poor wound healing,
- acute withdrawal syndrome (delerium tremens),
- agitation and self-harm,
- wound disruption,
- cardiovascular instability,
- bleeding varices.

Morbid obesity
Obesity is an increasing health problem worldwide. It is defined as having 25–30% greater than ideal body weight or body mass index (BMI) >30. The BMI is defined as weight (kg) divided by height (m) squared. Morbid obesity may be defined as being 100% greater than ideal body weight or BMI > 35. Morbid obesity is associated with a significant diminution of physiological reserve and an increase in associated pathological conditions including hypertension, coronary artery disease, diabetes and oesophageal reflux. Cardiovascular performance shows impaired diastolic filling and reduced rise in ejection fraction with exercise compared with non-obese patients. These associated medical conditions pose increased difficulties during surgery and anaesthesia. Osteoarthritis, hiatus hernia and gallbladder disease are common and frequently require surgery.

Perioperative problems associated with morbid obesity
Induction
- Venous access is often difficult and a central line may be required for access.
- Accurate BP monitoring is difficult and wide BP cuffs will be required if non-invasive monitoring is used. An arterial line may provide more reliable readings in this situation.
- Difficulty in intubation.

Intraoperative problems
- Patient positioning.
- Drug dosage to ensure adequate depth of anaesthesia.

Postoperative problems
- Respiratory insufficiency due to mass loading of chest wall and abdomen plus reduced vital capacity.
- The high incidence of OSA. Patients with morbid obesity and OSA have a 20–25% incidence of daytime hypoxia leading to pulmonary hypertension and 50% incidence of hypercarbia.
- Increased incidence of deep vein thrombosis (DVT).

Smoking
Smoking significantly increases perioperative risk. Elevated carboxyhaemoglobin levels due to inhaled carbon monoxide persist for up to 12 h after cessation of smoking and laryngeal irritability and bronchial reactivity are enhanced by smoking. Co-existing smoking-induced pathology is common and includes:
- hypertension,
- ischaemic heart disease and peripheral vascular disease,
- COAD.

Patients should be advised to cease smoking prior to surgery, however, compliance is poor and no decrease in postoperative complications has been found unless smoking is stopped >8 weeks prior to surgery. Careful assessment is necessary because symptoms of the presenting illness may mask those of other cigarette-induced disease processes, with angina, intermittent claudication and exertional dyspnoea being common examples.

Non-prescription drugs and substance abuse

The large number of 'recreational' and addictive drugs have implications for anaesthesia and surgery:

- Patients using injectable agents have an increased risk of blood-borne infections, including HIV, hepatitis and bacterial endocarditis.
- Withdrawal symptoms may appear and include violent and aggressive behaviour, or delusional and hallucinatory behaviour. A high clinical index of suspicion is necessary to diagnose drug withdrawal.
- Interactions between therapeutic and non-prescription drugs may complicate management, for example, opioid resistance in narcotics abuse, hypertension and tachycardia with amphetamine use and resistance to anaesthetic agents with sedative abuse.
- Venous access may be particularly difficult, especially in the hypovolaemic chronic drug user.
- Solvent inhalation sensitises the myocardium to arrhythmias especially with inhalational anaesthetic agents.

Herbal products

Because herbal products are not considered 'drugs' by most patients, the use of these products may not be volunteered at the preoperative interview. The use of these substances is increasing worldwide with up to 22% of patients (USA) taking some form of herbal supplement. Although most appear to have no effect on the conduct of surgery or anaesthesia, several can have significant effects (Table 1.7) and should be ceased

prior to surgery whenever possible. In addition, many may be taken as individually prepared preparations and hence the 'dose' consumed may vary widely.

CONCURRENT DRUG TREATMENT

Anticoagulants

Increasing numbers of patients are on long-term anticoagulation therapy because of chronic AF, pacemaker insertion or following valve replacement. The risk of embolisation if coagulation is withdrawn is used to guide perioperative management (Tables 1.9–1.11).

Antiplatelet drugs

Antiplatelet drugs pose a unique risk, especially with emergency surgery, because of the inability to reverse the effect of the commonly available antiplatelet drugs such as cliopidogrel or ticlopodidine. For elective surgery, cessation between 7 (clopidogrel) and 10 (ticlopidine) days prior to surgery is recommended.

Steroids

Adrenal suppression from oral steroid use (>2 weeks in the preceding 9 months) may cause a potentially fatal Addisonian crisis perioperatively if additional glucocorticoids are not given. Although there is no proven benefit from supra-physiological dosage, underdosage is disadvantageous. A *typical regimen* is hydrocortisone 100 mg IV twice daily tapering off by 25% per day over the next few days although lower doses are permissible with uncomplicated minor surgery (e.g. inguinal hernia repair).

Immunosuppressants

Immunosuppressant therapy poses several problems for the surgeon and anaesthetist:

- prolongs effect of suxamethonium,
- increases risk of wound infection,
- delays wound healing.

Table 1.7. Herbal products affecting anaesthesia or surgery.

Herb	Concern
Echinacea purpura (echinacea)	Immune suppression, chronic use hepatotoxic may decrease steroid effectiveness
Allium sativum (garlic)	↑ bleeding (affects platelet aggregation)
Ginkgo biloba (ginkgo)	↑ bleeding (patients on anticoagulants)
Panax ginseng (ginseng)	Low blood sugar, tachycardia, ?bleeding ↑ bleeding (patients on anticoagulants)
Glycyrrhiza glabra (licorice)	Hypertension, oedema, low K^+ contraindicated in renal/hepatic dysfunction
Goldenseal	Used as a diuretic, but water excretion predominates worsening hypertension
Piper methysticum (kava)	Prolongs anaesthesia
Mahuang (Ephedra sinica)	Arrhythmias, hypertension, death reported drug interactions
Hyperium perforatum (St John's wort)	↓ effect warfarin, steroids ↓ effect HIV protease inhibitors
Valeriana officinalis (valerian)	Prolonged anaesthesia, withdrawal syndrome
Vitamin E	Possible thyroid effect, may increase bleeding
Zimber officinale (ginger)	Antiplatelet effects

Table 1.8. **Drug interactions and anaesthesia.**

Drug	Effect
AIDs Rx	Increased sensitivity to midazolam and fentanyl
Angiotensin$_2$ blockers	May get hypotension at induction
Anticonvulsants	Liver enzyme induction may increase dose requirements for lithium may potentiate non-depolarising neuro-muscular blocking drugs
Diuretics	Hypokaelaemia may increase sensitivity to non-depolarising neuromuscular blocking drugs
MAOI	Pethidine may produce hypertensive crises
Platelet function drugs	Increased bleeding with spinal/epidurals

Table 1.9. **Risk of thromboembolism if anticoagulation is ceased.**

Low	AF/cardiomyopathy without stroke or systemic embolisation within 12 months
	Biological heart valves (after first 3/12)
	Post vascular stent insertion (after first 3/12)
	Non-recurrent systemic arterial emboli
	Venous thrombosis NOT within last 3/12 and without other risk factors:
	– hypercoagulable state
	– recurrent thrombosis
	– malignancy
	– preoperative immobility
High	AF/Cardiomyopathy with stroke or systemic embolisation within 12 months
	Biological heart valves (within first 3/12)
	Post vascular stent (within first 3/12)
	Mechanical aortic or mitral valve
	Recurrent systemic arterial emboli
	Venous thrombosis/pulmonary embolism in the last month*

*consider vena caval filter.

Tricyclic antidepressants

The complications associated with administering anaesthesia to a patient taking psychotropic drugs must be weighed against possible complications from their cessation.
- Antidepressants should only be discontinued in consultation with the treating psychiatrist.
- Monoamine oxidase inhibitors (MAOI): In general, following consultation with the treating psychiatrist, MAOI should be discontinued 2–3 weeks prior to surgery. This allows regeneration of adequate levels of monoamine oxidase, otherwise, excitatory effects, such as hypertension or convulsions, have

Table 1.10. **Recommendations for perioperative anticoagulation in the low-risk group.**

Day-4	Cease warfarin (if INR > 3.5 cease 5 days preoperatively)
Day-3, -2, -1	No anticoagulation
Day-0	Measure INR on morning of surgery. If INR > 2.0 postpone or transfuse FFP
Postoperative	Use heparin/LMWH (if indicated) for DVT prophylaxis
	Measure INR
	Re-commence warfarin when oral fluids tolerated and monitor INR

Table 1.11. **Recommendations for perioperative anticoagulation in the *high-risk* group.**

Day-4	Cease warfarin (if INR > 3.5 cease 5 days preoperatively)
Day-3 (full-dose UFH)	When INR < 2.0 commence UFH (treat as in patient) cease 6 h prior to surgery
Day-3 (LMWH)	When INR < 2.0 commence LMWH. Enoxaprin 1 mg bd (mechanical valves, >100 kg, extensive DVT), otherwise 1.5 mg daily
Day-2	As per Day-3
Day-1 (LMWH)	Do not give LMWH < 18 h prior to surgery (or <24 h spinal/epidural planned)
Day-0	Measure INR on morning of surgery. If INR > 2.0 postpone or transfuse FFP
Postoperative	Measure INR
	Re-commence warfarin when oral fluids tolerated and monitor INR
	Use UFH or LMWH until oral fluids tolerated
	titrate APTT to 50–70 s (48 h)
	then APTT 50–75 s until oral fluids tolerated

UFH: unfractionated heparin.

resulted from administration of pethidine to patients treated with MAOI. Hypertensive crises may occur when vasopressors are administered to patients on MAOIs. If surgery in patients on ongoing MAOI therapy is necessary or for emergency surgery, the following guidelines should be employed:
- Preoperative consultation with the treating psychiatrist.
- Benzodiazepine premedication.
- Avoid halothane, pethidine.
- If vasopressors are necessary, avoid indirect-acting pressors (metaraminol) and use fluids and posture wherever possible. Carefully titrate small doses of direct-acting vasoconstrictors (methoxamine or phenylephrine) if necessary.
- Suxamethonium effect may be prolonged due to decreased cholinesterase levels.

Oral contraceptives

The use of the progesterone-only pill poses no documented problems during surgery. However, the combination oestrogen-progesterone pill should be discontinued 6 weeks prior to elective surgery because of the increased risk of DVT, especially in women who smoke. When emergency surgery is necessary, additional thomboembolism prophylaxis is required. In all cases, the patient must be advised to use alternate forms of contraception as the reliability of oral absorption is affected by fasting, perioperative nausea and vomiting and any antibiotic-induced diarrhoea (Table 1.8).

PROPHYLAXIS OF THROMBOEMBOLIC DISEASE

Preoperative management of the surgical patient includes planning to avoid fatal complication of pulmonary thromboembolism. Clinically significant but non-fatal thromboembolism occurs in about 1 : 100 postoperative patients and fatal pulmonary embolism in 1 : 1000.

The origin of the pulmonary embolus is usually thrombosis in the veins of the calf muscles, but thrombosis may spread to the iliofemoral veins and the pelvic veins. The development of venous thrombosis in these veins is usually silent and may only manifest itself as an episode of pulmonary embolism. Hence the emphasis on prophylaxis to prevent this serious complication.

Many studies have defined a number of risk factors which predispose to the development of pulmonary embolism:
- age >40 years;
- obesity;
- immobilisation;
- previous DVT;
- general anaesthetic;
- major abdominal/orthopaedic surgery;
- pregnancy/postpartum;
- malignancy, particularly ovarian and pancreatic cancer;
- hypercoaguable states, for example, deficiency of antithrombin 3, protein C or protein S;
- medical illness, including myocardial ischaemia, respiratory insufficiency.

Surgical patients can be divided into low-, medium- and high-risk groups for venous thrombosis and pulmonary embolism.
A typical *low-risk* patient will be:
- aged <40 years;
- have surgery lasting <30 min, particularly avoiding general anaesthetic;
- rapidly mobilised postoperatively;
- have no other risk factors.

A typical *moderate-risk* patient will be:
- aged >40 years;
- show moderate obesity;
- need abdominal operation requiring general anaesthetic;
- have one other risk factor.

A typical *high-risk* patient will be:
- middle-aged or elderly, undergoing major surgery (orthopaedic or cancer surgery);
- need prolonged mobilisation;
- may have pelvic trauma or pelvic surgery;
- may have suffered orthopaedic trauma generally: for example, fractured neck of femur;
- have multiple risk factors.

All moderate- to high-risk patients should receive prophylaxis. It is not easy to categorise every patient and when in doubt prophylaxis against thromboembolism should be instituted.

Methods of prophylaxis
General
- early ambulation;
- use of venous support compression stockings, particularly where local venous insufficiency problems exist in the limbs;
- calf stimulation during operations under general anaesthetic.

These methods are sufficient prophylaxis for fit patients who fall in the low-risk group.

Moderate and high-risk patients

These patients require pharmacological intervention with antithrombotic drugs.
- *Low-dose subcutaneous heparin.* This has been shown to be effective in reducing thrombosis in the peripheral veins. It is given at a dose of 5000 units bd subcutaneously. The main complications are bruising and local wound haematoma if the injection is given close to the site of the operative wound. The heparin at this dose does not produce any alteration in standard coagulation screening studies. The main complication is the development of allergic thrombocytopaenia. This condition may be associated with thrombosis and heparin must be ceased.
- *Low-molecular-weight heparin (LMWH).* This may have a special place in orthopaedic surgery and is given as a single daily dose. It is as effective as heparin in preventing thrombosis and has fewer platelet side-effects. However, LMWH is expensive and is not routinely used for this reason.
- *Anticoagulants.* Use of the anticoagulant warfarin, either in low or full anticoagulation dose, has been shown to be effective in reducing thromboembolism. However, bleeding complications are common and accordingly warfarin is not in regular use for this purpose.
- *Antiplatelet agents.* Aspirin is an effective antiplatelet agent. However, it is ineffective as the sole agent to prevent DVT. Dextrans act as antiplatelet agents and have been shown to reduce the incidence of postoperative venous thrombosis. They are, however, expensive, must be given intra-venously and are more difficult to administer than subcutaneous heparin. Dextrans are not used routinely.

Post operative care
Part of the postoperative management of the surgical patient is to check the limbs on a daily basis for the development of

the early signs of venous thrombosis. These include calf tenderness and leg swelling. If there is any suggestion of the development of clinical venous thrombosis, a Doppler ultrasound and/or venogram is required to diagnose the peripheral venous thrombosis prior to the commencement of full anticoagulation.

PREADMISSION CLINICS

The economic and resource pressures in contemporary healthcare have resulted in a number of changes in clinical practice. These include increased use of day case (ambulatory surgery), various domiciliary post-acute care systems and the development of preadmission clinics to facilitate hospital admission on the day of surgery.

The aims of the preadmission clinic:
• reduction in bed occupancy and thus a shorter hospital stay;
• less disruption to patient's routine;
• development of guidelines for laboratory investigations to reduce ordering of unnecessary laboratory tests;
• adequate time exists between consultation and surgery for the relevant tests to be performed and the results obtained;
• fewer 'last minute' cancellations because of abnormal test results;
• education of patient (and family) regarding proposed surgery and preparation of a plan for anaesthesia and analgesia;
• to facilitate the use of the hospital for acute care only and to encourage the management of long-term health problems by community-based health services such as general practitioners or out-patient specialist appointments.

Where geographical distance precludes attendance of the patient at a central preadmission clinic, the process can be undertaken by a local medical officer or peripheral hospital with the information faxed or E-mailed to the central hospital where surgery is to be undertaken.

ROUTINE INVESTIGATIONS PRIOR TO SURGERY

The ordering of laboratory tests is still largely empirical with marked differences between hospitals and individuals. Evidence-based consensus guidelines have been developed to assist decision making (National Institute for Clinical Excellence – NICE http://www.nice.org.uk/pdf/cg3niceguidelinea4.pdf. Broad issues to consider in applying these guidelines are:
• age band,
• complexity of intended surgery,
• ASA classification,
• nature of co-morbidity present (ASA 2).

Some brief suggestions are listed in Table 1.12.

Biochemistry

Significant previously undetected abnormalities occur in <1% of cases, but occult diabetes and renal impairment are

Table 1.12. Routine preoperative tests for asymptomatic patients.

Chest radiograph	TB suspected
	Any change is symptoms/signs in patients with proven
	Lung or chest pathology
Coagulation	Clinical history of abnormal bleeding
	Cardiac, neurosurgery
ECG	Males >45 years, females >50 years
	Heart disease, hypertension, diabetes >35 years
	Significant respiratory disease (including OSA)
Full blood examination (FBE)	Females
	Major surgery where significant blood loss expected
	Anaemia suspected
Sickle cell test	Untested 'at risk' patients
Urinalysis	All patients (blood, glucose, protein)

frequently first detected on routine screening. Liver disease of sufficient severity to affect outcome from surgery will be detected clinically, and thus liver function tests are only indicated when clinically detectable disease is present. Routine biochemical testing is not indicated on asymptomatic patients <60 years of age.

Haematology

Routine haemoglobin estimation for clinically well patients undergoing minor surgery is unnecessary. For major surgery, haemoglobin estimation and 'group and save' is advised. The lowest level of haemoglobin at which elective surgery should *not* proceed has been strenuously debated with 7 g/dl being the lowest acceptable level in most studies (when major blood loss is not anticipated). Coagulation screening should only be done when clinically indicated or when undetected coagulopathy would be a major problem, such as in neurosurgery and heart surgery. Sickle cell status should be determined in patients at risk.

Chest radiograph

The chest radiograph is the most frequently over prescribed preoperative investigations. In the absence of clinical indications, the yield from this test is low. A chest radiograph (Fig. 1.1) should be performed only to confirm a suspected pathological condition likely to affect outcome from surgery, such as:
• cardiomegaly;
• suspected pulmonary metastases and mediastinal masses;
• suspected tuberculosis;
• significant known lung disease such as pneumonia, pulmonary oedema or atelectasis;
• suspected thoracic pathology such as fractured ribs, pneumothorax or pleural fluid accumulation.

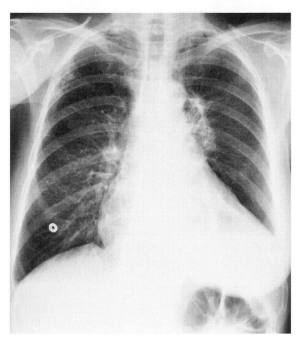

Figure 1.1. Chest radiograph showing an enlarged heart shadow.

ECGs

By contrast, the ECG often provides the initial information regarding several clinically 'silent' conditions which may impact adversely on the patient's perioperative outcome.

- myocardial infarction;
- arrhythmias:
  - atrial flutter or fibrillation,
  - ventricular ectopic beats;
- left or right ventricular hypertrophy;

- conduction problems:
  - arteriovenous block (1st, 2nd or 3rd degree),
  - Wolff–Parkinson–White syndrome,
  - atrial or ventricular ectopics,
  - prolonged 'QT' interval.

An ECG should be performed on all patients with known cardiovascular disease and on all asymptomatic patients >40 years of age.

Cardiac function tests

Nuclear medicine scanning provides valuable information of myocardial reserve in symptomatic patients. However, it should be remembered when assessing 'at risk' patients, that the presenting condition (e.g. arthritis requiring hip replacement) may mask cardiac symptoms by limiting the patient's exertion. TTE (if available) may provide valuable additional information regarding valve function and contractility.

Pulmonary function tests

Spirometry should be performed on patients with dyspnoea on mild to moderate exertion.

FURTHER READING

ACC/AHA Guideline update on perioperative cardiovascular evaluation for non-cardiac surgery. American Heart Association – www.americanheart.org

Carlisle J, Langham J, Thoms G. Guidelines for routine preoperative testing. *Br J Anaesth* 93; 2004: 495–497

Chassot PG, Delabays A, Spahn DR. Preoperative evaluation of patients with, or at risk of, coronary artery disease undergoing non-cardiac surgery. *Br J Anaesth* 89; 2002: 747–759

National Institute for Clinical Excellence – NICE http://www.nice.org.uk/pdf/cg3niceguidelinea4.pdf

2

Principles of Anaesthesia

Carlos MH Gómez[1] and John WW Gothard[2]

[1]Department of Anaesthesia and Intensive Care, Charing Cross Hospital, London and [2]Royal Brompton Hospital; National Heart and Lung Institute, Imperial College School of Medicine, London

CONTENTS

Definitions	16
Stages of clinical anaesthesia	16
Awareness	17
Assessment	17
History of previous anaesthesia	17
Past medical history	18
Drug history	18
Social history	19
Physical examination	19
Risk stratification	20
Premedication	21
Preoperative checks	23
Induction	23
Methods	23
Control of the airway	23
Control of breathing (ventilation)	24
Maintenance of anaesthesia	24
Anaesthesia (hypnosis)	24
Analgesia	25
Paralysis	25
Pharmacology of anaesthetic agents	25
Perioperative fluid management	28
Monitoring	29
Monitoring of the patient	29
Monitoring of the equipment	30
Recovery	30
Vasodilatation	32
Anaesthetic emergencies	33
Local anaesthetic drugs	34
Sedation	35
Regional anaesthesia	35
General Aspects	36
Specific techniques	36
Tourniquets	37
Ventilation	37
Further reading	38

Anaesthesia is a non-therapeutic intervention. It is particularly important, therefore, to determine potential benefits and estimated risks. Complications of anaesthesia are poorly tolerated and it is necessary to place safety before perceived efficacy.

DEFINITIONS

Anaesthesia

Anaesthesia is a reversible state of pharmacologically controlled sleep with reduction in cortical activity. At sufficient anaesthetic depth there is absence of conscious awareness and recall, and no sensory, motor or autonomic response to stimulation.

Balanced anaesthesia

This term is used to illustrate an equilibrium between the three constituents of an anaesthetic: anaesthesia (sleep), analgesia and paralysis. The three interact and the separation is more conceptual than clinical.

Sedation

Sedation is a state of sleepiness but preserved consciousness. Ideally, there is awareness and response to simple commands with verbal contact, but also a degree of amnesia and reduced anxiety.

STAGES OF CLINICAL ANAESTHESIA

In the 1920s four stages of progressively deeper anaesthesia were described in relation to inhalational induction. Drugs and techniques have changed considerably since and it is difficult to distinguish these stages clearly in modern anaesthesia.

Analgesia

This is the stage of inhalational sedation prior to loss of consciousness.

Excitement

The breathing slowly becomes more erratic; the airway is irritable. There may be uncontrolled movements of the limbs.

Surgical anaesthesia

Classically, this consists of four 'planes':

1. Small, pinpoint pupils; the tidal breaths are large and regular; the pharyngeal and vomiting reflexes are depressed.
2. Pupils are slightly larger; breathing remains regular; the corneal reflex is depressed.
3. Pupils are size 3–4; respiration becomes more diaphragmatic and the tidal volumes decrease; the lacrimation and laryngeal reflexes are depressed.
4. Pupils are dilated; respiration is irregular and shallow; the carinal reflex is depressed.

Surgery is normally conducted in plane 3 of surgical anaesthesia.

Overdose

The pupils are dilated and fixed; the brainstem reflexes are depressed and there is profound cardiopulmonary depression.

AWARENESS

The prime duty of the anaesthetist is to maintain the safety of the patient and to ensure that he/she is asleep, unaware and painfree. Awareness may cause considerable stress and psychological sequelae. For purposes of discussion, awareness can be divided into four categories:

1. *Conscious awareness with recollection*: This occurs when a patient remembers intraoperative events. It is very rare and is what most of us associate with being 'awake during an operation'. Awareness is often due to faulty anaesthetic technique or failure to check equipment [1].
2. *Conscious awareness without recollection*: There may have been response to intraoperative events but no recollection afterwards.
3. *Subconscious awareness without recollection*: A response to intraoperative events or commands may be triggered afterwards, say by hypnosis.
4. *No awareness or recollection*: This state is what most of us associate with being anaesthetised. However, some evidence suggests that patients are, to some degree, partially aware during anaesthesia but have no recollection.

ASSESSMENT

History of previous anaesthesia

Certain conditions are particularly relevant to anaesthesia.

Difficult intubation

Intubation is difficult in about 1–3% of cases and impossible in about 0.05–0.3%. It is an important cause of morbidity and mortality, especially in emergency anaesthesia, and is not always predictable.

Anaphylaxis [2]

Anaphylactic or anaphylactoid reactions to anaesthetic drugs are commoner amongst members of the same families, and may be more serious in atopic individuals or in those sensitive to other drugs. A history of collapse after induction requiring cancellation and/or postoperative intensive care is suggestive.

Malignant hyperpyrexia

This is a rare autosomal dominant condition triggered by inhalational anaesthetic vapours and probably suxamethonium. There is a certain predisposition in muscular dystrophy, strabismus and cleft palate. Malignant hyperpyrexia presents with acute cardiorespiratory collapse manifested by cyanosis, hypercapnia, muscle rigidity, acidosis, tachyarrhythmias and a huge temperature rise. Pathologically, there is uncontrolled muscle contraction and energy consumption by the sarcoplasmic reticulum. Treatment is by cardiovascular support and administration of dantrolene. Survivors and screened relatives may carry a 'medical alert' warning and will usually be aware of the condition.

Suxamethonium apnoea

Suxamethonium, a depolarising muscle relaxant, is metabolised slower than normal due to a recessive abnormality of the plasma cholinesterase enzyme. There is delayed recovery in breathing effort after surgery, requiring prolongation of anaesthesia (to avoid awareness) and ventilation.

Porphyria

This is a group of inherited disorders in haem synthesis. Some anaesthetic agents such as barbiturates (thiopentone), in addition to alcohol and sulphonamides, may precipitate crisis of abdominal pain, cardiovascular instability or neuropsychiatric manifestations.

Sickle cell disorders

This constitutes a group of autosomally inherited abnormalities in haemoglobin structure and function such that hypoxaemia triggers polymerisation of haemoglobin (Hb). This leads to a change in shape and a reduction in deformability of red cells which cause microvascular occlusion and haemolysis. Manifestations include haemolytic anaemia, susceptibility to infections, and ischaemic type pain and organ dysfunction, mostly in the lungs, spleen, vasculature and bone marrow. The genetic mutation is prevalent in sub-Saharan Africa, the Caribbean, parts of Asia and some parts of the south-eastern Mediterranean and the Arabian peninsula. It can be screened by an agglutination test and diagnosed by Hb electrophoresis.

A preoperative diagnosis is important, but should not delay life-saving surgery, when it is assumed that the at-risk patient has sickle cell disease. Anaesthesia during sickling crises has a high mortality and should be delayed.

The Hb electrophoresis distinguishes different Hb abnormalities and is the definitive diagnostic test. Sickle precipitation tests ('sickle dex', etc.) detect agglutination but cannot distinguish between the different variants (Tables 2.1 and 2.2).

Table 2.1. Sickle states.

	Normal	Trait	Disease	Hb SC
Electrophoresis	Hb AA	Hb AS	Hb SS	Hb SC
Clinical picture		Asymptomatic except in extreme hypoxaemia	Sickling crises	Sickling crises
Critical PO_2		2.5–3.5 kPa	5.5 kPa. Thus potentially constantly sickling at venous PO_2's	3.5 kPa
Hb S (%)	0	30	90	Variable (50%)
Anaemia	No	No	Yes	No
Sickledex	Negative	Positive	Positive	Positive

Table 2.2. Approach to surgery in sickle cell states.

	Yes/positive	No/negative	Unavailable
Patient at risk?	Do electrophoresis	Treat as normal	
Electrophoresis?	Diagnostic	Sickle disorders excluded	Do sickledex
Sickledex?	Check FBC, film	Sickle disorders excluded	Treat as sickle cell disease
Hb < 9 g/dl?	Probably sickle cell disease	Probably sickle cell trait, but beware of Hb SC (see Table 2.10)	Treat as sickle cell disease

Anaesthetic management is based on the evidence of factors known to precipitate sickling; these are hypoxaemia, dehydration and blood stasis, cold and acidaemia. Obviously, every anaesthetist tries to avoid these, but the margin of error is reduced in sickle disorders. It is recommended that tourniquets also be avoided. Postoperative complications include blood stasis and thrombosis, pain and opioid addiction.

Past medical history

The details for preoperative assessment are covered in Chapter 1. Specific day-to-day functional limitations which may affect the administration and recovery from anaesthesia are as follows:

Respiratory disease

Chronic airflow limitation, asthma and restrictive disorders have potentially great implications in anaesthesia. Cough, wheeze, haemoptysis and dyspnoea may seem 'normal' to some patients. Tolerance of everyday activities is a reliable gauge of severity. It is essential to detect active respiratory tract infection.

Cardiovascular disease

Questions should be directed towards the symptoms of ischaemic heart disease, valvular disease, congestive heart failure, arrhythmias, systemic hypertension and peripheral vascular disease. Detailed questioning should focus on angina, syncope, breathlessness, palpitations and tolerance of physical activity.

Gastrointestinal disease

The presence of hiatus hernia and peptic ulcer disease may require changes in anaesthetic technique to reduce the risk of regurgitation and aspiration. The character and timing of indigestion, heartburn and abdominal discomfort help determine if this is necessary.

Multisystem disease

Many different diseases affect anaesthesia. Diabetes mellitus, for example, is an important coexisting disease. Rheumatoid arthritis, osteoarthritis, ankylosing spondylitis, systemic lupus and scleroderma also have widespread effects relevant to the perioperative period.

Renal and liver disease

Questions should be directed towards the symptoms of anaemia, uraemia, bone disease, jaundice, coagulopathies, encephalopathy, nutrition and immunity; particular aspects of dialysis and vascular shunts may be relevant. Changes in body water, plasma protein and pH together with organ failure *per se* may affect drug kinetics.

Drug history

A detailed list of drugs, dosages and possible allergies is essential. Interaction with anaesthetic compounds is possible,

Table 2.3. Anaesthetic drug interactions.

Drug	Effect	Comments
Beta blockers	Potentiate cardiovascular depression; impair response to hypovolaemia	Continue, maintain normovolaemia; reverse with atropine and adrenaline
Nitrates	Vasodilatation, exacerbate hypovolaemia, tachyphylaxis	Continue, appropriate monitoring
Calcium channel blockers	Specific interactions with volatile anaesthetics can cause profound depression of heart rate, contractility and vascular tone	Continue but avoid specific volatiles; reverse if necessary
Diuretics	Electrolyte imbalance, arrhythmias, hypovolaemia	Continue, check electrolytes ECG
Angiotensin converting enzyme inhibitors (ACEI)	Potentiate cardiovascular depression, hyperkalaemia; may worsen renal function	Continue, monitor cardiovascular system, maintain normovolaemia
Anticoagulants	Bleeding	Withhold oral anticoagulants; may need heparin infusion
Aspirin and other antiplatelet drugs	Irreversibly inactivates platelet cyclo-oxygenase and inhibit platelet aggregation; Platelet half-life is about 7 days	Ideally stop 1 week before surgery; transfuse platelets
Monoamine oxidase inhibitors (MAOI)	Complex; potentiate sympathomimetics (including adrenaline present in local anaesthetics); decrease sympathetic system activity; potentiate opioids and barbiturates; pethidine may cause hypertension/hyperthermia	Ideally stop 2–3 weeks before surgery; avoid sympathomimetics and pethidine; extreme care in general
Tricyclic antidepressants	Cardiac arrhythmias, potentiate vasopressors, augment opioid effects	
Corticosteroids		Increase perioperatively
Diabetic drugs	See Table 2.9 and text	Insulin sliding scale

particularly with cardiovascular, respiratory, psychotropic and endocrine drugs (Table 2.3).

Social history

Symptoms of diseases associated with tobacco, alcohol and drug addiction should be sought.

Physical examination

There is agreement that a thorough history and physical examination are most important in assessing intercurrent illness.

Airway [3]

The following steps are helpful in predicting a difficult intubation (see also Table 2.4):
1. *Examination of the mouth* (Fig. 2.1) [4].
2. *Examination of the teeth*: Teeth can make intubation difficult. Teeth at risk of damage should be protected with a rubber tooth guard and false teeth must be removed. Features of special interest include:
   - crowns or loose teeth;
   - prominent upper incisors (buck teeth);
   - maxillary overbite.

3. *Examination of the neck*:
   - flexion of the neck (chin-to-chest manoeuvre);
   - extension of the head (with the neck flexed) is accomplished by extension of the occipito-atlantoid and atlanto-axial joints;
   - thyromental or Patil distance (anterior neck) should measure at least three finger breadths.

Upper respiratory tract

It may be necessary to examine the ears, nose and throat specifically for evidence of active infection, but also of bleeding or malignancy. Children presenting for anaesthesia who are pyrexial should have an ENT examination.

Lower respiratory tract

It is particularly important to seek evidence of active infection as well as acute deterioration in chronic conditions.

Cardiovascular system

Ischaemic heart disease may be silent. Nevertheless, positive physical findings can be very useful. The combination of gallop rhythm, expiratory crepitations, peripheral oedema

Table 2.4. Predictors of difficult intubation.

Factor	Severity	Points
Weight (kg)	<90	0
	90–110	1
	110	2
Head and neck movement	Over 90°	0
	90° ± 10°	1
	Under 90°	2
Jaw movement	Interincisor gap (IG) >5 cm (3 finger Breadths), or subluxation[†]	0
	IG gap <5 cm and neutral teeth	1
	IG gap <5 cm and no subluxation	2
Receding mandible	Normal	0
	Moderate	1
	Severe	2
Buck teeth	Normal	0
	Moderate	1
	Severe	2

From [4], with permission from the BMJ Publishing Group.
A total score of >2 points predicts 75% of difficult intubations, with 12.1% false alarms. A score of >4 points predicts only 42% of difficult intubations, but with a lower incidence of false alarms of 0.8%.
[†]Subluxation refers to the forward protrusion of the lower incisors beyond the upper incisors.

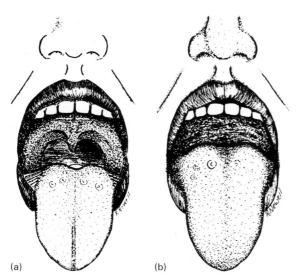

(a)   (b)

Figure 2.1. Maximal oropharyngeal aperture. (a) Good visualisation of faucial pillars, soft palate and uvula, Class 1. (b) Class 4: none of the structures seen. Class 2 (not shown): uvula not seen; pillars and soft palate seen. Class 3 (also not shown): uvula and pillars not seen; soft palate seen. Laryngoscopy is likely to be easier in classes 1 and 2 and difficult in classes 3 and 4. (From Mallampati SR, Gatt SP, Gugino LD et al. A clinical sign to predict difficult tracheal intubation: a prospective study. *Can Anaes Soc J* 1985; 32: 429–434, with permission.)

and venous engorgement suggests cardiac failure. Abnormalities of the pulses can contribute towards the assessment of arrhythmias, valvular conditions, atherosclerosis and congenital malformations. Diastolic murmurs and previously unrecorded systolic murmurs warrant further assessment.

Risk stratification

Many studies have provided data useful in establishing *a priori* categories of risk. Clearly, epidemiological conclusions made regarding patient populations cannot be extrapolated to individuals.

ASA status

The American Society of Anesthesiologists' (ASA) classification is shown in Table 1.1. Some have found it strongly predictive of mortality after general anaesthesia and surgery. Its limitations are based on the exclusion of age, sex and type of surgery in assessment [5].

Confidential enquiry into perioperative deaths reports [6]

The confidential enquiry into perioperative deaths (CEPOD) is a multispecialist investigation into perioperative fatalities in England and Wales (Table 2.5). Its recommendations constitute important guidelines regarding safety trends. Some of the more important points highlighted in recent years are:

- preoperative assessment and treatment;
- skill and experience;
- supervision of trainees;
- perioperative monitoring;
- prevention of thromboembolism;
- out of hours work;
- intensive care facilities;
- records and audit;
- postmortem examinations.

Table 2.5. CEPOD. Classification of operations.

Emergency	Immediate life-saving operations simultaneous with resuscitation. Surgery usually within 1 h.
Urgent	Surgery as soon as possible after resuscitation; operation usually within 24 h.
Scheduled	An early but not immediately life-saving operation. Surgery usually within 3 weeks.
Elective	Surgery to suit both patient and surgeon.

From [7], with permission.

Cardiac risk

Certain cardiovascular factors have been found to correlate with cardiac complications after non-cardiac surgery. They constitute a useful risk index (Table 2.6).

Table 2.6. Clinical Indicators of increased perioperative clinical cardiovascular risk (myocardial infarction, heart failure, death).

Major
- Unstable coronary syndromes
  - Acute or recent myocardial infarction with evidence of important ischaemic risk by clinical symptoms of non-invasive study
  - Unstable or severe angina (Canadian class III or IV)
- Decompensated heart failure
- Significant arrhythmias
  - High-grade aventricular block
  - Symptomatic aventricular arrhythmias in the presence of underlying heart disease
  - Supraventricular arrhythmias with uncontrolled ventricular rate
- Severe valvular disease

Intermediate
Mild angina pectoris (Canadian Class I or II)
Previous myocardial infarction history by pathologic Q waves
Compensated or prior heart failure
Diabetes mellitus (particularly insulin dependent)
Renal insufficiency

Minor
Advanced age
Abnormal ECG (left ventricular hypertrophy, left bundle-branch block, ST-T abnormalities)
Rhythm other than sinus (e.g. atrial fibrillation)
Low functional capacity (e.g. unable to climb a flight of stairs with a bag of vegetables)
History of stroke
Uncontrolled systemic hypertension

AHA guidelines [7].

Table 2.7. Risk of reinfarction following anaesthesia; relationship to previous myocardial infarction.

Interval between previous myocardial infarction and surgery (months)	Incidence of perioperative myocardial infarction (%)
0–3	36
3–6	26
7–12	5
No previous myocardial infarction	0.1–0.7

From [9], with permission.

The mortality following a perioperative myocardial infarction is between 40% and 60%. The risk of developing a perioperative myocardial infarction is exponentially related to the interval between a previous myocardial infarction [8], if there was one, and surgery (Table 2.7). It is therefore advisable to delay non-urgent surgery until at least 3 and preferably 6 months after a myocardial infarction. Patients who require surgery sooner should be considered individually and managed appropriately.

In men with coronary artery disease or who are at high risk of it, that is:
- age >65 years;
- hypercholesterolaemia (>6.2 mmol/l);
- current smoking;
- diabetes mellitus;
- sedentary lifestyle;
- hypertension.

Early postoperative myocardial ischaemia can occur in up to 40%, with up to a 2.8-fold increase in the odds of an adverse cardiac outcome [9]. Clearly, these patients require special management.

High-risk surgical patients

Certain factors are associated with a particularly high mortality in the perioperative period, often related to the development of multiple organ failure [10]:
- previous severe cardiorespiratory illness (acute myocardial infraction, stroke, chronic obstructive airway disease (COAD));
- extensive ablative surgery planned for carcinoma (oesophagectomy, gastrectomy, cystectomy);
- severe multiple trauma (>3 organs or >2 systems);
- massive acute blood loss (>8 units);
- age >70 years with evidence of limited physiologic reserve in one or more vital organs;
- septicaemia (positive blood cultures or septic focus);
- respiratory failure ($PaO_2 < 8$ kPa (60 mmHg), on an $FiO_2 > 0.4$, or mechanical ventilation >48 h);
- acute abdominal catastrophe with haemodynamic instability (pancreatitis, peritonitis, perforation, gastrointestinal haemorrhage);
- acute renal failure (urea >20 mmol/l, creatinine >250 mmol/l);
- late stage vascular disease involving the aorta.

These patients probably benefit from special anaesthetic and intensive care management, which is beyond the scope of this book.

PREMEDICATION

The objectives of premedication are to prepare the patient for anaesthesia and to help provide good conditions for surgery. In practice this involves a combination of the following:
- reduction of anxiety and pain;
- facilitation of intravenous (i.v.) access;

Table 2.8. Benzodiazepines: differential characteristics.

	Adult dose (mg)	Relative potency	Elimination half-life (h)	Active metabolite	Uses	Notes
Temazepam	10–30	0.5	4–10	no	Anxiolytic oral	Popular premedicant
Diazepam	5–10	1	20–30	yes	Anxiolytic sedation oral, IV	Long acting metabolites
Midazolam	1–10	2	1–4	yes	Sedation IV	Potent cardio-respiratory depressant
Lorazepam	1–3	16	10–20	no	Anxiolytic	

- reduction of excessive salivation, gastric contents and undesirable autonomic reflexes.

Preoperative fasting has traditionally been of great importance. There are several issues [11]. Anaesthesia involves the abolition of airway reflexes and an increased risk of vomiting and regurgitation, with subsequent lung aspiration. This potential is greater as the volume and acidity of stomach contents increase. The balance of risks is then established between the danger of aspiration and the danger of delaying surgery. For this reason, non-essential surgery with a full stomach is normally contraindicated.

Many departments have established protocols to deal with the issue of preoperative fasting. Most anaesthetists would accept a period of 4–6 h for solids and 2–4 for clear liquids in healthy adults and an even shorter period in small children.

Many factors determine the volume and acidity of the stomach contents. The most obvious is the time since the last meal. Other factors, like trauma, fear, pain, opioids and other drugs, and gastrointestinal disorders reduce stomach emptying and increase gastric contents up to 24 h after a meal. An excessively long starvation, conversely, has numerous metabolic consequences, including dehydration and protein catabolism, and potentiates nausea and vomiting. Some patients prefer not to have a premedication.

The commonest preparations are described below.

Benzodiazepines

These are excellent anxiolytics; benzodiazepines provide antegrade amnesia and light sedation. They are agonists at the gamma-aminobutyric acid (GABA) receptor. When administered orally 1–2 h before surgery they have only a small effect on cardiorespiratory function. i.v., particularly in frail patients, they cause profound cardiorespiratory depression. Large doses can interfere with the speed and quality of recovery. The differences between benzodiazepines are largely due to pharmacokinetic differences (Table 2.8).

Prokinetics

Metoclopramide (10 mg orally 1–2 h preoperatively) increases gastric motility and oesophageal sphincter pressure; these effects combine to reduce the risk of reflux. This also gives the drug a synergistic effect with the benzodiazepines, increasing their intestinal absorption. In addition, metoclopramide has antiemetic properties, an effect mediated by its antagonism at the central dopaminergic and 5-hydroxy-tryptamine Class 3 (5HT-3) receptors. It can produce dystonia and other extrapyramidal effects, more so when given intramuscularly (i.m.) or i.v.

Anticholinergics

Atropine (0.6 mg i.m.), the classical anticholinergic, is a tertiary amine; it is therefore more lipid soluble and penetrates the blood–brain barrier better, which confers more central activity. It has strong vagolytic action which protects against bradycardia, together with a moderate antisialagogue and weak sedative effect. Hyoscine (0.6 mg i.m.), also a tertiary amine, has strong sedative, amnesic and antisalivation properties. It is a moderately effective antiemetic and potentiates opioids. It is, thus, customary to prescribe i.m. atropine or hyoscine as a premedication, together with an opioid. Glycopyronium (0.4 mg i.m. or i.v.) is not usually administered in the premedication. It is a quaternary amine with little penetration of the blood-brain barrier and limited central action. It is a strong antisialagogue and protects against bradycardia.

Opioids

These are probably agents of choice as premedicants in the presence of acute pain (Table 2.9). In the absence of pain, however, some individuals may experience intense dysphoria. They also cause variable sedation (but not anxiolysis) and cardiorespiratory depression. All opioids cause nausea and vomiting which may overshadow their favourable effects. Most cause histamine release and can precipitate bronchospasm or anaphylaxis.

Topical anaesthesia

Eutectic mixture of local anaesthetic (EMLA) cream is a mixture of 2.5% lignocaine and 2.5% prilocaine in an emulsified and viscous white cream with an approximate density of 1 (1 g = 1 ml). It is used as a topical anaesthetic at the anticipated site of venepuncture. It should be administered between 1 and 3 h before anaesthesia. EMLA is contraindicated in children under 1 year old. Ametop is a topical 4% amethocaine gel which is applied 1 h before venepuncture. Hypersensitivity can occur.

Table 2.9. Opioids: differential characteristics.

	Adult IV dose (mg)	Elimination half-life (h)	Lipid solubility	Notes
Morphine	5–10	2–4	Low	Multiple routes
Pethidine	50–100	2–4	Low–moderate	Mild bronchodilator
				Smooth muscle (gut) relaxant
				Local anaesthetic effect
Fentanyl	0.025–5	3–4	High	Little or no histamine release
Alfentanil	0.25–10	1–1.5	Moderate	Less accumulation

PREOPERATIVE CHECKS

Before administering any anaesthetic the anaesthetist will want to verify that the equipment intended for use is available and functioning [12]. Some of the most important aspects are:

- trained assistance;
- airway equipment;
  - range of laryngoscope blades;
  - range of endotracheal tube sizes;
  - adequate suctioning;
  - intubation adjuvants, for example, bougie.
- oxygen and gases;
- anaesthetic machine and ventilator;
  - checked for safe gas delivery;
  - circuit checked for leaks or blockages;
  - ventilator functioning checked.
- drugs and accessories;
  - routine and emergency drugs;
  - i.v. cannula available.
- monitors and alarms; Minimum monitoring, as set out by the Association of Anaesthetists of Great Britain and Ireland, available in the anaesthetic room and theatre, namely:
  - ECG;
  - non-invasive blood pressure;
  - pulse oximetry;
  - capnography.
- operating table;
- identity of the patient, written consent and appropriate site of surgery (e.g. right or left) should be confirmed.

INDUCTION

Induction of anaesthesia should normally take place in the anaesthetic room, operating theatre or intensive care unit. After carefully positioning the patient on the operating table, monitoring is applied, normally an ECG, pulse oximeter and non-invasive blood pressure cuff. Other monitors may sometimes be indicated. Adequate i.v. access is secured.

Preoxygenation with 100% oxygen may be indicated; this increases the amount of oxygen in the lungs and tissues several fold [13]. It allows a longer period of apnoea and consequently more time before the development of hypoxaemia if difficulties arise. The disadvantages are that preoxygenation may exacerbate fear and anxiety. Furthermore, the longer period before hypoxaemia ensues may delay recognition of oesophageal intubation. Many anaesthetists do not preoxygenate healthy patients, but have a low threshold in other populations or when in doubt.

Methods

Intravenous induction

This is the commonest technique in adults and, since the widespread use of EMLA cream, is preferred by many for children. The i.v. induction is rapid, smooth and reliable but has the important disadvantages of loss of airway muscle tone and apnoea, which may occasionally make oxygenation difficult or impossible.

The chosen induction agent is administered slowly until the patient begins to lose consciousness; anaesthesia usually ensues within one arm–brain circulation time. Any amount administered, therefore, after loss of consciousness may result in overdose.

Inhalational induction

This is preferred by most anaesthetists for induction of anaesthesia in upper airway obstruction; some also prefer it for induction in children. It may also be indicated in bronchopleural fistula or empyema and when i.v. access is problematic. Airway muscle tone and breathing are normally maintained. However, inhalational induction is slow, requires some patient cooperation and can be associated with coughing, laryngeal spasm and bronchospasm, especially in the excitement stages of anaesthesia, also making oxygenation difficult or impossible.

Control of the airway

Intubation

Intubation of the trachea is performed with a cuffed tube in adults or a non-cuffed one in infants and small children.

In performing intubation, the position of the head and neck are vitally important. The neck should be flexed, supported by one or two pillows, and the head extended in the so-called 'sniffing the morning air' position. This is the best position for straight alignment between the mouth, pharynx and laryngeal glottis. If the neck is damaged or diseased it should not be moved and may require stabilisation. This may make intubation more difficult.

After consciousness is lost the chosen neuromuscular blocker is given. When full neuromuscular paralysis has developed, the laryngoscope is introduced between the tongue and hard palate. It is gently advanced, taking care not to damage the teeth, until lodged in the vallecular fossa, anterior to the epiglottis. Laryngoscopy is performed by lifting, not rotating, the laryngoscope; the mandible, tongue and epiglottis are thereby displaced anteriorly, revealing the laryngeal inlet. A tracheal tube of the appropriate size is placed between the arytenoids (posteriorly) and epiglottis (anteriorly), and guided into the proximal trachea. The view of the larynx may be facilitated by externally applied pressure on the anterior aspect of the larynx.

Intubation is the best, but not absolute, protection against aspiration into the airway. In addition, it enables positive pressure ventilation of the lungs. Some of its disadvantages are:

- delay or failure to intubate and ventilate may cause profound hypoxaemia;
- muscle relaxants can cause adverse effects;
- disconnection can cause hypoxaemia;
- sputum retention or lung collapse, especially in chronic obstructive airway disease, may lead to respiratory infection.

Laryngoscopy and intubation are invasive. They may produce tachycardia and hypertension, usually when insufficient anaesthesia and analgesia have been given, as well as local trauma. Conversely, stimulation of the pharyngo-larynx, especially in children, may produce profound bradycardia, and occasionally asystole, mediated by the vagus nerve.

Other methods

Other approaches involve maintaining airway patency with a face mask or a laryngeal mask airway (LMA) and allowing spontaneous ventilation to continue [14]. Neither a face mask nor an LMA seal the trachea and so do not prevent aspiration; their use is therefore only appropriate in patients with an empty stomach and no intestinal motility disorders. In many patients, however, once deep anaesthesia is established there is relatively little risk of regurgitation, which is normally a passive process in response to potent stimuli. During induction and recovery, providing the airway is handled with care and there is no undue surgical stimulation, there is also relatively little risk of laryngeal spasm or vomiting. This technique is used for many short procedures (<90 min) in reasonably fit patients undergoing non-major surgery where, in addition, muscle paralysis and controlled ventilation are not necessary.

Control of breathing (ventilation)

Controlled ventilation

Most commonly this is done through a tracheal tube and with muscle paralysis. In suitable patients undergoing suitable procedures, it can be performed through a laryngeal mask. Sometimes the relative relaxation provided by analgesic and anaesthetic drugs obviates the need for formal paralysis.

Controlled ventilation has the advantages of a reduction in the work of breathing, better control of arterial blood gases, reduction in anaesthetic concentrations and ideal conditions for surgery. Its disadvantages are need for tracheal intubation, possibility of disconnection, ventilator-induced barotrauma and the readjustment of blood gases to levels potentially very different from a particular patient's 'normal'.

Spontaneous ventilation

This is normally the case with a face mask or LMA technique. Spontaneous ventilation can also be allowed to resume after tracheal intubation, if controlled ventilation and paralysis are not required. This technique has the disadvantage of requiring high-anaesthetic concentrations which slows recovery.

MAINTENANCE OF ANAESTHESIA

Maintenance of anaesthesia involves constant vigilance of the patient's state of hypnosis, analgesia and paralysis, as well as attention to the condition of the airway, ventilation and cardiovascular system. Although no absolute monitor of depth of anaesthesia exists, several attempts have been made to provide some indication. One such monitor is bispectral index (BIS) monitoring, which is a mathematical interpretation of electroencephalogram (EEG) patterns to give a number between 0 and 100. The lower numbers refer to anaesthetised patients and higher numbers are in awake patients.

Anaesthesia (hypnosis)

Anaesthesia is maintained either by inhalational agents or by i.v. anaesthetic agents. The former is by far the commonest.

Inhalational anaesthesia

With continuous administration of anaesthetic drugs, a steady-state is reached where the partial pressures of anaesthetic in the breathing system, alveoli and brain are directly related. This occurs after about 20–30 min, depending mostly on the agent, breathing system and patient haemodynamics.

Clinical observation of sympathetic activity, pupil size, lacrimation and perspiration remains the commonest method of assessing anaesthetic depth. These signs may, however, be masked by many drugs and diseases. Therefore, it is customary to administer anaesthetic agents at concentrations known to provide unawareness, titrated according to individual response. Together with the use of nitrous oxide and allowing for premedication, induction agents and opioid analgesics, a properly conducted anaesthetic following these principles should produce hypnosis (see below).

The advantages of inhalational anaesthesia are that it is simple to administer and its extensive use over many decades has resulted in increased safety and efficacy. It has certain disadvantages:

- wash-in, wash-out times are relatively slow and there is some residual drowsiness;
- all inhalational agents are cardiorespiratory depressants.

Intravenous anaesthesia

This consists of the infusion of an i.v. anaesthetic agent, almost exclusively propofol. It can be commenced on or shortly after induction. Pharmacokinetic and pharmacological evidence has contributed to the development of safe infusion regimens. These vary depending on clinical observation and whether propofol is supplemented by other drugs. A common combination is propofol and remifentanil infusions in a Total Intravenous Anaesthetic (TIVA) technique.

The i.v. anaesthesia is smooth, stable, probably requires less muscle relaxation and provides a speedy recovery, perhaps with less residual drowsiness. It necessitates constant attention to the i.v. infusion site. There is greater interindividual variation in dose requirements than for inhalational anaesthesia.

Analgesia

It is difficult to separate anaesthesia from analgesia and most anaesthetists are cautious in this respect.

The i.v. opioids are the agents of choice. They are given on induction and during anaesthesia, depending on their pharmacokinetic properties and the patient's renal, hepatic and cardiovascular function. Other methods of analgesia include nitrous oxide, non-steroidal anti-inflammatory drugs (NSAIDs) and nerve blocks with local anaesthetics and/or opioids.

Paralysis

There are three groups of indications for neuromuscular paralysis:

1. intubation (usually) of the trachea (see above);
2. relaxation to facilitate positive pressure ventilation;
3. provision of ideal conditions for surgery, usually, for major abdominal, cardiothoracic and neurosurgical procedures.

Great interindividual variations make it difficult to predict how much muscle paralysis individual patients will need and the dose of muscle relaxant required to achieve this. In practice, it is customary to aim for the minimum paralysis which is clinically satisfactory and to monitor the neuromuscular block with a nerve stimulator.

The disadvantages of neuromuscular paralysis are:

- hypoxaemia due to failure to secure the airway;
- disconnection from the breathing system;
- unrecognised awareness;
- side-effects of neuromuscular blocking drugs.

Pharmacology of anaesthetic agents

Inhalational agents

Modern inhalational drugs are fluorinated hydrocarbons. Most are liquids at room temperature. Due to their high-saturated vapour pressure a significant proportion of the liquid is in the vapour or 'volatile' phase. Their lipid solubility, which is directly related to potency, is high. Their blood solubility is relatively low, and this is an advantage; see below.

Potency of anaesthetic agents is gauged by the minimum alveolar concentration (MAC). This is defined as the alveolar anaesthetic concentration that abolishes reflex response to a standard skin incision in 50% of subjects. MAC is expressed as a percentage of volume concentrations at atmospheric pressure in healthy adults not receiving other drugs. MAC is additive. About 1.5 MAC abolishes response in 95% of the population. At about 0.4 MAC amnesia ensues; awakening occurs at around 0.6 MAC. Many factors such as temperature, premedication, nitrous oxide and age influence MAC. MAC is a theoretical concept but useful in that it is intuitive and measurable.

Anaesthesia is directly related to partial pressure of anaesthetic drug in the brain. Blood acts as an inactive reservoir between the lung and brain. The greater the solubility in blood, the greater the amount required to generate a given partial pressure; this means the time to reach equilibrium (partial pressure alveolus–partial pressure blood–partial pressure brain) is greater and therefore that induction and recovery are slower. Inhalational anaesthetics are metabolised by the liver to a variable extent, but mostly eliminated unchanged by the lungs.

To different degrees the inhalational agents depress heart rate and contractility, dilate vascular smooth muscle, lower arterial blood pressure, and may alter the conduction system. Their effects on the respiratory system vary with the individual agent; in general their effects are bronchodilatation, airway irritability which may precipitate bronchospasm, and respiratory depression.

Although all modern volatile agents have similar characteristics, some differential features may occasionally prove clinically significant and are briefly discussed below.

Halothane (MAC = 0.75)

It is the classical fluorocarbon, in clinical use since the mid 1950's. It can cause depression of the sino-atrial node, leading to atrial or nodal bradycardias and ventricular ectopics. It is a potent depressant of myocardial contractility. Halothane provides a smooth induction of anaesthesia with little airway irritation, and is still preferred by many anaesthetists for inhalational induction in the difficult paediatric airway. Very rarely, its oxidative metabolites can induce immune mediated hepatic necrosis, which has dramatically curtailed its use. It is now rarely used in the UK.

Enflurane (MAC = 1.68)

It is probably the strongest depressant of cardiac output and of blood pressure. Prolonged administration of high concentrations yields fluoride metabolites potentially associated with renal tubular dysfunction. At high doses it can produce epileptiform-like EEG paroxysms. Most anaesthetists do not use enflurane in the presence of renal failure or epilepsy.

Isoflurane (MAC = 1.15)

It has less myocardial depressant than halothane or enflurane. It is a potent vasodilator and has been implicated in steal of blood from diseased rigid coronary arteries to more healthy ones. It is the agent of choice in neuroanaesthesia, as it is associated with least increases in cerebral blood flow and intracranial pressure. It is rather pungent and irritant to the airway; this makes inhalational induction more difficult and prone to laryngeal spasm.

Desflurane (MAC = 6.0)

Introduced into clinical practice over the last few years, it has the lowest blood solubility (0.4), and therefore the shortest equilibrium time. Its boiling point is 23.5°C, so near to room temperature that it requires a special vaporiser. It resembles isoflurane in its clinical performance.

Sevoflurane (MAC = 2.0)

It is also relatively new and almost as short acting as desflurane. It is not irritable to the airway, and is becoming an agent of choice for induction of anaesthesia in children.

Nitrous oxide (N_2O; MAC = 104)

Together with ether it is the oldest anaesthetic agent, dating back at least to 1846. Unlike the others it is a gas at room temperature (boiling point −88°C). Nitrous oxide is very insoluble in blood (0.47) and its equilibrium time is very short. It is a weak anaesthetic but a good analgesic and is therefore used as an adjuvant to the inhalational vapours in concentrations of up to 70% in oxygen.

Although relatively insoluble, nitrous oxide is nevertheless much more *soluble* than nitrogen. This is an advantage on induction as it diffuses out of the alveoli faster than nitrogen diffuses in, and increases the alveolar concentration of the remaining substances, oxygen and the volatile drug. During recovery, nitrous oxide diffuses into the alveoli quicker than nitrogen, causing a reduction in alveolar oxygen. This effect is known as diffusion hypoxia. A similar mechanism is responsible for its preferential diffusion into closed spaces such as the middle ear, pneumothorax, gut lumen, etc. In some circumstances, nitrous oxide is a potent cardiovascular depressant. Prolonged exposure may have deleterious effect on the metabolism of vitamin B12 and folic acid.

Intravenous anaesthetic drugs

Thiopentone

Thiopentone is a sulphur containing barbiturate administered at a concentration of 25 mg/ml. It is the most widely used induction agent in the world. It is highly lipid soluble and protein bound. It is smooth and predictable, inducing unconsciousness within 30–45 s. Awakening occurs after some 3–5 min due to redistribution from the brain to the skeletal muscle. It is metabolised mainly in the liver at a rate proportional to the dose administered. Its elimination half-life is around 11.5 h; after 24 h, some 30% of the dose still remains in the body. The induction dose is 2–6 mg/kg i.v. over 20–40 s and it is important to administer the drug slowly to avoid overshooting.

Thiopentone decreases the rate of GABA breakdown, leading to neuronal hyperpolarisation. It produces unconsciousness and inhibition of the reticular activating system and is a potent anticonvulsant. Thiopentone significantly depresses myocardial contractility; it also produces moderate vasodilatation. There is a baroreceptor mediated reflex tachycardia which is not sufficient to prevent an important reduction in arterial blood pressure. In those with cardiovascular compromise, even if only mild hypovolaemia, the fall in blood pressure may be profound and can induce cardiac arrest. Thiopentone produces apnoea and can induce laryngeal spasm, especially with early and abrupt manipulation of the airway. Recovery is normally associated with a hangover effect as a consequence of its lipid affinity and slow elimination.

Thiopentone can produce tissue necrosis if injected into subcutaneous tissue and arterial vasoconstriction leading to ischaemia if injected into an artery. For these reasons it is important, while injecting the drug slowly, to check for pain.

Contraindications to thiopentone include contraindications of i.v. induction in general, such as upper airway obstruction, and more specific ones, namely porphyria and known anaphylaxis.

Propofol

Propofol is a phenol derivative which comes in a white aqueous solution of egg phosphatide and soyabean oil, at a concentration of 20 mg/ml. It has gained enormous popularity since its introduction into clinical practice in the mid to late 1980's. Propofol has a higher lipid solubility, protein binding, and a larger volume of distribution than thiopentone. Metabolism is hepatic and probably also extrahepatic. Propofol produces a speedy recovery with less drowsiness. There is less accumulation of propofol after large doses or i.v. infusions, as its elimination remains relatively constant.

For induction of anaesthesia the dose of propofol is 1 to 3.5 mg/kg, administered slowly and titrated to response, but there seems to be considerable interindividual variation. For infusion as the primary anaesthetic the dose, after initial loading, is 6–9 mg/kg h. For sedation the recommended dose is 2–6 mg/kg h.

In addition to loss of consciousness, propofol produces amnesia, and has some antiemetic effect. Its effects on the cardiovascular system consist of a marked fall in peripheral resistance and a variable reduction in cardiac output; often propofol is associated with a bradycardia, particularly in young healthy patients who have been premedicated. Together these effects probably produce a greater fall in blood pressure than thiopentone. Apnoea ensues very rapidly after administration and at widely varying doses; readily available equipment for oxygenation is essential even if only 'sedation' is intended. Propofol produces greater depression of the laryngeal reflexes, making laryngeal spasm less likely.

Propofol, especially when injected rapidly into a small vein, frequently produces pain on injection. Propofol is safe in malignant hyperpyrexia and porphyria. There have been reports of epileptiform activity associated with its use in susceptible individuals and it is recommended that extreme care be exercised if it is to be administered in epileptic patients.

Etomidate

Etomidate is a carboxylated imidazole. It is less cardiodepressant than other agents, but not innocuous, and is associated with less histamine release. Many anaesthetists prefer it for induction of anaesthesia in cardiovascularly compromised patients and severe asthmatics.

Even one dose produces inhibition of the 11b and 17a hydroxylase enzymes involved in cortisol synthesis. It often produces excitatory type movements on induction. Etomidate has been associated with epileptiform EEG activity. It may be painful on injection and has a relatively high incidence of thrombophlebitis.

Opioids

Some of the more important locations of opioid receptors are the periaqueductal matter of the brainstem, hypothalamus, and substantia gelatinosa of the spinal cord. When stimulated they inhibit adenylate cyclase, which leads to hyperpolarisation of cell membranes and reduction in electrical discharge; this interferes with the release of Substance P and other pain mediators.

The effects of opioids on the central nervous system range, with progressively higher doses, from slight alteration of mood to deep unconsciousness. It must be emphasised that at ordinary clinical doses opioids act as supplements to anaesthesia, and if used on their own or with insufficient anaesthetic agent may be associated with awareness. Some important side-effects include miosis, increased smooth muscle tone (intestinal and sphincter of Oddi spasm), urinary retention and pruritus.

Morphine

A naturally occurring alkaloid, it is the standard opioid. It can be administered orally, i.m., i.v., subcutaneously, and also by the neuraxial (epidural, etc.) route. The i.v. dose is 0.1–0.2 mg/kg. It can be associated with histamine release and should probably be avoided in asthma.

Papaveretum

Papaveretum contains a mixture of morphine, thebaine and papaverine. Until recently it contained noscapine, which was eliminated because of potential teratogenic effects in animals. It causes more sedation and less smooth muscle spasm.

Fentanyl

A synthetic phenoperidine derivative of morphine, it is some 100 times more potent. Its short onset and redistribution times give it rapid onset and recovery after a single administration. Because of its high-lipid solubility, high doses or multiple administrations lead to accumulation in the lipid tissue, which acts as a reservoir; its action can be prolonged.

Fentanyl, even at high doses, has little effect on the cardiovascular system (small reduction in heart rate and blood pressure) and is considered an ideal drug for anaesthesia in those with cardiovascular compromise. The dose varies from 1 to 100 mg/kg. The higher doses ablate the stress response associated with surgery but do not guarantee abolition of awareness, and necessitate prolonged ventilation and observation.

Alfentanil

This is a synthetic derivative of fentanyl about 10–20 times more potent than morphine. It has a very rapid onset of action (1–2 min) despite less lipid solubility, as most of the compound is non-ionised. Its half-life and therefore recovery time is short; because of a relatively small volume of distribution, it shows less accumulation and hangover effect after large doses or i.v. infusions. Alfentanil has a more pronounced cardiodepressant effect than fentanyl. It is a potent emetic.

Remifentanil

A short acting, quick offset, synthetic opioid, used as an infusion typically at 0.01–0.03 μg/kg min as a sedative or to supplement anaesthesia. It has a 3–5 min half-life so does not accumulate, and facilitates rapid awakening. Supplementary analgesia is required if pain is expected once the remifentanil infusion is stopped.

Neuromuscular blocking drugs
Depolarising drugs

Suxamethonium (Succinylcholine) is a synthetic compound which depolarises the neuromuscular junction by mimicking the action of acetylcholine, the cholinergic transmitter; while the membrane remains depolarised muscle contraction cannot occur. The effect of suxamethonium ensues within 30–60 s of its administration and normally lasts a few minutes, until it is metabolised by plasma cholinesterase. Deficiencies in this enzyme cause suxamethonium apnoea.

Suxamethonium reliably provides the fastest and best conditions for intubation. The dose is 1–1.5 mg/kg after loss of consciousness. It is the drug of choice for emergency intubations. Some anaesthetists use it for difficult intubations in which ventilating the lungs is not likely to present a risk, as its rapid elimination facilitates the prompt return of breathing if intubation fails.

Suxamethonium has many side-effects. Hyperkaelemia, caused by the potent depolarisation, can be severe in extensive muscle damage, burns, peripheral neuropathy and paraplegia. Muscarinic stimulation can cause bradycardia. Fasciculations are thought to cause muscle pain. Anaphylactic or anaphylactoid reactions are more frequent than with other muscle relaxants and can be severe. Although it has traditionally been considered a trigger of malignant hyperpyrexia, there is now some doubt regarding this point. Nevertheless, anaesthetists avoid suxamethonium in susceptible patients.

Non-depolarising drugs

These agents bind reversibly to cholinergic receptors and prevent acetylcholine from activating them. Their onset time is 2–3 min. Their action is terminated by metabolism. The intricacies of neuromuscular pharmacology are outside the scope of this book.

The cholinergic block may also extend into other areas of the autonomic system. The differences between available drugs are due to their metabolism and degree of extranicotinic effects.

Pancuronium is an aminosteroid of moderate (1–2 h) duration; its sympathomimetic effect can cause tachycardia and a slight rise in cardiac output and blood pressure. It should be avoided in renal failure as it is partially excreted by the kidney.

Vecuronium is chemically very similar to pancuronium, but devoid of cardiovascular effect; it is shorter acting, and metabolised by the liver.

Atracurium has a time of onset and duration of action is similar to vecuronium. It may, however, release histamine. It is degraded by a process which is independent of liver and kidney function. Atracurium is the most suitable for i.v. infusion as it is subject to little accumulation.

Rocuronium is another steroid based compound. It was initially developed to be used in place of suxamethonium. Although faster in onset than other non-depolarising muscle relaxants (90 s), it still falls short of suxamethonium. It lasts longer than atracurium and vecuronium.

Perioperative fluid management

Guidelines for perioperative fluid administration (Table 2.10)

In principle, administration of fluids should be guided by estimations of existing deficits, maintenance requirements and ongoing losses:

1. *Deficit*: The usual preoperative starvation period (8 h) is likely to account for a water deficit of 800–1000 ml. This can be replaced by the appropriate volume of a crystalloid solution. Patients with gastrointestinal losses, for example, from fistulae or diarrhoea, are likely to have additional salt and potassium deficits.

2. *Maintenance*: The maintenance requirements can be met with an infusion of 50–150 ml/h of salt-containing solution.

3. *Losses*: Healthy adults have a circulating blood volume (CBV) of about 80 ml/kg or 4500–5000 ml. Blood losses beyond 15% of the CBV are normally replaced with blood. Increasingly, blood conservation methods are employed, such as cell salvage, in order to reduce the amount of donated blood used. Losses of less than this are normally replaced with equal volumes of colloid solutions. Alternatively, about triple volumes of crystalloid can be given, as these are distributed throughout the extracellular space, which is roughly three times greater in volume. Additional amounts of protein-rich fluid within the site of surgical trauma are sequestered from the extracellular space and lost into a metabolically inactive 'third space'. This fluid loss is variable but can be replaced by crystalloid or colloid solutions at rates of 1–10 ml/kg h.

Table 2.10. **Contents of common crystalloid solutions.**

	Na^+ (mmol/l)	Cl^- (mmol/l)	K^+ (mmol/l)	Osmolality (mosmol/Kg)	pH	Carbohydrates (g/l)	Calories (Kcal/l)
Sodium chloride 0.9%	154	154	0	308	5.5	0	0
Glucose 5%	0	0	0	278	4.1	50	188
Sodium chloride 0.18% with glucose 4%	31	31	0	284	4.5	40	150
Sodium lactate (Hartmann's)	131	111 HCO_3^-: 29 $Ca +2$: 2	5	281	6.5	0	0

MONITORING [19]

The best monitoring is provided by a trained anaesthetist applying continuous clinical observation skills throughout the entire anaesthetic. A patient with pink, warm and moist mucocutaneous membranes, a capillary refill of about 1 s, good strong regular peripheral pulses, adequate respiratory excursion of both hemithoraces and appropriate urine volumes is almost certainly in a stable condition and in no immediate danger.

In addition to good clinical judgement, there are technical devices which may provide early warning of problems; they constitute a much welcome aid to modern anaesthesia and have been associated with a reduction in legal claims and an increase in safety [18]. They help the anaesthetist to maintain the wellbeing of patients and reduce fatigue and stress. As a general principle, alarms must not be turned off out of habit, as this defeats their purpose. Rather, the abnormality setting the alarm off (e.g. tachycardia) should be addressed or the alarm limit adjusted accordingly, for example, in paediatric practice. Some of the more important instruments are discussed below.

Monitoring of the patient

Pulse oximetry

This is based on the physical principle of different but characteristic absorptions of light by oxygenated and deoxygenated Hb. Software developments have enabled separation of light absorption by blood (Hb) from that of skin and tissues.

Pulse oximetry measures blood oxygenation noninvasively. Indirectly it provides an indication of ventilation–perfusion match, heart rate and rhythm and peripheral perfusion. It warns of deterioration in oxygenation but does not indicate its aetiology. Abnormal Hb (carboxyhaemoglobin and methaemoglobin) can give false readings, as can severe hypoxaemia [20].

Expired CO_2

CO_2 analysers normally work by infrared gas analysis. This is based on the principle that gases with more than one atom in their molecule absorb radiation at a characteristic wavelength. It is most useful in children where the anatomical dead space, is small. In adults, because of the larger dead space, dilutional effects may make interpretation more difficult. The graph of concentration versus time can reflect the adequacy of ventilation. It is possible to detect rebreathing (high CO_2 during inspiration) and obstructive airways disease (delayed rise towards the expiratory plateau).

Expired CO_2 analysis is valuable in the detection of the following potentially lethal conditions:
- *Oesophageal intubation*: Even experienced anaesthetists can occasionally find oesophageal intubation very difficult to detect. Absence of CO_2 production after five consecutive 'breaths' is nearly pathognomonic of intubation of the oesophagus. It is an indication to remove the tube and oxygenate the patient by other means, that is, a face mask.
- *Disconnection*.
- *Deficiencies in ventilation*: Although airway obstruction or gas trapping have characteristic expiratory patterns, interpretation can sometimes be difficult and, if in doubt, it is best to obtain a sample of arterial blood for analysis of blood gases.
- *Detection of air or pulmonary embolism*: The increased deadspace created by ventilated but underperfused alveoli, causes a sharp decrease (by dilution) in expired CO_2 and in the ratio of expired/arterial CO_2. This is particularly useful in surgery where the position of the head is above that of the heart (head and neck surgery, neurosurgery, etc.). In general, a low cardiac output (impending cardiac arrest or cardiogenic shock, in addition to the causes discussed above) features an abnormally low perfusion, a high ventilation–perfusion ratio and, consequently, a low expired CO_2 (increased deadspace).
- *Malignant hyperpyrexia*: A frank increase in CO_2 often precedes other signs.

ECG

A three-lead ECG displays surface electrical activity of the heart; this is useful in the assessment of rhythm and rate, particularly in lead II. A CM5 configuration (negative lead, right sternal border; positive lead, same as V5) is the most sensitive in detecting intraoperative ischaemic events.

Non-invasive blood pressure

The cuff must be appropriate for the arm size. If the cuff is too small, it may give falsely high readings. All cuffs tend to be more inaccurate the lower the systolic pressure. Obviously arrhythmias and sudden changes in blood pressure may affect cuff accuracy.

Temperature gradient

It is easy to measure nasopharyngeal (core) and skin temperature. The gradient between the two provides a marker of peripheral perfusion and, indirectly and together with many other clinical signs, of vascular resistance and cardiac output.

Intra-arterial blood pressure

This provides accurate beat-to-beat measurement of blood pressure. It also provides useful information on rhythm and a gauge of the efficiency of individual beats, for example, in extrasystoles. In addition, it enables blood sampling. Careful cannulation of limb arteries is associated with a low incidence of side-effects. Before cannulating the radial artery, some anaesthetists routinely check for collateral flow from the ulnar artery.

Other monitors

Measurement of central venous pressure (CVP), pulmonary artery occlusion or wedge pressure (PAOP), cardiac output,

TOE, etc., are undertaken during complex surgery and/or in ill patients but they are outside the scope of this book.

Monitoring of the equipment

Inspired oxygen concentration

There are a multitude of oxygen analysers available based on several different electrophysical principles. They may be affected by water vapour and nitrous oxide and they must be calibrated regularly.

Volatile agent concentration

Monitors normally operate by infrared gas analysis. There can be a considerable difference between the vaporiser setting and the delivered concentration. Volatile agent concentration monitors should help to avoid excessively light or heavy anaesthetics.

Ventilator disconnect alarm

There are many different kinds and all are designed to detect an absence in cyclical pressure fluctuations within the breathing system rapidly. The two most important causes of this are disconnection and ventilator failure.

RECOVERY

Recovery from anaesthesia is considered to start when the patient is no longer under the direct care of an anaesthetist. It should take place in a specifically designated area.

The recovery unit should be staffed by appropriately trained personnel in a ratio of staff to patients of not less than one to one. It should have enough equipment and monitors to care for a wide range of patients, which will vary among different hospitals. Specifically, each patient should have dedicated oxygen and suction ports, a trolley or bed with head-down tilt, and similar monitoring to that used in theatre. In addition, every recovery unit must have a full range of anaesthetic and resuscitation equipment.

Communication between medical staff and recovery room personnel is extremely important. Anaesthetists must relay patient characteristics to the recovery nurses, and these in turn should keep anaesthetists informed of the patient's progress.

There are a multitude of potentially serious problems which can arise in the recovery room, many with little warning; some of the more common ones are discussed below.

Hypoxaemia

Hypoxaemia can be defined as low arterial oxygen content. It is a relative concept; nevertheless in healthy subjects breathing air an arterial saturation below 90% and/or a PaO_2 of less than 9 kPa normally represent hypoxaemia. In addition even moderate anaemia, say Hb below 10 mg/dl, causes significantly impaired oxygen carriage.

For purposes of discussion, hypoxaemia is divided into early, occurring up to 4 h postoperatively, and late, extending several days after surgery and anaesthesia.

Early hypoxaemia
Airway obstruction

This constitutes a spectrum which presents as respiratory distress characterised by inspiratory stridor, use of the accessory muscles of respiration, straining, and asynchrony between chest and abdominal excursion. In its most extreme form there is insufficient airflow to cause even these signs, with no air entering the lungs.

There are three main causes of airway obstruction. The first is loss of airway muscle tone, due to decreased consciousness or to residual neuromuscular paralysis. The second is laryngeal spasm caused by inappropriate stimulation of the pharyngo-larynx, or by blood, secretions, or stomach contents in the airway. Thirdly, surgical and anaesthetic factors, such as local haemorrhage, recurrent laryngeal nerve trauma, and foreign objects (throat packs, swabs, etc.) can cause airway obstruction.

Airway obstruction requires immediate treatment. Positioning the patient in the left lateral position may prevent posterior displacement of the tongue and collapse of the pharyngeal muscles. The chin lift and jaw thrust manoeuvres contribute to airway stability and may definitively solve the problem. An oropharyngeal airway may help to maintain the airway patent. However, in some patients, especially if they are too 'awake', an oropharyngeal airway may provoke coughing or laryngeal spasm. If all else has failed it becomes necessary to paralyse, intubate and ventilate the patient.

Alveolar hypoventilation

The causes of alveolar hypoventilation are respiratory depression, unresolved neuromuscular paralysis, and closure of lung units.

The latter has a complex mechanism but is very important. Anaesthesia causes a decrease in functional residual capacity (FRC), which often leads to closure of small airways while breathing within the tidal volume range. This reduction in alveolar volume causes relative underventilation of perfused areas, leading to venous admixture (low ventilation–perfusion ratio or shunt).

Low cardiac output

Common causes include hypovolaemia, poor ventricular function (see below), and cardiodepressant effects of anaesthetics, opioids, and other medications. In states of low cardiac output there is relative underperfusion of ventilated areas (high ventilation–perfusion) which creates alveolar dead space.

Diffusion hypoxia

This occurs minutes after discontinuation of nitrous oxide. It should be prevented by prompt administration of oxygen.

Increased oxygen consumption

When not compensated by increased extraction or increased cardiac output an increase in oxygen consumption, say in shivering or agitation, causes hypoxaemia. This may worsen the equilibrium between myocardial oxygen consumption and demand.

Late hypoxaemia

Respiratory dysfunction

Pain impairs the ability to cough efficiently, which can lead to sputum retention and consolidation. The postoperative reduction in lung volume already discussed, if allowed to persist unimpaired, leads to reduction in respiratory excursion and small lung volumes, which ultimately can cause lobar collapse.

In practice consolidation and collapse often coexist. They constitute a spectrum which presents clinically as pyrexia, purulent sputum, tachycardia and tachypnoea. Patients most at risk are smokers, the obese, those with chronic obstructive airways disease, and those undergoing high abdominal or thoracic surgery.

Treatment consists of close observation in an adequately staffed and equipped unit, oxygen therapy (see below) physiotherapy, analgesia, and appropriate antibiotics. Many anaesthetists consider epidural analgesia has certain advantages for this patient population; it provides effective analgesia and can reduce opioid requirements and side-effects.

Episodic desaturation

This is usually due to a decrease in airway muscle tone, which may persist up to 5 days postoperatively. In the first 48 h these muscle tone changes are thought to be related to opioids. From about 48 h onwards changes in sleep pattern, not unlike obstructive sleep apnoea, are implicated.

Postoperative oxygen therapy

Due to changes in lung mechanisms intrinsic to general anaesthesia, particularly a reduction in FRC, and to the diffusion hypoxia of nitrous oxide, most patients require at least a brief period of supplemental oxygen therapy. Many anaesthetists administer oxygen enriched air for a period equal to the duration of the operation, unless circumstances dictate otherwise.

Oxygen resolves the hypoxaemia of reduced minute ventilation, a common condition after surgery (Fig. 2.2). Administration of oxygen can maintain an adequate saturation even in serious hypoventilation [15], creating a false sense of well-being when, for example, a worsening hypercarbia is developing. Administration of oxygen to patients with chronic obstructive airways disease who rely on a certain hypoxaemic drive to stimulate their respiratory centre may abolish this stimulus and lead to apnoea.

In hypoxaemia of venous admixture (low ventilation–perfusion ratio or shunt typically caused by pneumonia, lung collapse, or pulmonary oedema) a high proportion

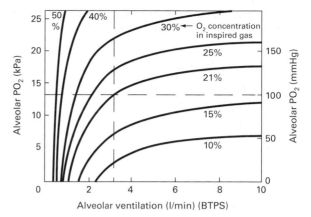

Figure 2.2

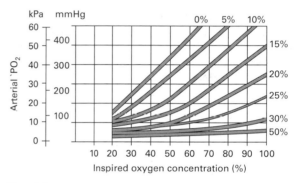

Figure 2.3

of the cardiac output bypasses functioning lung units creating a large alveolo-arterial oxygen gradient. Oxygen administered does not come into contact with pulmonary capillaries and may not completely reverse this hypoxaemia (Fig. 2.3).

The performance of different oxygen face masks depends on several factors. These are the flow of oxygen, the shape of the mask, total gas flow, and the respiratory pattern of the patient, in particular the peak inspired flow rate (PIFR). Face masks are divided into those of fixed or of variable performance.

Variable performance face masks

These masks (Hudson, M. C., nasal cannulae, etc.) provide an inspired oxygen concentration which varies breath by breath depending on the patient's PIFR and breathing pattern (expiratory pause). They are perfectly satisfactory for the majority of healthy patients undergoing non-major surgery. If there is any doubt about a patient's ability to maintain adequate oxygenation, they probably should not be used.

Fixed performance face masks

They provide a constant known inspired oxygen concentration, independent of the patient's breathing pattern. They are designed such that the jet of oxygen administered entrains a fixed proportion of air by the Venturi effect; this phenomenon is known as high air flow oxygen enrichment (HAFOE). The design also ensures that the total flow (oxygen dialed plus air entrained) is greater than the expected PIFR of patients likely to need oxygen therapy, normally 30 l/min; this avoids rebreathing gas poor in oxygen.

These masks are usually indicated for patients who require a constant and accurate oxygen concentration, usually those with ventilation–perfusion mismatch (shunt or dead space) or chronic obstructive airways disease. High concentrations of oxygen (up to 60%) can be used in the former; low concentrations (24–28%) are normally used in the latter.

Hypoventilation

In addition to hypoxaemia, hypoventilation also causes hypercarbia. Many of the factors involved are interdependent and have been already discussed. In the postoperative period reduced minute ventilation has two main aetiologies: reduced central respiratory drive and peripheral muscle weakness.

Hypotension

There are several important causes of hypotension.

Vasodilatation

Anaesthetic agents, opioids, phenothiazines, and other drugs often used have central and peripheral vasodilatory properties. The lack of efferent sensory stimuli under anaesthesia also contributes to a decreased sympathetic tone and vasodilatation. The treatment is adequate cardiovascular monitoring and intravascular volume expansion with i.v. fluids.

Low cardiac output

There are a multitude of causes of low cardiac output postoperatively and only the most important are discussed.

Myocardial depression

All anaesthetics and opioids are, to a variable extent, direct myocardial depressants and their effect can extend hours into the postoperative period.

Arrhythmias

Certain anaesthetic drugs, particularly halothane, can cause supraventricular, and very occasionally, ventricular arrhythmias, as can electrolyte imbalances, particularly potassium, calcium and magnesium deficits. Intraoperative events leading to hypoxaemia and/or hypercarbia, can cause serious arrhythmias which may extend into the recovery period. Some patients have pre-existing arrhythmias; others may have an irritable myocardium.

The detailed treatment of arrhythmias is beyond the scope of this chapter. The important issues are to assess the haemodynamic impact, to distinguish between supraventricular and ventricular arrhythmias, to determine and treat the cause, and to decide which drug, if any, to use. The most common and best tolerated antiarrhythmic agents are amiodarone, digoxin and lignocaine.

Hypovolaemia

Normally effective compensatory mechanisms to hypovolaemia (peripheral vasoconstriction, tachycardia) develop early and only quite marked hypovolaemia causes hypotension. Hypovolaemia should be diagnosed by looking for these earlier clinical signs before hypotension develops. Drugs given during anaesthesia can impair the sympathetic response and mask hypovolaemia.

A relatively low intravascular volume amidst anaesthetic induced vasodilatation is a common cause of cardiovascular instability and hypotension. Treatment is based on fluid administration in anticipation of these events.

Haemorrhage, most commonly from the operative site, may be difficult to detect in the recovery room and must always be considered.

Perioperative myocardial ischaemia or infarction

The diagnosis is made by suspicion in those at risk, exclusion of other causes of low cardiac output, clinical examination, ECG and serial enzyme changes. The importance of tachycardia, hypotension, hypoxaemia, shivering, and pain, as causes of myocardial ischaemia cannot be over-emphasised.

Sepsis

Even the most fulminant presentation of sepsis usually develops several hours after colonisation by the infective agent. Correspondingly, sepsis should be considered in those with potential entry sites of infection (peritonitis, trauma, compound fractures, skull fractures, abscesses, etc.).

Hypertension

Pain and anxiety on awakening are commonly associated with hypertension. Some patients may have preoperative hypertension, requiring target values to be adjusted accordingly. In addition, the late stages of hypoxaemia can cause a reflex mediated hypertensive response.

The cause of the hypertension must be addressed. For example, in a semiconscious patient hypertension and agitation may be due to pain; sedatives may worsen the situation. Conversely, hypertension and anxiety arising from partial paralysis will not respond to vasodilators or analgesics.

Pain

Pain after surgery is distressing; although common, it has until recently received little attention. Pain has been the subject of a report by the Royal Colleges of Surgeons and Anaesthetists [16]. It recommended regular assessment, prevention and treatment of postoperative pain, the establishment of dedicated multidisciplinary acute pain teams, staff training, and appropriate facilities.

Opioids constitute the drugs of choice for severe visceral pain. Unfortunately side-effects can limit their use. Some of the more important side-effects are nausea and vomiting, drowsiness and/or dysphoria, reduced intestinal motility, cardiovascular depression, especially in the frail, and respiratory depression. Opioids are customarily given i.v. or i.m. They can also be given by i.v. or regional (epidural) infusions, by patient controlled analgesia (PCA), or orally.

The NSAIDs can reduce opioid requirements. They are given rectally, orally, or i.v. Their side-effects are mediated by inhibition of cyclo-oxygenase and its deleterious effect on the prostacycline–prostaglandin–thromboxane ratio, which alters platelet aggregation, gastric mucosal protection and renal blood flow.

Paracetamol is an analgesic antipyretic with no clinically significant action on cyclo-oxygenase. It is therefore devoid of the side-effects but also of the anti-inflammatory properties associated with NSAIDs. At high doses it can cause hepatic necrosis. Many anaesthetists commence regular oral paracetamol or preparations of paracetamol with a weak opioid as soon as possible in an attempt to reduce the doses of stronger analgesics.

Epidural analgesia has established its place in surgery to the lower limbs, pelvis, upper abdomen and chest, as it can reduce i.v. opioid requirements and speed mobilisation. Most hospitals place patients receiving postoperative epidural analgesia in high dependency or intensive care wards.

Currently there is considerable interest on combining drugs and techniques. This should make it easier to adapt regimes to individual patient requirements and to minimise side-effects [17].

Postoperative nausea and vomiting

Postoperative nausea and vomiting (PONV) are amongst the commonest and disturbing complications of surgery and anaesthesia. Despite even the most effective regimes about 10–20% of patients suffer troublesome PONV. There are many causes; some easier to treat than others.

Anaesthetic drugs (opioids, nitrous oxide, and inhalational agents) and general anaesthesia *per se* cause emesis. Surgical factors, such as traction to the eyes, trauma and shock, peritonitis, and ENT, dental, upper gastrointestinal, and gynaecological surgery are associated with a higher incidence of emesis. Gastrointestinal conditions, such as delayed gastric emptying, oesophageal reflux, duodenal ulcers, and paralytic ileus are also associated with PONV. Finally, certain individuals are more susceptible to experiencing emesis, which also occurs more often in females.

Treatment may be difficult; it should involve the avoidance of predisposing factors, including excessive starvation and dehydration, together with the judicious use of the available antiemetics before, during and after surgery.

ANAESTHETIC EMERGENCIES

Rapid sequence induction

A rapid sequence induction is indicated when the stomach is not empty and therefore there is a high risk of vomiting or regurgitating on induction. This occurs in three groups of conditions. Firstly in emergency anaesthesia, when the condition precipitating the emergency is likely to also affect the emptying of the stomach; this also includes emergency as well as elective Caesarean sections. Secondly in primary gastrointestinal pathology necessitating surgery; this includes all forms of intestinal obstruction. Thirdly, many anaesthetists employ this technique in patients who have conditions known to be associated with significant delay in gastric emptying, such as hiatus hernia, reflux oesophagitis, autonomic neuropathy and severe uraemia.

After explanation and reassurance, the patient is preoxygenated and monitoring commenced. Before loss of consciousness, pressure is applied by a trained assistant to the cricoid ring. The cricoid is the only tracheal ring which completely encircles the trachea. Firm cricoid pressure, known as Sellick's manoeuvre, does not collapse the ring or trachea, but instead seals the cephalad end of the oesophagus by apposing it against the vertebral column posteriorly. The chosen i.v. induction drug is administered.

After loss of consciousness, suxamethonium is administered. Maximal relaxation occurs after the fasciculations have ceased and this is when the trachea should be intubated. The cuff is sealed and then cricoid pressure is released. Ventilation proceeds as usual. The entire procedure should take between 30 and 90 s; with adequate preoxygenation this should not produce serious hypoxaemia.

This technique fundamentally involves administering muscle relaxants before the airway is controlled. This entails a calculated risk which should be balanced against the risk of vomiting and aspiration. Patients thought likely to vomit on induction are at a similar risk on awakening, and should be extubated in the left lateral position when awake.

Failure to intubate

The primary objective of intubation is to facilitate oxygenation. When intubation proves difficult, too time consuming, or impossible, oxygenation, more than ever, remains the primary objective. Failure to understand and apply this essential principle can have disastrous consequences.

A difficult intubation can be made 'easy' and an impossible one 'possible' by meticulous attention to the following: effective preoxygenation, correct positioning of the head and neck, readily available auxiliary equipment such as different laryngoscopes, bougies, etc.; also, it is important to allow time for full muscle paralysis to develop.

Intubation should be considered to have failed after three attempts, or before serious hypoxaemia develops. If this occurs, anaesthetists should apply the 'failed intubation drill'; the first step of this drill is to communicate with the theatre personnel and to ask for additional anaesthetic help. It is impossible to state too strongly that the patient must not be repalarysed in order 'to have one more try'. This drill is designed to protect the airway, oxygenate the patient, and allow rapid awakening.

Failure to intubate and ventilate

Certain manoeuvres may make it easier to ventilate patients. These include proper control of the airway by lifting the chin and thrusting the jaw forward, if necessary with both hands while the assistant squeezes the reservoir bag; an oropharyngeal airway may be of use; gentle continuous positive pressure to the airway may help. The patient should be moved to the left lateral position, if, as is likely, there is risk of regurgitation; this may help ventilation. If these fail there is a good case for removing or repositioning cricoid pressure, if it was being applied. A LMA has been used successfully to ventilate patients in this situation.

If all these attempts fail to enable ventilation the situation is very serious and a difficult decision arises.

Many anaesthetists would then perform a cryco-thyroid puncture with a large bore (14 G or 16 G) cannula, and connect it to the plunger of a 2 ml syringe. The plunger can then be connected to the catheter mount of a 6 mm tracheal tube, which in turn connects to a standard breathing system.

Some would perform a tracheostomy or a retrograde intubation with the aid of a guide wire; these techniques are time consuming, technically difficult, and are not free of risks.

Hypoxaemia may cause multiple arrhythmias, including bradycardia and cardiac arrest. Clearly, drugs given as part of resuscitation will not be effective until the hypoxaemia resolves.

Cardiorespiratory collapse during anaesthesia

Rarely cardiac arrest develops without warning in healthy patients. Much more often, however, a spiralling loop of complications in a compromised patient finally leads to cardiac arrest. There is no substitute for careful observation and a high index of suspicion. Monitor alarms must not be cancelled and should not be assumed to represent technical faults until the patient's condition has been assessed.

In principle the management is to remove the cause, commence usual cardiopulmonary resuscitation [23] and call for assistance.

Primary cardiac arrest

The most likely causes are anaphylaxis to anaesthetic agents, arrhythmias, profound hypovolaemia, myocardial ischaemia, and electrolyte imbalances. Specific management priorities include securing the airway, by intubation if possible,

ventilation with 100% oxygen, and cardiac massage. In addition the following may be necessary:

1. *Adrenaline (1 mg bolus)*: Maintains organ perfusion to heart and brain and has positive effects on heart rate and contractility.
2. *Atropine (1 to 3 mg)*.
3. *Defibrillation*: Electrolyte imbalances causing ventricular fibrillation may not respond to DC cardioversion until the cause has been corrected.
4. *Fluids*: Anaphylaxis causes intense vasodilatation, which may require enormous volumes of intravascular fluids. The type of fluid is probably less important than the amount.

Primary hypoxaemia

The most important causes are as follows:

1. *Misplacement of the tracheal tube*: Oesphageal intubation can go undetected for some time, even to an experienced anaesthetist. If in doubt, the position of the tube must be confirmed by these methods: layrngoscopy, adequate ventilation, end expired capnography and fibreoptic bronchoscopy. The latter two are the only certain methods. In addition, a correctly placed tube may have been displaced from the trachea, for example during patient transfer.
2. *Upper airway obstruction*: Often caused by laryngeal spasm or by a blocked or kinked tracheal tube.
3. *Bronchoconstriction*: Can be caused by asthma and/or anaphylaxis.
4. *Pneumothorax*: This can be very difficult to detect. A pneumothorax may rapidly deteriorate with positive pressure ventilation, especially if nitrous oxide is used.
5. *Pulmonary or air embolism*.

LOCAL ANAESTHETIC DRUGS

Local anaesthetic agents reversibly block nerve conduction, predominantly by inactivating sodium channels, and prevent electrical depolarisation. Smaller nerve fibres are more sensitive so that increasing doses are required to block fibres transmitting sympathetic pain, temperature, proprioception and motor impulses. This phenomenon, known as differential conduction blockade, explains why patients may feel pressure but no pain and why a nerve block should be tested by checking for sharp pain or temperature. Furthermore, a limb which cannot be moved is quite likely to be painless.

Local anaesthetics are divided into those with an amide (-N-H-C-) or an ester (-C-O-) bond. The most commonly used drugs are amides. Termination of action is by redistribution into the intravascular space and by metabolism. Redistribution inversely affects duration and efficacy and directly increases toxicity. Vasoconstrictors, commonly adrenaline, reduce redistribution and toxicity and increase duration and efficacy.

Toxicity of local anaesthetics occurs by two mechanisms:

1. *Toxicity of the drug*: This is due to the result of absolute overdose or accidental intravascular injection; it causes excessive impairment of nerve conduction. Central nervous system toxicity is manifested, with increasing blood concentrations, by perioral numbness and paraesthesia, vertigo, tinnitus and muscle twitching and culminates in seizures. Cardiovascular toxicity occurs at relatively higher doses. The fall in vascular resistance and capacitance, poor myocardial contractility and a variety of arrhythmias may cause various degrees of cardiovascular collapse.

2. *Toxicity of the technique*: This includes sympathetic blockade and excessive cephalad spread of local anaesthetic which can affect the brain stem and cause apnoea, unconsciousness, convulsions and loss of vasomotor tone.

Allergy to local anaesthetics is mostly due to anaphylaxis to para-amino benzoic acid, a metabolite of most ester drugs. Genuine allergy to amide local anaesthetics is very rare. Local anaesthetic drugs probably do not trigger malignant hyperpyrexia.

Some of the more salient aspects of the common drugs are discussed below. Toxic doses are often quoted, but it is important to realise these vary greatly depending on the medical condition of the patient, site and rate of injection and use of a vasoconstrictor. The doses in parentheses are intended as a guide in standard patients without vasoconstrictor; the use of vasoconstrictors reduces toxicity.

Lignocaine (3 mg/kg)

This is the standard against which others are measured; it is also an antiarrhythmic.

Bupivacaine (2 mg/kg)

This is about four times more potent than lignocaine, which is of slower onset and longer duration. It has selective cardiac toxicity, particularly in pregnancy, often causing life-threatening ventricular arrhythmias which may be difficult to treat. Therefore, it should not be used for i.v. regional anaesthesia.

Ropivicaine

This is the newest amide local anaesthetic with similar potency and duration of action to bupivacaine. It appears less toxic to the cardiovascular and central nervous system than bupivacaine and is associated with less motor block.

Prilocaine

(5 mg/kg): this is equipotent with lignocaine and has a similar time of onset but a shorter duration. It has a wider margin of safety if the tourniquet becomes deflated during i.v. regional anaesthesia, for which it is the drug of choice. It can cause methaemoglobinaemia.

Cocaine

(7 mg/kg): one of the few ester local anaesthetics in use today, cocaine is also a vasoconstrictor. This makes it the drug of choice in ENT surgery. It is a drug of abuse worldwide; its vasoconstrictor effects can cause myocardial ischaemia, tachycardia and cerebral vascular accident.

SEDATION

The main objectives of sedation are:

- to reduce anxiety, awareness and psychological sequelae associated with diagnostic or therapeutic procedures;
- to induce amnesia;
- to enhance patient cooperation.

Sedation has important differences from anaesthesia. It is possible to arouse a patient by simple commands and sedation does not abolish response to pain.

Drugs can be administered intermittently, by continuous infusion, or by patient-controlled sedation. The most commonly used drugs are propofol, midazolam, fentanyl and alfentanil, nitrous oxide, isoflurane and occasionally ketamine. Many anaesthetists combine an hypnotic agent, to provide sedation and amnesia, with a short-acting opioid to provide analgesia and drowsiness. It is important to realise the differences between analgesia and sedation as the drugs which supplement one can potentially worsen the other. Patients undergoing sedation should normally receive supplemental oxygen.

Individual response varies enormously and sedation may end in excessive central nervous system and cardiorespiratory depression, with loss of airway, apnoea, hypoxaemia and hypotension. Equipment and monitoring should be comparable to that ordinarily required for a general anaesthetic on the same patient.

REGIONAL ANAESTHESIA

Regional anaesthesia constitutes the blockade and/or modulation of conduction in nerves supplying sensation to an anatomical region. Blockade of a nerve or plexus can normally be performed along its trajectory within the spinal cord, known as a central nerve block; at different points in a limb; or by infiltration of drug into an area, a technique termed field block. Regional anaesthesia can be performed on its own, supplemented by sedation or combined with general anaesthesia.

The preparation and assessment of the patient, as well as the equipment, assistance and monitoring should be the same as for general anaesthesia. This is particularly true for two reasons:

1. The local anaesthetic procedure may fail or be only partially effective and require 'conversion' to a general anaesthetic.
2. Treatment of toxicity or side-effects may require intubation, ventilation and resuscitation.

General aspects

Advantages

- *Avoidance of unconsciousness*: Regional anaesthesia does not normally interfere with consciousness and the ability to protect the airway is maintained.
- *Minimum interference with breathing*: There is therefore no need to intubate and ventilate and the disadvantages of these techniques are avoided. However, regional anaesthesia in patients known to be difficult to intubate can present problems if side-effects then make it necessary to intubate.
- *Postoperative analgesia*. Top-up boluses or infusions can provide good quality analgesia for days. This can reduce opioid consumption and aid early mobilisation. This has obvious benefits in lung conditions and in the prevention of thromboembolism.

Disadvantages

- *Sympathetic blockade*: This causes a fall in vascular smooth muscle tone which can lead to a precipitous drop in vascular resistance, blood pressure, venous return and cardiac output. If not treated effectively, it can lead to life-threatening hypotension and end-organ ischaemia, especially in patients with a fixed cardiac output. These effects can be partially prevented by volume loading and the use of vasoconstrictors such as ephedrine or phenylephrine; occasionally more aggressive treatment with potent inotropes may be necessary.
- *Toxicity of drug/adverse effect of technique*: As discussed above, this may cause loss of airway control in addition to convulsions and unconsciousness, apnoea and cardiovascular collapse. The combination of sympathetic block, surgical haemorrhage, incomplete block leading to partial analgesia, local anaesthetic drug toxicity and oversedation is particularly dangerous.
- *Motor block*: Although entirely reversible, this can be quite distressing to the patient. It should be discussed at the preoperative visit.

Indications

Every anaesthetist will assess each case individually and decide how to conduct anaesthesia based on advantages and disadvantages of general and regional techniques, experience and training, patient choice and surgical requirements. There is no conclusive evidence that either technique changes outcome. Some relative indications are:

- significant respiratory impairment;
- obstetrics: pain relief and Caesarian section;
- infraumbilical surgery: urological and orthopaedic procedures;
- analgesia in thoracic and upper abdominal surgery.

Contraindications

- local or generalised infection;
- bleeding diathesis;
- patient disapproval;
- hypovolaemia;
- extreme emergency;
- raised intracranial pressure.

Specific techniques

Intravenous regional anaesthesia (Bier's block)

A Bier's block consists of isolating a limb, usually the arm, with a pneumatic tourniquet and injecting local anaesthetic into a vein. The drug is distributed to the extravascular tissues, including the nerves. It is suitable for minor surgery to the distal upper limb and is commonly performed for reduction of wrist fractures. It is often performed in elderly patients, not uncommonly in Emergency departments after a fall or other accident. Great care must be taken in patient assessment; in particular, most anaesthetists insist that they are fasted. It is customary that one practitioner performs the block and cares for the patient while another performs the surgery.

Certain principles are particularly important [21]. Contralateral i.v. access is imperative. The tourniquet must be tested and known reliably to apply pressures of 50–100 mmHg above systolic. The area just distal to the tourniquet may not be completely anaesthetised; this may cause discomfort or pain about which the patient must be warned. The anaesthetist must be constantly vigilant during the procedure, in particular for deflation of the tourniquet and/or signs of drug toxicity. The tourniquet must not be deflated for at least 20–30 min; this should allow time for adequate redistribution of local anaesthetic and therefore safe blood levels upon deflation. Prilocaine is the drug of choice; its safety record, when used appropriately, is good and it has the widest safety margin. As for all regional anaesthetic techniques, monitoring and resuscitation facilities should be adequate.

Central nerve blocks

This includes subarachnoid or spinal and extra or epidural blocks; both can be performed with local anaesthesia and/or opioids. The most important differential characteristics are listed in Table 2.11. A caudal block consists of an extradural injection through the sacral hiatus, delineated by the sacral cornua.

Briefly, the technique of performing an epidural involves the detection of a characteristic loss of resistance as the needle enters the epidural space. A catheter is then threaded into the space. Before injecting the entire drug dose, it is imperative to administer a small 'test dose' to ascertain extradural and exclude subarachnoid placement.

The administration of opioids by spinal or epidural injections is aimed at reducing local anaesthetic doses and side-effects. Side-effects of central neural opioids include delayed respiratory depression, pruritus, nausea and urinary retention.

Some of the most important complications of central nerve blocks are:

- *Backache*: Back pain is more common after extradural anaesthesia in pregnancy, where the incidence is between

Table 2.11. Differential aspects of central nerve blocks.

	Subarachnoid (spinal); SAB	Epidural/extradural
Anatomy	Perforates dura and arachnoid	Perforates Ligamentum Flavum; superficial to dura mater
Dose	Low (1–3.5 ml)	High (5–25 ml). Increased systemic absorption
Onset/offset	Fast (min)	Slow (10–30 min)
Sympathetic block	Profound. Starts 1–2 segments cephalad to sensory block	Unpredictable distribution
Motor block	Profound. Starts 2 segments caudal to sensory block	May be patchy
Needle	Small (24 G)	Large (16–18 G)
Catheter	Very rarely used	Often used

8% and 15%. It is probably due to several mechanisms and a cause–effect relationship with epidural blocks has not been established.

- *Postdural puncture headache*: This is caused by cerebrospinal fluid (CSF) escape through a hole in the arachnoid. It has traditionally been described as a constant, sometimes incapacitating headache, worse on sitting, straining and often accompanied by photophobia and nausea. A postdural puncture headache, although very distressing, is not representative of a serious complication. An epidural, by definition, is not intended to pierce the dura and so a large needle is used. However, accidental dural puncture will cause significant CSF leak and is associated with a high incidence of headache, especially in young adults. In contrast, a subarachnoid block is intended to pierce the arachnoid and is therefore performed with a much smaller needle, often especially designed to reduce CSF leak; it is normally associated with a small incidence of postdural puncture headache [22].
- *Accidental total spinal block*. Essentially this occurs when the arachnoid is inadvertently punctured while attempting an epidural block; this leads to injection of an excessive amount of local anaesthetic, intended for the epidural space, into the subarachnoid space. The large dose can rapidly extend to the brain stem, affecting consciousness and the respiratory and vasomotor centres. It is a potentially serious complication which requires rapid action, normally in the form of intubation, ventilation and cardiovascular support.
- *Epidural haematoma or abscess*. These are both exceedingly rare; they require emergency neurosurgical assessment and probable surgical decompression without delay.
- *Meningitis.*
- *Arachnoiditis, myelitis, cauda equina syndrome.*

TOURNIQUETS

Tourniquets are used to isolate limbs from the circulation and reduce bleeding.

Technique

The limb is exsanguinated by elevation or with the use of an Esmarch bandage. Current cuffs are usually pneumatic; they must be regularly maintained. The cuff is inflated to about 30–50 mmHg and 70–100 mmHg above systolic pressure for the upper and lower limbs, respectively. Tourniquet inflation can be very painful. The limb must be appropriately padded; in addition, it is usually necessary to administer a general or local anaesthetic. During inflation it is essential to check cuff inflation constantly. Most surgeons and anaesthetists attempt to maintain the cuff inflated for not longer than 2 h.

Side-effects

In general the frequency and severity of side-effects is proportional to the duration of limb ischaemia. Ischaemia *per se* can cause nerve and muscle damage. There can also be damage to soft tissues. The tourniquet effectively reduces the intravascular compartment; thus the relative intravascular blood volume is increased. This causes a rise in venous return, which can increase the cardiac output and blood pressure. Circulatory stasis within the limb predisposes to thromboembolism.

Upon release of the tourniquet, anaerobic metabolites enter into the circulation. These metabolites, mostly CO_2, acids and potassium, cause a general vasodilation, not unlike reperfusion injury, which can be deleterious in the patient with poor cardiovascular reserve. There is also reactive hyperaemia which can increase bleeding.

Tourniquets are normally contraindicated in ischaemic peripheral vascular disease and sickle cell states.

VENTILATION

Intermittent positive pressure ventilation

This is almost universally the only technique used when applying controlled ventilation under anaesthesia. It consists of positive pressure applied to the airway during inspiration and passive exhalation of gas due to elastic recoil of the lungs. Two types of ventilators are commonly used:

1. *Pressure generators*: These ventilators operate at relatively low pressures and changes in compliance or resistance may affect the tidal volume delivered.
2. *Flow generators*: These ventilators operate at very high pressures (which are not transmitted to the patient). Changes in respiratory mechanics do not normally affect tidal volume.

End-expiratory pressure

There is normally no pressure gradient at the end of expiration between the airway and atmosphere. Rarely in anaesthesia but often in the intensive care unit, end-expiratory pressure is applied. It is termed positive end-expiratory pressure (PEEP) when ventilation is controlled (Intermittent positive pressure ventilation, IPPV) or continuous positive airway pressure (CPAP) if ventilation is spontaneous.

Some of its advantages include prevention of small airway closure and an increase in FRC with improved ventilation–perfusion matching; both of these allow a reduction in inspired oxygen concentration. Its deleterious effects are mostly caused by a raised intrathoracic pressure. This decreases venous return which may cause a fall in cardiac output; it may also further impair expiration, worsening air trapping in those with asthma and chronic obstructive airways disease.

Unusual forms of ventilation

Occasionally, especially during examination and surgery of the airway, other forms of ventilation are necessary. These include the ventilating bronchoscope, high pressure 'jet' ventilation and high-frequency ventilation.

FURTHER READING

Aitkenhead AR, Rowbotham DJ, Smith G. *Textbook of Anaesthesia*. Edinburgh: Churchill Livingstone, 2001

Lee JA, Rushman GB. *Lee's Synopsis of Anaesthesia*. Oxford: Butterworth-Heinemann, 1999

West JB. *Respiratory physiology-The Essentials*. Baltimore: Williams & Wilkins, 1999

3

Postoperative Management

Douglas M Bowley

Department of Colorectal Surgery, John Radcliffe Hospital, Headington, Oxford, UK

CONTENTS

Introduction	39
Preoperative physiological status	39
Operative severity	40
Provision of appropriate care	40
Recognition of the ill-surgical patient	40
Postoperative monitoring	40
Vital signs	40
Critical care	41
Goal-directed therapy	41
Intensive blood sugar control	42
Steroids in severe sepsis	42
Activated protein C	42
Blood transfusion	42
Allogeneic (bank) blood	42
Complications of blood transfusion	42
Autologous blood	43
Other blood products	43
Transfusion Requirements in Critical Care study	43
Postoperative pain	44
Pain pathways and mechanism	44
Postoperative pain management	44
Postoperative fluid and electrolyte balance	45
Assessment of the pre-existing circulatory deficit	45
An estimate of current status and likely ongoing losses (if any)	45
An estimate of maintenance fluid requirements	45
Choosing replacement and maintenance fluids	46
Postoperative complications	46
Haemorrhage	46
Respiratory complications	46
Cardiac complications	46
Wound complications	47
Fever	48
Urinary retention	48
Postoperative delerium and cognitive impairment	48
Venous thromboembolism	48
Postoperative nausea and vomiting, and ileus	49
Fast-track surgery	49
Conclusion	49
Further reading	49

INTRODUCTION

Outcomes after surgery are influenced by:
- preoperative physiological status,
- operative severity,
- the provision of appropriate care.

Surgeons can minimize the deleterious effects of the surgical insult by careful preoperative planning, meticulous intraoperative technique and by accurate postoperative care.

Preoperative physiological status

Preoperative co-existing medical problems translate into increased operative risk. The simplest tool to assess patient risk factors is the American Society of Anesthetists (ASA) scale. This is a subjective assessment of the patient's operative risk based on the presence and severity of co-existing medical problems, which are detected by routine history and physical examination.

The Physiological and Operative Severity Score for the enUmeration of Mortality and morbidity (POSSUM) was developed in 1991. POSSUM variables include physiological markers and other factors related to operative severity. These variables have been tested extensively and have resulted in a central database of over 200 000 patients. POSSUM scoring has been used to predict the outcome of patients undergoing a broad range of operations and has been recognized as being the most appropriate available score for assessing risk in surgical patients. However, POSSUM over-predicts mortality for those patients at the low-risk end of the spectrum. The

Portsmouth group revised the scoring and the so-called P-POSSUM is now widely used.

Operative severity

Surgery (or trauma from injury) has been shown to result in immune suppression and organ failure is the leading cause of death in surgical patients. A causal relationship exists between the extent of the surgical or traumatic injury, the postoperative metabolic and immunological changes, and the predisposition of patients to develop infectious complications and multiple organ dysfunction.

Provision of appropriate care

In a study in 2003, postoperative mortality was compared between centres in the UK and the USA with patients matched according to POSSUM criteria. The risk-adjusted mortality rates following major surgery were four times higher in the UK cohort. The reasons behind this difference are complex, but the authors speculate that the difference may be due to differences in the quality of patient care.

Higher-risk surgery performed independently by doctors in training correlates with poor postoperative outcomes. In the UK's National Confidential Enquiry into Perioperative Deaths (NCEPOD) published in 2000, of 1518 operations that resulted in postoperative death, 4.2% were conducted by a doctor with as little as 1 year of specialist training and 41% of the anaesthetics were administered by trainees.

The nature of postoperative nursing care is also important; in a study involving over 200 000 surgical patients in the state of Pennsylvania, higher patient to nursing staff ratios were associated with a higher-risk-adjusted postoperative mortality rate.

If we believe that high-dependency care is the optimum environment for an at-risk surgical patient then it is sobering to realize that over 50% of patients who die after surgery in the UK are never admitted to an intensive care unit (ICU).

Recognition of the ill-surgical patient

The ability to recognize an ill-surgical patient is a fundamental skill of a good surgeon and, unfortunately, can be harder than it might seem. History and examination remains the cornerstone, but understanding the definition of the systemic inflammatory response syndrome (SIRS) is helpful, because this physiological response can be amplified by several factors that can complicate surgery and lead to multiple organ failure. A postoperative surgical patient is said to be exhibiting SIRS if two or more of the following are present and action should be taken immediately:

- Temperature <36°C or >38°C.
- Respiratory rate >20 breaths/min.
- Pulse rate >90 beats/min.
- White blood count >12 ×10⁹/l.

POSTOPERATIVE MONITORING

The patient's response to a surgical procedure is assessed by measurement of vital signs. Observations that must be monitored by medical and nursing staff include:

- conscious state;
- temperature, pulse, blood pressure and respiratory rate;
- urinary output;
- drainage from the nasogastric tubes, T-tubes, or wound drains, stomas or fistulas.

More intensive monitoring may be needed for high-risk surgical patients and after major surgery; these include one-to-one nursing by highly trained nurses, continuous electro-cardiographical monitoring and invasive haemodynamic monitoring (arterial line, central venous pressure (CVP) monitoring and a method of monitoring cardiac output) in a high dependency or ICU.

Vital signs

Heart rate

Tachycardia is defined as a heart rate >90 beats/min. When premature ventricular contractions or other irregularities are present, the heart rate may be determined by auscultation at the apex; the difference between apical and radial rates represents the number of dropped beats. Tachycardia occurs with hypovolaemia, infection, anxiety, fear, fever and pain. Bradycardia (a heart rate <60 beats/min) may occur with heart block associated with myocardial ischaemia.

Blood pressure

Blood pressure falls after hypovolaemia due to blood or fluid loss, during cardiac failure from primary myocardial dysfunction or tamponade, or as a result of severe sepsis or anaphylaxis. Hypotension is often a late manifestation of shock, especially in children.

The pulse pressure is the difference between the systolic and diastolic pressures. A reduced pulse pressure may precede a fall in systolic pressure in a patient developing hypovolaemic shock and is a clinical sign of hypovolaemia. Mean arterial pressure (MAP) may be calculated from the formula: MAP = diastolic arterial pressure + pulse pressure.

Body temperature

Body temperature is measured orally, rectally or more commonly by use of a device that analyses the tympanic membrane. Temperature elevations are associated with infection, tissue necrosis, late stage carcinomatosis and malignant hyperthermia. Low-grade fever is also present after accidental or surgical trauma and particularly when haematoma, a foreign body, urinary extravasation, or stasis or bronchial secretions are present. Hypothermia (temperature <34°C) may occur in some patients with septic shock, reduced metabolism associated with a hypothyroid state, severe anaemia and exposure to cold. Hypothermia is of particular relevance to patients undergoing major operations. Muscle relaxants abolish the shivering response and the opening of a body cavity causes loss of large amounts of heat. Hypothermia causes platelet dysfunction, abnormalities of the enzymatic clotting cascade and can lead to a clinically relevant coagulopathy. Hypothermia also prolongs the action of neuromuscular blocking drugs.

Ventilatory monitoring

Clinical monitoring of ventilation consists of observation of the patient's colour, respiratory rate and adequacy of chest movements. Auscultation of both lungs should be performed to detect equality of air entry and the presence of secretions or consolidation. Pulse oximetry estimates the percentage of saturation of circulating haemoglobin. An arterial oxygen saturation of 95% represents a partial pressure of oxygen (PaO_2) value of approximately 85 mmHg. In the recovery period oxygen supplementation should be given to patients whose PaO_2 falls below 13 kPa (95 mmHg).

Urinary output

Urinary output is easily measured after bladder catheterization. The hourly rate of urine output is a rough marker of end-organ perfusion, and is typically used as a marker of the (in)adequacy of resuscitation.

Central venous pressure

A central venous catheter with the tip in the lower superior vena cava or right atrium provides valuable information concerning the volume status of the circulation. CVP monitoring can be used to guide fluid therapy after major surgery. A healthy person in the supine position typically has mean CVP values that range from 0 to 3 mmHg.

Arterial blood gases

Measurement of arterial blood gases is extremely useful to evaluate surgical patients: the first laboratory signs of early lung problems are arterial blood gas abnormalities, such as arterial PaO_2 values lower than 9.4 kPa (70 mmHg), arterial partial pressure of carbon dioxide ($PaCO_2$) values higher than 6 kPa (45 mmHg) and pH values <7.3 or >7.5. Respiratory failure is suggested by PaO_2 values lower than 6–7 kPa (50 mmHg) in a patient breathing room air.

Acute respiratory acidosis in the postoperative period is most commonly a complication caused by the respiratory depressant effect of anaesthesia and narcotics. Other causes are pneumothorax, airway obstruction (foreign body, laryngospasm, severe bronchospasm) and ventilator malfunction. Treatment of acute respiratory acidosis comprises adequate ventilation. In the case of respiratory depression, this may mean administering a narcotic antagonist (naloxone). Maintaining an adequate airway is critical and intubation and mechanical ventilation may be required. Respiratory alkalosis is due to hyperventilation and there is a decrease in $PaCO_2$. Hyperventilation can occur due to diverse causes (respiratory disease like pneumonia, pulmonary embolism or oedema, shock, pain, anxiety and disturbed ventilatory control). The treatment entails tackling the underlying cause.

Metabolic acidosis may be due to impaired perfusion of the tissues, as in hypovolaemic shock, or due to diabetic ketoacidosis or renal failure. It is critically important to recognize metabolic acidosis in a surgical patient.

CRITICAL CARE

Organ failure is the leading cause of death in surgical patients. Critical care is best provided by a multidisciplinary team focused on resuscitation, monitoring and life support. The fundamental goals of critical care are early restoration and maintenance of tissue oxygenation, and prevention and treatment of infection and multiple organ failure.

Multiorgan dysfunction syndrome (MODS) is a clinical syndrome characterized by progressive failure of multiple and inter-dependent organs. It occurs along a continuum of progressive organ failure, rather than absolute failure. The lungs, liver and kidneys are the principal target organs; however, failure of the cardiovascular and central nervous system (CNS) may occur. Specific therapy for MODS is currently limited, apart from providing adequate and full resuscitation, treatment of infection and general ICU supportive care.

Goal-directed therapy

After major trauma or surgical illness, hypoperfusion of tissues leads to cellular hypoxia and the initiation of the factors that lead to organ dysfunction. The fundamental defect is a failure of adequate delivery of oxygen to the respiring tissues. Traditional attempts at resuscitation have been guided by normalization of vital signs, such as pulse, blood pressure and urine output, and only when haemodynamic instability has been recognized has the patient been considered for invasive monitoring in a critical care environment. However, these vital signs fail to identify the important group of patients with occult hypoperfusion, whose outcomes are likely to be poor unless adequate oxygen delivery is restored.

Shoemaker and his co-workers from the University of Southern California discovered that survivors after major trauma had significantly higher cardiac output, oxygen delivery and oxygen consumption compared to those patients who died. This led them to introduce the concept of 'goal-directed therapy' in which they attempted to manipulate the circulation of patients and achieve target values for cardiac output, oxygen delivery and consumption. In a group of high-risk patients who had required major surgery for trauma, they were able to achieve significant reductions in mortality. However, other studies were unable to reproduce these results.

In 2001, a randomized-controlled trial of early goal-directed therapy compared to standard therapy was published in a group of patients arriving at hospital with severe sepsis or septic shock, but in whom organ dysfunction was not yet established. This study demonstrated significant survival advantage for the 'goal-directed group'. The conclusion that haemodynamic optimization as soon as possible in the perioperative period is helpful has been further strengthened by the publication of a meta-analysis, which has confirmed that optimization before organ failure has occurred leads to a substantial reduction in deaths in high-risk surgical patients.

Invasive monitoring is required in order to record the necessary haemodynamic variables; a pulmonary artery catheter is the traditional method of gathering these data, although less invasive techniques, such as oesophageal Doppler probes are now being used.

Intensive blood sugar control

Hyperglycaemia and insulin resistance are common in critically ill patients, even if they have not previously had diabetes. A recent prospective, randomized, controlled study randomly assigned adults admitted to a surgical ICU to receive intensive insulin therapy (maintenance of blood glucose at a level between 4.4 and 6.1 mmol/l) or conventional treatment (infusion of insulin only if the blood glucose level exceeded 11.9 mmol/l) and maintenance of glucose at a level between 10.0 and 11.1 mmol/l. Strict glycaemic control significantly reduced mortality during intensive care; the greatest reductions in mortality were in patients with a proven septic focus.

Steroids in severe sepsis

It is now well established that severe sepsis may be associated with reversible failure of the hypothalamic–pituitary– adrenal axis. In a randomized, double-blinded, placebo-controlled multicentre trial a 7-day treatment with low doses of hydrocortisone and fludrocortisone significantly reduced the risk of death in patients with septic shock and relative adrenal insufficiency without increasing adverse events stress doses of hydrocortisone (hydrocortisone 50 mg 6 hourly and fludrocortisone 50 μg tablet/day) are indicated in all inotrope-dependent patients with septic shock who have a stress (random) cortisol level of <25 μg/dl.

Activated protein C

Activated protein C, an endogenous protein that promotes fibrinolysis and inhibits thrombosis and inflammation, is an important modulator of the coagulation and inflammation associated with severe sepsis. Activated protein C is converted from its inactive precursor, protein C, by thrombin coupled to thrombomodulin. The conversion of protein C to activated protein C may be impaired during sepsis as a result of the downregulation of thrombomodulin by inflammatory cytokines. Reduced levels of protein C are found in the majority of patients with sepsis and are associated with an increased

risk of death. In a randomized, double-blind, placebo-controlled, multicentre trial, treatment with activated protein C significantly reduced mortality in patients with severe sepsis. Consistent with the antithrombotic activity of activated protein C, bleeding was the most common adverse event associated with the administration of the drug; serious bleeding tended to occur in patients with predisposing conditions, such as gastrointestinal ulceration. According to the trial results, one additional serious bleeding event would occur for every 66 patients with severe sepsis treated with activated protein C. However, one life would be saved for every 16 patients treated.

BLOOD TRANSFUSION

Allogeneic (bank) blood

Allogeneic blood is used after grouping and cross-matching, and is available for use in the postoperative period as:
• whole blood,
• packed red cells (plasma-reduced cells).
Red cells for transfusion are usually depleted of leucocytes as this is thought to reduce the possible immunological consequences of transfusion.

Blood stored at 4°C in a citrate–dextrose preservative solution has a shelf life of about 5 weeks; however, storage of blood causes abnormalities in red cell structure and function and results in a shortening of the red cell lifespan. These 'storage lesions' are caused by:
• a fall in 2,3-diphosphoglycerate (2,3-DPG) (which increases the red cells' affinity for oxygen);
• red cell membrane changes leading to spherocyte formation and leakage of potassium.

Upon transfusion, a proportion of the red cells in the transfused blood do not survive and this proportion increases in blood that has been stored for long periods (30% or even more are lost as the blood approaches the end of its shelf life).

The volume and rate of transfusion will depend on the clinical state. In general for a stable, euvolaemic adult patient, the transfusion of 1 unit of packed cells raises the haemoglobin concentration by 1 g/dl and each unit of blood should be transfused over 4 h. More rapid transfusion may be needed especially with cases of acute haemorrhage requiring blood transfusion in the postoperative period. If it is anticipated that more than 2 units of blood will need to be transfused, a blood warmer should be used to prevent hypothermia. Massive blood transfusion is defined as the transfusion of one or more times the patient's total blood volume within 24 h.

Complications of blood transfusion

To analyse the risks of transfusion, a confidential voluntary reporting system was instituted in the UK in 1996 entitled the Serious Hazards Of Transfusion (SHOT) initiative. Major morbidity and deaths were analysed and categorized into three major sections:

1. Incorrect blood or component transfused.
2. Immunological interaction between donor and patient.
3. Transfusion-transmitted infection.

Incorrect blood or component transfused

Major ABO incompatibility reactions and rhesus D sensitization in young female patients still occurs due to errors leading to failure to detect the correct identity of blood or patient. Collection of the wrong blood from the blood fridge is the most common primary error.

Immunological interaction between donor and patient

Immunological reactions were reported in five categories: acute and delayed transfusion reactions, post-transfusion purpura, transfusion-associated graft versus host disease and transfusion-associated acute lung injury. In addition, even in the absence of acute reactions, allogeneic blood transfusion leads to immunomodulation, which has been implicated in increasing the risk of postoperative infection, organ failure and worsened long-term survival after surgery for malignant disease.

Transfusion-transmitted infection

Transfusions may lead to infectious disease in the recipient if the component is contaminated during collection and storage, or if the transfusion unwittingly transfers a biological agent from the donor pool to the recipient.

Red cells are kept refrigerated, so bacterial contamination is usually by agents that survive at low temperature, such as *Serratia liquifaciens*. Platelets have to be kept at room temperature and so may be contaminated with skin organisms (*Staphylococci*) or coliforms. However, contamination by *Salmonella* species due to asymptomatic donor bacteraemia has been recorded, in one case the source of the *Salmonella* infection was the donor's pet boa constrictor.

The risk of transfusion-transmitted viral infections is primarily due to the failure of serological screening tests to detect recently infected donors in the 'window' phase of infection. Hepatitis B and C and HIV have all been transmitted by blood transfusion. A fatal case of cerebral malaria was also recorded by the SHOT initiative after blood transfusion. There is currently great concern about the possibility of transfer of prion proteins by blood transfusion.

Autologous blood

Autologous blood may be collected preoperatively or intraoperatively, and used for transfusion in the postoperative period. Some of the hazards of homologous transfusion are eliminated although these techniques also create problems of their own.

Preoperative autologous donation

In this technique, an otherwise fit patient who is to undergo an elective operation which is anticipated to need several units of blood, may donate up to 4 units of blood in the preoperative period. Recombinant erythropoietin may be used to restore a normal haematocrit in the interval between donation and surgery.

Intraoperative haemodilution

Up to 2 units of blood may be withdrawn from the patient after induction of anaesthesia and prior to commencement of the surgical procedure; intravascular volume is replaced with crystalloids or colloids.

Intraoperative blood salvage

Where it is anticipated that considerable bleeding is likely to occur intraoperatively (such as elective aortic aneurysm surgery), salvage of red cells with an apparatus such as the cell saver helps to reduce wastage of blood. In this system, blood shed into the intraoperative field is aspirated and washed to remove debris. The cells are then suspended in saline and re-transfused. Platelets and plasma proteins including clotting factors are lost during the washing process.

Other blood products

Platelet concentrates

The platelets recovered from a unit of freshly donated blood can be transfused into patients who are bleeding and who have a low platelet count. The risk of bleeding increases as the platelet count falls below $50\,000/mm^3$.

Fresh frozen plasma

This contains all the coagulation factors. It is used to reverse the effects of anticoagulation with warfarin and in patients who are bleeding and require transfusion. It provides Factors V and VIII, which are not present in banked blood. Each unit is 150–250 ml.

Cryoprecipitate

Cryoprecipitate contains Factors XIII, VIII, fibrinogen and von Willebrand's factor, and is used in cases of massive haemorrhage, disseminated intravascular coagulopathy (DIC) and fibrinogen deficiency. Each unit is 10–20 ml.

Transfusion Requirements In Critical Care study

An important trial (Transfusion Requirements In Critical Care (TRICC) study) was recently undertaken by the Canadian Critical Care Trials Group. Critically ill patients with euvolaemia after initial treatment were randomly assigned to either a restrictive or liberal strategy of transfusion. In the restrictive group red cells were transfused if the haemoglobin concentration dropped below 7 g/dl and thereafter haemoglobin concentrations were maintained at 7–9 g/dl. In the liberal group transfusions were given when the haemoglobin concentration fell below 10.0 g/dl and haemoglobin concentrations were maintained at 10.0–12.0 g/dl. The mortality rate during hospitalization was significantly lower in the restrictive-strategy group. This reduction in mortality was not seen among patients with clinically significant ischaemic heart disease.

POSTOPERATIVE PAIN

Pain as defined by the International Association for the Study of Pain is 'an unpleasant sensory and emotional experience associated with actual or potential tissue damage, or described in terms of such damage'. Nociception (perception of a painful stimulus) elicits physiological responses even in anaesthetized individuals and minimization of pain can improve clinical outcomes. An individual's response for months after injury may be determined by processes that occurred during the initial phases of the injury. Even brief intervals of acute pain can induce long-term neuronal remodelling and sensitization ('plasticity'), chronic pain and lasting psychological distress.

Factors which influence postoperative pain include the:
- site and size of the incision,
- anaesthetic management,
- psychological makeup of the patient,
- mental preparation (this includes a full explanation from surgeon and anaesthetist).

Pain pathways and mechanism

Injury causes the local release of bradykinin, arachidonic acid and prostaglandin derivatives, which stimulate peripheral receptors that in turn transmit impulses via peripheral afferent fibres (A and C) to the spinal cord where they terminate in the dorsal horn and synapse with second-order neurones. Modulation occurs in the spinal cord through the action of beta-endorphins and opiates and inhibitory interneurones (the Gate mechanism), which act to inhibit transmission of painful impulses. Fibres of the second-order neurones cross over to the contralateral spinothalamic tract and ascend to the midbrain (thalamus and other nuclei) where they synapse with the third-order neurones and are relayed to the sensory cortex where the location of pain is perceived.

Postoperative pain management

Pre-emptive treatment

There is evidence to suggest that a powerful stimulus such as an incision sensitizes the CNS to further stimuli and thus pre-incision analgesia should be beneficial. The majority of trials have shown that timing of analgesia does not affect postoperative pain control. However, a recent study has shown that multimodal treatment with opiates, anti-inflammatory drugs, local anaesthesia and a N-methyl-D-aspartic acid (NMDA) antagonist (ketamine) diminishes pain and analgesic requirement after hernia surgery. NMDA receptors are thought to mediate central sensitization pathways for pain.

Postoperative analgesia
Intramuscular opiates
Intermittent intramuscular opiates used to be the mainstay of postoperative pain therapy, but the quality of analgesia provided by this regime is often unsatisfactory and has generally been replaced by patient-controlled techniques.

Intermittent infusion of opiates: patient-controlled analgesia
In this technique, an infusion pump is used to inject a preset bolus dose of analgesic (morphine or pethidine) intravenously whenever the patient activates it. A 'lockout-interval' is incorporated in the system to ensure against accidental activation and opiate overdosage. A loading dose is needed, as is a maintenance dose. This technique provides very satisfactory control of pain in the postoperative period. Patient-controlled analgesia is widely used and improves patient satisfaction; however, meta-analysis has shown that PCA does not reduce postoperative morbidity compared to intermittent opioid therapy. Morphine is metabolized by the kidney and caution must be exercised in patients with renal impairment.

Non-opiate drugs
Non-steroidal anti-inflammatory drugs (NSAIDs) have an opioid-sparing effect of 20–30%, which may be important in reducing opioid-related side effects. NSAIDs act by inhibiting prostaglandin synthesis. Paracetamol acts centrally and has analgesic and antipyretic effects, but no anti-inflammatory activity. These preparations may be used alone for intermediate analgesic needs or combined with opiates and may be given orally or rectally.

Local, regional and epidural anaesthetic techniques
Local anaesthetic agents inhibit the sodium channels along nerve fibres. Commonly used local anaesthetic agents are *lignocaine*, which is short-acting (up to 2 h) and *bupivacaine*, which is longer-acting (up to 8 h). Bupivacaine (0.25% or 0.5%) is the drug of choice for peripheral nerve blockade and epidural block. The toxic systemic side effects of the local anaesthetic agents, particularly on the CNS (convulsions), and cardiac dysrhythmias limit the volume of agent that can be used.

Local anaesthetic infiltration
It is effective in reducing postoperative pain and subfascial infiltration is more effective than simple subcutaneous infiltration in operations where muscle has been divided.

Continuous epidural blockade

It reduces surgical stress responses and autonomic reflexes; in addition it has been shown to be the most effective method of providing dynamic pain relief (analgesia during patient movement, such a coughing) after major procedures. Epidural analgesia significantly reduces the incidence of postoperative ileus, with consequent reduction in respiratory morbidity and also allows earlier introduction of enteral feeding, which may be beneficial. In major abdominal and vascular procedures, epidurals lead to a significant reduction in pulmonary complications. Postoperative epidural analgesia, especially thoracic epidural analgesia, continued for more than 24 h reduces postoperative myocardial infarction (MI). Epidural analgesia has beneficial effects on the incidence of thromboembolic complications in lower limb procedures. In contrast, in an analysis of six randomized-controlled trials there was no significant difference in the incidence of thromboembolic complications in major abdominal and thoracic surgery with or without epidural analgesia.

A recent multicentre trial randomized 915 high-risk patients undergoing major abdominal surgery to intraoperative epidural anaesthesia and postoperative epidural analgesia for 72 h, or control. Mortality at 30 days was no different between the groups and only respiratory failure occurred less frequently in patients managed with epidural techniques. Postoperative epidural analgesia was, however, associated with lower pain scores during the first 3 postoperative days and there were no major adverse consequences of epidural-catheter insertion.

The risks in placement of an epidural catheter are low; nerve damage, epidural haematoma and infection of the CNS all have an incidence of less than 1/10 000. Permanent neurological injury is very rare (0.02–0.07%); however, transient injuries do occur and are more common (0.01–0.8%). Disturbances of micturition are a common accompaniment of epidurals, especially in elderly males. Hypotension is the most common cardiovascular disturbance associated with epidural blockade.

POSTOPERATIVE FLUID AND ELECTROLYTE BALANCE

Intraoperative fluid requirement is usually based on an assumption of maintaining a euvolaemic state. This requires assessment of:
- preoperative circulatory status (euvolaemic/dehydrated/overloaded);
- intraoperative losses of blood and insensible fluid loss during the operation.

Intraoperative monitoring of the circulation is used to determine fluid requirement. Postoperative fluid therapy can be difficult to judge and is often delegated to the most junior member of the surgical team. It is helpful to keep the following factors in mind:
- pre-existing circulatory deficit;
- ongoing losses (if any);
- daily maintenance fluid requirements.

Assessment of the pre-existing circulatory deficit

Each surgical patient should be assessed with the state of the circulation in mind. The patient should be asked if he or she is thirsty and physically examined with reference to their peripheral circulation and the state of hydration of mucous membranes. A review of vital signs and urine output, and an examination of jugular venous pressure, chest and abdomen, should enable the doctor to establish if the patient is euvolaemic, overloaded or dehydrated.

An estimate of current status and likely ongoing losses (if any)

The fluid chart must be examined to assess fluid input and output, including urine, nasogastric, stoma or drain losses. Full blood count and serum electrolytes should be ascertained. Tables 3.1 and 3.2 provide details of the approximate composition of some gastrointestinal secretions and typical intravenous fluids.

An estimate of maintenance fluid requirements

Maintenance fluid requirements are estimated for replacement of:
- insensible losses from the skin and respiratory system (about 750 ml);
- obligatory losses in urine (about 1 l).

A rough guide for maintenance fluid requirement for an adult is 30–40 ml/kg body weight/day. The following are approximate daily requirements of some electrolytes in an adult:
- 1 mmol/kg/day for sodium;
- 1 mmol/kg/day for potassium;
- 5 mmol/day for calcium;
- 1 mmol/day for magnesium.

Table 3.1. Electrolyte content of intravenous fluids (mmol/l).

Intravenous fluid	Na^+	K^+	Cl^-	HCO_3^-	Ca^{2+}
0.9% saline	150	–	150	–	–
0.18% saline + 4% dextrose	30	–	30	–	–
Hartmann's	131	5	111	29	2
Normal plasma	140	4.5	103	26	2.5

Table 3.2. Daily volume and electrolyte composition of gastrointestinal fluids.

Fluid	Volume (ml)	Na$^+$ (mmol/l)	K$^+$ (mmol/l)	Cl$^-$ (mmol/l)	H$^+$ (mmol/l)	HCO$_3^-$ (mmol/l)
Gastric	2500	30–80	5–20	100–150	40–60	
Bile	500	130	10	100		30–50
Pancreatic	1000	130	10	75		70–110
Small bowel	5000	130	10	90–130		20–40

Choosing replacement and maintenance fluids

For daily maintenance requirements 500 ml of Hartmann's solution and 1500 ml of dextrose 5% is sufficient to supply electrolytes and fluid, but it should be noted that it only provides 600 cal.

If the operation was a relatively straightforward procedure in a fit patient not involving the gastrointestinal tract, and associated with little blood loss and a short general anaesthetic, for example hernia repair, cystoscopy or pinning of a fracture, intravenous fluids may not be required at all. The patient may be allowed to drink when fully conscious after the operation and be able to have a normal diet as soon as convenient.

Dangers of potassium infusion: It should be noted that Hartmann's solution and Haemaccel contain potassium, and these should be used sparingly, if at all, in a patient whose urine output is reduced. It is not necessary to replace potassium if the anticipated need for intravenous fluids is likely to last for 1–2 days as the body's store of potassium (3000 mmol) is more than sufficient.

POSTOPERATIVE COMPLICATIONS

Haemorrhage

Haemorrhage is usually the result of a failure of technique but coagulation disorders may also play a role. Occult blood loss, for example postoperative haemoperitoneum, should be suspected when unexplained tachycardia, decreased blood pressure, decreased urine output and peripheral vasoconstriction occurs. A fall in the haematocrit is useful in making the diagnosis but this may not occur until quite late and consequently is of limited diagnostic help. The differential diagnosis of immediate postoperative hypotension includes MI, cardiac dysrhythmia, pulmonary embolism, pneumothorax, pericardial tamponade and severe allergic reaction. Infusions to expand the circulatory volume should be started as soon as other diseases have been ruled out. If hypotension persists, reoperation should be performed.

Respiratory complications

Postoperative respiratory complications (atelectasis and pneumonia) occur significantly more often than cardiac complications and are associated with significantly longer hospital stays. An accurate history and examination is central to the identification of patients at risk for respiratory complications. Approximately one-third of patients with respiratory complications will also have cardiac complications.

Risk factors can be patient or procedure related:
- Patient-related risk factors:
  - Chronic lung disease.
  - Current cigarette smokers even in the absence of chronic lung disease.
  - Morbid obesity.
- Procedure-related risk factors:
  - Surgical procedures lasting longer than 3–4 h.
  - General anaesthesia compared to regional anaesthesia.
  - The rate of complications is inversely related to the distance of the incision from the diaphragm.

Routine preoperative spirometry does not accurately predict the risk of postoperative pulmonary complications in individual patients; however, one simple tool to assess capacity is stair climbing. In a prospective study of patients undergoing thoracotomy or laparotomy, the incidence of postoperative cardiopulmonary complications unable to climb one flight of stairs was 89%. No patient able to climb seven flights of stairs developed a postoperative complication.

Treatment

Cessation of smoking, weight reduction and prophylactic treatment of at-risk patients is helpful; oral and inhaled bronchodilators, systemic steroids and antibiotics can decrease respiratory complications. Good postoperative analgesia, physiotherapy and provision of humidification to loosen secretions are vital; incentive spirometry can be helpful and chest physiotherapy is more effective if started preoperatively.

Cardiac complications

The normal physiological response to surgery is an increase in circulating catecholamines, which leads to an increase in heart rate, myocardial contractility and peripheral vascular resistance, all of which increase myocardial oxygen demand. Also, myocardial oxygen supply may be decreased by hypotension, tachycardia, anaemia and hypoxia. A patient with significant coronary artery disease may not be able to cope with this and may develop myocardial ischaemia. Most MI occur on the first postoperative night. Diagnosis of a perioperative MI can be difficult as the majority of postoperative myocardial ischaemic events are not associated with anginal pain. When present, features of perioperative MI include dysrhythmias, heart failure, hypotension and impaired mental status especially in the elderly.

In patients with significant ischaemic heart disease, coronary artery bypass grafting (CABG) prior to non-cardiac surgery is significantly protective against adverse cardiac events. The protection afforded by CABG appears to last for many years; however, the operative mortality of CABG is approximately 1%. Percutaneous transluminal angioplasty has also been advocated to alleviate myocardial ischaemia prior to non-cardiac surgery and also as an emergency intervention in perioperative patients with evolving acute MI in whom thrombolysis is clearly contraindicated.

Various interventions have been shown to reduce cardiac morbidity; a meta-analysis reported in 2001, showed that postoperative epidural analgesia, especially thoracic epidural analgesia, continued for more than 24 h reduces postoperative MI and maintenance of perioperative normothermia has also been shown to reduce cardiac morbidity in patients with known coronary artery disease undergoing major non-cardiac surgery.

In a randomized, double-blind, placebo-controlled trial comparing atenolol with placebo on overall survival and cardiovascular morbidity in patients with or at risk for coronary artery disease who were undergoing non-cardiac surgery, overall mortality after discharge from the hospital was significantly lower among the atenolol-treated patients than among those who were given placebo.

Heart failure

Heart failure is a syndrome where the cardiac output is insufficient for the body's needs. The best predictor for the development of postoperative heart failure is symptoms and signs of its existence preoperatively. However, heart failure can be precipitated by an increase in demand for cardiac output, such as anaemia, hypoxia and sepsis or through deterioration in pump function through MI, perioperative volume overload, pulmonary embolus or cardiac dysrhythmia. Treatment is directed at the primary cause and provision of medical therapy directed at normalizing intravascular volume and cardiac output.

Cardiac dysrhythmias

Cardiac dysrhythmias are common in the perioperative period; transient dysrhythmias are said to occur in approximately 80% of patients if continuous electrocardiographical (ECG) monitoring is employed, but only 5% are significant. Atrial fibrillation is the commonest rhythm disturbance seen in patients undergoing non-cardiac surgery, occurring in 10% of patients admitted to a surgical ICU.

The guiding principle in the treatment of perioperative cardiac dysrhythmias and conduction disturbances is that

Table 3.3. Analysis of infection rates related to wound types.

Wound type	Total number	Number infected	%
Clean	47 054	732	1.5
Clean contaminated	9370	720	7.7
Contaminated	442	676	15.2
Dirty	2093	832	40
Overall	62 939	2960	4.7

Note: From Cruse PJ, Foord R. The epidemiology of wound infection. A 10-year prospective study of 62 939 wounds. *Surg Clin North Am* 1980; **60**: 27–40.

the cause of the dysrhythmia should be identified and reversed if possible. Common causes include electrolyte disturbance, acid–base imbalance, acute volume depletion and alterations in autonomic tone.

Wound complications

Haematoma

Wound haematoma is almost always caused by imperfect haemostasis. Haematoma produces elevation and discolouration of wound edges, discomfort and swelling. At times, blood leaks through skin sutures. Small haematomas resolve but increase the incidence of wound infection. Treatment consists of gentle evacuation of clots under sterile conditions. Neck haematomas following operations on the thyroid and parathyroid may compress the trachea and need urgent evacuation.

Seroma

This is a serous fluid collection beneath the wound. Seromas often follow operations that involve elevation of skin flaps. Seroma delays wound healing and increases the risk of wound infection. A seroma may be gently expressed or evacuated by needle aspiration.

Infection

Wound infection has undergone a change in nomenclature and the term surgical site infection (SSI) is now used. SSI can be classified as (a) incisional or (b) organ space. Incisional SSI are further classified as superficial or deep.

Risks of SSI can be considered as patient or procedure related. The most important factor during the procedure is the degree of contamination (see Table 3.3).

Patient-related factors that increase risk of SSI include:
• comorbidity,
• malnutrition or obesity,
• smoking,
• steroid use.

Prophylactic antibiotics effectively reduce the rate of postoperative infection. One pre-incisional dose is usually sufficient, although a second dose is advised during surgery lasting more than 3–4 h. Prolonged antibiotic therapy should be avoided because of the cost and the increased likelihood of colonization and infection with antibiotic resistant bacteria.

Dehiscence and incisional hernia

Dehiscence of the wound is most often seen in abdominal surgical procedures. Systemic risk factors are old age, diabetes mellitus, uraemia, immunosuppression, jaundice, hypoalbuminaemia, cancer and obesity. Local risk factors are poor surgical technique of wound closure, raised intra-abdominal pressure due to obstructive airway disease and infection.

Wound dehiscence is commonly seen between the fifth and eighth postoperative day. The discharge of serosanguinous fluid is often the first warning of a disruption. In some cases, sudden dehiscence may occur on coughing or straining. Patients with wound dehiscence are returned to the theatre and the wound repaired.

Incisional hernia occurs in approximately 10% of laparotomy incisions; one important risk factor is the individual surgeon's technique and attention to detail; studies have shown no differences in the complication rate between different suture materials or between continuous and interrupted closure techniques but marked individual differences in wound complication rates between surgeons. A continuous big-bite closure (resulting in a 4 : 1, suture length: wound length ratio) with slowly absorbable monofilament suture has been found to be the optimal technique (see Chapter 6).

Fever

Fever is common in the postoperative period and it has diverse causes. Tissue trauma during surgery, with systemic release of pyrogenic substances, may be a major cause of early postoperative fever. Other non-infectious causes of early postoperative fever include drug hypersensitivity (including anaesthetic agents) and transfusion reactions.

Fever within 48 h after surgery is usually caused by atelectasis. Lung re-expansion causes the body temperature to return to normal. When fever appears after the second postoperative day, the differential diagnosis includes venous access site phlebitis, pneumonia and urinary tract infection.

Patients without an infection are rarely febrile after the fifth postoperative day. The onset of fever this late would suggest a wound infection, or less often, anastomotic breakdown and intra-abdominal abscess. Bacterial pneumonias are often precipitated by perioperative aspiration or early postoperative atelectasis and consequently tend to occur within the first week of surgery.

Urinary tract infections may appear at any time. They occur almost exclusively in patients with bladder catheterization or a previous history of urinary tract manipulation. Thrombophlebitis and pulmonary embolism are important causes of postoperative fever, which may occur either early or late.

Urinary retention

Urinary retention is common, especially after pelvic or perineal operations or operations under spinal/epidural anaesthesia and may require temporary catheterization. In a male patient if a catheter cannot be passed, a suprapubic cystotomy may be needed.

Postoperative delerium and cognitive impairment

Delerium, or acute confusional state, is a clinical syndrome characterized by acute disruption of attention and cognition, and it is associated with increased morbidity and mortality, longer hospital stays, higher costs, poor functional recovery and frequently leads to increases in dependency on carers after discharge.

Hypoxia must be excluded either by oximetry or blood gas estimation. A review of the anaesthetic chart or recovery room notes may reveal the cause. In most cases, of course, no cause is found. Management involves:

- the correction of metabolic disturbances;
- elimination or reduction of all non-essential medication;
- the presence of family members to provide emotional support;
- hypnotics, for example chloral hydrate (250–1000 mg orally at bed time) if sleep disturbance is severe or a short course of low-dose neuroleptic (oral or intramuscular haloperidol).

Lesser degrees of postoperative cognitive dysfunction, characterized by impairment of memory and concentration are common after major surgery in the elderly and symptoms may persist for months or years.

Venous thromboembolism

The pathophysiology of venous thromboembolism (VTE) involves three factors (Virchow's triad):
1. damage to the vessel wall,
2. slowing down of blood flow,
3. an increase in coagulability.

Clinical risk factors include the following: increasing age; prolonged immobility, stroke or paralysis; previous thrombotic disease; cancer and its treatment; major surgery (particularly operations involving the abdomen, pelvis and lower extremities); trauma (especially fractures of the pelvis, hip or leg); obesity; varicose veins; cardiac dysfunction; indwelling central venous catheters; inflammatory bowel disease; nephrotic syndrome and pregnancy or oestrogen use. For surgical patients, the incidence of VTE is affected by the preexisting factors just listed and by factors related to the procedure itself, including the site, technique and duration of the procedure, the type of anaesthetic, the presence of infection and the degree of postoperative immobilization.

Graded compression elastic stockings (ES) reduce the incidence of leg deep venous thrombosis (DVT). Intermittent

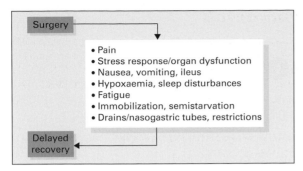

- Pain
- Stress response/organ dysfunction
- Nausea, vomiting, ileus
- Hypoxaemia, sleep disturbances
- Fatigue
- Immobilization, semistarvation
- Drains/nasogastric tubes, restrictions

Figure 3.1. Factors contributing to postoperative morbidity. (From Wilmore DW, Kehlet H. Management of patients in fast track surgery. *Br Med J* 2001; **322**(7284): 473–476. Reproduced with permission from the BMJ Publishing Group.)

techniques aimed at reducing surgical stress, optimizing recovery and reducing hospital stay. A multimodal combination of interventions, including thoracic epidural anaesthesia, avoidance of high abdominal incisions, early mobilization and enteral nutrition have been shown to attenuate the stress response to surgery, improve postoperative physical functioning and achieve highly significant reductions in hospital stay. The reproducibility of the 'Kehlet effect' has been proven in randomized-controlled trials (Fig. 3.1).

CONCLUSION

All surgeons will treat patients who develop complications. Recognition of risk factors and appropriate perioperative management can reduce the incidence and impact of these complications considerably.

pneumatic compression (IPC) is an attractive method of prophylaxis because there is no risk of haemorrhagic complications. In trials comparing IPC with prophylactic heparin, both agents produced similar reductions in DVT.

All surgical patients should be assessed for risk of VTE and appropriate prophylaxis established.

Postoperative nausea and vomiting, and ileus

Fear of postoperative nausea and vomiting (PONV) is a leading concern for patients about to undergo surgery. PONV is unpleasant and increases the risk of aspiration pneumonia; it is the leading cause of unexpected admission following planned day surgery. Several factors contribute to the aetiology of PONV:
- individual susceptibility;
- use of opioids in the perioperative period;
- gastrointestinal procedures;
- duration of surgery;
- intra- or postoperative hypoxaemia.

The incidence of postoperative vomiting may be reduced by preoperative administration of ondansetron, a 5-hydroxytryptamine 3 (5-HT3) receptor antagonist.

FAST-TRACK SURGERY

Kehlet and his co-workers in Denmark have developed the concept of 'fast-track' surgery. This involves a combination of

FURTHER READING

Annane D, Sebille V, Charpentier C *et al*. Effect of treatment with low doses of hydrocortisone and fludrocortisone on mortality in patients with septic shock. *J Am Med Assoc* 2002; **288**: 862–871

Bernard GR, Vincent JL, Laterre PF *et al*. Efficacy and safety of recombinant human activated protein C for severe sepsis. *New Engl J Med* 2001; **344**: 699–709

Hebert PC, Wells G, Blajchman MA, Marshall J, Martin C, Pagliarello G, Tweeddale M, Schweitzer I, Yetisir E. A multicenter, randomized, controlled clinical trial of transfusion requirements in critical care. Transfusion Requirements in Critical Care Investigators, Canadian Critical Care Trials Group. *New Engl J Med* 1999; **340**(6): 409–417

Mangano DT, Layug EL, Wallace A, Tateo I. Effect of atenolol on mortality and cardiovascular morbidity after noncardiac surgery. Multicentre Study of Perioperative Ischaemia Research Group. *New Engl J Med* 1996; **335**: 1713–1720

Poldermans D, Boersma E, Bax JJ, Thomson IR, van de Ven LL, Blankensteijn JD *et al*. The effect of bisoprolol on perioperative mortality and myocardial infarction in high-risk patients undergoing vascular surgery. *New Engl J Med* 1999; **341**: 1789–1794

van den Berghe G, Wouters P, Weekers F, Verwaest C, Bruyninckx F, Schetz M, Vlasselaers D, Ferdinande P, Lauwers P, Bouillon R. Intensive insulin therapy in the critically ill patients. *New Engl J Med* 2001; **345**(19): 1359–1367

Williamson LM, Lowe S, Love EM, Cohen H, Soldan K, McClelland DB, Skacel P, Barbara JA. Serious hazards of transfusion (SHOT) initiative: analysis of the first two annual reports. *Br Med J* 1999; **319**(7201): 16–19

4

Nutritional Support

Jason Payne-James

CONTENTS

Indications for nutritional support	50
Enteral and parenteral nutrition	52
Perioperative nutrition	52
Energy and nitrogen requirements	**52**
Monitoring nutritional support	53
Enteral nutrition	**53**
Types of enteral diet	53
Routes of administration	53
Techniques of administration	54
Complications	54
Total parental nutrition	**55**
Access	55
TPN nutrients	57
Monitoring	57
Metabolic complications	57
Nutritional support team	**57**
Further reading	**57**

Any form of physical injury, including major surgery, multiple trauma and sepsis, is accompanied by increased requirements for nitrogen and energy. Patients in these situations require nutritional repletion from an early stage, even when their pre-insult nutritional status is normal. The parenteral (intravenous) route was considered to be the main route of nutritional support in surgical patients for many years. Over the last two decades it was recognized that other routes of nutritional support may be as appropriate in surgical patients as they are in other patient groups. Sip feeds and oral diet supplementation are important and useful ways of increasing nutrient intake, particularly in postoperative patients, and reduce the incidence of complications. However, for many surgical patients oral feeding is not appropriate – either through inability to eat or swallow (e.g. following orofacial surgery) or because of gastrointestinal (GI) dysfunction (e.g. postoperative ileus). Artificial nutritional support (provision

of nutrient substrates by other than the oral route) is indicated for these patients. The two key options are – via the GI tract (enteral) or via the venous system (parenteral).

Malnutrition is a significant problem in hospitalized patients. Such malnutrition is of a mixed protein and energy deficit (protein-energy malnutrition (PEM)). Forty percent of patients are undernourished at the time of admission to hospital and over half of these have no nutritional data documented in their case notes. It is recommended that every hospitalized patient should have their nutritional status recorded in the medical notes at admission, and a simple screening tool has recently been devised to identify at risk patients. Once malnourished (or potentially malnourished) patients have been identified, the aim must be to correct or improve the nutritional status such that morbidity and mortality are minimized.

Patients who are malnourished have poorer outcomes because of impairment and eventual failure of physiological protein-dependent functions. These may be manifest by increased infection rates (e.g. chest, urinary, wound), slower wound healing, wound breakdown and dehiscence, and death. Assessment of patients to identify PEM is not always straightforward and a number of parameters have been used:

- biochemical (e.g. serum albumin, transferrin, retinol-binding protein);
- anthropometric (e.g. triceps skin-fold thickness (TSF), mid-arm muscle circumference (MAMC));
- immunological (e.g. lymphocyte count, delayed hyper-sensitivity skin testing);
- dynamometric (e.g. hand-grip strength).

These markers have poor sensitivity or specificity when used in isolation. Weekly weighing with a gradual increase in weight, is a simple and effective way of detecting a response to nutritional interventions.

INDICATIONS FOR NUTRITIONAL SUPPORT

All patients admitted to hospital, even for elective surgical procedures, should have a nutritional screening, the results of which should be recorded clearly in the notes, with a comment about whether nutritional support is required.

The routine history and clinical examination of a patient should enable patients to be placed in one of four groups:

1. Obvious severe malnutrition (recent or long term) (>10% recent weight loss; serum albumin <30 g/l; gross muscle wasting and peripheral oedema).
2. Moderate malnutrition (some nutritional parameters suggestive of depletion: dietary history shows impaired nutrient intake for preceding 2–4 weeks or more; there may be no obvious physical evidence of malnutrition).
3. Normal or near-normal nutritional status (but underlying pathology is likely to result in malnutrition if nutritional support is withheld, e.g. trauma patients, ventilated patients).
4. Normal nutritional status which is unlikely to be affected by illness.

There are specific aspects of bedside clinical assessment which assist with this nutritional classification. Height and weight must be recorded and compared with standardized charts. Protein and energy balance may be estimated from the dietary history and using the assumption that maximum requirements of protein and energy for hospitalized patients are 1.5 g/kg/14 h and 40 kcal/kg/24 h, respectively. Body composition studies suggest that when the 'finger–thumb test' (feeling the dermis between finger and thumb when pinching triceps and biceps skinfolds) is positive, the body mass is composed of <10% fat. If in the 'tendon–bone test', tendons are prominent to palpation and bony prominences of the scapula are apparent, patients have lost >30% of body protein stores. However a standard clinical history and examination will also identify loss of muscle power, peripheral oedema, skin rashes, angular stomatitis, gingivitis, nail abnormalities, glossitis, paraesthesia and neuropathy.

Nutritional support must be considered if the patient fits into one of the first three groups listed above. The best route of administration must then be chosen and for the last two decades much emphasis has been placed on the enteral route being considered first for all patients with a normal or near-normal functioning, accessible GI tract (Fig. 4.1).

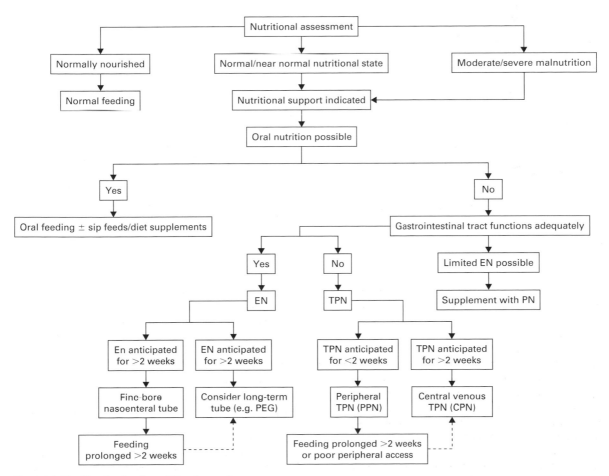

Figure 4.1. Algorithm for planning nutritional support.

Enteral and parenteral nutrition

The metabolic role of the GI tract in both fasting and stressed states is increasingly recognized. The GI tract can act as a reservoir for bacteria that may cause systemic infections, by allowing bacterial translocation across the gut wall. Gut-derived endotoxin may therefore be the link between GI failure and multiple organ failure in patients without overt clinical evidence of infection. The relationship between GI bacteria, systemic host defences and injury in the development of bacterial translocation is complex. Enteral nutrition (EN) appears to modify antibacterial host defences, blunt the hypermetabolic response to trauma, maintain gut mucosal mass, maintain gut barrier function and prevent disruption of gut flora. This potential benefit acted as a driver for EN in preference to parenteral nutrition (PN). However a number of recent studies comparing (in large randomized controlled trials) EN versus PN have shown that the theoretical benefits do not necessarily translate into practice. Indeed in one large study in surgical patients, patients receiving EN had a higher mortality with no differences in septic morbidity when compared with the parenteral route. This and other studies which also fail to show a significantly better outcome for enterally fed patients have resulted in a change in view by many nutritionists. This view can be summed up as 'neither of the two modes (enteral or parenteral) of nutrition confer significant advantages to the surgical patient with respect to either bacterial translocation or infectious complications, or overall complications or death' and thus the aim of therapy should be to optimize nutrition intake by whichever method works best.

The GI tract remains an appropriate and important route for nutritional support in if the gut is working adequately (inadequate function being manifest by abdominal distension, vomiting and large volume nasoenteral aspirates). Small intestine digestive and absorptive function is maintained in the postoperative period after abdominal surgery (the main sites of 'ileus' being the stomach and colon). EN may therefore be administered safely into the small bowel immediately after abdominal surgery (including major aortic reconstruction). It is often suggested that bowel anastomosis is a contraindication to EN in the early postoperative period, but studies have confirmed its safety. EN should be considered the first choice for feeding patients with severe head injuries and should be commenced early as aggressive nutritional support confers benefit on outcome.

Perioperative nutrition

Nutritional support (including supplementation and EN) should be used in the preoperative period in the following way:
1. If a patient is severely malnourished (e.g. >10% weight loss) give at least 10 days of:
   – dietary supplementation;
   if not possible
   – give EN;

if not possible
   – give PN, unless early surgery is clinically indicated.
2. If a patient is borderline or mildly malnourished, operation should not be delayed solely for nutritional support. Preoperative nutritional support should not be continued for so long that the patient's condition can deteriorate as a result of progression of the disease.

Postoperative nutrition should be considered for any patient who fails to have an adequate oral intake (as assessed by a dietitian) 5 days following surgery. Postoperative total parenteral nutrition (TPN) should be considered when oral feeding or EN is not anticipated within 7–10 days in previously well-nourished patients or within 5–7 days in previously malnourished or critically ill patients. For some patients it may be clear at the time of operation that adequate oral intake will not be possible (e.g. because of major oropharyngeal/maxillofacial surgery) for some time postoperatively, or that normal gut function will take more than a few days to recover (major upper GI resection). In cases such as these it may be advisable to insert access routes (e.g. gastrotomy, jejunostomy, central lines) while the patient is still in the operating theatre anaesthetized.

Each patient must be assessed individually. The reason for the operation, the degree of malnutrition and expected postoperative course are all important in deciding the route of nutritional support.

ENERGY AND NITROGEN REQUIREMENTS

Surgical patients most likely to need of nutritional support are metabolically stressed, septic or have been subject to trauma (accident or operation). These patients (particularly those with burns or head injuries) will be hypermetabolic.

Energy requirements for each patient may be determined from indirect calorimetry but this is not necessary nor practical for the vast majority of patients. Energy requirements are very rarely >2200–2400 kcal/24 h and at this or lower levels most surgical patients can achieve positive energy balance. Thus 35–40 kcal/kg/24 h energy will be appropriate for most patients, supplied as a mixture of carbohydrate and fat.

Nitrogen requirements are often considerably greater than normal, and in hypermetabolic, stressed and injured patients, nitrogen balance may be impossible to achieve until the primary pathology has been treated. Nitrogen intake should minimize net losses, permit maintenance of the patient's lean body mass, allow an adequate supply of nitrogen for repair and allow repletion of lean body mass in the previously compromised patient. Very few adult patients will require >14–16 g nitrogen/24 h. Those patients with increased energy needs will require increased nitrogen – up to 0.4 g nitrogen/ kg/24 h has been suggested. It is possible for nitrogen balance to be calculated from urinary and faecal nitrogen losses. There is a reasonable correlation between urinary urea excretion and total urinary nitrogen, with urea accounting for about 80%. Adjustments must be made for plasma urea levels and a figure of 2–3 g allowed for other routes of loss, including faeces. These figures are not appropriate for the severely ill patient, where the urinary urea may represent considerably <80% of the total nitrogen loss because of excessive excretion of ammonium and other non-urea nitrogenous compounds. Total urinary nitrogen is measured routinely by chemoiluminescence in many centres, obviating the need to estimate output from urea values.

Monitoring nutritional support

The most important parameters to be measured when monitoring nutritional support are:
- weight,
- diet charts,
- haematology,
- biochemistry,
- anthropometry,
- dynamometry.

Weighing is the simplest way to ensure that the nutritional regimen prescribed for a particular patient is satisfactory. A steady increase in weight of 1–2 kg/week suggests adequate nutrition in those requiring body mass repletion.

Diet charts (for patients on EN) enable an accurate record to be kept of the patient's actual versus prescribed intake. The charts allow intake problems to be corrected and are of importance if there is a changeover from enteral feeding to oral nutrition.

Basic *haematological* and *biochemical* parameters should be measured at the start of nutritional support. Close monitoring of the plasma potassium, phosphate and glucose are important at the beginning of nutritional support, particularly in the severely malnourished patient. In patients on long-term feeding, vitamin or trace element levels should also be monitored if clinically indicated. The plasma proteins albumin, transferrin and thyroid binding prealbumin are useful markers for measuring the response to nutritional support over a period of time.

Anthropometric and *dynamometric* measurements are often considered to be research tools, but they can offer sensitive and effective measurement of the efficacy of nutritional support.

ENTERAL NUTRITION

Types of enteral diet

There are three main types of nutritionally complete enteral diet appropriate for the surgical patient:
- polymeric,
- predigested (elemental or chemically-defined),
- disease-specific.

Polymeric diets

Polymeric diets are indicated for the vast majority (>90%) of patients with normal or near-normal GI function. They contain whole protein as a nitrogen source, energy derived from triglycerides and glucose polymers, while electrolytes, trace elements and vitamins are included in recommended amounts. Standard polymeric diets contain approximately 6 g nitrogen/l with an energy density of 1 kcal/ml. Other energy, nitrogen-dense diets (containing between 8 and 10 g nitrogen/l and an energy density of 1–1.5 kcal/ml) are used for those with higher requirements.

Predigested diets

In a small proportion of patients with very severe exocrine pancreatic insufficiency or with intestinal failure because of short bowel syndrome, intraluminal hydrolysis may be severely impaired, limiting diet assimilation. In such cases a predigested diet may be indicated. These diets have a nitrogen source derived from free amino acids or oligopeptides. Energy is derived from a glucose polymer mixture containing predominantly polymers of chain length >10 glucose molecules. The fat source consists of a combination of long- and medium-chain triglycerides.

Disease-specific diets

Specifically formulated disease-specific diets have been developed for patients with disorders such as encephalopathy associated with chronic liver disease, and respiratory failure. Malnourished patients with cirrhosis who present with encephalopathy, or who have a previous history of episodes of encephalopathy, present a difficult problem of nutritional management. Branched-chain amino acid-enriched diets have been advocated to normalize plasma amino acid profiles with the aim of improving nutritional state and preventing worsening of encephalopathy. Patients with respiratory failure on ventilators are adversely affected by diets with high carbohydrate loads which increase CO_2 production. Diets with a higher fat energy component allow earlier weaning from artificial ventilator support as a result of decreased CO_2 production and reduced respiratory quotient.

Research is being undertaken on the use of nutritional substrates or supplements such as fish oils, arginine, glutamine and nucleotides, designed to modify or modulate the immune and metabolic response to stress. As yet the clinical value of such diets is unclear and recommendations cannot yet be given on their use.

Routes of administration

The majority of patients need nutritional support for less than a month. For these patients the best method of enteral delivery is via a fine-bore nasogastric feeding tube. The most frequent complication (in <5% of patients) of these tubes is malposition when inserted, often into the trachea and bronchi. If this is not recognized, accidental intrapulmonary aspiration of feed may occur. This complication occurs most commonly in susceptible patients with altered swallowing, diminished gag reflex or who have had upper airway or

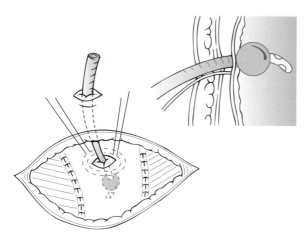

Figure 4.2. Stamm gastrostomy. An upper midline incision gives the best exposure and the catheter is placed laterally away from the incision. A Foley catheter is inserted into the gastric fundus through a double row of purse string sutures. The stomach around the tube anchored initially to the abdominal wall with sutures, becomes firmly adherent in about 10 days. Removal of the tube after this period is followed by rapid closure of the cutaneous orifice.

pharyngeal surgery. In patients who are alert and orientated, tube positioning may be confirmed by aspiration of gastric contents and auscultation of the epigastrum. If aspiration or auscultation is unsuccessful, radiograph confirmation of the position of the tube is essential, and must be undertaken routinely in all such susceptible patients. In some patients (e.g. diabetics with neuropathy, head injuries, postabdominal surgery and ITU/ventilated patients), nasogastric delivery of nutrients may not be appropriate because of increased risk of regurgitation and/or pulmonary aspiration of feed. All such patients and others with gastric atony or gastroparesis should be considered for postpyloric nasoduodenal or nasojejunal feeding. For the surgical patient for whom postoperative nutritional support is anticipated, placement at laparotomy is advised. In other cases a fine-bore tube may be introduced pernasally and, if spontaneous passage has not occurred after 12–24 h, endoscopic or fluoroscopic positioning is undertaken.

For longer-term feeding, pharyngostomy and oesophagostomy are used by some surgeons. Surgically placed gastrostomies are used for long-term administration of feed for patients with progressive deglutition disorders (motor neurone disease, multiple sclerosis). Stamm gastrotomy (Fig. 4.2) is simple to perform as a temporary procedure. The removal of the tube is rapidly followed by closure of the cutaneous orifice. The percutaneous endoscopically-placed gastrostomy (PEG) is now the technique of choice for long-term administration of EN. This technique has a lower morbidity and mortality, when compared with the conventional surgical placement. A needle catheter jejunostomy is shown in

Fig. 4.3. Jejunostomy by Witzel technique (Fig. 4.4) uses a 14 or 16 F catheter and is less likely to be occluded by the feeding solution. Either may be inserted as a separate surgical procedure or concurrently at the time of abdominal surgery. Needle catheter jejunostomy has been recommended for patients:
- malnourished at the time of surgery;
- undergoing major upper GI surgery;
- who may receive adjuvant radio- or chemo-therapy after surgery;
- undergoing laparotomy after major trauma.

Techniques of administration

Bolus feeding of enteral diets, where typically a volume of 200–400 ml of feed is instilled into the stomach via a nasogastric tube over a period ranging from 15 min to 1 h, was the standard method of administration for many years. This method has a high incidence of side-effects such as bloating and diarrhoea, in addition to which a considerable amount of nursing time is required and feeds may often be accidentally omitted. A continuous infusion either by gravity feed or by using a peristaltic pump is therefore the method of choice.

Starter regimens (diluting the feed or reducing the volume) limit the intake of diet in the first few days of feeding and thereby prolong the length of negative nitrogen balance. They should not therefore in general be used.

For those patients who are immobile or confined to bed, or with altered consciousness, the head of the bed should be elevated by 20° or 30° to help reduce the risk of regurgitation and pulmonary aspiration. In most adult patients with no other metabolic or fluid balance problems, between 2 and 2.5 l of diet are prescribed on a daily basis. This volume is infused from day 1.

Complications

The potential complications of EN are:
- *feeding-tube related*: malposition, unwanted removal, blockage;
- *diet and diet administration related*: diarrhoea, bloating, nausea, cramps, regurgitation, pulmonary aspiration, vitamin, mineral, trace element deficiencies, drug interactions;
- *metabolic/infective*;
- *infective*: diet, reservoirs, giving sets.

Tube blockage most commonly occurs after disconnection of the giving set from the feeding tube when the residual diet solidifies. This complication may be prevented by flushing the tube with water after disconnection.

Diarrhoea occurs in about 10% of patients. Its aetiology is multifactorial with a strong association with concomitant antibiotic therapy, and hypoalbuminaemia may have a role. Symptomatic treatment (with antidiarrhoeals such as codeine phosphate or loperamide) is appropriate and only rarely does enteral feeding have to be discontinued.

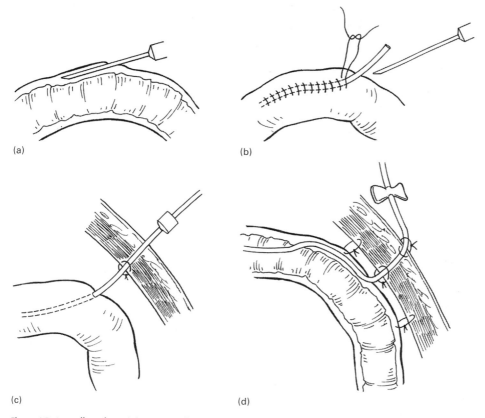

Figure 4.3. A needle catheter jejunostomy. This may be performed at the conclusion of the main operation. (a) A needle of the central venous catheterization type is inserted obliquely through the antimesenteric border of the jejunum about 15 cm distal to the ligament of Treitz. (b) A 30 cm, 16 gauge catheter is advanced about 10–15 cm into the lumen, the needle withdrawn and the catheter secured in place with a single 4, 0 silk purse string suture. (c) The needle is then passed into the abdomen from the skin surface and the extraluminal portion of the catheter is passed through the needle to the outside. (d) The catheter is secured to the skin and the jejunum tacked to the anterior parietal peritoneum of the abdominal wall.

Antibiotics that are no longer clinically indicated should be stopped. Nausea and vomiting rarely occur and may result from slowed gastric emptying. Antiemetics may be of benefit. The symptoms of bloating, abdominal distension and cramps most commonly occur following inadvertent too rapid administration of feed and are very similar to the symptoms described in association with bolus-type feeding. Enteral diets will interact with enterally administered drugs (e.g. theophylline, warfarin, methyldopa and digoxin). Failure of drug therapy in previously stable patients receiving EN support must be assumed to be feed related until proven otherwise.

TOTAL PARENTERAL NUTRITION

The successful use of TPN in maintaining body weight and allowing growth to progress normally was first demonstrated by Dudrick and co-workers in 1968. Up to 25% of patients in hospital requiring nutritional support need it administered via the parenteral route. TPN can be considered for all malnourished or potentially malnourished patients with a non-functioning and/or non-accessible GI tract, or those where there is concern that the GI tract is totally non-functioning.

Access

The high osmolality of TPN formulations results in rapid development of thrombophlebitis and line failure if infused into peripheral veins. This problem has been overcome by using central venous catheters to deliver TPN solutions into large veins, most commonly via the subclavian or internal jugular veins (see Chapter 3). Getting access to, and the presence of central venous catheters within these veins, can result in a number of complications:

- *insertion-related*: air embolism, arterial puncture, cardiac arrhythmias, catheter embolus, chylothorax, haemopericardium, haematoma, haemothorax, hydro/TPN-thorax, malposition, neurological injury, pneumothorax;

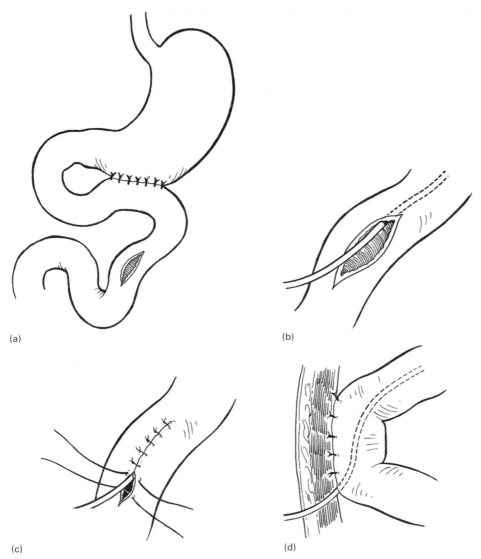

(a)

(b)

(c)

(d)

Figure 4.4. Witzel jejunostomy. (a) The site of insertion of the catheter into the jejunum is about 30 cm distal to the ligament of Treitz. (b) A fine-bore catheter is inserted through the seromuscular tunnel in the jejunal wall and fastened at the mucosal entrance by an anchor stitch. (c) The incision in the tunnel of the jejunal wall is closed over the catheter. (d) The jejunum is anchored to the anterior abdominal wall.

- *late complications*: catheter infection or sepsis, catheter displacement, central venous thrombosis, luminal occlusion.

Complications occur in up to 5% of catheter placements.

A variety of routes, catheters and techniques of insertion are available. The two main methods of insertion are blind percutaneous puncture of a vein or open surgical exposure. The advantages of the percutaneous technique in experienced hands are that insertion is quick and may be done under local anaesthesia at the patient's bedside as long as sterile procedure is observed. Open surgical exposure is done in an operating theatre and may require general anaesthesia.

This route of insertion should be used for patients with chronic respiratory disease, those on a ventilator, and those with severe clotting disorders because of the risks associated with development of complications. Strict catheter care protocols should be followed and monitored by an infection control or nutrition nurse to minimize the incidence of catheter-related sepsis. If a patient on TPN develops a pyrexia and leucocytosis in the absence of any other focus of infection, then the central venous catheter should be considered to be the source of infection. However, all other possible sources of infection should be considered and cultures of sputum, urine and other sites is mandatory.

TPN is increasingly administered by the peripheral route (peripheral parenteral nutrition (PPN)). A number of methods have been investigated to reduce the incidence of peripheral vein thrombophlebitis, including the use of heparin, in-line filtration, cortisol, buffering, locally applied glyceryl trinitrate patches and fine-bore cannulas. Reducing the osmolality by altering the formulation of carbohydrate energy components and nitrogen source may also have a role and specially formulated commercial mixtures have been shown in clinical studies to be suitable for PPN. Thrombophlebitis cannot be totally abolished, however, but it should be borne in mind that most courses of TPN rarely last more than 10–14 days. TPN can be administered peripherally if it is anticipated that support will be needed for <2 weeks.

TPN nutrients

Macronutrients consist of energy sources – carbohydrate (glucose) and lipid emulsions. Most regimens consist of a combination in proportions up to 50% : 50%. Nitrogen is provided as amino acid solutions. Micronutrients are electrolytes, trace elements and vitamins, deficiencies of which may present interesting clinical problems. PN requirements may be mixed together safely in a single container (generally made of ethyl vinyl acetate) – an All-in-One bag (AIO), the contents of which can be infused safely over 24 h. Ready-to-Use bags with set amounts of the key nutrients are becoming increasingly used. Many hospitals use a small range of formulations with different nitrogen and energy contents. The bag that most approximates the perceived requirements for the patient is then chosen. There is no evidence from randomized controlled trials that support the hypothesis that individually prescribed nutrient formulations provide any benefit in terms of clinical outcome.

Monitoring

TPN should be administered using infusion pumps or flow-control devices. In the 1st week of TPN administration, blood glucose should be measured 6-hourly, as many patients develop some degree of insulin resistance because of their underlying pathology and may require exogenous insulin administered by injection/infusion or included in the TPN regimen. Electrolytes should be measured daily to allow correction of initial electrolyte imbalance and fluctuations, and to detect changes before severe metabolic/biochemical changes can affect the patient's clinical status. Liver function tests should be monitored to observe changes in serum albumin, and to detect TPN-related hepatobiliary dysfunction.

Metabolic complications

A wide variety of metabolic complications can occur with TPN. In order of frequency:

- hyperglycaemia,
- hypoglycaemia,
- hypophosphataemia,
- hypercalcaemia,
- hyperkalaemia,
- hypokalaemia,
- hypernatraemia,
- hyponatraemia,
- other: particularly after long-term feeding – deficiencies of folate, zinc, magnesium, other trace elements and essential fatty acids.

A specific complication of TPN of multifactorial aetiology is the development of hepatic dysfunction. This is characterized by elevated hepatic enzymes, intrahepatic cholestasis and fatty infiltration of the liver. This is generally self-limiting and hepatic function returns to normal after cessation of TPN.

NUTRITIONAL SUPPORT TEAM

A multiprofessional nutritional support team is the best way of optimizing the nutritional care of hospitalized patients. The different members of the team can provide advice within their own expertise. Input to the team should come from clinicians, dietitians, pharmacists, nurses, chemical pathologists and microbiologists. The multiprofessional approach ensures the most appropriate administration of nutritional support and minimizes complications.

FURTHER READING

Kondrup J, Allison SP et al. ESPEN Guideline for Nutrition Screening 2002. *Clin Nutr* 2003; **22**: 415–421

Pacelli F, Bossola M et al. Enteral vs parenteral nutrition after major surgery. An even match. *Arch Surg* 2001; **136**: 933–936

Payne-James JJ, Grimble GK, Silk DBA (eds). *Artificial Nutrition Support in Clinical Practice*, 2nd edn. London: Greenwich Medical Media, 2001

Wicks C, Payne-James JJ. *Key Facts in Clinical Nutrition*, 2nd edn. London: Greenwich Medical Media, 2003

Woodcock NP, Zeigler D, Palmer D et al. Enteral vs parenteral nutrition: a pragmatic study. *Nutrition* 2001; **17**: 1–12

5

Surgical Sepsis: Prevention and Therapy

QM Nunes[1], CV Soong[2] and BJ Rowlands[3]

[1]Clinical Fellow in General Surgery, Queen's Medical Centre, Nottingham, UK [2]Department of General and Vascular Surgery, Queen's University of Belfast, Northern Ireland and [3]Queen's Medical Centre, University of Nottingham, UK

CONTENTS

Pathophysiology	58
Microorganisms	60
Mediators	61
Postoperative sepsis	62
Preventative measures	63
Definitive management of established sepsis	66
Resuscitation	66
Treatment of the primary pathology	67
Human immunodeficiency virus and viral hepatitis infection	69
Further reading	70

Table 5.1. **Comparison of admission sepsis score and mortality in ICU.**

Admission sepsis score	Mortality (%)
0–4	10
5–6	18
10–14	24
>15	22

Sepsis is defined as the development of a systemic inflammatory response syndrome (SIRS) as a result of an infective process. SIRS is characterized by two or more of the following conditions:

- temperature greater than 38.4°C or below 35.6°C;
- heart rate greater than 90 beats per minute;
- respiratory rate greater than 20 per minute or $PaCO_2$ less than 32 mmHg;
- white cell count greater than 12 000 cells per ml, or less than 4000 cells per ml or 10% immature (band) forms.

The above definitions of these different syndromes were made at a consensus conference jointly sponsored by the American College of Chest Physicians and the Society for Critical Care Medicine in 1991.

Severe sepsis may progress to multiple organ dysfunction syndrome (MODS), defined as organ dysfunction caused by systemic inflammation-induced damage in which homeostasis cannot be maintained without supportive measures. This may take the form of a primary insult (e.g. aspiration injury to the lung) or a secondary phenomenon (e.g. adult respiratory distress syndrome (ARDS) in severe pancreatitis). MODS was first described more than 20 years ago, following the observation that some patients succumbed to progressive organ system failure despite an initial phase of apparent stability. The phenomenon is a dynamic process which varies from patient to patient and even within the same patient at different times.

Despite better monitoring and supportive techniques in the intensive care unit (ICU), the mortality rate associated with sepsis remains high, especially when accompanied by shock and MODS. Mortality in the presence of organ failure is related to the number, duration and severity of organs that fail; the rate is <40% if one organ is impaired for 1 day and rises to 98% if >2 organs are affected for >5 days. The development of shock is associated with a three-fold increase in mortality. When the admission sepsis score is tabulated using the local and secondary effects of sepsis, pyrexia, laboratory data and a visual linear analogue scale ranging from mild to severe, a good correlation is found between the cumulative score and mortality (Table 5.1).

PATHOPHYSIOLOGY

The understanding of the various pathological mechanisms involved in sepsis and SIRS is continuously evolving. Many of the actions of the identified pleiotrophic mediators are

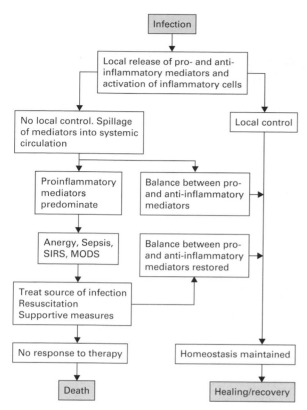

Figure 5.1. Local and systemic response to infection and progression either to successful resolution or deterioration/death. SIRS: systemic inflammatory response syndrome; MODS: multiple organ dysfunctional syndrome.

being unraveled while others remain poorly understood. It is known that an overwhelming release of these mediators occurs as a result of an inciting event such as trauma and infection. Usually, the initial injury causes a localized inflammatory reaction classically characterized by *rubor* (redness), *calor* (heat), *dolor* (pain), *tumor* (swelling) and *functio laesii* (loss of function). This is due to the activation of the coagulation and complement cascades, in particular C3–C5, the cleavage products of which are potent chemoactivators and attractants of macrophages, polymorphonuclear leukocytes and platelets. The release by the activated cells of more kinins, histamines, prostaglandins, cytokines, oxygen-derived free radicals and other products leads to increased capillary permeability and oedema. This chain of events is the natural defense of the host against invading organisms and is a prerequisite for normal healing. It is only when this response is exaggerated with systemic spillage of the mediators that a generalized inflammatory response occurs, resulting in sepsis, septic shock and MODS. A continuum of host reaction therefore exists in response to infection ranging from a localized inflammatory process to multiple organ dysfunction with its associated high mortality (Fig. 5.1).

Many factors predispose to the development of sepsis, SIRS or MODS, including:

- changes in the microenvironment;
- disruption of intestinal mucosal barrier function;
- ischaemia-reperfusion injury;
- blood loss and transfusion;
- malnutrition.

Changes in the microenvironment

In the small intestine, peristalsis, mucus secretions and resident flora help to minimize the growth of pathogenic species. The peristaltic waves discourage adherence of the organism to the bowel wall and prevent colonization with overgrowth. The normal reduction in motility from small intestine to colon accounts for the higher bacterial counts in the latter. The development of paralytic ileus and the formation of a blind loop leads to stagnation of intraluminal contents and the development of favourable conditions for microbial proliferation. In addition, the use of antibiotics causes a reduction in the normal colonization-resistant indigenous flora and an increase in number of the more noxious pathogenic species.

Disruption of intestinal mucosal barrier

Mucosal organisms or their breakdown products may permeate the intestinal wall if the mucosal barrier function is breached. This barrier may be compromised by many pathological states and processes. The mucosa at the tip of the villi are particularly prone to ischaemia due to the counter-current exchange mechanism of the vessels. Shunting of blood during low flow states may lead to ischaemia affecting the tips of the villi alone. Subtle mucosal damage, which is only detectable microscopically, may occur following mild ischaemia. In transient hypoperfusion or hypoxia, the mucosal injury is more pronounced during reperfusion when the oxygen supply is re-established. This is due to damage by the putative deleterious oxygen radicals which are generated mainly via the xanthine oxidase pathway. Xanthine oxidase occurs naturally as the dehydrogenase but in ischaemia it is converted by proteolysis to the oxidase form. This latter form then catalyses a reaction which utilizes oxygen to convert hypoxanthine to uric acid with the production of superoxide radicals. These free radicals may damage the mucosa directly due to their cytotoxicity or indirectly via the activation of neutrophils. The accumulation of neutrophils leads to sludging of capillaries, no reflow and worsening of the insult.

At the other extreme is complete disruption of the bowel wall which may occur with perforation or frank infarction. The severity of intestinal barrier function disruption dictates the mode of entry of intraluminal contents and organisms into the systemic circulation. If mild, the initial invasion is via the portal system with systemic bacteraemia delayed because of hepatic filtering. In cases with severe intestinal wall damage, direct peritoneal contamination may occur

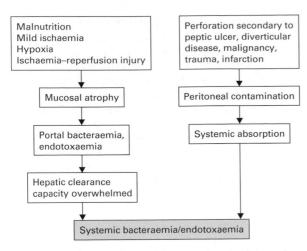

Figure 5.2. Development of systemic bacteraemia and endotoxaemia following disruption of mucosal barrier function.

allowing bacteria and endotoxin to enter the systemic circulation from the peritoneal cavity (Fig. 5.2).

Ischaemia-reperfusion injury

This phenomenon is not confined to the bowel as other organs and systems may also suffer when a reduction in blood flow is followed by revascularization or successful resuscitation. The release of mediators initially causes regional damage but with spillage into the systemic circulation other organs or systems are affected. Ischaemia-reperfusion injury to the lower limb may lead to non-cardiogenic pulmonary oedema and changes in intestinal morphology. Similarly, reperfusion of ischaemic bowel may damage the liver parenchyma and lungs. Such local and remote organ injuries may be abrogated by pretreatment with ibuprofen and mannitol, suggesting that the generation of oxygen-derived free radicals and the activation of the arachidonic acid cascade have important roles to play.

Blood loss and transfusion

Blood loss and shock have detrimental effects on the immune and hepatic cells, reducing their capacity to clear bacteria and endotoxin. In addition, blood transfusion can activate polymorphonuclear leukocytes which then sequestrate in various sites and have been implicated in the development of transfusion-related acute lung. Even autologous blood may have the same effect, leading to leukocyte activation and cytokine release.

Malnutrition

The nutritional status of the patient is important in determining the outcome following trauma and surgical disease (see Chapter 4). Patients may present with pre-existing malnutrition due to their inability to swallow, malabsorption, poverty, self-neglect, prolonged starvation in the ICU or

following surgery. As early as the 1930s, it was observed that patients with >20% weight loss have a significantly higher mortality following gastrectomy compared to those with less weight loss. In patients recovering from abdominal surgery, enteral feeding has been shown to improve muscle function and reduce morbidity and mortality. Although total parenteral nutrition (TPN) may improve outcome in those with intestinal failure and in the severely malnourished, it may lead to atrophy of the intestinal mucosa and a reduction in IgA antibody production. This is because the enterocytes and colonocytes are better supported by enteral intraluminal infusion, as opposed to parenteral feeding, especially if the enteral nutrition is enriched with glutamine and omega-3-fatty acid, which are important nutrients to enterocytes and colonocytes, respectively.

Microorganisms

The numbers and types of microorganisms involved in the development of sepsis are influenced by several factors, including site of intervention, immune and nutritional status of the patient, use of antibiotics and other comorbid states. Cutaneous infections are usually due to Gram-positive cocci. Staphylococci normally colonize the skin and integument and may lead to infection of surgical wounds, intravascular catheters and graft prosthesis. The organism is usually implanted at the time of the procedure but presentation may be delayed. Group A streptococci may also be inoculated during invasive procedures which breach the skin. Infection with this organism usually presents as spreading cellulitis but a more virulent strain, microaerophilic non-haemolytic, may produce a synergistic infection with aerobic haemolytic staphylococci giving rise to a rapidly progressive gangrenous ulceration which requires urgent extensive debridement of all affected tissue together with large doses of penicillin. Hospitalization, critical illness and possibly antibiotic usage may alter the cutaneous microorganisms, replacing the resident Gram-positive with Gram-negative ones.

Other organisms that may cause wound site infection include enterococci, *Escherichia coli* and *Pseudomonas aeruginosa*. The latter is one of the commonest organisms involved in nosocomial pneumonia. Many factors predispose critically ill patients to nosocomial pneumonia (Fig. 5.3). First, there is an increase in oropharyngeal colonization in critically ill patients due to the lack of mastication and salivation. Secondly, the routine use of therapies (e.g. H_2 antagonist and antacids) to neutralize gastric acid allows bacteria to colonize in the stomach. These organisms are found in increasing numbers within 24–96 h of admission to the ICU. The presence of a nasogastric tube leads to loss of lower oesophageal sphincter competence, allowing bacteria to ascend from the stomach to the upper airways where they may be aspirated. Thirdly, the presence of an endotracheal tube allows environmental organisms to gain entry into the airways and lungs. An association has been found between the duration

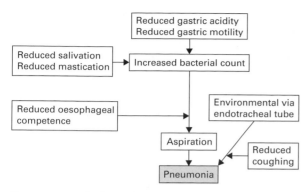

Figure 5.3. Factors leading to the development of pneumonia in the critically ill patient.

of endotracheal intubation and the incidence of pneumonia. Finally, the cough reflex is impaired in patients with a decreased level of consciousness and endotracheal intubation.

The Gram-negative bacteria, *Escherichia coli*, *Klebsiella*, *Enterobacter* and *Proteus* spp are normally associated with infections of the gastrointestinal and urinary tracts. These together with *Bacteroides* spp are found mainly in the distal ileum and colon and have been incriminated in Gram-negative sepsis. Although sepsis is predominantly caused by Gram-negative organisms, Gram-positive bacteria, viruses and fungi are becoming commoner. The incidence of Gram-positive bacterial sepsis in particular is gradually increasing and may be related to the increasing use of invasive monitoring devices in older and immunosuppressed patients and the development of resistant strains of organisms to routine antibiotics, for example methicillin-resistant *Staphylococcus aureas* (MRSA). Concurrent diseases such as cardiovascular, respiratory and renal disease may also contribute to the rise. Coagulase-negative staphylococci is the single commonest cause.

Mediators

Refer to Chapter 10 for overview.

The innate immune system is the first line of host defence against infection. Initially sepsis may be characterized by increases in inflammatory mediators, but with time there is a shift towards an anti-inflammatory immunosuppressive state.

Proinflammatory mediators

The presence of organisms or their breakdown products such as lipopolysaccharide (LPS) in both gram-negative as well as gram-positive bacterial infections, peptidoglycan, lipoteichoic acid, lipoarabinomannan, flagellin and fragments of microbial deoxyribonucleic acid (DNA) may initiate the release of inflammatory mediators such as tumor necrosis factor (TNF), interleukin-6 (IL-6), IL-8, and platelet activating factor (PAF). Important molecules in this process include

LPS-binding protein (LBP), soluble CD14 (sCD14), along with endotoxin docking molecules such as mCD14, CD11/CD18 complex and the Toll-like receptors (TLR) on the monocyte and macrophage surface. Various TLRs are involved in the recognition of different types of bacteria. CD14 cannot activate cells as it is attached to the cell membrane by a glycosyl-phosphatidyl-inositol (GPI) anchor and does not have an intracellular domain. There are a group of receptors, recently discovered which transduce the signal after contact with microbial structures intracellularly. TNF has been demonstrated to be partly responsible for the lethal effects of LPS which could be reproduced in animals if they were administered TNF.

Other cytokines such as IL-1 and IL-6 are also generated as a result of endotoxaemia and TNF release. Many of these inflammatory peptides act synergistically. IL-1 in particular mimics many of the properties of TNF as a pro-inflammatory mediator. The role of IL-6 remains controversial and may only represent an acute phase protein. It is, however, useful as a prognostic measure of outcome in various disease states. IL-1 has a naturally occurring antagonist, IL-1ra, which may have therapeutic potential in the management of septic patients.

Haemorrhage with resuscitation causes an elevation in TNF, IL-1 and IL-6 and may be associated with acute lung injury. An increase in the concentration of IL-8 has been demonstrated when shock complicates blood loss. The acute lung injury may be related to the sequestration of activated granulocytes in the pulmonary circulation. Elevation in concentrations of cytokines correlates with organ impairment following major vascular surgery. Sepsis induced activation of coagulation is initiated through the extrinsic pathway and is dependant on 'cross-talk' and feedback. Pro-inflammatory cytokines can activate endothelial cells and induce the release of tissue factor, which in turn activates factor VII and the coagulation cascade. Tissue factor and PAF can also be released by activated macrophages. PAF has now been established as a key signalling molecule with the capacity to trigger both thrombosis and inflammation. When these processes become systemic as in severe sepsis, it results in disseminated intravascular coagulation (DIC), impaired microcirculation and multiorgan failure. Proteins C and S and antithrombin play an important role in opposing procoagulant mechanisms. Protein C also has a potent anti-apoptotic effect on endothelial cells. The neutrophil is regarded as a double-edged sword in sepsis. When localized, it contributes towards the host defences against invading microbes. However, when its activation is overwhelming, it may produce deleterious effects in the local tissues and in organs remote from the initial site of insult. Many of the mediators produced in the systemic response are activators and chemoattractants of polymorphonuclear cells. Some of these plasma factors have been shown to be stable to heat and transfer even though their actual identities remain unclear. Studies have shown that neutrophil depletion may reduce the organ injury observed following trauma. However, a neutrophil-independent process may still occur which can cause both the local and remote organ injuries in the critically ill. The activated neutrophils probably exert their effect via the up-regulation of adhesion molecules such as CD-18 on cell surfaces, since antibodies directed against these can minimize the neutrophil-induced injuries.

Anti-inflammatory mediators

Anti-inflammatory mediators have been identified – IL-4, IL-10, IL-11, IL-13, transforming growth factor-b, TNF receptors and receptor antagonist to IL-1 – the actions of which are opposed to those of the proinflammatory mediators. Unfortunately, their activities and role in sepsis remain unclear as the plasma concentration of some such as the soluble TNF receptors are also elevated in many disease entities not related to sepsis, for example rheumatoid arthritis and systemic lupus, as well as in normal pregnancy.

A balance is required between pro-inflammatory and anti-inflammatory mediators to maintain homeostasis and facilitate recovery of the patient. If either response offsets the other, then SIRS with MODS and anergy with infection may occur. In addition to these anti-inflammatory mediators, studies have shown a reduction in antibody production, lack of delayed hypersensitivity and depression of lymphocyte activation following trauma and in the critically ill. This anergy may leave the patient susceptible to infective complications.

Antibodies to the core region of the endotoxin molecule can be detected and have been measured as an indicator of circulating endotoxin. A decrease in the concentration of these antibodies is proposed to reflect their consumption from current or recurrent exposure to endotoxin. In a study of patients undergoing major vascular surgery, a fall in antibody titres mirrored the elevation of TNF receptor status but only in those whose recovery was uncomplicated. The lack of correlation between endotoxin antibodies and TNF receptors in non-survivors may indicate an imbalance or inappropriate anti-inflammatory response leading to an overwhelming suppression of the immune system and patient demise, which supports the anti- and pro-inflammatory paradigm. Attempts have been made to correlate the levels of various pro and anti-inflammatory mediators with the final outcome with varying success. There is evidence to suggest that baseline serum IL-10 and TNF-α levels, together with IL-10: TNF-α ratio has a significant prognostic value, being significantly higher in patients who died.

POSTOPERATIVE SEPSIS

One of the commonest forms of postoperative infection is that of the surgical site. Factors that predispose to wound infection (refer to Chapter 6) may be categorized as follows:

• *Surgeon factors*:
  – poor handling of tissue;
  – inadequate haemostasis;
  – improper wound closure;
  – excessive electrocauterization;
  – incorrect drainage;
  – prolonged operation.
• *Patient factors*:
  – old age;
  – diminished local blood flow;
  – diabetes;
  – malnutrition;
  – uraemia;
  – jaundice.
• *Bacterial factors*:
  – high count;
  – high virulence.

The microbe is usually from an endogenous rather than exogenous source and the amount of contamination is dependent on the wound category (Table 5.2). Although usually superficial and overt, it may be deep and clinically difficult to diagnose. In the latter, radiological investigations are required to aid diagnosis and localization. In the era of prosthetic devices for implantation, graft infection is becoming commoner. In peripheral vascular bypass surgery, graft infection may occur in up to 3% of patients if the procedure involves dissection through the groin. Although presentation in such cases may be dramatic with haemorrhage, the signs may be subtle and diagnosis requires a high index of suspicion. Adjunctive investigations may be necessary including contrast-enhanced computerized tomography (CT) and radiolabelled white cell scans but these may not be absolutely accurate and are sometimes misleading.

Some patients need intensive monitoring and resuscitation. The use of invasive monitoring devices predisposes the patient to nosocomial infections. Urinary tract infection may result from bladder catheter placement, phlebitis and endocarditis from vascular cannulae and chest infection from nasogastric and endotracheal intubation. These techniques

Table 5.2. Classification of surgical wounds.

Clean wound	Wound in which the gastrointestinal tract or respiratory tract was not entered, no inflammation encountered and no break in aseptic technique.
Clean contaminated wound	Clean wounds that entered the gastrointestinal tract or respiratory tract but without significant spillage.
Contaminated wound	Acute inflammation without pus formation encountered or gross spillage from a hollow viscus occurred during the operation. Fresh traumatic wounds and operations during which a major break in aseptic technique occurred.
Dirty wound	Pus encountered. Perforated viscus.

together with the patient's reduced immunity inevitably lead to an increased susceptibility to infection.

In postoperative patients, especially those who are ventilated and already have MODS, the signs of infection may be subtle and difficult to recognize. Recovery may be slow and associated with prolonged ileus, general debility, anorexia and confusion. If the infection is severe or associated with SIRS, hypotension may occur. Patients may develop oliguria or biochemical evidence of renal impairment. Hepatic dysfunction may also be evident with elevation in transaminase levels or total bilirubin. Respiratory failure with the development of ARDS may develop. The resulting insulin resistance and increased production of glucagon may cause hyperglycaemia.

Investigation

Immunocompromised patients and those who have a depressed level of consciousness may not localize infection easily. A thorough examination is essential to determine the site of the infective process:

* surgical site must be inspected for inflammation, discharge and swelling;
* central intravascular catheters must not be overlooked and should be examined for infection along the track of the cannula or catheter;
* the chest must be examined for signs of pneumonia;
* a urine sample should be sent for analysis and culture;
* sputum, any effluent fluid from drains and wound swabs should be obtained if possible.

Further investigative procedures may be required to help establish the diagnosis:

* a chest radiograph will assist in the detection of chest infection and ARDS, especially when pneumonia may be difficult to diagnose in the ventilated patient;
* facial radiographs to diagnose sinusitis may be indicated in a patient with nasal discharge and a nasogastric tube *in situ*;
* ultrasound and CT scans may be used to look for evidence of fluid collection or abscess in the peritoneal cavity. The latter is more accurate in identifying collections in the extraperitoneal spaces, in the obese and in the presence of bowel gas.

Preventative measures

The most vital aspect of managing surgical sepsis is prevention. To reduce the incidence of wound site infection, strict aseptic techniques must be adhered to regardless of how minor a procedure may seem:

* *Reduction of bacterial count in patient*:
  – skin preparation: shaving immediately before surgery, preoperative shower, skin cleansing during surgery;
  – bowel preparation: purgatives, selective decontamination.
* *Reduction of contamination from medical staff*:
  – hand washing;
  – masks;
  – covering head and beards.
* *Surgical technique*:
  – adequate haemostasis;
  – gentle tissue handling;
  – non-strangulating sutures;
  – adequate debridement of devitalized tissues;
  – minimizing operating time.
* *Environmental*:
  – adequate ventilation system;
  – limit talking in the theatre;
  – minimum movements in and out of operating theatre.
* *Antibiotic prophylaxis*.
* *Minimizing hospital stay*.

Even superficial wound infections may lead to undue suffering for the patient and delay recovery which can prolong hospitalization and incur extra cost to the health service. In some, especially the elderly and those who are immunocompromised, it can lead to full-blown systemic sepsis.

Insertion of catheters

Catheter-induced sepsis is one of the commonest causes of nosocomial infection in the ICU but because intravascular cannulae and catheter placements for vascular access, monitoring and cardiac output measurements are now common practice, a sense of complacency has developed. Catheters must be inserted under sterile conditions; a proper surgical approach to skin preparation with gowning and glove donning is best, especially for critically ill and immunocompromised patients and if catheterization is planned for long-term use. As catheter infection is rare during the first 3 days of placement, it is suggested that catheter-related sepsis may be minimized by changing the catheter within 48 h. Unfortunately, this practice increases the risk of complications associated with catheter insertion. A single lumen catheter is preferred to a multilumen one as they require less manipulation and there is less temptation to use them for drug administration also, although there is no evidence that this practice reduces infection. Aftercare of central venous catheters is important. Sterile dressings are better than impermeable transparent occlusive dressings which promote bacterial growth. Similarly, urinary catheters must be inserted with care using the 'no-touch' technique if possible. The incidence of catheter-related urinary tract infection may be reduced by minimizing the duration of insertion and use of a closed drainage system.

Gut decontamination

Because the gut is a potent source of translocated gramnegative bacteria, the use of selective digestive decontamination (SDD) has been studied, on the theoretical basis that reduction of the intestinal bacteria will have a beneficial effect on the incidence of nosocomial infection. SDD aims to reduce potentially pathogenic bacteria and minimize the endotoxin load in the event of increased intestinal permeability. Many studies have demonstrated an effect on morbidity in multiple trauma patients. In cardiac patients gut decontamination has been found to reduce endotox-aemia and the plasma concentration of IL-6. Many different regimens are used; the combination of polymyxin, tobramycin and amphotericin is a popular one. SDD has not led to significant improvements in mortality in critically ill patients, although there have been reductions in acquired infections and a reduction in the incidence of infected necrosis in patients with severe pancreatitis. The routine use of SDD in clinical practice cannot be recommended on the basis of current evidence.

Nutrition
For more details refer to Chapter 4.

Hand hygiene
Hand hygiene is crucial in the general ward, intensive care and operating theatre, as cross-contamination and infection may result from bad practice. Hand washing with soap or detergent will remove most transient skin flora. Antiseptic formulations containing chlorhexidine and povidone iodine are slightly more effective than soap, especially if used repeatedly. However, to remove all transient flora and reduce detachable resident organisms during surgical scrubs, detergents containing 4% chlorhexidine or 7.5% povidone iodine are recommended. It is also important to remove dirt from behind the nails using a nail-brush before cleansing and disinfecting from elbows to hands. At the hands, both palms, dorsum, web spaces and fingers must be properly cleansed. A 2 min scrub is recommended with no advantage shown for longer scrubs. Proper drying and glove donning practices must be observed. The former is from the hand towards the elbow and the latter is a 'no-touch' technique, where gloving is performed with hands unexposed through the sleeves of the sterile gown. In addition to preventing wound contamination, gloves also protect and prevent the spread of communicable diseases such as human immun-odeficiency virus, hepatitis B and hepatitis C (see below). Complete penetration through piercing may be reduced sig-nificantly by double-gloving.

Skin preparation
Attempts to reduce the skin flora of the patient undergoing elective surgery should commence in the ward. Preoperative showering of the patient with hexachlorophene is associated with a 50% reduction in wound infection rate. Preparation of the operation site is important. Usual solutions include 60–80% alcohol, 0.5% chlorhexidine and 10% povidone iodine. The alcohol works rapidly while the latter may provide a more prolonged antimicrobial effect. Chlorhexidine has a cumulative effect, is effective against Gram-positive micro-organisms and is relatively stable in the presence of organic fluid. Povidone iodine has a broader spectrum of activity with some sporicidal and antifungal effect. The antiseptic solutions should be applied with a sterile gauze with friction

for 2 min. If hair needs to be removed, local clipping is less damaging than shaving and reduces the risk of postoperative wound infection. Shaving, if necessary, should be performed immediately before surgery. When using alcohol-based solu-tions, care must be taken to prevent pooling as burns may occur due to sparks from electrocauterization. As a conse-quence of this risk, many units have now stopped using inflammable antiseptics.

Draping
Towelling of the patient is performed with sterile cotton sheets or disposable prefabricated drapes. Some surgeons then apply a plastic adhesive film over the surgical site in an attempt to further reduce skin contact, especially if pros-thetic implants are to be used. However, there are reports of increased wound infection with their use because of bacter-ial proliferation under the plastic sheet. No difference in infection rate is observed between reusable and disposable drapes. When spillage of bowel contents is a real risk, especially when the bowel is to be transected or opened, the surround-ing tissues should be protected using chlorhexidine-soaked gauze or sterile towels.

Length of preoperative stay and duration of surgery
The length of preoperative stay in hospital directly correlates with the incidence of nosocomial infection. Another import-ant factor is the duration of surgery with the wound infection rate doubled for each additional hour of surgery. However, the duration of surgery may in fact be related to the severity of the disease state of the patient, which may result in malnourish-ment and immunosuppression. Increased blood loss and the need for transfusion may further reduce the resistance of the patient to infective pathogens.

Prophylactic antibiotics
Wound contamination is inevitable in surgery. This may be due to the patient's own skin flora, spillage of visceral contents, from the surgical team or other environmental contamin-ation such as surgical and anaesthetic instruments. Therefore, prophylactic antibiotics are commonly used to reduce the risk of this contamination developing into established infec-tion and sepsis. Indications include:
- gastrointestinal surgery, for example bowel resection, hepa-tobiliary operations, gastric surgery, palliative bypass pro-cedures for cancer;
- prosthetic insertion, for example vascular implants, ortho-paedic joint replacement, cardiac valve replacement;
- patients with prosthetic implants;
- patients with structural cardiac defects, for example valve or septal defects;
- immunocompromised patients.
Most surgeons normally give no prophylactic antibiotics to patients undergoing clean procedures (e.g. hernia repair without implant and breast surgery).

In bowel surgery when spillage is inevitable or in surgery when a prosthesis is inserted, prophylactic antibiotics are given in the hope of reducing the number of bacteria which may contaminate the surgical site. For antibiotic prophylaxis to be effective, it must be administered before the contamination occurs or shortly thereafter. It should be directed against the most likely organisms involved and given at a time when blood and tissue levels are highest for the duration of the contamination. Patients who are immunocompromised or who have prosthetic implants *in situ* should routinely be given antibiotic prophylaxis prior to any invasive procedures which disrupts the mucocutaneous lining. Infection of prosthetic implants, although uncommon, may have dire consequences:

- *Haemorrhage*:
  - graft to intestinal fistula, for example aortoduodenal fistula, aortoenteric fistula;
  - bleeding into surrounding space/tissue: haematoma, pneumoperitoneum; external haemorrhage.
- *Abscess*:
  - inflamed swelling;
  - discharging sinus;
  - pseudoaneurysm.
- *Thromboembolic phenomenon*:
  - septic emboli;
  - graft thrombosis.

Vascular graft infection may lead to fatal haemorrhage or limb loss.

The duration of administration of the antibiotics for prophylaxis varies between surgeons despite studies showing no benefit from prolonged administration over a single perioperative dose, even in colorectal surgery. Prolonged usage of antibiotics is not without complications and side-effects. Indiscriminate use can alter the indigenous bacterial population and give rise to infection with resistant strains, fungi and proliferation of normally insignificant organisms such as *Clostridium difficile* which is associated with pseudomembranous colitis. This is usually related to the prolonged usage of certain antibiotics, the commonest of which is ampicillin, although clindamycin has the highest incidence per course of therapy. Pseudomembranous colitis is associated with a non-specific hyperaemia, oedema of the mucosa and the formation of pseudomembrane. Histologically, epithelial debris, polymorphonuclear leukocyte infiltrate, chronic inflammatory cells and fibrin deposition is seen. Treatment consists of stopping the offending antibiotics and commencing vancomycin or metronidazole.

Good surgical techniques

It must be emphasized that antibiotic prophylaxis is no substitute for good surgical technique and a surgeon's obsessional attention to detail. Tissues must be handled with care and not crushed with forceps. Good haemostasis must be achieved to prevent haematomas. Wound approximation must be firm and not strangulating. All devitalized tissue must be excised. Electrocauterization should be used sparingly to minimize necrotic tissue. If drains are required, a closed system has been shown to cause less infection.

Sterilization of surgical instruments

Sterilization is the destruction of all microorganisms including spores. Various techniques are available to sterilize surgical instruments and equipment:

- *Heat sterilization*:
  - autoclaving (steam under pressure);
  - dry heat;
  - low temperature steam.
- *Cold sterilization*:
  - g-irradiation;
  - ethylene oxide;
  - glutaraldehyde.

The technique used depends on the heat sensitivity of the material to be sterilized and the risk of infection to the patient.

Chemical agents act by inducing a reaction with the organism which is dependent on temperature, chemical strength, freshness of the chemical, resistance of the organism and duration of contact. They work by oxidation, halogenation, poisoning of vital enzymes, hydrolysis or coagulation. Activated glutaraldehyde 2% will not corrode plastic or rubber and may be used for fibreoptic endoscopes. It is effective against bacteria, including mycobacteria, spores, viruses and fungi, depending on the immersion time. It is, however, important to ensure that all traces of the chemical are removed as it irritates mucous membranes, in particular those of the eyes. The instrument must be precleaned before immersion to allow good contact between agent and all parts of the instrument being sterilized. Disinfection takes approximately 10 min while proper sterilization requires up to 3 h.

The most effective method of sterilization is moist heat which destroys organisms by coagulation of the protoplasm. Heat-tolerant items such as surgical instruments, swabs, dressings and sutures may be autoclaved, that is exposed to high temperatures at supra-atmospheric pressures. Three main types of autoclaves are available:

- downward displacement sterilizer;
- prevacuum sterilizer;
- quickspeed sterilizer.

The exposure time to adequately sterilize an instrument depends on the temperature reached and should be taken from when the correct temperature of steam has reached all parts of the material being sterilized. The penetration times vary between different sterilizers and packing materials.

Ethylene oxide sterilization is slow, taking 4–6 h to complete the cycle. All residual air must be removed from the items sterilized as the gas is harmful when inhaled or absorbed. g-Radiation is used commercially for plastic items, sutures, prepacked sponges and gauze. Other techniques, that is boiling, pasteurization and low temperature steaming may suffice if there is only low or intermediate risk of infection.

Tests such as the bacterial spore strip may be carried out to ensure that sterilization is adequate.

Environmental factors

Circulation of the air supply to the operating theatre, apart from controlling temperature, humidity and ventilation for the occupants, minimizes the bacterial count in the atmosphere. Ideally, this air is filtered and flows from clean to less clean areas of the room. Unfortunately, this system may not function adequately when there is excessive movement of personnel in and out of the room. Masks should be worn to prevent bacteria-laden droplets from contaminating the patient's wound, although it has been shown that this does not occur with normal breathing and quiet talking. Studies in patients undergoing minor or intermediate general surgical procedures have demonstrated no difference between wound infection rate in those carried out by surgeons who wear masks and those who do not. However, this does not apply to major surgical procedures or those where implants are inserted. Hair and beards should be fully covered to prevent hairs being shed into the wound.

DEFINITIVE MANAGEMENT OF ESTABLISHED SEPSIS

Once sepsis is established, definitive management is required:
- *Recognition of sepsis*:
  - nature;
  - intensity;
  - speed of onset.
- *Resuscitation*:
  - restore organ perfusion and oxygenation.
- *Identification of possible primary pathology*:
  - history;
  - physical examination;
  - microbiological examination;
  - radiological investigation.
- *Treatment of primary pathology*:
  - antibiotics;
  - radiological drainage of abscess;
  - surgical drainage/debridement.

Therapeutic intervention depends on the severity of infection and whether there is associated systemic upset. If localized superficial wound infection is present, then treatment merely consists of providing local drainage which may just involve opening the wound. However, if sepsis develops with shock, then resuscitation to provide adequate tissue perfusion and oxygenation, followed by the provision of supportive measures to maintain haemodynamic stability, is necessary. The source of sepsis must be identified by radiological or surgical intervention and treated appropriately.

The extent of resuscitation depends on the severity of sepsis and the clinical status of the patient. If the patient responds promptly to minimal fluid resuscitation and remains stable, further management may be continued in a general ward with specially designated high-risk areas. If more intensive observation, treatment and nursing care is necessary, patients may be cared for in a high-dependency unit (HDU). In the HDU, facilities should be available for continuous monitoring of pulse, central venous pressure, arterial blood pressure and oxygen saturation. Although the nurse : patient ratio is higher than on the general ward, it is not 1 : 1 as on the ICU. The management of HDU patients must be supervised by experienced senior surgical staff. Patients with severe sepsis who are unstable, at risk from potentially reversible failure of two or more organs, or require ventilatory support, need ICU management where medical supervision is undertaken by dedicated medical staff with advanced life support skills. Although primary responsibility for care is assumed by the specialist team, optimal management requires a multidisciplinary approach. Continuous assessment and decision making by a multidisciplinary team, advice from microbiologists on antibiotic administration and the involvement of the nutrition team on matters pertaining to appropriate diet and route of administration are all essential.

Resuscitation

Fluid resuscitation

Hypotension should be reversed with the appropriate fluids to compensate for increased capillary permeability and vasodilatation associated with sepsis. There is no evidence-based support for one type of fluid over the other. Unfortunately, in some instances the hypotension is resistant to fluid infusion alone. This may be related to the generation of certain inflammatory mediators such as TNF and myocardial depressant factor. Dobutamine is the ionotopic drug of choice for patients with measured or suspected low cardiac output in the presence of adequate left ventricular filling pressure and adequate mean arterial pressure. Dopamine at low doses (3–5 mg/kg/min) has been suggested to increase renal blood flow via its dopaminergic receptors, although its effect on splanchnic perfusion remains controversial. Studies have shown that it may reduce mucosal perfusion and accelerate the onset of intestinal ischaemia in haemorrhagic shock and in patients with congestive cardiac failure. Higher doses may produce vasoconstriction by a-adrenergic stimulation off-setting the vasodilatory effect. If dopamine is inadequate, noradrenaline or dobutamine should be considered, although it must be emphasized that inotropes are no substitute for adequate fluid replacement.

Respiratory and ventilatory support

Respiratory insufficiency may occur in severe sepsis, especially if ARDS is present. Lung compliance is reduced in this syndrome due to the accumulation of interstitial fluid and alveolar oedema secondary to increased tissue permeability. It should be suspected if hypoxaemia persists despite increasing FiO_2 (inspired oxygen concentration) and there is evidence of pulmonary infiltrates on chest radiograph. The patient is usually tachypnoeic, dyspnoeic and confused because of hypoxia. Oxygen saturation and arterial PaO_2 are reduced.

There is no specific treatment for ARDS and the main aim of therapy is to provide adequate oxygenation and, if necessary, ventilatory support with positive end expiratory pressure. However, oxygenation should first be provided with the administration of humidified oxygen by face mask or nasal catheters and mechanical ventilation only used if this fails to provide adequate oxygenation. Typically, the lungs are stiff and high inflation pressures may be needed. The goal is to achieve an acceptable PaO_2 level using the minimum of pressure. Unfortunately, mortality is high even with optimal management.

Assessment of tissue oxygenation

Information on oxygen delivery and the degree of shunting due to ventilation/perfusion mismatch in the lung may be obtained from blood gas measurements and the inspired oxygen concentration. Lactic acidosis identifies tissue hypoperfusion in patients at risk who are not hypotensive. A recently popularized device which has been shown accurately to indicate tissue perfusion is the silicone tonometer. The principles of the tonometer are based on the assumption that the partial pressure of CO_2 within the bowel is similar to that of the lumen, and the concentration of standard bicarbonate within the tissues is the same as that of arterial blood. The tonometer measures the intramucosal pH of the bowel which has been shown to correlate well with diminished perfusion once oxygen delivery falls below a critical level. The fall in gastric intramucosal pH following cardiac surgery is associated with a higher incidence of morbidity and mortality, and tonometric measurement of gastric pH is now an accepted means of monitoring systemic oxygenation and outcome in ICU patients. Sustained acidosis beyond 2 h is highly predictive of mortality and the occurrence of major complications in aortic surgery. Intramucosal acidosis may therefore be an early warning of an impending complication and therapy guided by these measures may significantly improve outcome in critically ill patients.

Treatment of the primary pathology

Following resuscitation and stabilization of the patient, further investigations must be carried out to establish the primary pathology and cause of sepsis. Occasionally, the disease process, such as necrotizing pancreatitis, diverticular abscess or limb gangrene, may already be recognized. In these situations, definitive drainage, debridement or excision should be carried out once the patient is stabilized. Re-exploration may be required in some patients with further debridement but prognosis in these patients is poor and worsened by each exploration.

In many instances the diagnosis may not be clinically obvious and radiological investigations are obligatory to help identify the cause. If an abscess or collection is found, ultrasound- or CT-guided percutaneous drainage may be performed. Diagnosis may prove elusive in some despite the use of sophisticated imaging techniques. When this occurs, supportive measures with optimal antibiotic therapy are all that can be offered. The latter should be directed by laboratory information on microorganisms cultured from drainage fluid, blood, urine and sputum.

Antibiotic therapy

When considering antibiotic therapy, the efficacy, toxicity, dosage, route of administration, duration of treatment and whether a mono- or multi-agent regimen is required all need to be carefully evaluated. In sepsis, therapy is commonly commenced without the benefit of microbiological information on culture and sensitivities of the organism and empirical regimens are usually started as soon as life-threatening infection is diagnosed or suspected. The antibiotic used depends on the most likely source of infection and the organisms that commonly originate from it. It is important that a good history is obtained and physical examination undertaken to determine the most likely source of infection. Symptoms and signs of respiratory distress may point to a pulmonary origin. The abdomen must be examined for evidence of intra-abdominal sepsis and urinary symptoms may indicate a urinary source. Previous health problems must not be overlooked as certain chronic conditions may predispose to sepsis. However, if the correct regimen is used the patient should improve. If not, a careful review of the clinical symptoms and signs should be performed and laboratory and radiological investigations may need to be repeated. When bacteriological data become available, treatment should be corrected accordingly or additional antimicrobial agents supplemented if necessary.

The antibiotic of choice for the different organisms causing infection at various anatomical sites and their dosages are well established. Many are currently available and the choice is usually dependent on the practice of the particular unit with the exception of certain well-documented regimens.

Penicillin

Penicillins are popular but resistant strains are increasingly recognized, that is penicillinase-producing and methicillin-resistant staphylococci. They are bactericidal and act by disrupting the peptidoglycan of the bacteria cell wall. The natural penicillins are indicated for treatment of pneumococcal chest infection, cellulitis and mild throat infections. Until laboratory data indicate otherwise, the penicillinase-resistant group (such as methicillin, oxacillin and cloxacillin) is now recommended as initial therapy against Gram-positive coccal infections, due to the growing incidence of penicillinase-producing strains. Ampicillin is used commonly for infection due to *Escherichia coli*, *Proteus mirabilis* and *Haemophilus influenzae* but is ineffective against *Pseudomonas aeruginosa* and klebsiella species. The carboxypenicillins carbenicillin and ticarcillin are active against pseudomonas but not klebsiella which is sensitive to the ureidopenicillins, that is mezlocillin, azlocillin and piperacillin.

Cephalosporins

This group of bactericidal agents is conveniently divided into three generations depending on their activity. The first-generation cephalosporins are the most effective against Gram-positive cocci. The second- and third-generation cephalosporins have broader Gram-negative cover. Although suggested to be effective as monotherapeutic agents, they are normally used in conjunction with an aminoglycoside and metronidazole to provide adequate cover for enteric organisms and anaerobes in intra-abdominal sepsis.

Aminoglycosides

Aminoglycosides are poorly absorbed by the gut and adequate serum concentrations can be obtained only by parenteral administration. They are rapidly cleared by the kidneys. Their most feared side-effects are nephrotoxicity and ototoxicity. Traditionally, they are administered in two or three daily divided doses and peak and trough levels checked after the third. A once daily maximum dose is now recommended and does not require the laborious task of level monitoring, except in patients with renal impairment. The high peak and low trough of this method of administration have been shown to be efficacious with low nephrotoxicity. Aminoglycosides are usually used in combination with a penicillin or cephalosporin and metronidazole because binding to active sites on the cell membrane does not occur with streptococci or anaerobic organisms. There is also a delay in achieving therapeutic levels in patients with intra-abdominal infection which may be secondary to the expansion in extracellular fluid.

Vancomycin

This agent was introduced primarily to treat penicillinase-producing staphylococci infection but this use has now largely been replaced by cephalosporins and vancomycin is therefore only used as a second-line agent. It is effective against Gram-positive organisms and resistance is uncommon. It is the treatment of choice for methicillin-resistant strains of staphylococcal infections and in pseudomembranous colitis resulting from overgrowth of *Clostridium difficile*.

Carbepenems

Carbepenems such as imipenem-cilastatin have a broad antimicrobial spectrum and are effective against Gram-positive and Gram-negative aerobes as well as anaerobes, including bacteroides. It is therefore used for gynaecological infections and in life-threatening infections as an alternative to the aminoglycosides. In view of its wide range of microbial cover, it is suitable as a monotherapeutic agent for intra-abdominal infection.

Quinolones

The most commonly used quinolone is ciprofloxacin. They are active against enterobacteriaceae, *Haemophilus influenzae*, *Neisseria gonorrhoeae* and *Pseudomonas aeruginosa*. The quinolones are also effective against staphylococci, including the methicillin-resistant strains. However, they are not effective against streptococci, anaerobic cocci and bacilli.

Anti-anaerobic antibiotics

These include clindamycin, metronidazole, chloramphenicol, imipenam and cefoxitin. An antianaerobic agent is usually included in a treatment regimen if lower intestinal organism are potential pathogens. Metronidazole is probably the most commonly used in view of its relative safety.

Newer therapies

Despite advances in critical care management, mortality from sepsis remains high. Newer therapies have therefore been developed in the hope that outcome in patients suffering from sepsis may be improved. Therapeutic strategies aimed at reducing the production of cytokines and improving outcome in sepsis remain controversial. Endogenous cytokine production is part of the normal reaction to injury and inflammation. Together with other cascades they form part of the natural defenses against invading microorganisms and are essential in the healing process following injury.

Anti-LPS antibodies/LPS inhibitors

The concept of passive immunotherapy is receiving some revival though the avidity of these antibodies against LPS is weak and non-specific. SCD14 can transfer LPS into high-density lipoproteins (HDL) and low levels of HDL have been associated with a higher mortality.

Anti-cytokine antibodies

Antibodies against TNF, IL-1 (IL-1 RA – receptor antagonist) have been found to be beneficial. However a recent meta-analysis has found TNF neutralization to be of little benefit in lowering mortality. This is probably because TNF and IL-1 reach peak concentrations as early as a few hours after the onset of sepsis and decline with time. Administration of antibodies against C5a decreases bacteraemia and apoptosis.

Bactericidal/Permeability increasing protein

It has LPS-neutralizing and antibacterial properties and is currently being tested.

Activated protein C/Tissue factor pathway inhibitor/Platelet-activating factor acetylhydrolase

These are currently being studied for their potential benefits. Recombinant human activated protein C (rhAPC) is recommended in patients at high risk of death. It inactivates factors Va and VIIIa, thereby preventing thrombin formation. It also has direct anti-inflammatory properties. Blocking cell adhesion and cytokine production. Tissue factor pathway inhibitor (TFPI) is a useful adjuvant in sepsis therapy. PAF acetylhydrolase is a naturally occurring enzyme which is currently being studied.

Corticosteroids

High doses of corticosteroids does not improve survival among patients with sepsis. However, patients who are extremely ill and have persistent shock requiring vasopressors and prolonged mechanical ventilation may benefit from 'physiologic' doses of corticosteroids.

Intensive insulin therapy for hyperglycemia

Its protective mechanism is unknown. The phagocytic function of neutrophils is impaired by hyperglycemia. Insulin is also anti-apoptoic.

HUMAN IMMUNODEFICIENCY VIRUS AND VIRAL HEPATITIS INFECTION

The viral infections which are of interest to clinicians, and especially surgeons, are human immunodeficiency virus (HIV) and hepatitis B and C viruses (HBV and HCV). This stems from their transmission risk from patient to healthcare worker or vice versa. Guidelines for reducing the risk of transmission of HIV, HBV and HCV are available for healthcare workers. Their main objective is to minimize exposure of any individual to blood and body secretions regardless of infective status of the second individual involved. Routine serological testing for HIV is not recommended. The debate over testing has not been made easier by the finding that prior knowledge of HIV status does not decrease the risk of transmission. In addition, a negative test does not exclude HIV infection as a seroconversion window exists which may last up to 3 years and during which a person may have circulating antigen but has not yet produced the antibody. If testing is required, consent must be obtained and, if positive, counselling provided and confidentiality ensured. In HIV-infected patients with sepsis, the CD4 count does not correlate with in-hospital mortality, though higher acute physiology and chronic health evaluation (APACHE) II scores are associated with a poor outcome.

The prevalence of hepatitis seroconversion for surgical personnel in a high-risk area is thought to be about 3%, although in the United Kingdom (UK) overall it may be as low as 0.3%. Known cases of seroconversion have occurred following deep penetration by hollow bore needles. It is estimated that the risk of seroconversion for HBV is between 6 and 30% following percutaneous injuries involving patients positive for the e antigen. The infectivity of HBV is greater than HIV because of the persistently higher count of transmissible particles in body fluids in the former.

Patients who are infected with HIV, HBV or HCV need not be isolated unless they:
- are actively bleeding or likely to bleed;
- have open wounds;
- have surgical drains;
- are incontinent of urine or faeces;
- have active chest infection;
- have diarrhoea and vomiting;
- are unconsciousness;
- are uncooperative.

When dealing with such patients, personnel should wear gloves, fluid-impervious gowns or aprons, shoe covers and fluid-impervious leggings, masks, head covering and goggles. Hands must be washed before and after such contact and needles must not be recapped or removed from the syringe before being discarded into sharps boxes.

The risk of transmitting HIV or hepatitis from healthcare workers to patients is extremely remote. Although HBV infection has occurred from surgeon to patients this risk is low. Studies have shown that the seroconversion rate to hepatitis exposure is similar in patients operated on by infected and non-infected surgeons. Therefore, these data are difficult to interpret and the true incidence is unclear. Nevertheless, every precaution must be taken, regardless of infectivity status of the individual patient or clinician.

If needle-stick injury occurs, antibody testing for HIV should be performed. If this is negative, the test should be repeated at 6 weeks, 3, 6 and 12 months after exposure to determine if transmission has occurred. Every Trust or other health care setting should develop a post-exposure policy and protocol. A case control study amongst health care workers exposed to HIV has found that the administration of zidovudine after exposure was associated with an 80% reduced risk of seroconversion. It is assumed that a combination of two or three drugs may be even more effective than zidovudine at blocking HIV infection. It is recommended that post-exposure prophylaxis commence within 24–36 h of injury, and preferably within a few hours of exposure.

If medical personnel are accidentally exposed to the body fluids of a potentially infected patient, the hepatitis B status of both parties needs to be determined. If the source is negative, no additional action needs to be taken. If the source is positive, then further action will depend on the hepatitis status of the person exposed. If the latter has had only one dose of hepatitis vaccine pre-exposure, the course of vaccination should be accelerated, that is doses spaced at 0, 1 and 2 months. In addition, a dose of antihepatitis B globulin antibody should be given. If the exposed person has had two doses of vaccine, then one dose of hepatitis vaccine followed by a further dose should be given. If the exposed person is fully vaccinated with good response, then a vaccine booster should be administered. However, if the exposed person has not responded to a previous vaccination course, the antihepatitis B globulin should be given in addition to the booster dose of hepatitis vaccine. If the source is not tested and has unknown hepatitis infectivity status, then the exposed person should have his vaccination course accelerated if only one dose of vaccine has been given. The patient should be given one dose of vaccine if two have already been given. No action is necessary if the patient is fully immunized with antihepatitis B surface antibody >100 miu/ml and antihepatitis globulin has been given plus a booster dose of vaccine, if the person has not responded to a previous vaccination programme.

FURTHER READING

ACCP/SCCM Consensus Conference Committee. Definitions for sepsis and organ failure and guidelines for the use of innovative therapies in sepsis. *Crit Care Med.* 1992; **20**: 864–874

Bone RC. Sir Isaac Newton, sepsis, SIRS and CARS. *Crit Care Med.* 1996; **24**: 1125–1128

Dellinger RP, Carlet JM, Masur H, Gerlach H, Calandra T, Cohen J, Gea-Banacloche J, Keh D, Marshall JC, Parker MM, Ramsay G, Zimmerman JL, Vincent JL, Levy MM; Surviving Sepsis Campaign Management Guidelines Committee. Surviving Sepsis Campaign guidelines for management of severe sepsis and septic shock. *Crit Care Med.* 2004; **32**: 858–873

Gluck T, Opal SM. Advances in sepsis therapy. *Drugs.* 2004; **64**: 837–859

6

Surgical Techniques and Technology

RM Kirk

Department of Surgery, Royal Free Hospital, London, UK

CONTENTS

Skin preparation	71
Local anaesthesia	72
Topical	72
Local infiltration	72
Nerve blocks	72
Intravenous regional anaesthesia	73
Regional nerve block	73
Incisions and their closure	73
Incisions	73
Closure	74
Haemostasis	78
Explosion and fire hazards	79
Pathophysiology of wound healing	79
Modifying factors	80
Classification of surgical wounds	81
Open	81
Closed	81
Wound management	81
Primary closure	81
Secondary healing	82
Infected wounds	82
Penetrating and missile wounds	82
Burns	82
Scars and contracture	83
Scars	83
Contracture	83
Wound dehiscence	83
Abdominal wounds	84
Excision of cysts of the skin and subcutaneous tissues	84
Biopsy and cytological sampling	85
Biopsy	85
Cytological sampling	86
Drainage of superficial abscesses	86
Basic principles of anastomosis	87
Digestive tract	87
Vascular anastomosis	88
Further reading	88

SKIN PREPARATION

Traditionally patients were bathed the day before operation, the operative area was shaved and, especially before orthopaedic operations, the area was cleaned with antiseptic solution and then bound with sterile bandages. Many of these firmly held practices have been discarded. Hair removal should be avoided unless the hair will interfere with the operation. If it is to be removed, depilatory agents cause least damage. Shaving or clipping should be performed as close to the time of the procedure as possible, so that the abraded and scored skin cannot become contaminated with microorganisms.

Before starting the procedure, the skin of the operative site is cleaned with an antiseptic. Iodine in the form of povidone–iodine (10% in 10% alcohol) is popular; however, some patients are allergic to it and a test on a remote area of skin 24 h beforehand will exclude any resulting hyperaemia. Where there is a suspicion of hypersensitivity, chlorhexidine (0.5% or 0.5% in 10% alcohol) or 10% alcohol on its own can be used. Due to the danger of causing an explosion, it is essential that the alcohol is allowed to evaporate from all areas of skin before diathermy is used.

A sterile swab soaked in antiseptic solution is wiped along the line of the proposed incision, gradually extending the cleaned area centrifugally in ever-widening circles so that the incision line is not contaminated with a swab that has touched skin at the periphery.

Sterile skin towels are applied to isolate the incision line, held together with towel clips that do not grip the skin. Alternatively, a sterile plastic adhesive dressing is applied to cover the area.

LOCAL ANAESTHESIA

(For more details refer Chapter 2 for dosage and toxicity).

The required equipment and knowledge to carry out resuscitation must be available. Adrenaline solution 1 in 1000 should also be to hand. Except for the most trivial procedure, an adequately trained assistant should be present. The volume of local anaesthetic agent used, and any reactions to it, must be recorded.

Local anaesthesia may be combined with premedication drugs such as triazolam up to 0.5 mg or temazepam up to 20 mg for adults. However, they may blanket the effects of local anaesthetics and should be used sparingly, especially in day case surgery, so that the patient can achieve early full recovery.

Topical

Lignocaine 4% and prilocaine 4% are effective when applied to mucous membranes within the mouth, urethra, conjunctival sac and also in wounds.

Local infiltration

Lignocaine 0.5–2% is often used but it is effective in more dilute solution. The effect is prolonged if it is given in adrenaline solution, up to 1 in 200 000, which causes vasoconstriction and also reduces bleeding. No more than 3 mg/kg body weight should be used, except when given with adrenaline, in which case up to 7 mg/kg body weight may be given. However, adrenaline must be avoided if the local blood supply is prejudiced. Lignocaine anaesthesia lasts up to 90 min. This may be extended by adding 0.25% bupivacaine to 0.5% lignocaine.

If the operation site is painful or tender, a bleb is first raised in normal skin a short distance away, such as 1 cm. The needle is inserted and anaesthetic gently injected as the tender area is approached. The local anaesthetic spreads ahead of the needle. Initially the solution is infiltrated superficially to produce a wheal along the line of the proposed incision.

If the exposure is deepened, infiltration is taken progressively deeper to create a field block. The injection is given slowly to avoid pain caused by hydrostatic pressure. Each time the needle is in a new area, aspiration is performed to guard against intravenous injection. It is often wise to inject deeper progressively as the operation proceeds, rather than attempt a complete field block at the beginning.

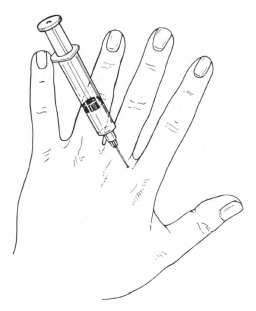

Figure 6.1. Blocking digital nerves in the web space to avoid raising tissue tension.

Local infiltration of anaesthetic agent is commonly used to enable the manipulation of fractures. Perhaps the commonest such use is for setting recently acquired Colles' fracture of the wrist. The level of the fractured radius is identified and infiltration of the fracture haematoma with 10–15 ml of plain, 1% lignocaine can begin. After 10 min, the fracture may be reduced.

The amount of anaesthetic agent used should be checked constantly to ensure the maximum amount has not been exceeded. The patient should be asked to report pain or untoward symptoms and signs of cerebral toxity such as drowsiness and slurred speech, and myocardial depression, such as slowing or irregularity of the pulse, should be closely monitored.

Sufficient time (5–10 min for lignocaine and up to 20 min for bupivacaine) should be allowed for the anaesthetic to act before starting the operation. It should be explained to the patient that touch sensation remains after pain sensation has been abolished, but discomfort or pain should be reported as soon as it is felt. Additional anaesthetic should be retained to use if there is discomfort.

Nerve blocks

These reduce the amount of local anaesthetic that needs to be used and they can sometimes be injected at a distance from the operation site.

Digital nerve block can be injected from the dorsal surface of the fingers and toes. There is a risk of ischaemia if the circumferential tension is raised by injecting a large volume or from digital artery spasm if adrenaline is added and as such, adrenaline must never be used. The nerves in the web space are blocked so the tension does not rise (Fig. 6.1). As an extra precaution an ampoule of hyalase, the spreading enzyme, may be added to the local anaesthetic; this reduces the volume of fluid needed to achieve anaesthesia and encourages the fluid to spread and be reabsorbed quickly. The two dorsal nerves are injected first, on either side of the first phalanx; the injection is then deepened from the dorsum to catch the palmar branch on either side.

The pain of a fractured rib can be alleviated for several hours by injecting 1–2 ml 0.25% bupivacaine posteriorly beneath the affected rib to block the intercostal nerve. Aspiration is carried out before injecting it to avoid intravascular injection.

When carrying out certain operations, nerve block can be combined with field block. A common example is in repair of inguinal hernia under local anaesthesia. Field block is augmented by infiltrating around the ilioinguinal and iliohypogastric nerves as they lie between internal and external oblique muscles about 2 cm medial to the anterior superior iliac spine.

Intravenous regional anaesthesia

This is also known as Bier's block and is valuable for producing anaesthesia in a limb. The limb is exsanguinated using an Esmarch bandage or rubber roller sleeve, or simply elevated. A proximal tourniquet is then inflated to higher than systolic pressure to isolate the blood vessels of the distal limb. Dilute local anaesthetic is injected through a previously placed intravenous cannula and perfuses the venous system, producing anaesthesia. This should not be attempted without special training and appropriate equipment and assistance (refer to Chapter 2).

Regional nerve block

This entails injecting local anaesthetics proximally into the nerves supplying a region or a limb. It requires a special knowledge of the anatomy, the specialized technique and the dangers (refer to Chapter 2).

INCISIONS AND THEIR CLOSURE

Incisions

These may be made for procedures on the skin or through the skin to reach deeper structures. They require careful planning and placement. Whenever possible incisions should be made along tension lines, not across them. The tension lines on the face can be identified by getting the patient to smile or grimace. Critical incisions may be marked with ink before incision.

For most incisions a scalpel with a large blade is used and the belly of the knife is drawn along in a smooth line, cutting at right angles to the skin surface. For very small and crucial incisions, it may be better to use a small bladed scalpel held

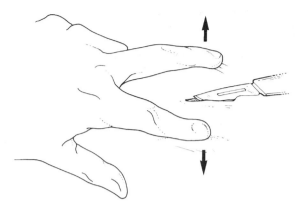

Figure 6.2. Steadying the tissue when making an incision and separating the edges with the fingers of one hand.

like a pen. Skin is elastic and the drag of the knife distorts it. To avoid this, the skin is fixed with the non-dominant hand and the edges slightly separated as the knife cuts through (Fig. 6.2).

The depth of cut is as important as the line. A fold of skin can be picked up to estimate its thickness. When making the incision, the correct depth should be reached as soon as possible and cutting then continued at that depth. One of the crucial surgical skills is the knowledge of tissues and tissue planes. The plane that has been reached must be carefully identified.

Bleeding is encountered as the incision is made and can be reduced or abolished in several ways:

- For very fine surgery of the extremities, the blood may be drained and a tourniquet applied.
- The skin and subcutaneous tissues can be infiltrated with a weak (e.g. 1 in 250 000) solution of adrenaline, which produces vascular constriction.
- Simple pressure on the cut edges for a few minutes usually controls small vessel bleeding. Neurosurgeons traditionally apply the tips of fine haemostatic forceps to the dermis and evert the edges to slightly compress them and control bleeding. Haemostatic forceps can be applied to individual vessels which may be sealed by compression, by twisting or by ligature.

Cutting diathermy is becoming increasingly popular for making skin incisions. Avoid using coagulation diathermy near the skin surface for fear of causing burns that heal slowly and leave ugly scars. Bleeding from small vessels can also be avoided by using a laser beam to cut through the skin; the depth of cut determines the choice of laser.

Deep exposures

To approach deep regions, intermediate structures must be divided or displaced. There are standardized approaches to various parts of the thorax, abdomen and pelvis, joints, bones, nerves, blood vessels, the central nervous system and special sense organs. There are well-documented anatomical anomalies that should be remembered and pathological processes that can distort the normal anatomy.

Closure

Healing will take place and produce the best scar if the wound edges, retaining a good blood supply, are apposed accurately, without tension or trauma, in the absence of infection, and with the minimum foreign material present.

Healing cannot take place if the blood supply is deficient. Ischaemic edges must be cut back until bleeding is seen at the cut edges and the colour appears normal. As in many circumstances in surgery, good and absent blood supply make decisions easy. It is in the 'grey areas' between these extremes that difficulty arises. In case of doubt it is usually best to leave the wound open until the viability of the edges is clear; if they then appear healthy, delayed primary suture is appropriate. If the blood supply is poor, the skin edges can be cut back until they appear healthy and the defect closed with a flap or skin graft.

Traumatized or crushed skin may show little evidence of non-viability at the time of repair but will subsequently die and scar. Rough handling and grasping the skin with dissecting forceps will add to the trauma; rather the closed blades of the forceps should be used to move the skin and exert counterpressure, or use skin hooks. Suture material mounted in eyeless needles should be used.

Tension not only pulls the wound edges apart but also aggravates any deficiency of the blood supply. In wounds that are oedematous, closure should be deferred until the oedema has resolved. If the blood supply is good, the tension can be spread by undermining the edges in the subcutaneous tissue, or by forming a flap that can be swung in. Very occasionally after undermining, a relieving incision can be made so that the defect is transferred to a more convenient area – in some instances the relieving incision may further prejudice the blood supply of the skin which has already been undermined. Sometimes skin tension can be reduced by drawing together the deeper layers of the wound.

Infection or heavy contamination are inimical to good wound healing. It is much safer to leave the wound open and wait until the tissues are clean and healthy before closing it. Local antiseptics and antibiotics are usually of less benefit than exposure. In some circumstances, appropriate systemic antibiotics may be indicated. Foreign material causes tissue reaction that retards healing and the material may harbour, or form a suitable nidus for, infecting organisms. In this context dead tissue is foreign material. For this reason, when dealing with wounds, every particle of dead or foreign material must be removed, relying on gentle exploration. Foreign material in the form of sutures should be kept to a minimum.

When closing a simple, straight incision made along tension lines, apposition is easy but for more complex closures, the progression should be planned carefully. If the edges are not of similar length, the extra length of one edge should be evenly distributed along the whole length of the wound. This can usually be achieved by inserting stitches across the middle of the wound, then halving this and continuing until the wound is closed (Fig. 6.3).

Perfect apposition implies the edges are united across the gap so that the living layers are brought together. Overlapping brings together dissimilar layers. Inversion of skin apposes dead, keratinized layers. The method of uniting the edges influences the perfection with which they are apposed.

Stitches

Stitches vary in type and size, and in the distance from the edges and from each other, depending upon the circumstances. For closing the skin of large abdominal wounds, they may be 2/0 nylon or polypropylene, placed 5 mm apart,

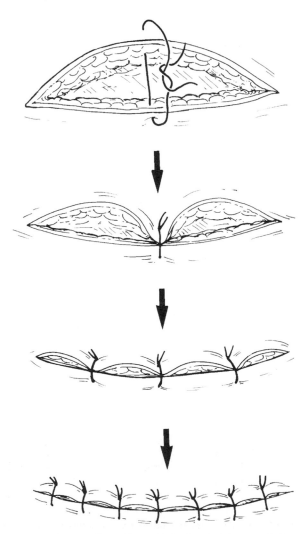

Figure 6.3. Accommodating disparity in the length of the wound edges by successively halving the wound with sutures.

up to 5 mm from the wound edges. In cosmetically important areas they may be 4–6/0 nylon or polypropylene, placed 2–3 mm from the edge and 2–3 mm apart. The thread is usually mounted in a half circle cutting edge, eyeless needle, held in a needle holder. Each stitch must cross the wound exactly at right angles and emerge at the same distance from the edge as it entered on the opposite side. It should be tied with a reef knot, and an extra half hitch added to form a reef knot with the second hitch. The first hitch should be tightened just sufficiently to appose the edges, the second just to secure it, and the third tightly, otherwise the first hitch will be overtightened, with consequent ischaemia. The ends should be cut short so they do not interfere with subsequent stitches. Stitches may be interrupted or continuous. Each

type has advantages and disadvantages; the use of one or the other is a matter of personal choice.

If the skin edges tend to invert, they can be everted using mattress sutures. These are double stitches that may cross the wound parallel to each other (horizontal mattress, or in the same line) vertical mattress (Fig. 6.4). These stitches must be removed at varying times. On the face they can often be removed after 48 h to avoid producing ladder-type marks across the scar. On the other hand, abdominal wound skin stitches are sometimes left in for 8–10 days.

Subcuticular stitches avoid the cross marks that may mar a scar sutured conventionally (Fig. 6.5). Non-absorbable monofilament nylon or polypropylene is inserted through the skin about 5 mm from one end of the wound to emerge through the deeper part of the skin in the angle of the wound. It then takes horizontal bites of the deep epidermis on alternate sides until the far end is reached. The needle is then passed through the far angle to emerge on the surface about 5 mm from the end of the wound. The two ends of the suture are then drawn apart to tighten the stitch and draw the skin edges together. The suture ends can be taped to the skin at each end. When the suture is to be withdrawn, it is gently tautened and freed by gently drawing on the ends alternately, then pulling through intact from one end.

Absorbable subcuticular sutures, for example, metric 1 or 1.5 (5/0 or 4/0) multifilament polyglactin 910 or polyglycolic acid, do not need to be removed. A subcuticular stitch at one end, uniting both sides, begins the process, then a knot should be tied, which will be buried. The subcuticular suture is then inserted until the other end is reached, a loop being retained before the last encircling stitch is inserted, catching both sides. This loop is then tied to the thread end, forming a knot that will be buried.

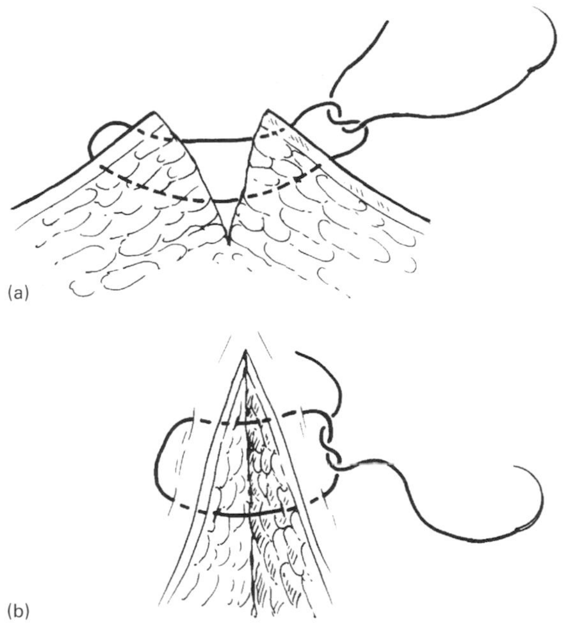

Staples

Staples are useful in some circumstances but are not as versatile as sutures. Although they can be inserted rapidly, the time required to appose the skin edges accurately takes as long as it does with stitching. Staples are now usually dispensed from a

(a)

(b)

Figure 6.4. Everting mattress sutures. (a) vertical section through a longitudinal mattress suture. (b) View of a longitudinal mattress suture.

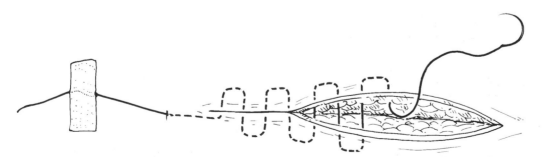

Figure 6.5. Subcuticular stitches inserted in the deep dermis. A non-absorbable suture is inserted a short distance from the end of the wound to emerge within the wound and then the edges are picked up alternately. When drawn taut, as shown on the left, the edges are opposed. The ends of the non-absorbable suture are fixed using adhesive tape as shown on the left. The ends can be freed and drawn out.

cartridge which thrusts the ends of a U-shaped metal staple into the apposed edges on each side of the wound, then deforms the shape into a nearly closed 'O'. These staples are expensive and no more effective than Michel clips that were formerly used from a rechargeable gallery mounted on toothed dissecting forceps. The toothed clips are drawn from the gallery with a second pair of forceps with specially shaped jaws, applied across the wound and squeezed into place.

Adhesive strips

Adhesive strips can often be used to avoid stitching when the edges lie accurately together. Make sure the skin surface is absolutely dry. Adhesion is improved if a plastic spray is first applied and allowed to dry. Alternatively, paint the edges with Whitehead's varnish. Place the strips across the wound at right angles, pressing them into place. These strips may be spaced or placed contiguously, forming a dressing for the wound.

Abdominal wound closure

Most abdominal wounds incorporate peritoneum, muscles, aponeuroses, subcutaneous tissues and skin. In the past these have been closed as individual layers – and this is still appropriate for many incisions. Catgut was the traditional suture material but has now been virtually abandoned. Peritoneum can be sutured with size 3 or 3.5 metric absorbable synthetic suture and the muscles and aponeurotic sheaths with metric size 4 non-absorbable monofilament polyamide or size 4 or 5 monofilament or multifilament braided absorbable synthetic suture. A continuous suture at least 4 times the length of the abdominal incision is loosely inserted through peritoneum, aponeuroses and muscles but not the subcutaneous tissues and skin. Wound dehiscence is virtually abolished. The subcutaneous tissues are sometimes apposed using fine metric 3.0 or 2.0 (3/0 or 4/0) catgut, or metric 1.5 or 1.0 (4/0 or 5/0) multifilament synthetic absorbable suture and the skin is closed with 2/0 (metric size 3) black silk, fine polyamide, polyester or metal clips.

Suture and ligature materials (Table 6.1)

All known threads have been used in surgery, including silk, cotton and linen and are all only partially destroyed by the tissues. They can be twisted or braided. These materials are easy to handle and knot reliably. For many years monofilament or multifilament stainless steel was used because of its strength and because it causes little tissue reaction but it is difficult to handle and later tends to fragment.

The classic absorbable material is catgut, which is composed of twisted strips of the submucous coat of sheep's or cow's intestine. It soon loses strength within days. Plain catgut is rapidly, but irregularly, absorbed. If the protein is denatured by tanning, usually with chromic acid, absorption is delayed.

Natural threads cause inflammatory reaction, may harbour infection and lose their strength capriciously and have largely been replaced by synthetic materials. Among the

Table 6.1. Metric suture material sizes.

Metric gauge (mm)	Previous gauges	
	Catgut	Non-absorbables Synthetic absorbables
0.1		
0.2		10/0
0.3		9/0
0.3		8/0 virgin silk
0.4		8/0
0.5	8/0	7/0
0.7	7/0	6/0
1.0	6/0	5/0
1.5	5/0	4/0
2.0	4/0	3/0
3.0	3/0	2/0
3.5	2/0	0
4.0	0	1
5.0	1	2
6.0	2	3&4
7.0	3	5
8.0	4	5

non-absorbable threads are polyamides, polypropylene and polyesters produced as monofilaments or braids. The monofilamentous threads often have 'memory' – they tend to return to their original shape after being deformed, as in a knot. They cause very little tissue reaction and retain their strength reliably. However, they are very susceptible to weakening by surface damage. Never grasp any part except the ends with a metal instrument and never snatch or snag them.

Absorbable polymer threads have been synthesized which cause relatively little tissue reaction, retain their strength and are absorbed slowly and reliably by hydrolysis rather than by inflammatory reaction. They are also produced in monofilament and multifilament, braided forms. Polyglyconate (Maxon) and polydioxanone (PDS) are monofilaments; polyglactin 910 (Vicryl) and polyglycolic acid (Dexon) are multifilaments.

Ligatures

Traditionally, ligatures have been made of catgut because they remain in the body, but have the disadvantage that in the presence of infection they may be rapidly digested and lead to secondary haemorrhage. For this reason, important vessels are often ligated with silk. The reliability of synthetic absorbables has made these ligatures increasingly popular.

The vessel to be ligated is preferably isolated and doubly ligated in continuity before being divided between the ligatures. Alternatively the isolated vessel is doubly clamped with haemostatic forceps, divided and then doubly ligated. When a vessel is already divided, it should be carefully picked up with haemostatic forceps and then ligated.

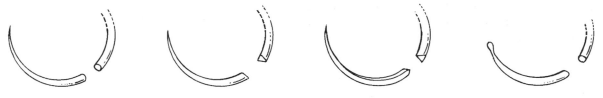

Figure 6.6. From left to right, round bodied, cutting, reverse cutting and blunt pointed needles.

Sutures

Suture threads are also made from silk, linen, cotton or catgut. Those that are to be removed, such as skin sutures, are made from non-absorbable silk or synthetic polyamide, polyethylene or polyester. These sutures are usually dyed so that they are easily seen against the skin.

Buried sutures of catgut are still popular and extensively used in economically poor countries but increasingly the synthetic materials are employed because of their reliability. The braided synthetic absorbable materials do not retain their strength as long as monofilament PDS which retains its strength for about 50 days and takes about 6 months to be reabsorbed.

Where permanent retention of sutures is important, then synthetic non-absorbable sutures are usually chosen because they evoke little tissue reaction. Polyamide, polypropylene and polyester are frequently used. Monofilaments are less likely to retain microorganisms because they have a smooth exterior surface. Strong threads are ideal for abdominal wound closure and for uniting fascia and tendons. Fine synthetic materials are used for vascular sutures.

Needles

Nearly all needles are now 'eyeless', the thread having been attached to the needle during manufacture. This is done either by swaging or crimping the needle onto the thread, or drilling a hole into the shank of the needle and inserting the thread end after first dipping it into an adhesive substance.

In the past, many surgeons used hand-held straight or curved needles with incomparable facility. Unfortunately, the risks of needlestick injury and consequent viral transmission make hand-held needles dangerous. In addition, many such needles were of large cross-section and produced large stitch holes. All needles should now be held in a needle holder and for this reason, the majority are curved needles.

Round-bodied needles penetrate soft tissues that can be dilated by the passage of the needle and then close around the thread to form a leak-free stitch. For this reason they are used for intestinal and cardiovascular sutures. Cutting needles penetrate tough tissues such as aponeuroses, tendons and skin. These needles are triangular in the cutting section, with edges laterally and on the inside of the curvature. If such needles carry through threads that need to be tied under tension, the suture may tear towards the edge. Reverse cutting needles have the third cutting edge on the outside of the curvature to avoid this (Fig. 6.6). Other shapes include trocar-, spear- and spatula-pointed needles. In the hope of reducing the number of needlestick injuries, modified blunt-pointed needles have been introduced and these penetrate the tissues remarkably well but do not easily penetrate surgical gloves.

Dressings

Wound dressings serve many functions but not necessarily all of them on every occasion. A dressing should be chosen to suit the need.

Seal

A clean, dry, perfectly apposed wound seals itself rapidly and often requires no dressing if on an area where it is not exposed to damage, such as the face. For extra protection such wounds can be sprayed with a plastic sealant or painted with Whitehead's varnish. Proprietary adhesive strips of thin porous material can be applied over the wound; they allow moisture to evaporate through them.

Protection

It may be necessary to protect the wound from inspection or picking by the patient or from inadvertent damage during movement or activity. The amount of protection varies. A neonate or infant cannot easily be restrained; an active boy who is not in pain soon forgets that he has a wound; an elderly, confused person may attempt to remove the dressing. A cotton gauze pad can be laid over the wound and held with adhesive plaster. Additionally, a pad of cotton wool can be applied and held with elastic, adhesive plaster or an encircling crepe bandage. In a few cases, a part can be temporarily immobilized by binding it; for example, an arm can be bound to the body with an encircling bandage to protect a wound over the shoulder that might be stretched and torn. Hand wounds can be protected by placing a large pad or roll of wool in the palm and binding the fingers over it in the shape of a fist, with crepe bandages.

Pressure

Some wounds require compression if oozing of blood, collection of tissue or joint fluid, or oedema are likely. Compression must be applied evenly without producing constriction. Seal the wound and protect it with a cotton dressing. Apply evenly laid cotton wool or compression wool. Depending on the circumstances, compression may be applied using crepe bandage, stretch adhesive plaster, elastic corset or other methods.

Absorbance

Throughout the operation every effort should be made to prevent bleeding, collection of pus or tissue fluid. If, in spite of this, considerable oozing or discharge is expected, drainage or the application of a stoma-type bag should be considered. Controlled and closed collection is better than incurring the risk and inconvenience of soaked dressings that need to be changed frequently.

When the discharge is likely to be minimal and temporary, the wound is covered with material that will protect the skin and allow the discharge to pass through into an absorbent. Traditionally, this was achieved using tulle gras (literally, greasy net) onto the wound. The original *tulle gras* tends to make the tissues soggy; proprietary non-adherent preparations are available that allow the skin to remain healthy. Now apply absorbent cotton gauze followed by cotton wool, held in place with adhesive plaster, crepe bandage or a corset. Ensure that the thickness of absorbent cotton is sufficient to last until the next projected dressing or the cotton wool will become soaked and produce an uncomfortable caked, wet pack.

Cavities and raw areas

Whenever there is a raw area, some exudation takes place, whether or not there is infection. The raw area can be covered with a layer of non-adherent net to allow the discharge to pass through and be absorbed in layers of cotton gauze. In the presence of infection, unhealthy granulation tissue, or necrotic tissue that has been excised, gauzes soaked in flavine emulsion, or Edinburgh University solution of lime (Eusol) alternating daily with hypertonic saline dressings, are often used. Eusol is considered to be harmful to the tissues but many surgeons still prefer it.

New wound dressings such as alginate hydrophilics, hydrogels and hydrocolloids absorb or transmit fluids and exudate and maintain a moist environment. Some proprietary preparations are impregnated with antibiotics.

It is sometimes important to keep a cavity open while it granulates up from the base, rather than allowing the skin to bridge across. It can be packed with a dressing. Alternatively, it can be packed with a plastic material that sets into a polymerized foam which can be washed and reapplied.

Haemostasis

Having anticipated the possibility of abnormal bleeding preoperatively, great care must be taken to prevent bleeding at operation by using good technique. Hoping for the best is not enough. Stagnant blood separates tissues that are intended to unite. It attracts infection and creates tissue tension, resulting in anoxia.

Prevention

- A *tourniquet* safely prevents bleeding in the distal limbs provided there is no ischaemia or venous thrombosis. This offers a bloodless field for very fine surgery. A tourniquet is applied proximally. The limb is elevated and can then be further exsanguinated by winding an Esmarch or Martin bandage from the extremity, proximally. The tourniquet is inflated above systolic pressure by 50–70 mmHg in the arm and 90–100 mmHg in the leg. The constricting bandage is then unwound. The tourniquet is released after a maximum of 1 hour in the arm and 1.5 h in the leg. The tourniquet should not be re-inflated for at least 30 min. At the end of the procedure, the tourniquet should be released before closing the wound, so that missed open vessels can be identified and sealed.
- *Fluid infiltration* of the tissues with sterile physiological saline increases the local tissue pressure and bulk so that blood vessels are easily visible. If adrenaline diluted even as much as 1 : 400 000 is added, it produces vascular constriction.
- *Diathermy* current seals vessels by coagulation.
- *Laser*, which is a high-energy coherent light beam, vaporizes tissues while simultaneously coagulating small vessels.
- *Ligature*. Intact blood vessels can be isolated, doubly ligated and then divided between the ligatures. Alternatively, apply two haemostatic forceps across the vessel, divide it between the haemostats and ligate it. Secure very major vessels using a double ligature or suture–ligature which impales the vessel and is then tied as a ligature which is thus prevented from slipping off.

Control

- *Pressure* between finger and thumb, against a firm base with a finger or swab, or gentle compression using a non-crushing clamp stops bleeding. Sometimes a confined region can be packed with one or more swabs to compress one or several bleeding vessels. If bleeding is severe, pressure should not be relaxed for 5 min, timed by the clock. Arterial bleeding that is difficult to reach can often be controlled by compressing the proximal supplying vessel.
- *Ligature* control of a divided vessel must be preceded by capture with a haemostatic forceps.
- *Sutures* can be used to constrict a vessel that is difficult to isolate. They are also useful to appose oozing surfaces after completing all other appropriate measures.
- *Diathermy* current can also be applied once a small vessel is captured with a forceps.
- *Coagulating agents* may be applied over areas of capillary oozing. Gelatine foam, absorbable gauze and powdered collagen are usually effective, or a small piece of excised, crushed muscle can be sewn over the area.

Diathermy

This is a high-frequency alternating current which produces heat, not by the effect of electrical resistance but by oscillation of the ions in the tissues. A pulsed high-frequency alternating current coagulates the tissues with minimal disruption. Continuous output disrupts the tissues because an arc is struck between the electrode and the tissues. It produces only minimal coagulation. A blended current of cutting and coagulation frequencies improves haemostasis, but beware of using coagulation current close to the skin surface for fear of causing burns.

Monopolar diathermy machines have one large electrode attached, with good contact to the skin, usually of the thigh. The other electrode is small and is applied directly or indirectly to a blood vessel to coagulate and seal it. A bipolar machine discharges current through the tissues only between two closely adjacent electrodes, usually the tips of dissecting forceps, so that current does not have to pass through the body of the patient.

The use of diathermy coagulation of blood vessels entails risks. If the large plate of a monopolar diathermy does not make good contact, or its lead is broken, current can flow through alternative routes, including any metal in contact with the patient, and cause burns. Explosions have occurred when alcoholic substances have been used to prepare the skin followed soon afterwards by the use of diathermy, which may produce an electric arc. Similarly, bowel gases may explode when polyps are diathermized at colonoscopy. Anaesthetic vapours such as ether can also explode if ignited by a diathermy spark.

When used through metal cannulae during minimal access surgery, a phenomenon called capacitance coupling may develop, resulting in burns, even though the diathermy lead is well insulated.

Laser

The name is an acronym for Light Amplification by Stimulated Emission of Radiation. The atoms of a medium, often a gas, are excited so that the electrons reach a higher-energy state. As they revert to their lower-energy state, they emit photons which cause further photons to be emitted. The photons are reflected back and forth between two opposed mirrors, which amplifies the light until some of it escapes as a coherent beam. The coherent beam of high intensity light vaporizes tissues and simultaneously coagulates small blood vessels.

There are several mediums, such as argon, CO_2 or neodymium yttrium aluminium garnet (NdYAG), resulting in beams of differing wavelengths and therefore different tissue absorptions. Argon and NdYAG laser light can be transmitted through optic fibres. NdYAG light is used to destroy lesions in the gastrointestinal tract and urinary bladder through endoscopes and in ophthalmology to destroy a thickened lens capsule and to treat lesions of the retina. CO_2 laser light has very low penetration and can be used to act at a surface, such as the destruction of cervical and vulval lesions in gynaecology. It may be passed into diseased, blocked blood vessels to perform laser angioplasty. Ruby laser light is valuable for the destruction of certain skin lesions.

Excimer laser light is used in ophthalmology to reshape the cornea to correct myopia. The name excimer derives from a contraction of the words 'excited dimer'. Dimers are molecules that can unite and dissociate. When they dissociate they emit high-energy photons which break surface molecules – photoablation, because this is non-thermal, no deep damage is caused.

Dangers

When using lasers there is danger of damaging tissues that lie in the path of the beam. This is a particular risk during minimal access surgery since the field of view may be limited. Another risk with penetrating laser light is that deep tissues may be damaged or perforation of vessels or hollow viscera may ensue.

The operator must take precautions not to accidentally expose his or others skin or eyes to damage by laser light.

Lasers are classified by their manufacturers by the degree of risk they engender. Wherever these instruments are used there must be proper supervision by a trained Laser Protection Officer and only nominated, properly trained people may use them.

EXPLOSION AND FIRE HAZARDS

Since operating theatres contain inflammable and often explosive substances, vapours and gases, together with electricity and sparks, they have the potential for explosions and fire. In the past inhaled anaesthetic gases were exhaled into the operating theatre atmosphere. In particular, ether is explosive. Sparks resulting from the build up and discharge of static electricity can cause explosions. Metal stools are covered with antistatic so that sparking does not occur when the surgeon's cotton theatre gown brushes against the bare metal and induces a static charge. Diathermy current with the attendant risk of sparking adds a further risk of explosions of anaesthetic gas. To a great extent the free exhalation of potentially explosive anaesthetic gases has been eliminated.

Two frequent risks remain:

1. Many skin cleansing agents contain alcohol spirit which evaporates to create a potentially explosive vapour. If sparking occurs from the use of diathermy current for cutting or coagulation, an explosion may occur, with the possibility of a flash burn of the patient's skin.
2. Bowel gases are also potentially explosive. At sigmoidoscopy and colonoscopy it is usual to remove polyps with a snare and the base of the polyp may be sealed to prevent bleeding by connecting the snare to a diathermy machine. If bleeding occurs after a lesion has been removed with a snare or forceps, the base may be coagulated with diathermy current. In both cases a spark may ignite the bowel gas and cause an explosion with the danger of colonic rupture.

PATHOPHYSIOLOGY OF WOUND HEALING

Whatever the mechanism of damage to the tissues, the reaction is essentially similar. It is conventional to divide the responses into phases, as though they occur in sequence, but this is only a convenient method of describing them, because they actually occur in parallel.

Inflammatory phase
This lasts about 3–5 days.

Vascular response
If the injury causes bleeding, the response is vasoconstriction and activation of the coagulation cascade that results in the conversion of fibrinogen to fibrin. Together with platelet adhesion, this seals the open blood vessels. Active amines are released which increase vascular contraction and capillary permeability to proteins; the colloid osmotic pressure of the proteins within the extracellular compartment retains filtered fluid and electrolytes causing oedema. Serotonin and histamine released by mast cells dilate the venules and also increase capillary permeability. There is a period of vasodilatation which together with the increase in tissue fluid, and the effect on the nerve endings of injury and raised tissue tension, produces the cardinal features of inflammation – swelling, redness, heat and pain.

Cellular response
Leukocytes attracted by chemotactic factors migrate from the axial stream to the periphery of the capillaries and by active movement (diapedesis), migrate through the walls into the damaged areas releasing hydrolytic enzymes to break down debris and any bacteria, and ingest the products of injury. They are assisted by local macrophages. The macrophages release growth factors stimulating the proliferation of fibroblasts and blood vessels, and cytokines which are chemoattractants and activators of white cells and endothelial cells.

Fibroblasts synthesise large protein-polysaccharide complexes called proteoglycans whose function is obscure. They also release fibronectin, a polymorphic glycoprotein, which is important in the adhesion of cells with each other and with the matrix; fibronectins provide binding sites for receptors on a wide variety of cells. Epithelial cells in intact skin do not bind to fibronectins but if the skin is deficient the epithelial cells have a fibronectin receptor and so migrate across the defect.

Lag phase
The only strength in the injured area initially is the fibrin clot. Only as the inflammatory response subsides is collagen laid down and then the strength of the repair begins to rise. This period is not truly a lag in activity but a short period of 1–2 days during which there is intense preparation for the next phase.

Proliferative phase
For about 3 weeks the epithelial and connective tissue cells undergo hyperplasia. One stimulus is platelet-derived growth factor, although other cells such as macrophages also

synthesise the factor. Epidermal growth factor, also released by platelets, acts in association with transforming growth factor. Epithelial cells respond to absence of contact with a contiguous epithelial cell by undergoing mitosis and spreading across the denuded area until they meet other epithelial cells to complete the skin envelope.

Wound contraction
Fibroblasts proliferate. Some of them appear to have the dual properties of fibroblasts and smooth muscle cells although they contain actin and not myosin. They have the ability to attach themselves to fibronectin which links them to collagen fibres, and then shorten, drawing the opposing sides of the wound area together. This is termed wound contraction and is a normal process.

Wound contracture
Collagen is extruded as fibrils by the ordinary fibroblasts in greater amount than will eventually remain. As collagen matures the fibres shorten and become insoluble. If healing is delayed excessive collagen is produced and shortening results in the pathological condition of wound contracture, which may lead to restriction of movement and deformity.

Granulation tissue
Vascular cells grow out from the torn and sealed capillaries to form loops which are at first solid and then become patent, extending, with associated fibroblasts into the damaged area. They are attracted into the fibrin/fibronectin gel by chemoattraction. When seen from above in a raw area, the apices of the vascular loops appear granular, like minute cobblestones, which explains the name given to the tissue formed, that is, granulation tissue. This tissue fills in the defect as phagocytes remove the debris. If the epithelium has not yet covered the injured area, the granulation tissue forms the pink, granular, vascular bed over which it will extend.

The collagen fibres that have been laid down irregularly are gradually removed and replaced with fibres laid down in response to the local stresses. Collagen, which has produced the bulk of the resulting scar, gradually diminishes and softens.

Modifying factors

Nutrition
There is no evidence that administration of nutrients to a previously healthy individual improves or speeds healing. Protein deficiency retards healing and lowers resistance to infection. Although vitamin C is essential for collagen synthesis, giving supplements to a well nourished person has no beneficial effect. Vitamin A deficiency retards epithelialization and collagen synthesis.

Oxygen
Adequate oxygenation is essential to wound healing, especially for fibroblast replication and collagen synthesis. Therefore,

vascular disease, both reduced arterial supply and venous stasis, and cardiorespiratory deficiency prejudice wound healing.

Infection

Elderly, diabetic, immune deficient patients and those suffering from advanced cancer or major trauma, are susceptible to infection. Locally, heavy contamination, especially with virulent microorganisms, dead tissue, ischaemia and anoxia and haematoma, all raise the likelihood of infection and consequent inability of the local defence mechanisms to cope with the competing needs of fighting infection and wound healing.

Steroid hormones

Glucocorticoids inhibit healing and fibrosis.

Wound type
First intention healing

A clean surgical wound in which haemostasis is perfect and that has been meticulously repaired so that the apposing layers are brought into contact, will heal with minimal scarring.

Second intention healing

If there is a defect between the tissues after wounding, or if some has been removed, then the defect fills with granulation tissue composed of capillary loops with accompanying fibroblasts. The granulation tissue is accompanied by macrophages and polymorph leukocytes to remove debris and bacteria. Wound contraction occurs because of the effect of the myofibroblasts. Chronic delay in healing allows collagen laid down by fibroblasts to mature, when it shortens, resulting in contractures. If there is a skin defect, epithelial cells proliferate at the edges and spread across the granulation tissue to complete the skin cover.

CLASSIFICATION OF SURGICAL WOUNDS

(For more details refer Chapter 7.)

There are many ways of classifying surgical wounds; early and late, closed or open, the open into tidy and untidy, clean and contaminated. Burns form a separate category. These divisions are only of value in order to make decisions for diagnosis and treatment.

Open

- A tidy, cleanly cut wound may result from a surgical scalpel, accidentally while carving a joint, from broken glass or from a violent attack.
- In a lacerated wound the skin has been stretched and subjected to a shear effect.
- Gross avulsion and degloving injuries result in full thickness skin loss.
- Contusion suggests crushing of the skin to split it.

- A flap wound implies that the skin has been stripped, so that it may be lacerated or contused.
- Puncture wounds may occur from window or windscreen glass, accidental penetration of nails, wood splinters or thorns, and missile and stab wounds.
- Deep penetrating wounds may have trivial openings as following a fall on a spiked fence.
- Missile wounds are caused by bullets, shrapnel – fragments from an exploding shell or bombs.
- The wound may be seen within 6 h – early, intermediate or late – after 12 h.
- Any of these may be clean, contaminated, or heavily infected.

Closed

- Contusion may be a simple bruise, which is extravasation of blood through ruptured blood vessels diffusely into the tissues, or involve crushing of the tissues.
- A haematoma is a localized collection of blood usually within a tissue plane. Fluctuation can usually be detected.
- An abrasion implies partial wearing away or shearing away of the superficial layers of the skin.

WOUND MANAGEMENT

Before embarking on local treatment of the wound, a survey of the patient should be carried out to determine if there are other injuries and if there are any incidental health considerations such as cardiovascular disease, diabetes, psychological or legal implications. It must be established whether the patient has been immunized against tetanus or has had a 'booster' of tetanus toxoid within the last 10 years; if not, tetanus immunoglobulin may need to be given together with prophylactic penicillin.

Primary closure

Before embarking on the treatment of wounds, consideration should be given to the possible consequences in terms of the anatomy of the region. Local structures, such as nerves, tendons and blood vessels, should be identified.

Success depends upon early restoration of anatomy with good blood supply, perfect haemostasis and absence of tension. Success is prejudiced if there is any dead material included, ischaemia or anoxia, or imperfect haemostasis. If there is contamination, closure can still sometimes be accomplished successfully after assiduous removal of all foreign material, washing with antiseptics and prophylactic systemic antibiotic treatment.

If tissue has been lost, primary closure is still often possible. Split skin grafts can sometimes be applied. Tissue repair and cover can be achieved using a skin flap or a vascularized free graft.

Delayed primary closure

It is often difficult to decide which tissues are viable and which should be excised. It is easy to decide between pink healthy tissue that is bleeding and black necrotic tissue, but most decisions are in the grey area between these extremes. The decision can be delayed for up to 72 h by applying saline or hydrogel dressings to keep the tissues moist and then examine the wound daily to decide if the tissues are viable and excise areas that have declared themselves necrotic. If there were oedema when the wound was first seen, primary closure might result in ensuing tension. By leaving the wound open for 24–48 h, the oedema may resolve, particularly if the part can be elevated.

Secondary healing

Primary closure may not be possible, or may not be carried out when tissue has been lost. In this case, healing will occur by granulation. Granulation tissue consists of fibroblasts and capillary loops. Wound contraction occurs followed by contraction when the collagen fibrils laid down by the fibroblasts mature and shorten. At this stage, if the skin has not covered the wound, skin grafts may be applied.

Infected wounds

Late wounds that have been heavily contaminated with foreign material carrying virulent microorganisms and have necrotic or ischaemic tissue must *not* be closed. The wound must be carefully explored and extended if necessary to ensure that every part can be inspected. Carefully and gently remove every particle of foreign material. All dead tissue should be identified and carefully excised. The wound should be left open and packed with saline-moistened dressings or hydrogel dressings which contain a starch polymer matrix, or hydrocolloid dressings, both of which absorb exudate. The use of enzymes to digest dead tissue has been tried with streptokinases but collagenases offer great promise. Wound irrigation is also used but presents problems in containment of the irrigating fluid. For hollow wounds that have a tendency to spontaneous closure yet are producing much exudate, synthetic foam may be poured in and allowed to set. This absorbs exudate and can be cleaned and re-inserted. Alternatively repack the wound with dressings such as moist saline or flavine-soaked packs.

For many years sugar paste or honey have been sporadically popular as applications to wounds; they appear to promote the growth of granulation tissue. Recently there has been a revival of interest in the use of fly larvae to digest necrotic tissue.

When, by means of the various methods (surgical excision and local applications) the wound becomes clean, pink and healthy and free of necrotic material, it can be closed. During the time taken to reach this stage, wound contraction and contracture will have taken place and once the wound is clean, it may rapidly heal itself. If necessary, it can be closed by split skin grafting or other types of graft.

Penetrating and missile wounds

The care of these wounds demands an intimate knowledge of anatomy in order to estimate the risk to deep structures. In some cases there is an exit wound which indicates the line of penetration. A careful history should be taken to determine the cause of the injury and its likely force and direction, and then the patient carefully examined to assess the damage, in particular to nerves, blood vessels, tendons and bones. In some cases when the injury has been made cleanly and there are no abnormal physical signs, the superficial wound can be closed. In the majority, however, it is important to explore the wound.

Exploration usually entails extending the wound carefully, to allow access, while ensuring that the exposure does not increase the damage to important structures. The whole wound is gently examined, excising crushed, avascular or ragged tissue and foreign material while carefully preserving important structures. Any adherent material is washed off using sterile saline or hydrogen peroxide solution.

The injury caused by a missile depends upon its velocity and the amount of kinetic energy released by it. A high-velocity bullet may produce little surrounding damage if it passes only through soft tissues that do not obstruct it. However, if, for example, it strikes bone, its effect is like that of an explosion within the body, causing a shock wave that homogenizes and kills muscles, may cause endothelial damage in nearby blood vessels, and sends off splinters of bone that act like shrapnel. The bullet velocity carries particles of clothing into the tissues with attendant microorganisms. It is vitally important to explore and assiduously clean these wounds. Every visible particle of dirt and dead tissue must be removed. The vitality of muscle can be gauged by gently pinching it to see if it contracts and cutting it to see if bleeding occurs.

Burns

The local management of burns cannot be separated from the general care of the patient. The mechanism of the burn is important, since the temperature and time in contact with the skin are important in determining the depth. As a rough guide, the patient's palm covers 1% of the body area. Adults with 15% and children with 10% of body surface burned, need to be admitted. The severity of through and through electrical burns is greater than is immediately apparent. Fluid is lost because heat damage to capillaries increases their permeability. In extensive burns, fluids, electrolytes and protein must be replaced.

If burns are red, blistered and painful, they are superficial. They should be burst, but not removed. The area should then be covered with non-adherent gauze overlaid with cotton wool and crepe bandage compression applied if possible.

Partial thickness burns in which the deep dermis is preserved may blister. They are often painless, but needle pricks can usually be felt. These burns, and those with indeterminate or mixed partial and full thickness loss can either be dressed or left open, depending upon the area burned and the facilities available. Partial thickness burns should heal within 2 weeks. Any residual unhealed areas are then shaved with a skin graft knife until healthy oozing tissue is reached, followed by split skin grafting.

Deep burns are often obvious and painless and needle pricks cannot be felt. There is no virtue in waiting; as soon as possible the dead tissue should be excised to reveal healthy, bleeding tissue and the area then grafted with split skin.

In an emergency, deep circumferential burns that will compress and impair the distal circulation should be released. Escharotomy, longitudinal incisions on both sides of a limb throughout the length of the burn, should be performed. Since the burns are full thickness, no anaesthetic is needed.

SCARS AND CONTRACTURE

Scars

Scarring is a normal part of tissue repair except during fetal and early neonatal life. Whenever there is damage, fibroblasts are attracted and they multiply and align themselves before extruding collagen fibrils which mature and undergo shortening. As a result of this, a longitudinal incision often shortens over a period of months unless it is subjected to excessive strain, when it stretches. The collagen is remodelled in order to adjust the alignment of the fibrils to strains exerted on them, but it never reaches the strength of the unwounded tissue.

Hypertrophic scars

Infection, presence of foreign material, repair of irregular wounds, burns and trauma during the healing phase provoke the production of dense, eosinophilic collagen in the dermis with hypertrophy of the scar. It stands proud and red but usually flattens and pales over a period of 1–2 years. A frequent cause of hypertrophy is overtightened stitches that are left too long. They form a 'ladder pattern'.

Keloid scars

Keloid scars differ from hypertrophic scars in that they extend outside the area of the original wound. Keloid scars tend to develop more commonly in those of African ancestry, and in certain parts of the body, notably over the shoulders, upper back and sternum. They are prone to develop following ear piercing. Their development is reduced if continuous pressure is exerted on the wound during healing and for up to 12 months afterwards; elastic compression devices must be individually designed. Radiotherapy to the healing wound also diminishes the laying down of collagen but the safety of this has been questioned. Triamcinolone, a

potent steroid, can be injected through a fine needle into the scar until it pales, this is quite painful. The injection can be repeated after 6 weeks.

Contracture

Wound contracture

This results from the maturing and shortening of collagen fibrils. If a wide area of skin is lost, successive fibrils of collagen are laid down and mature so that the skin margins are gradually drawn together, sometimes bringing about large shifts of skin. For example, in extensive untreated burns of the neck, webbing, deformity and restricted movements result. Similarly, burns of the chest and axilla restrict abduction at the shoulder.

Contractures following nerve damage

When muscles are paralysed, they contract as they atrophy and undergo fibrosis. Contracture of the flexors predominates so that unless active measures are taken to maintain full passive movement, the limbs are retracted.

Volkmann's ischaemic contracture

This occurs in the forearm and distal leg. Prolonged constriction of limbs by plasters or tourniquets, swelling within the inelastic fascial compartment or arterial obstruction provoke microvascular occlusion and fibrosis of the muscles with consequent shortening of the musculo–tendinous complex. There may also be a neurological component. It causes severe pain. The condition can be prevented only by early recognition, removal of the constriction, fasciotomy and overcoming the vascular occlusion.

Dupuytren's contracture

There appears to be a familial susceptibility. Diabetes, epilepsy or its treatment are also associated. The palmar and plantar fascia undergo thickening and contracture. In the foot the pressure of walking and standing maintain the foot's normal shape. In the hand, the medial side is most affected so that the little finger is held flexed. The condition can usually be considerably improved by excising the palmar fascia and carrying out Z-plasty on the overlying skin, since the tendons are not shortened.

WOUND DEHISCENCE

Wound healing depends upon optimal local levels of oxygen, pH and nutrients, so that blood supply is paramount. There is a zone of several millimetres close to the healing edge which is metabolically active and remains weak until full healing has taken place. Complete healing may take several months. Tension at the healing edges is poorly tolerated. Infection is a potent inhibitor of healing. The metabolically active zone close to the healing edge widens. The presence of a haematoma or seroma, and imperfect apposition or overtight sutures that strangulate the tissues, may contribute to rupture. Immunosuppression, diabetes, jaundice, advanced neoplasia and major operations prejudice wound healing.

Abdominal wounds

In the past the deep tissues of abdominal wounds were often sutured in layers with catgut. There was an accepted rate of wound dehiscence. There were two possible reasons for the failures. The sutures were often inserted close to the edge in the metabolically active but weak zone. Another, perhaps even more potent cause, was the use of catgut. Catgut loses its strength rapidly, often before the wound is sufficiently strong.

The likelihood of abdominal wound rupture has been greatly reduced by the work of Terence Jenkins. He showed that dehiscence is almost completely eliminated by following simple rules. He advocated non-absorbable sutures. The length of the suture material should be at least 4 times the length of the wound. The abdomen is stitched with mass sutures – large stitches placed well away from the wound edges, catching all the layers except the subcutaneous fat and skin. The stitches are inserted loosely, producing apposition but not constriction.

Management of burst abdomen

It is sometimes possible to anticipate impending wound dehiscence. Bowel sounds and gut activity are late in returning. A little serosanguinous fluid discharges from the suture line. Finally the wound ruptures, usually when the patient coughs or strains. It is not usually painful but is often distressing. There may be full dehiscence or even partial disembowelment, or the skin and superficial layers may remain intact.

The patient must be reassured. Sterile packs and a corset or roller towel are applied. Immediate resuture in the operating theatre is a priority. Although resuture can be performed using local anaesthetics, it is usual to carry it out under general anaesthesia. The wound is gently reopened and the sutures examined to note any breakages or cutting out through the tissues. Infection, leakage, discharge or adhesions are looked for. Wound swabs should be sent for culture and sensitivity to antibiotics. If a predisposing cause is found, it should be dealt with, otherwise the wound is sutured in the manner previously described. It is remarkably rare for a wound to rupture a second time.

Anastomotic leak

The causes of leakage following anastomosis of the bowel have been well studied. The essentials for safe anastomosis are good blood supply, absence of tension and perfect apposition. Infection, distal obstruction, continuation of a disease process (such as ileitis or neoplasm) and the presence of foreign material must be eliminated.

Leakage from an anastomosis of the gastrointestinal tract within the abdomen may cause general or local peritonitis, but postoperative complications do not produce typical clinical features. The leak may produce gas shadows outside the bowel or it may be revealed by contrast studies. The patient's general condition deteriorates with features of sepsis. The most urgent need is to drain the leak and any collections of pus. The patient will not improve until the sepsis is controlled.

If a discrete track develops rapidly so that the remainder of the peritoneal cavity is not contaminated or if the leak can be brought to the surface, the leak can be treated conservatively, in many cases by applying a base plate onto the skin around the stoma of karaya gum or a commercial preparation. A stoma bag is applied over this.

When sepsis is controlled and metabolic needs met, if necessary by total parenteral nutrition, the leak often seals spontaneously. In some cases enteral nutrition can be given distal to the leak.

In some cases, when there is minimal sepsis, early exploration is appropriate. In a few cases it is possible to insert further stitches but as a rule it is necessary to defunction the leak by means of a bypass or external stoma, when the leak often closes spontaneously.

Vascular leaks

As most vascular anastomoses are performed on diseased vessels, sutures may cut out and leakage occur. To obtain a smooth lining the vessel walls are everted. If the apposition of the everted endothelial surfaces is not perfect, leakage is likely. Temporary leakage may also occur through the stitch holes. It usually ceases following gentle pressure for 5 min timed by the clock. If it continues, consider whether there is a clotting defect.

EXCISION OF CYSTS OF THE SKIN AND SUBCUTANEOUS TISSUES

The commonest subcutaneous cysts encountered are epidermoid, often called sebaceous cysts. They are most frequently seen on the scalp, face and scrotum and are sometimes infected. The only indication for operation on an infected epidermoid cyst is if it forms an abscess that needs draining; otherwise the infection should be treated first. True dermoid cysts are seen at the outer end of the eyebrows or in the midline. Implantation dermoids occur where skin has been driven deeply as occurs in the fingers of seamstresses.

Before excising a simple, uninfected epidermoid cyst, written, informed consent must be obtained and all the required materials and instruments and good light secured. If hair interferes with the procedure, it should be shaved or trimmed. The skin is cleaned. A short distance from the normal skin near the cyst, 0.5% or weaker lignocaine is injected through a fine needle, raising a wheal extending to and over the cyst. The crown of the cyst where the punctum lies should be avoided in order not to penetrate the cyst and burst it. The injection is then extended around and under the cyst. The hydrostatic pressure should separate the cyst from all its attachments except at the punctum.

Five minutes is allowed for the local anaesthetic action of lignocaine to take effect. An incision is then made over the cyst, to one side of the crown, and extended a few millimetres at each end beyond the cyst, taking care to avoid opening the cyst. Control of bleeding is achieved by simple pressure. The two sides of the incision are separated with the tips of haemostatic forceps and the white cyst is now visible, free of attachments. Using the forceps blades as levers, the cyst is gently mobilized and freed until it is attached only at the punctum. Once free, the intact cyst is removed by cutting its attachment to the skin. If the cyst is ruptured, sebaceous material should be carefully removed, the cyst wall identified and dissected free.

Simple pressure is applied or persistent bleeding vessels picked up and tied. The wound is carefully sutured using fine metric 1. 5 or 1 (4/0 or 5/0) black monofilament polyamide or similar material. The wound usually requires only a plastic spray seal. The sutures can be removed after 4–5 days.

BIOPSY AND CYTOLOGICAL SAMPLING

Always fully explain the procedure and its implications to the patient and obtain consent.

Biopsy

This implies a viewing of living tissue but dead tissue is also included. Specimens are taken for examination, usually histologically. Those for routine histology should be placed in 10% formalin but not those for electron microscopy. Some specimens are later divided so that part can be sent for microbiological or chemical investigation. Advice should be taken from the laboratory staff and the correct specimen bottles and media used and the correct forms filled in.

Elliptical biopsy
This entails removing a full thickness boat-shaped specimen of skin. If it is an excision biopsy, ensure the ellipse is completely clear of the margins of the lesion. The ellipse is aligned with the skin tension lines. With the scalpel cutting vertically into the skin, crossing the cuts at the ends is avoided (Fig. 6.7). Some normal skin is included, together with the junctional tissue at the edge of the lesion. For potentially malignant lesions, ensure that you have adequate clearance in depth.

To close the ellipse, the skin edges may be gently undermined. The wound is sutured to bring the edges together, forming a linear scar. It is often valuable to place the first stitch across the centre of the ellipse where the gap is greatest and insert the other stitches subsequently. If the first stitch is now lax, it can be removed and a replacement inserted. If the ellipse is short and wide, closure will be difficult. Long, narrow ellipses are easy to close and produce the best scars.

Wedge biopsy

This is indicated where the lesion is near an edge such as a lip or an ear. It can be used to remove part of a lesion or as an excision biopsy. It can be closed as a linear scar (Fig. 6.8).

Needle biopsy

This allows for a core of tissue to be removed at a depth. The most usual needle is the Trucut (Travenol) instrument (Fig. 6.9). The lesion and its depth must be confirmed. Adjacent important structures must not be at risk. The skin is cleaned and a bleb raised with local anaesthetic. A nick is then made with a sharp-pointed scalpel at the insertion point of the needle. With the fingers of one hand, the lump is fixed, if necessary, while inserting the closed needle into it. The cannula is held still while the stylette (which has a flattened area behind the sharp tip into which some tissue bulges) is advanced. The stylette is held still and the needle advanced over it, cutting off a thin core of tissue that bulges into the flat part of the stylette. The needle is kept closed and withdrawn to reveal the excised core of tissue which is gently placed in the fixative. As a rule the entry point in the skin requires a simple dressing only.

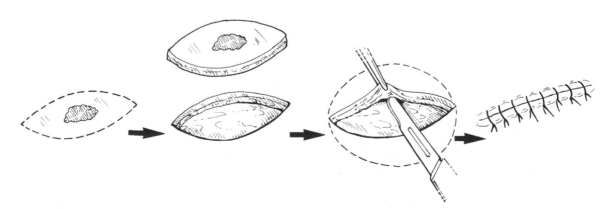

Figure 6.7. Elliptical biopsy. On the left, an ellipse is marked out with its long axis parallel to the skin tension lines. A boat-shaped full-thickness specimen is excised. If necessary, the edges are undermined to allow linear closure without tension.

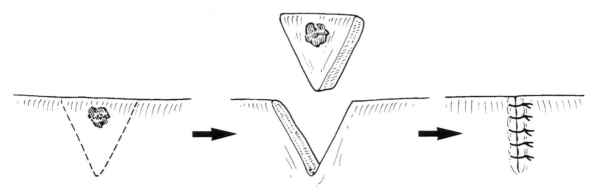

Figure 6.8. A wedge biopsy removed near an edge, followed by linear closure.

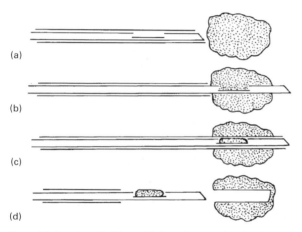

Figure 6.9. Trucut needle biopsy. (a) The stylette, enclosed within a hollow needle, has a thinned segment. (b) when the needle reaches the lesion, it is held still while the stylette is advanced into the lesion. (c) The stylette is then held still while the needle is advanced, cutting off the tissue that has bulged into the thinned segment. (d) The closed needle and stylette are withdrawn, the needle is drawn back, freeing the biopsy specimen.

Cytological sampling

In a number of areas, diagnosis can be made from specimens of cells. An example is the simple aspiration of ascitic fluid in the abdomen that may on cytology reveal metastatic carcinoma, sparing the patient extensive, distressing investigations of no further benefit. After the skin is cleaned, a size 12 needle is gently inserted through the full thickness of the abdominal wall in one quadrant. Fluid is aspirated and the syringe emptied into a container that will be sent immediately, with a completed form, to the cytology laboratory. If necessary, aspiration is performed in each of the four quadrants. This technique can be used wherever there is fluid that may contain diagnostically important cells. Sometimes

elusive fluid can be identified and aspirated using imaging by ultrasound or CT.

Cells may be removed from solid lumps for cytological examination. A well-developed technique is used for breast lumps. The fixative pot and microscope slides should first be made ready. After the skin is cleaned and the patient made aware of the procedure, the lump is fixed with the fingers of the non-dominant hand. A fine, for example, 23-gauge needle attached to a 10 ml syringe is advanced into the lump. The syringe plunger is strongly withdrawn while the needle tip is jerkily moved within the lump. The technique is facilitated by fitting the syringe into an apparatus that allows it to be controlled with one hand. The syringe and needle is withdrawn, the contents ejected onto several prelabelled microscope slides and fixative immediately applied. Finally, some fixative is drawn up into the syringe through the needle and the contents emptied into a specimen bottle for centrifugation. The specimen and completed form are sent immediately to the cytology laboratory.

DRAINAGE OF SUPERFICIAL ABSCESSES

An abscess is a collection of pus confined within a cavity. Sometimes the abscess resolves spontaneously; a 'blind boil' is an example. Abscesses may also become chronic and remain static. If the abscess is superficial it causes local swelling and inflammation. The fact that it contains fluid can be detected by fluctuation. Others track towards internal or external surfaces. The tracking of an abscess to the external surface is described as 'pointing'. There is often a swelling with central tenderness. The centre of the swelling softens and often turns white, later becoming necrotic and turning black, and may break down so that the contained pus can discharge. If the overlying skin is macerated by applying moist dressings, this facilitates the breakdown and discharge of pus. Abscesses in some places increase the dangers; an example is the 'danger triangle' between the root of the nose and the corners of the mouth where infection may spread via the veins to the cavernous sinus.

Abscess cavity walls are relatively impervious to systemically administered antibiotics. If an abscess is localized and superficial but does not show signs of pointing, it is usually best to drain it. It is important to know the anatomy and be aware of important structures in the region. The necessary instruments and materials, including receptacles for collecting the pus for culture, should be available before the procedure is started.

Aspiration

The contents of a very soft abscess may be fluid, in which case a large bore needle can be introduced under local anaesthesia and the pus aspirated. This can be repeated if necessary. This method is often successful provided there is no continuing cause.

Incision

Superficial abscesses can be incised under local anaesthesia. Infiltration is started a short distance from the central, tender spot. A bleb in the skin is raised and the needle is gradually advanced. The anaesthetic is injected into the skin over the crest of the swelling. Five minutes is allowed for the local anaesthetic to take effect.

A small incision is made over the crest of the swelling and a specimen of the pus collected for culture and determination of antibiotic sensitivities. The inside of the cavity is then explored. If it is small, closed dissecting forceps or sinus forceps should be used. If it is large, a gloved finger may be inserted to examine the inside.

The contents of the abscess cavity are emptied using gentle suction, flushing with physiological saline or by swabbing. In some cases, such as a perianal abscess, a portion of the abscess wall is removed for histology, to aid in determining the cause of the abscess.

The *hand* offers particular difficulties in diagnosis and treatment. The pus may lie beneath thick, tense tissues through which it is difficult to detect the relatively small abscess. The tension causes severe pain, especially in the distal pulp space. It may be necessary to rely on finding the most tender spot. However, paronychia is obvious, as are web space infections. Subungual infections can often be drained by cutting or drilling a panel or hole out of the nail. Palmar space abscesses often produce oedema of the dorsum of the hand or tendon sheaths; these demand expert treatment.

BASIC PRINCIPLES OF ANASTOMOSIS

In surgery anastomosis is usually union between tubes, especially the digestive tract, blood vessels or other ducts. These may be united end-to-end, end-to-side or side-to-side (Fig. 6.10).

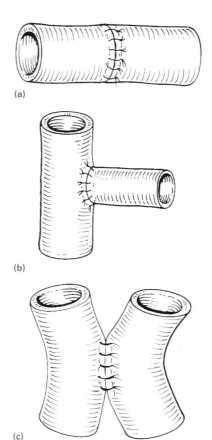

(a)

(b)

(c)

Figure 6.10. (a) end-to-end (b) end-to-side and (c) side-to-side anastomosis of tubes.

Digestive tract

Anastomoses are used to reconnect bowel after resection of a segment or to bypass a diseased portion. It was shown by Lembert that if the serous (visceral peritoneal) coats of bowel are apposed, they fuse and seal the junction. From this developed the convention of inverting bowel ends when they are united with a seromuscular stitch. The important stitch holding the bowel is an all-coats stitch which picks up the strong, collagenous submucosal layer (Fig. 6.11). Conventionally, the anastomosis is performed in four successive layers. The bowel ends are apposed and their back layers united with a continuous seromuscular suture of metric 3 or 2 (2/0 or 3/0) size synthetic absorbable thread. The back layers are united a second time, either as a continuous or interrupted stitch. This is then continued onto the front wall to complete the union. Finally, the seromuscular stitch on the back wall is continued onto the front wall as an inverting suture to complete the encircling and inverting anastomosis.

It has been shown that single layer can be as safe as two layer anastomoses. Edge-to-edge union is also safe; in theory,

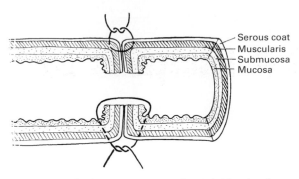

Figure 6.11. Lembert's inverting seromuscular stitch (above) and all-coats intestinal stitch (below).

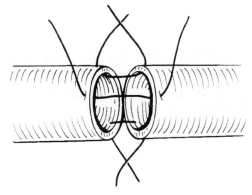

Figure 6.12. Triangulation method of performing vascular anastomosis.

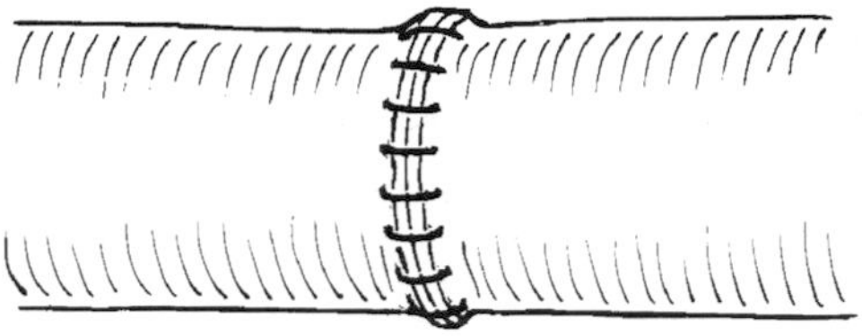

bringing together the layers that will unite seems sensible. Finally, many surgeons exclude the mucosa from the traditional all-coats stitch. The technique that can best be applied to all gastrointestinal anastomoses is a single layer of extramucosal interrupted sutures of synthetic absorbable thread, with edge-to-edge union.

Mechanical circular *stapling devices* have been developed that insert a double row of titanium staples across the inverted edges of the two pieces of bowel that are to be united, and then cuts off any excess bowel edges. They produce a conventional inverted anastomosis.

Vascular anastomosis

The union of blood vessels must be carried out not by inversion but by eversion, in order to bring into apposition the inner endothelial layers. If this is not done, clots form at the anastomosis and block the lumen. Classically, the ends of vessels are first united by three stay sutures that divide the circumference into thirds (Fig. 6.12) . A running stitch of fine (metric 0.7–0.4) monofilament polyamide or polypropylene suture is then carried round the circumference of the stoma (Fig. 6.13).

Very small vessels can be united but this requires an entirely different technique. The anastomosis is carried out using very fine instruments and the procedure is performed using an operating microscope. It is not possible to evert the vessels; instead, the anastomosis is formed using a series of interrupted sutures bringing the ends together, edge-to-edge.

Figure 6.13. Everted edges in vascular anastomosis to bring the inner, endothelial surfaces into contact.

FURTHER READING

Amid PK, Shulman AG, Lichtenstein IL. Local anaesthesia for inguinal hernia repair; step by step procedure. *Ann Surg* 1994; **220**: 735–737

Jenkins TPN. The burst abdominal wound: a mechanical approach. *Br Med J* 1976; **131**: 130–140

Kirk RM. *Basic Surgical Techniques*, 4th edn. Edinburgh: Churchill Livingstone, 1994

MacGregor IA, MacGregor AD. *Fundamental Techniques in Plastic Surgery*, 9th edn. Edinburgh: Churchill Livingstone, 1995

Kirk RM, Mansfield AO, Cochrane J (eds), *Clinical Surgery in General*, 2nd edn. Edinburgh: Churchill Livingstone, 1996

Memon AA. Surgical diathermy. *Br J Hosp Med* 1994; **52**: 403–408

7

Trauma: General Principles of Management

C Macutkiewicz and ID Anderson

Department of Surgery, Hope Hospital, University of Manchester, School of Medicine

CONTENTS

Prevention and pre-hospital management	90
Immediate hospital management (the golden hour)	90
Organisation of hospital trauma care	90
The injured patient	91
History of injury	92
Blunt and penetrating injuries	92
Investigations and definitive care	93
Head injury	93
Spinal injury	95
Penetrating neck injuries	97
Chest injuries	97
Abdominal trauma	98
Pelvic fractures	101
Injuries to the bony skeleton	102
Vascular injuries	103
Missile and blast injuries	103
Burns	103
The pathophysiology of trauma	106
The response to injury	106
The early response to injury	106
Neuroendocrine	107
The late response to injury	110
Summary	110
Further reading	110

Trauma is the leading cause of deaths in patients under the age of 40 years and consequently is the leading cause of loss to productive years of life. More than 7 000 patients per year die from trauma in the UK (more deaths than from cancer of the stomach or pancreas) and up to 7% of all hospital care and UK National Health Service (NHS) expenditure is due to trauma care. These figures show the importance of trauma as a health problem but the true scale of the problem only begins to become clear when it is appreciated that approximately 10 times more patients do not die but are temporarily incapacitated as a result of injury. Much of current surgical practice has its roots in the surgery of trauma and as such many of the principles of management have been well defined for many years. However, it has been well documented that for each new advance, there has been a tendency to forget some of the previously established principles, often with disastrous consequences, particularly in times of war. This chapter therefore focuses more on the general principles of management than on the treatment of specific injuries, although both will be covered. One of the most basic principles of management is the importance of prompt treatment and, given the magnitude of the trauma problem, it will be seen that organisation of trauma services form an important part of these considerations. Unfortunately, injured patients undergo a series of systemic pathophysiological changes as a consequence of their injury and this makes the provision of adequate and timely treatment more difficult. These pathophysiological principles will be covered and again these encompass new research as well as established and sometimes forgotten basic principles.

Deaths following injury occur at *three principal times* and the causes of death differ between the three groups. Consequently, the underlying principles are different at each time point. These principles, in turn, underpin attempts to achieve more successful management:

1. Deaths can occur very shortly after injury as a result of *catastrophic injury* to the central nervous system and to the great vessels. Virtually all these deaths take place at the scene of the accident and, with the exception of the occasional death due to airway obstruction, there is no active treatment that will alter outcome.

2. Patients with serious injuries may die, largely from *haemorrhage* or *hypoxia* during the first 1–2 h following injury. These injuries are potentially survivable provided optimal and rapid care is provided; the time period during

which this care must be given has become known as the '*golden hour*'.

3. Patients may die during the days or weeks following the initial resuscitation. This most often occurs from multiple organ failure as a result of *infectious complications* (*sepsis*) and it is generally believed that the seeds of later septic deterioration are sown at the time of initial resuscitation.

Recent years have seen great improvements in the treatment of injury during the golden hour and consequently later septic deaths have become relatively more important. As this has happened, the importance of understanding the complex pathophysiological changes which underlie injury has become all the more clear (see below).

PREVENTION AND PRE-HOSPITAL MANAGEMENT

Up to 50% of deaths following injury occur at the scene, mostly as the result of overwhelming injury to the central nervous system and great vessels. Except for occasional cases where the patient can be transported directly to a major hospital, there is virtually no chance of survival and prevention of injury is the only means whereby this percentage can be reduced. Prevention has usually required legislation and in the most advanced countries (such as Australia), this legislation has been driven forward by the surgical profession rather than relying on pressure groups within the population. Such legislation has included safety at work measures (e.g. hard hats, safety ropes and belts, equipment and machinery checking procedures), control of firearms and other weapons and, most prominently, road traffic legislation, with mechanisms such as:

- drink driving campaigns,
- front seat belts,
- rear seat belts,
- child safety seats,
- rollbars,
- airbags,
- traffic calming measures,
- cycle helmets,
- pedestrian precincts,
- cycle lanes.

Some legislation, for example, drink driving and seat belt laws, have significantly changed the number and patterns of certain injuries and brought about a culture change within society whereby adverse behaviour is no longer tolerated even in the absence of legislation. The impact of trauma prevention therefore cannot be underestimated.

The *retrieval of injured patients* from the scene of an accident has developed greatly in the last few years with the establishment of a paramedic-trained ambulance service. A small but consistent proportion of deaths do occur at the scene due to uncorrected problems such as external haemorrhage or obstruction of the airway and the ability to manage these promptly is undoubtedly of value. What is less

clear is whether involved interventions (e.g. intravenous (i.v.) access) at the scene are more effective than a 'scoop and run' ambulance policy. It is accepted that most field interventions are inevitably more difficult and less successful than those that are carried out in the resuscitation room and it is important that resuscitative efforts are not unduly prolonged before transfer to hospital. Two principles are thus embodied here:

1. Immediately life-threatening events must be managed as they occur.
2. Definitive treatment of injuries, as can only be offered within a hospital setting, is the major determinant of outcome subsequently.

IMMEDIATE HOSPITAL MANAGEMENT (THE GOLDEN HOUR)

The hospital phase of management of injured patients can be divided usefully into:

- Immediate management which is undertaken to diagnose and treat life-threatening injuries.
- Identification of other injuries and arrangements for their definitive care on a priority basis.
- Recovery (and subsequent rehabilitation).

The second (definitive care) phase is considered later. In many cases there is overlap between the first and second stages. Aspects of immediate management may need to be undertaken urgently on the ward or high-dependency unit at a later stage as, even with optimal care, not all injuries may be identified immediately. It is essential, therefore, that senior members of the relevant subspecialties are involved with the care of the injured patient from the earliest possible time, and that close senior review is maintained once the patient leaves the emergency department for the ward.

Organisation of hospital trauma care

Salvaging patients with injury before they die from haemorrhage or hypoxia requires assessment and treatment as quickly as possible and this requires a suitable degree of organisation and training before injured patients arrive. Resuscitation rooms should be laid out so that all necessary equipment is readily to hand. Appropriate doctors from a range of necessary specialties should be called to the resuscitation room, preferably before the injured patient arrives. This will require the hospital trauma team to be alerted by the ambulance crew by radio. For a trauma team to work efficiently it is essential that they all follow similar principles in an identical order. Such consensus management is made possible by the adoption of a training system, such as the *Advanced Trauma Life Support* (*ATLS*) *system*. To say that the widespread adoption of ATLS in the UK and, indeed, in many countries throughout the world has been a major contributor to the revolution that has taken place in the management of injured patients over the last decade does not overstate matters. Before the adoption of this type of system, some 20–30%

of all patients who died in hospital from their injuries did so unnecessarily. Contemporary figures show that not only can avoidable deaths be prevented but that almost all injured patients who reach hospital alive can be resuscitated sufficiently to enable them to reach the intensive care unit and for the definitive care stage of management to begin (see below).

The establishment of an ATLS-trained trauma team can be achieved in any general hospital but it remains debatable whether the creation of trauma centres further improves care of the injured. Experience from the USA demonstrates quite clearly that the centralisation of the care of major injury to large hospitals with round-the-clock specialists on hand is associated with greatly improved outcomes. To date, it has been difficult to show the same advantages in the UK given the different healthcare system, level of funding, pattern of injury and the other changes (e.g. ATLS training) which have occurred in the interim. Notwithstanding this, it remains clear that all the surgical management of complex injuries is best carried out by those who see them relatively frequently and who have the necessary support available on site.

The injured patient

When an injured patient arrives, vital functions are rapidly assessed for abnormalities which pose an immediate threat to life. Systems are assessed in the order in which they pose the most urgent threat (i.e. ABC, *airway* then *breathing* then *circulation*) and any life-threatening abnormalities are dealt with as they are identified. Usually, all patients receive full treatment but when multiple casualties arrive simultaneously and overwhelm local resources, it may prove necessary to implement a system of triage, again based on the ABCs, where the treatment of patients with unsurvivable injuries is downgraded such that the greatest number of survivors can be obtained.

Airway management, administration of high-flow oxygen and cervical spine stabilisation

Airway patency is rapidly assessed, achieved and maintained by a hierarchy of interventions. A conscious, talking patient can maintain his own airway. Failing this, the following manoeuvres should be employed:
- *Clear the airway*:
  - suction,
  - chin lift,
  - jaw thrust.
- *Maintain the airway*:
  - oropharyngeal airway,
  - nasopharyngeal airway.
- *Definitive airway*:
  - endotracheal tube.
- *Surgical airway*:
  - needle cricothyroidectomy,
  - surgical cricothyroidectomy.

These techniques can be learned on courses such as the ATLS course, and remember, *high-flow oxygen should be given to all patients*.

The great majority of patients sustaining at least moderate injury will have been exposed to the risk of injury to the cervical spine. This can be missed, particularly in those with obtundation or airway compromise, so it is essential that the risk of cervical spine injury is considered in every patient because of the catastrophic possibility of causing or aggravating an injury to the cervical spinal cord and thereby causing paralysis or death. This is particularly so in patients who have sustained injury to the head and neck, who are unconscious, who have suffered a significant fall or a marked deceleration. The cervical spine is immobilised by the application of a semi-rigid collar and by supporting the head with sandbags on either side and by securing the forehead with tape. Similar immobilisation can be achieved by managing the patient on a specially designed spine board which incorporates these features. Spinal immobilisation should be maintained until adequate cervical spine films (including the C7/T1 junction) have been seen and cleared by a competent radiologist or spinal surgeon.

Breathing and respiratory function
Even with a patent airway, lung function can be critically compromised by a range of injuries. For example:
- *Tension pneumothorax*: attempt needle decompression, or insert a chest drain.
- *Massive haemothorax*: site i.v. infusion and insert a chest drain.
- *Flail chest*: support ventilation adequately.
- *Pericardial tamponade*: attempt a pericardiocentesis, or perform a pericardiotomy.
- *Open chest wound*. apply a flap dressing to the wound, and insert a chest drain at a remote site.

Foremost amongst these is the *tension pneumothorax*. This is characterised by hypoxia, distress, loss of breath sounds, tracheal deviation and possibly hyperresonance. Immediate needle thoracocentesis should be followed as soon as possible by placement of a chest drain using a cut down technique, using the trocar to decrease the possibility of iatrogenic impalement injury of vital structures.

Pericardial tamponade is a particularly difficult diagnosis to make and is often associated with other injuries. It is commonest with penetrating injury although the entry wounds may lie posteriorly (usually between the shoulder blades) or at an even more remote site. It is occasionally seen after blunt injury. Diagnosis in the doubtful case can be confirmed by urgent ultrasonography but often there is no time to obtain this and a high index of suspicion for this diagnosis should be followed by a pericardiocentesis.

Circulatory support and haemorrhage control
The key step in maintaining the circulation is to stop haemorrhage and to replace blood already lost. Obviously, any external haemorrhage should be controlled and this can always be achieved by direct pressure without a need for vascular clamps or tourniquets. Heart rate and blood pressure are poor indicators of the presence or absence of haemorrhage (see below) and it is a safe policy to establish large-bore vascular access at

two sites in injured patients and to obtain blood for rapid cross matching. Usually, a fluid bolus is administered directly and 1–2 l of warmed crystalloid solution given immediately is a reasonable starting point. It should be remembered that many patients will have lost 1500 ml or so of blood by the time they show signs of hypotension and they will require 4–5 l of crystalloid infusion just to restore the circulating volume. Individual responses vary and repeated reassessment is vital. Should any patient fail to respond as expected, then a further search for continuing haemorrhage must be made.

As part of the assessment of the cardiovascular system, the chest, abdomen, pelvis and thighs are examined as potential sources of internal haemorrhage. Considerable volumes of blood can be lost around femoral fractures (1–2 l) and progressive exsanguination around a pelvic fracture is by no means uncommon. Large volumes of blood can be lost into the abdomen or chest with very little in the way of physical signs and clinical examination may need to be supplemented with chest radiography or abdominal investigation (see below). When any source of haemorrhage is identified, it should be dealt with directly and it is not unusual for the initial assessment of the patient to be interrupted and for the patient to be taken to the operating theatre to have major internal haemorrhage dealt with surgically. Systematic assessment of the patient's injuries should be resumed in the operating theatre and in the recovery room thereafter.

The relative importance of stopping haemorrhage as opposed to supporting the circulation with i.v. fluids has been highlighted by an investigation of patients suffering penetrating injuries in Texas. Patients given i.v. fluid early had a worse outcome in terms of complications than those who received no i.v. fluids until they reached the operating theatre. The reason for this is believed to be that the i.v. fluids expand the circulation and provoke further haemorrhage from the sites of injury and thus a greater overall blood loss. This treatment policy should not be applied to patients suffering blunt injury (who constitute the majority in many countries), but nevertheless the importance of stopping haemorrhage is clear.

Massive transfusion, particularly of cold fluids, results in *coagulopathy* and in the patient entering a spiral of continued haemorrhage from multiple sites which can be impossible to break. It is worthy of re-emphasis therefore that all patients should be repeatedly assessed for their response to any i.v. fluids to ensure that the expected response has not only been achieved but is also maintained. It is understood that even in the face of a normal blood pressure, vital organs can be underperfused and this may set off the enzyme and cytokine cascades which ultimately contribute to *multiple organ failure* at a later stage.

Neurological disability

Rapid assessment of the degree of apparent injury to the central nervous system is made by assessing the patient's response to verbal and painful stimuli and by examining the pupils. Abnormalities of the cardiorespiratory system or the

presence of hypoglycaemia, alcohol or drugs can also suppress central neurological function.

Finally, the patient should be exposed such that full and complete examination can be undertaken, but at each stage the patient should be protected from hypothermia. Once this first rapid assessment of the patient's condition has been made, his condition should have begun to stabilise, although continued close observation is needed to ensure that further deterioration from a missed injury does not occur. It is only at this stage that initial radiographs (usually chest, cervical spine, pelvis) and basic monitoring (pulse oximetry, electrocardiogram (ECG), urine output) are instituted. Thereafter, a full top-to-toe reassessment of the entire patient is undertaken and specific investigations arranged as clinically indicated.

The use of a system of patient assessment such as that outlined above has many advantages. It can be undertaken promptly by a single doctor or synchronously and without interspecialty conflict when several surgeons are available. A system also makes it less likely that major areas will be omitted with the potential for missed injuries and avoidable mortality.

History of injury

Obtaining the history of the accident or injury is an essential step. This can be obtained from the patient, ambulance crew or bystanders. This information gives an understanding of the magnitude and direction of forces sustained by the patient and therefore the likely magnitude of injury. Many injuries will be self-evident but the true value of the history of injury lies in alerting the surgeon to injuries that he might otherwise have overlooked. This may then prevent him from underestimating a severe injury which appears to be minor at initial presentation. Typical pointers to severe injury in road accidents include:

- death of other occupants of the car,
- expulsion of the injured patient from the vehicle,
- marked deformation of the passenger compartment of the car.

The history of injury may indicate specific injuries also, for example, a car passenger on the impact side of a vehicle should be examined closely for evidence of broken ribs or injury to the lung or abdominal viscera on that side. Likewise injuries tend to run in certain patterns. A patient with injuries to the right side of the head, the right arm, fractured ribs on the right side and a fractured right femur should be reassessed very carefully to see whether or not there are signs of liver injury!

Blunt and penetrating injuries

For more details refer to Chapter 6.

Blunt and penetrating injuries can cause different management problems, although the principles of immediate resuscitation, rapid diagnosis and definitive treatment apply to both. Blunt injury accounts for about 80% of major injuries in surgical practice in the UK but only about 50% of injuries in metropolitan trauma practice in the USA. Blunt injuries are associated with greater surrounding tissue damage. This damaged tissue contributes to the systemic response to injury (see below), but in addition considerable volumes of extracellular fluid, as well as blood, can be lost into this tissue and require i.v. replacement. Clearly, the proportion depends on the environment. Often injuries have both blunt and penetrating components. For example, following a road traffic accident, a fractured rib end can penetrate lung or liver and similarly, following a typical penetrating injury (knife or gunshot), blunt injuries may have been caused by other blows, a fall or a blast.

Blast injuries from explosives have their own particular problems. Injuries are seen due to the blast wind (which can cause pneumothorax or eardrum perforation in addition to gross bodily disruption) and burns can also occur from the heat of the blast.

Gunshot injuries cause their own particular problems also. Bullets or other missiles (shell fragments, pellets) follow an unpredictable course through the body, depending on the flight of the projectile, the point of entry and internal ricochets. The speed of the missile is also a major determinant of the amount of injury caused. High-velocity missiles (typically a rifle bullet) cause a phenomenon known as cavitation around the missile track. The energy dissipated from the bullet creates a temporary space damaging viscera in its path and a vacuum occurs within this temporary space sucking in debris and clothing. The consequence of this is that there is an unpredictable area of dead tissue around the obvious missile track and it is almost inevitable that this dead tissue will be infected. It is therefore necessary to clean this track adequately and to excise the dead tissue. This may take several operations in addition to adequate antibiotic and antitetanus therapy. It should be emphasised that antibiotics cannot replace the role of surgery here and this lesson has had to be relearned at the expense of many soldiers' lives during times of conflict.

INVESTIGATIONS AND DEFINITIVE CARE

The aim of trauma management is to treat all injuries definitively at the ideal time and in many cases this means as quickly as possible. In progressing beyond this general principle, it will be clear that some injuries require *immediate* intervention at the time of diagnosis (e.g. tension pneumothorax), others require *prompt surgery* perhaps following selective investigation (e.g. surgery for a bleeding spleen diagnosed by peritoneal lavage), whereas the treatment of others (e.g. complex plastic reconstruction) may be able to wait some hours or even days. In general terms, however, prompt surgery reduces haemorrhage, restores the individual towards recovery at an earlier stage and thereby reduces mortality and morbidity.

The most seriously injured patients have, or are suspected of having, multiple injuries and it is often necessary to conduct investigations to diagnose all the relevant injuries. Some investigations will be needed to confirm or exclude diagnoses that are considered likely in a particular patient. A focused multidisciplinary approach remains necessary at this stage because priorities differ between individual patients. A diagnostic test used in any situation will have to be tailored to the facilities and degree of urgency of the case. Although it is unusual for a diagnostic test or operation to harm the patient directly, the performance of a low priority procedure at the wrong time can be detrimental to the patient because other more pressing injuries will be left untreated at that time. An example of this might be performing a negative laparotomy for suspected abdominal haemorrhage while bleeding continues steadily into the chest or into major long-bone fractures.

Head injury

For more details refer to Chapter 19.

Head injury is common and accounts for 125 000 hospital admissions each year in the UK. It is a common cause of death among patients with multiple injuries. Head injuries and their management raise a number of principles of trauma care but perhaps the most notable is the phenomenon of secondary injury. *Primary injury* denotes the damage caused to the patient by the accident itself whereas *secondary injury* refers to further tissue damage which takes place at a later stage as a result of *tissue hypoxia*. Without good management, this is a common problem in head injury (and in many other forms of injury) and can, on its own, convert a moderate injury into a fatal one.

Only a minority of head injuries are open, that is, a wound that penetrates all the layers of the skull and exposes the brain. By their nature, these tend to follow penetrating injury and may be caused by a sharp stone corner, knife or bullet. The survivable injuries tend to be localised and damage limited. The patient is often conscious and requires referral to a neurosurgeon to have the defect closed under antibiotic cover in order to prevent infection. Brain scarring (gliosis) occurs and post-traumatic epilepsy is common. Prophylactic anticonvulsant therapy may be needed.

Closed head injuries comprise the majority. These can be subdivided into:
- The commoner form, *concussional injury*, where the brain is contused or even lacerated following a blunt blow to the head. The brain is additionally injured when it moves and strikes the opposite side of the skull as a result of the force imparted by the original blow (*contrecoup injury*). There may simply be tissue swelling around contused areas or, alternatively, a significant degree of haemorrhage may result. This intracranial bleeding can occur in a number of well-defined sites and causes its own particular problems due to rapid rises in intracranial pressure.
- *Diffuse axonal injury* (*DAI*) occurs when deceleration forces cause a shearing injury to the brain tissue, usually in a car accident and sometimes without any direct head trauma. This is diagnosed when there is an absence of focal damage

on computed tomography (CT) scan but obviously a degree of DAI can coexist with contusions under appropriate circumstances. DAI is seen in 40–50% of all severe head injuries and perhaps one-third of these patients will die.

Pathophysiology

The brain is particularly prone to secondary injury for two reasons:

1. Neurones are exquisitely sensitive to hypoxia.
2. The rigid confines of the cranium expose the neural tissue to a number of related risks from elevated intracranial pressure after injury.

Neural tissue reacts to injury (primary or secondary) by swelling. Being a rigid box, the skull has a fixed volume and under normal circumstances there is relatively little free space around the brain within the skull. When brain swelling occurs, the only compensatory mechanisms that delay a rise in intracranial pressure are the expulsion of cerebrospinal fluid (CSF) or diminution in blood volume. *Retention of CO₂*, perhaps due to depressed conscious level, results in *cerebral vasodilatation* and will tend to increase cerebral blood volume. Similarly hypoxia, from whatever cause, will lead to secondary brain injury and more severe oedema. Although hypovolaemia from other injuries might appear to exert a protective effect, in fact the *autoregulation* of the brain preserves cerebral blood flow to the point where further hypovolaemia results in diminished neural perfusion with aggravation of secondary injury. Thus, with the exception of displacement of CSF, there is little that can be done to delay an increase in intracranial pressure. As intracranial pressure rises, there is a *reflex increase* in systemic arterial blood pressure (*Cushing's reflex*) in order to maintain cerebral perfusion. If intracranial pressure increases further, it ultimately becomes impossible for cerebral perfusion to be maintained and the state of brain death is entered.

More commonly, localised tissue damage results in local elevations of intracranial pressure which cause herniation of brain tissue either from side to side beneath the falx or downwards and out through the foramen magnum. These focal elevations of intracranial pressure may be caused by contusion, but most commonly, they are caused by an intracranial haematoma. *Intracranial haematomas* may be classified as extradural, subdural or intracerebral depending on their anatomical location but all exert a mass effect. The effects, particularly of an extradural haematoma are quite typical. *Extradural haematomas* occur most commonly in the region of the middle meningeal artery, where the artery has been disrupted by a fracture to the temporal bone. The haematoma compresses the lateral aspect of the brain forcing the ipsilateral uncus of the temporal lobe downwards through the central gap in the tentorium which is usually occupied by the midbrain. This compression of the midbrain results in disturbances of consciousness as well as abnormalities of respiration and contralateral motor weakness. The third nerve runs around over the edge of the tentorium ear and

will be compressed, resulting in dilatation of the ipsilateral pupil. Whatever the cause of intracranial pressure, once massive herniation of the vital structures of the hypothalamus and brainstem are forced downward through the foramen magnum (a process known as *coning*), death results.

Interventions must obviously be undertaken to prevent intracranial pressure reaching this level and these depend on whether the elevation is focal or generalised:

*   *Focal swellings*, such as an extradural haematoma, need immediate diagnosis and prompt surgical evacuations (see below).
*   *Generalised elevations* of intracranial pressure, such as may occur following multiple contusions or DAI, need systemic measures to try and manipulate the homeostatic mechanisms. It is essential that:
    *   Any secondary injury is reversed or at least limited by the correction of *hypoxia* and *hypovolaemia*.
    *   Any *hypercarbia* is eliminated by, if necessary, the institution of mechanical ventilation. The CO_2 level is returned to normal.
    *   Existing brain swelling is limited by the administration of *mannitol* which is an osmotic diuretic.

During the phase of assessment of a patient with raised intracranial pressure an urgent CT scan will have been obtained to ensure there is no focal lesion. In Western practice, it is now customary to insert a transcranial catheter to measure intracranial pressure such that further interventions can be undertaken to limit any further increases which might cause a perilous reduction in cerebral perfusion pressure. Certain expert units have advocated a more precise measurement of cerebral perfusion by assessing jugular venous bulb oxygen content.

Criteria for admission, investigation and referral
Admission

Many patients present to hospital with a history of head injuries and only a minority require admission. Indications for admission are:

*   patients who cannot be adequately assessed or discharged to the care of an appropriate adult;
*   patients who are unwell or who have a risk of later deterioration from an intracranial haematoma;
*   patients who are confused or have a depressed level of consciousness at the time of examination;
*   patients who lost consciousness or who have suffered amnesia of >5 min duration;
*   presence of abnormal neurological findings;
*   the existence of other diseases such as diabetes;
*   skull fracture.

Most patients will recover completely within 24 h and it is usual that complications show themselves within this time, so patients can usually be discharged after this period. The presence of a *skull fracture* mandates admission and any patient with significant scalp contusion should have a skull X-ray series because fractures are associated with an increased risk of intracranial haematoma. Patients who have a fracture will require admission and either a CT scan or a longer period of observation. A lower threshold is maintained for the admission and investigation of children as they are harder to assess and the linkage between skull fracture and intracranial haematoma is less clear-cut. When any patient is discharged after a head injury, the adult assuming responsibility for them is given a head injury warning card which details warning symptoms and signs for which they should look.

Investigation

The primary aim of CT scanning following head injury is to diagnose intracranial haematomas and thereby allow their treatment as quickly as possible.

Head-injured patients are assessed serially using the Glasgow Coma Score (GCS) scale (Table 7.1). Severe head injury is defined as a GCS 8 or less. Urgent CT scanning is required for all patients who have:

- moderate (GCS 9–12) or severe (GCS ⩽ 8) head injury;
- focal neurological signs;
- sustained an epileptic fit following injury;
- a fractured skull or penetrating injury.

Patients who continue with a depressed conscious level for >6 h and any patient who suffers a deterioration of a GCS by ⩾2 points should undergo immediate reassessment and a further CT scan.

Referral

CT scanning is available in most hospitals but neurosurgical support is usually centralised. Neurosurgeons will usually wish to know about any patient who has any of the following features (see also Chapter 19):

- abnormal CT scan,
- depressed conscious level >6 h,
- deterioration in conscious level,
- fractured skull with persisting symptoms or signs including seizures or CSF leakage,
- penetrating wounds,
- any compound fracture.

Before transferring a patient it is obviously essential to ensure that there is no other life-threatening event which will kill the patient en-route, such as continuing haemorrhage or an insufficiently protected airway. Most patients who are ill enough to require neurosurgical transfer need to undergo intubation and ventilation before leaving the referring hospital but this will depend on other injuries and should be discussed with the neurosurgeon.

The outcome from head injury depends on the severity of the primary injury and on the development of any complications. *Extradural haematomas* have received much attention because they are a fatal condition which is often associated with relatively little underlying damage to the brain. Typically, the patient will have sustained a modest head injury with perhaps a brief period of unconsciousness. They then recover before lapsing into progressive coma as the haematoma swells. These occur in perhaps 2% of all severe head injuries but the prognosis is good so long as the condition is recognised and treated promptly.

Subdural haematomas carry a much higher mortality of perhaps 50%. This is because these are associated with more severe primary injuries. *Intracerebral haematomas* are seen as a result of laceration and contusion of the brain itself and also carry a higher mortality. Blood may also be seen within the subarachnoid space but is not itself a particularly bad prognostic feature. Overall some 40% of patients with severe head injuries die.

Spinal injury

For more details refer to Chapter 19.

Injury to the spine is of importance primarily because of the potentially catastrophic effects of damage to the spinal cord. It is by no means always accompanied by neurological damage, but because of the severe and usually permanent effects of neurological injury, it is essential to assume that the possibility of spinal instability exists in almost all injured patients until this can be satisfactorily excluded. Occasionally, neurological injury can occur, particularly in children, without there being an associated spinal fracture.

Most spinal injuries are caused by road traffic accidents, falls or during sport. Many patients sustain a whiplash injury to the soft tissues and ligaments following road accidents, but bony and neurological injuries are more likely when the occupant has been ejected from the vehicle or suffered head injury. Falls from a height, either onto the head or feet, can cause spinal injury, whilst swimming (particularly diving) and horse riding, in addition to contact sports, give rise to a significant number of spinal injuries each year.

Table 7.1. GCS is the sum of the best eye, motor and verbal response.

Best eye response (4)	1. No eye opening
	2. Eye opening to pain
	3. Eye opening to verbal commands
	4. Eyes open spontaneously
Best verbal response (5)	1. No verbal response
	2. Incomprehensible sounds
	3. Inappropriate words
	4. Confused
	5. Orientated
Best motor response (6)	1. No motor response
	2. Extension to pain
	3. Flexion to pain
	4. Withdrawal from pain
	5. Localising pain
	6. Obeys commands

The spine can be injured by any excessive abnormal motion, be it flexion, extension, lateral movement or rotation. Direct compression can also cause bony damage during a fall from a height. Whether or not the spinal cord is injured depends on the severity of the original trauma, the instability (and hence degree of movement of the fragments) of the bony injury and the anatomical site at which the injury occurs. Certain patterns of bony injury, particularly those associated with disruption of anterior and posterior ligaments or fractures of the vertebrae which involve the bony columns in front of and behind the spinal cord, are more likely to be unstable, but a detailed account of this is beyond the scope of this book and it is safest for the inexperienced to assume that all injuries are unstable to begin with.

The cervical spine is the site most commonly injured on account of its exposed position and the leverage applied by sudden movement of the head relative to the body. There is, however, more room around the spinal cord within the cervical spine and this protects against some damage. The thoracic spine is strong and rigidly held by the supporting ribs but when fracture does occur, concomitant neurological damage is seen more frequently. The spinal cord ends at the level of the *second lumbar vertebra* and injury below this will only damage the *cauda equina*. These are lower motor neurone fibres and as such have the capacity to regenerate.

Clinical features

Patients with spinal injury may present complaining of localised pain, limitation of movement or distal neurological signs. More commonly, however, the patient is unconscious or obtunded and is unable to recount any symptoms. The onus is then on the clinician to maintain a high index of suspicion. Patients particularly likely to have suffered cervical spine injury include those who:

- are unconscious,
- have sustained a significant head or facial injury,
- have local complaints or signs regarding the neck,
- have abnormal neurological findings distally.

Clinical features suggesting spinal injury include bogginess or swelling, particularly posteriorly, while a step or gap may be felt in the normally orderly progression of vertebral spinal processes. Neurological findings include distal weakness or abnormal sensations. There may be a clear sensory cut-off with numbness below a certain dermatomal level, which indicates the level of damage to the spinal cord:

- When injury occurs above the level of C3, all ventilatory muscles will be paralysed and the patient will die.
- When injury occurs in the lower cervical cord, only diaphragmatic breathing will be possible.

Certain incomplete patterns of spinal cord injury are seen and these usually carry a better prognosis. Typical clinical findings include sparing of sensation in the sacral and perineal area. When the cord is damaged, the autonomic nerve supply is also injured. This results in vasodilatation and this in turn aggravates hypotension causing neurogenic shock. This will often be compounded by hypovolaemia from concomitant injuries. Urinary retention may occur and, on occasion, priapism is seen.

Investigation

The usual minimum investigation of the cervical spine is a three-film series, including:

1. a lateral view which shows the upper border of the first thoracic vertebra;
2. an anteroposterior view;
3. a view of the odontoid peg.

When the upper border of T1 cannot be seen using conventional imaging, a special axillary view (swimmer's view) can be used; alternatively a CT scan of the cervical spine may be required. Anteroposterior and lateral views of the thoracic and lumbar spines are obtained as clinically indicated.

Management

As the great majority of patients with cervical spine injury present either unconscious or with multiple injuries, the accepted safe management policy is to immobilise at least the cervical spine of all patients who are at risk. This is achieved either by:

- manually maintaining the head in the neutral anatomical position relative to the body;
- protecting the cervical spine in a semi-rigid collar of appropriate size and fixing the head by supporting it on either side by sandbags and immobilising it with stout tape across the forehead.

Increasingly, entire spinal immobilisation is practised using custom-made spinal boards. The cervical and, if necessary, the whole spine is kept immobilised until adequate radiological imaging has been examined by a competent specialist and considered normal.

This rigorous approach to spinal immobilisation is necessary in order to prevent the catastrophe of secondary injury occurring. This is where a patient with an unstable cervical spine but as yet no neurological damage, suffers neurological injury during resuscitative attempts. This is particularly likely to occur during:

- extrication at the scene of the accident;
- injudicious attempts at intubation with excessive movement of the cervical spine;
- inappropriate handling or mobilisation at a later stage.

In patients with a suspected cervical spine injury, the airway can be opened using a gentle jaw thrust manoeuvre but expert help should be obtained for intubation whenever possible. The safe technique of 'log-rolling' the patient minimises the risk of further injury.

No specific neurological treatments exist for established injury although steroids may help limit damage. The patient should thus be resuscitated according to standard principles and adequate oxygenation and perfusion maintained. Bony injuries will require stabilisation and in some cases operative fixation.

Penetrating neck injuries

The neck is an exposed but confined anatomical area which contains several vital structures in close proximity. These factors make stab wounds a relatively common clinical problem. Many knife wounds fail to penetrate the *platysma* and as such, do not damage vital structures. Wounds which have penetrated more deeply, may or may not cause vital damage and the signs of important internal injuries may or may not be obvious at presentation.

Management is along the prioritised guidelines outlined above. *ABC* must be corrected and maintained by whatever methods necessary and then a subsequent detailed search made for other injuries as clinically appropriate:

- Obvious open injury to the airway (*larynx or trachea*) may require intubation if possible or, occasionally, emergency cricothyroidotomy or tracheostomy below the site of injury. Knife wounds in the neck may pass downwards to cause *pneumothorax* or *haemothorax*, the latter through injury to the subclavian vessels which are notoriously difficult to control either by external pressure or at surgery, because of their protected course behind the clavicle.
- *Haemorrhage* is more commonly due to injury to the jugular vein or carotid artery or branches thereof. This may present as brisk or exsanguinating haemorrhage or as an expanding haematoma. Venous bleeding may show itself as dark blood rapidly welling from the depths of a wound when it is exposed or explored injudiciously in the emergency department. Open wounds of the jugular veins also expose the patient to the risk of air embolus. *Haemorrhage* and *embolism* are both prevented by simple pressure. Due to these risks it is usual for neck wounds to be briefly inspected in the emergency room. If they clearly penetrate the platysma then further exploration in the operating theatre is necessary.

Penetrating wounds of the neck may also injure the many *nerves* within the neck, the *thoracic duct* or the *oesophagus*. These injuries may be obvious or may be suspected from relevant clinical signs, for example, haematemesis or dysphagia in the case of oesophageal injury. Unstable patients are transferred to the operating theatre for further management. Stable patients can undergo urgent but selective investigation of systems which are believed to be injured. This might include angiography, gastrografin swallow or laryngoscopy. It is a general principle of trauma care that unstable patients are not subjected to prolonged investigation in the relatively unsafe environment of the radiology department.

Patients with deep neck wounds but without signs of specific visceral damage can be treated conservatively. If worrisome signs do not appear following a period of observation (24 h), then it is safe to discharge these patients. Wound toilet would have been carried out at an early stage but a further principle of trauma management is illustrated here, namely that multiple investigations to look for theoretically possible but not clinical suspected injuries are not necessary.

Chest injuries

For more details refer to Chapter 16.

Chest injuries are very common, being seen in roughly 50% of multiply injured patients. Chest injuries cause problems via three mechanisms:
1. hypoxia,
2. haemorrhage,
3. obstruction to circulatory flow (cardiac tamponade).

Chest injuries can be caused by either blunt or penetrating mechanisms and the pattern of visceral damage varies accordingly. Treatment principles remain very similar and in summary comprise:

- provision of supplementary oxygen,
- prompt drainage of any collection of pleural blood or air,
- aspiration of any pericardial fluid,
- performance of a thoracotomy for continuing massive haemorrhage.

This last intervention is relatively rarely required and simpler interventions are all that will be required in the great majority of patients, provided these are carried out with sufficient speed.

The two principal diagnostic techniques are firstly clinical evaluation and re-evaluation, and secondly the chest radiograph. Acquiring a system by which chest radiographs can be assessed quickly when under pressure is well worthwhile.

Rib fractures

Many patients present with fractured ribs: the range of severity is wide. When uncomplicated by visceral damage, fractured ribs cause the same problems as chest wall contusion, that is, *hypoxia* and *retained pulmonary secretions* as a result of painful breathing. Adequate analgesia (e.g. from intercostal blockade) is used with physiotherapy to facilitate sputum clearance. Supplementary oxygen will be necessary and even two or three simple fractures can cause major difficulties for patients with chronic lung disease.

Open injuries to the chest wall create their own problems, particularly when the defect is more than a few centimetres in diameter. Here, air enters preferentially through the abnormal hole and a tension-type pneumothorax may develop, impairing the mechanics of breathing. This is known as a *sucking chest wound* and immediate treatment by placement of a chest drain at a remote site and covering the hole with flap valve dressing is needed.

Rib fractures also serve as a marker for *underlying visceral damage*. Laceration of an intercostal artery associated with rib fractures is one of the commonest sources of continuing intrathoracic haemorrhage necessitating thoracotomy (see below). The upper ribs are short and difficult to break and fracture indicates severe injury and carries with it a likelihood of damage to major vessels in the root of the neck or mediastinum. Fractures of the middle ribs (4–9) suggest damage to the lung (contusion, pneumothorax, haemothorax), while injuries to the lower ribs are often associated with damage to the abdominal viscera, particularly the liver and spleen.

When more than three adjacent ribs are broken at two sites, the intervening section of the chest wall becomes loose and moves independently. This is known as a *flail segment* and even a small flail segment can greatly compromise the mechanics of breathing resulting in hypoxia and intrapulmonary blood shunting. When ventilation is compromised, artificial ventilation is employed both to support the work of breathing and also to make the flail move in unison with the rest of the chest wall. This permits healing to take place.

Pulmonary contusion

Not surprisingly blunt injuries to the chest wall are often associated with pulmonary contusion. The cardinal feature of pulmonary contusion is that radiographic signs are minimal at the time of initial assessment. Radiological and clinical features only appear over the ensuing 24–72 h and this can result in 'sudden' deterioration once the period of most intensive observation has passed. There is *no specific therapy* and the routine supportive methods of oxygen supplementation, analgesia, physiotherapy and adequate ventilatory support are the mainstays of treatment. The impact of any pulmonary contusion depends on the presence of any pre-existing lung disease. This is also worsened by lung congestion as may occur with pulmonary oedema due to over-transfusion or, more commonly, due to post-traumatic or septic *adult respiratory distress syndrome* (ARDS).

Pneumothoraces

The importance of immediate treatment of a tension pneumothorax by needle and then formal chest tube drainage is described above. Simple pneumothoraces are much more common and should, in general, be treated by placement of a chest drain following injury. Simple pneumothoraces are particularly prone to 'tension' during general anaesthesia or air transport. Whenever possible, drains should be inserted in the anterior axillary line at about the 4th or 5th interspace and the use of a trocar to insert the drain is completely unacceptable because of the risk of impalement injury. Occasionally, the lung will not re-expand despite adequate placement of a chest drain and in these cases a major bronchial injury must be suspected. This may require the placement of a second drain, with both attached to low-grade suction. Ventilatory support will be needed while arrangements are made for bronchial repair.

Haemothoraces

A haemothorax may exist on its own or in conjunction with a pneumothorax depending on the cause. Common sources of haemorrhage include:
- intercostal vessels,
- the lungs,
- the major vessels of the mediastinum.

It is advisable to obtain vascular access before draining a clinically suspected haemothorax. If bleeding continues after drainage of >1 l or if slower haemorrhage continues (100–200 ml/h for >2–3 h), or if the patient remains shocked with no other source of haemorrhage, then a thoracotomy is advisable. In general, a lateral thoracotomy should be undertaken on the side of the injury but expert help should be obtained whenever time and circumstances permit.

Aortic transection

Aortic transection occurs quite commonly, particularly following *high-speed vehicle accidents* in which there is *sudden deceleration*. Only 10–20% of patients reach hospital alive but in these patients the rupture is contained and surgical repair is feasible. The diagnosis is suspected primarily from the widening of the mediastinum seen on the chest X-ray and a definitive diagnosis is made by arch aortography. There is some urgency about aortic repair as these patients are not stable and delayed rupture does occur. However, a balance must be struck between over hasty intervention and delay and some experts now favour a semi-urgent operation in cases where there is benefit to be gained from a more prolonged period of stabilisation of other injuries.

Blunt thoracic injury may also rupture the *oesophagus* or *diaphragm* or cause *myocardial contusion*. The latter may present with hypotension, dysrhythmia or sudden arrest. Penetrating injuries may also damage any of these viscera. While knife tracks are usually predictable, those of missiles are often less so. This makes the surgical approach to the chest difficult to plan as, unlike the abdomen, the incision greatly influences the access obtained. In certain gunshot injuries, further imaging may help to plan surgery but this is, of course, only feasible in the stable patient. *Penetrating injuries* also account for the great majority of *pericardial tamponades* (see above). On occasion thoracotomy will be necessary in the resuscitation room to save life. This rule only applies to patients who have sustained penetrating wounds (usually stab injuries) to the chest and who arrive with signs of life. If these patients undergo cardiac arrest within the resuscitation room, then opening the chest will permit haemorrhage, usually from the heart, to be controlled digitally until the operating theatre can be reached, sutures can be placed or expert help arrives. Opening the chest of patients with blunt thoracic trauma outwith the operating theatre is not usually associated with survival.

Abdominal trauma

For more details refer to Chapter 12.

Injury to the abdomen can cause death rapidly from *haemorrhage* or at a later stage from *sepsis*. It is unusual for abdominal injury to cause death before arrival at hospital and a window of opportunity for treatment therefore exists in most patients. Problems arise, however, because the diagnosis of abdominal injury is often less than straightforward.

Clinical signs can be misleading in 30–50% of cases and consequently a range of investigative tools have developed to assist the surgeon in achieving a diagnosis. It should be stated clearly, however, that when unequivocal evidence of abdominal injury in an unstable patient is found, laparotomy should usually be undertaken without further delay, that is, for:

- gunshot wound of the abdomen,
- gastrointestinal perforation,
- hypotension or shock due to abdominal injury,
- protrusion of viscera through a stab wound.

Patients shown to have abdominal injury by the investigations described below should also usually undergo operation.

Before considering the various investigative modalities, it is pertinent to recall the anatomy of the abdomen. The abdomen extends up as far as the nipple or fourth costal interspace and a significant proportion of the commonly injured abdominal viscera lie within the confines of the bony thorax. Thus injuries to the chest and abdomen frequently coexist and one may complicate the other. Fractured lower ribs are indicative of abdominal trauma. Similarly, the abdomen extends down within the bony pelvis and injuries to the buttocks or perineum can involve abdominal viscera. Although many of the organs are clothed in peritoneum, the retroperitoneal organs can also be damaged and because of their position may not cause free bleeding or leakage of contents into the peritoneal cavity and this will therefore be missed by certain investigations. Although injuries to the anterior abdominal wall predominate, it must be remembered that injuries also occur to the flank and back where there are thicker protective layers of body wall but where injuries may be harder to diagnose, but with no less serious consequences if overlooked.

When there is doubt about the presence or absence of abdominal injury, further investigation is indicated. This doubt may arise because of equivocal clinical signs, inability of the patient to respond on account of injury, drugs or anaesthesia or where the future inaccessibility of the patient (by prolonged non-abdominal operation or interhospital transfer) makes the firm exclusion of suspected abdominal injury necessary.

Investigation
Diagnostic peritoneal lavage
Diagnostic peritoneal lavage (DPL) is the best studied investigation. This involves the instillation of 1 l of warmed saline into the adult abdomen to look for the presence of blood or intestinal contents. The fluid is siphoned out after a few minutes and inspected. Clear criteria for a positive test exist:

- >10 ml of free blood on opening the peritoneum;
- >100 000 red blood cells/mm^3 or >500 white blood cells/mm^3 in the aspirated lavage;
- bowel contents in the abdomen.

Criteria other than these reduce the sensitivity and specificity of the test. DPL is extremely sensitive to the presence of blood within the abdominal cavity. Indeed, as many minor injuries to the liver and spleen cause a small amount of haemorrhage which then stops spontaneously, the test is oversensitive and may prompt unnecessary laparotomy to stop further bleeding in 20–30% of cases. A further drawback of DPL is that it cannot assess the retroperitoneal viscera. These problems aside, DPL remains useful because it can be quickly performed in almost any setting and is sometimes useful in rapidly defining priorities in an unstable and multiply injured patient. A positive DPL indicates the need for prompt laparotomy.

Ultrasound
Ultrasound scanning of the abdomen is safe, cheap and quick but suffers from the principal drawback of undue reliance on the ultrasonographer's experience and ability. Ultrasound is really only able to identify the *presence or absence of fluid* within the abdomen and specific injuries can seldom be seen. Ultrasound is also associated with a modest rate of missed significant injuries (2–10%). Ultrasound can be useful in identifying significant volumes of abdominal fluid where injury is suspected and thus direct priorities, but extreme caution should be observed in permitting the findings of a single ultrasound scan to override other clinical pointers.

Computed tomography
In many ways CT scanning is the best investigation for the *stable trauma patient*. CT can identify specific organ injury and the presence of free blood and can image the retroperitoneum and the pelvic viscera. The principal limitation of the technique is the need to move the patient to an often isolated and potentially hazardous part of the hospital. CT scanning is therefore only indicated in otherwise stable patients.

Laparoscopy
Laparoscopy has gained popularity in recent years for many surgical procedures and it has been used in an attempt to diagnose abdominal injury. It has even been used on occasion to repair diaphragmatic stab wounds. Although local anaesthetic techniques using mini-laparoscopes have been described, these have not gained widespread popularity and the limitation of the technique is the need to administer a general anaesthetic to otherwise stable patients. Again laparoscopy is really only indicated in stable individuals and its main use has been in identifying whether or not equivocal stab and gunshot wounds have reached the peritoneal cavity. This remains controversial and the true role of laparoscopy for trauma has yet to emerge.

Laparotomy
Laparotomy should be used sparingly as a method to detect abdominal injuries that would otherwise be missed. Laparotomy itself can cause complications but of more concern is that carrying out a negative laparotomy will divert attention from the injuries that are the true source of a

patient's deterioration and thus expose the patient to a greater risk of death and complications.

Management

Abdominal gunshot wounds should be treated by routine laparotomy because of the high (>90%) incidence of visceral damage.

The same cannot be said of stab wounds. Anterior abdominal stab wounds clearly require operation if there are signs of shock, peritonitis or visceral protrusion (omentum excluded). In the equivocal case, the choice lies between serial clinical examination and further investigation. The investigations of choice are exploration of the local wound to see if the peritoneum is breached and if so, DPL or one of the other investigations mentioned above:

- Wound exploration should be undertaken by a surgeon competent to carry out a laparotomy should this be necessary and blind probing of the wound is uninformative and dangerous. If wound exploration is carried out, it should be performed under adequate anaesthesia, in an appropriate environment and through an adequate incision.
- The sensitivity of DPL in stab wounds is somewhat lower, at 91%, compared with 98% in blunt trauma, but this is obviously still a valuable pointer. Stab wounds of the flank or back are less likely to cause signs of peritoneal irritation or injury and are less commonly associated with visceral damage, but serious injuries do occur. This possibility should be remembered and the indications for operation are the same as for anterior abdominal wall stab wounds.
- Investigation by triple contrast CT scan (oral, rectal, i.v.) can help in the diagnosis of retroperitoneal injury to the duodenum, great vessels or colon.

Not all abdominal injuries show themselves in the 'golden hour' and an essential part of surgical management therefore is *frequent reassessment* of the patient with an injured abdomen following admission to hospital.

Stable patients may show clinical features or injury patterns that suggest particular injuries. These can be investigated using specific techniques. Examples are:

- *Water-soluble radiological contrast* examination of the upper gastrointestinal tract to look for duodenal rupture in a patient with blood in the nasogastric aspirate.
- *Ascending urethrography* to look for urethral damage in patients with clinical signs suggestive thereof (blood at the external meatus, perineal bruising, boggy prostate on rectal examination, certain pelvic fractures).

Serum *amylase* should be checked in all patients with abdominal injury as this is an indicator of, but not diagnostic for pancreatic or duodenal trauma. The investigation of pancreatic and duodenal trauma is notoriously unreliable and CT scanning in stable patients remains the best option. Apart from indicating urethral damage, rectal examination may show evidence of spinal cord damage (sphincter paralysis) or gastrointestinal bleeding.

The history of the injury mechanism and the pattern of associated bony injuries can both provide valuable pointers to abdominal visceral damage. For example, fractured lower ribs are associated with damage to the liver and spleen; lumbar spinal fractures suggest pancreaticoduodenal injury; and patients with injuries to the left arm, left chest and left leg are extremely likely to have injury to viscera on the left side of the abdomen (spleen!).

Once the indication for laparotomy has been established, it is important that this is carried out expeditiously. Priorities for intervention need to be discussed between all doctors involved in the care of a patient but it is often the case that thoraco-abdominal injuries take precedence over neurosurgical and orthopaedic injuries simply because the patient is likely to die more rapidly from these.

A *long midline incision* provides the access of choice and it is usual to evacuate the free blood and place packs in each area of the abdomen before removing these sequentially. If the patient is in extremis then the packs can be left in place while the anaesthetist catches up with some of the blood loss. Severe arterial haemorrhage can be controlled by clamping the aorta at the aortic hiatus or, on rare occasion, by accessing the descending thoracic aorta through an emergency left thoracotomy. The abdomen should be fully explored, including opening the lesser sac. Depending on the individual case, it may be necessary to mobilise the right or left colon in order to access the vena cava, the renal pedicles or other retroperitoneal structures.

It is important to avoid unduly prolonged operations in unstable patients as the combined effects of massive transfusion, injury and the open abdomen lead to hypothermia, coagulopathy and acidosis. These combine to precipitate organ failure and it is now recognised that the concept of '*damage-control surgery*' has much to offer. This means that in multiply injured patients the least operative intervention immediately necessary is undertaken in order to stabilise the patient. This might mean controlling haemorrhage by packing and simply closing perforations rather than resecting damaged intestine. The abdomen is temporarily closed and the patient transferred to the intensive care unit for correction of the systemic derangements mentioned above. The patient is then returned to the operating theatre within 24–48 h for definitive surgical intervention.

Certain injuries to the liver, spleen and kidney stop bleeding spontaneously and this has led to the selective adoption of a *conservative treatment* programme in certain patients. Provided other indications for laparotomy are not present and the patient can be easily stabilised, when these injuries are diagnosed by CT scanning the patient can be treated without operative intervention provided haemorrhage does not continue. This conservative management must be an active process in that the patient must be managed in an intensive care unit with immediate access to the operating theatre should the patient deteriorate or haemorrhage briskly or in a prolonged fashion. Using this technique, many expert centres have been able to avoid laparotomy in 75–90% of such patients.

Patients who have a laparotomy for *liver injury* are often best treated by perihepatic packing for several reasons. First, some complex liver injuries will stop bleeding when packed for 36–48 h. Secondly, the delay permits correction of coagulopathy and hypothermia, and thirdly it becomes possible to transfer the patient to a specialist liver surgeon. When the patient arrives at the liver unit, he may undergo hepatic angiography and possible embolisation before removal of the packs. Some of the more severe liver injuries, particularly those that involve the retrohepatic vena cava, are not amenable to packing. One possible intervention here is to insert a vascular shunt from the infrahepatic cava into the right atrium in order to isolate the liver while repair is attempted. Not surprisingly, this is successful in <10% of cases, even in expert hands.

Whereas conservative management of liver injury is pursued on account of the morbidity and mortality associated with liver debridement or resection, conservative treatment of *splenic injury* is favoured because of the rare but dramatic effect of post-splenectomy sepsis. Patients who have had their spleens removed, particularly children, are prone to overwhelming infection by *encapsulated bacteria* such as pneumococci. When conservative management is inappropriate, splenic repair (splenorrhaphy) or partial splenectomy is favoured when the operator is familiar with the necessary techniques. Patients who require *splenectomy* should be protected from infection by the prescription of oral penicillin and by immunisation against the relevant bacteria 6 weeks after operation.

Duodenum and pancreas
The duodenum and pancreas are usually injured during road traffic accidents by *compression* of the seatbelt against the vertebral column. The second part of the duodenum may rupture and the pancreas may split across the neck of the gland. Diagnosis of duodenal injury is suspected in patients with blood-stained nasogastric aspirate and is confirmed by water-soluble contrast examination. Pancreatic injury is suspected by raised serum amylase and confirmed by operation, CT scanning or endoscopic retrograde cholangiopancreatography (ERCP). The techniques of surgical intervention for pancreatico-duodenal trauma are beyond this text but suffice it to say that resection carries a formidable mortality and various techniques of repair, diversion and tube drainage are preferred, when possible.

Intestine, rectum and anus
The small intestine can be simply managed by repair or resection as needed but colonic injury may be more taxing. Injuries to the retroperitoneal colon can be easily overlooked, whether caused by blunt trauma or by penetrating flank or back wounds. Exteriorisation is the *procedure of safety* and should certainly be performed when there is delay in operating, devitalised tissue or significant contamination. Rectal injuries may be caused by pelvic fracture, penetrating wounds or the insertion of foreign bodies through the anus. Contrast radiological examination can confirm rectal perforation in the doubtful case and treatment consists of *defunctioning* by

sigmoid colostomy, rectal lavage and presacral drainage. Injury to the anal sphincters should be treated similarly by defunctioning and cleansing and definitive repair undertaken thereafter by a coloproctologist.

Kidney, bladder and urinary tract
For more details refer to Chapter 17.

Most injuries of the kidneys are minor and result from blunt trauma to the loin. Minor haematuria which resolves quickly does not need further investigation. More severe haematuria or loin haematoma can be investigated in the resuscitation room by a single-shot i.v. urogram (primarily to show the presence of a contralateral functioning kidney) or, more commonly, by contrast-enhanced CT scanning. CT scanning has the advantage of showing both structure and function. Kidneys avulsed from their vascular pedicle usually need to be removed but occasionally can be salvaged by rapid surgery. Most minor and moderate injuries to the kidney can be simply observed with follow-up imaging conducted by ultrasound as necessary.

Bladder injury is particularly likely in the inebriated individual with a *full bladder* who has an accident on the way home from a bar and the rupture may be either intraperitoneal or extraperitoneal. The diagnosis can be confirmed by cystography. The ruptured bladder should be repaired and the bladder drained using a suprapubic and urethral catheter.

Similarly, the *urethra* can be injured in two principal sites. Injury in the *prostatic urethra* is usually a complex injury which proves difficult to repair and manage subsequently because of the incidence of late stricturing. In these injuries the prostate may no longer be palpable on rectal examination (*high-riding prostate*). A proportion of these posterior injuries are of partial degree when the patient first presents and it is important that injudicious attempts at catheterisation do not convert this to a full thickness injury which is harder to treat. By contrast injuries to the *bulbous urethra* are usually simpler to treat because the area is more accessible and any subsequent stricturing is also more easily dealt with.

Pelvic fractures
For more details refer to Chapter 20.

Pelvic fractures exemplify a number of basic principles of trauma care:
- there may be difficulty in diagnosing the presence or severity of injury;
- the injury may be trivial or rapidly life-threatening;
- a pelvic fracture may be associated with injuries to other body areas;
- a number of therapeutic options exist;
- interdisciplinary collaboration is essential.

Minimally displaced injuries to the pelvic rami are often minor although fracture to all four rami can be associated with *posterior displacement* and *bladder injury*. The more *major injuries* involve the lateral and posterior elements of the pelvis and these fractures are often associated with *major haemorrhage* from the *small veins* within and around the bone. This haemorrhage can be of enormous magnitude and can, on occasion, be very difficult to arrest. Intrathoracic and intra-abdominal haemorrhage need to be excluded in patients with pelvic fracture who present in shock. DPL is less sensitive in the presence of a pelvic fracture and can only really be regarded as positive if there is free blood present upon initial entry to the peritoneum. It is preferable not to open the pelvic haematoma for fear of infection and an early therapeutic step, often required during initial resuscitation, is the application of an *external fixator* to realign certain pelvic fractures. Other short-term manoeuvres include the application of a tight bandage around the pelvis or the internal rotation of the hip joints, again secured by strapping the legs together. Where haemorrhage continues, further treatment options include angiographic embolisation or pelvic packing.

Injuries to the bony skeleton

For more details refer to Chapter 20.

Certain basic principles run commonly through the wide range of operative procedures available in the management of bony injury.

Blood loss

Bony injury may be associated with very considerable blood loss. Compound wounds may cause external haemorrhage. Massive haemorrhage from pelvic fractures is discussed above but even apparently simple, closed long-bone fractures can cause very considerable blood loss and shock. For example, a fractured femur can be associated with loss of 1–2 l, a fractured tibia with loss of 500 ml to 1 l and, obviously where multiple injuries coexist, there will be a loss of a similar scale at each site. Knowledge of the degree of blood loss expected at the common fracture site is important because if the degree of blood loss cannot be accounted for, the injured patients must have a missed injury which requires prompt identification.

Skin wound management

The principles of skin wound management are straightforward. They involve adequate cleansing, removal of dead tissue and skin coverage at a safe time. Thus, clean incised recent wounds may be closed primarily, whereas contaminated wounds which require debridement will usually be left to heal by second intention or can be closed at 4–5 days providing they remain clean (delayed primary suture). Compound fractures and deep muscular wounds require antibiotic prophylaxis in addition to local cleansing. Appropriate *antitetanus cover* must also be given.

With certain bony injuries the viability of the covering skin may be compromised. This is particularly likely in markedly displaced ankle fractures and in certain fractures of the tibia and fibula. Where possible, judicious emergency realignment should be undertaken at an early stage in order to preserve skin cover.

Neurovascular supply

Bony injuries can compromise the blood and nerve supply to the part of the limb beyond and examining the adequacy of distal neurovascular supply is an integral part of assessment. Loss of adequate distal vascularity is clearly an emergency, the artery usually being occluded by kinking around the fracture site. The commonest example of this is the supracondylar fracture of the humerus in children. Where the blood supply is not restored promptly, irreversible ischaemic damage will occur to the muscles of the forearm, leaving the child with a useless limb.

Nerve damage can occur in three forms:

1. *Neuropraxia* (*or bruising*): a condition which recovers spontaneously within a few weeks.
2. *Axonotmesis*: more severe damage to the axons of the nerve but the overall structure of the nerve remains intact and regeneration of the axons can occur. This is a slow process (1 mm/day) but return of function can be expected.
3. *Neurotmesis* is the severest form of nerve injury where the nerve is actually destroyed by division or scarring and here, resuture or nerve grafting may be needed. The outcome is much less predictable.

Soft tissue injury

Soft tissue injury, with or without an associated fracture, results in swelling of the soft tissues and when this occurs within an enclosed fascial compartment, for example, in the lower leg or forearm, a *compartment syndrome* may occur. This can occur from crushing injury in association with any type of fracture or as a result of a comatose patient lying in an unusual position. As the pressure within the compartment rises, the vascularity of the muscles are compromised and ischaemia and contracture may result. Typical symptoms and signs include *pain* on passive stretching of involved muscle groups, reduced *distal sensation*, *weakness* of involved muscles and intense *swelling* of the area. This is an urgent condition and a generous *fasciotomy* is necessary to prevent permanent muscle damage. Where concern exists, tissue pressure can be measured and measurements >35–45 mmHg suggest impairment of vascular supply.

Fat embolism

Major fractures may be associated with the fat embolism syndrome. This is where *globules of fat* are dislodged from the *marrow* and are embolised around the circulation. This can occur at or shortly after the time of injury or during operative intervention for fractures. The fat globules usually lodge in the lungs and may cause a syndrome similar to *ARDS*. The diagnosis should be considered in patients who are hypoxaemic or dyspnoeic following injury or surgery for orthopaedic trauma. Treatment entails adequate support of respiratory function.

Reduction and fixation

Reduction of the fracture and support of the broken bone forms the mainstay of treatment. The realignment of bony fragments is essential for maintaining limb length and for setting the scene for the most important subsequent event, namely rehabilitation to full function. The means whereby the bones are held reduced range from the simple *Plaster of Paris backslab* to complicated *operative techniques* where the bones are held either *internally* by a variety of metal pins and plates or, increasingly, by *external fixation*. This technique permits rigid early fixation and gentle realignment of the bones without the same infection risk associated with full internal fixation. It is important that some form of reduction and fixation is undertaken early in the management, particularly of the multiply injured patient, because the longer the fractures are unfixed, the greater the incidence of subsequent sepsis and other complications.

Vascular injuries

Arterial injuries can present with major exsanguinating haemorrhage or with an expanding or pulsatile haematoma, often associated with a bruit. The arterial injury is usually associated with distal ischaemia, which is a further important clinical sign, especially when there has been no major haemorrhage from the injured artery but where a flap of intima has completely or partially occluded the arterial lumen. This last point indicates that not all arterial injuries are easily recognised and a high index of suspicion should be maintained in order to diagnose these and prevent late ischaemic sequelae. Diagnosis is usually made by angiography and treatment is by surgical repair.

When the patient presents with exsanguinating haemorrhage or when this occurs during the course of another operative procedure, it is important to recall that all haemorrhage can be controlled with simple manual pressure and that the blind placement of forceps in an attempt to control spurting arteries is often fruitless and always hazardous. It is best to maintain manual pressure while help is sought and until the patient is transferred to the operating theatre and proper proximal and distal control of the injured artery obtained. Repair may be achieved by suturing, the use of a vein patch or by insertion of a prosthetic graft.

Missile and blast injuries

Missiles (bullets, shrapnel, etc.) cause injury by two mechanisms:

1. The track of the missile will injure a range of viscera. It is important to understand that the track will often not be a straight line as the missile will ricochet off solid structures and can thus follow a remarkably tortuous course.
2. Higher-velocity missiles also cause tissue damage as a result of the process of cavitation. High-velocity bullets in particular cause a sizeable cavity along their track, injuring or destroying adjacent tissue which becomes contaminated with dirt and debris. The size of the cavity may be

reflected in the exit wound (if present) which is often considerably larger than the entry wound.

Treatment consists of adequate surgical intervention to control haemorrhage or damaged vital structures. The wound must be cleaned adequately and, particularly with higher-velocity missiles, this may require several trips to the operating theatre for further debridement as the extent of devitalised tissue becomes clear. Surgical debridement is the mainstay of treatment and here an undue reliance on antibiotics (although part of the treatment protocol) is dangerous.

Blast injuries occur during explosions and the patient may be injured by a number of mechanisms. Apart from the blast itself, he may suffer injury from burning or from conventional blunt or penetrating trauma as a result of striking or being struck by other objects. The blast wave itself causes pressure injuries to the lungs and eardrums. Victims close to the blast may suffer traumatic amputations but mortality is obviously very high close to the source.

BURNS

Burns can be caused by thermal, chemical, ultraviolet irradiation or electrical energy. This section will deal with burns caused by thermal injury.

Pathophysiology

Burns can occur through direct contact with hot objects, flames, steam or hot liquids. At temperatures above 40°C and particularly above 45°C, heat coagulates proteins and damages enzyme systems leading to cell death. The burn injury as classically described by Jackson has three zones – a central zone of coagulation (3rd degree or *full thickness*), surrounded by a zone of stasis (2nd degree or *partial thickness*) and peripherally a zone of hyperaemia (1st degree or simple *erythema*). The zone of stasis is the site of the most activity after a burn and in this zone the cells, although injured, are potentially salvageable. Thermal injury results in an *acute inflammatory response*. This consists of an initial fleeting period of *vasoconstriction* followed by *vasodilatation* and increased *microvascular permeability* for 1–3 h during which time local oedema rapidly occurs. Patchy areas of ischaemia develop as the microcirculation fails and wound perfusion generally then decreases for a period of 12–24 h. Following this is a period of *transformation* and subsequent *wound repair*.

The acute inflammatory response is related to the extent and severity of the burn. When the burn is large it may cause an *acute systemic inflammatory response* which is characterised by failure of the normal homeostatic mechanisms and which can itself cause further systemic injury.

Fluid shifts

Fluid losses are greatly increased after a burn. Fluid is lost from the damaged microcirculation and enters the interstitial tissues causing oedema. In addition evaporative water losses are increased because of loss of normal skin. The rate of fluid loss is proportional to the size and depth of the burn and when full thickness burns of greater than 20% occur, homeostatic mechanisms become unable to compensate for these losses. The circulating volume is then reduced and shock can ensue.

During the first 24 h, and particularly during the first 3 h, fluid losses are rapid due to the *increased microvascular permeability*. During the second 24-h period the rate of fluid loss decreases as the capillary permeability returns to normal. Subsequently evaporative fluid losses continue from the burn and the rate of fluid loss remains high until the wound is closed. However, 48 h after the burn, interstitial fluid is reabsorbed into the intravascular space. During this period oedema fluid which can amount to several litres, is reabsorbed and the reabsorption of this fluid may be associated with a diuresis.

Heat loss

A significant increase in heat loss largely through increased evaporation occurs after a burn as a consequence of loss of normal skin. Evaporative water losses in ml/h can be calculated from a formula:

$$\text{Loss ml/h} = (25 + \text{per cent body surface area (\%BSA) burn}) \times \text{BSA}$$

Since the latent heat of vaporisation is 0.58 kcal/ml of water an adult with a 40% burn losing 100 ml/h may lose 1000–1500 kcal as a result of increased evaporation alone.

Alterations in metabolism

After a burn the metabolism of the cells in the region of the burn wound becomes altered. For reasons which are not yet clear, the cells utilise *anaerobic* rather than aerobic pathways of metabolism. This less efficient mode of metabolism requires more substrate to release the same amount of energy as aerobic metabolism. The burn wound thus consumes *large quantities of substrate* (*glucose*) and particularly during the wound repair period the blood flow to the wound is greatly increased to provide sufficient substrate to meet this need. Large quantities of *lactate* and *pyruvate* are produced and these can contribute to a metabolic acidosis.

The metabolic rate of the burns patient is also greatly increased and may be increased 2–2.5 times normal. There is increased catabolism of proteins, lipolysis and gluconeogenesis. The reasons for this increased rate of metabolism have not been fully explained although part of the reason is the need to generate more heat to compensate for the increased losses from the burn wound.

Circulatory changes

Cardiac output falls immediately after a significant burn as a result of loss of plasma volume. After adequate resuscitation the cardiac output in the flow phase is greatly increased and may be more than twice the normal cardiac output.

Infection

Wound infection remains a major cause of mortality in patients surviving the initial thermal injury. The burn wound is initially sterile but later becomes colonised by microorganisms from the surrounding environment. In the first week Gram-positive organisms, especially *Staphylococcus aureus* predominate but by the second week Gram-negative organisms particularly *Pseudomonas aeruginosa* become important. Defects in the immune system in both cell- and humoral-mediated immune responses, are important in contributing to wound infection.

Smoke inhalation injury

Smoke inhalation injury is more likely to occur when the burns victim has been trapped in an enclosed space. The injury occurs as a result of inhalation of:

• hot gases which cause thermal damage particularly to the upper airways;
• toxic fumes including carbon monoxide (CO) and cyanide from burning materials, particularly plastics;
• hypoxia from inhaling air with a low oxygen content within an enclosed space;
• particulate matter.

Clinical features

As with all trauma patients, a primary survey should be performed to assess an ABC and determine if life-threatening conditions are present. This is followed by a detailed secondary survey to identify any other injuries or concomitant illnesses.

Assessment of severity

The American Burn Association classifies the severity of a burn into three groups: major burn, moderate burn and minor burn. This is based on the size and depth of the burn and whether so-called primary areas (face, neck, hands, feet) are involved, as well as whether inhalation and other associated injuries are present.

• *Burn size*
  In the rule of nines the head and each upper limb correspond to 9% of the BSA whilst the lower limbs and anterior and posterior surfaces of the trunk each correspond to 18% of the BSA. The perineum is 1% of the BSA. In children the proportions of the head trunk and limbs is dependent on the age and Lund and Browder charts are usually used to estimate the area of the burn. The palmar surface of one hand corresponds to approximately 1% of the BSA and can also be used to estimate smaller burns. Note that only areas of full and partial thickness are counted, areas of erythema are ignored.
• *Depth*
  The depth of the burn can be difficult to assess and in addition it may not be uniform. A number of methods of classifying the depth of a burn have been devised and the

terminology can be quite confusing. Four commonly used systems are summarised below.

Wound infection
Diagnosis of infection of a burn wound can be difficult to make clinically and sometimes a bacterial count from a full thickness biopsy of the burn wound is needed.

Smoke inhalation injury
The presence of facial burns, nasal singeing, stridor and wheezing suggest the possibility of smoke inhalation injury. Laryngoscopy and broncoscopy can reveal the extent of the burn, but the immediate priority is to secure the airway with an endotracheal tube before oedema occludes the airway. Pulmonary parenchymal injury can result in atelectasis and pulmonary oedema.

Management
Moderate and severe burns will require admission to hospital and, where available, transfer to a Burns Centre.

Fluid replacement
The fluid replacement regime should aim to replace deficits and ongoing losses as well as to provide sufficient fluids to meet the daily requirements. A number of formulae and regimes have been devised and these can be grouped into those which use colloids only, crystalloids only, a mixture of colloids and crystalloids and finally those which use hypertonic saline. The formulae used depend on knowledge of the patient's weight and per cent total body surface area (%TBSA) burn to calculate the amounts to be infused. Examples of fluid replacement regimes and formulae are listed below:

- Colloids only

  Muir and Barclay formula
  - Six 'rations' of plasma to be given over the first 36 h where one ration in ml = (%BSA burn × weight in kg)/2.
  - Three rations in the first 12 h, two rations in the second 12 h and one ration in the third 12 h.
- Crystalloids only

  Parkland formula
  - Ringer's lactate 4 ml/kg per %BSA burn per day. Half to be given in the first 8 h.
- Colloids and crystalloids

  Brooke formula
  - Colloids (plasma/dextran) 0.5 ml/kg/%BSA burn.
  - Crystalloids (Ringer's lactate) 1.5 ml/kg/%BSA burn.
  - Water (dextrose 5%) 2000 ml/day.
- Hypertonic saline 250 mmol/L sodium – volume of replacement fluid needed is titrated to maintain blood pressure and urine output.

When crystalloids are used the fluid does not remain in the intravascular space for long and it is soon lost through the burn wound or into the interstitial tissue. Large volumes of crystalloid are therefore needed. When colloids are used as replacement a much smaller amount is required to restore the circulating volume than if crystalloids only were to be used. However, colloid, especially plasma is expensive and in addition this regime is associated with fluid accumulation in the lungs. The increased extravascular lung water can lead to complications. A mixture of colloids and crystalloids is a popular compromise. When hypertonic saline is used smaller volumes of fluid replacement are needed but it has been demonstrated to be associated with an increased occurrence of renal failure and a higher mortality rate.

Often the weight of the burns patient cannot be obtained on arrival, particularly in the patient with extensive burns since the patient may be too ill to stand on a weighing scale(!) and the estimate of %BSA burn may not be very accurate. Thus formulae should only be used as a *guide* to therapy and the fluid regime should be regularly reviewed. Volume infused should aim to produce a urine output of 0.5 ml/kg/h, pulse rate of 120/min and a systolic blood pressure of about 100 mmHg.

Nutritional support
Calorie requirements can be calculated from the Harris–Benedict equation:

Male BMR $= 66 + (13.7 \times W) + (5 \times H) - (6.8 \times A)$
Female BMR $= 665 + (9.6 \times W) + (1.7 \times H) - (4.7 + A)$

where W is weight in kg, H is height in cm and A is age in years.

Since the BMR in a patient with moderate or major burns will usually be twice the normal rate, double the daily caloric intake should be supplied. This can be supplied in the form of glucose and fats. Large amounts of protein (at a rate of 1.5–2.5 g/kg/day) should also be supplied.

The preferred method of delivery is through the oral route via a nasogastric tube and this should be initiated as early as possible. However, in the presence of significant ileus the pareneteral route via peripheral veins can also be used but lipids should be infused with caution.

Wound management
- *Immediate management*

  Circumferential burns of the limbs may result in a tight constricting eschar which can compromise the blood supply and *escharotomy* should be performed to relieve the constriction. Circumferential burns to the chest can similarly restrict breathing and escharotomies should also be performed here.
- *Conservative treatment/preparation for grafting*

  This involves the prevention of wound infection and the promotion of healing by secondary intention. The techniques include the open, semi-open and closed techniques. Topical antibacterial agents such as silvasulphadiazine and silver nitrate can reduce the extent of bacterial colonisation.

- *Excision and grafting*
  - Excision and grafting of the burn wound removes necrotic tissue and provides skin cover.
  - Full thickness burns – excision and skin grafting.
  - Partial thickness burns – tangential excision and skin grafting.

Smoke inhalation injury

If carbon monoxide (CO) inhalation is suspected, oxygen should be administered to displace the CO. Cyanide toxicity should be treated with sodium nitrite and sodium thiosulphate.

Results and long-term management

The results of management of burns have shown progressive improvement over the last 30 years (Fig. 7.1). Currently, the burn size lethal to 50% of young adults is 80% of the TBSA compared to 60% of the BSA 30 years ago particularly from burn shock and infection.

Factors important today include:
- Size of the burn.
- Age of the patient (Fig. 7.1). Patients in the age group 5–20 years old have the best chance of survival. After age 20, the mortality rate rises with age and is highest in the elderly (>70). Infants up to the age of 2 years also have a higher mortality rate.
- The presence of smoke inhalation injury.

Rehabilitation often takes time and in addition, hypertrophic scars and keloids may require repeated surgery to regain function particularly in primary areas. In children there is a drastic reduction in growth rate in the first year after a major burn and it may take several years for the child to fully recover.

Future possibilities

It may be possible to modify the (largely catabolic) endocrine response to a burn using an anabolic hormone such as growth hormone (GH). In addition GH has been demonstrated to improve healing at donor skin graft sites. Attempts to modify the ischaemia–reperfusion injury with high-dose Vitamin C also appears promising. Vitamin C which is an antioxidant may decrease the damage caused by oxygen free radicals and minimise the oxidant-mediated injury and hence reduce the capillary permeability.

THE PATHOPHYSIOLOGY OF TRAUMA

Despite advances in the early treatment of trauma, it remains one of the major causes of death and disability in the UK. The adaptation of the ATLS® framework has had a huge impact on the management of trauma in the UK, with the aim of identifying and managing immediately life-threatening conditions and the prevention of a cascade of metabolic events that can lead to the deterioration in a patient's condition. The understanding of the pathophysiology of severe

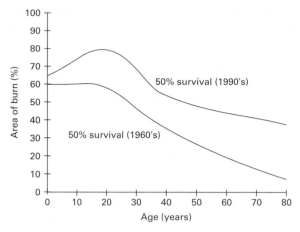

Figure 7.1. Improvement in survival of burns patients over the last 30 years.

trauma is *vitally important* in the management of the injured patient, as early recognition and correction of abnormalities are pivotal to preventing complications such as sepsis and secondary brain injury that become apparent after the initial management is successful and the patient is moved to the intensive care unit. Sepsis remains a major cause of mortality and is an area into which a lot of research is being focused and the understanding of the pathophysiology of trauma is helping in the search for future treatment modalities.

The pathophysiology of severe trauma is a multisystem response to local and systemic stimuli with interactions between the sympatho-adrenal system, hormones, cytokines and vascular endothelium. The majority of the metabolic changes occur in order to conserve energy and redirect energy sources to vital organs. The emphasis in initial management of the trauma patient remains on correcting hypovolaemia, acid-base disturbance and hypoxia. In the longer term, the maintenance of enteral nutrition, wound care and the prevention of infection take over.

The response to injury

The purpose of the injury response is to mobilise stored fuel and other tissue components and transport them to:
- vital organs to optimise function,
- immunologically active tissue to support cellular function and replication,
- wounds to support the healing process.

Classically, the patient enters a state of *catabolism* following severe injury that can last from days to weeks depending on the severity and duration of the injurious event.

The early response to injury

The early stage after injury includes the pattern of physiological and metabolic changes associated with the preparation for '*fight or flight*' on which are superimposed the responses to *fluid loss* from the circulation and/or tissue damage associated with injury. It may be transient or persist for 24 h or more. The changes are designed to preserve life in the short term. If the patient survives this phase of catabolism, then the body enters a state of anabolism, with increased protein synthesis and a return of lean body mass and strength as recovery takes place.

The manifestations of the response are determined by a number of factors (Table 7.2). In general, responses are dampened at the extremes of age, and in patients over 70 years of age, who have suffered severe trauma, the response is also limited by a decrease in their cardiac output and loss of muscle mass.

Emphasis during resuscitation must be on the provision of *adequate oxygen* and *volume resuscitation* to restore intravascular volume and correct hypovolaemia. This response has several components including acute phase, neuroendocrine, sympathetic and metabolic.

Neuroendocrine

A neural and endocrine response to injury is elicited by signals reaching the hypothalamus and causing subsequent release of pituitary hormones and activation of the sympathetic nervous system.

Hypothalamo-pituitary-adrenal axis

The hypothalamo-pituitary-adrenal axis is perhaps the most thoroughly investigated example of such a response to injury. The hormones released from the hypothalamo-pituitary-adrenal axis have three major roles:

1. To increase catabolism by mobilising substrates for energy.
2. To initiate a mechanism to retain salt and water and help maintain intravascular volume.
3. To control the effects of systemically released cytokines, which stimulate local and systemic inflammatory responses.

Regulatory peptides arise from the hypothalamus and are transported through the capillary plexus of the *hypophyseal portal system* to the anterior pituitary. This results in the release of the following into the bloodstream:

- adrenocorticotrophic hormone (ACTH);
- growth hormone (GH);
- thyroid stimulating hormone (TSH);
- luteinising hormone (LH);
- prolactin.

Following trauma, there is a prompt increase in ACTH whereas the other pituitary hormones are generally suppressed. This suppression is augmented by the therapeutic administration of infused catecholamines and dopamine. The posterior pituitary gland increases its secretion of antidiuretic hormone (ADH), which is important for water conservation.

Table 7.2. Factors affecting the injury response.

Patient related	Age
	Sex
	Co-morbidity
	Nutritional status
Trauma related	Severity of injury
	Time course of injury
Management related	Steroids
	Drugs
	Operations
Post 'injury' related (after the initial insult and management)	Nutrition and feeding
	Temperature control
	Nutrients (e.g. glutamine, selenium)

ACTH and cortisol: ACTH stimulates the adrenal cortex to produce *glucocorticoids*, in particular cortisol. The relationship between cortisol release and injury is complex and the normal *negative feedback* mechanism is lost after trauma and surgery. Plasma cortisol concentrations, both free and bound, are higher after injuries of moderate severity than after minor trauma, but more severe injuries are associated with lower concentrations. This cannot be attributed to low ACTH levels as after severe injury plasma ACTH levels are raised to around the concentration needed for maximal stimulation of the adrenal cortex: reduced perfusion of the adrenal cortex may be important. The effects of cortisol are mainly *catabolic*. It promotes gluconeogenesis and lipolysis, but also inhibits the use of glucose by cells, dampens the acute phase response and alters the vascular endothelial response.

Aldosterone acts on the *distal convoluted tubule* and *collecting ducts* of the renal tubules to increase sodium reabsorption and potassium secretion, thereby helping to maintain *intravascular volume*. The levels of aldosterone rise after trauma due to a number of stimuli. The release of ACTH stimulates aldosterone secretion in the short term and the renin–angiotensin system (which is stimulated by hypovolaemia and increased sympathetic afferent activity, resulting in increased aldosterone levels) has influence in the longer term.

ADH production is increased following trauma. It acts on the *distal convoluted tubules* and *collecting ducts* to increase the reabsorption of water, thereby helping to preserve intravascular volume. It also acts on the liver to stimulate glycogenolysis and gluconeogenesis and acts on the splanchnic bed as a powerful *vasoconstrictor*.

GH secretion is stimulated by the release of GH-releasing hormone (GHRH) from the hypothalamus and in response to low plasma glucose levels. In addition to its role in growth regulation, it also has important metabolic actions, which are attenuated after injury. Its effects are mediated through insulin-like growth factor-1 (IGF-1) released from liver, muscle and other tissues. Operations and major injury result in a marked fall in IGF-1 and this coincides with *muscle breakdown*. There is also evidence of GH resistance in critically ill patients.

Sympatho-adrenal system

The actions of the sympatho-adrenal system are *central* and *peripheral*, direct and indirect, with the release of noradrenaline from peripheral nerve ganglia and the release of both adrenaline and noradrenaline from the adrenal medulla. The rapid rise in plasma catecholamine concentration produces its effect via α- and β-adrenergic receptors. Cardiovascular changes occurring in the early response to injury result in the redistribution of blood from the skin and viscera (α) to the vital organs (β2) and increased contractility of the heart (β1).

Glycogenolysis, gluconeogenesis and *lipolysis* are the main metabolic changes occurring in direct response to stimulation of the sympatho–adrenal system. For example, plasma insulin concentrations are often acutely low after severe injuries despite a marked hyperglycaemia and this is a result of a suppres-sion of insulin secretion by adrenaline acting on pancreatic α-adrenergic receptors. In contrast, the secretion of glucagon is stimulated by raised catecholamine concentrations through a β-adrenergic receptor mechanism. The peak hormonal response occurs within a few hours and usually declines rapidly.

The system eventually becomes *hyperdynamic*, with increased cardiac output in order to satisfy the demands of increased metabolism, changes in the thermoregulatory system and wound healing. The magnitude of the changes in metabolic rate varies depending on the injury. Treatment with aggressive fluid resuscitation and inotropic support may include additional catecholamines to maintain the body's response to injury. The induced hypermetabolic state peaks at 5–10 days after the injury at the height of inflammation, and returns to normal as wounds heal.

Metabolism and utilisation of energy substrates

The catabolic phase of severely injured patients is characterised by the *mobilisation* of fuel stores, that is, increased glycogenolysis, gluconeogenesis and lipolysis, and breakdown of proteins. The main stimulus for the breakdown of glycogen in both skeletal muscle and liver is *adrenaline*, although glucagon and vasopressin may also have a role in the liver. This glycogenolysis leads to hyperglycaemia either directly due to liberation of glucose from the liver, or indirectly, via the Cori cycle, from lactate released from skeletal muscle. It should always be remembered that raised plasma lactate concentrations can reflect this increase in skeletal muscle glycogenolysis as well as tissue hypoxia. The *hyperglycaemia*, which is directly related to the severity of the injury, is potentiated, after severe injuries, by the reduction of glucose utilisation in skeletal muscle following the inhibition of insulin secretion by raised adrenaline levels and by the development of intracellular

insulin resistance. Plasma concentrations of *non-esterified fatty acids* (*NEFA*) and *glycerol* are also raised after injury reflecting the mobilisation of triacylglycerol stores in adipose tissue. The patterns of fuel mobilisation do not seem to be modified by the site of injury but the age of the patient may influence the changes seen. For a given severity of injury, there is a suggestion that the plasma concentrations of lipid metabolites (NEFA, glycerol and ketone bodies) are higher in elderly patients. At the other extreme, children show an exaggerated hyperglycaemia acutely after head injury and burns.

Protein metabolism

Unlike carbohydrates and fats, proteins are not a stored fuel. Proteolysis results in the loss of structural and functional components of living organisms and therefore results in weight loss and muscle wasting, as proteins are transferred from skeletal to visceral tissues. During the *catabolic phase*, protein breakdown is dramatically increased and synthesis is normal or only slightly elevated. Protein loss can be measured indirectly by determining urinary losses, as little protein is excreted in faeces. Nitrogen balance is the difference between nitrogen intake and nitrogen losses. Following injury, there may be large nitrogen losses despite normal or increased protein feeding regimens (Table 7.3).

The amino acids released from skeletal muscle are predominantly *alanine* and *glutamine*. Alanine is an important precursor for glucose and therefore a fuel source. Glutamine, as well as being gluconeogenic, is a primary substrate for immune cells and enterocytes and serves as a precursor for *glutathione* (an important antioxidant). The net effects of protein catabolism are loss of *muscle bulk*, decreased *wound healing* and *prolonged convalescence*. The use of *glutamine supplements* in feeding regimens has been shown to reduce infection rates following trauma and *decrease mortality* in elderly patients with gastrointestinal sepsis.

Although the major changes in protein metabolism following injury are associated with the 'flow phase', the *acute-phase plasma protein response* is initiated soon after injury. A number of plasma proteins increase in concentration (e.g. C-reactive protein (CRP) and fibrinogen), although there is always a lag of approximately 6 h before changes are seen. The cytokine *interleukin-6* (*IL-6*) may be responsible for inducing the hepatic synthesis of such acute-phase proteins. Such a delay is not seen for the proteins that show an acute phase decrease in concentration after injury. The rapid fall in, for example, albumin concentration cannot be attributed to a reduction in its rate of synthesis but is due to changes in its distribution between intra- and extravascular compartments secondary to an increase in microvascular permeability.

Heat production and thermoregulation

In experimental studies, a fall in heat production is seen after severe haemorrhage and can be ascribed to a failure of oxygen delivery. This is not the case after tissue injury where

Table 7.3. **Estimates of nitrogen losses in the first 10 days following 'injury'.**

Mechanism of injury	Cumulative nitrogen loss (g)
Major burn	170
Multiple injury	150
Peritonitis	136
Simple fracture	115
Untreated pneumonia	59
Major operation	50
Minor operation	24

Table 7.4. **The main features of the acute phase response.**

Fever*
Malaise*
Headache*
Musculoskeletal pains*
Granulocytosis*
Activation of immune system
Release of ACTH and Cortisol
Activation of clotting cascades
Increase in erythrocyte sedimentation rate (the ESR)
Production of acute phase proteins in the liver
Increase in CRP
Increase in fibrinogen
Increase in α_2-macroblobulin
Increase in caeruloplasmin
Increase in transferrin
Decrease in albumin
Decrease in circulating levels of iron and zinc

*Encourage energy conservation.

nociceptive impulses from the site of injury bring about changes in thermoregulation within the brain. The situation is less clear in man but body temperature is reduced acutely after injury and the reduction is directly related to injury severity. Furthermore, patients do not shiver despite having low body temperatures and also the appreciation of thermal comfort following injury is modified.

Acute phase response

The initiation of the acute phase response occurs early in the response to injury and its effects are both local and systemic. The local inflammatory response is mediated by granulocytes, mononuclear cells, fibroblasts and endothelial cells. These cells produce cytokines, which have mainly paracrine effects.

The main features of the acute phase response are the symptoms and signs that we, as clinicians witness every day in the injured patient (Table 7.4).

Cytokines: the main cytokines released are IL-1, IL-2, IL-6 and tumour necrosis factor-alpha (TNF-α). More recently IL-8 and IL-10 have been discovered to have a role in the acute phase response.

IL-1 and TNF-α released from macrophages and monocytes *initiate* the acute phase response. These in turn stimulate the release of more cytokines (in particular IL-6). *IL-6 is the main cytokine responsible for inducing the systemic inflammatory response syndrome (SIRS)*. For a patient to qualify as having SIRS, they must have *two* of the following components:
- *Temperature derangement*: <36°C or >38°C (rectal).
- *Tachycardia*: >90 bpm.
- *Tachypnoea*: respiratory rate >20 bpm or $PaCO_2$ <4.3 kPa.
- *Abnormal white cell count*: <4 or >12 × 10^9/L.
  The effects of IL-1, IL-6 and TNF-α include:
- Induction of a hypermetabolic state.
- Disruption of thermoregulation, with upregulation of the central reference temperature, leading to a rise in core temperature by peripheral vasoconstriction and hypermetabolism.

Severely injured patients usually have a *low-grade fever*. It is therefore beneficial to manage an injured patient in a warm environment as is reduces thermoregulatory drive and hypermetabolism. The use of warming devices for prolonged surgery has been linked with *decreased morbidity* and the absence of a febrile response is usually correlated with a poor outcome.

In contrast, IL-10 depresses other cytokines, macrophages, T-cells and natural killer cell function. It is thought to play a major role in modulating the cytokine network in trauma patients as a 'cytokine synthesis inhibitor factor'.

The complement cascade also plays a key role in the sequence of the trauma response. It acts via the alternative pathway, releasing substrates such as the anaphylatoxins C3a, C4a, C5a and the C5–C9 complex, which in turn act upon granulocytes, causing their activation. Complement also has actions through chemotaxis, opsonisation and phagocytosis.

Acute phase reactants have already been mentioned and are produced in the *liver*. They are present under normal conditions but their concentrations can be increased or decreased in response to trauma. Examples include CRP (increase in response to injury) and albumin (decrease in response to injury).

Vascular endothelium

Endothelial cells are affected by a number of noxious stimuli, including:
- bacteria,
- endotoxins,
- cytokines,
- platelet aggregating factors,
- complement,

- hydrogen peroxide,
- oxygen free radicals.

During the catabolic phase, *leukocytes* adhere to endothelial cells via *adhesion molecules* such as E-selectin and P-selectin and intercellular adhesion molecule-1 (ICAM-1). These interactions result in endothelial cell injury leading to changes in vascular permeability and oedema. This can manifest as acute respiratory distress syndrome (ARDS) and may be responsible for gastrointestinal bacterial translocation.

Nitric oxide is A potent *vasodilatator* released from endothelial cells, macrophages, neutrophils, Kupffer cells in the liver, and renal cells. It causes local changes in vasomotor tone and its actions are opposed by endothelins, which are potent vasoconstrictors released by thrombin, cytokines, endotoxins, hypoxia and catecholamines. Platelet activating factor (PAF) and prostaglandins are also involved, causing vasoconstriction and vasodilatation respectively.

The interaction between inflammation and coagulation is a complex one. The normal fibrinolytic process is disrupted in sepsis, which may be mediated by interactions between endothelial cells. Decreased levels and activity of coagulation inhibitors (e.g. activated protein-C, antithrombin-III) and insufficient fibrinolytic activity have been identified in multiple organ dysfunction syndrome (MODS). A procoagulant state may ensue, characterised by local clotting and the development of deep venous thrombosis (DVT), which can eventually consume the clotting factors and lead to micro-haemorrhages, typically seen in meningococcal septicaemia.

The late response to injury

The late response to injury is characterised by an early and late anabolic phase. The transition from catabolism to anabolism is marked by a decrease in nitrogen loss, diuresis of retained water and an improvement in the patient's overall condition. The early anabolic phase occurs over a period of several months and the nitrogen gain gradually equals the nitrogen lost in the catabolic phase. Nitrogen balance is achieved in the late anabolic phase, as the body's protein structures are repleted. Fat stores will be restored if the caloric intake is greater than caloric expenditure.

Unfortunately, in many patients who have sustained severe trauma, an overload of inflammatory cytokines and an overactive vascular endothelial response lead to an increase in metabolism and the inability of the cardiac output to maintain a hyperdynamic circulation. These in turn lead to anaerobic metabolism, organ failure and death and prompt resuscitation and treatment of injuries is one way to try to limit this.

A significant catabolic phase is observed in critically ill patients as part of the stress response. The advantages of instigating early enteral feeding are thought to include maintenance of the mucosal barrier of the gut, limiting the alteration of commensal flora in the gut, minimising the catabolic response, and boosting the immune system. Enteral feeds, particularly those supplemented by L-arginine, omega-3 fatty acids, L-glutamine (the enterocyte's primary energy source) or branched amino acids, have been shown to decrease infective complications and intensive care unit (ICU) stay after major trauma.

An interesting avenue of research is into bacterial translocation and the development of sepsis. Glutamine enteral nutrition has been shown to decrease this phenomenon, but isolation of specific protein involved in bacterial translocation, and their antagonism, may be possible future therapeutic options. In the future, care of the severely injured patient is likely to undergo some exciting changes, with the emergence of combination antioxidant therapy, activated protein-C trials, and blood substitutes, which may improve outcome and ultimately survival.

Summary

Trauma encompasses a multitude of mechanisms of injury (which include pain (nociception), tissue damage and hypovolaemia) and components of trauma are seen in patients undergoing major surgery to those with severe infections. The body's response to trauma is generally *proportional* to the severity of injury and an understanding of the pathophysiology of major trauma will contribute to the initial investigation, management and subsequent long-term outcome of the patient.

FURTHER READING

Russel RCG, Williams NS, Bulstrode CJK. *Bailey & Love's Short Practice of Surgery.* 24th Ed. Arnold. 2004

Burnand KG, Young AE, Lucas JD, Rowlands BJ, Scholefield J. *The New Aird's Companion in Surgical Studies.* 3rd Ed. Churchill Livingstone. 2005

8

Intensive Care

Angela Neville[1] and Aljafri A Majid[2]

[1]Department of Surgery, University of Southern California, Los Angeles, USA [2]University Hospital, Kuala Lumpur, Malaysia; Department of Surgery, University of Malaya; Royal College of Surgeons, Edinburgh, UK

CONTENTS

Cardiovascular system   **111**
Cardiac anatomy   111
Physiology   113
Invasive monitoring   115
Interpretation of special investigations   118
Cardiovascular support   118
Cardiac arrest and resuscitation   121
Arrhythmias   122
Cardiac tamponade   123

Shock   **124**
Definition   124
Diagnosis   124
Types of shock   124
Resuscitation   125
Cardiogenic shock   125
Hypovolemic shock   126
Obstructive shock   126
Distributive shock   127

Respiratory system   **128**
Physiology   128
Interpretation of special investigations   129
Respiratory failure   131
Artificial airways   132
Mechanical ventilation   134
Pulmonary embolism   137

SIRS, sepsis, and multi-organ dysfunction syndrome   **138**
Definitions   138
Pathophysiology   138
Treatment   139
Acute lung injury and ARDS   139
Acute renal failure   141
Acute liver failure   143
Infections in the ICU   144

Principles of intensive care   **145**
Organization and staffing   145
Indications for admission and discharge   146
Scoring systems   147

Further reading   **148**

CARDIOVASCULAR SYSTEM

Cardiac anatomy

The heart has four chambers, four valves, and specialized conduction tissue. It is generally referred to as having left- and right-sided chambers, but in humans the interatrial septum and inter-ventricular septum are located in a plane some 45° from the sagittal plane (Fig. 8.1). The right atrium and ventricle are therefore located anterior and to the right of the corresponding left atrium or ventricle. It is useful to bear this in mind when visualizing the cardiac chambers through echocardiograms (ECHO) or when assessing traumatic injuries to the chest wall.

Cardiac valves

The aortic and pulmonary valves are similar in structure and function, and consist of three components:
1. three-valve leaflets or cusps;
2. a three pronged fibrous annulus;
3. three dilations of the aortic/pulmonary wall (sinuses of Valsalva).

The aortic valve leaflets are referred to by clinicians as the left coronary, right coronary, and non-coronary leaflets. The fibrous annulus is shaped like a three-pronged coronet from which the valve leaflets are suspended. Valve stenosis may arise when the valve leaflets are fused or stiff and the annulus narrows; valve incompetence results from abnormalities of the valve leaflets and/or dilation of the annulus. The sinuses of Valsalva are important for initiating valve closure. They prevent the valve leaflets from being pressed flat against the aortic wall during systole, and eddy currents within the sinuses help initiate valve closure in diastole.

The mitral and tricuspid valves each consist of an annulus, leaflets, chordae tendineae, and papillary muscles. They prevent backflow of blood into the atria during systole. Regurgitation can be caused by annular dilation, chordal elongation or rupture or papillary muscle dysfunction. Both leaflet fusion and narrowing of the annulus can contribute to valve stenosis.

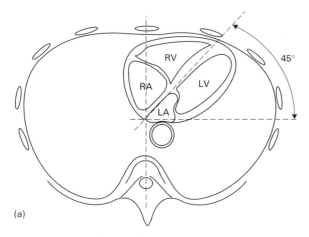

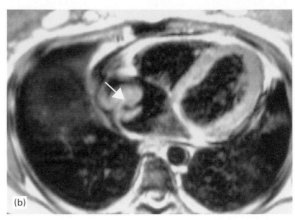

(a)   (b)

Figure 8.1. Position of heart in thoracic cavity. (a) The intra-atrial and intra-ventricular septae are located 45° from the sagittal plane. Anterior penetrating thoracic wounds are more likely to injure the right atrium or ventricle than the 'left-sided' chambers. (b) MRI demonstrates the position of the intra-ventricular septum. In addition, this figure shows a right atrial myxoma (arrow). MRI: magnetic resonance imaging; RV: right ventricle; LV: left ventricle; RA: right atrial; LA: left atrial.

Coronary arteries

The heart is perfused by right and left coronary arteries arising directly from the take off of the thoracic aorta. There are some differences in the nomenclature used by anatomists and clinicians when describing the coronary arteries. The left coronary artery leaves the aorta and is referred to as the 'left main stem' before its bifurcation. It then divides into the circumflex artery and an anterior branch, the anterior inter-ventricular artery or 'left anterior descending' (LAD) artery. The branches of the circumflex artery are referred to as obtuse marginal (OM) branches and individual branches as OM1, OM2, etc. (Fig. 8.2).

Classically, the right coronary artery gives rise to the marginal branches of the right ventricle (RV), before terminating as the posterior inter-ventricular artery referred to by clinicians as the 'posterior descending artery' (PDA). There are some anatomic variations in size and extent of distribution of the right coronary artery and not all right coronary arteries terminate as a PDA. In 10–15% of cases the right coronary artery is small and the PDA may arise as a terminal branch of the left circumflex artery. When the PDA arises from the left circumflex, it is referred to as a left dominant circulation. If the right coronary artery gives rise to the PDA, the right coronary is said to be dominant. It should be noted, however, that regardless of the origin of the PDA, the bulk of the blood supply to the heart is still borne by the left coronary artery.

Coronary blood flow, which amounts to about 225 ml/min at rest, can increase to just over 1 l/min with exercise. During systole, particularly during the phase of isovolumetric contraction, the intra-myocardial coronary arteries are compressed and coronary flow is reduced. Coronary blood flow thus occurs mainly during diastole. Conditions which result in a low diastolic blood pressure or which increase the intra-myocardial

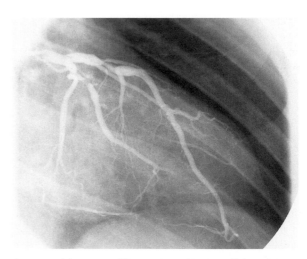

Figure 8.2. Right anterior oblique angiographic view of left coronary artery and major branches. Note the stenotic lesion in the LAD and the obstructed OM artery arising from the circumflex. The PDA, which in this case arises from the right coronary artery, is filled in a retrograde fashion by dye from the LAD.

tension during diastole (e.g. an increase in end-diastolic pressure) can compromise coronary blood flow. In these situations, the subendocardial muscle is particularly vulnerable.

Cardiac muscle

Cardiac muscle consists of specialized striated muscle cells with an intrinsic, involuntary ability to contract, know as automaticity. Pacemaker cells within the sinoatrial node establish the heart rate and are influenced by innervation from the autonomic nervous system. Cardiac cells are dense

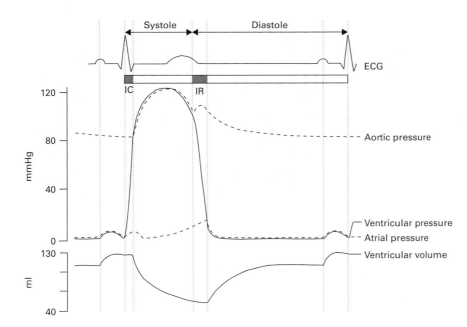

Figure 8.3. The cardiac cycle.
IC: isovolumetric contraction; IR:
isovolumetric relaxation.

in myofibrils consisting of sarcomeres and their actin and myosin components. The cells are branched, intertwined and in tight communication via gap junctions and desmosomes. This arrangement allows depolarization to occur rapidly throughout the heart such that it acts as single unit or snycytium.

Cardiac troponins (cTn) have received significant attention for their use in evaluating acute coronary syndromes. The cTn 'complex' regulates cardiac muscle contraction and consists of three protein subunits: Ca^{2+} binding (cTnC), inhibitory (cTnI), and tropomyosin binding (cTnT). In the absence of calcium, the troponin–tropomyosin complex inhibits cross-bridge formation between actin and myosin filaments. When calcium binds to the troponin complex, its conformation is changed. Consequently, formation of cross-bridges between the filaments is facilitated and cardiac contraction occurs.

While the majority of cTn is within the myofibril, a small fraction of cTnI and cTnT is found within the cardiac cytoplasm. When cardiac cells are injured, cytoplasmic troponin is immediately released. As cTn is specific to cardiac cells, serum assays cTnI or CTnT can provide early, sensitive information about cardiac injury. Troponin levels stay elevated for days because of ongoing breakdown of the structural elements. Both cTnI and cTnT assays are available for evaluation of acute coronary syndromes.

Physiology

Cardiac cycle

The cardiac cycle is divided into two phases: systole and diastole (Fig. 8.3). *Systole* begins with a period of isovolumetric contraction during which the intra-ventricular pressures rise

until the aortic and pulmonary valves open. A period of ejection follows and ends when the aortic and pulmonary valves close. *Diastole* commences with a period of isovolumetric relaxation which lasts until the atrioventricular valves open. This is followed by a period of rapid inflow of blood into the ventricle, diastasis, and atrial systole. Atrial contraction is important and contributes up to 25% of the filling of the ventricle.

For optimal cardiac function, the mitral valve must remain shut during systole, whereas the aortic valve must remain shut during diastole. To prevent regurgitation, the mitral valve withstands the systolic pressure and the aortic valve the diastolic pressure. The mitral valve is thus normally subjected to a higher-pressure load than the aortic valve.

Cardiac output

The purpose of the heart is to effectively pump blood to the body to meet its metabolic demands. We describe such cardiac work as 'cardiac output' (CO), which is the volume of blood pumped from the heart each minute. It is a function of stroke volume (SV) and heart rate (HR):

$$CO = SV \times HR$$

Stroke volume is the amount of blood ejected from the heart during each systole. It is defined by end-diastolic volume (EDV; full heart) minus the end-systolic volume (ESV; empty heart):

$$SV = EDV - ESV$$

It follows that increasing either the stroke volume or the heart rate will increase cardiac output. It should be noted that it is 'impossible' to measure heart volumes. Thus stroke

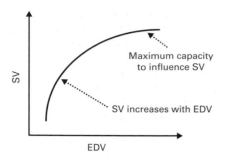

Figure 8.4. The Frank–Starling curve.

volume is usually a calculated number based on measuring the patient's cardiac output and heart rate:

$$SV = CO/HR$$

The body modulates cardiac output both intrinsically and extrinsically. Intrinsically, the output is affected by the Frank–Starling mechanism (Fig. 8.4). Starling found that 'the energy of contraction is a function of the initial length of the muscle fiber'. The ascending limb of the Starling curve was initially attributed solely to the length–tension relationship of the sarcomeres – the greater the overlap of the thick and thin filaments, the greater the force of contraction. It is now realized that myofilaments become more easily activated when they are stretched and that this also increases the contractile force. Extrinsic regulation of the heart is performed by the autonomic nervous system. Input from baroreceptors and chemoreceptors alter cardiac output by impacting the sympathetic and parasympathetic discharges to the heart.

Using these concepts, we have found ways to modulate cardiac output. Improving cardiac output involves either increasing heart rate or stroke volume. Heart rate manipulation is limited. The body's ability to increase heart rate decreases with age. Maximum heart rate (MHR) is approximated by a simple formula: MHR = 220 − age. Thus, for an 80-year-old, their MHR is only 140. This is useful to remember in that heart rates greater than a patient's MHR generally reflects pathologic arrhythmias (such as atrial fibrillation, etc.). Another point to consider is that with increased heart rate, diastolic filling time decreases. Above a heart rate of 160 beats/min (bpm), the diastolic filling time decreases to a point that the stroke volume diminishes and cardiac output begins to drop.

Stroke volume is impacted by three factors: preload, afterload, and contractility. Preload is the 'load' or quantity of blood that is entering the heart from the venous circulation. Its value is reflected by the central venous pressure (CVP) (see invasive monitoring section). To increase cardiac output, one of the first things often done is to optimize preload by giving fluid challenges. As intra-vascular volume increases, preload increases, EDV increases, and cardiac output improves. Alternatively, situations such as heart failure may be improved by 'off-loading'

the heart. Here, preload can be decreased by using venodilators such as nitrates (nitroglycerin and isosorbide dinitrate). By decreasing venous tone, blood is redistributed peripherally, and the amount of blood returning to the overloaded heart is diminished.

Afterload is the 'load' or impedance that the heart must pump against during systole to deliver its stroke volume. Afterload is estimated by the patent's systemic vascular resistance (SVR). SVR is a calculated value that depends heavily on the patient's mean arterial blood pressure (MAP). The calculations for these are as follows:

$$SVR = (MAP - CVP)/CO$$

$$MAP = P_{diastolic} + 1/3(P_{systolic} - P_{diastolic})$$

To make this easier to conceptualize, notice that MAP relies heavily on the diastolic blood pressure. The higher the resting diastolic blood pressure, the more difficult it is for the heart to generate a pressure to open the semi-lunar valves and deliver its volume. The result is a decreased stroke volume. By decreasing afterload, the heart is able to pump a larger volume without needing to generate such a large pressure. Afterload reduction is a significant way in which clinicians can help augment cardiac output. Agents that decrease arterial pressure, particularly arterial dilators, are useful in this regard. Pure arterial dilators include hydralazine and minoxidil. Mixed arterial and venodilators are also available (e.g. sodium nitroprusside, angiotensin converting enzyme (ACE) inhibitors, and calcium channel blockers).

Enhancing the heart's contractility is the final way in which we can manipulate cardiac output. Optimizing preload and taking advantage of the cardiac muscle's intrinsic contractile properties (Starling's law) should be the first mechanism employed to improve cardiac output. Once the heart has been optimally filled, inotropes can be utilized to further augment cardiac output. Inotropes are agents that increase cardiac contractility by increasing intra-cellular calcium. They are discussed further in the section on cardiovascular support.

Oxygen delivery

At the most basic level, the function of the heart is to deliver enough blood (and therefore oxygen) to meet the demands of the body. Often in critical illness, particularly in shock, there is disruption of this balance. Our role as clinicians is to help restore it, but understanding the physiology of oxygen delivery is needed.

Oxygen delivery (DO_2) is defined as the amount of gaseous oxygen delivered to the body per minute. It is determined by the cardiac output and the oxygen content of the blood (CaO_2):

Oxygen delivery (ml O_2/min) = cardiac output (ml blood/min) × oxygen content (ml O_2/dl blood)

$$DO_2 = CO \times CaO_2$$

The oxygen content of the blood is the amount of oxygen that is carried by the blood. It includes both the oxygen that is bound to hemoglobin (Hb) and that which is dissolved in the blood:

Oxygen content (CaO_2) = oxygen bound to Hb + oxygen dissolved in the blood

The amount of oxygen bound to hemoglobin will depend on the patient's hemoglobin, the oxygen saturation (SaO_2), and a constant which reflects the amount of oxygen in milliliters carried by a gram of fully bound hemoglobin:

Oxygen bound to Hb (ml O_2/dl) = SaO_2 × Hb (g/dl) × 1.34 ml O_2/g saturated Hb

The amount of oxygen dissolved in the blood is relatively insignificant, as oxygen is not very soluble in blood. Nevertheless, it is determined by product of the partial pressure of oxygen in the blood (PaO_2) and the solubility coefficient of oxygen:

Oxygen dissolved in blood (ml O_2/dl) = PaO_2 × 0.0031

To summarize:

CaO_2 = (SaO_2 × Hb × 1.34) + (PaO_2)(0.0031)

Oxygen delivery then can be augmented either by increasing cardiac output or oxygen content. Improving cardiac output was explained in the above section. As is evidenced by the formulas, oxygen content can be improved by primarily by increasing the hemoglobin (transfusion) or by providing additional oxygen.

Oxygen consumption

Oxygen consumption (VO_2) is the volume of gaseous oxygen consumed by the body per minute. It is a calculated value that is obtained by knowing how much is oxygen is delivered to the tissue (DO_2) and how much oxygen is returned to the heart by the venous blood. The volume of oxygen returned to the heart in venous blood is referred to as the venous oxygen content (CvO_2). Its equation is identical to that of the arterial oxygen content, except that a venous hemoglobin saturation and partial pressure of oxygen is obtained:

CvO_2 = (SvO_2 × Hb × 1.34) + (PvO_2)(0.0031)

Obviously, different organs extract oxygen in different quantities. For example, the heart extracts much more oxygen from the same quantity of blood than does the resting bicep muscle. Drawing venous blood from the arm then might not give a true representation of the body's consumption. The most sensitive sample of venous blood to detect the amount of oxygen being utilized by the entire body would be a sample coming from the right heart itself. This technique is indeed used in critically ill patients. Venous samples can be drawn from catheters that sit in the pulmonary artery (PA; see invasive monitoring section). These 'mixed venous' oxygen saturations (SvO_2) are utilized to most accurately determine the body's CvO_2. Normal SvO_2 is 75%, because about 25% of oxygen delivered to the body is utilized.

Putting these factors together, we conclude:

Oxygen consumption = oxygen delivered − oxygen returned to the heart in venous blood

VO_2 = DO_2 − oxygen returned to heart
VO_2 = (CO × CaO_2) − (CO × CvO_2)
VO_2 = (CO) (CaO_2 − CvO_2) × 10 dl/l

Oxygen extraction ratio

Knowing how much oxygen the body is utilizing and how much oxygen the cardiovascular system is delivering allows us to calculate a ratio. The oxygen extraction ratio (O_2ER) is determined by comparing oxygen consumption to oxygen delivery:

O_2ER = VO_2/DO_2

Normally, the body consumes approximately 25% of the oxygen that is delivered. Thus, the normal O_2ER is 0.25. When oxygen delivery decreases, in order maintain a constant level of tissue oxygenation, cells extract more oxygen from the available blood than usual. The result is a decreased mixed venous saturation and increased oxygen consumption. Improving oxygen delivery to normalize the mixed venous saturation (and O_2ER) is an important goal of resuscitation.

A summary of the above hemodynamic variables, their formulas, and normal values are provided in Table 8.1. Of note, because of variation in patients' size and shape, most variables are indexed to their body surface area (BSA).

While there seems a multitude of equations, awareness of the concepts of oxygen consumption and delivery are fundamental to the understanding of critical care. If the patient consumes more oxygen than the circulatory system can deliver, the patient is in oxygen debt. If this persists, the end result will be cellular hypoxia and by definition, shock. Understanding that cardiac output and oxygen content are the two ways in which we can improve oxygen delivery allows for a systematic way of treating the shocked state.

Once these concepts are grasped, it is a matter of filling in equations with values. Many of these values would not be obtainable without the assistance of invasive hemodynamic monitoring. We will focus on this in the following section.

Invasive monitoring

Arterial catheterization

Indications for arterial lines include the need for continuous blood pressure monitoring (e.g. shock or hypertensive crisis)

Table 8.1. Hemodynamic variables, formulas, and reference ranges.

	Abbreviation	Formula	Reference range	Units
Measured variables				
Cardiac output	CO		4–8	l/min
Central venous pressure	CVP		0–6	mmHg
Mixed venous saturation	SvO_2		75%	
Calculated variables				
Arterial oxygen content	CaO_2	$(Hb \times SaO_2 \times 1.34) + (PaO_2 \times 0.003)$	18–20	ml/dl
Mean arterial pressure	MAP	$DBP + 1/3 (SBP - DBP)$	70–110	mmHg
Oxygen consumption	VO_2	$(CaO_2 - CvO_2) \times CO \times 10$	100–280	ml/min
Oxygen delivery	DO_2	$CaO2 \times CO \times 10$	640–1200	ml/min
Oxygen extraction ratio	O_2ER	VO_2/DO_2	0.22–0.30	
Stroke volume	SV	CO/HR	60–130	Ml
Systemic vascular resistance	SVR	$[(MAP - CVP) \times 80]/CO$	800–1400	$dyn/s/cm^5$
Venous oxygen content	CvO_2	$(Hb \times SvO_2 \times 1.34) + (PvO_2 \times 0.003)$	13–16	ml/dl
Indexed variables				
Cardiac index	CI	CO/BSA	2.8–4.2	$l/min/m^2$
Oxygen delivery index	DO_2I	DO_2/BSA	500–600	$ml/min/m^2$
Oxygen consumption index	VO_2I	VO_2/BSA	120–160	$ml/min/m^2$
Stroke volume index	SVI	(CO/HR)/BSA	40–60	ml/m^2
System vascular resistance index	SVRI	$[(MAP - CVP) \times 80]/CO/BSA$	1700–2400	$dyn/s/cm^5/m^2$

or frequent arterial blood gases (ABGs) (e.g. diabetic ketoacidosis (DKA) or respiratory failure). Continuous blood pressure monitoring allows the clinician to closely track responses to interventions.

As of waveform physiology, as the stroke volume is ejected from the heart, there is a progressive increase in systolic blood pressure and decrease in diastolic blood pressure as blood moves peripherally. For this reason, MAP provides the most accurate measurement of systemic pressure. MAP is often calculated within the equipment and available on constant display.

While the usual site of insertion of arterial catheterization is the radial artery, the dorsalis pedis, femoral, and rarely brachial artery can be used. The most significant complications of arterial lines are thrombosis and infection. When a radial line is planned, an Allen's test should first be performed to test for collateral flow to the hand via the ulnar artery and palmar arch. Multiple punctures, catheters greater than 20 G, and prolonged line duration should be avoided to minimize the risk of thrombosis. Cannulation of the brachial artery has a significant risk of distal emboli (5–41%) and should be avoided if at all possible.

Central venous catheterization

Central venous catheters are placed in one of the major veins leading to the heart: subclavian, internal jugular, or femoral. Indications for central venous lines include continuous monitoring of the CVP, infusion of multiple medications or vasoactive drugs, need for parenteral nutrition, or inability to secure peripheral venous access. Complications of central venous catheters include infection, venous thrombosis, arterial puncture, bleeding, and air embolism. Pneumothorax is complication of subclavian and internal jugular line insertion.

Central venous pressure

The CVP is a pressure reading obtained from a central venous catheter whose tip is ideally situated in the vena cava at the level of the right atrium. Subclavian and internal jugular lines are usually employed for such measurements, and location placement (as well as ruling out pneumothorax) should be confirmed with a post-procedure chest X-ray (CXR). A pressure transducer is then attached such that readings of the CVP may be performed.

The CVP reflects the adjacent right atrial pressure (RAP). As blood is in continuity between the heart and the cava, the CVP reading is useful in helping gauge intra-vascular volume and cardiac filling. Intuitively, CVP is directly proportional to venous return and inversely proportional to cardiac contractility. It follows that CVP can be used to guide fluid replacement.

In order for the CVP to be an accurate guide for the management of fluid replacement, the patient's heart should be normal with RV function paralleling left ventricular (LV) function. Starling's law indicates that cardiac output is optimized as LV filling is optimized. As we cannot measure ventricular EDV, we rely on the ventricular end-diastolic pressure (VEDP). When the heart is normal, RV filling parallels that of the left. Furthermore, in a normal heart, right VEDP (RVEDP) equals RAP (as the tricuspid valve is open in diastole). Thus, RVEDP = RAP = CVP. To summarize, in the normal heart, CVP can be used as a guide to resuscitation because it ultimately reflects left VEDP (LVEDP).

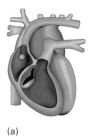 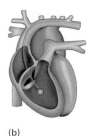 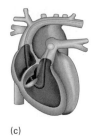 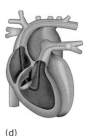

(a)   (b)   (c)   (d)

Figure 8.5. Floating a PA catheter. The catheter is introduced through a central vein and the balloon inflated. The flow of blood pulls the balloon and thus catheter via the right atrium and RV to its final resting position in the PA. As the catheter is floated, its position can be followed by evaluating pressure tracings on the monitor. Once the balloon has 'wedged' itself in the PA, the balloon should be deflated to avoid complications such as a ruptured PA or pulmonary infarct.

The problem is that the vast majority of critically ill patients do not have normal hearts. Thus, as an absolute value, CVP can be unreliable for a variety of reasons. CVP will be elevated in any situation where the intra-thoracic pressures are increased (mechanical ventilation). Pulmonary vascular disease, RV disease, LV failure, or valvular heart disease will also affect the CVP reading. Keeping such limitations in mind, looking at the dynamic changes in the CVP in response to fluid therapy can be very useful. If the CVP remains low in a hypotensive patient after receiving a fluid challenge, they may need more fluid. If the CVP rises rapidly in response to a fluid challenge, it implies the patient may already be appropriately filled.

PA catheterization

PA catheters are long catheters which are introduced through large bore central venous lines usually in the subclavian or internal jugular veins. The catheters have a balloon at their tip which allows them to be carried via the flow of blood or 'floated' to their resting position within the PA (Fig. 8.5). The catheter has a distal lumen which allows for measuring PA pressures and obtaining mixed venous (SvO_2) blood samples. A proximal lumen permits fluid infusions and manometric measurement in the right atrium.

PA catheters allow for measurement of a number of hemodynamic parameters which can be useful in characterizing a patient's illness and guiding therapy. These are summarized in Table 8.2. Indications for PA catheterization thus include: characterizing a hemodynamically unstable patient (trying to discern type of shock), distinguishing cardiogenic and non-cardiogenic pulmonary edema, and assistance with goal directed therapy.

PA catheters measure cardiac output via a technique known as thermodilution. A small bolus of cold 5% dextrose is quickly injected into the right atrium via the proximal lumen of the PA catheter. The injectate mixes with the blood and causes a fall in temperature which is recorded by a temperature probe at the catheter tip. The change in temperature over time is recorded as a curve. Cardiac output is inversely proportional to the area under the curve and is calculated using the Hamilton–Stewart equation (performed by

Table 8.2. Measurements and derived variables attainable from PA catheterization.

Measurements	Derived variables
Cardiac output	Stroke volume
Mixed venous saturation	Oxygen consumption
Pressures	Oxygen delivery
RAP	SVR
RVP	Pulmonary vascular resistance
PAP	
PAWP	

RAP: right atrial pressure; RVP: right ventricle pressure; PAP: pulmonary artery pressure; PAWP: pulmonary artery wedge pressure.

computer software). A modification of this technique, allowing more frequent measurements, utilizes a heating filament located in the right atrium. The filament is intermittently heated causing a change in temperature of the blood which will be measured in the PA.

Along with measuring PA pressures and cardiac output, PA catheters also estimate LVEDP via a measurement known as the PA wedge pressure (PAWP). To obtain this reading, the balloon at the tip of the PA catheter is inflated and occludes the vessel. The pressure in the vessel distal to the balloon then equilibrates through the pulmonary vasculature with the left atrial pressure (LAP). In end diastole, the mitral valve is open, such that end-diastolic pressure equals LAP. Thus, as there is a continuum of blood, what we have is the following:

LVEDP = LAP = PAWP

As was previously discussed, LVEDP is our best measurement of cardiac filling. Thus, PAWP can be used to guide fluid resuscitation. As with the CVP, there are significant limitations to these readings. Diagnostically, the PAWP can be useful in distinguishing cardiac versus non-cardiac pulmonary edema. Patients with left heart failure will have an elevated LAP and thus an elevated PAWP. This is not the case in patients with non-cardiogenic pulmonary edema.

While no one will dispute the utility of cardiac output and even PAWP measurements in certain critically ill patients, less invasive methods are becoming available for use. Complications of PA catheters include arrhythmias, pulmonary infarction, pulmonary embolism (PE), PA rupture, infection, and knotting of the catheter within the heart. Furthermore, with regard to patient outcome, multiple studies have failed to show either a benefit or a detriment to PA catheter use. These studies are difficult to perform and interpret because of the complexity of patients and their illnesses. Suffice it to say that PA catheterization should be used judiciously in the treatment of the critically ill patient.

Pulse contour cardiac output

Pulse contour cardiac output (PiCCO) is a novel method of hemodynamic monitoring that employs a specialized femoral or axillary arterial line and a central venous catheter. PiCCO uses analysis of the pulse contour (obtained via the arterial catheter) in conjunction with a thermodilution technique to estimate variables such as cardiac output, stroke volume, and SVR. Unlike the thermodilution technique utilized with the PA catheter, PiCCO depends on transpulmonary thermodilution. The injectate is administered via the central venous line, travels through the heart (and lungs), and is analyzed at the specialized arterial line site. Hemodynamic values obtained from PiCCO technology correlate well to conventional PA catheterization and avoid the complications associated with catheterizing the right heart.

Interpretation of special investigations

Doppler ultrasound

Doppler ultrasound is utilized in some intensive care units (ICUs) to provide a less invasive way of monitoring cardiac output. A Doppler probe positioned in the suprasternal notch or in the esophagus is used to detect a change in frequency of ultrasound waves caused by reflection from the blood moving through the ascending aorta (suprasternal notch) or descending aorta (esophagus). From an analysis of the velocity waveform and the aortic diameter, an estimate of the stroke volume and hence cardiac output can be made.

Echocardiography

ECHO has become an increasingly utilized modality in ICUs. An ultrasound beam is transmitted to the heart and the reflections are analyzed, and integrated to create an image or ECHO. Two methods of imaging are available, transthoracic ECHO (TTE) or transoesophageal ECHO (TOE). In TTE, the ultrasound probe is placed on the chest wall and ultrasound waves are emitted through the intercostal spaces. TOE obtains images with a transducer on the end of a flexible endoscope in the esophagus; it is useful for visualizing the thoracic aorta as well as the heart.

In the ICU, ECHO can be utilized to assess cardiac filling and correlate this observation to pressure readings. ECHO is useful in characterizing right and left heart interactions. For example, in a patient with right heart failure, ECHO can help determine whether this is secondary to a failing left heart or otherwise. Measurements of ventricular size and function (ejection fraction) can be made. ECHO can identify myocardial ischemia, pericardial effusion, and valvular abnormalities. When ECHO is used in conjunction with Doppler technology, intra-cardiac blood flow can also be studied. This is particularly useful in characterizing valvular abnormalities or septal defects. Doppler ECHO can also estimate cardiac output.

Radioisotope scans

Radioisotope scans have limited use in the ICU but are occasionally used to assess myocardial perfusion in patients with coronary artery disease. The degree to which thallium or technetium radioisotopes are taken up by the myocardium can help delineate myocardial perfusion. They can also be used to follow the progress of myocardial infarction (MI) which is detected as a cold spot.

Cardiovascular support

Cardiovascular support can be both pharmacologic or invasive. The goal is restore perfusion to physiologic levels. Adding cardiovascular support usually occurs in a stepwise fashion, such that the least invasive modalities are employed first.

Inotropes

Inotropes are drugs that work directly on the heart to increase its output by increasing the heart rate and contractility. Inotropes fall into two broad categories:
1. Cyclic adenosine monophosphate (cAMP) dependent (beta-adrenergic agonists and phosphodiesterase (PDE) inhibitors).
2. cAMP independent (alpha-adrenergic agonists and digoxin).

The vast majority of inotropes are cAMP dependent; their primary action is to increase second messenger cAMP. In the heart, cAMP activates a protein kinase which opens a sarcolema calcium gate allowing calcium to influx into the cytoplasm. Calcium then binds troponin C and cardiac muscle contraction is facilitated (see physiology section).

Importantly, cAMP activation causes the opposite effect in vascular smooth muscle. In smooth muscle, cAMP leads to calcium uptake by the sarcoplasmic reticulum and resultant smooth muscle relaxation. These contrasting effects of cAMP account for the inotropy and systemic and pulmonary vasodilation (inodilation) seen with a majority of inotropes.

Adrenergic receptor agonists (catecholamines)

Naturally occurring catecholamines and synthetic amines act via beta-adrenergic and alpha-adrenergic receptors. The different amines have varying affinities for the receptors leading to their variable effects.

Table 8.3. **Catecholamines, adrenergic activity, and clinical effects.**

Catecholamine	Property	Beta-1	Beta-2	Alpha-1	Clinical effect
Norepinephrine	Endogenous catecholamine	++	−	++	Predominantly increases MAP. Increase in SVR limits inotropic effects.
Epinephrine	Endogenous catecholamine	++	++	++	Predominant effect is inotropy at low doses and vasoconstriction at high doses. May cause tachyarrhythmias.
Dopamine	Endogenous catecholamine	++	−	++	Dose dependent. 2–5 (μ/kg/min): dopaminergic receptor activation increases splanchnic blood flow. 5–10: predominant beta/inotropic effect. >10: predominant alpha/vasoconstrictor effect.
Dobutamine	Synthetic catecholamine	++	++	−	Potent inotrope. May cause significant hypotension, particularly in hypovolemic patients.

++: potent agonist; +: moderate agonist; −: minimal agonist. SVR: systemic vascular resistance.

Beta-1 adrenergic receptors in cardiac muscle account for 80% of inotrope activity. Catecholamines bind beta-1 receptors on the cardiac muscle sarcolema. The beta-1 receptor acts via a G protein to activate adenylate cyclase and convert adenosine triphosphate (ATP) to cAMP. As described above, increased cAMP ultimately causes enhanced cardiac muscle contraction. Beta-1 receptor activation also causes an increase in sinoatrial node firing (chronotropy), an increase in atrioventricular conduction, and a decrease in the muscle cell excitation threshold.

Beta-2 and alpha-adrenergic receptors also exist in the heart and likely contribute to inotropy. Beta-2 receptors also work via cAMP dependent pathways. They have an important role in patients with chronic heart failure who have persistently elevated levels of catecholamines and thus downregulation of their beta-1 receptors. Alpha-adrenergic receptors are cAMP *independent*. The alpha-receptor is linked to the phospholipase C, GTP, inositol phosphate pathway. Ultimately, calcium is released to aid in cardiac muscle contraction, but cAMP is not required.

Catecholamines used for inotropic support include dobutamine, dopamine, epinephrine, and norepinephrine. These catecholamines, their receptor affinities, and primary clinical effects are listed in Table 8.3.

PDE inhibitors
PDE is responsible for the breakdown of cAMP. PDE inhibition then limits the breakdown of cAMP and thus increases cardiac contractility (and vascular smooth muscle relaxation). PDE evokes the same physiologic response as the beta-1 pathway, but is independent of beta-1 receptor occupation. Thus, PDE inhibitors can be particularly useful in patients who are likely to have downregulation of their beta-1 receptors (chronic failure). It is useful to note that there are a variety of PDE inhibitors available; PDE III is the active PDE in the heart, thus agents specific to PDE III are used for inotropy.

Amrinone, milrinone, and enoximone are examples of PDE III inhibitors. Amrinone was the first PDE used for inotropic support, but it has fallen out of favor as the result of causing gastrointestinal (GI) side effects and thrombocytopenia. Milrinone is currently the most widely used PDE inhibitor.

Digoxin
Digoxin increases intracellular calcium and thus cardiac contractility via inhibition of a sodium/potassium membrane pump. Digoxin is of limited use in the critically ill patient because of its narrow therapeutic index and increased potential for toxicity (electrolyte disturbances, hypoxia, and acidosis).

Vasopressors
Vasopressors are agents that cause vasoconstriction of the peripheral vasculature. Their main purpose is to increase MAP. This is done predominantly via alpha-adrenergic mechanisms.

Catecholamines
As previously discussed, catecholamines vary in their receptor activity. Those which strongly influence alpha-receptors (norepinephrine, high-dose epinephrine, and dopamine) can be used to support a failing blood pressure.

Phenylephrine
Phenylephrine is a strong vasopressor with almost exclusive alpha-receptor activity. It has minimal beta activity and only at very high doses. Its primary use is treating refractory hypotension in patients with neurogenic shock (loss of pure alpha-mediated vasomotor tone).

Vasoregulatory agents
Vasoregulatory agents are endogenous mediators that have a role in maintaining vascular tone. In sepsis and multiple organ dysfunction syndrome (MODS), there can be loss of the body's responsiveness to these agents.

Vasopressin

Vasopressin is a peptide hormone normally secreted by the posterior pituitary. It helps regulate intra-vascular fluid volume by facilitating water re-absorption by the renal collecting tubules (hence its other name – anti-diuretic hormone), but it also has direct vasoconstrictor effects. Decreased vasopressin levels have been noted in patients in septic shock. Vasopressin infusions have been shown to decrease catecholamine requirements in patients with septic shock. Vasopressin's effect on mortality outcome has not yet been established.

Steroids

Stress dose steroids (200–300 mg hydrocortisone per day) improve vascular responsiveness to catecholamine infusion in patients with septic shock. They are now recommended as a treatment in patients with septic shock. The adrenocorticotrophin stimulation test can also be done in such patients to assess if they have an element of hyopadrenalism.

Intra-aortic balloon pump

The intra-aortic balloon pump (IABP) is an invasive device utilized to increase cardiac output and myocardial perfusion. The IABP consists of a balloon which is connected to a long catheter. The catheter is inserted via the femoral artery and positioned such that the balloon sits in the descending thoracic aorta (Fig. 8.6). The balloon is also connected to a pump that allows it to be inflated and deflated at designated intervals.

The pump is synchronized with the electrocardiogram (ECG) so that the balloon is deflated in systole and inflated in diastole. When the heart ejects in systole, rapid deflation of the balloon creates an 'empty space' in the aorta, thus decreasing afterload and hence myocardial work. This improves cardiac contractility and output. During diastole, inflation of the balloon displaces a volume of blood equal to the volume of the balloon. Some of the blood will be pushed 'forward' and by this means the output of the heart is further augmented. As coronary blood flow occurs largely during diastole, inflation of the balloon during diastole also displaces blood 'backward' and thus enhances coronary blood flow.

Use of the IABP is indicated in selected cases of cardiogenic shock. It is particularly used for support of cardiac failure after coronary artery bypass graft (CABG) and as to a bridge to intervention for patients with acute coronary syndromes, mitral regurgitation, or septal defects. The device is not useful at very rapid heart rates (>150 bpm), since there is insufficient time for inflation and deflation of the balloon. It is contraindicated in aortic regurgitation as it exacerbates valvular insufficiency and heart failure. The IABP is also not useful in children because of their relatively rapid heart rates and because the major vessels in children are more distensible than in adults; inflation of the balloon in diastole simply distends the aorta without augmenting flow.

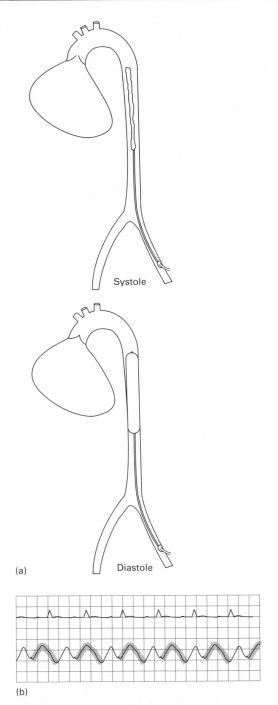

Systole

Diastole

(a)

(b)

Figure 8.6. IABP. (a) The IABP *in situ*. (b) The arterial waveform showing augmented diastolic blood pressure (highlighted section of the trace).

Extracorporeal circulation

Extracorporeal circulation use in the adult ICU is extremely rare. The most common setting in which extracorporeal circulation is utilized is in intra-operative cardiopulmonary bypass

(CPB). Still, familiarity with the process is useful in caring for patients post-operatively.

Indications for extracorporeal circulation include:

- cardiac surgery (valve replacement or repair, coronary bypass grafting);
- operation on the aortic arch or ascending aorta;
- heart or heart–lung transplantation;
- cardiopulmonary support;
- hypothermia.

CPB is performed by the following technique. After anticoagulation with heparin, venous blood is drained from the right atrium or from both vena cavae by special cannulae into the CPB circuit. This circuit consists of a reservoir, heat exchanger, oxygenator, and a pump. The reservoir collects the blood. The heat exchanger allows the patient's body temperature to be controlled, usually employing a moderate degree of hypothermia (25–28°C) in order to reduce the metabolic rate. (Deep hypothermia (18–20°C) significantly reduces metabolic rate so that bypass can be temporarily interrupted. This technique, known as circulatory arrest, is useful for the surgical treatment of aneurysms of the aortic arch.) The oxygenator facilitates gas exchange. The pump maintains a blood flow rate of around 2.4 and 2.8 l/min/m²; perfusion pressures are usually around 60 mmHg providing adequate tissue perfusion and oxygenation. On completion of the operative procedure, the patient is warmed and bypass is discontinued by allowing the heart gradually to take over the circulation. Anticoagulation is reversed by means of protamine.

Although CPB diverts returning venous blood from the systemic circulation away from the heart, coronary blood flow continues and the heart continues to beat. A dry, still, operating field is achieved by cross-clamping the aorta and inducing diastolic arrest by perfusing the heart with a special cold potassium-rich cardioplegia solution. Cessation of mechanical activity and low temperature reduces the rate of myocardial metabolism so that ischemia can be better tolerated. Cardioplegia infusions are repeated half-hourly and ice is applied topically to the heart to keep its rate of metabolism low. Ischemia times of up to 2 h are generally well tolerated although longer ischemia times increase the chance of damaging the myocardium.

CPB is now routinely performed with a much lower morbidity than in the past. It does, however, evoke systemic effects including: activation of the systemic inflammatory response, platelet destruction, dilution of clotting factors, red cell hemolysis, transient renal and hepatic insufficiency, and elevated amylase levels (usually without symptoms of pancreatitis).

Cardiac arrest and resuscitation

Cardiac arrest is sudden cessation of the pumping action of the heart (loss of heartbeat) resulting in the loss of effective circulation. Causes include:

- cardiac arrhythmias, conduction disturbances, MI;
- respiratory failure;
- shock;
- metabolic and electrolyte disturbances – hyperkalemia, metabolic acidosis;
- hypothermia, especially below 32°C.

Clinical presentation

When patients arrest, they almost immediately lose consciousness. If the arrest occurs whilst the patient is being monitored in the ICU or operating theater, an arrhythmia or asystole may be seen on the monitoring screen.

Three situations are possible:

1. ventricular fibrillation (VF)/pulseless ventricular tachycardia (VT);
2. pulseless electrical activity (PEA);
3. asystole or severe bradycardia.

Resuscitation

Well developed guidelines have been established by the European Resuscitation Council for patients with sudden cardiac arrest. Advanced life support guidelines mandate that patients with a witnessed arrest be given a single precordial thump before moving quickly to the algorithms of resuscitation.

Adult basic life support

When cardiac arrest occurs, basic life support should be initiated immediately. Briefly, after ensuring lack of responsiveness and administering a pre-cordial thump, the health care provider should begin the ABCs. In the hospital setting, it is crucial to attach a defibrillator monitor as soon as possible:

- *A – Airway*: Tilt the head backwards, lift the chin and clear the airway. If need be, consider an oro-pharyngeal airway. Begin preparations for formal tracheal intubation; however, this usually will be performed once cardiopulmonary resuscitation (CPR) has been initiated.
- *B – Breathing*: A bag-valve-mask is available on any code/crash cart. It should be connected to high flow oxygen and rescue breaths administered.
- *C – Circulation*: Once the absence of a carotid pulse is confirmed, chest compressions are initiated.

CPR combines external cardiac massage (cardio) with intermittently administered breaths (pulmonary). Cardiac massage involves compression of the chest in the lower third of the sternum. Current recommendations for both one and two person CPR are 15 chest compressions for 2 breaths. Once the patient's airway is secured, uninterrupted chest compressions should be done at a rate of 100 times per minute. For compressions to be effective the patient should be lying on a firm surface, and on the ward a board will need to be placed under the patient.

External cardiac massage usually results in an output sufficient to achieve systolic pressures between 50 and 100 mmHg. Though higher pressures may be achieved by greater compression, the risk of myocardial contusion is increased. Diastolic pressures during CPR are low (0–20 mmHg). This has implications for blood flow to all organs; it means that perfusion will occur largely during systole and that the mean perfusion pressure will be low. Coronary blood flow, which usually occurs in diastole, now must also occur in systole. As VF raises intra-myocardial tension and increases the resistance to blood flow, the heart is particularly vulnerable to ischemia.

Bag-valve-mask ventilation should be performed until tracheal intubation is possible. Tidal volume recommendations are 700–1000 ml via bag-valve-mask (air only); once high flow oxygen is available, tidal volumes can be reduced to 400–600 ml. Of note, the tidal volume should be sufficient to make the chest visibly rise. Once tracheal intubation is established, ventilation at approximately 12 breaths/min is recommended. Again, at this point, uninterrupted chest compressions are recommended to allow for higher coronary perfusion pressures. Laryngeal mask airway (LMA) is an acceptable alternative to tracheal intubation if the health care provider is more familiar with this type of airway.

Throughout resuscitation, evaluation of potentially reversible causes of arrest should be sought and corrected. These include the four 'H's (Hypoxia, Hypovolemia, Hypothermia, and Hypo/hyperkalemia, hypocalcemia, and academia) and the four 'T's (Tension pneumothorax, Tamponade, Thrombo-embolic event, and Toxic/therapeutic substance overdose). As such, administration of intravenous (IV) fluids, high flow oxygen, checking for clinical signs of pneumothorax and tamponade, an ABG to evaluate for acidosis or electrolyte disturbance, and review of the drug chart are essential components of any arrest situation.

Adult advanced life support

Advanced life support modifications of the BLS protocol were discussed above. It is critically important that the defibrillator-monitor is attached to the patient as soon as possible. Once attached, the patient's rhythm should be immediately established as either:

- shockable: VF or pulseless VT;
- non-shockable: asystole or PEA.

Ventricular fibrillation/Ventricular tachycardia
Defibrillation with up to three sequential shocks (200, 200, 360 J) should be applied as needed. Between each shock, the ECG trace should be checked for a change in rhythm. If VT/VF persists after three shocks, then CPR is resumed for the next 1 min and 1 mg adrenaline given. Airway and venous access should be secured here. If patient still remains in VF/VT, then Amiodarone 300 mg may be administered. Amiodarone administration should not delay further defibrillation however. Three more defibrillations (360 J) should be repeated, followed by an additional 1 mg adrenaline. Rhythm assessment, three attempts at defibrillation, and 1 min of CPR should take 2–3 min. One milligram adrenaline is administered every 3 min. This cycle repeats itself until

defibrillation is achieved – either in the form of a survivable rhythm or asystole.

Asystole/PEA
CPR should be administered while the cause of the arrest is sought and corrected (see above). Airway and IV access should be secured. One milligram adrenaline should be administered. CPR should be paused and the rhythm re-assessed every 3 min. Adrenaline can be administered at these 3 min intervals. A single 3 mg dose of atropine should be considered for patients with asystole and PEA. Sodium bicarbonate can be given to correct a severe acidosis (pH < 7.1) or a suspected acidosis in sustained arrest situations (20–25 min). Pacing has a role in bradyarrhythmias; its role in asystole is less established, but it may be considered.

Arrhythmias

Sinus rhythm is initiated by the sinoatrial node and is recognized by the presence of a P-wave, a QRS complex, and a T-wave. In sinus rhythm, the heart rate is between approximately 60 and 100 bpm. Occasionally, other 'ectopic' foci within the heart will discharge spontaneously, causing a premature heartbeat. Atrial ectopy is frequent, occasionally symptomatic, and usually benign. It is characterized by an abnormal P-wave followed by a normal QRS complex. Treatment is re-assurance, avoiding caffeine, and occasionally beta- or calcium blockade. Junctional ectopy has a normal looking QRS complex but is not necessarily preceded by a P-wave; the P-wave may immediately precede, follow or be located within the QRS complex. Ventricular ectopic beats lack a P-wave and often have a bizarre, wide QRS complex. Such premature ventricular contractions usually also occur in the absence of any cardiac pathology, are self-limited, but may be treated with beta-blockade if patients are severely symptomatic.

Tachycardia

Sinus tachycardia is a fast heart rate (>100 bpm) that is generated by the sinoatrial node in response to autonomic or catecholamine stimulation. By definition, a normal P-wave should precede each QRS. It is a 'benign arrhythmia' in that there is no intrinsic abnormality of the heart. However, sinus tachycardia is a response to physiologic stress, be it exercise and anxiety or hypotension, anemia, sepsis, PE, etc. Thus, in any patient with sinus tachycardia, a pathologic source of stress should be sought and treated.

Supraventricular tachycardias are arrhythmias initiated above the A–V node resulting in a narrow QRS complex on the ECG. They include atrial fibrillation, atrial flutter, and varying conduction or re-entry abnormalities that are often grouped together broadly as 'supraventricular tachycardias' (SVTs). Atrial fibrillation is characterized by rapid, random depolarizations of the atria (up to 600 bpm) which are irregularly transmitted to the ventricles. This accounts for the lack of a P-wave as well as the irregular rate and rhythm. Treatment of atrial fibrillation depends on patient stability as well as duration of the arrhythmia. Expert help should be sought in any unstable patient (HR > 150 bpm, chest pain, poor perfusion) as cardioversion is recommended. A complex algorithm for further management of atrial fibrillation is provided in the European Resuscitation Council Guidelines which are referenced at the end of this chapter. Suffice it to say that amiodarone has gained prominence as a means of medical cardioversion, but that rate control is still an option in patients with no history of heart disease and atrial fibrillation of uncertain duration. Patients with other narrow complex tachyarrhythmias are often categorized together for treatment purposes. Pulseless narrow complex tachycardia requires immediate cardioversion. In patients with a pulse, initial treatment involves vagal maneuvers and adenosine administration. If the patient fails to convert to sinus rhythm, expert advice should be sought; less stable patients may need cardioversion, whereas stable patients may benefit from amiodarone, beta- or Ca^{2+} channel blockade, or digoxin.

VT is recognized by bizarre QRS complexes which occur at a rate of 100–200 bpm. A patient with VT who is pulseless need be treated by the arrest algorithm that was discussed in the previous section. VT in the unstable patient (chest pain, heart failure, hypotension) is treated with cardioversion and amiodarone. VT in the stable patient is treated with amiodarone (and potentially cardioversion). Expert evaluation is critical as certain patients may benefit from automatic implantable cardiac defibrillators (AICDs). Potassium levels should be checked in all cases, keeping in mind that potassium and magnesium supplementation may be indicated.

Bradycardia

Bradycardia is defined as a heart rate of less than 60 bpm. While this may be normal in a well-trained athlete, it may be pathologic in others and not allow for a sufficient cardiac output. Bradycardia usually results from either sinus node dysfunction or from atrioventricular (heart) block. First-degree heart block is characterized by a prolonged PR interval (>0.21 s). In second-degree heart block, there is failure to conduct all atrial impulses to the ventricle. In Mobitz I, the PR interval increases until there is a dropped beat. In Mobitz II, there is a normal PR interval but not all atrial impulses are conducted to the ventricle such that the ratio of atrial to ventricular beats may be 2 : 1 or 3 : 1. Third-degree heart block is also known as complete heart block; P-waves and QRS complexes occur independently as no atrial impulses are transmitted to the ventricle. Patients showing adverse signs of bradycardia should be given a trial of atropine if unstable. Subsequently, external pacing should be considered (or low-dose adrenaline if pacing is not available). Expert advice is recommended to determine if the patient is a candidate for more permanent pacing options.

Cardiac tamponade

Cardiac tamponade is compression of the heart due to fluid accumulation within the pericardial space. When fluid or blood accumulates within in the pericardial cavity, the intra-pericardial pressure rises and compresses the heart. The lower pressure atria are most vulnerable to this increased pressure; their compression leads to impaired venous return and decreased cardiac filling. Compression of the heart as a whole also impairs diastolic filling.

Surgical causes include penetrating cardiac wounds, blunt trauma to the chest, or post-operative accumulation after open heart surgery. Tamponade can also occur as a complication of central line placement. Medical causes include malignancy, pericarditis, post-MI ventricular rupture, and uremia.

Clinical presentation and diagnosis

Presentation may be acute when fluid or blood accumulates in the heart very rapidly or it may be late when the rate of fluid accumulation is slow and compression occurs only after a period of time. Beck's triad of muffled heart sounds, hypotension, and elevated jugular venous distension may be evident particularly in the acute setting. Hemodynamically compromised patients are tachycardic and hypotensive. In the acute setting, they may be sitting up and extremely anxious. Evidence of right heart failure with jugular venous distension and hepatomegaly may be apparent. Decreased heart sounds or a pericardial friction rub may be noted in up to a third of patients.

Pulsus parodoxus is a classic finding in patients with pericardial tamponade. It is defined as an exaggerated fall in arterial systolic pressure (>10 mmHg) during inspiration (Fig. 8.7). Kussmaul described this 'paradox' by noting a disappearance of the pulse during inspiration, although the heartbeat was still audible. Here is how it works. During inspiration, intra-thoracic pressure falls and allows for increased venous return, and increased RV filling. However, in tamponade, because the heart is compressed and there is no room to accommodate the increased RV filling, the intra-ventricular septum becomes displaced to the left. The bulge of the septum inhibits LV filling, and as a result, stroke volume decreases with a subsequent decrease in cardiac output and arterial pressure.

In the acute setting, diagnosis should be suspected clinically. In a post-operative cardiac patient, hypotension, tachycardia, and low urine output should put the surgeon on instant alert. Diagnosis is now made quickly and easily with ultrasound. Bedside ultrasound is becoming increasingly available, even in Accident and Emergency (A&E) departments. In the absence of ultrasound, pericardiocentesis may be performed as a diagnostic and potentially therapeutic measure. Nevertheless, pericardiocentesis has associated risks (arrhythmias, cardiac laceration, coronary artery laceration, tamponade, and pneumothorax) and is ideally

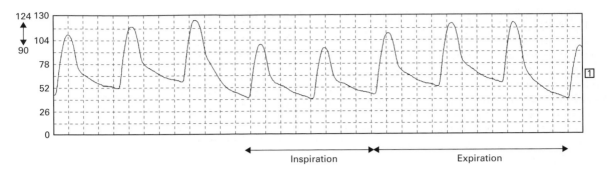

Figure 8.7. Pulsus paradoxus. Arterial waveform of a patient with pulsus paradoxus. Note the exaggerated fall in systolic pressure (>10 mmHg) seen on inspiration.

performed only once pericardial fluid is confirmed or very highly suspected.

Management

Management involves draining the cause of tamponade. In a patient who has undergone cardiac surgery, emergent sternal re-opening and evacuation of blood may be life saving. Patients with penetrating chest wounds and tamponade should be taken for immediate sternotomy. Incidentally, these patients are rarely stable and often will require emergent thoracotomy (and opening of the pericardial sac) in A&E. Pericardiocentesis has a role in providing urgent symptomatic relief in tamponade due to more chronic conditions such as uremia or malignancy. It should be performed with the patient sitting up and a needle introduced just to the left of the xiphoid, at a 15° angle to the skin, and directed slowly toward the left shoulder. Ultrasound guidance is now the norm. Surgical creation of a 'window' or small hole in the pericardium to communicate with the pleural space is a useful option for draining chronic pericardial effusions causing tamponade.

SHOCK

Definition

Shock is defined as circulatory failure resulting in inadequate tissue perfusion and thus end-organ/cellular hypoxia. Shock occurs when the circulatory system (heart, blood vessels, and blood) is unable to deliver a necessary amount of oxygen to meet the demands of the body. While initially a simple definition, shock can arise from a variety of causes, making the diagnosis and treatment quite complex.

Diagnosis

Patients in shock will demonstrate evidence of end-organ hypoperfusion. Thinking of this systemically will allow one not to be fooled by less obvious signs. Confusion or altered mental status may be one of the most subtle and least appreciated signs of cerebral hypoxia; in the late stage, shocked patients are often obtunded. Patients are tachypneic and show increased

work of breathing as they attempt to meet body's oxygen demands. Their extremities may be cool and they may appear 'clamped down' with delayed capillary refill as the periphery vasoconstricts to divert blood flow to the more important splanchnic organs. Urine output diminishes as the kidneys are hypoperfused. Ultimately, cells receiving inadequate oxygen resort to anaerobic metabolism and systemic lactic acidosis results.

Patients in shock may have a low blood pressure and compensatory tachycardia. These can be very misleading signs for a variety of reasons and thus should not be used to define shock. For example, in a usually hypertensive elderly patient, a 'normal' blood pressure may not provide adequate tissue perfusion. Likewise, a patient on a beta-blocker may not be capable of mounting an expected tachycardia. It is important not to count on these classic signs when approaching a patient with suspected shock.

Types of shock

Thinking of shock as either pump (cardiac) failure or peripheral circulatory failure can be a useful starting point in approaching the shocked patient. With this in mind, four main types of shock have been defined (Table 8.4):

1. *Cardiogenic*: The heart intrinsically is not providing the output to meet the demands of the body.
2. *Hypovolemic*: The heart is under filled because of an inadequate circulating blood volume and thus not able to deliver adequate output to the body.
3. *Obstructive*: The heart itself is healthy and there is adequate blood volume, but the heart is still not able to deliver adequate output because of impedance. This is due to either inflow obstruction (e.g. pericardial tamponade, constrictive pericarditis) or outflow obstruction (e.g. pulmonary or air embolism).
4. *Distributive*: Loss of systemic vascular tone results in decreased venous return to the heart and decreased cardiac output.

It should be noted that patients may have more than one type of shock at any given time. While the initial management of the shocked patient is the same regardless of its cause, early

Table 8.4. **Classification of shock.**

Cardiogenic shock	Hypovolemic shock	Obstructive shock	Distributive shock
Heart failure	Hemorrhage	Pericardial tamponade	Sepsis/SIRS
MI	Fluid depletion	Constrictive pericarditis	Neurogenic
Arrhythmia	(vomiting, diuretics,	Tension pneumothorax	Anaphylaxis
Valvular failure	diarrhea fistula/	PE	
Cardiac contusion	stoma losses)	Air embolism	

SIRS: systemic inflammatory response syndrome.

recognition of the type of shock affecting the patient is paramount to providing further appropriate treatment. In the following sections, we will first discuss early resuscitation of the shocked patient followed by a look at strategies for managing the particular types of shock.

Resuscitation

The treatment of shock begins with the ABC model of treating any critically ill or injured patient. Airway and breathing may be intact, but this is not always the case. Obtunded patients or hemorrhaging, severely injured patients may need airway protection and control. Intubation is sometimes necessary in ventilatory failure and may also decrease work of breathing thus decreasing the body's oxygen demands.

Improving circulation and perfusion is the cornerstone of shock treatment. It begins with early goal directed fluid resuscitation which has been shown to improve survival. Fluids should be administered immediately with the goal of improving deranged physiologic parameters. In its initial stages the clinician should aim for mental status improvement, urine output increase, lactic acidosis correction, normalization of capillary refill, and blood pressure rise.

Fluid administration can be in the form of crystalloid (normal saline or Hartmann's solution) or colloid (albumin, gelofusine). While there was some concern that colloid solutions might lead to a slightly increased mortality (*Cochrane Review, Br Med J* 1998), a larger and more recent meta-analysis (MM Wilkes, *Ann Intern Med* 2001) disputed this claim. Furthermore, a well-designed multi-center randomized controlled study of critically ill patients failed to find a difference in outcome in patients resuscitated with normal saline versus albumin (SAFE Investigators, *New Eng J Med* 2004). Thus, it is the appropriate administration of fluid rather than the fluid itself that is important. Blood and blood products may also be judiciously used as resuscitative fluids in patients in shock. Certainly, blood replacement should accompany fluid replacement in an actively hemorrhaging patient. Red blood cell transfusion can also be useful to increase oxygen delivery.

After fluid resuscitation begins, the clinician should quickly assess the patient's response. In addition to improvement, patients should also be monitored for any signs of volume overload (such as pulmonary edema or increased jugular venous distension). If physiologic markers are not improving, then more objective parameters and invasive monitoring will likely be needed to guide further therapy. CVP monitoring or ECHO can be very useful in determining fluid status. ECHO has the additional benefit of looking at cardiac function. Cardiac output monitoring may be necessary for shock that in unresponsive to treatment and may aid in determining the type of shock encountered (please refer to invasive monitoring section).

Vasoactive drugs should not routinely be part of initial resuscitation efforts. Vasoconstrictors increase blood pressure and thus may cause clinicians to prematurely limit needed fluid resuscitation. Such drugs should be utilized when patients remain shocked despite adequate filling and often should be used with invasive monitoring.

In the following section, we will address the major categories of shock. A summary table of the hemodynamic disturbances associated with each type of shock is provided for a reference in Table 8.5. Recognizing trends is important in helping to distinguish a patient's type of shock and administering appropriate treatment. Nevertheless, it should also be recognized that patients may have several etiologies for their hemodynamic compromise (e.g. cardiogenic and hypovolemic shock). Keeping an open mind and frequently re-assessing responses to therapy ideally will ensure the best outcome in this critically ill group.

Cardiogenic shock

Cardiogenic shock refers to pump failure, or failure of the heart to generate a sufficient cardiac output despite adequate filling (preload). Cardiogenic shock may be due to variety of causes including MI, cardiac contusion (trauma), arrhythmia, or valvular abnormality. In cardiogenic shock, patients' extremities are cold and have delayed capillary refill. Patients often will demonstrate clinical signs related to

Table 8.5. **Summary of hemodynamic variables in different types of shock.**

	Cardiogenic shock	Hypovolemic shock	Obstructive shock (tamponade)	Obstructive shock (PE)	Distributive shock (neurogenic)	Distributive shock (sepsis/SIRS)
HR	↑→↓	↑	↑	↑	↑→↓	↑
BP	↓	↓	↓	↓	↓	↓
CVP	↑→	↓	↑	↑→	↓	↓
CO	↓	↓	↓	↓	↑	↑
PAWP	↑	↓	Equalization of diastolic pressure with CVP	↑→↓	↓	↓
SVR	↑	↑	↑	↑	↓	↓

↑ : increased; →: decreased; ↓ : neutral; ↑→↓ : variable. SIRS: systemic inflammatory response syndrome; BP: blood pressure.

the etiology of their cardiac failure. They may have an elevated jugular venous pressure (RV failure), pulmonary crackles (LV failure), an irregular heartbeat (arrhythmia), or murmur. Invasive parameters reveal a decreased cardiac output and increased SVR (a reflection of their compensatory increase in diastolic blood pressure). CVP varies, but is generally elevated as the heart fails and can not adequately distribute the venous return.

The classic cause of cardiogenic shock is systolic dysfunction or LV heart failure. With LV failure, left heart stroke volume is diminished and there is subsequent increase in LAP and PA pressure. This manifests clinically as pulmonary edema, but will be demonstrated as an increase in the PAWP in patients with PA catheters. Acute coronary syndromes (ischemia) are the most common cause of such dysfunction with cardiogenic shock occurring in up to 10% of patients sustaining an acute MI. If possible, early revascularization either by interventional cardiology or surgery has demonstrated survival benefits.

Treatment

- Ensure adequate preload. Central venous or PA catheter may be needed for guidance of fluid resuscitation.
- Inotropes.
- Reduction of afterload.
- Intra-aortic balloon counterpulsation.
- Correction of the cardiac abnormality. Modalities may include early revascularization (ischemia), correction of the valvular abnormality (valvuloplasty, valve replacement), anti-arrhythmic, etc.

Note: Inotropes and IABP are discussed in detail in the cardiovascular support section.

Hypovolemic shock

Hypovolemic shock occurs as a result of hemorrhage or severe dehydration. Patients at highest risk of dehydration are children and the elderly. Causes of dehydration may include diarrhea, vomiting, heat (including burns), diuretic use, prolonged

operation, and fistula losses. A patient in hypovolemic shock will have cold extremities with delayed capillary refill. They are often initially anxious and later somnolent. Invasive monitoring demonstrates a low CVP, a high SVR, and a low CO.

Hemorrhagic shock has been divided into four classes based on the amount of blood lost and the body's compensatory response (Table 8.6). Of importance, the body has significant ability to compensate for blood loss; hypotension is a late sign of hemorrhage, not occurring until 30–40% of the circulating blood volume is lost. Compensatory mechanisms include baroreceptor reflexes leading to an increase in myocardial contractility, tachycardia, and peripheral vasoconstriction. Humoral mediators (vasopressin, aldosterone, and rennin) are released in attempt to stabilize intra-vascular volume.

On-going bleeding should be treated with blood replacement and surgical control of the source. If there is difficulty or delay in controlling hemorrhage, initial compensatory mechanisms begin to fail. Myocardial depression occurs and vasomotor reflexes are lost. Hypoxic cells develop an altered membrane potential, allowing sodium and water influx into the cell and subsequent edema. Organ failure may follow. A vicious triad of metabolic acidosis, hypothermia, and coagulopathy begins to perpetuate itself ultimately leading to arrhythmia and death.

Treatment

- Fluid replacement.
- Blood replacement in hemorrhagic shock. Of note, if massive transfusion (greater than 10 units of blood or more than one blood volume in a 24 h time period) is needed to control hemorrhage, patient should be assessed for coagulopathy. Often times such patients will also require platelets and/or fresh frozen plasma transfusion.
- Surgical control of the bleeding source.

Obstructive shock

In obstructive shock, the heart is not able to deliver adequate output because of impedance of either blood inflow

Table 8.6. **Classification of hemorrhagic shock.**

	Class 1	Class 2	Class 3	Class 4
Estimated blood loss (ml)	<750	750–1500	1500–2000	>2000
Estimated blood loss (% total blood volume)	10–15%	15–30%	30–40%	>40%
Respiratory rate	14–20	20–30	30–40	>35
Heart rate	<100	>100	>120	>140
Blood pressure	Normal	Normal	Decreased	Decreased
Urine output (ml/h)	>30	20–30	5–15	Negligible
Mental status	Slightly anxious	Anxious	Anxious, confused	Confused, lethargic
Fluid replacement	Crystalloid	Crystalloid	Crystalloid + blood	Crystalloid + blood

Modified from Committee on Trauma of the American College of Surgeons, *Advanced Trauma Life Support.*

or outflow. As the end result is a low cardiac output, the patient will be cold and clamped down. SVR will be increased with a compensatory tachycardia.

Inflow obstruction (tamponade and tension pneumothorax)

Inflow obstruction is primarily due to pericardial tamponade or tension pneumothorax. In tamponade, CVP will be dramatically increased as there is impedance to inflow and back up of venous return. As the heart is being compressed externally, all of the pressures within the heart at rest (diastole) will all be the same. Such 'equalization of pressures' is reflected by the PAWP (a reflection of LAP), PA pressure, RV pressure, and RA (or CVP) being the same in diastole. This finding is highly suggestive of pericardial tamponade. Please refer to the previous section for the causes, diagnosis, and treatment of pericardial tamponade.

Tension pneumothorax is another source of inflow obstruction. In tension pneumothorax, the positive intrathoracic pressure pushes the heart toward the opposite side of the chest (away from the pneumothorax), distorting anatomy and impairing venous return. Treatment involves emergent needle thoracostomy followed by thoracostomy drain placement.

Outflow obstruction (thrombo-embolism and air embolism)

Outflow obstruction is usually secondary to a pulmonary embolic event. In outflow obstruction, the right heart outflow tract or pulmonary arteries are obstructed with emboli. This leads to impaired emptying of the right heart and right heart strain. Invasive monitoring will demonstrate an increased CVP. The PAWP is highly variable in this situation and is in no way diagnostic. Venous thrombo-embolism is the most common cause of outflow obstructive shock; it is discussed in detail in the following section.

Of note, air embolism is another embolic phenomenon seen in surgical patients. Air embolism is seen when a bolus of air travels through the venous system and becomes lodged in the RV outflow tract. This bolus can occur if pressurized gas is forced into a body cavity, or it can occur when there is disruption of the venous system above the level of the heart. In this last situation, the pressure differential causes air to be 'sucked' into the vasculature. Air embolism most commonly occurs in the setting of neurosurgery or head and neck surgery when patients are in a seated operative position. Nevertheless, it can also be seen in penetrating vascular trauma or as a complication of central venous access. Approximately 50 ml of air is needed to cause hemodynamic compromise; the lethal dose is probably around 100–300 ml of air. Treatment of air embolism is to first suspect it. Next, the patient should be positioned in the head down and left lateral decubitus position (Durant's maneuver) such that the bolus of air drifts to the apex of the RV away from the outflow tract. After this, the aims are to prevent further air entry, if possible aspirate the air versus give it time to reabsorb, and provide hemodynamic support. Some authors recommend a trial of aspirating the air from a central venous catheter positioned at the level of the right atrium.

Distributive shock

There are three types of distributive shock; they are neurogenic, anaphylaxis, and sepsis/systemic inflammatory response syndrome (SIRS). The clinical picture of distributive shock differs from other forms of shock as the mechanism is loss of peripheral vascular tone causing pooling of blood peripherally and thus a diminished preload. Patients tend to be peripherally warm and may even have an increased capillary refill. Their diastolic blood pressure is classically low. The heart compensates by increasing its rate and contractility, thus resulting in a high cardiac output state. Invasive monitoring demonstrates a low CVP, low SVR, and a high CO. Of note, there is a small subset of septic patients who demonstrate myocardial depression; the reason behind this is still uncertain.

Neurogenic shock

Neurogenic shock occurs because of disruption of sympathetic innervation to peripheral vessels leading to venodilation and venous pooling. It is seen in severe stress states, in high spinal anesthesia, and more commonly in injury to the cervical or high thoracic spinal cord. Most patients will demonstrate reflexive tachycardia; however, injuries of the cervical cord tend to be associated with sinus bradycardia. Neurogenic shock occurs immediately after a spinal cord injury and is self-limiting, generally resolving several days after the insult.

Treatment

- Volume expansion to fill the expanded intra-vascular space.
- Vasopressors. This is the one shock state where a pure alpha-agonist (phenylephrine) may be judiciously used to counteract the loss of vascular tone. Adequate filling should be ensured prior to initiation of such agents.

Anaphylactic shock

Anaphylactic shock is the severest form of an allergic reaction in which a sensitized individual releases histamine in response to antigen exposure. This response leads to peripheral vasodilation and potentially hemodynamic instability (shock). Other symptoms include wheezing and respiratory distress, swelling of the throat and mucous membranes, itching, and urticaria.

Treatment

- ABCs (patients may have airway and breathing compromise as well).
- Volume expansion to fill the expanded intra-vascular space.
- IV epinephrine.
- Anti-histamines.
- Steroids.

Septic shock

Septic shock is the extreme end of the spectrum in the entities of systemic inflammation. It is defined as hypotension not responsive to fluid resuscitation or requiring the use of inotropes or vasopressors in a patient with a severe inflammatory response to a source of infection. Please refer to the section on SIRS, sepsis, and MODS for a detailed discussion of the definition, pathophysiology, and treatment of these complicated disorders.

RESPIRATORY SYSTEM

Physiology

Work of breathing

During quiet respiration, inspiration occurs through diaphragmatic contraction decreasing the intra-thoracic pressure and drawing air into the respiratory tree. This pressure must be great enough to overcome airway resistance and the compliance of the lung and chest wall. Elastic recoil

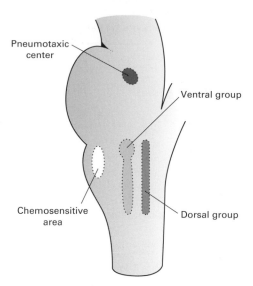

Figure 8.8. The respiratory center. Note the location of the three regulatory groups of neurons (dorsal, ventral, and pneumotaxic) within the pons and medulla.

is responsible for expiration and the whole process of breathing utilizes very little energy, only 1–2% of the total body oxygen consumption. During active respiration, the accessory muscles are used for inspiration and the abdominal muscles and internal intercostals are used for expiration. Much more energy is required and the work of breathing may consume as much as 25% of the body's total oxygen consumption. It is little wonder that compromised patients quickly fatigue with such an increased work of breathing.

Regulation of respiration

The respiratory system supplies O_2 and removes carbon dioxide (CO_2) over a wide range of metabolic demands. Control is exercised by the respiratory center located in the medulla oblongata and pons. It is divided into three groups of neurons (Fig. 8.8). The dorsal group functions during quiet respiration and also acts as the pacemaker by initiating inspiration. The ventral group is more important during active respiration. The pneumotaxic center responds to stimuli by increasing the rate of respiration.

The respiratory center receives input from higher brain centers and from chemo- and mechanoreceptors. In short, there are two major stimuli to breathe – hypoxia and acidosis. Central chemoreceptors are located in the medulla and are sensitive to acidosis in the form of CO_2 (as hydrogen ions can not cross the blood–brain or blood–CSF barriers directly). CO_2 crosses the blood–brain and blood–CSF barriers to reach the medulla. The CO_2 binds with water and produces hydrogen ions which act on the pacemaker (dorsal group of neurons) and stimulate respiration. Peripheral chemoreceptors are located in the carotid and aortic bodies and respond to a fall in partial pressure of arterial oxygen (PaO_2) below 60 mmHg

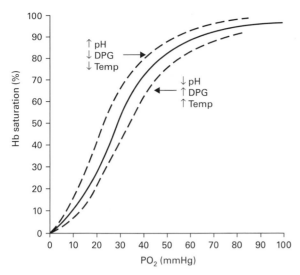

Figure 8.9. The hemoglobin dissociation curve. Note the effects on pH, DPG, and temperature allowing for alterations in oxygen unloading at a given PO$_2$. A shift of the curve to the right indicates that hemoglobin will remain less saturated for a given PO$_2$.

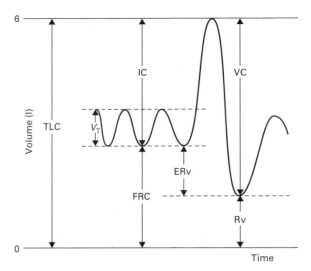

Figure 8.10. Spirometric tracing of lung volumes. ERV: end residual volume; IC: isovolumetric contraction.

(8 kPa). They provide input to the higher brain centers and brainstem to increase respiration. Mechanoreceptors include stretch receptors, irritant receptors, and juxtacapillary (or J) receptors. Stretch receptors inhibit the level of inspiration and juxtacapillary receptors are thought to be important in the sensation of dyspnea.

Hemoglobin dissociation curve

There are four iron atoms in a hemoglobin molecule and each can bind one molecule of oxygen in a reversible interaction. As hemoglobin binds oxygen it changes its conformation and takes up oxygen more readily. This accounts for the sigmoid shaped hemoglobin dissociation curve (Fig. 8.9). As demonstrated by the curve, hemoglobin binds oxygen rapidly to a PaO$_2$ of 8 kPa (60 mmHg) and then levels off, requiring higher partial pressures of oxygen to remain fully saturated. Another way of looking at it is that a PaO$_2$ of 8 kPa is required to maintain saturations above 90%. This is important physiologically, because it allows for the easy off-loading of oxygen in the peripheral capillary beds where oxygen is needed (i.e. if the PaO$_2$ is low in the periphery, hemoglobin gives up its oxygen molecule easily). Factors such as acidosis, increased temperature, and increased 2,3-dihydroxyphosphoglycerol (2,3-DPG) shift the hemoglobin dissociation curve to the right resulting in easier unloading of oxygen for a given PaO$_2$.

Interpretation of special investigations

Pulmonary function tests

Lung volumes are measured by spirometry and once quantified can be compared against predicted values for the size,

age, and gender of the patient. An example of a spirometry tracing is provided in Fig. 8.10 and an explanation of these volumes is provided below:
- Tidal volume (V_T) is the volume of air inspired or expired per breath.
  Normal tidal volume = 500 ml
- Minute ventilation is the volume of air inspired or expired over 1 min.
  Minute ventilation = V_T × respiratory rate
  Normal minute ventilation = 5–7 l/min
- Total lung capacity (TLC) is the volume of air in the lungs after maximal inspiration (6 l). TLC equals the sum of the vital capacity (VC) and the residual volume (Rv).
- VC is the maximal volume of air that can be exhaled after a maximal inspiration. It depends on the strength of the respiratory muscles and the resistance of the lungs and chest wall. Normal VC is approximately 4.8 l.
- Forced expiratory volume in 1 s (FEV$_1$) is the volume of air that can be forcibly exhaled in 1 s.
- Functional residual capacity (FRC) is the volume of air left in the lungs after exhalation (2.2 l). It is a critical volume because it allows for gas exchange throughout the entire respiratory cycle. FRC decreases with anesthesia, obesity, surgery (particularly thoracic and abdominal), and increasing age. When the FRC is too low, atelectasis occurs resulting in hypoxemia. Recruitment maneuvers to open alveoli (e.g. positive end-expiratory pressure – PEEP) are aimed at increasing FRC.
- Rv is the amount of air remaining in the lungs after a maximal expiration (1.2 l).

Diffusion capacity of carbon monoxide (DL$_{CO}$) is the ability of CO to diffuse across intact alveoli. This study is often performed in conjunction with spirometry. The patient inhales a small known quantity of CO, holds his breath for 10 s, and then exhales. The expired gas is analyzed for CO. A low DL_{CO} implies that there is a ventilation/perfusion (V/Q) mismatch and is often seen in disorders that disrupt normal alveolar architecture (emphysema or pulmonary fibrosis). It can also be present in severe anemia. Alternatively, DL_{CO} may be increased in patients with polycythemia.

Measurements of VC and FEV_1 are useful in determining whether obstructive, restrictive, or mixed airways disease is present. FEV_1 is also one of the best predictors of outcome for patients about to undergo pulmonary resection (e.g. in lung cancer). In general, a patient with a FEV_1 greater than 2 l or 60% predicted and $DL_{CO} > 60\%$ is at low risk of complications even for pneumonectomy.

Pulmonary compliance

Compliance reflects the distensibility of an elastic structure, like the lung. Pulmonary compliance is defined as the change in pulmonary volume (in milliliters) produced by a given change in pressure (in mmHg or kPa or cmH_2O):

Compliance = change volume/change in pressure

Pulmonary compliance changes in diseased states, and calculating compliance helps us understand both the intrinsic properties of the lungs and the work needed to ventilate a patient. Conceptually, patients with fibrotic lungs (pulmonary fibrosis) or a significant consolidation process (acute respiratory distress syndrome, ARDS) will need to generate large pressures to create enough force to draw in relatively small tidal volumes; such patients are said to have low compliance or stiff lungs. On the other hands, patients with emphysema have destroyed parenchymal architecture; their lungs fill easily when a breath is drawn in, and they have highly compliant lungs.

We often measure pulmonary compliance in patients undergoing mechanical ventilation. The ventilator allows us to easily obtain values to determine compliance:

Dynamic compliance $(C_{dyn}) = V_T/(\text{PIP} - \text{PEEP})$

where V_T = tidal volume (change in volume); PIP = peak inspiratory pressure (highest inspiratory pressure generated); PEEP = positive end-expiratory pressure (pressure at end expiration, note this would be zero for a non-ventilated patient).

The normal value for a non-ventilated adult would be 500 ml/(68 cmH_2O − o) = ~60–80 ml/cmH_2O. In a patient with decreased compliance, such as in ARDS, the compliance is generally 40 ml/cmH_2O or lower. For example, 500 ml/(30 − 10) = 25 ml/cmH_2O. Noting improved compliance in a ventilated patient with ARDS implies that the lungs are recovering.

Pulmonary perfusion

Abnormalities in pulmonary perfusion can be visualized using radioisotope perfusion scans. Combined V/Q scans can demonstrate areas of V/Q mismatch where areas of the lungs are ventilated, but not perfused. The classic example of this is PE where a thrombus obstructs the pulmonary vasculature but the lung is still being ventilated.

Areas of the lung that are ventilated, but not perfused are called dead space. In the normal lung, 'physiologic' dead space includes the upper airways and bronchials where air is present, but no gas exchange occurs. As CO_2 comes from the alveoli (and not the dead space) and because arterial pressure of CO_2 ($PaCO_2$) very closely approximates alveolar (exhaled) PCO_2, we can calculate physiologic dead space. This calculation is made based on the Bohr equation:

$$V_D/V_T = PaCO_2 - \text{expired } PCO_2/PaCO_2$$

where V_D is the dead space volume and V_T is the tidal volume. Expired CO_2 can be measured by infrared absorption spectrometry. In an intubated patient a CO_2 sensor is attached to the endotracheal tube (ETT) and the CO_2 in the expired gas is measured. When CO_2 is recorded over time, a 'capnogram' is produced.

Capnography

As noted above, capnography is a continuous measurement of the CO_2 in expired gas. A value known as the end-tidal CO_2 ($ETCO_2$) can be determined from capnography. $ETCO_2$ is the measurement of CO_2 at the end of expiration, just before inspiration is initiated.

In normal subjects, the $ETCO_2$ closely reflects the $PaCO_2$, though there should be a difference of 2–5 mmHg (1 kPa). A blood gas is done at the time that capnography is set up to see how the two correlate. The $ETCO_2$ should always be slightly lower then the $PaCO_2$ because there is mixing of the alveolar air with the air in the physiologic dead space (i.e. basis of the Bohr equation). The difference between the arterial CO_2 and the $ETCO_2$ reflects V/Q mismatch.

While there is always a small degree of physiologic V/Q mismatch, lung pathology exacerbates V/Q mismatch. This will be manifest by a change in $ETCO_2$. For example, if a patient suddenly develops a mucous plug and stops ventilating several segments of lung, the $ETCO_2$ will decrease and difference in arterial CO_2 and $ETCO_2$ increase as a result of the V/Q mismatch. $ETCO_2$ also changes with alterations in cardiac output and pulmonary blood flow; decrease in cardiac output/pulmonary blood flow will cause a decrease in $ETCO_2$. Evaluation of the capnographic waveform can give clues to alterations of the ventilator circuit or airway obstruction. Overall, $ETCO_2$ monitoring can contribute significantly to evaluating minute-to-minute cardiopulmonary changes in a ventilated patient.

Alveolar gas equation

V/Q mismatch can be detected by looking at the difference in alveolar oxygen pressure (PAO_2) and arterial oxygen pressures (PaO_2). Normally, the difference between alveolar and arterial oxygen pressures is relatively small. However, when V/Q mismatch occurs, as fraction of inspired oxygen (FiO_2) (and PAO_2) is increased, PaO_2 does not increase accordingly.

PAO_2 is calculated by the alveolar gas equation. The partial pressure of oxygen within the alveoli equals the amount of oxygen inspired minus the amounts of water and CO_2 within the alveoli. The equation is as follows:

$$PAO_2 = [FiO_2 (P_{atm} - P_{H20})] - PaCO_2/0.8$$

From here, the alveolar to arterial (A–a) gradient can be determined:

$$A\text{–a gradient} = PAO_2 - PaO_2$$

The normal A–a gradient is age dependent and is estimated by the equation (Age + 10)/4. Thus, for ease of recollection, a normal A–a gradient is <25 mmHg. A gradient is >25 mmHg indicates a significant V/Q inequality. It is important to note that the A–a gradient increases 5–7 mmHg for every 10% increase in the FiO_2, and this should be considered when analyzing the gradient.

Oxygen delivery and consumption

Concepts of oxygen delivery and consumption were discussed in detail in the cardiovascular section of this chapter and should be reviewed here. Simple estimates of oxygenation can be made using pulse oximetry or transcutaneous monitoring.

Pulse oximetry

Pulse oximetry is used to estimate the arterial oxygen saturation. It utilizes a spectrometric method in which light of two known wavelengths is transmitted through a pulsating vascular bed. Light of one wavelength is absorbed by oxyhemoglobin and the other by deoxyhemoglobin. The amount of light of each frequency transmitted through the vascular bed will depend on the relative proportions of oxyhemoglobin and deoxyhemoglobin present. By evaluating the amount of light transmitted, it is possible to obtain an estimate of the relative proportion of oxygenated hemoglobin (i.e. saturation). Fingers, toes, earlobes, and the nosebridge have good vascular beds that can be used for pulse oximetry.

Transcutaneous oxygen monitoring

Electrodes applied to the skin can estimate PaO_2 (and $PaCO_2$) in a non-invasive manner. The electrodes are heated inducing a local hyperperfusion, partial pressure of oxygen (PO_2) readings are obtained, and calibration and correlation to formal blood gasses are established. Good correlation between transcutaneous PO_2 and PaO_2 are found in neonates who have very thin epidermal layers; thus, this technology has been utilized for years in neonatal ICUs. Thicker epidermal layers in adults have lead to increased variability in readings and blood

gas correlations, making it a less utilized and reliable tool in adult ICUs. Any one caring for a neonate utilizing this technology should be aware of the potential for skin injury at the measuring site.

Arterial blood gas

An ABG is probably one of the most important and heavily utilized tests in the ICU. It provides information about the patient's respiratory status (oxygenation and ventilation), acid base status, and often times even provides a rapid assessment of hemoglobin and electrolyte levels. An ABG can be withdrawn from any artery and should be analyzed immediately (or immersed in iced water) to provide accurate information before leukocyte and reticulocyte metabolism ensue.

The normal values for ABGs from a healthy young adult are:
- pH   7.35–7.45
- PO_2 10–13 kPa (75–100 mmHg)
- PCO_2 4.8–6.1 kPa (36–46 mmHg)
- Actual HCO_3 22–26
- Base deficit   0–2.5

Acidemia occurs when the hydrogen ion concentration in the blood rises above the normal range and alkalemia when it falls below it. Acidosis and alkalosis are the processes which lead to acidemia and alkalemia, respectively. Arterial hypoxemia occurs when the PaO_2 is <8 kPa (60 mmHg) and arterial hypercapnia when the $PaCO_2$ is >6.7 kPa (50 mmHg).

Actual bicarbonate is calculated from the Henderson–Hasselbach equation. Standard bicarbonate is the value obtained after correction of the PCO_2 to 5.3 kPa (40 mmHg). This correction is performed in order to remove any respiratory component. The base deficit is the amount of base needed to return the pH to 7.4.

Interpretation of the blood gases should be performed systematically. First, the arterial pH indicates whether the patient is acidemic or alkalemic. Next the PCO_2 and the standard bicarbonate are inspected. PCO_2 will be elevated in a respiratory acidosis and will be decreased in a respiratory alkalosis. Standard bicarbonate is low when there is metabolic acidosis and is elevated when there is metabolic alkalosis. The primary acid base disturbance will generally be accompanied by a compensatory response. For example, if a primary respiratory acidosis occurs, the body responds by increasing bicarbonate re-absorption and metabolic alkalosis results. However, not uncommonly in severely ill patients, compensatory mechanisms may be weak and there may be more than one reason for an acidosis. For example, a patient who has a cardiac arrest may have both a metabolic and respiratory acidosis, the metabolic acidosis occurring as a result of the absence of perfusion and the respiratory acidosis from the absence of respiration.

Respiratory failure

The respiratory system has two major functions: provide oxygen to meet the metabolic demands of the body (oxygenation) and remove CO_2, the byproduct of metabolism,

Table 8.7. Causes, pathophysiology, and examples of respiratory failure.

V/Q mismatch	Shunt	Hypoventilation	Diffusion abnormalities
Ventilation to areas of lung which are not adequately perfused	In essence, blood bypasses alveoli such that gas exchange does not occur	Decreased ventilation due to a variety of causes	Thickened alveolar membrane impairs diffusion
PE	Pulmonary consolidation (pneumonia, edema, ARDS)	Neurologic event	Pulmonary fibrosis
		Drugs/narcotic overdose	ARDS
Obstructive airway disease	Atelectasis	Muscular weakness	
	Cardiac R → L shunt		

from the body (ventilation). As such, respiratory failure is the failure of oxygenation or ventilation (or both).

Hypoxemic respiratory failure is failure of oxygenation. It is characterized by a $PaO_2 < 8$ kPa (<60 mmHg). There are four causes of hypoxemic respiratory failure (Table 8.7). The most common cause of hypoxemia is V/Q mismatch. Pathologic V/Q mismatch occurs when ventilated portions of the lung are not being perfused or when perfused portions of the lung are not being ventilated. V/Q mismatch affects oxygenation more than ventilation. As CO_2 diffuses much more easily (and quickly) than oxygen, when hypoxia causes respiratory stimulation and increased minute ventilation, CO_2 is rapidly removed. Thus, PCO_2 may be normal or decreased.

In discussing hypoxemic failure, the term 'V/Q mismatch' is usually reserved for a situation in which the lung is being ventilated, but not in areas which are being perfused. Theoretically, V/Q ratio will approach infinity at a point when there is no longer pulmonary perfusion. Alternatively, 'shunting' refers to a situation in which the alveoli are perfused, but not ventilated. This can occur because the alveoli are collapsed (atelectasis) or full of fluid (pneumonia or pulmonary edema). Intra-cardiac defects that result in blood flow from the right to left heart bypassing the lungs are also a form of shunt. In shunting, the V/Q ratio equals zero in the absence of ventilation. Hypoxemia due to V/Q mismatch improves with the administration of supplemental oxygen. On the other hand, in shunting, deoxygenated blood essentially bypasses alveoli. Thus, supplemental oxygen is much less useful in correcting hypoxemia secondary to shunt pathology. In an absolute shunt (when the V/Q ratio equals zero) hypoxia cannot be corrected by the addition of supplemental oxygen.

Hypoventilation is a less common cause of respiratory failure, but it always associated with hypercapnia. Additionally, because the alveolar and arterial relationship is maintained, there is no difference in the alveolar–arterial gradient (as there will be in V/Q mismatch). Hypoxia due to hypoventilation responds to supplemental oxygen as it increases the alveolar PO_2.

Hypercapnic respiratory failure is failure of ventilation. It is characterized by a $PaCO_2 > 6.7$ kPa (>50 mmHg). As was just discussed, hypoventilation tends to cause both hypercapnia and hypoxemia. Hypoventilation may be caused by

central nervous system (CNS) depression (drugs, opiates) or by pathology of the brainstem (infarction, compression). Peripheral nervous system involvement (spinal cord injury, myasthenia) and respiratory muscle or chest wall abnormalities may also cause ventilatory failure.

It should be noted that in late stages of any cause of respiratory failure combined failure – oxygenation and ventilation is the norm. Thus, even causes of primarily hypoxemic respiratory failure (ARDS, chronic obstructive airways disease (COAD)) will lead to hypercapnia as the disease progresses.

Patients who develop acute respiratory failure are often anxious and complain of feeling short of breath. Alternatively, they may be confused or even somnolent. On examination, signs of respiratory failure include cyanosis, use accessory muscles, and stridor. Patients may be tachypneic or hypoventilating. Tachycardia is also a common sign. Work-up of a patient with acute respiratory failure involves a thorough history and physical examination, chest radiograph, ECG, and ABG. Supplemental studies such as computed tomography (CT) scan, bronchoscopy, and V/Q scan can be done at the evaluator's discretion.

Artificial airways

Endotracheal intubation

Endotracheal intubation may be performed via the orotracheal or nasotracheal route; however, orotracheal intubation is by far the most common mechanism. Orotracheal intubation involves using a laryngoscope or fiberoptic bronchoscope to visualize the vocal cords and direct the endotracheal into the trachea. In the intensive care or emergency setting, orotracheal intubation is usually done via a technique known as rapid sequence intubation/induction (RSI). RSI allows for rapid, safe intubation in patients who have a potentially full stomach and are at risk for aspiration.

RSI involves using a short-acting sedative (etomidate, midazolam, fentanyl, ketamine) to relax the patient followed by a short-acting neuromuscular blocker (succinylcholine, vecuronium) to disable the patients reflex to fight intubation. Before administering medications, patients are pre-oxygenated with 100% oxygen to a goal saturation of 100%. The medications are then given. Once neuromuscular blockade is in place, intubation is attempted. Applying cricoid pressure (Sellick maneuver) to compress the esophagus and prevent aspiration is essential throughout the entire procedure until tracheal intubation is confirmed. Children undergoing RSI can develop profound reflex bradycardia (to vagal stimulation, hypoxia, medications), thus pre-medication with atropine is essential. Fiberoptic assistance may be needed in difficult airways.

Nasotracheal intubation involves directing an ETT through the nasal passage and into the trachea. It can be done blindly or with a fiberoptic bronchoscope. It is done without the assistance of a laryngoscope and has been advocated by some to be the method of choice in cervical spinal cord injury where manipulation of the neck is to be avoided. Its primary indication is for rapid awake intubations (e.g. decompensating COAD) where sedation would be undesirable. Other indications for nasotracheal intubation include elective oral surgery or limited mouth opening (e.g. temporo-mandibular joint (TMJ) dysfunction). It is contra-indicated in severe facial trauma to avoid placement of the tube through the cribiform plate, which has happened! Advantages of nasotracheal intubation are ease of communication for the patient (and potentially less need of sedation), easier mouth care, avoidance of occlusion of the tube by biting down (good in pediatrics or head injury). Disadvantages are that a smaller tube is needed, making procedures such as bronchoscopy difficult. It also is associated with a higher incidence of sinusitis, nasal trauma, and epistaxis.

ETTs are usually made of an inert material and have a low-pressure cuff which is blown up in the trachea creating a seal. This allows for positive pressure ventilation without an air leak. Uncuffed tubes are usually used in infants and small children to reduce the risk of damage to the tracheal mucosa. The size of the internal diameter of the tube is written on the outside. For most women a 7.5–8.0 mm ETT is appropriate; for men an 8.0–9.0 mm ETT is used. The diameter of the little finger can be used to size pediatric ETTs; an alternative is the calculation, child's age divided by four plus four. The ETT is guided into place under direct vision and then immediately checked for placement in the lungs. Visualization of placement, ETCO$_2$ detectors, and auscultating for bilateral breath sounds are all indicated to ensure the trachea is intubated (and not the esophagus). The tube is then secured and a chest radiograph done to confirm proper placement of the end of ETT approximately two finger breadths above the tracheal bifurcation. In addition to the standard single lumen tubes, double lumen ETT are available to allow each lung to be ventilated separately. These are used during thoracotomy or for independent lung ventilation.

Alternatives to endotracheal intubation

Laryngeal mask airway
LMA is becoming an increasingly utilized method for short-term airway management. It consists of a tube with a large cuff that is inflated within the pharynx. In the critical care setting, LMA can be an appropriate alternative during a difficult intubation, as it is often easier to insert for the experienced clinician. Later on, it can be used to assist in placement of a definitive ETT. In fact, there is a modified LMA, called Fastrach, which is designed precisely for this purpose. Of note, an LMA does not block the lungs from aspiration (no tracheal cuff).

Combitube
The Combitube is a double lumen tube with two balloons which allows for blind orotracheal intubation. If the tube is placed into the trachea (15% of the case), the pharyngeal balloon is blown up and standard ventilation initiated. It the Combitube intubates the esophagus, both esophageal and pharyngeal balloons are inflated allowing for satisfactory ventilation of the trachea.

Cricothyroidotomy
Cricothyroidotomy is a procedure done to gain control of the airway in an emergency situation. A small incision is made in the cricothyroid membrane, dilated, and a tracheostomy tube inserted. Cricothyroidotomy is a life saving procedure in patients with severe maxillofacial trauma who require an emergent airway and in patients who have failed all other forms of airway access. A temporary alternative to cricothyroidotomy is to place a needle in the cricothyroid membrane and connect a jet ventilator. This technique, known as needle cricothyroidotomy, can allow for life saving oxygenation. It has limited use in adults; however, as they will quickly develop hypercapnia due to the size of the needle. Importantly, needle cricothyroidotomy is the preferred method of emergent airway control in children who are at significant risk of tracheal complications with formal cricothyroidotomy.

Tracheostomy
A tracheostomy is a surgically created opening within the trachea through which a tracheostomy tube is inserted to allow for mechanical ventilation. Indications for tracheostomy tube insertion include:

- Prolonged ventilatory insufficiency (>2 weeks). May be secondary to prolonged pulmonary insufficiency (multiple chest injuries or ARDS), long-term unconsciousness (coma), or paralysis (spinal cord injury).
- Airway obstruction (e.g. maxillofacial trauma, pharyngeal edema).
- Post-laryngectomy or pharyngo-laryngectomy.
- Paralysis of the swallowing apparatus to prevent aspiration (e.g. bulbar palsy).
- Facilitate weaning from mechanical ventilation.

Tracheostomies have certain advantages over ETTs. They improve patient comfort and decrease sedation requirements, allow for easier pulmonary toilet, and facilitate ventilator weaning. Tracheostomies can be performed at the patient's bedside or in the operative theater. Options include a standard open technique or a percutaneous technique.

In either situation, the tracheostomy is ideally positioned between the second and third tracheal cartilage. In the open method, the skin and strap muscles are divided. Once the trachea is exposed, it is incised and the tracheotomy tube inserted. In the percutaneous technique, the trachea is accessed with a needle. The Seldinger technique is then utilized to sequentially dilate a stoma and insert the tracheostomy tube. Complications of tracheostomy placement include bleeding, injury to local structures, misplacement of the tube, and loss of airway. Long-term complications are tracheitis, tracheal stenosis, tube dislodgement, and tracheo-innominate artery, or tracheo-esophageal fistula.

An alternative to a formal tracheostomy is a mini-tracheostomy. Mini-tracheostomies are 4 mm uncuffed tubes which are inserted through the cricothyroid membrane into the trachea. They are useful for secretion removal/suctioning in patients whose cough effort is weak, but they are not made for mechanical ventilation.

Mechanical ventilation

Indications for mechanical ventilation include:
- Inadequate oxygenation Hypoxemic respiratory failure – $PaO_2 < 8$ kPa (<60 mmHg) despite supplemental oxygen.
- Inadequate ventilation Apnea, or hypoventilation resulting in $PaCO_2 > 8$ kPa (>60 mmHg). An relative risk (RR) > 35 breaths/min with a diminished tidal volume (rapid shallow breathing; $V_T < 5$ ml/kg) indicates inadequate ventilation and fatigue.
- Elective ventilation post-operatively in high-risk surgical cases.
- Airway protection
  - Airway obstruction (trauma/edema).
  - Loss of ability to protect airway due to neurologic event (cerebrovascular accident, CVA/head injury).
- Decrease work of breathing.

The clinical objectives of mechanical ventilation are to support a patient who is unable to meet the demands of the respiratory system due to a variety of reasons (as described above). Generally, mechanical ventilation should relieve respiratory distress and decrease the patient's work of breathing. While achieving this, it should normalize oxygenation and ventilation to physiologic levels. Finally, it should support the patient so that the underlying cause of respiratory failure can be identified and corrected.

Modes of mechanical ventilation

There are three classes of ventilator:
1. volume cycled,
2. pressure cycled,
3. time cycled.

The term 'cycling' refers to the way the ventilator changes from inspiration to expiration. Volume-cycled ventilators change over when a preset volume has been delivered, pressure-cycled ventilators when a preset pressure level has been reached, and time-cycled ventilators after a preset time has elapsed. Many ventilators are controlled by micro-processors which allow more than one method of cycling to be used. Keeping these fundamentals in mind, there are four main modes of mechanical ventilation:

Controlled mechanical ventilation

Controlled mechanical ventilation (CMV) is a volume-cycled ventilatory mode in which tidal volume and rate are set. In this mode all breaths are delivered by the ventilator. The patient does not contribute to ventilation. CMV is used for ventilation of the completely apneic patient. This usually means that CMV is reserved for anesthetized or paralyzed patients. CMV is very poorly tolerated by a conscious or even moderately sedated patient who attempts to breathe on his own. CMV does not respond to spontaneous respirations, but systematically delivers its preset tidal volume. Modes that detect a patient's respiratory efforts and allow the patient to inspire between preset breaths are much better tolerated and have made CMV an obsolete mode in the ICU setting.

Assist control ventilation

In this mode a breath is delivered when triggered by the patient's inspiratory effort or after a preset time if the patient does not breathe. Assist control (A/C) is available in volume-cycled pressure limited '*volume control*' or pressure-targeted '*pressure control*' modes. In the former, minute volume and rate are preset and a fixed tidal volume is delivered with each breath. Any patient breaths above the preset rate will also be supported. This mode of ventilation is better tolerated by conscious or semi-conscious patients.

Pressure control ventilation

Pressure control ventilation (PCV) is pressure cycled. Rate and airway pressure are set and the ventilator delivers a volume of air to achieve the preset pressure. PCV is useful when there is a need to restrict the upper airway pressure. The ventilator delivers gas at a preset pressure by precisely controlling flow through the inspiratory valve. Inspiration ceases after the pre-selected time interval. Thus, in PCV, tidal volume may change based on pulmonary compliance. As lung become more compliant, a larger tidal volume will be administered per the same pre-select pressure. PCV is preferred by some for the ventilation of small children in conjunction with an uncuffed tube in order to reduce the risk of barotrauma.

Intermittent mandatory ventilation and synchronized intermittent mandatory ventilation

Intermittent mandatory ventilation (IMV) and synchronized intermittent mandatory ventilation (SIMV) are volume-cycled modes, thus a tidal volume and rate are set. IMV delivers a preset tidal volume according to the rate that is set, and it allows for additional spontaneous breaths between the mandatory breaths. In SIMV, mandatory breaths are programmed to be delivered at regular time intervals which are synchronized with the patient's respiration. Thus, if the patient initiates an inspiratory effort, the ventilator will deliver its mandatory breath for that time interval. Additional patient breaths may be taken in between mandatory breaths. IMV and SIMV were originally designed to function as weaning modes in that the number of mandatory breaths could be slowly reduced allowing the patient to assume more and more responsibility for the work of breathing. The difference between A/C and SIMV is that in A/C, each spontaneous breath is fully supported. In SIMV, only the preset number of breaths are fully supported; additional patient breaths are on their own.

Setting up mechanical ventilation

In setting up mechanical ventilation, a mode of ventilation should be chosen. Mode selection depends on the amount of support that a patient requires, pulmonary mechanics, patient sedation/co-operation, and underlying pathology.

Ventilator settings are determined with optimization of oxygenation and ventilation in mind. Once a patient is intubated, initially a high FiO_2 is administered. An ABG is done after 20 min to determine the adequacy of oxygenation. Subsequently, FiO_2 should be reduced to the lowest possible level to maintain a $PaO_2 > 8$ kPa (>60 mmHg) or saturations above 92%. This is important in reducing complications of oxygen toxicity. PEEP is generally added to prevent atelectasis, and may be increased to help decrease oxygen requirements (see below).

Adequate ventilation is based on appropriate minute ventilation. Minute ventilation depends on tidal volume and respiratory rate, both which can be manipulated in mechanical ventilation. A normal tidal volume in a spontaneously breathing individual is about 5 ml/kg. While this volume is generally too small in mechanical ventilation (due to increased dead space), large tidal volumes have been associated with alveolar injury. Setting initial tidal volumes in the 7–8 ml/kg range is appropriate. Respiratory rates can be adjusted to obtain appropriate PCO_2 levels but can be started in the 10–14 breaths/min range.

Aside from the standard modes of ventilation, additional amounts of pressure support can be given to patients undergoing mechanical ventilation. These are discussed below.

Pressure support ventilation

Pressure support ventilation (PSV) is supplemental positive pressure administered to assist the spontaneously ventilating patient. When the patient makes an inspiratory effort, the fall in airway pressure triggers the ventilator to begin inspiration. The ventilator then supplements the patient's effort by supplying inspired gas to a pre-selected pressure until the flow rate decreases and the expiratory cycle then begins. Importantly, as its name suggests, PSV supports ventilation. It can be administered on its own or be incorporated

into other modes of ventilation. For example, isolated PSV may be used for ventilator weaning; support is gradually withdrawn as the patient assumes more of the work of breathing. Alternatively, in SIMV with pressure support, a patient's spontaneous, unsynchronized breaths will be augmented with pressure support.

Positive end-expiratory pressure

In this technique, airway pressures are maintained above atmospheric pressure at the end of expiration. This is done by attaching a valve to the expiratory end of the ventilator circuit to create resistance and prevent the end-expiratory pressure from reaching zero. PEEP means that a positive pressure is administered even during expiration. PEEP recruits alveoli, increases the FRC, and thus improves oxygenation. PEEP can supplement the previously discussed modes of mechanical ventilation. Addition of PEEP often allows for decreased levels of FiO_2.

Auto-PEEP refers to the phenomenon of air-trapping. This can occur in patients with obstructive physiology or when rapid ventilatory rates (>20 breaths/min) are used. As the rate of ventilation quickens, the time available for expiration decreases and gases are incompletely exhaled. The result is increased air within the alveoli and an end-expiratory pressure rise. Treatment of auto-PEEP is to prolong the expiratory time and decrease the inspiratory time.

Continuous positive airway pressure

Continuous positive airway pressure (CPAP) is a continuous positive pressure administered through the ventilator circuit. It is essentially, pressure support (inspiratory positive pressure) plus PEEP (expiratory positive pressure). CPAP provides supplemental pressure to patients who are breathing spontaneously. Patients can be weaned from the ventilator using steadily decreasing levels of CPAP.

Other considerations
Humidification and warming of inspired gases

The gases supplied to the ventilator are cold and dry. Such gasses can desiccate secretions and depress ciliary activity. Since artificial ventilation bypasses the upper airways, some means of humidification and heating of the gases is needed to avoid this phenomenon. Heat and moisture exchangers are useful for short-term ventilation (<72 h), but for longer-term humidification, heated water humidifiers are used. A problem with the latter is that considerable water condensation can occur along the tubes. This can be overcome by having water traps.

Prevention of atelectasis and pneumonia

Chest physiotherapy using percussion and vibration together with postural drainage are important. If secretions are plentiful, frequent suctioning may be needed. Elevating the head of the patient's bed to at least 40° has been associated with a decreased incidence of ventilator associated pneumonia (VAP).

Analgesia and sedation

Analgesia to control pain caused by the underlying injury or operation is often administered by continuous parenteral infusion in the ICU. Epidural opioids or local anesthetics are useful, particularly for control of pain after chest injuries, thoracotomies, and abdominal operations. Benzodiazepines are useful for sedation and are administered as bolus doses or by infusion. Short-acting drugs such as midazolam or lorazepam are preferred. Sedation should be interrupted daily in critically ill patients to assess level of cognition, ensure that drug levels are not accumulating, and potentially allow for daily spontaneous breathing trials.

Complications of mechanical ventilation

Complications of mechanical ventilation include:
- Ventilator-induced trauma (see below):
  - barotrauma,
  - volutrauma.
- Hemodynamic instability (decreased venous return, especially with moderate PEEP > 15).
- Respiratory muscle dysfunction and wasting with prolonged periods of mechanical ventilation.
- Nosocomial infections.
- Mucus plugs and atelectasis.
- Technical complications (tube dislodgement, kinking, disconnections).

Ventilator-induced lung injury

While mechanical ventilation is critical to the supportive care of patients with respiratory failure, it is not without its own complications. Animal and human studies have found that mechanical ventilation can actually cause lung injury. This has been termed ventilator-induced lung injury (VILI).

VILI is likely secondary to over-distension of the alveoli caused by the volume of air that is delivered. This mechanism of injury is referred to as 'volutrauma'. The previous notion that VILI was related to ventilatory pressures ('barotrauma') is being challenged. Animal studies in which the chest wall is banded and high airway pressures, but low tidal volumes, are maintained do not result in lung injury. Thus, low tidal volume ventilatory strategies are being studied with increased interest and have become standard of care in the treatment of ARDS (see ARDS management). Low tidal volumes result in lower minute ventilation and will cause an increase in CO_2 if the respiratory rate is not adjusted. Allowing the PCO_2 to rise in order to accommodate lower tidal volumes for lung protection is called permissive hypercapnia. Under these circumstances, hypercapnia above 50 mmHg may be accepted provided the pH can be kept above 7.30.

Additionally, shear injury is becoming implicated as a contributing factor to VILI. Shear injury occurs during the respiratory cycle as a mechanically generated volume of air is delivered. Imagine a completely collapsed alveoli being popped open by a positive pressure volume of air and then collapsing on itself in expiration. This repeated popping open and collapse ultimately causes injury to the delicate alveoli and can lead to their disruption. Adding a baseline PEEP helps keep the alveoli from completely collapsing at the end of expiration and has been shown to help reduce shear-related injury.

Discontinuation of mechanical ventilation

The daily evaluation of any intubated patient should include the thought: is the patient ready for extubation and if not, why not. Seeking and reversing any contributing factors to ongoing respiratory failure is an important part of the ventilatory discontinuation process.

Discontinuation of mechanical ventilation should be considered when the patient displays:
- Evidence of reversal for the underlying cause of respiratory failure.
- Adequate oxygenation (PaO_2/FiO_2 ratio > 27, PEEP < 5–8 cmH$_2$O, $FiO_2 \leqslant$ 40–50%).
- Adequate ventilation and correction of acid base status (pH $\geqslant$ 7.25).
- Hemodynamic stability.
- The capability to initiate an inspiratory effort.
- The capability to clear secretions.

Accurately determining whether or not a patient still requires mechanical ventilation is important. If discontinuation is initiated too early, it will result in failure and likely re-intubation. Delaying mechanical ventilation discontinuation subjects the patient to further discomfort and the risks associated with ventilation (infection, tracheal stenosis, prolonged bed rest, etc.) Multiple predictors have been evaluated to help estimate the likelihood that extubation will succeed or fail. There is currently no reliable predictor of weaning success. Several of the most promising predictors of successful extubation include a respiratory rate <38 breaths/min and a rapid shallow breathing index (RSBI) of <105 breaths/min/l. RSBI is calculated as a ratio between the patent's spontaneous breathing rate and his spontaneous tidal volume (RSBI = rate/V_T). Intubated patients who breathe spontaneously at a lower rate and a larger tidal volume have greater extubation success than those who exhibit rapid, shallow breathing.

Patients who have been ventilated for a prolonged period of time (even >48 h) may require a process of 'weaning' or gradual removal from the ventilator. Several techniques for weaning are available:

1. *T-piece trials*: A T-piece consists of tubing that connects to the ETT or tracheostomy and provides a continuous flow of oxygen. The patient breathes entirely on his own and no ventilatory support is administered. Patients can be placed on a T-piece for a variable amount of time and thus have a 'spontaneous breathing trial'.

2. *PSV*: Patient remains on the ventilator, with positive support. The support is gradually decreased as the patient

assumes more and more of the work of breathing, ensuring that the tidal volume and respiratory rate is adequate.

3. *IMV*: Patient remains on the ventilator with a set volume and frequency of ventilator administered breaths. The number of ventilator administered breaths is decreased as patient assumes more and more of the work of breathing. Studies have shown that daily spontaneous breathing trials are associated with a shorter weaning duration. Ultimately, PSV and daily spontaneous breathing trials are appropriate weaning modalities. IMV is least likely to result in successful extubation and requires longer weaning protocols.

Pulmonary embolism

Pulmonary emboli primarily originate from lower extremity deep venous thrombosis (DVT), but embolization from the vena cava or upper extremity (axillary/subclavian), iliac, and pelvic veins does occur. Risk factors for PE are listed in Table 8.8. Surgical critically ill patients are at particularly high risk and daily prophylaxis with either subcutaneous heparin or low molecular weight heparin is in order.

Clinical presentation and diagnosis

Patients with PE most commonly present with acute shortness of breath and hypoxia, with or without associated pleuritic type chest pain. They may have a new onset tachycardia and low-level pyrexia is not uncommon. Clinically, patients tend to have unremarkable examinations unless they have new findings of right heart failure. Mindful auscultation may notice a new split S2, accentuated pulmonic valve closure

Table 8.8. Risk factors for PE.

Immobilization	Pregnancy	Surgery
Bed rest	Increasing age	(particularly
Trauma	Obesity	orthopedic,
Spinal cord injury	Central venous access	pelvic, and
Malignancy	Hypercoagulable states	abdominal)

sound, or murmur of tricuspid regurgitation. Occasionally, unilateral leg swelling will be supportive of the diagnosis.

ECG most commonly shows sinus tachycardia or non-specific ST changes. Right heart strain with the classic S1Q3T3 pattern may be seen with a large PE (Fig. 8.11). CXR findings vary widely. A peripheral wedge shaped infiltrate may suggest pulmonary infarction, yet non-specific cardiomegaly, infiltrates, effusions, or atelectasis may also be seen. Incidentally, a normal CXR in the presence of new hypoxemia may be one of the most suggestive sings of a PE. Thus, the major role of the ECG and CXR in the evaluation of PE is to exclude other primary cardiopulmonary pathology.

D-dimer assays have become an important tool in the evaluation of PE. The test is highly sensitive with studies revealing normal D-dimer levels in less than 10% of patients with a proven PE. Unfortunately, D-dimer assays are of limited use in post-operative patients or surgical trauma patients who already have an increased level of fibrinolysis present due to their primary insult. Thus while a positive result is essentially meaningless in this patient group, a negative D-dimer does virtually exclude PE as a cause of sudden onset hypoxia.

Diagnostic modalities include V/Q scanning, CT angiography, or pulmonary angiogram. V/Q scans are reported as high, intermediate, or low probability of PE. High probability scans offer a reliable result in patients with a good clinical history. Unfortunately, only a minority of patients will have a high probability scan. Conversely, patients with a low probability scan and low clinical suspicion have a low probability of PE. The vast majority of patients, however, fall into a 'non-diagnostic' category with intermediate probability scans or low probability scans and higher clinical suspicion. These patients will require further imaging. Lower extremity Doppler is an easy and useful study to begin with because treatment for DVT and PE are the same. Other options are CT or pulmonary angiogram.

Helical (spiral) CT scan is becoming an increasingly popular diagnostic modality. CT has good specificity, but its sensitivity (ability to detect a true positive) ranges from around 50–70%. Improved technology and the ability to perform

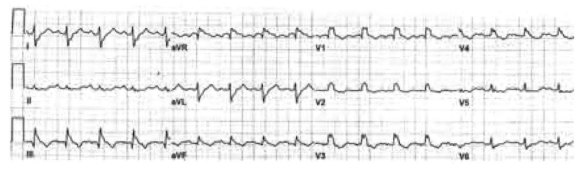

Figure 8.11. ECG findings in acute PE. The S1Q3T3 findings represent the volume and pressure overload experienced by the obstructed RV ('right heart strain'). The S-wave in lead I represents a complete or incomplete bundle branch block. The strain on the RV leads to conduction abnormalities which account for the Q-wave, mild ST-segment elevation, and T-wave inversion seen in lead III.

digital reconstructions are improving diagnostic accuracy. Pulmonary angiogram is still considered the gold standard modality of assessing for PE. PE is indicated by a filling defect or a vessel cut off sign. It is a reliable study for up to a week from the onset of symptoms, even after the initiation of anticoagulation.

Treatment

Anticoagulation is the treatment for PE and should be initiated at the clinician's discretion, but ideally once the thrombo-embolic event is suspected. A heparin infusion (goal prothrombin time (PTT) 1.5–2.0 above control) or therapeutic dose subcutaneous low-molecular-weight heparin (LMWH) is recommended to prevent further embolization. Once diagnosis is confirmed, long-term anticoagulation with Warfarin (International Normalized Ratio (INR) > 2.0) or an LMWH should be organized. Thrombolytic therapy is an alternative for patients with hemodynamic instability or severe hypoxia. Surgical embolectomy may be considered in the unstable patient who has contraindications to or failure of thrombolytic therapy.

SIRS, SEPSIS, AND MULTI-ORGAN DYSFUNCTION SYNDROME (MODS)

Definitions

In 1992, a consensus conference of the American College of Chest Physicians and the American Society of Critical Care Medicine published definitions of the SIRS and sepsis syndromes (Table 8.9). These definitions have been adopted worldwide and provide a universal language through which clinicians can discuss, research, and improve outcomes in of one of the most significant entities affecting critically ill patients.

Sepsis is the most common cause of mortality in critically ill patients. Mortality approaches 40% in patients with severe sepsis and 80% for patients with septic shock and multi-organ dysfunction syndrome (MODS). The pathophysiology of SIRS and sepsis is still being intensively studied in hopes of developing new and effective therapies.

Pathophysiology

The prevailing theory in SIRS and sepsis has been that the body initiates an exaggerated inflammatory response to an insult (Table 8.10) or organism. Inflammatory mediators such as tumor necrosis factor alpha (TNF-alpha) and cytokines (interleukins (IL)-1, IL-6, IL-8) have been implicated in perpetuating this response. While such mediators clearly have an immunomodulatory role, the notion that they cause uncontrolled inflammation is now being challenged. For example, TNF antagonists have been associated with increased mortality in sepsis. Furthermore, septic patients demonstrate features of immunosuppression – loss of delayed hypersensitivity, failure to clear infections. Thus, the concept of a compromised

---

Table 8.9. Classification of the SIRS.

SIRS:
- Two or more of the following:
  - Temperature >38°C or <36°C
  - Tachycardia – HR > 90
  - Tachypnea – RR > 20 breaths/min or $PaCO_2 < 4.3$ kPa (32 mmHg)
  - White cell count >12 000 or <4000 or >10% immature (band) cells

Sepsis
- SIRS + established focus of infection

Severe sepsis
- Sepsis + associated organ dysfunction and hypoperfusion as evidenced by one of the following:
  - Acute mental status change
  - Systolic blood pressure <90 mmHg or decrease normal systolic pressure by >40 mmHg
  - Oliguria
  - Lactic acidosis

Septic shock
- Severe sepsis and
  - Hypotension not responsive to IV fluid resuscitation *or*
  - Need for inotropes or vasopressors to maintain blood pressure

---

Table 8.10. Non-infectious causes of systemic inflammation.

Pancreatitis	Burns
Ischemia	Hemorrhagic shock and transfusion
Trauma	

---

immune system (at least in some patients) is emerging. On-going research will hopefully more clearly elucidate this complicated interplay of immune mediators and the systemic inflammatory response.

MODS is the culmination of inflammatory events associated with SIRS and/or sepsis which leads to organ failure. It is characterized by the sequential failure of organs, usually starting with the lungs and progressively involving other organ systems. The mortality rate is high and increases with the number of organs involved: 30% when one organ fails and 100% when four organs fail.

Although a number of different terms have been used to describe this syndrome (e.g. multi-organ failure, multi-system organ failure), MODS is currently accepted as the most appropriate terminology. The term dysfunction rather than failure is considered more appropriate since the process starts with derangement of function and then progresses to failure.

Multiple insults are likely needed for the development of MODS. An initial insult primes the immune/inflammatory response, and a second insult may push the patient to organ dysfunction. Many mechanisms are suggested as contributing factors. One postulate is that injury stimulates mononuclear cells (particularly macrophages) to produce excessive cytokines. Humoral and cellular cascades are then activated causing systemic effects. Alternatively, endothelial cell ischemia, followed by reperfusion, results in the release of toxic free radicals. Such microvascular injury can contribute to the inflammatory response. Furthermore, TNF and IL-1 change the endothelial cell from a non-inflammatory to a pro-inflammatory state. Pro-inflammatory endothelial cells can activate the extrinsic clotting pathway and promote leukocyte adherence, resulting in focal microvascular thrombosis and further leukocyte-mediated endothelial injury. Finally, there may be loss of the intestinal mucosal barrier leading to systemic spread of bacteria or endotoxin, a process termed bacterial translocation. Once in the circulation; the bacteria or endotoxins further stimulate an inflammatory reaction. It is possible that each of the above mechanisms may be involved to greater or lesser degrees in the genesis of MODS.

Treatment

Significant research into the pathophysiology and treatment of sepsis is slowly leading to improved outcomes in afflicted patients. The evidenced-based recommendations for the treatment of severe sepsis were summarized in a recent consensus publication (2004). The 'surviving sepsis campaign' is being adopted by ICUs globally. The recommendations are summarized below. Of note, the major components of treating sepsis are: resuscitation, source (infection) control, antibiotics, and supportive care:

- Resuscitation should begin immediately with the following goals: CVP 8–12 mmHg, MAP $\geq$ 65 mmHg, urinary output (UOP) $\geq$0.5 ml/kg/h, and mixed venous O_2 saturation $\geq$70%. Resuscitation fluids can be either crystalloid or colloid.
- Antibiotics should begin win the first hour of recognizing severe sepsis. Before starting antibiotics, cultures of blood and any other potential source of infection should be obtained. Initial coverage should be broad and then narrowed as culture results become available.
- Controlling the source of infection is a critical part of the sepsis treatment. This includes catheter removal, tissue debridement, abscess drainage, etc.
- Vasopressor therapy (norepinephrine ore dopamine) should be introduced when fluid challenge fails to restore blood pressure and perfusion.
- Dobutamine may be added in patients with a low cardiac output despite fluid resuscitation.
- Patients who require vasopressors despite fluid replacement should be given hydrocortisone 200–300 mg/day in three or four divided doses (or continuous infusion) for 7 days.
- Activated protein C (Xigris) is recommended in patients at high risk for death (sepsis-induced multi-organ dysfunction or septic shock) with no contraindication for bleeding. Activated protein C is the first licensed therapy for the treatment of severe sepsis and associated multi-organ failure. Studies found an absolute mortality reduction of 6.1% (from 31% to 25%) in patients receiving activated protein C.
- Red blood cell transfusions should be administered to target a hemoglobin between 7 and 9 mg/dl.
- Maintain blood glucose <150 mg/100 ml using continuous insulin and glucose infusions as needed. This simple intervention significantly reduced in hospital mortality. It also resulted in significant decreases in length of ICU stay, duration of ventilatory support, need for renal replacement therapy (RRT), incidence of septicemia, and incidence of polyneuropathy.
- Manage mechanical ventilation with low tidal volume strategy and implement daily spontaneous breathing trials as appropriate (refer to ARDS and mechanical ventilation sections).

While these guidelines were written for sepsis, they translate well to the prevention and treatment of MODS. Prevention of MODS may be achieved by early resuscitation and control of the source of sepsis. Once established, treatment of MODS involves supportive care. Manifestations of MODS are expanded on in the following organ specific sections.

Acute lung injury and ARDS

Acute lung injury (ALI) and ARDS are *sudden onset inflammatory-mediated* conditions of the lungs resulting in *pulmonary edema* and subsequent hypoxia. In 1994 the American–European Consensus Conference Committee established clinical criteria to define these conditions.

ARDS is defined by the following:

1. acute onset;
2. bilateral pulmonary infiltrates on chest radiograph (Fig. 8.12);
3. PAWP < 18 mmHg or absence of clinical evidence of left atrial hypertension;
4. PaO_2/FiO_2 ratio $\leq$ 27 kPa (200 mmHg).

Evaluating these criteria closely, the bilateral pulmonary infiltrates on CXR are the clinical manifestation of pulmonary edema. The critical aspect of the definition is the requirement that the pulmonary capillary wedge pressure (PCWP) is less than 18 mmHg or that there is lack of clinical evidence of left atrial hypertension. These criteria eliminate heart failure as a cause of the observed edema, and thus point to an inflammatory etiology.

The resultant pulmonary edema leads to tissue hypoxia. Normally, an individual has a PaO_2 of 13 kPa on 21% FiO_2 (room air). The PaO_2/FiO_2 ratio then is 13/0.21 or 62. In ARDS, the pulmonary edema and disruption of the pulmonary

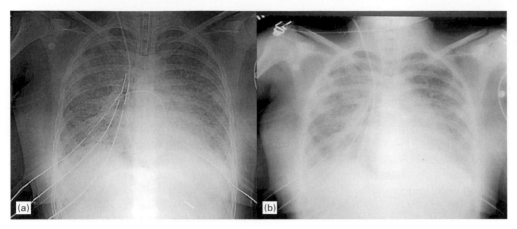

Figure 8.12. Chest radiographic findings in ARDS. (a) Note the bilateral patchy infiltrates necessary to make diagnosis of ARDS. (b) This CXR is of the same patient 12 h later. It emphasizes how rapidly such patients can deteriorate and helps illustrate why oxygenation can be extremely difficult.

architecture is so profound that gas exchange is severely impaired. Oxygenation is poor despite increasing oxygen requirements. Thus the PaO_2 decreases, while the FiO_2 increases, driving down the ratio to less than 27. For example, a patient with ARDS may require a FiO_2 of 70% to get a PaO_2 of 10 kPa. The PaO_2/FiO_2 ratio is $10/0.70 = 14$. ALI implies a less severe form of lung injury and shares the definition of ARDS with the exception that the PaO_2/FiO_2 ratio is ≤40 kPa (300 mmHg).

Etiology

ARDS is seen in both medical and surgical patients and has an extensive list of causes. The most common cause of ARDS is sepsis; sepsis may be pulmonary related (pneumonia), but any septic focus can trigger the cascade leading to ARDS. Other causes of ARDS in surgical patients include aspiration, inhalation injury, transfusion, pancreatitis, and trauma.

Pathogenesis

Regardless of the inciting factor for ARDS, the lungs respond characteristically. Normally, the alveoli are comprised of an epithelial cell layer lying adjacent to a capillary endothelial cell layer. These thin layers permit necessary diffusion of oxygen and CO_2. A prominent feature of early ARDS is epithelial and endothelial cell injury. Endothelial injury leads to a markedly increased vascular permeability and the influx of a protein-rich fluid into the alveolar space. Injured epithelial cells are unable to remove such edema and do not make needed surfactant. As these cells are sloughed, denuded alveolar surfaces are lined by a thick hyaline membrane. Fluid filled alveolar spaces and disruption of the alveolar architecture explain the problem with gas exchange seen in these patients. This phase of ARDS is known as the acute or *exudative* phase and generally lasts 1–3 days.

A complex interplay of cytokines and inflammatory cells likely both causes this alveolar disruption as well as helps to resolve it. Neutrophils are prominent in early ARDS. Cytokines (such as IL-1, IL-6, IL-8, IL-10, and TNF-alpha) are secreted by macrophages and activate neutrophils. Inflammatory mediators also stimulate fibroblast activity and can lead to increased collagen deposition in the interstitial spaces.

While some patients quickly resolve their lung injury after the acute phase, others may go on to develop fibrotic lung changes and move into what is know as the *proliferative* phase of ARDS. In these patients at approximately 5–7 days, mesenchymal cells proliferate and there is increased collagen deposition in the alveolar spaces. This histologic finding is known as fibrosing alveolitis and is associated with an increased mortality.

Ultimately, the injured alveoli enter a complicated process of repair. Type II alveolar epithelial cells must differentiate into Type I cells to repopulate the alveolar lining. Fluid and protein are cleared form the alveolar space. Inflammatory cells are removed most likely by a combination of apoptosis and phagocytosis. Finally, remodeling of the fibrosis must be done in attempts to re-establish normal alveolar architecture. While this is process is successful in some patients, others are left with areas of lung tissue destruction, emphysema, and fibrosis. The mechanisms explaining this complicated process of recovery, who will progress to long-term lung injury, and how to prevent it are still unknown.

Management

Management involves treating the underlying cause and supportive care. Mechanical ventilation is necessary in the majority of patients with ARDS because of problems with oxygenation. In recent years, there has been considerable focus on identifying ventilatory strategies which will optimize outcomes in patients with ARDS. The biggest breakthrough in the management of ARDS to date came in 2000 in a landmark multi-center, randomized controlled trial put forth by the NIH-funded ARDS Network of 10 centers in

Table 8.11. Causes of ischemic ARF.

Hypovolemia	Decreased 'effective' intra-vascular volume	Hypotension	Renal vascular disease	Medications
Bleeding	Cirrhosis	Shock	Renal artery cross-clamp	IV contrast
Renal losses	Heart failure	Medication related	Malignant hypertension	NSAIDs
GI losses	Third spacing (pancreatitis)		Renal artery thrombosis	Cyclosporine

NSAIDs:non-steroidal anti-inflammatory drugs.

24 hospitals and 75 ICUs; 861 patients were randomized to either a conventional ventilatory strategy of a 12 ml/kg body weight tidal volume or a low tidal volume strategy of 6 ml/kg. Of importance, in the low tidal volume group, airway pressures were maintained below 30 cmH$_2$O. Mortality was 39.8% in the conventional group and 31% in the low tidal volume group, a reduction of 22% ($P = 0.007$). The trial was stopped early because of the significant findings, and low tidal volume ventilation has become standard of care in the ventilatory management of ARDS. Studies evaluating optimal PEEP, prone positioning, recruitment maneuvers, and alternative ventilation styles are ongoing.

Fluid management can be complicated in ARDS patients. As the central pathology is pulmonary edema, some people have advocated fluid restriction. The caveat to this is that the majority of these patients are systemically unwell and fluid restriction may come at the cost of reducing preload, cardiac output, and thus organ perfusion. Current recommendations are to maintain intra-vascular volume at the lowest possible level to maintain adequate tissue perfusion. Future investigations will hopefully identify optimal fluid strategies and allow for improved outcomes.

Acute renal failure

Acute renal failure (ARF) is the sudden development of renal insufficiency resulting in the body's inability to excrete nitrogenous waste and maintain fluid and electrolyte balance. While a straightforward concept, defining renal failure in the clinical setting remains more challenging. Novis et al. reviewed 26 studies of post-operative renal failure and found no two studies utilized the same definition. That being said, commonly used definitions include: an increase in serum creatinine by 20–50% over baseline, a creatinine clearance of less than <50%, or the need for RRT.

The incidence of ARF thus varies depending on the definition used. Based on the definition of a raised serum creatinine, up to 15–35% of critically ill patients will develop ARF. However, only approximately 1% will need RRT. Development of ARF in critically ill patients is a poor prognostic indicator, associated with up to a 50% mortality rate. Despite major advances in critical care, this mortality rate has not changed in the past 50 years.

Etiology

The causes of ARF are classified as pre-renal, renal (intrinsic), or post-renal (obstructive). Seventy-five percent of ARF is related to renal hypoperfusion resulting in the reversible 'pre-renal' state or acute tubular necrosis (ATN). Renal hypoperfusion can come from a variety of sources in the surgical patient (Table 8.11) and many patients in the ICU will demonstrate a combination of these.

Pre-renal ARF

Although the kidney has an auto-regulatory mechanism to maintain the glomerular filtration rate (GFR), when renal perfusion decreases below a critical level the GFR decreases and urine output falls.

Intrinsic ARF

ATN may occur after prolonged hypoperfusion or as a result of the toxic effects of certain drugs or pigments. Histologic examination reveals multiple areas of focal necrosis along the nephron with rupture of the basement membranes and occlusion of the lumen by casts.

Post-renal ARF

Obstruction anywhere along the urinary tract may cause post-renal ARF. Common causes include calculi and prostatic hypertrophy.

Diagnosis

The diagnosis of ARF is usually made either because of oliguria or derangement of laboratory values. Non-oliguric ARF (>400 ml urine/day) is often seen in ARF secondary to contrast or aminoglycoside toxicity. Alternatively, anuric ARF (<100 ml urine/day) is often seen in complete obstruction, severe ATN, glomerulonephritis, or vascular injury. While the amount of urine output ranges in any type of ARF; anuric renal failure is associated with a worse outcome.

As a vast majority of ARF (particularly in surgical patients) is secondary to renal hypoperfusion, the next important diagnostic dilemma is determining whether the patient has pre-renal failure or ATN. Pre-renal failure is reversible if perfusion to the kidney is restored promptly. In the pre-renal state, the still functioning kidney actively absorbs sodium and urea in an attempt to retain as much water (and thus intra-vascular

Table 8.12. Diagnosis of ARF. The most sensitive and specific determination of ARF is the FENa.

	Pre-renal	ATN
Urea/Cr ratio	>15–20:1	<15:1
Urine Na (mmol/l)	<20	>30
Urine osmolality (mosmol/l)	>350	<350
FENa (%)	<1	>1

FENa: ratio of the amount of sodium excreted to the amount of sodium filtered = (urine Na/serum Na)/(urine Cr/serum Cr).

volume) as possible. This results in an increased urea: creatinine ratio, a decreased urinary sodium, a high urine osmolality, and a decreased fractional excretion of sodium (FENa). Conversely, when the kidney has been subjected to prolonged ischemia and ATN ensues, the kidney loses its concentrating ability. The urinary sodium increases, urine osmolality decreases and the FENa raises. A summary of these parameters is available in Table 8.12.

Of note, while the FENa is the most sensitive and specific tool for evaluating ARF, the urinary sodium is a quick and reliable test to begin assessing a patient with suspected ATN. Evaluating urinary sediment may also be an easy adjunctive test in patients with ARF. Patients with pre-renal failure will often have bland hyaline casts. On the other hand, 80% of patients with ATN will have brown casts and tubular epithelial cells.

Treatment

As was previously mentioned, despite medical advances of the past 50 years, the mortality of patients developing ARF in the ICU has remained unchanged. Likely this is because there are still no real treatments for ARF. The two mainstays of therapy in ARF are: appropriate volume expansion and avoidance of any further nephrotoxic insults. What is appropriate volume expansion in a patient whose kidneys are failing and is oliguric? Excellent question. Optimizing tissue perfusion (see shock section) without pushing the patient into fluid overload is the main objective. If the patient's renal failure progresses to acidosis, hyperkalemia, fluid overloaded, and/or severe uremia, then RRT will be required.

Two potential therapies, dopamine and loop diuretics, which have received intensive study in past years are worth mentioning. Dopamine has potential advantages in ARF because it increases renal blood flow, increases the GFR, and increases sodium and water excretion (diuretic property). Nevertheless, a multitude of studies have consistently found that dopamine does not prevent ARF in at risk patients, nor does dopamine change the outcome (particularly mortality, need for RRT) in patients with ARF. Thus, at this time, there is a growing consensus that dopamine should not be utilized for either the prevention or treatment of ARF.

Loop diuretics have also received considerable attention. They have the potential advantages of decreasing oxygen consumption in tubular cells (by inhibiting sodium transport), and thus limiting cellular injury, causing vasodilation of arterial vessels to improve oxygenation, and augmenting tubular flow via their diuretic function and thus decreasing tubular obstruction. Nevertheless, studies have also failed to find diuretics beneficial in either the prevention or treatment of ARF. In fact, one well-designed, prospective, cohort study found that diuretics were actually associated with an increased risk of death and non-recovery of renal function. Thus, at this time, the use of diuretics in ARF cannot be advocated.

Many novel therapies for ARF continue to be studied. We are learning that ARF in humans is more complicated than originally thought and that sublethal cell damage and apoptosis play a predominant roll. The fact that most previous animal models were those of wide spread necrosis may explain why promising interventions in animal models have not awarded the same success in human studies.

Renal replacement therapy

When the kidneys ultimately fail, RRT is needed. There are generally two forms of RRT utilized in the intensive care setting: hemodialysis and hemofiltration. In hemodialysis, blood is pumped through a semi-permeable filter which is bathed in a dialysate fluid. Electrolytes and fluid move down a concentration gradient into the dialysate fluid and it is removed, carrying off potassium, phosphate, urea, water, etc. Hemodialysis utilizes rapid blood flow rates over a 2–4 h duration and is performed on a daily or every other day basis. As such, it is felt to be associated with hemodynamic instability and large fluid shifts, which may not be tolerated in an unstable patient. That being said, slower forms of dialysis (sustained low-efficiency dialysis, SLED), which occurs over a longer time period, up to 12 h, is now being utilized in some centers. Peritoneal dialysis is generally not utilized in the ICU.

In hemofiltration, blood is pumped through highly permeable fibers with hydrostatic pressure driving water, urea, and electrolytes out to be collected as an 'ultrafiltrate.' There is no concentration gradient, so it is based on pressure. Generally, 1–6 l of ultrafiltrate are generated each hour. At the same time that ultrafiltrate is being drawn off, fluid and electrolytes (in the amount the clinician determines) are added back to the now highly concentrated blood before its return to the body (Fig. 8.13). The blood flow for hemofiltration is approximately 200 ml/h (slower than hemodialysis) and thus has the potential advantage of providing more hemodynamic stability. Proponents have also advocated that it provides better control over volume status and that it may help clear inflammatory mediators hastening the recovery of SIRS/sepsis. The disadvantages of hemofiltration is that it is a continuous 24 h process. This makes it work intensive and difficult for mobilizing a critically ill patient who may need studies, return to surgery, etc.

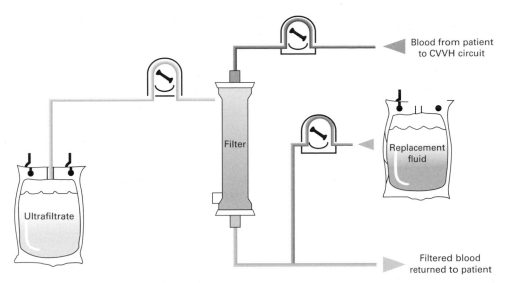

Figure 8.13. Schematic of CVVH. Blood is pumped from the patient through a filter while ultrafiltrate is removed and discarded. Replacement fluids are added to the concentrated blood before it is returned to the patient.

Hemofiltration was initially done by withdrawing blood from the arterial side and returning it to the venous side (continuos arterial venous hemofiltration – CAVH). This was fraught with complications such that continuous veno-venous hemofiltration (CVVH) is now the standard mechanism of filtration. A counter-current of dialysate fluid can also be run though the CVVH circuit to enhance electrolyte clearance. This is know as CVVH dialysis (CVVHD).

Prognosis

ARF is associated with a mortality rate of 50% in critically ill patients. A 25% mortality rate is seen in patients with non-oliguric ARF, but rates as high as 70% may be seen in patients with oliguric ARF. The cause of ARF also influences outcome. ARF related to trauma, abdominal sepsis, or burns has an associated mortality of 70–90%. Conversely, aminoglycoside or contrast-induced ARF is associated with a mortality rate of 25–30%.

If the patient with ARF survives, recovery of renal function is common (75–95%). Approximately half of these patients will have long term, asymptomatic, minor reductions in GFR or renal concentrating abilities. The typical clinical course of ARF is a 10–14 day period of oliguria. This may be followed by a 'diuretic phase,' lasting 3–7 days, in which concentrating ability is impaired. During this phase, patients may require fluid support, but dialysis can often be discontinued. Complete renal recovery is generally complete by 30 days, but may take as long as 60–90 days.

Acute liver failure

Acute liver failure is the sudden development of liver parenchymal injury resulting in coagulopathy (INR > 1.5) in a patient who lacks underlying chronic liver disease. Progression to encephalopathy in such a patient is known as fulminant hepatic failure (FHF).

The etiologies of acute liver failure include:
- *Viruses*: Hepatitis viruses A, B, C, D and E, rarely herpes simplex, varicella-zoster, and CMV.
- *Drugs/toxins*: Paracetamol, isoniazid, phenytoin, halothane, carbon tetrachloride, mushrooms (*Amanita* spp.).
- *Ischemia*: Blood flow to the liver may be reduced in shock, resulting in hepatocellular damage.
- *MODS*: Ischemia and endotoxemia stimulate Kupffer cells to produce cytokines which then act on the hepatocytes resulting in injury.

The leading causes of FHF, in order of frequency, are paracetamol toxicity, cryptogenic (unknown), other drug toxicity, hepatitis B, and hepatitis A.

Clinical features

Patients with acute liver failure are jaundiced as the liver fails to conjugate and excrete bilirubin. Their laboratory values demonstrate marked transaminase elevation (AST and ALT in the range of 1000–5000), as liver cells are injured. Synthetic function is compromised and coagulopathy occurs as a consequence of clotting factor depletion. Disseminated intravascular coagulation (DIC) can also contribute to clotting abnormality.

Life threatening hypoglycemia may develop secondary to impaired gluconeogenesis and depletion of glycogen stores.

Hepatic encephalopathy is a key feature of FHF. Four clinical grades are recognized:
- Grade 1: Awake, mild confusion, altered personality.
- Grade 2: Awake, agitated, disoriented, hallucinations.
- Grade 3: Stuporous, but may be aroused.
- Grade 4: Comatose, but with intact pupillary reflexes and usually ability to withdraw to pain.

Importantly, hepatic encephalopathy in the acute setting differs from that of encephalopathy related to cirrhosis and chronic liver failure. In chronic hepatic failure, encephalopathy is related to increased ammonia levels. Conversely, encephalopathy in FHF is related to cerebral edema. Thus, worsening of encephalopathy in patients with FHF is a sign of progressive edema and a poor prognostic indicator. Progression to central herniation is possible in these patients.

Management

The cornerstone of management of acute hepatic failure is treating the source of failure (if possible) and systemic support. Liver transplantation is indicated in patients with FHF and Grade 3 or 4 encephalopathy. Only 10–20% of these patients will survive without transplant; transplant improves survival to 60–80%.

Supportive care for less severe acute hepatic failure or as a bridge to transplant for those awaiting transplant can be quite intensive. These patients may be hemodynamically compromised, thus close monitoring of CVP, arterial pressure, oxygen saturation, and urine output may be needed to ensure optimal tissue perfusion. Vitamin K administration is used to correct coagulopathy; transfusions should be restricted to patients with active bleeding. Glucose infusions are often needed to correct hypoglycemia. Early, aggressive treatment of sepsis with antibiotic therapy is recommended. Oral lactulose and reduction of dietary may reduce the load of nitrogen metabolism and assist in management of encephalopathy. Even though encephalopathy in FHF is related to cerebral edema, ammonia may play a role in the development of this edema. Management of cerebral edema is critical in encephalopathic patients; mechanical ventilation may be needed for airway protection and an intracranial pressure (ICP) monitor placed to guide therapy. Liver support devices such as the extracorporeal liver assist device (ELAD) are still being developed and evaluated.

Prognosis

Prognosis in acute liver failure is related to the cause of the failure and the severity of the failure. Patients with acute liver failure due to paracetamol toxicity demonstrate an overall 50% survival rate. Liver failure caused by hepatitis A or B have survival rates in the 30–50% range. Finally, in FHF secondary to non-A, non-B, non-C hepatitis or Wilson's disease the survival rate may be less than 10%. Progressive encephalopathy is associated with a worse prognosis. Metabolic acidosis, renal failure, severe jaundice, or marked coagulopathy also suggest a worse prognosis.

Chronic liver disease

Superimposed acute hepatic failure also occurs in patients with chronic liver disease. Often times an event such as a new infection (spontaneous bacterial peritonitis) or GI bleed will tip a previously stable cirrhotic into fulminant liver failure. Treatment is supportive as described above. Generally such patients may have already been candidates for liver transplant, and this acute event may increase their priority on the organ recipient waiting list. Each health care system must prioritize organ allocation to those individuals who most urgently need it.

Infections in the ICU

Infections are common in the ICU and are a significant cause of mortality. Critically ill patients are particularly vulnerable to infection because their immune responses may be impaired (trauma, burns, malignancy, diabetes) or suppressed (cytotoxic agents, steroids). Extremes of age, malnutrition, and co-morbid diseases also render patients more susceptible to infection. Finally, ICU care involves invasive procedures and indwelling devices which disrupt anatomic and physiologic barriers further predisposing patients to infection.

The widespread use of broad-spectrum antibiotics in the ICU setting has contributed significantly to the appearance more virulent and drug resistant organisms. These strains may arise by mutation or by the transfer of codes for resistance through plasmids and phages. Infection control teams, including intensivists, microbiologists and infection control nurses, play an important role in prevention and control of infection in the ICU. Through surveying infectious trends, they can help guide empiric therapy, knowing the types of organisms encountered in the ICU and their antibiotic sensitivities.

Surgical patients come to the ICU with their own unique causes of infection. Many are admitted with a primary surgical infection (cholangitis, peritonitis, diverticulitis). Furthermore, post-operative patients are at risk for infectious complications including anastomotic leaks, wound infections, abscesses, and foreign body (mesh, grafts) infections. This being said, critically ill surgical patients are afflicted by nosocomial infections the same as anybody else. Pneumonia and catheter-related infections are major causes of morbidity and mortality in the intensive care setting.

Pneumonia

Nosocomial pneumonia is a common, serious condition in critically ill patients. Ten percent of patients requiring post-operative ICU care will develop pneumonia. Intubated patients are at increased risk of pneumonia, with the chance of developing pneumonia increasing the longer the patient is ventilated. Risk of VAP is 3% per day for the first 5 days of ventilation, 2% per day for days 5–10, and 1% per day for days 10–15. The mortality rate of VAP ranges from 25% to 50%.

Microorganisms involved in nosocomial pneumonia are mainly the Gram-negative bacteria, such as *Pseudomonas aeruginosa, Enterobacter, Klebsiella pnuemoniae, Acinetobacter,* and *Serratia.* Gram-positive infections with *Staphylococcus aureus* in particular are becoming increasingly more common however. If the patient has received prior antibiotic therapy, the risk of infection with drug resistant species such as *P. aeruginosa*, *Acinetobacter*, and methicillin-resistant *S. aureus* (MRSA) is increased.

Several factors contribute to the high mortality rate seen in nosocomial, and particularly VAP. H_2-receptor blockers are frequently used to prevent stress ulceration in ICU patients. Consequently, the pH in the stomach lumen rises and allows it to be colonized by Gram-negative organisms. In intubated patients, upper respiratory defense mechanisms are bypassed and the mucociliary transport mechanism in the lower respiratory tract is depressed by the use of opiates, high FiO_2, and insufficient humidification. The cough reflex may be depressed by sedative drugs and is impaired intubated patient. Positive pressure ventilation delivers potential pathogens deep into the lungs while these other factors prevent their removal. Host factors such as age, malnutrition, hemodynamic instability, and immunocompromise also predispose patients to nosocomial pneumonia.

The diagnosis of VAP is based on both clinical and radiologic findings. The patient should have at least two of the following clinical signs: fever >38°C, leukocytosis, purulent tracheal secretions, or worsening oxygenation. Additionally a new or progressive infiltrate should be apparent on chest radiograph. Once VAP is suspected diagnostic tests can be done. Endotracheal aspiration can be useful, but is likely to identify non-pathogenic organisms. Broncho-alveolar lavage has been advocated by some with growth of 10^4 organisms consistent with a diagnosis of pneumonia.

A fundamental concept in the treatment of VAP is that patient outcomes are optimized when the initial antibiotic therapy accurately treats the responsible pathogen. Another way of stating this is that patients do worse when they are started on inadequate antibiotics, even if the antibiotics are later tailored to the culture results. Thus, it is important for clinicians to know the organism trends in their hospital and begin empiric therapy accordingly. Nosocomial pneumonias can be very difficult to treat since the organisms found in the ICU are likely to be multiply resistant. If Gram-negative bacilli are found, an extended-spectrum penicillin (ticarcillin, pipracillin) in combination with an aminoglycoside or third-generation cephalosporin may be indicated. If Gram-positive cocci are seen, and MRSA is suspected, vancomycin is the drug of choice.

Several preventative measures have been advocated for preventing VAP. These include: positioning the patient with the head of the bed above 40°, using ETTs that allow for subglottic secretion drainage, careful handling and regular changing of ventilator circuits, and the use of non-invasive ventilation (rather than intubation) whenever possible.

Intra-vascular catheter-related infection

Intra-vascular catheter-related infections may occur when peripheral IVs, central venous lines, arterial lines, and PA catheters are used. It is estimated that about 5% of patients with central venous cannulae and 1% with arterial cannulae develop serious infections related to the cannulae. Bacteria may gain entry to the circulation through the site of cannula insertion, be introduced through the hub of the catheter, or be directly infused (in the case of contaminated solutions). Diagnosis should be made by drawing peripheral blood cultures and cultures through the line (if possible). The line should also be inspected for any signs of inflammation. Generally, if a catheter-related infection is suspected, the line should be taken out immediately and the catheter tip sent for culture. Diagnosis of a catheter-related infection is supported if the same organism is isolated from both the catheter tip and from the blood.

Coagulase-negative staphylococci, *S. aureus*, and *Candida* are the most commonly encountered pathogens. Decisions regarding type and duration of antibiotic therapy depend on the patient's clinical condition, the organism grown, and the type of catheter. Whether or not a permanent line need be removed in the presence of a suspected infection can be a difficult decision. In the case of a suspected catheter-related infection, it is best to seek the diagnosis and request microbiology consultation for guidance of empirical therapy.

Urinary tract infections

Colonization of the urinary tract occurs quite commonly in the ICU. Almost all patients in the ICU have a urinary catheter and the risk of colonization increases with the duration of catheterization (estimated incidence is 5% per day). About 20–30% of patients go on to have a urinary tract infection. Differentiating colonization from infection in a critically ill patient is not easy. The presence of pus cells is important, but their absence does not exclude infection. With regard to bacterial counts, whilst the presence of colony forming units of $>10^5$/ml are significant, in critically ill catheterized patients counts of $>10^3$/ml can rapidly increase and therefore should not be dismissed. In addition, it is not unusual for more than one organism to be cultured from critically ill patients and such a result should not be interpreted merely to represent contamination of the specimen. When suspected clinically, cultures should be sent from the urine and antibiotics tailored to organism sensitivities. Catheters should be removed if possible, otherwise, changing the catheter (to remove the bacterial biofilm) is recommended.

PRINCIPLES OF INTENSIVE CARE

Organization and staffing

In 2000 an expert panel supported by the UK's Department of Health put forth an executive summary on adult critical care services. In this manuscript, recommendations for the organization and delivery of critical care were made. They recommended a classification of critically ill patients according to their clinical need (examples provided for readers understanding and are not part of the recommendations):

- *Level 0*: Patient needs can be met on normal ward care in an acute hospital.

– Example: Post-operative 4–6 hourly observations, patient-controlled analgesia (PCA), IV fluids, and medications.
• *Level 1*: Patient is at risk of a deteriorating condition or has recently relocated from a higher level of care. Patient needs can be met on an acute ward with support from the critical care team.
  – Example: Abnormal vital signs, observations more than 4 h, tracheostomy or epidural care.
• *Level 2*: Patient requires more detailed observation or intervention. Patient may need support for a single failing organ system, post-operative care, or 'step down' from a higher level of care.
  – Example: Non-invasive ventilation, invasive monitoring, infusion of vasoactive drug.
• *Level 3*: Patient requires advanced respiratory support or basic respiratory support plus support of at least two other organ systems. This includes all complex patients requiring support for multi-organ failure.
  – Example: Mechanical ventilation with vasoactive drug infusion and RRT.

These new recommendations provide a framework that may ultimately replace the traditional division of high dependency and ICUs, emphasizing the level of care required rather than patient location. Consultants with specialized training in Intensive Care Medicine should be responsible for directing patient care. Medical, nursing, and support staffing should be available on a 24-hour, 7-day a week basis according to workload and patient need.

Ideally, critically ill patients should be located in a unit which is in close proximity to diagnostic facilities, operating theaters, and the emergency department. The number of ICU beds varies with the workload the hospital is expected to handle – for a busy district general hospital, it has been estimated that just over 2% of the total number of acute beds in the hospital should be ICU beds, that is, 10 beds for a hospital with 500 acute beds.

Indications for admission and discharge

Since intensive care is limited and expensive, it is useful to have guidelines for admission and discharge to such units. The most recent guidelines put forth by the Department of Health are from 1996. Formulation of guidelines is difficult and the aforementioned executive summary recommended that these be reviewed and revised. At the present time, the following algorithm (adapted from the Department of Health guidelines) should be used to consider admission to high dependency or ICUs.

In general, patients are candidates for intensive care when they are unstable and require multi-organ monitoring and support. These patients should have a reversible illness, an anticipated meaningful quality of life, and limited co-morbidities. Patients with anticipated poor outcomes or

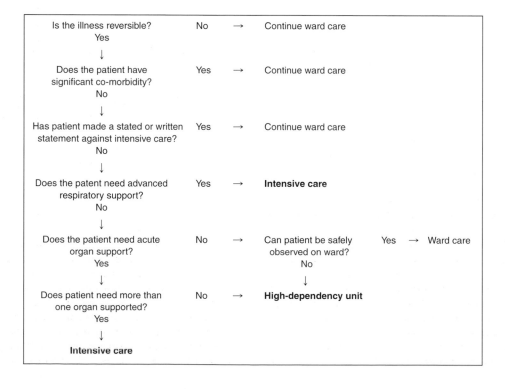

significant co-morbidities are likely not intensive care candidates. These can be difficult decisions and often require dialog between primary and ICU consultants as well as discussions with patients or their family members.

Discharge from intensive care occurs when the patient's condition has been treated or when it is felt that the patient can no longer benefit from the available treatment. Ideally, patients will be stabilized, no longer require respiratory support, and have their underlying illness corrected. If the patient is not improving and organ support is only deferring death, if the patient enters a persistent vegetative state, or if the patient or the family wish to pursue palliative care, then discharge from intensive care should be considered. Sometimes discharge from intensive care will mean a step down in the level of care and transfer to a high dependency unit. Other patients are well enough to be transferred directly to ward care.

Scoring systems

A number of scoring systems have been developed for use in the ICU. In general, scoring systems are used to help assess the degree of patient illness and predict patient outcome.

Scoring systems can be broadly grouped as follows:

- *Assess severity of physiologic derangement.* The acute physiology and chronic health evaluation (APACHE) score is a physiologically based score used to measure illness severity. The APACHE II score, a modification of the original, is based on 12 acute physiologic variables (acute physiology score), a chronic health score, and the patients age (Table 8.13). Scores are totaled providing a value between 0 and 71; the higher the APACHE II score, the more severe the illness. APACHE II remains the most widely studied and used illness scoring system. APACHE III is refinement which includes more variables and is still being evaluated. Another example is the simplified acute physiology score (SAPS) II.
- *Assess severity of injury.* The injury severity score (ISS) quantifies a patient's anatomic injury. The revised trauma score (RTS) looks at physiologic parameters (Glasgow Coma Score (GCS), systolic blood pressure, and respiratory rate) to assess injury severity.
- *Predict outcome.* The mortality prediction model (MPM) has undergone a number of modifications but essentially uses variables available at the time of admission to the ICU to predict the probability of hospital mortality. APACHE II has been shown to be a good predictor of mortality outcome in large patient groups, but a poor one in individual patients and some subgroups that were not represented in the original database (e.g. acquired immune deficiency syndrome (AIDS) or trauma patients). APACHE III was established using a larger database and has demonstrated improved mortality prediction.
- *Assess utilization of resources.* The therapeutic intervention scoring system (TISS) was originally devised to quantitate

Table 8.13. **APACHE II.**

Acute physiology score (APS)
Normal values score 0, abnormally low or high values score from 1–4 (except creatinine and GCS).

	Scores
1. Score temperature	0–4
2. Mean blood pressure	0–4
3. Heart rate	0–4
4. Respiratory rate	0–4
5. Oxygenation	0–4
6. Arterial pH	0–4
7. Serum Na^+	0–4
8. Serum K^+	0–4
9. Serum creatinine	0–8
10. Hematocrit	0–4
11. White cell count	0–4
12. Neurologic score obtained by subtracting the GCS score from 15	
Age $\leqslant 44 - \geqslant 75$ score range from	0–6

CHS

Surgical cases

	Score
• Elective admission to ICU post-operatively	2
• Admission to ICU after emergency surgery	5

Medical cases
- Admission to ICU with any of the following: 5
  1. cirrhosis
  2. chronic heart failure
  3. chronic hypertension
  4. dialysis dependent renal disease
  5. immunosuppression

APACHE II score	Approximate hospital death rate (%)
0	2
10	10
20	30
30	70
40	µ95
>40	100

CHS: chronic health score.

the intensity of care and the severity of illness of critically ill patients; it has since been found to be more useful as an index of utilization of resources. Points are assigned for the complexity of interventions, for example, 1 for ECG monitoring, 2 for a central venous line, 3 for intercostal drainage, and 4 for dialysis or ventilation. Points are totaled and patients grouped into four classes: class I – routine post-operative care; class II – observation; class III – considerable nursing care; class IV – intensive multi-disciplinary care.

- *Assess outcome of ICU care.* An example is the perceived quality of life (PQ$_O$L) score. This is a questionnaire that gauges patients' satisfaction with life after they have left the ICU.

While scoring systems can be used to evaluate patients individually, no scoring system is accurate enough to predict the outcome of a given patient and should not be used as such. Scoring systems have greater merit in evaluating patient populations. They can serve as an important research tool by helping stratify patients for randomized clinical trials. Scoring systems also help standardize illness severity in patients with highly complicated and varying disorders; this allows for comparisons between predicted and actual outcomes.

FURTHER READING

A Collective Task Force Facilitated by the American College of Chest Physicians; the American Association for Respiratory Care; and the American College of Critical Care Medicine. Evidence-based guidelines for weaning and discontinuation of ventilatory support. *Chest* 2001; **120**: 375S–396S
Review of several thousand articles in world literature to address issues of ventilator discontinuation.

De Latorre F, Nolan J, Robertson C et al. European Resuscitation Council Guidelines 2000 for Adult Advanced Life Support. *Resuscitation* 2001; **48**: 211–221
Public access to these guidelines, and their algorithms for cardiac arrest and arrhythmias, is available on the European Resuscitation Council web site.

Dellinger RP, Carlet JM, Masur H *et al.* Surviving sepsis campaign guidelines for management of severe sepsis and septic shock. *Crit Care Med* 2004; **32**: 858–873
Extensively referenced and researched guidelines for management of severe sepsis and septic shock. On line access to these guidelines is available by searching surviving sepsis campaign.

Department of Health. *Guidelines on Admission to and Discharge from Intensive Care and High Dependency Units*. London: Department of Health, March 1996

Department of Health. *Comprehensive Critical Care: A Review of Adult Critical Care Services*. London: Department of Health, May 2000

Hotchkiss RS, Karl IE. Medical progress: the pathophysiology and treatment of sepsis. *New Eng J Med* 2003; **348**: 138–150
Comprehensive review of the most recent developments surrounding pathophysiology and treatment of sepsis.

Mermel LA, Farr BM, Sherertz RJ *et al.* Guidelines for the management of intravascular catheter-related infections. *Clin Infect Dis* 2001; **32**: 1249–1272
Detailed review of infections related to vascular catheters and recommendations for treatment.

Ware LB, Matthay MA. Medical progress: the acute respiratory distress syndrome. *New Eng J Med* 2000; **342**: 1334–1349
Review of diagnosis, pathophysiology, and treatment of ARDS.

9

Principles of Cancer Management

A Patrick Forrest[1] and Mark S Duxbury

[1]University of Edinburg, Edinburgh; Department of surgery, Welsh National School of Medicine, UK

CONTENTS

The genetic code	149
Cell signalling pathways	150
The cancer cell	152
Cell cycle	152
Telomeres	152
Apoptosis	153
Molecular genetics of cancer	153
Oncogenes	154
Tumour-suppressor genes	154
Carcinogenesis	155
Chemical carcinogens	155
Diet	155
Viruses	157
Radiation	158
Reproductive factors	158
Cancer inheritance	159
Investigation of the hereditary trait	159
Genetic testing	161
Mechanisms of invasion and metastases	162
Epidemiological studies	163
Descriptive epidemiology	163
Analytical epidemiology	165
Screening for cancer	166
The disease	166
The screening test	166
The screening programme	168
Cost	169
Continued evaluation	169
Staging of cancer	169
TNM staging	169
Tumour markers	171

Principles of cancer treatment	173
Curability	173
Local treatment	173
Systemic treatment	175
A new paradigm and novel therapies	176
Relief of cancer pain	178
Palliative care	178
Principles of cancer pain control	178
Evaluation of the patient	178
The analgesic ladder	179
Quality of life and age	181
Quality of life	181
The elderly	182
Further reading	182

THE GENETIC CODE

Little more than 50 years have passed since James Watson and Francis Crick reported the structure of deoxyribose nucleic acid (DNA) in an understated article in the journal *Nature*. This discovery ushered in a new era of discovery in the biological sciences that continues at an ever-increasing pace.

The growth and differentiation from a single fertilized ovum into a functional organism requires around 2000 proteins, many of which are enzymes that catalyse chemical reactions directly or via intermediates. Other proteins have structural roles, contribute to cell membranes, bind ions or act as hormones. Proteins consist of polypeptides chains, each built from unique sequences of 20 amino acids into chains of between 30 and 3000 amino acids (primary structure). The chains are folded into conformations containing active sites that allow allosteric interaction between enzyme and substrate. Enzymatic reactions require energy, which is supplied by the breakdown of food molecules coupled to the phosphorylating system. Unlike sugars, which are synthesized by repeating blocks of similar composition and therefore require

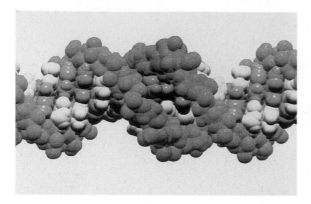

Figure 9.1. The double helix.

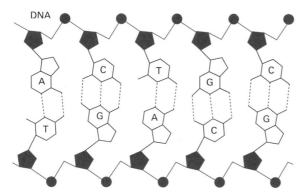

Figure 9.2. Base-pairing of double-stranded DNA.

a limited number of enzymes, proteins are uniquely irregular, each coded for by a template of DNA, which carries a specific genetic code.

DNA is composed of two strands, each with a deoxyribose sugar 'backbone' to which are attached sequences of two purine (adenine and guanine) and two pyrimidine (cytosine and thymidine) complementary nucleotides. As the 'backbones' are on the outside of the molecule, the complementary purine and pyrimidine bases of opposing strands face each other and are loosely attached by hydrogen bonds: A to T (two H-bonds) and G to C (three H-bonds). The whole molecule is supercoiled into a double helix (Figs 9.1 and 9.2). This arrangement allows a complementary 'negative' strand to be available for replication of the original molecule.

Triplets of bases (codons) form a unique code for each of the 20 amino acids required for the synthesis of proteins (e.g. TGG for tryptophan and AAG for phenylalanine). The code is described as 'degenerate' because from four separate bases, 64 (4^3) 'triplet' sequences can be constructed, a greater number than that required to synthesize 20 amino acids; that is, each amino acid can have more than one codon. Some code for the same amino acids while others (TAA, TAG and TGA) provide 'stop' signals for the synthetic process. The first two

bases are most critical in determining the appropriate amino acid. There is a degree of 'wobble' in that the third base of the codon may differ and yet code for the same amino acid.

Proteins are synthesized by the ribosomes within the cell cytoplasm. DNA cannot pass through the nuclear membrane but ribonucleic acid (RNA), which is of similar composition except that uracil is substituted for thymidine, freely transgresses it. The code from a positive strand of DNA is transcribed into a complementary RNA molecule through the action of DNA–RNA polymerase and is transported to the ribosomes. On the surface of the ribosomes, the RNA strand meets strands of transfer RNA (tRNA), which are chemically linked to amino acids to which they give a genetic identity. By moving over the surface of the ribosome, the RNA recruits amino acids in the required sequence to synthesize a specific protein, the process of 'translation' (Fig. 9.3).

The human chromosome contains some 30 000 functional genes, but 90% of the genome is made up of 'spacers' of 'junk' DNA. Not all the sequences of bases within a gene actively code for amino acids. They are divided into 'exons' which code and 'introns' which do not. As transcription yields an mRNA strand longer than that required to transfer the genetic code, the unnecessary segments are excised and the ends spliced. Recently, it has been recognized that so-called 'junk' DNA may serve distinct and important regulatory functions. Furthermore, RNA species have been shown to have regulatory roles. MicroRNA (miRNA) and small-interfering RNA (siRNA) have been shown to regulate gene expression. Introduction of siRNA complementary to a target mRNA sequence into a cell induces highly specific and potent post-transcriptional silencing of gene expression. Although poorly understood, this phenomenon appears to contribute to genomic stability by suppressing potentially damaging destabilizing elements such as transposons and may act as an antiviral defence mechanism. Gene silencing induced by antisense oligonucleotides and siRNA have shown therapeutic potential in early preclinical studies.

CELL SIGNALLING PATHWAYS

Cells communicate with each other, exchanging stimulatory and inhibitory signals (Fig. 9.4). These may be autocrine (affecting one cell), paracrine (between neighbouring cells) and endocrine (acting at a distance). Cell functions are modified by an enormous number of molecules, ranging from small and diffusible polypeptides to large protein complexes that act at the cell surface. Gap junctions between cells allow the passage of small molecules; cell-specific receptors are required for distant actions. These may lie on the cell membrane externally, within the cytoplasm or within the nucleus.

The largest group of cell membrane receptors function as protein tyrosine kinases which phosphorylate tyrosine residues on target proteins, altering their function. The prototype cell surface receptor has three 'domains': an external domain on the cell surface to which the agonist (ligand)

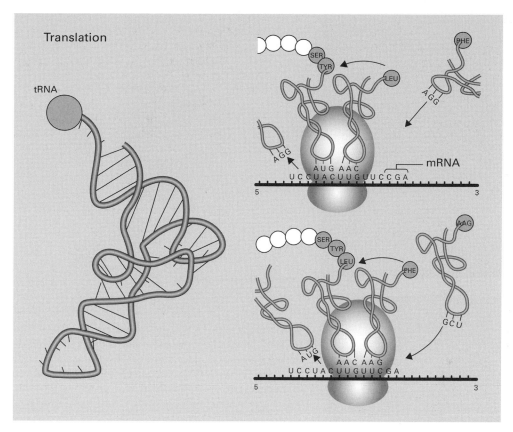

Figure 9.3. The process of translation – each of the 20 amino acids which form a protein have a specific genetic identity which is 'called up' by the triplet sequences of codons transcribed onto mRNA.

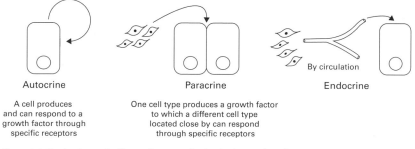

Figure 9.4. Mechanisms of cell-to-cell communication by humeral mediators.

binds, a transmembrane domain and an internal domain, which on receiving the stimulus modulates intracellular enzymatic activity, either directly or via 'second messenger' systems (Fig. 9.5). A major class of cell-surface receptor exist whose transduction processes are linked to G-proteins (guanine-nucleotide-binding proteins), which translocate between the membrane and cytoplasm and can modulate a diversity of intracellular targets.

'Second messenger' systems activated by the signals transmitted across the cell membrane may induce cytoplasmic metabolic processes directly or act via transcription factors on nuclear DNA to activate gene expression and growth control. An example is stimulation of cell growth due to activation of the cytoplasmic enzyme serine/threonine protein kinase C (PKC) which is widely distributed in normal tissues and stimulates DNA synthesis. DNA-binding proteins acting as transcription factors may also be activated through cAMP–protein kinase, a second messenger system.

Specialized receptors for lipid-soluble hormones reside in the nucleus. When bound to their specific hormone they act

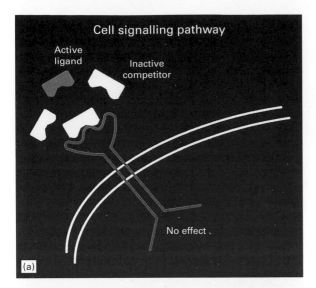

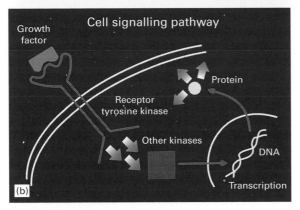

Figure 9.5. Cell signalling pathways.

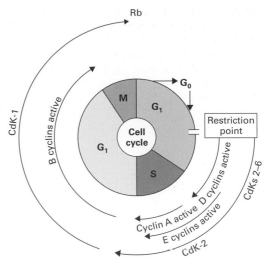

Figure 9.6. The cell cycle engine.

as transcription factors, side-stepping cell-membrane receptors and cytoplasmic second messengers. These nuclear receptors are related by homologous sequences and form a 'superfamily' of hormone receptors.

Each of these signal transduction mechanisms have been shown to be dysregulated in cellular transformation and malignant progression.

THE CANCER CELL

Cell cycle (Fig. 9.6)

All cells of the human body are derived from a single cell, the zygote, by a series of cell divisions following which they progress along a large number of differentiation pathways to acquire specialized functions. Specialized cells occupy a unique differentiation compartment within the organism, and once 'committed' to that lineage generally cannot change to another cell type. A limited number of progenitor 'stem

cells' occupy each compartment and are genetically controlled to proliferate continuously and repopulate it. As differentiating genes take over control, proliferative activity usually decreases. Once fully differentiated, cells enter a third sequence of genetic events, that of apoptosis or programmed cell death.

A characteristic of neoplastic cells is their unregulated progression through the cell cycle. It is now known that this cycle is driven by a family of proteins, cyclins, which form complexes with cyclin-dependent protein kinases. The most important trigger for mitosis occurs during the G1-phase of the cycle, which is effected by cyclins A, D and E in combination with a range of regulatory protein kinases, of which cdk 2 is particularly important. Once the cells pass through the synthetic phase and reach G2 they are committed to mitosis, which is initiated by the action of cyclin B complexed to cdk 1.

Regulatory steps, termed check-points, occur between G1 and S and G2 and M which, should there be damage to DNA allows time for repair so that errors in replication are avoided. Repair of DNA is brought about by topoisomerase I and II, enzymes which unwind the helix, and realign the strands. Inhibition of these enzymes causes cell death.

Chemotherapeutic drugs are now classified according to their cell-cycle specificity. Type 1 drugs, which include alkylating agents and platinum derivatives act by complexing DNA to cause irreparable damage by intercalation. Type 2 drugs specifically inhibit the 'engine' driving the cycle and are termed antimetabolites.

Telomeres

There has been recent interest in the repeat sequences of TTAGGG which form 'tails on the ends of human chromosomes and protect them against enzyme digestion, stopping end replication and loss of DNA. As a cell ages, the length of these telomeres shorten. Telomeres are constructed by reverse transcription from RNA by the enzyme telomerase, which is expressed in highly proliferative cells, such as those of the basal epithelium of the small intestine, sperm and marrow stem cells. Although not expressed by mature normal cells, it is expressed by 80% of cancers, when it may be detected as a marker of early malignant change or used as a target for novel therapies.

Apoptosis

Like cell growth, cell death or apoptosis (shedding of leaves), other than that caused through necrosis or degeneration, is an active phenomenon which programmes cells towards their self-execution. This phenomenon was first recognized in basal cell cancers of the skin, which grow slowly despite the presence of plentiful mitotic figures indicating active proliferation.

Unlike necrosis or degeneration, which affect groups of adjoining cells, apoptosis characteristically affects single cells scattered throughout a tissue. The earliest recognizable changes are compaction of the nuclear chromatin into finely granular masses which become distributed peripherally close to the nuclear membrane. The cytoplasm also becomes condensed, so that cell density is markedly increased. The nuclear membrane convolutes and breaks up into segments, which enclose small fragments of nucleus and are extended from the cell as buds or clusters of 'apoptotic bodies' which include cytoplasmic organelles. They are rapidly ingested by nearby cells and degraded. Unlike necrosis, apoptosis does not evoke an inflammatory response.

The changes of apoptosis apparently start with the cleavage of double-stranded nuclear DNA into fragments of decreasing size, preventing intact genetic material from being transferred into the engulfing cells. The mechanisms responsible for the condensation of the cell cytoplasm are poorly understood, but it is suggested that extension of apoptotic bodies is due to convulsive movements of the cell surface caused by contractions of the cytoskeleton.

Expression of a number of genes and their protein products have been linked with both stimulation and inhibition of apoptosis. These include the proto-oncogenes c-*myc*, c-*fos* and *bcl*-2, and the p53 tumour-suppressor gene, suggesting that mitosis and apoptosis may share signalling pathways.

The importance of apoptosis in the control of normal tissue growth during development is well established in both slow and fast proliferating tissues. In the latter, such as intestinal epithelium and spermatogonia, shedding of cells from the surface accounts for the greater part of cell loss, but in those which proliferate slowly, mitosis and apoptosis balance each other. Apoptosis counts for a number of involutional processes (e.g. that of the lactating breast) and can be recognized in virtually all untreated malignant tumours.

Apoptosis is enhanced by ionizing radiation and chemotherapy, particularly in stem cells, possibly to prevent transfer of mutant DNA. It may have a role in drug resistance, the effects of hyperthermia, withdrawal of trophic hormonal stimulation and immune-cell killing on cancer.

A subset of apoptosis termed *anoikis* (Greek: homelessness) is induced by depriving cells of adequate or appropriate adhesion to substrate. Resistance to anoikis is a characteristic of malignant cells and increases the ability to invade and metastasize *in vivo*.

MOLECULAR GENETICS OF CANCER

The transformation of a normal to a malignant cell is a multistage process during which the orderly processes of proliferation and differentiation become uncoupled and the balance between proliferation and cell death is disturbed. Cancer cells proliferate unceasingly and do not proceed along normal maturation pathways. Cells cultured in the laboratory undergo two changes in phenotype (physical characteristics) during the route to malignancy:

- *Immortalization*: when the cells continue to proliferate true to type but maintain inhibition of growth when contact is made with other cells.
- *Transformation*: when contact inhibition is lost and proliferation becomes unlimited.

Fully transformed cells are biologically 'malignant' but not necessarily 'tumourigenic' or 'metastatic' in an experimental animal. To be so, additional changes of phenotype are required. Clinically, a 'benign' neoplasm, although continually growing, is limited to its primary site. A 'malignant' neoplasm may either form an *in situ* cancer, showing only unrestrained growth, or invade and metastasize. Only an invasive cancer is truly malignant to its host. Cancer is now regarded as a multifactoral disease of the cell genome which undergoes a series of 'multiple hits' each of which contributes towards the cell's progress from normality to malignant cell type.

Knowledge of the genetic cause of cancer stemmed from studies of hereditary cancers and of the mutagenic activity of ionizing radiation and mustard gas which were associated with chromosomal deletions. On restoring these by fusing normal to malignant cells, the hybrids proceeded along a normal differentiation pathway. With the discovery that the transmissible agent which caused the Rous sarcoma in chickens was a virus, it was recognized that viral genes introduced into normal cells could actively promote uncontrolled growth in a dominant fashion. Most of the known chemical carcinogens which transform cells form adducts with DNA leading to mutations and abnormal gene function.

Viral genes and carcinogens act in a dominant and positive fashion to induce excessive proliferation and growth. But the absence or mutation of genes which normally inhibit proliferation also leads to tumour formation. Two types of cancer gene are now defined:

1. *Oncogenes*, which directly stimulate proliferation.
2. *Tumour-suppressor genes*, which normally inhibit excessive proliferation and growth.

Oncogenes

Oncogenes function by altering transcriptional events either directly or through control of the cell-signalling pathways.

Both DNA and RNA viruses can harbour oncogenes, which transform cells in a dominant fashion:

- *DNA viruses*: Of the three classes of DNA tumour viruses – adenovirus, papilloma virus and simian SV40 virus, only the papilloma virus is tumourigenic in man. When the genes of DNA tumour viruses are incorporated into the genome of normal cells, viral-specific proteins are encoded and these push the cell into a continuous synthetic phase which is of benefit to the virus. The proteins expressed during the DNA synthetic phase also stimulate viral replication. The oncogenes incorporated in the genome of DNA viruses are not derived from genes within the human genome and are foreign to the host.
- *RNA viruses*: Retroviruses are small viruses which contain only about 10 genes in a single strand of RNA. Through the action of reverse (RNA–DNA) transcriptase they copy their genetic material into the DNA of the host cell. Unlike the transforming genes of DNA viruses, those of RNA tumour viruses are not of viral origin but have been 'hijacked' from normal host cells in which they existed as 'proto-oncogenes' which normally regulate cell growth. The proto-oncogene may be incorporated in the virus genome in an incomplete or mutated form which, when re-inserted into the host genome, may lead to the expression of abnormal protein products. Alternatively, re-insertion of the oncogene into a region of the genome different from its normal proto-oncogenic site may bring it under the control of genes which stimulate overexpression of its normal protein product so that it is permanently 'turned on'.

Nuclear oncogenes

Nuclear oncogenes regulate transcription and other interactions within the growth control network. As proto-oncogenes they are the original developmental genes for proliferation and differentiation in normal cells but when mutated or inappropriately expressed (i.e. 'jammed on') they cause uncontrolled cell division and transformation. Examples are *myc, jun, fos* and *erb-A*.

Cytoplasmic oncogenes

A number of classes of cytoplasmic oncogenes have been described. Some are homologous to growth factors, for example *sis* and platelet-derived growth factor (PDGF), *his* and *int-2* and fibroblast growth factor (FGF); others activate growth factors, for example *ras* and TGF-α, a member of the epidermal growth factor (EGF) family. Some have receptor tyrosine kinase activity, the most prominent of which is *erb-B2* which codes for the EGF protein; others may code for non-receptor PKCs. Most have no role in human cancers; three, *ras, erb-B2* and *abl*, have been implicated in colon and breast cancer and leukaemia.

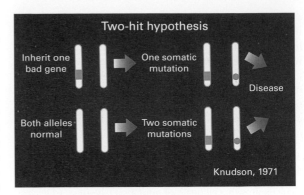

Figure 9.7. Retinoblastoma gene showing difference between hereditary and sporadic forms.

Tumour-suppressor genes

Activated proto-oncogenes act on the cell in a dominant fashion. Mutation of one copy of the gene can drive a cell towards malignancy, even when the other copy is normal. Recognition that loss of genetic material through chromosomal deletions might also be associated with the development of cancer, implicated a second set of cancer genes whose normal function is to suppress growth.

The first suggestion that human cancer might be associated with loss of suppressor genes came from studies of the genetic epidemiology of retinoblastoma, a highly malignant tumour of the retina. Retinoblastoma occurs in hereditary and sporadic forms. Hereditary tumours occur at an earlier age and are multifocal: sporadic cases occur later as a single focus in one eye. Studies of affected families suggested that two 'hits' were required, each affecting one allele of the suppressor gene. In the inherited form of the disease, the first-'hit' mutation or loss of a single allele occurs in the retinal germ cells, predisposing daughter cells to neoplastic growth. Tumour formation occurs only with a second 'hit' causing mutation or loss of the remaining normal allele which takes place during the time of maximum proliferation of retinal cells. In the sporadic form of the disease, both inherited alleles are intact, so that their disruption requires two somatic events. This explains occurrence in older individuals and single-site distribution. Discovery of the Rb gene confirmed this 'two-hit' action of tumour-suppressor genes (Fig. 9.7). Although inherited in dominant fashion, their biological action is recessive, one normal copy of the gene being sufficient to maintain normal function.

Mutations or loss of tumour-suppressor genes have now been identified for a number of hereditary tumours (Table 9.1). Loss of p53, a tumour-suppressor gene, is one of the commonest genetic defects observed in human tumours.

It is evident that the conversion of a normal to a cancer cell does not occur in a single step, but requires a number of sequential genetic and possibly 'epigenetic' events, which do not involve structural changes in the genome. Accessibility of biopsy material for genetic analysis during the evolution of

Table 9.1. Mutations of tumour-suppressor genes associated with rare hereditary tumours.

Tumour	Gene	Chromosome	Frequency
Retinoblastoma	Rb	13q14	1:20 000
Li–Fraumini syndrome	p53	17p13	Very rare
Wilms' tumour	WT1	11p15	1:10 000
Neurofibromatosis	NF1	17q22	1:3000
Polyposis coli	APC	5q21	1:8000

colon cancer from hyperplasia to adenoma, adenoma to *in situ* carcinoma and finally to invasion has revealed mutations of one or more proto-oncogenes (including K-*ras* and in inherited forms, the AP gene), loss of tumour-suppressor genes (DCC and p53) and the epigenic event of DNA hypermethylation.

CARCINOGENESIS

Although chemicals, ionizing radiation and viruses are able to cause cancer in experimental animals their precise role in human cancer is still largely undetermined:

Chemical carcinogens

The natural history of experimental tumours caused by chemical carcinogens consists of three phases:
1. *Initiation*: An irreversible interaction between the chemical carcinogen and stem cells, so that the carcinogen is 'fixed' by proliferation and replication of the cells.
2. *Promotion*: Regular development of a tumour requires an additional 'promoting' agent such as for example for experimental skin tumours, croton oil. Unlike initiation, promotion is reversible and ceases when the promoting agent is no longer applied. This effect is analogous to the hormone dependence of experimental mammary tumours. Promotion is modulated by the frequency with which the agent is applied and by environmental alterations such as diet and age.
3. *Progression*: Includes such changes as increase in growth rate, invasiveness and metastatic potential, which imply increasing genetic instability.

Initiating carcinogenic chemicals act by forming DNA adducts or electrophilic intermediates which interfere with DNA repair mechanisms. Promoting agents act through mediation of receptor mechanisms and gene expression. The changes which occur as a tumour progresses have also been explained in genetic terms due to environmental agents acting on gene integrity and expression. These three separate events in the development of experimental cancer are of doubtful relevance to human cancer which implicates a whole cascade of genetic activity.

Endogenous and exogenous chemical agents are the cause of the majority of human cancers. Lifestyle, diet and reproductive history, although not appearing to fall under the heading of chemical carcinogenesis, exert their carcinogenic effects through chemical processes. Of the estimated 10 million existing chemical compounds only 50 have been identified as carcinogenic to man. Those to which exposure occurs in the workplace include benzene, chromium compounds, coal tar, mineral oils, nickel and various solvents used in the rubber industry. Their effects are site related: coal–tar and mineral oils cause cancer of the skin, lung and bladder; nickel of the nasal sinuses and lung; and arsenic of skin, lung and liver. Improvements in industrial hygiene since the Second World War with constant surveillance for potential 'clusters' of cases of cancer around factories has greatly reduced these hazards. As the latent period between exposure and cancer is generally long, the hazard may have disappeared before its association with cancer can be identified.

Chemical carcinogens may be related to cultural habits. *Tobacco* is by far the most important, causing in the UK each year approximately 100 000 male and 50 000 female cancers. While cancer of the lung receives greatest prominence, tobacco use is also associated with buccal, pharyngeal, oesophageal, pancreatic and urinary cancers. Cigarette smoke contains over 3000 chemicals of which tars and nicotine are the most hazardous. The duration of tobacco use is critical to cancer risk. On ceasing to smoke, the risk for lung cancer does not continue to increase but persists at its predetermined level. Inhaling snuff carries a risk of lung cancer; chewing tobacco on its own or with betel nut can cause oral cancer. While tobacco consumption has fallen rapidly in developed countries, increasing consumption in developing countries in which subliminal marketing strategies are being applied is of concern. *Alcohol* also is related to cancer. Workers in the drinks industry are at increased risk of oral cancer and habitual consumers of strong alcoholic drinks have an increased risk of cancer of the oesophagus. While this may be due to a promoting effect of ethanol through cytochrome p450 enzyme systems, initiation from aromatics in alcoholic drinks cannot be ruled out.

Diet

Much attention has been paid to dietary factors in human cancer. Initially, only toxic food additives came under suspicion, but the potential carcinogenic role of all macro- and micronutrients in the normal diet is now under scrutiny. These do not necessarily act as direct carcinogens but also through other modulating (promoting) mechanisms. For example, a high intake of dietary fat increases the availability of circulating oestrogens, which may promote breast and endometrial cancer; a high intake of fibre reduces the intestinal content of the carcinogen deoxycholic acid which may reduce the risk of colon cancer. Accurate studies of dietary intake are difficult to achieve. Day-to-day and seasonal variations of diet are common and modification of one constituent is likely to be associated with change in another: for example an increase in protein intake with a reduction in that of fat and carbohydrate.

Only two direct carcinogenic agents have been identified in foodstuffs: aflatoxin and bracken fern. Aflatoxin has greatest relevance to human cancer and is produced by a fungus which affects grain and ground-nuts stored in the damp, a situation commonly found in the developing world. It is a possible cofactor to hepatitis B virus for liver cancer in Africa and Asia. N-nitroso compounds, proven to be carcinogenic in experimental animals, can occur in the primary form in bacon and other smoked foods and are potential causes of nasopharyngeal and gastric cancer. Nitrosamines may also be formed in the mouth or stomach by bacterial action, which combines secondary and tertiary amines in the diet with dietary or endogenous nitrites. These reactions are enhanced in the achlorhydric stomach, providing an explanation for an increased risk of gastric cancer in pernicious anaemia. Ascorbic acid lowers the intragastric formation of N-nitroso compounds.

Variations in the normal constituents of the diet may explain the international differences in the incidence of such common cancers as breast and colon, which are positively correlated with the intake of dietary fat. Migration from a country of low cancer risk to one of high risk alters the incidence of certain cancers in migrants. The time-scale may vary: for breast cancer the effect of migration is delayed but for cancer of the colon it is immediate.

Fat, protein and calories

Evidence for a positive interaction between dietary fat and cancer (particularly of the colon and breast) is supported by experimental studies and geographical correlations between fat intake and incidence, but large cohort studies of detailed dietary habits provide little support. Individual fatty acids may be more relevant than total fat intake. A high intake of monounsaturated fatty acids is associated with a reduced risk of breast cancer, which possibly explains the low incidence of breast cancer in Mediterranean countries where olive oil is widely consumed. α-linoleic acid is also believed to have a protective effect on breast cancer risk.

In animal models, reduction in total caloric intake explains much if not all of the potentiating effect of dietary fat on experimental tumour induction. Low-calorie diets inhibit tumour formation and this is possibly one reason for the lower incidence of breast and colorectal cancer in those of poorer socioeconomic status. There is increasing evidence that nutrition in early life may be an important factor for human breast cancer risk: a strong positive correlation between height and breast cancer risk has been observed. Foetal development within the uterus may also influence breast cancer risk.

There is little evidence that the quantity of protein in the diet affects cancer risk. Although the intake of meat is positively correlated with the risk of breast and colon cancers in Japan, it is now believed that this is more dependent upon total caloric intake than on individual macronutrients.

Although some experimental studies suggest that carbohydrates may modulate the later stages of cancer, non-starch polysaccharides provide fibre which may have protective effects. For example, the high fibre content of the Finnish diet may counteract the enhancing effect of the high dietary fat on the risk of breast and colorectal cancer, the incidence of which is surprisingly low.

Fibre

The term fibre covers a large variety of non-starch polysaccharides with different physical properties. Suggestions of an inverse relationship between the intake of dietary fibre and colon cancer risk in Africa were based on possible dilution and faster transit of dietary carcinogens through the colon. Fat-derived bile acids reaching the gut through the enterohepatic circulation were also diluted and less likely to contact colonic epithelium. Subsequent studies have failed to confirm the benefit of fibre as a means of providing bulk and the chemical composition of a specific fibre type is now regarded as more relevant.

Vegetables

Vegetables may protect against cancer, not through their fibre content, but as a result of a number of potential anticancer agents that they contain (e.g. phytoestrogens for breast, ovarian and endometrial cancers). Phytoestrogens include isoflavinoids and lignans. Isoflavinoids are diphenolic compounds found in leguminous vegetable – soya and other beans, chickpeas and plants; lignans, which are also diphenolic compounds, are formed by microflora in the gut from complex precursors found in vegetables. Both contain a number of conjugated weak oestrogens which, following ingestion, are deconjugated to active forms which are absorbed and excreted in the urine and faeces. As their concentration in body tissues is many times greater than that of endogenous oestradiol, they successfully compete for binding to the oestrogen receptor, suppressing endogenous oestrogen action. Dietary diphenolics are antioxidants and scavenge-free radicals.

Brassicas such as cauliflower, cabbage and spinach contain indolic compounds (indol-3 g-methylglucosinates), the metabolites of which induce C2 hydroxylase activity. During its metabolism, endogenous oestradiol follows two competing pathways of hydroxylation at the 2 or 16 carbon atom position. As only the 16-hydroxy metabolite has oestrogenic activity, indoles act as antioestrogens.

Micronutrients

Green-yellow vegetables – pumpkin, carrot, spinach, green lettuce and green asparagus, contain over 600 mg of β-carotene/100 g. This may protect against cancers of the lung, stomach and breast by directly restraining proliferation and promoting differentiation through antioxidant activity. Similar properties have been reported for the retinoids, synthetic analogues of vitamin A, which are under trial for the chemoprevention of breast cancer.

There is some evidence that lack of 1-2,5-dihydroxy-vitamin D may promote carcinoma of the prostate and that vitamin E may enhance epithelial cell adhesion. Trace elements such as selenium may be protective against cancer.

Viruses

It is estimated that 20% of human cancers are associated with viruses. These include the following:
- Genital cancer with human papilloma viruses (HPV).
- T-cell leukaemia with human T-cell leukaemia virus type 1 (HTLV-1).
- Burkitt's lymphoma and nasopharyngeal cancer with Epstein–Barr virus (EBV).
- Liver carcinoma with hepatitis type B and C viruses (HBV and HCV).

A number of specific tumour types are also associated with human immunodeficiency virus (HIV). Although in experimental systems infection by virus can directly transform a cell, it is unlikely that in humans this is the sole event. It is more likely that viral infections initiate a cascade of events which include activation of cellular oncogenes and loss of tumour-suppressor genes. Virus can also act in an indirect fashion, increasing susceptibility to malignant disease, as in those rendered immunodeficient.

Retroviruses

The family of retroviruses consists of three groups: spumaviruses, lentiviruses (of which HIV types 1 and 2 are members) and oncogenic viruses. Oncogenic viruses are further divided into acutely transforming and slow-transforming viruses. The genome of acutely transforming retroviruses contains an oncogene, originally hijacked from a host cell, which on re-insertion in mutated form or under novel transcriptional control disrupts normal growth control mechanisms. While the discovery of oncogenes has been central to the understanding of the mechanism of transformation, there is no record of a human cancer being caused in this way. Slow-transforming viruses do not contain a classical oncogene, but exert their effect through the insertion of viral material (pro-virus) into the host genome near to the coding region of a cellular proto-oncogene, which leads to overexpression of normal gene products. However, the only related human cancer is T-cell leukaemia.

DNA viruses

These contain double-stranded DNA. A number of groups, the hepadana viruses (hepatitis B), papilloma viruses (HPV) and herpes viruses (EBV) are associated with hepatocellular carcinoma, uterine cervical cancer, Burkitt's lymphoma and nasopharyngeal carcinoma, respectively.

Hepatocellular carcinoma

Liver cancer, the eighth commonest cancer worldwide, is particularly prevalent in sub-Saharan Africa, China, Japan and East Asia. Cholangiocarcinoma, although commonest in Asia (where it is associated with parasitic infections), does not present on the same scale as hepatocellular cancer which in China alone causes 100 000 deaths each year. More prevalent in males, 80% of cases develop in livers affected by multinodular cirrhosis.

Carriers of HbSAg have higher rates of both multinodular cirrhosis and hepatocellular carcinoma than non-carriers. Viral antigens have been identified in the liver cells of affected patients and the viral genome in cancer cells, suggesting that viral DNA may play a central role in the transforming process.

The exact mechanism underlying this process is unknown, but promotion by later exposure to mycotoxins (e.g. aflatoxin) or alcohol excess has been implicated. Unlike in the Western world, in which infection with HBV occurs through contact with blood and blood products or sexual activity (horizontal transmission), in the East it is transmitted vertically from mother to child during the first year of life. As 250 million humans worldwide are chronic carriers of the virus (10% of the population in some endemic areas), the scale of the problem is immense.

Eradicating HBV infection is obviously of huge importance. Large-scale programmes of vaccinating newborn infants, using a recombinant vaccinia virus carrying the HBV gene, are being evaluated. Exposure to aflatoxin is also being addressed.

Carcinoma of the cervix

HPV have small double-stranded circular genomes of DNA which cause benign infective skin warts. They infect basal cells during their proliferative phase which on full differentiation complete the life cycle of the virus. Genital warts, the third commonest form of sexually transmitted disease, are also due to infection by HPV, and are associated with carcinoma of the cervix. Some 30% of all women are infected with HPV and DNA sequences from this have been identified in the majority of cervical carcinomas. Over 70 types of HPV are known to infect genital sites but only a few (predominately types 16 and 18) are associated with neoplasia. Cofactors are smoking, infection by herpes simplex virus and, possibly, oral contraceptives.

Burkitt's lymphoma and nasopharyngeal cancer

EBV is a member of the herpes virus group. Its primary human target is the B-cell lymphocyte in which it establishes a latent infection. It may also infect cells of the nasopharynx, the parotid gland and the uterine cervix and is present in saliva and cervical secretions. Person-to-person spread by saliva during adolescence (e.g. by kissing) is probably the most important method of transmission in the West. In Africa and Asia, infection occurs during the first year of life causing a non-specific fever. The associated neoplasms, Burkitt's lymphoma and nasopharyngeal carcinoma, are uncommon in the Western world.

Burkitt's lymphoma first presented as a maxillary tumour, initially believed to be a localized granuloma or round-cell sarcoma, but with recognition that deposits were present also in kidneys, adrenals and ovaries, the condition was identified as an unusual form of lymphoma. The tumour occurs only in a belt north and south of the equator where there is a high rainfall and very high levels of malarial infections. The discovery of EBV in cells cultured from Burkitt's lymphoma suggested that this was the causative agent, but the disease can occur in its absence. Furthermore, EBV infection affects >95% of the world population. The restricted geographical distribution of Burkitt's lymphoma implicates a cofactor and this is believed to be constant antigen stimulation from malarial infection stimulating the continuous recruitment of new B-cells which, under the influence of virus, avoid programmed cell death.

Nasopharyngeal cancer, an undifferentiated epithelial cancer of the nasopharynx, is common in southern China, Hong Kong and amongst the Chinese in South-East Asia. EBV DNA can be detected in most tumour samples. Its restricted geographical distribution again indicates the importance of cofactors which are believed to be related to smoking and a diet of salt-cured fish and preserved meats rich in nitrosamines.

Human Immunodeficiency Virus

Certain types of cancer are more likely to occur in immuno-suppressed patients, indicating a protective role of the immune system against tumour formation. Immuno-suppressed patients following organ transplantation are more susceptible to lymphomas, Kaposi's sarcoma, and in the female, cancer of the cervix. Infection by the HIV types 1 and 2 has similar effects.

In AIDS patients, Kaposi's sarcoma occurs 20 000 times more frequently than in the general (HIV seronegative) population. The initial stimulus for transformation is a specific viral protein (tat) to which is added cell proliferative factors (cytokines) released from activated T-cells and possibly from the Kaposi cells themselves. As the risk of Kaposi's sarcoma is greater in those infected by AIDS as a result of sexual rather than other forms of contact, an additional sexually transmitted agent may be a cofactor.

Radiation

Many pioneers of radiation research, including Madame Curie, died from cancer. In the 1930s a high incidence of osteosarcomas was reported in luminous watch-dial painters who ingested radium from licking brushes. During the following decade a high incidence of leukaemia and skin cancer was observed amongst radiologists. A variety of cancers follow radiotherapy for benign conditions, most notably those of breast, thyroid and liver and following irradiation for ankylosing spondylitis.

In Hiroshima and Nagasaki there has been an excess mortality from cancer as a result of the nuclear weapons detonated over these cities. Leukaemia accounts for half of all cancer deaths, but a small but significant increase in the incidence of tumours affecting lung, gastrointestinal tract, bladder, breast and ovaries has also been recorded. Radiation exposure during early life is particularly hazardous for breast cancer and leukaemia.

Ionizing radiation includes electromagnetic irradiation, X-rays and γ-rays and subatomic particles (α particles, neutrons and electrons). As X-rays and γ-rays liberate electrons, their final effects are the same through direct damage to DNA or indirect damage as a result of the formation of free radicals (e.g. OH•). Neutrons interact with atoms within tissues to liberate ionizing protons and other nuclear particles. The ionizing properties of these various types of radiation and their damaging effects vary according to penetration and absorption in tissues and the capacity for tissue repair.

The biological effects of radiation on tissues include loss of proliferative capacity, gene mutations, chromosomal abnormalities and neoplastic transformation. These have been extensively studied in experimental systems, but the variation in sensitivity of different tissues prevents a uniform approach. The potential dangers of chronic exposure to low-dose radiation, such as that around nuclear establishments, from diagnostic investigations, from cosmic radiation and from low-frequency electromagnetic radiations emitted from power cables and electrical appliances, are of current concern. Ultraviolet radiations as a cause of melanoma in white-skinned individuals is well recognized.

Other physical forms of tissue damage may lead to the development of cancer. Burns or gravitational ulcers predispose to skin cancer, and asbestos, silicates and synthetics to lung and pleural cancers.

Reproductive factors

Sexual behaviour affects cancer risk through the acquisition of sexually transmitted infections. Transmission of HPV and the HIV predispose to cancer of the uterine cervix, Kaposi's sarcoma and some other tumours. Cancer of the uterus is commoner in women cohabiting with men who have multiple sexual partners. Cancer of the penis is not associated with sexual activity but is commoner in the uncircumcized and those with poor hygiene.

It is now 100 years since George Beatson, a Glasgow surgeon, first reported that removal of the ovaries of a young female could reverse the progress of recurrent breast cancer, and there is now unlimited evidence that deprivation of oestrogens in both pre- and post-menopausal women can alter the progress of the disease. In young women, oestrogens are secreted by the thecal cells of the ovary, but following the menopause, oestrogens are synthesized from precursors of adrenocortical origin in liver and fat through the action of aromatase enzymes.

Active ovarian function is a necessary prerequisite for the development of breast cancer. Women who have an artificial menopause before the age of 35 years have one-third the incidence of breast cancer compared to women whose ovaries remain intact until their natural menopause. The younger the age at menarche and the older that at menopause the greater is the risk of breast cancer, this being related to the number of ovarian cycles during the reproductive years. The sooner a woman has her first full-term pregnancy, the lower the risk, but whether this effect is due to interruption of ovarian cycles or to differentiation of stem cells during full lactational development of the breast is unclear. Multiple pregnancies reduce risk as does prolonged lactation.

Knowledge that the development of breast cancer is dependent upon functioning ovaries has led to a number of preventative strategies which aim to reduce endogenous oestrogen in those women believed to be at greater risk from breast cancer, for example those with a first-degree relative with the disease. These include the administration of the antioestrogen tamoxifen, reduction in dietary fat, increase in intake of vegetables and the administration of the retinoid fenretidine. Knowledge that maximum proliferative activity in the breast occurs during the luteal phase of the ovarian cycle has led to the suggestion that both oestrogen and progesterone are concerned with the development of breast cancer, leading to a feasibility study of reversibly ablating ovarian function in young women with gonadotrophin-releasing hormone agonists. A small 'titrable' amount of oestrogen, which on its own is believed to be safe, is given to maintain good health. Endometrial and ovarian cancer share some of the factors associated with breast cancer.

It is likely that cancer of the prostate is similarly dependent upon the male hormone testosterone but there is a lack of good epidemiological evidence of a direct association with risk. Unlike the female ovary, the male testis continues to secrete testosterone until old age, and it can also be synthesized from adrenal precursors. Orchidectomy and adenalectomy are effective treatment for metastatic prostatic cancer. 5α-reductase drugs, which prevent the conversion of testosterone to its active metabolite 5α-hydroxy-testosterone are now available.

CANCER INHERITANCE

The physical appearance or phenotype of an organism, whether plant, animal or human, is determined by its genetic composition or genotype. The mechanism of inheritance was explored by Gregor Mendel who, from observations on the propagation of peas in a monastery garden, is credited with suggesting that the qualities of the parent were transmitted to offspring in 'units' – now known to be genes, and not, as was then believed, 'blended' together. Genes were defined as being 'dominant' or 'recessive'. A 'dominant' gene exerts a specific phenotypic effect but there may be <50% chance of inheritance depending on the degree of

'penetrance' of the gene. The function of a 'recessive' gene is suppressed by a normal copy, two identical (homozygous) copies being required to alter phenotype. Tumour-suppressor genes, although inherited in a dominant fashion, function biologically in a recessive manner, one normal copy being insufficient to maintain normal function. Unlike plants, family units are small and their reproduction time long, which constrains studies of human genetics; however, the long lifespan of humans allows greater time for variations in phenotype to become evident.

A number of diseases are due to a unique single chromosomal abnormality which is inherited according to classical Mendelian laws. Mutational alterations of enzyme structure are responsible for many 'inborn errors of metabolism' (e.g. cystic fibrosis).

Although one or two inherited genes play a major role in the causation of some rare cancers, this is not so for the majority of common cancers which are due to a cascade of abnormal genetic events. Interactions between them and the environment produce a complex background which confounds genetic analysis.

Investigation of the hereditary trait

The cancer family

Initial recognition that an inherited trait is associated with a cancer usually comes from knowledge of 'cancer families' in which the incidence exceeds that of the normal population. Historical examples are Napoleon's family, in which Napoleon, his father and sister all died from cancer of the stomach (and which was suspected also in two more sisters, his brother and a grandfather) and the family of the French surgeon Paul Broca in which 10 of 24 female members spanning three generations died of breast cancer. While single-site tumours may form family clusters, multiple tumours, such as carcinoma of the colon and endometrium (hereditary non-polposis colorectal cancer (HNPCC syndrome)), soft tissue sarcomas, cancer of the breast and brain and leukaemia (Li–Fraumini syndrome), and carcinoma of the breast and ovary (BRCA1) may also occur. Any patient with cancer is more likely to have a closely related family member affected by the disease than is expected by chance.

The larger the kindred available for study the greater is the likelihood of determining precise familial relationships. The Utah Population Database, which combines three data sources – a geneology of the Utah pioneers and their descendants, the Utah Cancer Registry and Utah death certificates, includes approximately 1 million individuals with 180 000 supporting family records and is a unique facility.

Segregation analysis

While inspection of the pedigrees of a few affected families may allow the mode of transmission to be determined, a more comprehensive statistical analysis – segregation analysis – is used to determine the 'best fit' of the distribution of the cancer phenotype to a number of modes of inheritance, and also the concentration of gene frequency and penetrance. It determines whether the observed pattern of distribution of cases is consistent with Mendelian inheritance, whether it is due to an autosomal dominant, autosomal recessive or sex-linked gene or whether it is likely to be due to environmental or other epigenic factors.

Family members tend to be brought up in similar environments, which may affect the risk of cancer. Demographical, cultural, and behavioural factors (e.g. smoking) may be transmitted from parent to offspring and mimic true inheritance. Studies of twins and parent–child pairs allow the separation of genetic from environmental influences. Identical twins have the same genetic structure and differences between them are likely to be environmental: non-identical twins can be used as controls. Ideal are twins who had been reared apart. Parent-natural and parent-adopted child pairs can also be studied.

Linkage analysis

Having established that a cancer is familial, the next step is to identify the gene which governs susceptibility. The most practical approach is by 'linkage analysis', in which the segregation of a defined 'genetic marker' in affected and unaffected family members is compared. During meiosis there is considerable crossing over of genes between chromosomes, which are reassorted and recombined. Genes on different chromosomes segregate independently, so that four possible combinations of alleles appear with equal frequency in the gametes (Fig. 9.8). If a disease and marker gene lie close together on the same chromosome, they will segregate together and be 'linked' in the daughter chromosomes (Fig. 9.9). There is a between state when the distance between disease and marker gene allows some degree of separation and independent segregation. Those that break the link and are reassorted independently are known as 'recombinants'; their proportion in the total pool is the 'recombinant fraction' (Fig. 9.10), and the size of this allows assessment of the likelihood of linkage. Having identified the distribution of the marker gene in each family member, the probability that the observed pattern occurs by chance can be calculated. This is represented by a function known as the 'lod' score, 1 of +3 or more demonstrating significant linkage.

There is generally no functional relationship between the disease and marker genes and different alleles of the marker gene may be associated with the disease gene. Even if a strong linkage can be demonstrated between a marker and disease gene in one family, it does not follow that this will cross family boundaries or be suitable for population screening. Only a few functional marker genes have been identified, such as that coding for glutamic-pyruvic-transaminase which is linked with breast cancer (BRCA1).

Linkage studies may concentrate on individual suspect chromosomes or on areas of the genome in which 'candidate'

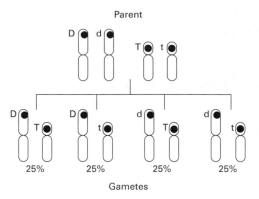

Figure 9.8. Independent segregation of genes to form combinations with equal frequency.

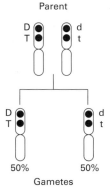

Figure 9.9. Linkage of disease on markers genes, which being closely related segregate together.

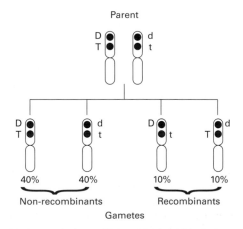

Figure 9.10. Breakage of link to form 'recombinants'.

genes are suspected. The discovery of DNA restriction fragment length polymorphisms (RFLPs) has made thousands of different 'anonymous' polymorphic genetic markers available for gene testing.

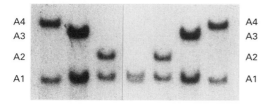

Figure 9.11. A 'Southern blot' demonstrating loss of one allele (one of a pair) of a likely tumour suppressor gene in DNA from a human cancer.

Restriction fragment length polymorphisms

Restriction enzymes, isolated from bacteria and fungi, cleave DNA into fragments of different lengths. Each of these enzymes digests a specific sequence of bases so that they 'cut' the double DNA strand into fragments of different sizes. These fragments can be separated by electrophoresis in an agarose gel. To provide a solid support for the DNA fragments, they are transferred as single strands from the gel onto nitrocellulose paper (or other membrane) by a process known as Southern blotting. Although 'western' – and 'northern' blots employ a similar technique to tRNA and antibody fragments onto a solid matrix, the original 'Southern blot' took its name from its inventor (Dr EM Southern) and not from the cardinal point (Fig. 9.11).

Particular sequences of nucleotides within these fragments are identified by DNA or RNA 'probes' which are prepared by inserting a particular sequence of nucleotides or fragment of DNA in a plasmid, a virus-like vector which is replicated in a bacterial host to provide millions of copies. The 'cloned' DNA is labelled with a radioactive nucleotide by a procedure called 'nick translation' which enzymatically induces breaks (nicks) in the DNA strand through which a radioactive nucleotide can be inserted. The labelled probe hybridizes with complementary sequences on the 'blot' to produce a band for each allele on autoradiography.

The large amount of 'junk' DNA present in the genome means alterations of its sequence of bases can readily occur without functional effect. These alterations change the position of the sites which are cut by restriction enzyme, so that fragments of different size (RFLPs) are found within the same genome and which on account of the stability of the cleavage sites are inherited according to Mendelian laws. Such 'anonymous' DNA probes have provided a huge resource for linkage studies. Once an RFLP has been found to be linked with a disease gene, probes for adjacent 'flanking' markers can be used to 'walk' up or down the genome to define specific portions of DNA containing the disease gene which can then be sequenced.

Genetic testing

As a result of the identification of a number of mutated genes in hereditary non-polyposis colon cancer – MSH2, MSH1,

PMS1 and PMS2, and in breast and ovarian cancer – BRCA1 and 2, the genetic testing of individuals for common cancers has become a reality. As over 20% of all cases of breast cancer have a family history (usually only a mother or aunt with the disease), breast cancer has become the spearhead for genetic testing. In the study of a family with a suspected inherited genetic disorder, it is best to define the mutation of the disease gene which, as it may only affect one base-pair, requires sequencing of the whole gene from an index case. For a large gene such as BRCA1 this is impracticable, but likely sites of mutation have been identified on which limited sequencing can be performed. Having identified the specific mutation, it can be sought in other members of the family. For the genetic testing of 'familial' rather than dominantly inherited cancer: for example those with one or two first-degree relatives affected, a less specific test seeking alterations in the expressed product (e.g. a 'protein trunction test') can be used.

The indiscriminate use of genetic testing is to be avoided. Young women, knowing that they have a family history of breast cancer, must be made aware of the benefits and risks before having a test and care should be taken to minimize psychological distress, stigmatization and discrimination. This has led to the development of the genetic clinic where a geneticist with the support of a nurse counsellor will compile a detailed family pedigree, recognizing that most people have knowledge of at most two generations. At this clinic the woman should be fully informed about the concept of inheritance, the extent to which this contributes to general population risk and the benefits and risks of genetic testing. This should include the nature of the gene to be tested, its mode of inheritance and associated cancer risk, and the advantages and limitations of the test to be used. The implications of a positive test must be fully described, in particular the effect it might have on employment and insurance. Potential monitoring or preventative measures should be explained.

Emotional and psychological support may be necessary at this first session. Should serious anxiety be identified, a psychiatric assessment may be advised. Blood may be collected at this first attendance, recognizing that if the patient is uncertain and wishes further counselling before agreeing to have the test, the specimen can be stored.

In some clinics this initial attendance is followed up by a letter which reviews the information which has been given, reinforces the concept of inheritance, the benefits and risks of genetic testing and likely recommendations should the test prove positive. If blood has been collected at the first visit, consent for the test to proceed may be given at this stage.

Once the result of the test is known, further counselling is necessary. The risks to the woman and her female offspring and other close relatives is reviewed. Should the test prove positive, alternative measures to monitor the breasts and the possibility of prophylactic surgery are explained. Consultation with a surgeon can be arranged so that the pros and cons of prophylactic mastectomy can be assessed, recognizing that even this cannot completely remove all risk.

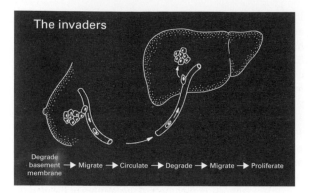

The invaders

Degrade basement membrane → Migrate → Circulate → Degrade → Migrate → Proliferate

Figure 9.12. The metastatic cascade.

MECHANISMS OF INVASION AND METASTASES

Metastases do not develop passively, but as a result of a cascade of tumour–host reactions caused by a series of genetic and epigenetic events which cause the cancer cells to detach from their neighbours, migrate through the interstitial tissues, intravasate through a blood or lymphatic vessel wall, survive the mechanical stress of circulating in the blood stream, target a new capillary and invade new host tissues where they proliferate and grow (Fig. 9.12). Normal cells can also invade (e.g. trophoblast and vascular endothelium), but this is a regulated process during which arrival cues are sensed. Only a very small fraction of cells in a tumour are able to survive in the circulation and even fewer are capable of forming metastases. These cells can be regarded as having accumulated the essential phenotypic changes required for invasion and metastasis.

Cells normally adhere to each other by a macromolecular 'glue' which binds to specific adhesion receptors. Inadequate or inappropriate adhesion between cell and substrate induces anoikis, a specific form of apoptosis. Under normal circumstances, anoikis prevents ectopic cellular proliferation, maintains tissue architecture and guards against metastasis. Resistance to anoikis is a characteristic of transformed cells. Several families of cell adhesion molecule have been described which mediate cell-to-cell and cell-to-matrix binding. These include integrins, cadherins, the immunoglobin superfamily, hyaluronate receptors and mucins. Best characterized are the integrins, which are transmembrane glycoproteins and provide a functional and structural chain between extracellular matrix molecules, for example collagen, fibronectin and laminin, and cytoskeletal components within the cell. Before the cells can separate the ligand–integrin interactions must be disrupted enzymatically or by inhibitors. This event is critical to both invasion and metastasis.

To gain access to the interstitial tissues the cells must penetrate the basement membrane and become mobile. The basement membrane is a specialized layer of extracellular matrix

containing proteoglycans (chondroitin and heparin), matrix proteins (laminin and fibronectin) and type IV collagen. The cell first attaches to the basement membrane through surface laminin receptors. Release of proteolytic enzymes, such as calcium- and zinc-dependent metalloproteinases, type IV collagenase, cathepsin and stromolysin from cancer and neighbouring fibroblasts degrade the matrix allowing the cell to migrate by active contractions of its cytoskeleton. By pushing out pseudopodia, studded with matrix receptors which act as a 'sense organ', the cell advances by attaching and subsequently releasing itself from the matrix proteins of the interstitium. Motility-stimulating cytokines (autocrine motility factors, AMF) have been identified.

Some tumours (e.g. sarcomas) contain large primitive vascular spaces which can readily be penetrated by tumour cells; most gain access to the intact capillary network of the interstitial tissues, by deforming and squeezing their way between the endothelial cells. Tumours do not contain lymphatics, which are penetrated only following invasion of the interstitium.

Once in the blood or lymphatic systems, tumour cells are free to circulate. As the lungs receive 100% and the liver 73% of the cardiac output, these organs are first encountered by the tumour cell. In order to survive, tumour cells must resist anoikis, surviving to become attached to the capillary endothelium but only a few cells adhere and grow. Most freely circulating cells are arrested at points of vascular branching to be destroyed by host defence mechanisms (see Chapter 11) but some continue their onward passage to other sites.

Having targeted a capillary in a new site, the malignant cells attach to its endothelial wall. As cells within a clump are relatively protected by the outer layer, they are more likely than single cells to proliferate within the capillary and burst out into the interstitial tissues and degrade the subendothelium of the capillary. Having migrated through the tissues of the new host site, the cells initially receive nourishment by diffusion but their growth is limited to a spheroid of 1–3 mm in size. For further proliferation they must acquire new vessels (neovascularization), which are formed through release of angiogenesis factors from stromal cells. Those of greatest significance are PDGF and FGF. The tumour must also be supplied with autocrine and paracrine factors which enhance cell division and growth.

Considering the complexity of this metastatic cascade, and the hazards that the tumour cells encounter at every step, it is not surprising that only a few of the millions of cells that are shed from a tumour survive to form metastases. Many aspects of this process are ill-understood, including the varying distribution of metastases in different types of cancer, the long periods of time that may pass before they become clinically evident and the mechanism by which they cause death in the absence of obvious organ failure. A number of 'check-points' in the metastatic process (e.g. inhibitions of cell surface and secreted proteins) offer sites for regulatory restoration by novel therapies.

These various processes are under the genetic control of 'metastasis-promoting' genes which may have dominant positive effects. Metastases-suppressor genes also have been identified, of which nm23 on chromosome 17q has received particular attention. This gene, which was first isolated from murine melanoma cell lines of high metastatic potential, is closely homologous to a fruit fly gene associated with normal wing development. Its expression in human tumours interacts with aggressiveness.

EPIDEMIOLOGICAL STUDIES

Epidemiology is the study of the distribution and determinants of disease in humans and the application of the results to potential prevention and control. It is a science based on the measurement of disease within a population and the identification of associated risk factors. Unlike an experimental study, which considers the effect of altering risk factors, an epidemiological study starts by measuring effect and then investigates risk. Two major types of epidemiological study are described: descriptive and analytical.

Descriptive epidemiology

Descriptive studies examine differences in the distribution of a disease with respect to the population, its age, sex, place (geographical area) and time. The most informative estimates of the frequency and distribution of cases of cancer come from the cancer registry which records all newly diagnosed cases of cancer in the general population.

Cancer registration

Cancer registries may be national, regional or local. The first national cancer registry was established in 1941 in Denmark, to be followed by national registries in other Nordic countries. Although in England and Wales attempts to monitor the incidence of cancer were made in the 1920s, it was only in 1947 that a national cancer registry was proposed for the UK. Fourteen regional registries were established in England and Wales, and one each in Scotland and Northern Ireland. However, as a result of the lack of personal identifiers and dependence upon hospital clinical and administrative staff for completion of registration forms, only a small proportion of the total number of new cancers were enumerated. This situation has greatly improved as a result of culling records from hospital medical record departments, pathology departments, death certificates and general practitioners, and by establishing direct computer links between registries and National Health Service databases. The cancer registry in the UK is now the largest in the world. The minimal dataset for all cancers includes personal identifier, site and type of primary tumour, initial treatment, country of origin, occupation and marital status. Date of death is provided later through linkage with death certification.

Similar regional registries have been combined to produce national figures in a number of countries. However, in some, including the US, these do not cover the whole country and national incidence data is not available. In 1972 the US National Cancer Institute set up the Surveillance, Epidemiology and End Results (SEER) programme which combines the data from 10 state and urban registries and allows cancer incidence and survival experience to be related to demographical and social characteristics of the population. Although only 11% of the total US population is sampled, the geographical distribution of these registries facilitates extrapolation of national trends. Local cancer registries, based on religious groups (Mormons, Seventh Day Adventists), health insurance plans and other community health schemes, have also been instituted.

The International Classification of Disease (ICD) is used universally to code cancer data. This classification is largely organized on an anatomical basis, on the premise that the organ involved by a cancer may be specific to a cause (e.g. lung cancer and smoking). Location of the cancer also affects its histological type and treatment. A specialized adaptation for cancer (ICD-Oncology) provides code numbers for topographical location, histological type, behaviour (e.g. invasive or *in situ*) and parts of an organ affected (e.g. of the colon).

Cancer registries worldwide publish an annual report in which incidence is presented as rates per 100 000 population, determined by the number of cases diagnosed during that year divided by the population at risk. This crude rate takes no account of the age at which the cancer is diagnosed or the age structure of the population. To take account of age at diagnosis, 'age-specific rates' are compiled, usually for 5-year age groups. For rare cancers, or when the ages of the population are not known, longer time intervals are used. As the age structure of the population varies greatly between countries, crude rates do not allow comparisons. This is taken into account by compiling 'age-adjusted rates' by which age-specific rates are adjusted to a world standard population derived from the age structure of 46 countries. The age-adjusted rate is most accurate for the age group 35–64 years, which is presented as the 'truncated standard rate'. A cumulative rate is also calculated to estimate the probability of developing a specific cancer over a defined period of life. This is presented as between 0 and 64 and 0 and 74 years of age.

The accuracy of determinating rates depends not only on the incidence of the cancer (numerator) but also on the confidence with which the population can be measured (denominator). Although vital statistics – births, deaths, etc. are collected in many countries on an annual basis, these are usually available only locally and do not take account of variations in age between those migrating between urban and rural areas. Five-year national census data are preferred.

Each 5 years the data from the annual reports of regional and national cancer registries are compiled into a volume, *Cancer Incidence in Five Continents*, which is published jointly by the International Agency for Research on Cancer and the International Association of Cancer Registries. This provides data for each ICD code of cancer listed as age-specific incidence in 5-year age groups, age-standardized rates for world and truncated world populations, cumulative rates for ages 0–64 and 0–74 years and, for selected cancers, divisions of topographical site. The most recent volume (VI), published in 1992, provides standardized data up to the year 1987 for 136 populations in 50 countries, from which regional and national differences can be determined.

Death certification

Owing to the variable prognosis of different cancers, mortality cannot be taken as a surrogate measure of incidence, except for those cancers from which death is invariable, for example those of lung or pancreas. However, mortality statistics are relevant to many analytical studies and the mechanism of death certification should be understood.

It is generally accepted that death certificates provide more accurate statistics than does cancer registration, but errors between the underlying cause of death on the death certificate and that on postmortem examination vary from 20% to 40%. Similar errors occur between clinical and autopsy causes of death. These errors are less likely to occur for cancer deaths as a clinical diagnosis of cancer tends to be accurate.

Towards the end of the last century, certification of the cause of death became obligatory in many countries. Statutory registration of deaths replaced parish registers in England and Wales in 1837 and in Scotland in 1885. However, it was only in 1956 that comparative data on cancer mortality in different countries first became available through the World Health Organization.

The statutory death certificate consists of two parts. In Part I, the sequence of events leading to death are recorded, the immediate cause of death being listed first, followed by one or two antecedent conditions. The cause that is listed last is the 'underlying cause' of death. Part II lists unrelated conditions which may have adversely affected the outcome.

Internationally agreed rules for identification of the underlying cause of death have been laid down by the World Health Organization. The general rule states that the underlying cause of death is either that which has been listed alone in Part I, or should more than one condition be entered, that which was entered last. This underlying cause of death is underlined by the registrar on the certificate and is recorded as its ICD code. Should it appear improbable that the last entered condition led to the sequence of events leading to death, the registrar will first seek clarification from the person who completed the certificate and if this is not possible, he may apply three subsidiary rules which allow him to select the most likely underlying cause of death from those listed.

Other measures

The success of treatment is often monitored by survival rates over periods of 5 years, but as these are biased by the time at which the diagnosis was made (lead-time bias) and by the form of treatment given, better estimates of outcome are mortality rates based on the population at risk. The 'gap' between age-specific incidence and mortality may be taken to provide a rough guide to the success of treatment, but this may be biased by overdiagnosis of a cancer; for example through the institution of a screening programme or by errors in death certification.

Relative frequency

Relative frequency expresses the frequency of cancer at a single site as a proportion of all cancers. A high relative frequency of one cancer does not necessarily indicate a high incidence; it may be due to a relative absence or low frequency of other cancers. The relative frequency is most commonly derived from biopsy series, which themselves may be biased by the practice of the surgeon and threshold of suspicion of the pathologist, especially in borderline and *in situ* lesions. It is useful only to define which cancers are most common to a specific population.

Time Trends

Changes in the incidence and mortality of a cancer over periods of time can have great significance, but artefacts in short-term changes may arise from the sudden availability of a backlog of records or greater public awareness. A good example was the sharp increase in incidence of breast cancer in the US following its diagnosis in the wives of the president and vice-president. To be of significance, a steady increase or decrease over time must be observed.

Time trends are usually presented graphically by calendar period. As changes in incidence over time may first be observed in younger age groups, it is important that these are standardized for age. They may also be presented as age-specific rates for each birth cohort, representing the experience of cancer in those born at one point in time. This takes account not only of increasing age and the time of diagnosis, but of the effect of a specific year of birth.

Cancer Maps and Charts

A recent trend is to present data on the distribution of cancer as a 'cancer map'. However, distribution may be distorted by large areas with small populations, arbitrary boundaries and regional deficiencies in registration. An unusual distribution (cluster) within a restricted geographical area; for example around a potential source of exposure to a carcinogen such as a factory or rubbish dump, may point to a potential cause, but great care is required to eliminate all possible confounding factors.

Migration

Changes in cancer incidence following the migration of populations from one area of the world to another may provide information on the environmental effects. It is important to determine the time sequence of changes in incidence following migration. When this is immediate, as in colon cancer, a promoting influence may be responsible, whereas when it is delayed, as in breast cancer, it may point to a more fundamental initiating effect. Migrants do not represent a random sample of their 'home' population but may be selected through culture or occupation which introduces selection bias.

Correlation Studies

Studies of the incidence and locality of a cancer in a country can be correlated with environmental factors, for example diet (fat and colon cancer), occupation (asbestos workers and mesothelioma) or climate (melanoma and exposure to the sun). However, such correlations tend to be crude as they can only consider factors which affect the whole population and not its individual members.

Analytical epidemiology

Analytical studies consider relationships between exposure to risk factors and disease outcomes. Two types of studies are described – experimental (interventional) and observational.

In an *experimental or interventional* study, individuals are randomly allocated to be included in a study group, which is exposed to a factor under study or allocated to a non-exposed control group. Such studies offer the most direct and conclusive method of establishing a causal relationship between a risk factor and a cancer. Although the introduction of a suspected risk factor may happen opportunistically, as in irradiation following the atomic bombs in Japan, the introduction of harmful measures (or withdrawal of beneficial ones) from random sections of the population is not ethical. Although this study design is standard for assessing the effects of treatment, it is applicable only to epidemiological studies of primary or secondary prevention; for example vaccination against hepatitis B or screening for breast cancer. Such large and expensive population studies will become more frequent as chemoprevention becomes a reality.

In *observational* studies, the investigator has no control over likely causal relationships or disease outcomes. He can only compare groups of individuals with or without the diagnosis of cancer either proceeding from effect (the cancer) to potential cause (the 'case–control study') or commencing with suspected causes and proceeding to effect (the diagnosis of cancer) (the 'cohort study'). These two methods are complementary and can be combined in a 'nested' study.

Case–control study

In a case–control study, those diagnosed to have a cancer are selected as the 'cases' and those without as controls, allowing comparison of suspected present or past risk factors related to cancer development. The 'relative risk' of the disease between those exposed and those not exposed to such factors is calculated. Cases may be identified from a variety of sources (e.g. hospital admission records) cancer or death registers, and may be institutional or population based. They may consist of all cases diagnosed during a specified time period or, if these are numerous, a random sample. Incident (new cases) are preferred to prevalent (existing) cases as they are less likely to introduce selection bias.

The control population must be carefully chosen to avoid bias, usually by matching controls to each case by a number of factors unrelated to the cancer under study, for example age, sex, place of residence, same class at college, etc. For large population studies random selection of controls is preferable. As the size of the population determines the power of the study, this can be enlarged by selecting a number of controls (advisably not >4) for each case.

An advantage of the case–control study is that it allows the simultaneous study of a number of potential risk factors, some of which may have produced their effects many years previously, and interactions between them. As the researcher is dependant upon past records for information, only risk factors that are readily ascertained can be studied. There is a high susceptibility to bias owing to improper ascertainment, faulty diagnosis of cases or non-comparability of control groups.

Cohort study

Two types of cohort study are described – prospective and historical (retrospective). In a prospective study, potential risk factors for a specific cancer are identified in a selected population at the 'present' time. The population is then followed up over time to ascertain the incidence of the cancer. It may take many years for a sufficient number of cancers to be diagnosed (90% follow-up over 20 years is advised) and losses from follow-up can pose problems. Large populations are required to yield reasonable risk estimates of even common cancers, which is expensive. As incidence rates can be calculated in those exposed or not exposed to a particular risk factor, differences can be directly demonstrated. A great advantage of the prospective cohort study is that biological materials can be stored for later analysis.

The historical (retrospective) cohort study looks back in time, possibly for 20 years or more, to define a population exposed to specified risk factors whose cancer experience is determined to a specified date. As the period of follow-up has already taken place, results can be rapidly achieved, but only if suitable records of past experience are available. The incidence of cancer in those exposed to a risk factor can then be matched against cancer registration or mortality records and expressed as standardized incidence and mortality rates (SIR and SMR) compared to those expected to occur in the general population of the same age and sex during the same period of time. Such studies are constrained by the quality of the historical information available which in these days of non-preservation of records may not readily be ascertained. Biological samples are not likely to be available.

Nested case–control study

Due to the long period of time and scale of resources necessary to conduct a prospective cohort study and difficulty in measuring potential risk factors in a retrospective study, incorporation of a case–control study within a cohort is now popular. The cohort component identifies the population and ascertains information on exposure and disease experience during the follow-up period, while the case–control component is used to assess risk in the most informative group of individuals; that is, those with cancer and controls within the same cohort.

Monitoring and surveillance studies

In a comprehensive National Health Service, such as that in the UK, information held in patient data-banks (e.g. the use of prescriptive medicines) can potentially be used to conduct follow-up studies from which effects can be determined. Computerized 'linkage' between hospital and population data-sets, such as the cancer registry, can facilitate this. It is important that in conducting such studies individuals in the two registers are accurately matched for a number of identifying factors.

Meta-analyses

Statistical methods have long been available to pool the results from a number of different studies. While still taking account of individual variability, these increase the statistical power of the analysis through the acquisition of larger numbers of values. Usually performed on published data, meta-analyses have the disadvantage of 'publication' bias, which arises from the likelihood that positive results are more frequently published than negative ones.

An alternative method of combined analysis, the 'overview', considers not only published data but also all studies that have been carried out and for which basic data (deaths, recurrences) can be reascertained. This was the method used by the Early Breast Cancer Triallists Collaborative Group which has pooled data from all trials conducted on selected forms of therapy. The most accurate method of pooling the results of trials conducted by different investigators is to design an agreed protocol with central analysis of the results.

SCREENING FOR CANCER

The fundamental premise for screening a normal population for cancer is that diagnosis and treatment during the presymptomatic phase results in a better outcome than when symptoms develop. Screening is not diagnostic but only defines a group of individuals who are test positive and require further investigation. The principles which underlie a population-screening programme are as follows:

- The cancer must present an important health problem. Its natural history must be adequately understood, including the course of its development from 'latent' (preclinical) to 'declared' (symptomatic) disease.
- A suitable validated and acceptable test should be available to recognize this latent stage.
- An acceptable method of treatment must be available for the detectable earlier stage which has been proven to improve outcome.
- Facilities must be available for the diagnosis and treatment of those with screen-detected abnormalities.
- Benefits must be greater than costs and must give equal value for money to those of other health needs.

The initiation of a screening programme for cancer involves a series of phases. First, the development and evaluation of a test which can detect the cancer at a presymptomatic, preinvasive or, if invasive, premetastatic phase. The tests used to investigate screen-detected abnormalities must also be evaluated. There must be proof that treatment of the screen-detected cancer results in a reduction in the mortality from the disease and that the cost to the individual, the population to be screened and to the tax payer is justified. Established screening programmes in the UK have been initiated for cancers at two sites only – cervix and breast, but consideration is being given to screening for colorectal, ovarian and prostatic cancer.

The disease

For screening to be cost-effective, the cancer must constitute a major health problem. This usually implies a high incidence, or for uncommon cancers, a high fatality rate. As incidence rates vary with age, target age groups in whom screening is most likely to be effective should be defined. The age distribution of a cancer also affects the frequency of screening. A single test in early life may only be required to detect the majority of childhood cancers; for example neuroblastoma or Wilms' tumour or to define an identifiable premalignant state such as colonic polyps during middle age. Repeat screens are necessary for the early detection of the majority of cancers whose incidence continues to accumulate with advancing years.

It is now generally accepted that invasive cancer is preceded by a sequence of events which includes excess proliferation, the development of atypical features, transformation of normal into cancer cells, and the formation of *in situ* disease. These events are time dependent; as a preinvasive cancer increases in size, it is more likely to become invasive; as the size of an invasive cancer increases so does the likelihood of metastases. Screening goes back in time but as it is not always certain that had the cancer remained undetected it would have progressed to a later stage, some degree of overdiagnosis is inevitable.

The screening test

The suitability of a screening test is determined by three standard measures (Fig. 9.13):
1. sensitivity,
2. specificity,
3. predictive value.

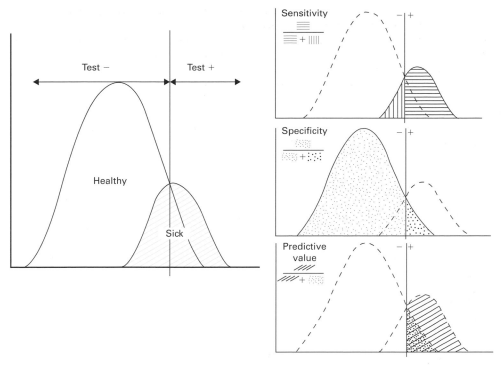

Figure 9.13. Models of estimates of efficiency of screening. sensitivity and specificity relate to healthy and sick populations. Predictive value relates to the validity of the test.

The value of a test used for diagnosis cannot be extrapolated to the screening situation. A diagnostic test provides information which is complementary to that of a number of other tests. A screening test has to stand-alone.

The *sensitivity* of a test defines the proportion of those with cancer in whom a positive test has been recorded. Both the number who are test positive and those with false negative tests need to be known so that the total number of cancers can be calculated. As it is impracticable to fully investigate those with a negative test for the presence of cancer, the number of cancers which 'surface' spontaneously during a defined period after a negative screening test, so-called 'interval cancers', are taken to represent those missed by the screening test. The number of interval cancers is expressed as the proportion of the estimated incidence of the disease, allowing the number of those whose diagnosis has been advanced by the screening test to be estimated. If interval cancers account for 20% of the expected incidence, it is assumed that screening has advanced the diagnosis of the other 80% (Table 9.2).

The *specificity* of a screening test is the reciprocal of the false-positive rate and is the proportion of all those without cancer who were correctly classified as negative by the screening test. As all persons with a positive test will be further investigated, the actual number of false-positive tests is known.

Sensitivity and specificity are inversely related. Although ideally they should each approach 100%, this is unrealistic. There is a 'trade-off' which depends upon the threshold for an abnormal test. If this is set so that no cancers are ever missed, the test will have a high sensitivity, but as a greater number of tests will be falsely positive, a low specificity. Conversely, if the threshold is set so that false-positive tests are minimized (high specificity), sensitivity will suffer. The relationship between sensitivity and specificity is represented by relative operating characteristic (ROC) curves, which are used to set the most suitable threshold for a test (Fig. 9.14). The more efficient a screening test, the greater will be the yield of cancers and the lower the false-positive rate.

The third criterion used to define the validity of a screening test is the *positive predictive value*. This represents the proportion of those with a positive test who are subsequently proven to have cancer. This measure is largely dependent on the specificity of the test but also on the underlying prevalence of the cancer in the population to be screened. When this is low the number of true positive tests decreases while, as there are more healthy persons, false-positive tests increase and the positive predictive value falls.

The acceptability of the test must clearly be evaluated before its use is extended to population screening.

Table 9.2.

| | | True Disease State | |
		Cancer Present	Healthy (Cancer Absent)
Screening test	Positive	a	b
	Negative	c	d

$$\text{Sensitivity} = \frac{a}{a + c} \qquad \left[\frac{\text{positive test in those with cancer}}{\text{all who have cancer}}\right]$$

$$\text{Specificity} = \frac{d}{b + d} \qquad \left[\frac{\text{negative test in healthy}}{\text{all who are healthy}}\right]$$

$$\text{Positive predictive value} = \frac{a}{a + b} \qquad \left[\frac{\text{positive test indicative of cancer}}{\text{all who have a positive test}}\right]$$

a = true positive; b = false positive; c = false negative; d = true negative.

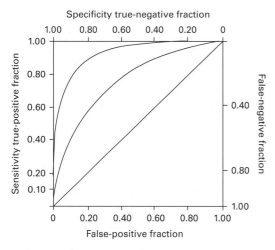

Figure 9.14. Relative operating characteristic curves showing the 'trade-off' between sensitivity and specificity.

The screening programme

The introduction of a programme of screening is complex. First, the target group needs to be identified from those who, for a variety of reasons, should not be screened. It is essential for success that compliance is high and the best form of invitation, the most acceptable system of appointments, the most convenient method of performing the test, its interpretation and the notification of results all need to be explored. Those to be invited for screening should be aware of its objectives, provided with background information on the test and the implications of a positive result, including the nature of further investigations.

It is best that facilities for additional diagnostic tests should be provided within the programme. In the UK breast-screening programme, the further assessment of women with abnormal mammograms is carried out by members of a multidisciplinary team who have the expertise and experience to perform the necessary tests efficiently and pleasantly in minimum time. Counselling by trained personnel is included.

During the development of a programme, it is likely that a number of pilot studies will have been conducted to define the best options for the final programme. However, before a programme can be instituted, it must be demonstrated beyond doubt that death or other event from the cancer concerned are beneficially affected by its earlier diagnosis and treatment.

It is best to conduct a randomized controlled trial in which subjects are randomized either to be invited for screening or to be included in non-screened control group. A longer duration of survival for screen-detected cancers cannot be taken as evidence of benefit owing to two types of bias. *Lead-time* bias is due to screening by advancing the time at which the cancer is diagnosed, and extending the time between the date of diagnosis and death, even if death occurs at the same time as in the absence of screening. *'Length bias'* also prolongs apparent survival due to the tendency of screening to detect slow-growing cancers which spend longer in their preclinical detectable (sojourn) phase and have a better prognosis irrespective of treatment. To eliminate these biases, cancer-specific mortality rates in study and control groups must be calculated using the total number of subjects at risk as denominator. On account of non-acceptance of the invitation to attend for screening, the observed reduction in cancer-specific mortality may underestimate the true effect of screening. Tests designed to reduce disease-specific mortality in one section of the population cannot be expected to have a significant effect on all-cause mortality.

Ideally, the subjects to be included in a trial should be individually randomized but this is not always feasible in large population studies. Randomizations of 'clusters' or geographical units may be used. As those who accept or refuse an invitation to be screened may consider themselves to be at higher or lower risk of a cancer than the general population ('*selection*' *bias*), incidence rates must be monitored in non-attenders who must be included in comparisons of mortality.

It has been proposed that a number of 'surrogate' outcome measures of mortality may give an earlier indication of effectiveness. These measures include tumour size, nodal status and grade.

An alternative to the randomized trial is the case–control study, which does not require a control population and can be carried out within a population which has been offered screening. The relative risk of death from a cancer in those who were screened is compared with unscreened controls. Case–control studies are particularly liable to 'selection' bias.

Cost

Before introducing a programme of screening, it must be shown that this is cost-effective compared to other health promotion and interventional policies. This is generally done by comparing 'life-years saved' adjusted for quality of life (QALYS). Financial costs must be calculated for the whole programme, including assessment, treatment and follow-up. These may in part be offset by the cost of treating advanced disease in the unscreened population. Non-financial costs such as potential harmful effects of the screening test, false reassurance from a negative test or unnecessary concern from a false-positive test and unnecessary treatment must also be considered. The anxiety of having to live longer with a disease, which might remain indolent, must be balanced against assurance of the majority that they are free from the cancer and the possibility of using more conservative treatment.

Continued evaluation

If a population-screening programme is to be instituted there must be rigid monitoring of quality. This requires the institution of a quality assurance network at regional and national level. A programme must be continually audited and regular reports provided on such performance indicators as compliance, reliability of test performance, cancer detection rates and characteristics of screen-detected cancers. The desired end point, a reduction in cancer-specific mortality within the population, may not be seen for many years. Mathematical models have been constructed by which expected performance can be defined.

STAGING OF CANCER

TNM Staging

Development

The TNM system for the classification of malignant tumours was developed during the 1950s (Table 9.3). It had five stated objectives to:

1. aid the clinician in the planning of treatment;
2. give some indication of prognosis;
3. assist in the evaluation of the results of treatment;
4. facilitate exchange of information between treatment centres;
5. contribute to the continuing investigation of human cancer.

Its original purpose was to allow clinical experience to be conveyed to others without ambiguity, mainly concentrating on the anatomical extent of the disease at the time of initial presentation. It was not designed to 'stage' the disease for prognostic purposes, for which many other variables have to be taken into account. The division of the disease into stages was an attempt, by crude merging of TNM factors, to define groups which are more or less homogeneous in terms of the extent of the disease.

In its initial form, the same basic principles were applied to all sites and coded as T to classify the extent of the primary tumour, N to determine the condition of the regional nodes and M to indicate the presence or absence of distant metastases. The minimum information required to allow comparisons to be made was clinically based and was simple, as were the subdivisions of each category. The subdivisions were:

- four degrees of primary tumour (T1–4) depending on size and local extent;
- four degrees of node status (N0–3) representing increasing involvement;
- two degrees of distant metastatic disease (M0–1) indicating absence or presence.

Although in the initial classification attention was paid to the penetration, extent and histological grade of the primary tumour and also to the histology of the lymph nodes, this was used in a restricted way so that emphasis remained on the clinical findings. It was primarily a clinical classification.

Several revisions have taken place since. With realization that the relationships between clinical findings and outcome are not firm and do not reflect those found on pathological examination, the system of classification became more complex. Account was taken of the results of increasingly refined investigations to assess the extent of the disease, the sites of metastatic involvement, and findings at operation and those determined histopathologically, and pre- (cTNM) and post-operative (pTNM) categories were introduced. A number of additional and somewhat ambiguous factors have also been

Table 9.3. **TNM Clinical Classification.**

Categories used to determine for all sites of disease are based on evidence from physical examination, imaging, endoscopy, biopsy, surgical exploration and other relevant examinations.

T – Primary tumour
>   TX – primary tumour cannot be assessed
>   T0 – no evidence of a primary tumour
>   Tis – carcinoma *in situ*
>   T1, T2, T3, T4 – increasing size and/or local extent of the primary tumour

N – Regional lymph nodes
>   NX – regional lymph nodes cannot be assessed
>   N0 – no regional lymph node metastases
>   N1, N2, N3 – increasing involvement of regional lymph nodes

M – Distant metastases
>   MX – presence of distant metastases cannot be assessed
>   M0 – no distant metastases
>   M1 – distant metastases which are further specified according to their site

It should be noted that a number of subdivisions of some main categories are available to allow greater specificity.

TNM Pathological classification

For the pathological classification similar categories are used with subdivisions for those requiring greater specificity. In addition histopathological grading may be recorded as

GX – grade of differentiation cannot be assessed
>   G1 – well differentiated
>   G2 – moderately differentiated
>   G3 – poorly differentiated
>   G4 – undifferentiated

Additional descriptors

Additional optional descriptors can be applied to tumours assessed following multimodal therapy (y), to recurrent tumours (r), to the certainty or validity of the classification (C-factor) and to the likelihood of residual disease (R).

C – factor definitions are based on evidence obtained by:
>   C1 – standard diagnostic means (inspection, palpation, imaging, endoscopy)
>   C2 – special diagnostic techniques (CT, MRI, cytology)
>   C3 – surgical exploration including biopsy
>   C4 – pathological examination of the surgical resected specimen
>   C5 – autopsy

R – category is based on the perceived presence or absence of residual tumour after treatment:
>   RX – presence or absence of residual tumour cannot be assessed
>   R0 – no residual tumour
>   R1 – microscopic residual tumour
>   R2 – macroscopic residual tumour

added: the 'y symbol' (for cases in which surgery has followed treatment by other methods); the 'r symbol' (for the classification of recurrent disease); the 'C factor' which attempts to determine the certainty with which the findings have been recorded at different sites; and the 'R factor' which defines the likelihood of residual disease. For each cancer the methods of clinical assessment to define each TNM category and for some, but not all, cancers, the criteria used for pathological staging have been defined.

As there were variations in the extent to which these criteria were applied in various countries, the 1987 revision was accepted by all national TNM committees, by the American Joint Committee on Cancer and by the European Organization for Research on Treatment of Cancer (EORTC) as a standard classification which will remain unchanged until major advances determine that a further revision is necessary.

Current system

The basis of the TNM system remains the assessment of three components, the extent of the primary tumour (T), the presence or absence of metastases in regional lymph nodes (N) and in distant sites (M), these being separately classified for pre- (cTNM) and post-operative (pTNM) treatment. Following determination of each category, they are grouped into stages, the limits of which are stage 0 representing *in situ* cancer and stage 4, distant metastases. As the extent to which detailed clinical, surgical and pathological findings contribute to the stage varies, there is a regrettable lack of uniformity for staging cancers at different sites. For some cancers (e.g. thyroid), simple clinical findings are still used, whereas for others (e.g. uterine, cervix or prostate), detailed pathological findings predominate.

The suggestion that the clinical stage is of primary importance to select and evaluate therapy, while the pathological stage provides the most precise data to estimate prognosis and calculate end results, is an oversimplification. Recognition of the frequency of early systemic spread of cancers in many sites has led to acceptance that the clinical stage is an insufficient indicator of the need for systemic treatment for which pathological staging (e.g. that based on regional lymph node findings) has become the hallmark. Similarly, in the absence of information on the biological type of the tumour, which now may include the results of sophisticated immunological and molecular genetic studies, the pathological stage of the disease may give erroneous information on prognosis. For example, the presence of lymph node metastases does not necessarily determine a poor outcome for the individual patient with a well-differentiated cancer. Many consider that those who developed the current TNM system have compromised their efforts by including, for some cancers, the sophisticated staging practice used in highly specialized cancer units which are not available to the general surgeon or oncologist who still treats most cases of cancer.

Tumour markers

A tumour marker can be defined as a quantitative change, or other form of deviation from normal, of a molecule, substance or process which is associated with a tumour that can be detected by some type of assay in tissue or body fluid. Markers have potential value for screening and diagnosis, assessing the likely natural history of the disease and its outcome, predicting the most appropriate form of treatment and for monitoring its success.

Histological examination of a tumour is the model. Not only does the histological appearance of a tumour provide a definitive diagnosis, but knowledge of its type and grade, indicating its degree of differentiation, reflects its natural progress and likely prognosis. Histological examination of surrounding tissues for lymphovascular or perineural invasion and regional lymph nodes for metastases offers the most reliable method of determining the likelihood of micrometastatic disease. The completeness of primary excision can be determined, or should the neoplasm remain *in situ*, as in leukaemia, lymphoma and some solid tumours, its response to systemic treatment can be monitored. The application of immunohistochemistry, *in situ* hybridization

and other molecular methods of investigation of the tumour can predict the likely outcome of treatment.

Circulating markers

The surgeon is primarily concerned with the use of tumour markers as diagnostic and monitoring tools. It was a forlorn hope that specific markers for individual tumours, when liberated into body fluids, would allow sensitive diagnostic assays. Even if such 'tumour-specific antigens' were secreted into the circulation, their minute concentration would defy the most sensitive of methods. However, there are a small number of tumour products present in serum or urine in sufficient quantity to be of value for diagnosis and for monitoring the effect of treatment when their steadily rising concentration on sequential assays may give the lead-time for clinical relapse.

Some of these products are appropriate to the tissue of origin of the tumour (e.g. endocrine tissue). Cortisol, aldosterone and catecholamines may be secreted in excess by adrenal tumours, calcitonin by medullary carcinoma of the thyroid, insulin by pancreatic islet adenomas and human chorionic gonadotrophin (HCG) by chorioncarcinoma. Peptide hormones may also be secreted inappropriately by tumour tissue; for example corticotrophin or antidiuretic hormone by bronchial carcinomas and HCG by testicular teratomas.

Human chorionic gonadotrophin

HCG is produced by both the cytotrophoblast and syncytiotrophoblast and can be detected in the maternal urine about 5 days after conception, providing a useful diagnostic test for pregnancy. It is a glycoprotein composed of α and β subunits. The subunit is common to other peptide hormones, whereas the β subunit is specific to HCG. While a range of tumours can produce HCG, its main clinical use has been in monitoring malignant trophoblastic tumours. This has proved to be particularly useful for gestational tumours and the selection of patients with hydatidiform mole for aggressive treatment by chemotherapy.

α-fetoprotein

alpha;-fetoprotein (α-FP) is an α_1 globulin produced during a normal pregnancy in the foetal yolk sac and liver and can be detected in maternal serum from approximately 6 weeks after conception. Its production is increased in neural tube defects and its concentration in maternal serum and/or amniotic fluid is used as a prenatal diagnostic test. α-FP is also secreted by a variety of adult tumours but is of clinical value only in hepatocellular carcinoma and to a lesser extent in malignant testicular or ovarian teratomas. It is not used for screening.

Carcinoembryonic antigen

Carcinoembryonic antigen (CEA) is a glycoprotein present in foetal gut, pancreas and liver and expressed by a variety of human tumours (e.g. colon, stomach, pancreas, lung, breast and liver). In non-malignant adult tissues it is found only in very low concentrations. Its clinical use has generally been restricted to the monitoring of treatment of carcinoma of the colon and rectum, either to determine the completeness of surgical removal or to predict impending clinical relapse during follow-up. It is also insufficiently sensitive for use as a screening test. Other CEA-related cell adhesion molecules (CEACAM) family members play diverse roles in oncogenesis and have shown early promise as potential tumour markers and targets for therapeutic intervention.

Carbohydrate antigens
Carbohydrate antigens such as CA19.9 and CA125 have clinical application as markers in pancreatic and ovarian cancer, respectively.

Prostate-specific antigen
The only circulating tumour marker to be used for screening is prostate-specific antigen (PSA). PSA is a glycoprotein and serum protease, which is apparently produced exclusively by the epithelial cells lining the acini and ducts of the prostatic gland. Its assay in serum has been widely used in the US for the early detection of prostatic cancer, which undoubtedly has led to the detection of an increased proportion of clinically and pathologically localized cancers of the prostate. However, as its specificity is low, this is at the expense of false-positive results. PSA may be elevated in benign prostatic hypertrophy, prostatitis and following prostatic manipulation. As early-stage prostatic cancer may progress slowly, there is a risk of overtreatment by radical prostatectomy and radical radiotherapy which can have serious side-effects. Although current PSA estimations do not have the required sensitivity and specificity to be used for population screening, the large health problem posed by prostatic cancer has stimulated the initiation of a number of trials.

Circulating tumour cells and DNA may also have application as tumour markers. Polymerase chain reaction (PCR) techniques are particularly useful for detecting single tumour cells or tiny amounts (of the order of pg) of abnormal genetic material against a background of normal cells or DNA.

Tissue and cellular markers
As indicated above, histopathology provides surgeons with a readily available and interpretable model for tumour markers. This cannot be said of the profusion of other markers which have been identified by the assay of amplifications, deletions and mutations of DNA, overexpression and mutations of RNA and overexpression, abnormal structure and abnormal cellular location of expressed proteins. These are divided into two main groups – prognostic and predictive.

Prognostic markers
Prognostic markers predict the future behaviour of the disease independent of the effect of treatment. They can be grouped as:

- *Markers of proliferation*, such as the thymidine labelling index and Ki-67 immunoreactivity. Alternatively, flow cytometry can be used to determine the proliferation rate from the proportion of cells which are in the DNA synthetic phase (S-phase) of the cell cycle. Many tumours have an abnormal DNA content with disturbance of the normal diploid content of chromosomes (aneuploidy). This is primarily a marker of genetic instability, which is associated with disease of poor prognosis.
- *Markers of receptor and growth factor activity*. An example is the observation that human breast cancers which contain oestrogen-receptor protein have a more favourable prognosis than those that are oestrogen-receptor negative. Other receptors and growth factors with prognostic significance include EGF and its receptor (EGFR), the c-erb B2 and H-ras oncogene products, insulin-like growth factor and the vitamin D receptor. Basic FGF, by promoting angiogenesis, is also related to tumour progression.
- *Markers of invasiveness*, such as pro-cathepsin D, heat shock proteins and laminin receptors.
- *Markers of suppressor functions*, for example the products of p53 which regulate cell cycle arrest, and of nm23, the antimetastatic gene.

A number of miscellaneous markers of uncertain significance have also been identified. Application of genomic- and proteomic-screening techniques may facilitate panoramic analysis of tumour gene expression. More meaningful prognostic information may be provided by simultaneously profiling a large number of markers in a high-throughput manner.

Predictive markers
Predictive markers are those that determine the outcome of treatment. They have usually been defined in terms of survival, but increasingly their relationship to the quality of life following treatment and even to the costs of healthcare is being considered. The prototype for a predictive marker is the oestrogen receptor assay, which like several other markers of hormonal sensitivity of a breast tumour (EGFR, c-erb B2, pS2 expression), is also an index of prognosis. Equally reliable markers of sensitivity to chemotherapy are not yet available, although there would appear to be some relationship between cell proliferation markers and response. There is hope that the product of the mdr-1 gene, P-glycoprotein, may provide a marker for pleomorphic drug resistance, but this will be relevant only to treatment by anthracyclines and vinca alkaloids.

Reliability
If tumour markers are to be clinically useful, they must be detectable by a reliable assay which is widely available and easily interpreted by the clinician. This requires the performance of pilot and confirmatory studies which take many years and cannot keep pace with the number of new

markers being identified. In an endeavour to clarify what has become a chaotic situation and establish a consistent and objective process to evaluate new markers, a group of investigators from 10 cancer centres in the US have designed a Tumour Marker Utility Grading Worksheet (TMUGS) to allow the precise characteristics of a marker to be defined in a standard way. Factors include a marker's precise designation, the manner in which it is altered from normal, the method of assay and reagents used, the type of specimen required and the neoplasm for which it is being evaluated. A series of utility scales has been developed by which each variable can be described. To determine the potential clinical usefulness of each marker, its association with risk assessment, screening, differential diagnosis, prognosis and monitoring of the clinical course following treatment is also included. The 'bottom line' is that the availability of marker data to the clinician should contribute to his decision-making and result in a better outcome for the patient.

PRINCIPLES OF CANCER TREATMENT

Curability

The logical objective of the treatment of cancer is destruction of all cancer cells. The disease is then eradicated and the patient 'clinically cured'. This definition of clinical cure is impractical as it can only be proven by a complete search for asymptomatic deposits of tumour on death. However, clinical cure should follow the complete removal of all non-invasive cancers, and also a number of small invasive cancers, particularly in superficial sites, which have not metastasized.

Life is personal and freedom from recurrence of the cancer during the remainder of a patient's lifetime constitutes 'personal cure'. This does not rule out the possibility that the disease is present in asymptomatic form and is clearly dependent upon the duration of life following its diagnosis. By this definition, the patient who is killed in a road accident on the way home from hospital following the palliative resection of an incurable gastric cancer is 'cured'!

A third definition of cure is 'statistical cure'. Those achieving such cure form a group of disease-free survivors whose annual death rate from all causes is the same as that of a group of the normal population of similar sex and age distribution. The time at which they can be expected to be statistically cured depends on the natural history of the disease. For aggressive cancers such as those of lung, few patients will survive for >5 years, whereas for those which are chronic, excess mortality from metastatic disease may persist for >30 years (Fig. 9.15). Only if the disease is aggressive and rapidly progressing can 5-year survival rates be regarded as a valid index of cure.

Whichever definition of cure is used, the objective of treatment is to cure the disease. Traditionally the only hope of curing a cancer is to 'cut it out'. With the discovery of anaesthetics, antiseptic and later aseptic surgery, operations became more extensive, partly on account of the advanced

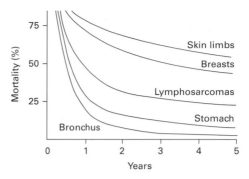

Figure 9.15. Mortality curves for some common cancers.

stage at which many tumours presented to surgeons, but also because it was believed that there were two distinct stages in the natural history of a cancer: a 'primary stage' when the cancer is confined to its organ or other site of origin and their regional lymphatics, and a 'secondary stage' when it is disseminated to distant sites. Only when the natural defences of the lymph nodes draining the primary site is overridden was such secondary spread believed to occur. Haematogenous spread was regarded as a late phenomenon. This concept has been replaced by evidence that invasive cancer disseminates early in its course by both lymphatic and blood systems to form micrometastases in regional lymph nodes and in systemic organs and tissues. Although it may be many years before these micrometastases become clinically evident, the effective treatment of invasive cancer now includes not only the control of local disease by surgery and/or radiotherapy but also of systemic disease by chemotherapy and, in a few hormone-dependent cancers, antiendocrine measures. The objective of systemic treatment is eradication of micrometastases.

Local treatment

Surgery

Primary tumour

The main methods of local treatment of the primary tumour are surgery and radiotherapy. As these can cure only disease localized to its primary site, the objectives of local treatment in most invasive cancers is to provide local control of the disease and to prevent its local recurrence. The removal or irradiation of normal tissues beyond that necessary to establish local control, as was widely practised during the era of radical surgery, only increases morbidity.

The extent of removal of normal tissues was planned on anatomical principles and on the belief that wide removal of surrounding normal tissue was necessary to prevent local recurrence. It is now generally recognized that the extent of surgical excision of a primary tumour depends upon:
- *Natural history of the tumour*, including the likelihood of multifocal deposits and the liability to local recurrence.

It has been generally believed that the more aggressive the tumour the greater is the need for wide excision or adjuvant radiotherapy, but some benign tumours (e.g. pleomorphic adenomas of the parotid and phylloides tumours of the breast) are equally prone to recurrence.

- *Anatomy of the involved part*, recognizing that in some sites, because of nearby vital structures, excision must be less than ideal.
- *Morbidity of the operative procedure* and its effect on the quality of life.

Guidelines on the extent of removal can come only from well-conducted clinical studies, including randomized trials. However, local treatment must be adequate; local recurrence of tumour is devastating and tumour must be removed completely with a margin of microscopically normal tissue. The completeness of removal must be determined with the histopathologist post-operatively.

Regional lymph nodes

The belief that cancer cells spread primarily along lymphatic channels and are trapped for variable periods of time in regional lymph nodes led to their resection or irradiation as an accepted part of local treatment despite lack of evidence of involvement. Radical and mutilating operations to remove all regional lymphatic pathways were commonly performed as a routine, such as amputations for skin melanoma, radical and superradical mastectomy for breast cancer and neck dissections for cancer of the tongue. Realization that the presence of cancer cells in lymph nodes is a marker for micrometastatic disease in other sites, and that removal of normal lymph nodes serves no purpose, led to a more conservative approach. Except in those sites in which removal of normal nodes causes no morbidity (e.g. within the abdomen and to a lesser extent in the axilla), regional lymph nodes are now generally resected or irradiated only when there is proof of involvement.

Radiotherapy

During the period of radical surgery, radical radiotherapy frequently followed surgery to 'sterilize' the tissues of regional cancer cells. Post-operative radiotherapy is also now used more discriminately and only when there is a high likelihood of residual disease or when the potential problems associated with recurrence exceed the morbidity caused by irradiating normal tissues. The radiosensitivity of a tumour is also relevant. Some primary tumours are better managed by radiotherapy than by surgery.

Radiotherapy acts differently from surgery. Radiation tends to fail at the centre of a tumour where the cells are hypoxic. Surgery is more likely to fail at its perimeter, due to the need to preserve anatomical boundaries.

Ionizing radiations are composed of packets of energy (photons) which cause ejection of an orbital electron. In clinical practice they are generated as X-rays (roentgen rays) by machine or as γ-rays from a decaying radioactive source. The amount of energy absorbed by tissue is known as the 'absorbed dose' which is measured in γ-rays, each Gy equalling 100 rads. The intensity of radiation varies inversely to the square of the distance from the source (inverse square law).

Beams of ionizing radiation are described as superficial if their energy lies between 10 and 125 kV, orthovoltage if between 125 and 400 kV and megavoltage if over 400 kV. As the energy increases so does the penetrating power. For orthovoltage therapy, the skin is the limiting factor; while megavoltage radiations are skin sparing, the maximum dose being delivered to tissues below the surface.

Radiotherapy can be delivered by applying the source within or near to the tumour (brachytherapy) or from a distance (teletherapy). Radium needles were first used for interstitial and intracavitary radiotherapy, but have been superceded by iridium-192, caesium-137 and cobalt-60 which emit γ-rays and yttrium-90 which emits β-rays. These sources are normally 'after-loaded' into plastic tubes or receptacles which are implanted at the time of surgery. Electrons, which like β-radiations have rapid fall-off, are also used for local therapy.

For teletherapy of other than superficial sites, beams of 4–8 MeV from cobalt-60 sources are normally used. Higher-energy beams can be generated from a linear accelerator.

In planning treatment, the radiotherapist must ensure accurate localization of the beam to the tumour site, modifying its intensity and shape by the use of filters, and develop a treatment plan to give the best distribution and homogeneity of the radiation. This is tested on a simulator which utilizes superficial radiation to reproduce the effect of treatment on radiographs or through an image intensifier. The fields are marked in indelible ink on the patient and the treatment usually given in a series of fractions spread over several weeks.

The important target molecule for radiation is DNA, but reaction between electrons and water produces free radicals which also may cause cell damage. As the effect of radiation varies during the cell cycle, not all cells are killed; others evoke repair mechanisms. There is also recruitment of new cells. Fractionation of the total dose of radiation achieves higher cell kill while sparing normal tissues from excessive radiation.

The effect of radiation on normal tissues is variable. Tissues which do not require renewal, such as muscle, nerve, bone and liver, are relatively resistant compared to the skin, gastrointestinal tract, reproductive organs and exocrine glands which are constantly repopulated and most sensitive to damage. Tissues such as the lung fall in between. Adverse effects include inhibition of the immune response, mutagenesis and, through damage to cell membranes, oedema.

Tumours contain areas of anoxic cells which require greater doses of radiation for 'kill' than do well-oxygenated cells. In the belief that these anoxic cells are likely to cause relapse, treatment during exposure to hyperbaric oxygenation at 3–4 atm was introduced, but was found to have a beneficial effect only when the radiation was given as a small number of fractions. Other radiosensitizers such as halo-genated pyrimidines and nitroimidazoles are also used.

The ataxia-telangectasia (AT) gene is autosomal recessive and one defective gene is carried by 1.4% of the population. In those who are homozygous for the gene there is a high incidence of new cancers in childhood and adolescence and an exquisite sensitivity to radiation which causes lethal necrosis of normal tissues.

Photodynamic therapy

Photodynamic therapy (PDT) utilizes a combination of light and photosensitizing drugs to treat accessible deposits of cancer. First used in Germany in 1903 with a combination of eosin and light to treat skin cancer, in its modern form it uses low-energy lasers and a synthetic photosensitizer, derived from the blood of cows and pigs (Photfrui). The drug is injected intravenously when it is concentrated in all cells. However, unlike normal cells which only retain the drug for several hours, tumour cells retain it for several days. If they are exposed to low energy they are destroyed. Initially used to treat metastatic tumour deposits on the skin, extending the laser source using fibreoptic cables allows light to be applied to oesophageal, bronchial and gastrointestinal cancers. The mechanism of action is not fully understood, but apparently a toxic form of oxygen is released and this damages cell membranes and other cellular components, particularly in the blood vessels feeding tumour cells.

To date the main use of PDT has been as palliation for advanced or metastatic cancers and as an adjuvant to surgery for mesothelioma and brain tumours. Recently, it has been used as primary treatment for lung cancers, to eradicate multiple skin cancers in the basal cell naevus syndrome, and to treat premalignant lesions such as Barrett's oesophagus.

The main advantage of PDT over other forms of treatment is its relative mildness. Its only side-effect is to render the skin hypersensitive to the sun. A new generation of photosensitizers is being developed which are cleared from normal cells within minutes and this prevents this side-effect and offers the possibility of repeated treatments. A disadvantage of current photosensitizers is that they absorb light best in the red area close to that of haemoglobin and melanin, which limits the penetration of light. New agents with different spectra for light absorption allow greater depths of light penetration.

Systemic Treatment

Adequate local treatment of the primary tumour and its lymph nodes is an essential part of the total treatment of cancer. Exceptions are those in which systemic therapy leads to complete remission of the local disease, as with lymphomas. However, once a cancer has disseminated, effective systemic therapy is essential. This is generally given as an 'adjuvant' to local treatment. 'Neoadjuvant therapy' is the administration of systemic therapy before local treatment, reducing the bulk of the primary tumour before surgery or radiotherapy. In sites where the size of a tumour may be measured, response to systemic treatment may be assessed and if ineffective changed.

Chemotherapy

Although in Western countries the administration of chemotherapy lies within the province of the non-surgical oncologist, all surgeons must be aware of its advantages and shortcomings. Initially used for the palliation of advanced cancers, the first critical evaluation of the role of chemotherapy in early cancer arose from the observation that the course of acute lymphoblastic leukaemia in children, a uniformly fatal disease, could be dramatically altered by the administration of the folic acid antagonist aminopterin. Although early hopes of 'cure' were not realized, the development of new agents that could be given in combination, recognition of the principles of their action and the ability to objectively monitor response by the marrow aspiration, led to successful and often curative treatment. Although this success has been extended only to a small number of solid tumours – lymphomas, testicular and ovarian cancers, the principles are equally applicable to other forms of cancer and should be understood.

Effective drugs

Administered drugs must be effective against the tumour. During early experience in the management of leukaemias it became apparent that achieving a complete remission of disease is an essential factor in prolonging survival and that the duration of remission is a critical determinant of survival time. Prolongation of the state of complete remission became a prime objective of treatment and led to the use of combinations of drugs to which cross-resistance does not develop. A wide range of cell-cycle specific and non-specific drugs are now available.

Pharmacological Sanctuaries

During the management of acute leukaemias it was recognized that there are pharmacological 'sanctuaries' in which leukaemic cells continue to proliferate despite remission of disease in other sites, for example within the CSF compartments where, as the drugs fail to cross the blood–brain barrier, sheets of leukaemic cells continue to grow on the meninges and invade the CSF. Intrathecal methotrexate with low-dose radiation is effective treatment but causes brain atrophy. Intensifying the dose of systemically administered methotrexate with folic acid rescue is preferred treatment and also combats disease in the testicular sanctuary. Vinca alkaloids must never be administered intrathecally as they induce fatal neurotoxicity.

Dosage

Experimental studies in mouse leukaemia indicated that chemotherapy acted in a logarithmic fashion on cancer cells according to 'first-order kinetics'. A given dose of drug kills the same fraction, not the same number, of cells. The fractional reduction of tumour cells following chemotherapy is constant, irrespective of the size of the tumour burden. The amount of treatment required to effect a 99% reduction of a tumour of 1 mg (from 10^6 to 10^4 cells) is the same as that for one of 1 kg (from 10^{12} to 10^{10} cells). This finding suggests that the induction of an apparent complete remission is only the first step in treatment. To eradicate all leukaemia cells and maintain remission, more intensive, prolonged and potentially lethal therapy is required. This in turn requires measures to counteract its effects.

Marrow transplantation

The potentially lethal problems associated with intensive chemotherapy are infection and haemorrhage due to destruction of marrow cells. Initially these were countered by intensive antibiotic treatment, laminar-flow isolation and granulocyte and platelet transfusions, but with the development of marrow transplantation a more lasting solution evolved. Supralethal cytoreductive therapy followed by salvage allogeneic marrow transplantation, when practised during the initial remission of acute leukaemia, results in a high proportion of disease- and treatment-free survivors.

During developmental studies in experimental animals it was noted that stem cells from the buffy coat of the peripheral blood, when injected into recipients, can repopulate marrow spaces. Following the discovery of the colony-stimulating factors, CSF and GCSF, which control the proliferation of granulocytes, monocytes, macrophages and related haemopoietic cells in human marrow, it became practical to 'shift' stem cells from the marrow into the peripheral blood, from where they could be harvested and stored for re-infusion at a later date. Peripheral stem-cell rescue has now largely replaced marrow transplantation in the initial management of leukaemias and lymphomas and increasingly in other cancers in which high-intensity dose regimens of chemotherapy are being used. However, as chronic graft-versus-host reaction may attack the host's leukaemic as well as normal cells of skin, liver and/or intestinal tract, allogeneic marrow transplantation still has a place in the long-term management of this disease.

Resistance

Combinations of chemotherapeutic drugs are more effective than single agents and their scheduling is of primary importance to the duration of their effect. Resistance to cytotoxic chemotherapy is well established in the laboratory and it is believed that similar mechanisms may operate in some human tumours.

In the clinical situation resistance may be temporary due to physiological barriers such as the blood–brain and blood–testicular barriers already referred to. Temporary resistance may also follow sojourning of the cells in the G0 (resting) phase of the cell cycle when they are no longer sensitive to cell-cycle specific drugs. Permanent resistance implies

alteration of the phenotype of the cancer cell. Drug-resistant phenotypes may be inherent in the initial cell population so that only sensitive cells are eliminated but these more commonly develop due to mutations in the genetically unstable cells. As the mutated pool of cells increases so does the resistance of the tumour. Such mutations may be spontaneous or, as in laboratory situations, result from continuous exposure to the relevant drug.

Although developed *in vitro* by exposure to a single agent such as doxorubicin, resistance to anthracyclones is characteristically shared with other seemingly unrelated agents (e.g. vinca alkaloids and colchicine). This 'pleomorphic' drug resistance is due to overexpression of a 170 kDa protein, P-glycoprotein, which forms a molecular marker for resistant cells. The gene encoding this protein, *mdr-1*, has been sequenced. It belongs to a superfamily of genes which are highly conserved in plants, bacteria, insects and mammals, and express ATP-dependent transport proteins.

P-glycoprotein spans the cell membrane. An internal ATP-binding domain couples the energy to pump a number of diverse hydrophobic compounds through transmembrane ion channels to the exterior of the cell. It is normally expressed in the adrenal, gravid uterus, colon and capillary endothelium of the brain where, as in the testicle, it may be concerned with blood–brain barrier function. Overexpression in tumour cells may be due to amplification of the *mdr* gene or to abnormal transcriptional or translational events.

The *mdr* gene is not responsible for resistance to alkylating agents or to methotrexate. Intracellular glutathione (a ubiquitous tripeptide of glycine, glutamic acid and cystine) has detoxicating actions through the formation of glutathione conjugates with organic ions which are transported from the cell by a specific membrane pump. Intracellular glutathione is a major factor in resistance to those anticancer drugs that produce electrophilic reactive compounds such as alkylating agents and *cis*-platinum. Glutathione-*S*-transferase, which is responsible for their conjugation, is overexpressed in some drug-resistant cell lines. Methotrexate and other antimetabolites (fluoropyrimidines, thiopurine and cytosine arabinoside) inhibit nucleic acid synthesis and are dependent for their action on inhibition of dihydro-folate-reductase. Resistance may be due to altered affinity for the enzyme or to its overexpression.

The calcium channel blocker verapamil and cyclosporin A are known to reverse the action of P-glycoprotein and ethacrynic acid to inhibit that of glutathione-*S*-transferase. Their potential role to reverse drug resistance is under study. Other enzymes such as ribonucleotide reductase also appear to play important roles in determining chemoresistance to agents such as gemcitabine and represent potential targets for therapy.

A new paradigm and novel therapies

The current model for treating cancer is based on the belief that cure can be achieved only by the eradication of each and every cancer cell. This model, which is derived from the need to destroy invading microorganisms, may not necessarily apply to cancer cells which are derived from their host. It has been suggested that the malignant cell should be regarded as part of a biological communications network where processes of cell growth, division and migration take place in an environment of impaired regulation. While conventional antineoplastic approaches, such as surgery, radiation therapy and cytotoxic chemotherapy, still play a part in treatment, the essential need is to reassert normal controlling mechanisms so that re-regulation of critical processes in the growth, invasion and metastatic process can occur. This will entail reversal of inducing and promoting events, blocking the action of defective or false transmitters, overriding inefficient enzymes or receptors and inducing alternative metabolic pathways.

Over 100 separate protocols for 'gene therapy' are now under investigation worldwide. These do not necessarily indicate a direct attack on a defective gene; rather current use investigations of 'gene therapy' rather have focussed on the use of DNA constructs to augment existing therapies. Examples of such strategies include the following:

- The infusion of genetically modified immuno-competent cells which overexpress cytokines (e.g. interleukin-2, IL-2) and mount an exaggerated immune response against the tumour. Initially it was believed that those lymphocytes found within the tumour (tumour-infiltrating lymphocytes, TIL cells) would prove ideal for this purpose, as they could be readily extracted from the tumour, their population expanded in laboratory culture, transfected with an IL-2 gene and re-infused. However, subsequent studies in which a 'marker' gene was inserted into TIL-cells indicated that they were not selectively taken up or retained by the tumour. Alternative strategies include the use of autologous tumour cells transduced with a cytokine gene as a vaccine; or tumour cells which have been genetically modified (e.g. by transfection with HLA genes) to increase their immunogenicity.

- The enhancement of protection against the toxic effects of chemotherapeutic agents by the insertion, into normal cells, of a drug-resistance gene. This applies particularly to bone-marrow stem cells into which the *mdr*-1 gene can be inserted. Through stimulation of the P-glycoprotein efflux pump, daughter cells expressing this gene are protected against the cytotoxic effects of the drug which can then be given in higher dose.

- The development of strategies to enable tumour cells to selectively activate a 'pro-drug', normally inert, into a highly toxic metabolite. An example is the insertion of the thymidine kinase gene, the product of which can convert ganciclovir into its cytotoxic triphosphates. This gene can be inserted into neurological tumours using a herpes simplex virus vector.

- The synthesis of 'antisense' DNA oligonucleotides which have complimentary coding to mRNA but which, being inert, block the normal process of translation (Fig. 9.16).

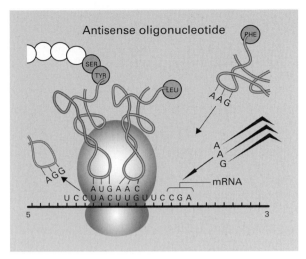

Figure 9.16. Mechanism of action of antisense oligonucleotides.

- siRNA which potently inhibits gene expression at a post-transcriptional level which an apparently high degree of potency and specificity.

- The development of inhibitors of enzymes such as topoisomerase and telomerase which are concerned with repair and integrity of the genome. Drugs which override the check-points in the cell cycle apparently sensitize the cells to DNA damaging agents.

It is obvious that the ideal form of gene therapy is that which allows replacement or correction of a defective oncogene or tumour-suppressor gene which is causally associated with the cancer in question. But difficulties arise in the delivery of the replacement gene, which must be transduced into the tumour cells by a suitable vector. To date most attention has focussed on the use of virus vector, particularly retrovirus, but alternative non-viral vectors are also being studied. These include liposomes, synthetic molecular complexes as well as 'naked' and modified oligonucleotides. It is hoped that by the attachment to these vectors of ligands, which bind to tumour cell antigens, selectivity can be achieved.

Other forms of non-genetic biological therapy are under study. These include the use of monoclonal antibodies (Fig. 9.17) specific for tumour antigens, which carry a radioactive isotope (e.g. yttrium-90) or a cell toxin (e.g. saporin) which can penetrate the cell membrane. Inhibitors of those 'downstream events' that affect the metabolism, proliferation of the cancer cell and its invasive properties are also being developed. Examples are antagonists to growth factors, collagenase activity and angiogenesis. The promotion of apoptosis is another area of interest.

The development of new cytotoxic drugs is an ongoing process leading to new effective agents such as taxol, suramin and imatinib.

Whatever the outcome of research into these approaches, the 'take-home' message is that, unlike infecting parasites

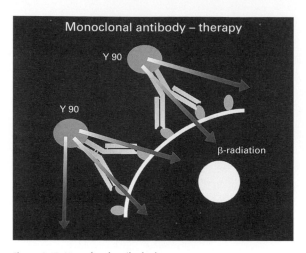

Figure 9.17. Monoclonal antibody therapy.

and microorganisms, cancer cells are not new invaders but aberrations of the proliferation, growth and migration of normal host cells.

RELIEF OF CANCER PAIN

Palliative care

Palliative care, is commonly regarded as synonymous with terminal care; that is, the management of patients with advanced disease for whom curative treatment is not appropriate and who are approaching death. It has been converted from a passive form of care practised as an alternative to radical or curative care to one that includes active measures to counteract symptoms and provide support. At times, this may include aggressive treatment, for example by chemotherapy or surgery. Palliative care is now 'holistic' and all embracing and therefore requires a multidisciplinary approach.

Four broad domains of palliative care are described – physical, psychological, social (cultural) and spiritual. Of these physical needs are most likely to concern the surgeon, whose services may be required to relieve a mechanical dysfunction. He must also understand the principles of modern pain control.

Principles of cancer pain control

Pain at diagnosis is experienced by 20–50% of cancer patients. By the time the disease is advanced, this proportion has risen to 75%. Considering that worldwide some 7 million new cases are diagnosed every year and that 8% of all deaths are due to cancer (25% in developed countries), some 4 million persons require treatment of cancer pain at any one time.

Pain may be acute or chronic. *Acute* pain is severe, may be catastrophic and accompanied by autonomic and psychological responses, drawing attention to an acute pathological process which needs to be remedied. *Chronic* pain is continuous, recurring at intervals of months or years, and is associated with vegetative disturbances such as lack of sleep, anorexia, decreased libido and personality change. Unlike acute pain it does not serve any useful purpose.

Pain associated with cancer may be caused by the cancer itself, when it may be somatic or visceral in origin, or due to associated factors such as muscle spasm, bedsores, constipation or complications of treatment. It may also arise from an unrelated disorder. Cancer pain can be differentiated from other forms of pain by its chronicity and by overwhelming associated features of insomnia, reduced appetite, irritability, depression, rage and spiritual or social disturbance. It is described as 'total pain' (Fig. 9.18). A number of typical cancer pain syndromes have been described for particular sites of primary or metastatic disease, which must be recognized.

The mainstay of the successful treatment of cancer pain is the use of non-opioid, opioid and a number of adjuvant drugs. The WHO 'ladder' ascends from the prescription of non-opioid drugs, through 'weak opioids' to 'strong opioids' as control is lost (Fig. 9.19). Opioid is a generic term which refers to codeine, morphine and other natural and synthetic drugs which act on specific receptors in the central and peripheral nervous systems. With correct administration of appropriate drugs, pain can be controlled in 90% of cases. In the remainder, it will be reduced to acceptable proportions. Inappropriate use of opioids is due to lack of availability or incorrect prescribing by physician or surgeon who may equate need with the prescription of opioids for benign conditions. Unwarranted fear of addiction and lack of knowledge of alternative remedies also contribute to this.

Patient factors may constrain appropriate pain control. Believing that cancer pain is inevitable and untreatable, a patient may put on a brave face to their doctor who then falsely believes that their pain is well controlled. Non-compliance with prescribed medication may be a problem, either because of adverse effects or a desire to keep 'strong drugs' for a time when things get worse. The key to successful control is that the dose and duration of opioid treatment is determined solely by the needs of the patient. Peripheral nerve blocks, cordotomy and intrathecal blocks are now required only for drug resistant or certain specific forms of pain.

Evaluation of the patient

As with all forms of patient management, diagnosis and evaluation of symptoms must precede treatment. This requires knowledge of the pathological processes that give rise to pain, sites of referral and the anatomy of the central and peripheral nervous systems. When evaluation is complete, the physician or surgeon should have ascertained

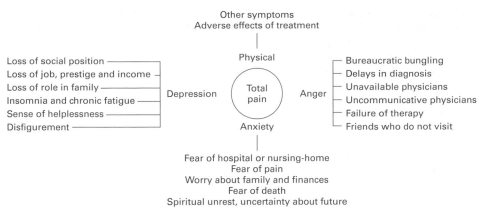

Figure 9.18. Total pain as described by Twycross (1994).

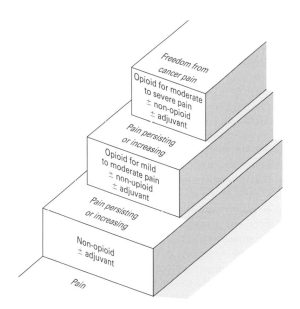

Figure 9.19. WHO 'ladder' for treatment of pain.

whether the pain is caused by the cancer or another (possibly remedial) disorder, whether it constitutes a specific cancer pain syndrome and whether it is of somatic or visceral type. He also should recognize neuropathic pain due to irritation or compression of central or peripheral nerves.

A specific plan should be identified for each patient, which must be fully discussed with him and his family. The aim of treatment and the risk of adverse effects should be explained. Optimum requirements for non-opioids and opioids, laxatives and psychotropic drugs are planned. As these will require adjustment, continuing assessment is necessary. A particular pathological process (e.g. bone metastases) may respond to direct treatment by radiotherapy or bisphosphonates. Mobility

must be preserved. Muscular spasm and other pains associated with immobility can be as severe as cancer pain.

The analgesic ladder

The World Health Organization ladder for the relief of cancer pain consists of three steps at each of which the right drug is given in the right dose and at the right time intervals for a particular patient. For other than transient pain, analgesics should not be used 'as needed' but prescribed at time intervals appropriate to their duration of action. To allow pain to re-emerge before the next dose causes unnecessary pain and encourages tolerance. At each step a number of adjuvant drugs are included to relieve the adverse effects of pain control.

Step 1: Non-opioids

The basic drugs used in this step are the non-steroidal anti-inflammatory drugs (NSAIDs, of which aspirin is the parent drug) and paracetamol. The analgesic effects of NSAIDs are believed to be due to their ability to inhibit cyclo-oxygenase with reduction in tissue prostaglandins, which sensitize pain receptors to noxious stimuli. NSAIDs also have a central analgesic action through release of endorphins. A variety of preparations of aspirin and of non-acetylated salicylates are available. A single dose is usually effective for about 6 h. A wide range of NSAIDs other than aspirin and salicylates are available which can be given in modified-release tablets. They are all rapidly absorbed by mouth and topical preparations for transdermal administration are available.

Symptoms of hypersensitivity can occur within minutes. Gastroduodenal erosions with haemorrhage follow the ingestion of aspirin in unbuffered form and buffered or enteric coated aspirin are preferred for long-term administration. Aspirin and other NSAIDs alter the composition of gastric mucus and ingestion, in any form, may be associated with chronic duodenal ulceration. This may be prevented by the administration of the H_2 receptor antagonists cimetidine or ranitidine or the prostaglandin-E1 analogue misoprostol. Inhibitors of type 2 cyclo-oxygenase offer the theoretical benefit of inducing fewer gastrointestinal side-effects.

Paracetamol, a synthetic, is now the most widely used analgesic. In therapeutic doses, paracetamol is the safest analgesic available and a single dose is effective for 4–6 h. As with aspirin, allergic reactions may occur and occasional cases of cholestatic jaundice have been reported. An overdose (15 g) can cause fatal hepatocellular necrosis but intravenous acetylcysteine and methionine (both precursors of glutathione) are effective antidotes if given within 10–12 h.

Step 2: Weak opioids

The weak opioids most commonly used are codeine, dihydrocodeine and dextropropoxyphene. Pentazocine, although an effective analgesic, may have psychotic effects and is better avoided in the cancer patient. Due to the constipating effects of codeine and dihydrocodeine, dextropropoxyphene hydrochloride (combined with paracetamol as co-proxamol) is initially preferred. As a weak opiod should be added rather than substituted for a step 1 non-opioid, compound preparations are available (Table 9.4). 'Kangarooing' between one weak opioid and another is not advised.

Step 3: Strong opioids

Morphine is the main active constituent of opium and the strong opioid of choice for control of cancer pain. Its analgesic effect is mediated by the mu 1 opioid receptor in the cerebral cortex. Binding to the mu 2 receptor is responsible for its adverse effects (respiratory depression, gastrointestinal and urinary stasis).

Morphine is readily absorbed by all routes of administration, but its potency varies according to route (oral: subcutaneous 1:2; oral: intravenous 1:3) as does plasma half-life (oral dose 2–2.5 h compared to 1.5 h following parenteral administration).

The availability of controlled-release tablets of morphine sulphate allows pain to be controlled by twice-daily administration which is particularly convenient for home use. A range of different strengths of tablet (from 10 to 200 mg) are

Table 9.4. **Compound preparations.**

Preparation	Weak opioid	Non-opioid
Co-codaprin	Codeine 8 mg	Aspirin 400 ng
Co-codamol	Codeine 8 mg	Paracetamol 500 mg
Solpadol-Tylex	Codeine 30 mg	Paracetamol 500 mg
Co-drymol	Dihydrocodeine 10 mg	Paracetamol 500 mg
Remedeine	Dihydrocodeine 20 mg	Paracetamol 500 mg
Remedeine forte	Dihydrocodeine 30 mg	Paracetamol 500 mg
Co-proxamol	Dextropropoxyphene 32.5 mg	Paracetamol 325 mg

available. It is recommended that for the initial titration of dose against pain, ordinary oral tablets or solutions should be given 4 hourly, and in a hospice setting this is the preferred long-term practice. As long as a patient is able to swallow by mouth and is not vomiting repeatedly, morphine should be given by mouth. If vomiting is a problem, the vaginal or rectal route can be used or morphine may be administered by subcutaneous infusion. A number of inexpensive portable infusors are available. If pain is resistant to oral morphine, changing to the subcutaneous or intravenous route of administration will not provide relief. However, epidural or spinal infusions may prove effective.

A range of alternative strong opioids to morphine (methadone (Physeptone), pethidine, levorphanol (Dromoran) papaveretum (Omnopon)) are available but have no advantage over morphine. Diamorphine (heroin) is a semisynthetic derivative of morphine which, as its solubility in fat is greater, crosses the blood–brain barrier more readily than morphine. When given parenterally it is 2.5 times more potent than morphine, but when given by mouth it is equipotent. As it is a pro-drug for release of morphine, and does not itself bind to opioid receptors, its only advantage over morphine is that its greater solubility in water allows smaller volumes to be used when parenteral medication is required. Such traditional remedies as the Brompton cocktail (morphine or diamorphine, cocaine and alcohol), Schlessinger's solution (morphine, ethylmorphine and hyoscine) and nepenthe (alcoholic tincture of opium) are no better than oral morphine sulphate in controlled-release form.

The commonest complications of morphine administration are nausea, vomiting, constipation, drowsiness and confusion. Difficulty with micturition, ureteric spasm and antidiuresis and a variety of autonomic effects may also occur. Large doses of morphine can cause respiratory depression and hypotension, leading to circulatory failure and deepening coma. Unless there is a definite reason for not doing so, a laxative should be prescribed for all patients receiving morphine. Best is a combination of a contact laxative (e.g. senna) and a faecal softener (e.g. docusate). Some patients may develop severe faecal retention and require suppositories, enemas or manual evacuation.

Vomiting must be controlled. Haloperidol or fluphenazine are preferable to prochlorperazine which is more likely to cause drowsiness. Vomiting secondary to delayed gastric emptying or to a 'functional' opioid-induced intestinal ileus usually responds to metoclopramide.

Drowsiness and a feeling of being 'drugged' can be troublesome. It should be confirmed that this is not due to causes other than morphine administration, for example renal failure, hypercalcaemia, cerebral metastases or the administration of psychotropic drugs. When caused by morphine, tolerance will usually develop, but if intractable psychostimulants, for example dexamphetamine can be used cautiously. Delirium and unsteadiness of gait may be problems in the elderly. Respiratory depression is not usual unless the patient has chronic obstructive airways disease. Intravenous naloxone blocks morphine receptor sites and can be used to counteract respiratory depression or morphine overdosage.

Opioid-resistant pain

A number of measures are available to treat opioid-resistant pain. Local anaesthetics administered either orally or by intravenous injection may have a general analgesic effect. The α-receptor antagonist clonidine administered transdermally, orally or by injection, either alone or combined with morphine may provide relief. Subcutaneous infusions of the dissociative anaesthetic ketamine may be used.

A variety of non-drug treatments are also available for the management of intractable pain. These may consist of simple counter-irritation with cold compresses, hot water bottles or ointments. Transcutaneous electrical nerve stimulation (TENS) is of benefit in a wide range of conditions causing localized pain, particularly of muscle origin. This is believed to be due to stimulation of large nerve fibres which release the inhibitory neurotransmitter γ-aminobutyric acid (GABA) in the dorsal horn. A similar effect may account for the success of acupuncture whether by deep needling alone or combined with electrostimulation. A number of psychological methods of pain relief (e.g. relaxation therapy) are also employed.

As a result of the use of oral morphine, spinal analgesia and improved psychosocial support, neurodestructive procedures are now rarely required for the management of pain due to advanced cancer. A local anaesthetic block may give temporary relief of localized pain arising from a myofascial 'trigger point', rib metastases, sacroiliac joint or other local site. More permanent destruction of nervous tissue can be achieved by phenol, alcohol, thermocoagulation or cryodestruction. Abdominal visceral pain can be relieved by coeliac plexus block or somatic pain by intrathecal lysis of nerve roots, but at the risk of producing bladder and anal dysfunction. Percutaneous and open cordotomy are now rarely used as their effect is transient. Pituitary ablation, apart from its effect in relieving pain through the induction of remission of hormone-dependent cancers, may relieve other forms of cancer pain but is now rarely used.

Other symptoms

In the palliation of advanced cancer a number of other symptoms which may have a crescendo effect on pain, such as dyspnoea, mouth infections, skin ulcers, constipation and vomiting, require relief.

Stomatitis and mucositis due to infection with *Candida albicans* is improved by an antifungal antibiotic such as ketoconazole or fluclonazole. Gastric distension can be relieved by metoclopramide and intestinal colic or an irritable bowel by anticholinergic antispasmodics such as dicyclomine. Corticosteroids may improve appetite and well-being.

About half of all patients with advanced cancer have psychological symptoms including anxiety, depression, personality disorders and confusion which can cause great distress to their family. Boredom, loneliness and feeling a burden all contribute to a general state of unhappiness. Psychotropic drugs are commonly prescribed, some of which may apparently have an additive analgesic effect. Neuroleptics (phenothiazines), anxiolytic sedatives (benzodiazepines), antidepressants (particularly amitriptyline) and psychostimulants (dexamphetamine) and are used as indicated. They should not be prescribed routinely other than for night sedation.

QUALITY OF LIFE AND AGE
Quality of life

During the past decade there has been increasing concern that the success of treatment of cancer cannot be measured only in terms of freedom from disease and survival. Of equal importance to the patient is the quality of well-being during remaining life. This is of particular importance to those with advanced cancer, in whom the unpleasant side-effects of treatment must never exceed potential benefit. The advent of adjuvant cytotoxic chemotherapy has made quality of life assessment relevant in early disease.

A number of self-completing questionnaires have been developed to assess the functional quality of the day-to-day life of the cancer patient. These include the Functional Living Index for Cancer (FLIC), the Cancer Rehabilitation Evaluation System (CARES) as well as the more traditional Karnovsky Performance Status and General Health Questionnaire. Profiles of mood states and scales for global adjustment to illness are also available.

In 1986 the EORTC initiated a research programme whose long-term objective was to develop an integrated measurement system for use in clinical trials. This used a modular approach to combine a sufficient degree of generalizability for comparisons across the various trials but with a level of specificity by which research questions relevant to a particular trial could be addressed. The resulting questionnaire (EORTC QLQ-C30) incorporates five functional scales (physical, role, cognitive, emotional and social), three symptom scales (fatigue, pain and nausea and vomiting) and a global health and quality of life scale. In addition, there are a number of single items to assess commonly reported symptoms (dyspnoea, appetite loss, sleep disturbance, constipation and diarrhoea) and to uncover the perceived financial impact of the disease and its treatment. A tumour-specific questionnaire module and selected scales for performance status and toxicity are added. The reliability and validity of this approach has been confirmed by a study of the quality of life in patients with cancer of the lung in 13 countries composed of three language– cultural groups, and inclusion of the questionnaire in therapeutic trials is likely to become standard European practice. Completion of the questionnaire takes 11 min.

To allow quantitation of quality of life with survival, a novel approach has been developed by the International Breast Cancer Study Group, the quality adjusted survival analysis or Q-TWisT. TWisT refers to Time without Symptoms and Toxicity, which is calculated by subtracting from the survival time that time during which the patient has experienced toxicity, local and systemic relapse of the disease. A function has been developed for quality-adjusted survival related to TWisT, which includes evaluation of the state of health during periods of toxicity and relapse and provides a numerical value that can be used in standard survival analyses.

The elderly

Following the age of 25 years, the risk of developing cancer doubles every 5 years and 50% of all cases of cancer occur in those older than 65 years. While some believe that the two processes – ageing and the development of cancer, are fundamentally different, others consider that a common set of genetic alterations underlies both. These may affect patterns of oncogene or tumour-suppressor gene expression or such epigenetic processes as methylation of DNA. Experimental evidence in favour of such common mechanisms comes from the action of so-called 'genoprotector' drugs which prolong lifespan and reduce the incidence of spontaneous cancers in experimental animals.

Whether there is a true interrelationship or not, the combination of cancer and age does not necessarily act in the interests of the patient who, because they are 'elderly', may not be offered the full range of available diagnostic and therapeutic measures. For example, those older than 65 years are seldom the target for health promotional or screening activities, so that the disease frequently is diagnosed at a later stage than in younger persons, as has been documented for cancers of the breast, ovary, uterus and bladder and melanomas. Owing to avoidance of more extensive staging procedures, the true stage of a cancer may not be recognized. Such 'down-staging' of a cancer may lead to the choice of a less intensive approach, so that treatment becomes inadequate for the true stage of the disease.

Chronological age should not be regarded in isolation as a guide to the choice of treatment. Of greater relevance is functional or physiological age and the extent to which 'co-morbidity' from concomitant chronic illness affects this. Aged patients are more exposed to other chronic diseases, such as diabetes, hypertension, heart or lung insufficiency, which may complicate the clinical course of cancer and impair their ability to withstand long or complicated treatment. It cannot be assumed that an elderly patient does not wish to undertake aggressive treatment and his preferences must be sought following a clear explanation of the benefits and costs of a particular regimen. In many instances the risks of radical surgery and acute discomfort of intensive chemotherapy that preserve hope may be preferable to the prospect of a slow and lingering final illness to which the intolerance of feeling unwell only adds further anguish.

Quality of life is no less important to the elderly. Physical function may be particularly cherished as its compromise may result in loss of independence, which, to an elderly person, may represent critical failing. Psychological function is equally important, but this may already be compromised by drug therapy, on top of which anticancer chemotherapy may impose an intolerable burden. The elderly tend to adhere to predetermined patterns of behaviour and upset in normal habits and relationships can cause embarrassment and loss of confidence. Fear of becoming a burden to others can lead to depression; although despite this and other fears, the elderly can often tolerate toxic treatment more readily than the young. Suggestions that the elderly should have less appropriate treatment are unwarranted. Modifications of standard treatment should be considered only after all such factors have been taken into account.

An area of difficulty in the elderly is the lack of objective evidence about best treatment. There is a reluctance to include older patients in randomized therapeutic trials and such subgroup analyses as may be available do not necessarily reveal the truth. Specifically designed trials for elderly patients should be instituted.

From a socioeconomic point of view, age is often associated with retirement and economic non-productivity. In a developed society these factors should never affect the delivery of appropriate care.

ACKNOWLEDGEMENTS

Figs 9.3 and 9.16 are adapted from illustrations in Watson et al. 1990; Fig. 9.6 from Langdon et al. 1997; Figs 9.13 and 9.14 from Forrest 1990; Fig. 9.7 from Vile 1992; Fig. 9.8 from Yates and Connor 1986; Fig. 9.18 from Twycross 1994 and Fig. 9.19 from WHO technical report 804 (1990). The authors are grateful to Mrs Dorothy May for secretarial assistance and to Mr Eugene Chang and Mrs Anne McNeil for illustrations.

FURTHER READING

Much of the information reported in this chapter has come from the series *Accomplishments in Cancer Research* which have been produced annually since 1979 by the General Motors Cancer Research Foundation, edited by JG Fortner and JE Rhoads (latterly JG Fortner and PA Sharp) and published by Lippincott-Raven (Philadelphia and New York) and from reviews and reports in the *Journal of the National Cancer Institute*, the *New England Journal of Medicine*, the *Lancet* and *British Medical Journal*.
Other sources for further study include:
Aaronson NK, Ahmedzai S, Bergman B et al. for the European Organisation for Research and Treatment of Cancer Study Group on Quality of Life. The European Organisation for Research and

Treatment of Cancer QLKQ-C30: a quality of life instrument for use in international trials in oncology. *J Natl Cancer Inst* 1993; **85**: 365–376

Chaganti RSK, German J. *Genetics in Clinical Oncology*. New York: Oxford University Press, 1985

Chamberlain J, Moss Berlin S. *Evaluation of Cancer Screening*. Hiedelberg: Springer-Verlag Ltd, 1996

Cancer Pain Relief and Palliative Care Report of WHO Expert Committee World Health Organisation Technical Report Series 804: Geneva, 1990

Fentiman IS, Monfardini S (eds). *Cancer in the Elderly: Treatment and Research*. Oxford University Press, UK 1994

Forrest AP. *Breast Cancer: The Decision to Screen*. The Nuffield Provincial Hospital Trust, UK 1990

Hayes DF, Bast RC, Desch CE et al. Tumour marker utility grading system: a framework to evaluate clinical utility of tumour markers. *J Natl Cancer Inst* 1996; **88**: 1456–1466

Higginson J, Muir CS, Munoz N. *Human Cancer: Epidemiology and Environmental Causes*. Cambridge University Press Syndicate, 1992

Knudson AG. Hereditary cancers: clues to mechanisms of carcinogenesis. *Br J Cancer* 1989; **59**: 661–666

Langdon SP, Miller WR, Berchuck A (eds). *Biology of Female Cancers*. New York: CRC Press, 1997

Parkin DM, Muir CS, Whelan SL, Gao YT, Ferlay J, Powell J. *Cancer Incidence in Five Continents*. IARC Scientific Publications No 120: Lyon International Agency for Cancer Research, 1992

Twycross R. *Pain Relief in Advanced Cancer*. Edinburgh: Churchill Livingstone, 1994

Vile RG (ed). *Introduction to the Molecular Genetics of Cancer*. Chichester: John Wiley and Sons, 1992

Watson JD, Tooze J, Kurtz DT. *Recombinant DNA. A Short Course*. New York: Scientific American Books, 1990

Yates JRW, Connor JM. Genetic linkage. *Br J Hospital Medicine* 1986; **36**: 133–136

www.nci.nih.gov/cancertopics

www.cancerresearchuk.org

10

Ethics, Legal Aspects and Assessment of Effectiveness

SJ Leinster

Department of Surgery, Norfolk & Norwich Hospital, Norwich, UK

CONTENTS

Ethics and medicine 184
Ethical analysis 185
Ethical decision-making 186
Ethical committees 186
Ethics of animal experimentation 187
Ethics of resource allocation 187

Legal considerations 188
Consent 188
Confidentiality 189
Complaints 190
Negligence 190
Coroner's court 191

Assessment of effectiveness 191
Clinical audit 191
Clinical research 192
Critical reading 197

Further reading 198

If surgeons are to be more than highly trained technicians, they must have an understanding of the wider issues which affect the practice of surgery. The discipline of ethics allows surgeons to examine and justify their actions in relation to accepted standards of moral behaviour and a knowledge of the law as it affects medical practice is essential if they are to remain within the legal boundaries of practice. In order to fully debate the ethical and legal implications of surgical practice, a solid grasp of the scientific evidence behind it is necessary. Surgeons must know that their actions will benefit the patient in the long term and this requires an understanding of statistical methods, including clinical trial design and interpretation which is the basis for the current emphasis on *evidence-based medicine*. This chapter, somewhat improbably,

attempts to give an overview of these themes. Wider reading on each of the themes is recommended and suitable starting points are suggested in the reading list.

ETHICS AND MEDICINE

There is an increasing emphasis in society on the *rights* pertaining to particular groups and individuals. On joining the medical profession the doctor accepts a number of *duties* which are defined and debated under the heading of medical ethics. Traditionally, these duties were regarded as taking precedence over the doctor's own rights.

The common understanding of medical ethics has changed with time. For many years acceptance of the Hippocratic Oath, or at least of the underlying principles contained in it, was regarded as the basis for medical ethics. There was a tacit assumption that in any situation there was a right course of action on which there would be universal consensus and departure from that consensus was regarded as unethical. At the same time, many matters which were really a matter of etiquette rather than morality became subsumed under the heading of ethics.

With the drift in society away from a universally accepted, absolute standard of morality, ethics has moved from being a system which indicates what should be done in a given situation to a system which gives a rational and effective framework for analysing the options in that situation. Ethics, therefore, defines the problem rather than prescribing the solution. Certain concepts such as justice, honesty, beneficence, autonomy and legality are fundamental to the practice of ethical reasoning. These general ethical principles apply in any situation and traditionally have been enshrined in moral codes. Specific ethical principles are those interpretations of the general principles applied to a given field, in this case, medicine. These specific principles are contained in ethical codes which depend for their authority on the acceptance of the underlying values behind them. This causes difficulties in obtaining consensus among groups with different moral codes and within groups when the basic assumptions undergo change. From the practical point of view, the arbiters of acceptable practice are the professional registration bodies in each country (in the UK this is the Professional Misconduct Committee of the General Medical Council).

The oldest ethical code applied to medicine is the Hippocratic Oath which originates from the 4th century BC. Over time it became accepted as the customary basis for the regulation of medical practice. The religious overtones sound odd to modern ears and must always have been a stumbling block to physicians from the monotheistic faiths, but the underlying emphasis on the sanctity of life found wide acceptance. The main principles can be summarised as:
- to do no harm;
- not to assist suicide or administer euthanasia;
- not to procure abortion;
- to refer patients for specialist treatment;
- not to abuse professional relationships, especially for sexual motives;
- to keep the patient's confidences.

As the underlying theistic assumptions lost hold on the profession, a number of attempts were made by the World Medical Association to revise and modernise the medical ethical codes. The most widely recognised is the revision of the clear prohibition, 'I will not give a woman an abortive remedy' to the much more flexible 'I will maintain the utmost respect for human life from the time of conception'. The implications of the Declaration have been spelled out in the International Code of Medical Ethics.

The Declaration of Geneva attempts to govern the whole scope of medical practice. Other Declarations have been adopted which deal with more specific issues. The Declaration of Helsinki (revised 1975) sets out the conventions governing clinical research and human experimentation. Among the most important propositions in this Declaration, is the need for a clearly formulated protocol describing the proposed research to be agreed by an independent committee.

Less well known is the Declaration of Tokyo (1975) which deals with the doctor's approach to torture and other cruel, inhuman or degrading treatment or punishment in relation to detention and imprisonment. The final clause of this Declaration reads, 'The doctor shall in all circumstances be bound to alleviate the distress of his fellow men, and no motive – whether personal, collective or political – shall prevail against this higher purpose'. The Declaration of Oslo (1970) deals with the question of abortion and is a clear example of the possibility of codes of conduct, which are based not on absolute values but on consensus opinion, changing with time.

Ethical analysis

For the practising doctor, the niceties of definition of ethical issues are less important than the practical application of the ethical standards in practice. In many circumstances, the ethical question never becomes explicit. There is a standard of behaviour which is accepted by the profession and the public without question. This is not to say that there are no ethical dilemmas within this situation, just that they are never raised. In other circumstances there is fierce public debate about an issue, often leading to polarisation of views within the profession itself. It is clearly desirable in both types of situation that there is an understanding of the proper process of ethical analysis and that this process should be pursued before a position is accepted.

The first question to be asked is whether there is an ethical issue at all. The establishment of a hospital formulary may be an ethical issue raising questions about limiting the autonomy of the doctors to choose the treatment which they think best. A dispute about which drugs should be included in a hospital formulary, once the principle of having a formulary is accepted, is largely a technical issue, unless the problem of shortage of resources dictates the substitution of a less effective but cheaper drug for the drug of choice. It is, usually, inappropriate to conduct the debate on content of the formulary on ethical grounds.

Once it is clear that there is an ethical issue to be addressed, the next stage is to determine which ethical components are involved. This is a two-stage process. First, the area of ethical concern should be identified. What is the nature of the ethical problem? Secondly, which ethical principles are to be applied in this situation?

Faced with a novel situation the first question to be asked is whether or not a proposed course of action is *legal*; that is, is it permitted under the laws of the country. Clearly, an action may be legal in one country and illegal in another. For example, abortion is (under certain defined circumstances) legal in the UK but illegal in Ireland. It is also possible for an action to be legal but immoral as when torture is approved by the state. On the contrary, actions can be illegal but morally obligatory as shown by protesters who have broken the law and in retrospect have been recognised to have taken the right course. A decision on the legality of a course of action does not necessarily determine an individual's response but it should inform it. It should be noted that if involvement in an illegal act is detected, professional discipline (including ejection from the profession) may ensue. It is the responsibility of the individual doctor to be aware of the law as it affects his or her practice.

The principle of *autonomy* defines the individual's freedom to take decisions about his or her actions. This has been recognised for many years in the practice of obtaining the patient's consent before treatment. There has been an increased emphasis on the patient's right to choose with much attention being focused; for example, on the right of a woman to have an abortion. It is clear, however, that this right to choose must also extend to the doctor who may refuse to undertake a given line of treatment.

The doctor has a duty to maintain an attitude of *beneficence* to the patient. The implication of beneficence is that whatever action the doctor takes will always be in the best

interests of the patient rather than in the interests of the doctor. This is essential if the relationship between doctor and
patient is to be one of trust. The corollary of beneficence is
non-malficence which is traditionally expressed in terms of
the obligation 'First to do no harm'.

Honesty is another fundamental requirement for any
interaction between individuals which is to be based on
trust. This implies not only that the doctor does not lie to the
patient but that the doctor will keep any promise (tacit or
explicit) which might be made to the patient. Some would
regard *confidentiality* (the implied promise not to give information about the patient to a third party without the
patient's consent) as part of the duty of honesty.

The other major principle governing medical practice is
justice. While the main emphasis of the other principles is on
the interaction between the doctor and an individual
patient, justice takes a wider view and includes the effects of
the doctor's actions on other members of society.

Ethical decision-making

Once the nature of the decision is clear, debate as to the correct decision can take place. Different people will reach different conclusions about what that decision should be and
even for an individual the decision may be very finely balanced. There may be a conflict of two ethical principles and
it may be necessary to give precedence to one over the other.
When such conflicts arise a number of factors determine the
action that will be taken.

For some people certain principles are absolute and will
always take precedence. The clearest example of this is the
view of some members of the Pro-Life campaign that abortion is wrong in all circumstances because of the principle
that life should be respected from the time of conception.
No matter what other principles (e.g. autonomy or beneficence) seem to indicate, they will never perform an abortion. This type of decision has been called a '*through way*'
because it by-passes all the difficult issues faced by someone
who does not hold a similar viewpoint.

When such a through way does not exist for the decision-
maker, it is appropriate to consider the consequences of the
available decisions. It requires a certain amount of imagin-
ation to explore all the consequences of a given course of
action, but it is necessary if a valid decision is to be made. In
considering the significance of the identified consequences,
several principles may be taken into account.

Double effect

There are many actions in surgery where the intended good
effect of the surgery is accompanied by inevitable bad effects.
It is wrong to cause suffering and pain, but all surgery is
accompanied by pain after the event. Mutilation of another
person is wrong but in order to save a person's life it may be
necessary to carry out an amputation. The classical example
which is quoted is the administration of powerful analgesics

to relieve pain in the knowledge that it will shorten the patient's
life. This is not a good example to take as it is not clear that
pain relief does shorten life. It may even be that adequate doses
of opiate analgesia prolong life in the terminally ill. Nevertheless, the problem is one which needs to be noted because
it does affect day-to-day practice. Notice that the justification
is not that the action undertaken does not lead to consequences which are considered to be wrong or undesirable,
but that the good to be achieved outweighs the bad.

Lesser of two evils

In some circumstances the consequences of two courses of
action may both be undesirable. Consider a situation where
a boy of 14 years is admitted with multiple injuries and
requires an intensive care unit (ICU) bed. All the beds within
a reasonable radius are full and none of the patients is fit to
move out. In one bed is an 81-year-old who is on obligatory
ventilation after the repair of a ruptured aortic aneurysm.
What should the doctor do? Inevitably, he will have to make
a choice between the two and the prognosis for the untreated
patient is very poor. Effectively, one of the patients is being
condemned to die. In this case, the decision must be based
on what is perceived to be the lesser of the two evils.

There is a risk that if such decisions have to be made repeatedly, the actions will come to be regarded as right rather than
wrong but unavoidable. This is undesirable and it is necessary
from time to time to examine even the most time-honoured
customs to determine if there is a better way of doing things.

Slippery slope

When considering the consequences of a given action it is
important that the long term as well as immediate consequences are considered. If a fixed boundary is removed, the
range of acceptable behaviour may change markedly. This
is described as the 'slippery slope'.

One of the concerns about legalising voluntary euthanasia
is that when it becomes the accepted norm, there will be
pressure to extend euthanasia to groups who are not in a
position to give consent (e.g. an elderly patient with dementia who develops cancer). This phenomenon is reported as
happening in the Netherlands where the legal system has for
some time permitted voluntary euthanasia. It is possible to
imagine that the criteria would then extend to other groups
who might be actively opposed to the idea of euthanasia but
who were decreed to be better off dead. Such a change in
public attitude has already been seen for abortion in the UK
where the original, strictly defined criteria of who could have
an abortion are now interpreted to mean that any woman
has the right to choose to have an abortion, because only she
can determine whether or not she is going to suffer severe
mental disturbance as a result of the pregnancy continuing.

Ethical committees

When the action under consideration relates to a research
project, there is a clear procedure to be adopted. All research

projects which involve human subjects, whether physio-logical experiments or clinical trials of a new form of treat-ment, must conform to the Declaration of Helsinki. The detailed protocol for the study must be put to a properly constituted committee containing lay representatives as well as members of the medical profession. The committee will form its conclusions based on a number of considerations:

1. *Is the proposed experiment necessary?* An acceptable study should be expected to produce a significant improvement in the management of patients.
2. *Is the proposed experiment scientifically valid?* The methodology described should be capable of answering the question that has been set. For example, the proposed numbers of patients in a clinical trial should be shown stat-istically to be adequate to produce a reliable answer.
3. *Is there any alternative method of determining the answer to the question without experimenting on humans?*
4. *Is the information to be given to the subjects full, accurate and understandable?* The information should include the risks to the subject and emphasise the subject's right to withdraw from the study at any time.
5. *Is valid consent to be obtained from the participants?* Valid consent must be freely given without duress and should be witnessed by a third party.

It is unethical to carry out a study on human subjects in order to answer a trivial question. It is equally unethical to carry out a poorly designed study which is not capable of answering the question which has been posed.

Ethics of animal experimentation

The majority of the medical profession feels it is right to use animals as alternatives to experimentation on humans. In most countries the use of animals in live experimentation is strictly controlled, although the mechanisms of control and the nature of the experiments which are considered to be acceptable varies greatly from country to country. In the UK, the control of animal experiments lies with the Home Office which has appointed inspectors to supervise all such experi-ments. Anyone who is using live animals in experiments must hold a Personal Licence permitting them to carry out the necessary procedures defined in the protocol and there must be a Project Licence for each experiment which is issued if the inspector approves the protocol. The inspectors are also responsible for ensuring that the facilities in which the animals are housed meet an acceptable standard.

There is an increasing lobby against the use of live animals in any form of study, coupled with the demand that alterna-tives methods of research be found. Sometimes a technical question is to be answered by research and, with thought, an alternative experiment avoiding the use of animals can be found. Where this is the case it seems right to suggest that the ethical approach would avoid the use of animals. In other circumstances, there may be no alternative to the use of animals. The decision whether or not to proceed will then depend on such things as the importance of the question to be answered and the relative value placed on animals as against humans.

Ethics of resource allocation

Most of the decisions doctors are called upon to take seem to be concerned with individual patients but there is often an underlying problem of resource allocation determining the nature of the dilemma. In the example above of the two patients requiring an ICU bed, the dilemma would not have arisen if there had been no limit on the provision of ICU beds. Clearly, it is unrealistic to expect that all possible health care needs will always be met and decisions on the allocation of resources must be taken. These decisions have an ethical component and should be analysed with regard to the justice of the alternative lines of action. This is a larger question than just the distribution of resources within the health services and includes how national governments partition their resources among health, education, welfare, defence, etc.

So far, no satisfactory approach has been found. In free mar-ket economies, the distribution is based on what the individ-ual can afford so that the wealthy have the latest and best technology while the poor have nothing. In government-financed systems, what is available to a given patient may depend on the idiosyncrasies of the local medical personnel. In both systems rationing occurs without any explicit public debate as to who should be treated and which services should be provided. When debate does occur it is often centred on specific cases and driven by emotion rather than careful analysis.

A just allocation of resources can take place only when the costs and consequences of various alternative interventions are accurately known and can be overtly compared with one another. A difficulty arises in attempting to define outcomes. Improvement in survival can be accurately quantified, but how is an improvement in quality of life to be quantified and how is an improvement in quality of life to be compared with an improvement in survival? This is a difficult enough deci-sion when it concerns one individual, but is even more diffi-cult when the comparison is between the survival of one patient and the improvement in quality of life of another. Attempts have been made to overcome these problems using quality-adjusted life years (QALYs) but this is only partly successful. While the QALY gives a figure which can be manipulated by the health economists, it is not as objective as it at first appears since the value of the QALY is dependent on the assessment of quality of life which is still, despite great efforts, a subjective judgement. The QALY is concerned with the 'average' patient and does not take account of indi-vidual differences between cases. It is very sensitive to minor changes in the estimates of the duration of benefit and the outcome.

An attempt was made in Oregon State in the USA to pro-duce explicit criteria for resource allocation based on a prioritised list derived from modified QALYs. The weightings for quality of life were derived from a telephone survey of local citizens. This experiment has not proved to be effective in practice. Some of the results were distinctly odd, with cosmetic breast surgery being rated as more important than the treatment of a compound fracture of the femur. The attempt was shelved when the Federal Government intervened.

LEGAL CONSIDERATIONS

Increasingly, medical practice is governed by law as well as ethics. It is essential that surgeons have a grasp of those aspects of the law which directly affect their practice. There are three areas in particular which are important: consent, confidentiality and negligence.

Consent

The legal position with regard to consent to treatment is summed up in a famous American judgement:

Every human being of adult years and a sound mind has the right to determine what should be done with his own body; and a surgeon who performs an operation without his patient's consent commits an assault for which he is liable to damages.

This position has been extended in the UK in the Patients' Charter, which states that as a patient you have the right:

to be given a clear explanation of any treatment proposed, including any risks and any alternatives before you decide whether you will agree to treatment.

The concept of giving the patient's a clear explanation of any treatment proposed is generally regarded as being equivalent to obtaining *informed consent*. This latter concept arose in the USA in the late 1950s and is the legal corollary of the ethical concept of autonomy. Closer examination suggests that the concept of informed consent is flawed although the aim set out in the Patients' Charter is entirely laudable. Leaving aside the fundamental question whether consent has in any sense to be informed in order to be valid, there is a problem in defining 'informed'. Two approaches have been taken. In North America, the tendency is to use the test of what the 'prudent patient' would wish to know; in the UK, the test is the 'professional standard'. When using the prudent patient test, the question is what information would a reasonable person wish to know in order to make a decision. The doctor should disclose the 'material risks' of the procedure to the patient and failure to do so is negligent unless the doctor can show that revealing the risk would harm the patient. The argument as to what constitutes a material risk varies from case to case. The professional standard test (known as the Bolam test) requires that the doctor only

practices measures that are accepted as proper by a responsible body of medical opinion. This was accepted in the case of *Sidaway v Board of Governors of the Bethlem Royal Hospital* in the House of Lords but strictly speaking applies only to information that the doctor volunteers and failure to answer properly any questions that the patient asks may still be regarded as negligent. That is to say, the level of information that is, when volunteered by the doctor, regarded as being adequate, may be considered to be inadequate if given in response to direct questions by the patient.

A particular problem arises in the case of randomised-controlled trials where the patients must be informed that they are being entered into a trial. The difficulty of explaining the basis of and the rationale for randomisation may lead to patients refusing to enter the trial. This may lead to unexpected biases in the trial if all the trial refusers have a certain set of characteristics not shared by the patients who agree to enter the trial.

Forms of consent

Although surgeons tend to think of consent in terms of a signed consent form, consent may be implied, verbal or written. All forms of consent are equally valid in law and a written consent form is not necessarily proof that valid consent was obtained as the patient can claim that the signature was obtained under duress or that the explanation of the proposed treatment was flawed, either of which would invalidate the consent. If a conscious patient allows a doctor to carry out a procedure without question or protest, then consent has been implied. The presence of a third party who can testify that the patient did not protest would strengthen the case that consent was effectively given. Similarly, if a patient agrees verbally to a procedure, consent has been given. These forms of consent are the ones most usually obtained for simple matters like examination of the patient (which does require the patient's consent) or taking a blood sample.

Written consent, like the other forms of consent, must first of all be appropriate. A blanket consent to: '*any surgical procedure*' would not be valid. Ideally, the explanation of the treatment to be undertaken should be given by the surgeon who is going to carry out the procedure, although in practice this task is often delegated. Certainly, the person obtaining the consent must be able to answer relevant questions about the treatment and the expected outcomes and should consciously give the patient the opportunity to ask questions. The consent must be given without undue pressure, it must be given within 24 h of the operation and it must be witnessed. The weakest part of the customary consent forms used in the UK is that the patient's signature is witnessed by the doctor who is seeking to obtain the patient's consent. It would be better if a third party were to witness the signature and also to state that the consent was given after adequate explanation and without undue pressure. Such consent forms are accepted as standard for patients entering clinical trials.

Patient criteria for giving consent

Age

There is widespread misunderstanding about who is entitled to give consent to treatment. Clearly, if the patient is able to understand what is proposed, the patient can give (or withhold) consent. In British law, anyone over the age of 18 years is regarded as potentially able to give consent. When the patient is a minor (under 16 years of age), the parents (or another adult acting *in loco parentis*) can, by law, give consent to treatment and, until the *Gillick* case it was assumed that the minor could not. In *Gillick*, the House of Lords decided in a majority judgement that under certain circumstances, a minor under 16 years could consent to treatment without the parent's knowledge. For young people of 16 and 17 years the situation is also rather muddled. The *Family Law Reform Act* gives this age group the right to give valid consent to treatment (but not to participation in research projects), but does not remove the right of the parents to consent. Conflicts could arise because of this parallel right to consent and the situation has yet to be resolved in law.

The courts have made exception in dealing with the children of parents who refuse essential treatment for their child. The most prominent recurrent example is the refusal of Jehovah's witnesses to accept blood transfusion on religious grounds even when it would be lifesaving. A child is not in a position to make informed choices and if it is felt that the parents are not acting in the best interests of the child, the doctor treating the child can apply for the child to be made a ward of court. This can be done at any time and the court can then give permission for treatment.

Physical condition

If the patient is incapable of giving consent because of a physical condition (e.g. unconsciousness) and has not previously said anything to indicate that treatment would be unacceptable, the senior doctor caring for the patient can recommend that treatment should proceed. This is justified because of the doctor's common law duty of care to the patient. Specific 'consent' forms are used which call for the doctor to certify that the patient is not able to take the decision but that, in the opinion of the doctor, the proposed treatment is essential. The patient's next of kin cannot give consent to treatment. It is a matter of courtesy to inform them of the need for treatment (if they can be contacted) and they may be able to give some insight into what the patient's views would be, but they are not able to authorise or prevent treatment.

Mental health

Patients with some psychiatric conditions may refuse treatment, even when that treatment is lifesaving. In the UK, under the *Mental Health Act 1983*, severely disturbed patients can be detained and treated without their consent, but only their psychiatric condition can be treated. Treatment of a physical disorder cannot be undertaken without the patient's consent.

The hope is that the psychiatric disorder can be brought under control sufficiently quickly to allow the patient to consent to the other treatment. Some argue that the doctor's common law duty of care could be evoked to allow treatment to be carried out against the patient's will but this is a difficult position to sustain.

Patients who are educationally subnormal (ESN) pose special difficulties. Although their mental age may be below 16 years, they are regarded as adults and their consent to treatment must be obtained. The major difficulties have arisen when sterilisation has been proposed for sexually active ESN patients. The permission of the courts has usually to be sought, and has been given, but considerable unease still exists.

It has until recently been considered that an adult has the absolute right to refuse any form of treatment provided that they understand the consequences of that refusal. Two court cases have thrown doubt on that concept. Both involved pregnant women who had previously had a Caesarean section and who were demanding to be allowed to attempt natural childbirth. In both cases the court gave permission to the medical team to carry out the operation against the patients' wishes, presumably acting on behalf of the unborn child. This has raised serious questions which have yet to be resolved.

Confidentiality

There is an ethical and common law duty on the doctor to maintain the confidentiality of anything that is discovered about a patient in the course of the consultation unless the patient gives consent to disclosure. Problems can arise when the doctor's duty to the patient of confidentiality comes into conflict with an overriding duty to society or even duty to another patient. A patient may be found to be suffering from an inherited but treatable disorder. If the patient refuses to allow his relatives to be informed so that they can be screened and treated, the doctor may have a duty to break the patient's confidentiality. There may be a legal obligation on the doctor to breach confidentiality such as the statutory duty to notify specified infectious diseases, or when called upon to do so by a Court Order. Certain Acts of Parliament (e.g. *Road Traffic Act 1972*, *Prevention of Terrorism Act 1984* and *Police and Criminal Evidence Act 1984*) specifically lay down that access to medical records and other excluded material can be granted by order of a circuit judge.

The commonest breach of confidentiality, which has become hallowed by custom, is the practice of giving bad news about the patient's diagnosis or prognosis to the relatives rather than the patient. This is particularly a problem with cancer patients. This procedure is wrong and no information should be divulged about the patient without the patient's express consent unless the patient is incapable of giving that consent.

Hospital notes are the property of the hospital authorities. It has been common practice in the past to deny patients access to their notes. This situation has been altered by statute and the *Access to Medical Records Act* now gives patients the right to see their notes. They may be required to make formal application and the medical staff have the right to edit the notes to remove material which they believe may be harmful to the patient before the patient is allowed access to the notes. Medical records should only be divulged to a third party with the patient's permission and it is wise to have this in writing with the exception that Courts of Law can subpoena patients' notes and order disclosure to a patient's legal representative. Records held on computer are a special case and are governed by the *Data Protection Act 1984*. These records must be divulged unedited if the patient requests them. The *Freedom of Information Act 2000* also applies to the National Health Service (NHS) and it is possible that in the future applications for disclosure of medical records might be made under this Act.

Complaints

Mistakes occur and patients may be dissatisfied with the way they have been treated. Complaints are, therefore, inevitable. Complaints about non-clinical matters can, if unresolved, be referred to the Health Service Commissioner (the Ombudsman) who is an independent official responsible to Parliament. Clinical complaints are handled under the procedures set out in Appendix B to Circular MC(88)57.

All hospitals now should have a formal procedure for handling complaints. When a complaint is received, the appointed officer of the hospital will attempt to ascertain the facts of the case. It is important that all members of staff involved in the case (especially the medical staff) should produce written statements of the facts as soon as possible. The appointed officer will then write a reply to the complainant setting out the hospital's view of the case. This should contain an explanation of the events which led to the complaint and, if necessary, an apology along with a statement of the steps that will be taken to ensure that a similar situation does not arise in future. If the complainant is not satisfied, and the complaint is about a clinical matter, the manager will arrange a meeting between the complainant and the consultant in charge of the case, usually in the presence of a senior manager. If this meeting fails to resolve the problem, the Clinical Complaints Review Procedure will be invoked. The Regional Director of Public Health will invite two independent consultants from the same speciality to consider the case. After studying the notes the assessors meet with the complainant and clarify the details of his complaint. They then interview all the doctors concerned and discuss their view of the complaints. Having formed a view of whether the complaint is justified or not, the assessors meet again with the complainant and explain their opinion which is then delivered to the Regional Director of Public Health as a formal report. If errors have been made, the assessors will recommend the steps that should be taken to avoid similar

problems in the future. The report is forwarded to the Chief Executive of the Trust who will initiate whatever action is necessary.

The process is designed to resolve complaints in the fairest and most efficient way possible. If the complainant is not satisfied, recourse to legal action is still possible. The commonest civil claim against doctors is one of negligence.

Negligence

Negligence is defined in law as a failure to act in a manner appropriate to a practitioner of similar training and experience. It is often said that most alleged claims for negligence arise as a result of poor communication on the part of the doctors when complications arise. The evidence for this statement is largely anecdotal, but it is true that some cases appear to arise as a result of misunderstanding by the patient of the expected outcome of their treatment. The formal complaints procedure is intended to reduce such cases to a minimum.

The usual defence against a claim of negligence is that the outcome which occurred is one which would be expected in the clinical situation. If the outcome is of sufficient seriousness (e.g. a facial palsy following parotid surgery) the doctor who failed to warn the patient could be considered to be guilty of negligence, although the development of the facial palsy is not evidence of negligence.

It is difficult to refute a claim of negligence if there are no contemporaneous notes. If a patient develops a pulmonary embolism (PE) postoperatively, it is not sufficient to state that the unit policy is always to administer subcutaneous heparin as prophylaxis if the notes do not record that this did in fact happen. If the notes record that heparin was administered in an acceptable dose schedule, then the PE was an unfortunate accident. If the notes do not record the fact, then it is presumed that such administration did not take place and the doctor is guilty of negligence, since responsible medical opinion holds that prophylactic heparin is essential. The other reason for negligence claims succeeding is the failure of a doctor to attend when called, unless some other more pressing duty prevented it (e.g. being involved in the treatment of another patient who could not be left).

Claims for negligence arising as a result of employment by a hospital authority in the UK fall under the *NHS* Indemnity scheme. If a notice of an action for negligence is received, the doctor should immediately notify the hospital management who will request the help of their legal adviser. The matter will usually be referred to the *NHS Litigation* Authority who will decide whether the case can be defended or should be settled. The doctor should cooperate fully with the legal adviser by producing statements without delay. There is no point in refusing to allow the plaintiff's solicitors access to the records as a Court Order can be obtained which will force access. The delaying tactic will merely raise the suspicion that the medical team have something to hide. If the doctor is a member of a medical defence organisation, it is advisable to inform them as well so that they can hold a watching brief to ensure that the doctor's interests are protected.

The plaintiff's solicitor will submit the notes to an independent medical expert who will report his opinion as to whether there has been any negligence in the management of the case. The defence solicitors will similarly seek independent expert advice. Under the terms of the *Wolfe* report the independent medical experts have a duty to the court to submit an impartial report-based solely on their professional opinion backed by appropriate evidence. The duty to the court supersedes their duty to the instructing solicitor or their client. Where there is disagreement between the experts, they are required to meet to reach an agreement and to produce a joint report. Both sides will then consult with counsel who will advise whether or not a court action is likely to succeed. If each counsel advises their respective clients that an action is likely to be successful, it is probable that the hospital will attempt to settle the claim out of court. If the plaintiff's counsel thinks the action is likely to succeed but the defence counsel thinks the case could be successfully defended, then the case will probably go to court. If it does the doctors involved will be called as witnesses to fact and should confine their testimony to the facts of what happened. Independent medical experts will be called as expert witnesses and they will be expected to give their opinion on the case and supply the court with relevant evidence with regard to accepted medical practice.

Coroner's court

The coroner in the UK is a public official (holding either a medical or a legal qualification) who is empowered to hold inquests into cases of unexpected or violent death. When a doctor is called upon to certify the cause of a death which falls into one of these categories, the coroner should be informed. The coroner has the discretion as to whether or not to hold an inquest and whether that inquest should be before a jury. The doctors involved may be called upon to give evidence at the inquest. Once again, their main purpose is to state the facts of the case as they know them, but as expert witnesses are unlikely to be called the doctor may be called upon to give background information and opinion. The coroner's verdicts range from death by natural causes through accidental death to unlawful killing.

ASSESSMENT OF EFFECTIVENESS

Although factors other than effectiveness of different treatments need to be taken into account when deciding on ethical and legal issues, it is clear that measures of effectiveness are essential if reasoned decisions are to be taken. The use of ineffective or unproven treatments is unethical on the grounds of failure of beneficence (the doctor is not acting in the patient's best interests if the treatment is not known to be effective); lack of autonomy (the patient cannot take a valid

decision in the absence of information on the treatment); lack of honesty (the doctor cannot pretend that a treatment will work in the absence of evidence to that effect) and lack of justice (the resources consumed in the ineffective treatment might have been used to deliver an effective treatment for a different condition to someone else).

There are two methods of determining clinical effectiveness. The first is *clinical audit* and the second is *research*, usually in the form of clinical trials. It is important to note that a treatment is not proved to be effective just because it has been used for a long time and is regarded as the standard approach. Mastectomy was regarded in the UK for many years as the only acceptable treatment for breast cancer but when the question was examined in clinical trials it was found that breast conservation was an acceptable alternative. This raises questions over the increasing trend towards the development of clinical guidelines which are often derived on the basis of consensus, unless that consensus is based on independent verifiable evidence.

Clinical audit

Participation in audit has been recognised by the profession as desirable for many years but it is now mandatory in the UK. Much that has passed for audit in the past has been ineffectual, consisting of an enumeration of the procedures that had been carried out in a unit in a given time span, with a note of the complications and deaths. Unless action is taken as a result of the enumeration no purpose has been served.

The requirements for audit are:
- accurate, prospective data collection;
- recognition of variation in case-mix;
- clearly defined outcome measures;
- a system for introducing changes;
- re-evaluation of the system after change.

Accurate data collection is very often the weakest point in the clinical audit system. In the best systems the data which is recorded as an essential part of the hospital administration (patient's name, age, date of admission, date of discharge, etc.) forms the basis for the audit database and can be used to verify that all the patients who have been treated in a given period are included in the audit. The diagnoses, treatment and complications should be entered contemporaneously by the doctor responsible for the patient. It is best if the surgeon who carries out an operation enters the details either directly on to a computerised database or at least on to a specific audit proforma. Codes can be used but it is possible to get so involved in the refinement of codes that the purpose of the audit is lost and free text is workable for most practices. In principle, the same database can be used for patient administration, the production of discharge summaries and letters, and audit. Unfortunately, few such systems are in operation at present.

A correct interpretation of audit data (such as the Department of Health league tables) requires a knowledge of the case-mix of the unit concerned. While outcomes do depend on the abilities of the surgeon, they depend to a greater extent on the fitness of the patient being treated. Attempts have been made to develop methods of taking the variation in patients into account. One of the most successful of these has been the Physiological and Operative Severity Score for Enumeration of Mortality and morbidity (POSSUM) scoring system developed by Copeland. This assesses the patient's preoperative physiological status and the nature and severity of the surgical procedure to produce a score which can be used to predict from a nomogram the expected morbidity and mortality. As the score cannot be calculated until the operation has been undertaken, it cannot be used to exclude a patient from undergoing surgery but it does allow a more informed appraisal of the outcome. The POSSUM score is particularly helpful in comparing the performance of different units or the performance of a single unit at different points in time. For example, two units within a region had different mortalities for aortic aneurysm surgery. This was initially ascribed to one of the units being a specialist vascular unit but when the POSSUM scoring was applied it was found that the entire difference could be accounted for by the difference in the age and general condition of the patients admitted to the two units.

One of the most difficult aspects of clinical audit is the defining of realistic outcome measures. The real outcome measures for a surgical procedure are long term – the survival of a cancer patient or the incidence of recurrence following hernia repair – but the immediate requirement is for a surrogate measure that will allow prompt corrections of any shortcomings to be made. In practice there is a tendency to select variables on the basis of their ease of measurement rather than their utility so that average length of stay for a given procedure or percentage of cases done as day cases become critical measures, although both are influenced by factors other than the performance of the surgical team. In some circumstances, it may be better to monitor the process rather than the outcome and this approach has been adopted by the National Health Service Breast Screening Programme in the UK. A detailed set of guidelines has been developed for each aspect of the service and regionally based Quality Assurance teams monitor the achievement of these targets by the screening units. This approach does beg the question of whether adherence to accepted procedures will always result in the expected outcome but is likely to become more widespread as purchasers attempt to ensure that they are getting the best value for their contracts.

When a defect in the system is detected through audit, changes have to be made. The nature of these changes should be decided by reference to the literature. When the literature does not provide a satisfactory solution, it is necessary to set up a formal research study to provide the answer. What must not happen is that a solution is adopted because it appears superficially to be a logical approach. Once changes have been implemented, the audit should be repeated to establish that they have been effective.

Clinical research

Clinical studies may be *observational or experimental*. As the name implies, observational studies record what is happening without any intervention on the part of the researcher. Care must be taken that the observations do not perturb the situation. If participants (doctors or patients) are aware that they are under observation they may modify their behaviour to such an extent that the study is invalidated. In experimental studies, the researcher deliberately alters one of the variables and observes the outcome.

Sources of error

All forms of study are subject to various sources of error. The most serious of these are systematic errors (*biases*) which may lead to invalid conclusions being drawn:

- *Selection bias* arises when the study group and the control group differ systematically in some important characteristic which affects the outcome. A comparison of the outcome of a new treatment for myocardial infarction (MI) would be seriously flawed if the treatment group were drawn from patients with MI treated at home and the control group from patients with MI who were hospitalised.
- *Confounding bias* arises when confounding variables are present in the dataset. A confounding variable is one which differs between the test and control groups and is later found to affect the outcome. For example, if in a clinical trial of hormone therapy for breast cancer, the control group were younger than the test group, age would be a confounding variable as the response rate to hormone therapy increases with increasing age.
- *Information bias* will lead to incorrect conclusions being drawn from a study but will not be eliminated by randomisation. This bias arises from the collection of incorrect data as a result of faulty questionnaires, misunderstanding by observers of what they should be recording or incorrect answers being given by the respondents. The latter can arise from a desire to give the answer which it is thought the interviewer wants to here, or an avoidance of giving an answer which would be embarrassing to the respondent.

Sensitivity and specificity

Errors in interpretation may also arise because the variable used to identify subjects as cases or non-cases has a *false positive* or a *false negative* rate. The *sensitivity* of a test is the number of true positives which are correctly defined by the test and is equal to 1 minus the false positive rate. The *specificity* of the test is the number of true negatives which are defined by the test and is equal to 1 minus the false negative rate. There is an inverse relationship between the two measures. Altering the test criteria to improve one will lead to a reciprocal change in the other. This consideration is important when screening tests are being developed. Too many false positives (a low specificity) will lead to an unnecessarily high workload for the assessment team and unnecessary anxiety for a large number of patients. In contrast, too many false negatives (a low sensitivity) will reduce the effectiveness of the screening programme by missing cases which need treatment.

Regression to the mean

When measurements of a given parameter (e.g. blood pressure) are repeated, the extreme values will tend to move towards the mean value. Patients who had a high blood pressure will be found to have a lower blood pressure, whereas it will tend to increase in those who had a low blood pressure. This phenomenon has also been found within populations so that tall fathers have shorter sons and short fathers have taller sons. The practical implication of this phenomenon is that treatments must be tried on a whole range of patients. If only those patients lying at the extremes of the range are treated an apparent effect will be detected purely as a result of regression to the mean.

Observational study

Cross-sectional study

Cross-sectional studies are the simplest to perform as the data is collected at a single point in time with the subjects being contacted only once. When the data collected is purely descriptive (e.g. the use by surgeons of routine perioperative anticoagulation), a cross-sectional study is often described as a survey. It is possible to use a cross-sectional study to explore relationships between variables, such as the relationship between cigarette smoking and benign breast disease. The data may be collected by postal questionnaires which allows a wide sample to be taken, but the response rate may be a problem with 50–80% response rates being common. Often the characteristics of responders and nonresponders is different, which affects the interpretation of the results. The problem is compounded where the population under study is too large for every member to be approached. Sampling is then necessary and sampling in a cross-sectional study has the same problems as sampling in other forms of study.

Case–control study

A common approach to observational studies is the case–control study. This is usually a retrospective study in which a patient with a given condition is compared with one or more controls, matched as far as possible for characteristics other than the disease under investigation. Putative risk factors for the disease are then examined in the two groups. If the cases show a higher frequency of the risk factor than the controls, then it can be deduced that the risk factor is indeed related to the disease. Note that a case–control study does not establish causation, it merely establishes association. Both the risk factor and the disease may be related to a third unidentified factor.

The identification of a suitable control group is not as simple as it first appears. For example, if a study of cigarette smoking and lung cancer had drawn controls from a group (say patients from the same ward in hospital) which contained a high percentage of patients with myocardial ischaemia or peripheral vascular disease, the relationship between smoking and lung cancer would be obscured since the diseases in the control group are also smoking related. A further problem arises when an attempt is made to match the controls with the cases for certain important variables (e.g. age and sex). The study cannot then be used to explore the relationship between the matched variables and the condition under investigation.

Even when the problem of the control group has been satisfactorily resolved, other difficulties exist.

An important drawback to case–control studies is *recall bias*. It is accepted that the recall of risk factors may be different between the control group and those who have the condition, especially if the possibility of the risk factor being involved has been publicised. Patients with the condition are more likely to remember exposure to the putative risk factor than those who do not have the condition. Even when this bias does not exist the collection of retrospective data is likely to be inaccurate. This is particularly true of attempts to collect information such as dietary information directly from patients, but is also true of attempts to collect information from hospital records, many of which are incomplete.

Detection bias may also be a problem. Patients who perceive themselves to be at risk of a given condition (e.g. because of a family history) may ask for more regular screening with the result that an excess of cases may be found.

As with the cross-sectional study, even when all the biases have been eliminated, the case–control study identifies an association and not a causal link.

Cohort study

The most informative of the observational studies is the cohort study in which a group of subjects is identified and then followed up long term. Theoretically, a cohort study can be based on retrospective data (the *historical cohort study*), but it is rare for adequate data to be available for such a study to be mounted and the majority of cohort studies are prospective. As the data are collected prospectively they can be tightly controlled but only those data identified at the start of the study will be available. The endpoint, or event of interest, should be identified before the study starts (e.g. death or onset of a particular disease). If this endpoint is a rare event very large numbers of subjects must be entered into the study.

Subject selection is especially important in a cohort study. The probability of the endpoint occurring may be determined by the population under study. If a study is to be undertaken of the long-term sequelae of gallstones, it is likely that a different result will be obtained if the patients studied are those who have been admitted to hospital with an attack of acute cholecystitis rather than all the people in a defined community who are found to have gallstones in a population screening exercise. The answer obtained might still be clinically important but the conclusions drawn should be limited to the type of patient studied. Failure to differentiate the type of patients who had been studied led in the past to the recommendation that all patients with gallstones should undergo cholecystectomy because patients with symptomatic gallstones have a high rate of developing complications.

A specific difficulty of the cohort study is *loss to follow-up*. There may be many reasons for this and it is important to ascertain that the reason for dropout does not affect the conclusions of the study. Suppose, for example, that the incidence of pancreatitis in patients with untreated gallstones increases with the number of attacks of acute cholecystitis. If all patients who have a single attack of acute cholecystitis undergo immediate cholecystectomy, the relationship will never be identified. A successful cohort study demands that great efforts be made to keep the subjects under review. If the endpoint is death, and the registration of deaths in the country of the study is good, registration data can be used to ensure complete follow-up to this endpoint. Similarly, if there is national registration of cancers, studies in which the endpoint is the development of cancer can be completed from registration data.

Cohort studies are also prone to *surveillance bias* because the group thought to be at highest risk of a condition may be followed up more closely, with a consequent increased detection of cases of the disease under investigation.

Experimental study

In experimental studies, the researcher carries out some intervention and observes the outcome. In the clinical setting these are usually called *clinical trials*. Clinical trials are now regarded as obligatory before the introduction of new drugs, with regulatory bodies in most countries demanding evidence of safety and effectiveness before licensing the drug for release onto the market. Surgical procedures are much less likely to be rigorously tested before coming into general use, but this is gradually changing.

The first stage in the use of a new drug in human subjects (after appropriate toxicology and efficacy studies in animals and *in vitro*) is the Phase 1 clinical trial. To confirm the toxicity and to determine the clinical pharmacology the drug is given in escalating doses to end-stage patients who have had all conventional forms of treatment. If there is unacceptable toxicity or there is no effect, drug testing will not proceed. If some effect is noted the drug will then be subjected to a Phase 2 study. This, too, is an open study with no control group receiving an alternative therapy. The purpose is to evaluate the correct dose of the drug, to estimate the likely level of response and to detect major unwanted side effects. If the drug passes the Phase 2 study by showing an apparent useful effect with tolerable toxicity, the next stage is the Phase 3 study which is a controlled trial with a properly constituted control group. Assignment to the control or test

group is random and ideally neither the subject nor the researcher should know which treatment group the subject is in (double-blind).

Randomisation is essential to reduce the various errors to which clinical trials are prone. Randomisation does not mean the selection of subjects haphazardly. Each subject must have the same chance of receiving a given treatment as every other subject and this can be assured only by formal randomisation procedures using random number tables or a random number generator on a computer. Other methods of selecting subjects for a given treatment such as order of entry into the study, or year of birth (e.g. odd numbers receive treatment A; even numbers receive treatment B) may give rise to systematic errors. For example, if on the basis of the selection method it is known which treatment the subject is going to receive, the researcher might choose not to enter a given patient into the trial because of prior beliefs about the efficacy of one of the treatments. This will affect the overall results. Randomisation should eliminate this and other forms of selection bias where the outcome of the trial is a result of the differences between the patients in the groups rather than the treatments themselves. Even when randomisation has been carried out it is necessary to check the balance between the groups of important characteristics which might have a bearing on the outcome.

If the treatment group to which the patient belongs is known to the participants and the experimenter, the results of the trial will be distorted. Phase 2 studies, in which it is known that the patient is receiving a novel treatment, tend to give an optimistic estimate of the effectiveness of the treatment. Ideally, neither the patient nor the observer should know which treatment the patient is receiving. This condition is known as a *double-blind* trial. When a new treatment is being tested against no treatment, it is good practice to administer a *placebo* to the control group. This should be identical in appearance and presentation to the active treatment. Considerable argument has developed around the use of placebos. There are few conditions where treatment is desirable which can, at the same time, be deliberately left without treatment while the trial proceeds. For that reason, it is now common practice to compare a new treatment with the current standard therapy. This does have problems since the difference between the two treatments is likely to be smaller than the difference between treatment and placebo which means that the study has to be larger in order to be sure of detecting the difference.

Cross-over studies, where both groups receive both treatments but are randomised to receive them in different orders, may be possible when the condition to be treated is chronic (e.g. breast pain). Such studies reduce the number of patients who must be recruited. A *matched pairs design* may also be used to reduce the number of patients needed.

It is important that the sample size for the trial is calculated before the trial is started. In the past, statistical testing concentrated on ensuring that any positive result found was not the result of chance. A small sample size is more likely to miss a real difference when it does exist (a Type II statistical error). Calculations can be made to determine the power of the trial to detect a predetermined difference between the groups if it exists. It is common to establish a target trial size which will give a 90% chance of detecting the expected difference. If that difference is 10%, then the trial will need a minimum of 500 pairs of patients. In order to achieve this entry in a reasonable time, most trials are conducted as multicentre trials.

The introduction of a new form of operation without full evaluation should be as unacceptable as the introduction of a new drug without evaluation but ensuring blinding is difficult when surgical procedures are being tested. This is especially true when there is a considerable difference between the treatments (e.g. abdominoperineal resection versus low anterior resection). The problem is mitigated if there is a clear-cut endpoint such as absolute survival. Softer endpoints such as disease-free survival are more of a problem as the detection of recurrence may be more difficult with one of the groups and an apparent advantage for one treatment may merely represent delay in diagnosis of recurrence. When the morbidity of two procedures (e.g. return to work after laparoscopic versus open hemiorrhaphy) is being compared, the problem is even greater, especially since there are likely to be a number of confounding variables such as the patient's occupation and financial circumstances. Occasionally, it is possible to overcome the problem by the use of a blinded observer if the patient cannot readily distinguish which treatment they have had (e.g. a comparison of different suture materials for wound closure) but it is better to define hard endpoints where possible.

Statistical considerations

If research studies are to be interpreted correctly, an understanding of the principles of statistics is needed.

Variability

Medicine, by one definition, is applied biological science and biological systems are characterised by *variability*. Three major types of variability are recognised:
- within individual,
- between individuals,
- with time (as a result of growth or decay).

If the serum sodium concentration is measured in the same individual on different occasions it will be different on each occasion, although lying within a fairly narrow range. The same phenomenon is found with many other parameters. Similarly, if the same parameter is measured in different individuals on the same occasion, a marked variation will be noted. Height is an obvious example. The existence of such variability means that care must be exercised to ensure that differences between readings before and after treatment or between different treatment groups are not just a result of natural variation.

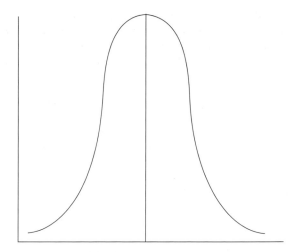

Figure 10.1. A normal distribution curve.

Where variability exists, the individuals within the sample can be arranged into a frequency distribution, showing the number of observations at different values or within certain ranges. When the sample is large enough, the frequency distribution will approach that of the population and will form a smooth curve with high frequencies at the centre of the distribution (*peak*) and low values at the ends (*lower and upper tails*). Many biological variables are described by a symmetrical distribution, known as a *normal* or *Gaussian distribution* (Fig. 10.1), but other distributions are also found. Many of the commonly used techniques of statistical analysis are based on the assumption that the data being tested is normally distributed. If this is not the case, the deductions made from the statistical analysis will be incorrect. Checks for normality of data should be made before using these statistical tests, or else alternative, non-parametric tests should be used. Non-parametric tests are less sensitive but more robust.

Quantitative data can be summarised by two measurements: one indicating the average value and the other the spread of the values. The commonest measure of the average value is the *arithmetic mean* which is usually referred to simply as the *mean*. This is calculated as the sum of the observations divided by the number of the observations. The *median* is the value that divides the distribution in half. When the distribution is skewed the median is a better estimate of the average value than the mean. When the distribution is normal the two values coincide. The *mode* is the value which occurs most frequently but it is seldom used.

The simplest indicator of variability is the *range*, which is the difference between the highest and lowest values. It does not give any indication of how the observations are arranged between the extremes and a single extreme reading can lead to a very large range. It is better to express variation in terms of deviation from the mean. This value, the *variance* is calculated as the average of the squares of the differences of each observation from the mean. The variance is useful in statistical theory but for understanding the relevance of the observations (in terms of the units of measurement), it is customary to take the square root of the variance, which is known as the *standard deviation*. For a normal distribution approximately 70% of the results lie within 1 standard deviation and 95% lie within 2 standard deviations. What has been measured is the mean and standard deviation of the sample. This will almost certainly differ from the mean and standard deviation for the population from which the sample is drawn and ultimately it is the results for the population which actually matter. If a sufficient number of samples is taken, a frequency distribution of sample means will be obtained. The mean of this distribution would be the *population mean* and the standard deviation of this distribution is the *standard error of the mean*, which gives an estimate of how close to the population mean the sample mean is. The standard error of the mean can be calculated without taking multiple samples and is equal to the standard deviation divided by the square root of the number of observations. The standard error of the mean takes into account the size of the sample as well as the variability.

It is possible to calculate a range of likely values for the true population mean based on the sample mean and the standard error of the mean. This is usually expressed as the *95% confidence interval* and is now regarded as the preferred way of expressing results.

Correlation

The second important statistical concept is the determination of the relationship of one variable to another. This can be examined graphically in a *scatter plot* and tested more formally by testing for *correlation*. There may be no correlation, a positive correlation (as A increases and B increases) or a negative correlation (as A increases and B decreases). The correlation coefficient measures the closeness of the association between the two variables. When two variables are correlated, a *linear regression* equation can be calculated which allows the calculation of the value of one variable when the value of the other variable is known. It is important to note that a correlation demonstrates association and does not say anything about causation.

In clinical practice, one variable (e.g. the risk of developing breast cancer) may be related to a number of other variables. *Multiple regression* allows examination of the effect of several independent variables on the dependent variable simultaneously. If more than one variable is likely to affect the dependent variable, then multiple regression should be performed rather than a series of linear regressions as there may be interaction between the independent variables which will not otherwise be detected. Often a variable will have an association in univariate analysis but will not be found to be significant in the multivariate analysis because its effect is contained within the effect of another variable.

Probability

The third important statistical concept is *probability*. The common definition of probability used in statistics is the proportion of times an event would occur in a large number of similar repeated trials. It has a value between 0 and 1. This is known as the *frequentist* definition in contrast to the subjective definition which is used in everyday speech where 'probability' represents the degree of belief that an event will occur. This approach corresponds to the *Bayesian* approach to statistics in which a *prior probability* of an event is decided by the investigator. After collection of the data, the probability is modified to give a *posterior probability*. This approach is not widely used in medical statistics but is becoming more common.

Any research project should begin with an hypothesis. An experiment is then designed to disprove the hypothesis and data is collected and analysed. For most biological data it is necessary to carry out statistical testing to decide if there is any difference between the experimental groups as a result of an intervention in one group. As the experiment attempts to falsify the main hypothesis, the assumption is made that there is, in fact, no difference between the groups and that any apparent difference between them occurred by chance. Somewhat confusingly, this assumption is called the *null hypothesis* (this has nothing to do with the main hypothesis of the study but refers to the basis on which the statistical analysis is done). The statistical tests are designed to show whether or not any difference between the groups could have occurred by chance. This is expressed as the *probability (p) value.*

A p-value of 0.5 means that the result obtained will occur by chance on 50% of the occasions on which the test is repeated and, therefore, there is no difference between the groups. A p-value of 0.05 means that the result obtained will occur by chance only once in every 20 times the test is repeated. By convention, $p = 0.05$ is taken to mean that the result obtained is real and is not a chance finding. This is commonly expressed in the statement that the result is *statistically significant*. As this is often referred to simply as *significant*, misunderstanding of the term is frequent with statistical significance being interpreted on many occasions as meaning important. An improvement in response rate to a new therapeutic agent from 30% to 35% may be statistically significant but does not represent a huge leap forward in treatment unless the new agent is different in its mode of action from the old, and thus may open an entirely new approach to treatment. Conversely, the new treatment may improve the response rate from 30% to 60% (which represents a major breakthrough) but the trial may be too small for a p-value of 0.05 to be attained. (This implies poor trial design, but does emphasise the problems of interpreting a p-value in isolation.)

Selecting the right statistical test

Most textbooks of statistics set out to describe how to carry out the many available statistical tests. In the era of

Table 10.1. Appropriate statistical tests for given datasets.

Type of data	Normal	Non-parametric or small numbers
Comparison of 2 independent groups		
Interval	Unpaired *t*-test	Mann–Whitney
Ordinal		Mann–Whitney
Nominal, with order		Chi-square
Nominal, without order		Chi-square
Dichotomous		Fisher's exact test
Comparison of same group under different conditions		
Interval	Paired *t*-test	Wilcoxon signed rank test
Ordinal or nominal		Sign test
Dichotomous		Matched pairs test (McNemar or Liddell)
Relationship between 2 groups		
Interval versus interval	Simple linear regression; Pearson's product moment correlation	Linear regression; Kendall's or Spearman rank correlation
Interval versus ordinal or nominal	One way analysis of variance	Kruskall–Wallis test
Ordinal versus ordinal		Kendall's or Spearman rank correlation

Note:
- Interval data has a scale with fixed and defined intervals (e.g. time or temperature).
- Ordinal data is arranged in scores from low through to high (e.g. pain scores on a visual analogue scale).
- Nominal data with order is arranged in discrete categories but with some order imposed (e.g. mild, moderate, severe). It can be difficult to distinguish from ordinal data.
- Nominal data without order is arranged in discrete categories (e.g. blood group).
- Dichotomous data comprises two distinct categories.

computer-based statistical packages it is more important to know how to select the right test for the dataset. Table 10.1 outlines the commonly used simple tests and their indications but it is always wise to consult a statistician, preferably before undertaking a study. Failures in data collection may lead to subsequent problems in analysis.

Meta-analysis

The realisation that clinically important results might be being obscured because trials were too small led to the development of new statistical techniques to allow the results from trials to be combined. It is not possible to take the results of different trials and merely add them together but the sample means are normally distributed around the population mean so, given a large enough number of sample means, it is possible to calculate the true mean and standard deviation of the population. This technique has been very successfully applied to adjuvant chemotherapy for breast cancer and is now being widely used in other settings. Once again, care must be taken in the interpretation of the results. Statistical significance does not necessarily mean clinical importance.

Critical reading

While the above discussion concerns the design and execution of research studies, a more common problem is the assessment and evaluation of published studies. In so far as is possible, clinical management should depend on evidence rather than dogma. The best evidence is that which is obtained from randomised-controlled clinical trials. When this is not available, the evidence from large, consecutive series may give some guide.

There is currently a fashion for developing consensus guidelines and it is being recommended that management decisions should be based on these guidelines. Unless these guidelines are backed by proper studies, they may do more harm than good and may actually inhibit progress. After all, the consensus in the UK until the 1980s was that mastectomy was the only safe procedure for women with primary breast cancer.

Some system for deciding the quality of evidence presented in any published report is necessary. Certain standard questions should be asked about any published study:
- Is the study of any clinical importance?
- Is the population from which the study subjects were drawn well-defined? Is the sample used representative of the population?
- Are the inclusion/exclusion criteria clearly defined and are they satisfactory? Is the sample size adequate?
- What happened to refusers/dropouts?
- Are the data from the refusers/dropouts included in the report? Are concurrent controls used?

- Is the method of allocation to treatment groups described and is it satisfactory? Is the treatment well-defined?
- Are the outcome criteria clearly defined?
- Were the therapists, assessors and patients blinded as to which treatment the patients were receiving?

These questions allow judgements to be made about the reliability and significance of a study. If the answers are satisfactory the evidence from that study can then be weighed against the evidence from other sources in order to determine the appropriate clinical action.

Different weight must be given to different types of study when deciding on action or developing guidelines. The US Agency for Health Care Policy and Research have suggested the following categories:

- Ia: Meta-analysis of randomised trials
- Ib: At least one randomised trial
- IIa: Controlled, non-randomised study
- IIb: Other quasi-experimental study
- III: Descriptive studies
- IV: Consensus views.

The greatest weight should be given to the highest form of evidence available. Guidelines can be classified on the basis of the type of evidence on which they are based.

Guidelines

- A: Directly based on Cat 1 evidence
- B: Directly based on Cat 2 or extrapolated from Cat 1
- C: Directly based on Cat 3 or extrapolated from Cat 1 or 2
- D: Directly based on Cat 4 or extrapolated from Cat 1, 2 or 3b.

Clinicians have are expected to follow the most up to date guidelines but should also be striving to improve the evidence on which their practice is based.

FURTHER READING

Ethics and law

Baxter C, Brennan M, Coldicott Y. *A Practical Guide to Medical Ethics and Law*. Manchester: PasTest, 2002

Beauchamp TL, Childers JF. *Principles of Biomedical Ethics*. London: Oxford University Press USA Inc., 2001

Brazier M. *Medicine, Patients and the Law*. London: Penguin Books, 2003

Seedhouse D. *Ethics: the Heart of Health care*. London: John Wiley and Sons Ltd, 1998

Statistics

Bland JM. *An Introduction to Medical Statistics*. Oxford: Oxford Medical Publications, 2000

Campbell MJ. *Statistics at Square Two*. London: BMJ Books, 2001

Harris M, Taylor G. *Medical Statistics Med Easy*. London: Taylor and Francis, 2003

Kirkwood RB, Sterne JAC. *Essentials of Medical Statistics*. Oxford: Blackwell Scientific Publications, 2003

Swinscow TDV, Campbell MJ. *Statistics at Square One*. London: BMJ Books, 2002

11

Haemopoietic and Lymphoreticular Systems: Anatomy, Physiology and Pathology

Dirk C Strauss[1], Abraham J Botha[2] and Irving Taylor[3]

[1] Department of Upper GI Surgery, [2] Department of Upper GI and General Surgery, St Thomas' Hospital and [3] Department of Surgery, University College London Medical School, London, UK

CONTENTS

Introduction	199
Anatomy	**200**
Bone marrow	200
Circulating cells	200
Tissue cells	203
Physiology and the normal response to surgery	**205**
Intercellular communication	205
Haemopoiesis	207
Oxygen carrying	207
Haemostasis	208
Immunity	210
Response to surgery in normal patients	214
Pathological states and surgical implications	**214**
Disordered haemopoiesis/bone marrow failure	214
Transfusion of blood products	215
Transfusion-related acute lung injury	218
Red blood cell/haemoglobin disorders	218
Disordered haemostasis	218
Immune deficiency disorders	220
Acquired immune deficiency syndrome	220
Auto-immune diseases	222
Cancer	224
Approach and differential diagnosis of lymphadenopathy	225
Splenic disorders	225
Organ transplantation	227
Further reading	**229**

INTRODUCTION

Whereas blood is something that most surgeons prefer not to see too much of whilst operating, we all depend heavily on normal quantities and qualities of the various components of circulating blood to ensure a successful outcome after surgery and to prevent peri-operative complications. The main functional components of blood that are important to the surgeon are:

- oxygen (O_2) carrying (haemoglobin);
- haemostasis (endothelial cells, platelets, coagulation, fibrinolysis);
- inflammation (granulocytes, humoral mediators, endothelial cells, fibroblasts);
- immunity (lymphocytes, macrophages, antibodies).

On some occasions surgery is performed on patients with known deficiencies in one or several of their blood components and it is important to be aware of the potential intra- and post-operative problems which constitute a risk.

In this chapter the anatomy and physiology of the haemopoietic and lymphoreticular systems, and abnormalities of these systems relevant to surgical practice are reviewed.

The haemopoietic system refers to the blood-forming aspects of the bone marrow and the released circulating cells. The lymphoreticular system refers to the secondary lymphoid tissues such as the spleen and lymph glands, as well as blood cells resident in the tissues such as macrophages, lymphocytes and mast cells. Although this is a somewhat artificial anatomical classification, it separates the functional components of blood cell formation (haemopoiesis) and blood cell function (immune response). Blood cells from both anatomical

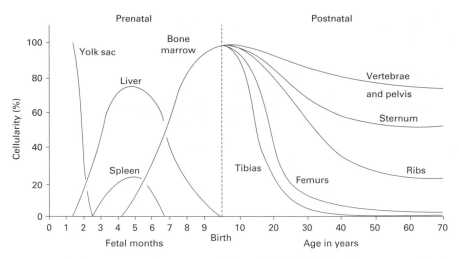

Figure 11.1. The change in organs of haemopoiesis before and after birth. After birth haemopoiesis takes place in the bone marrow, and with increasing years predominantly the marrow of the central skeleton (from Jandl, 1996).

compartments interact and are involved with both haemopoiesis and immunity.

ANATOMY

Bone marrow

In the foetus the yolk sac, liver and spleen contribute to haemopoiesis, but at birth the bone marrow harbours all the pluripotent stem cells (stem cells from which all blood cells originate) and is the sole producer of non-lymphocytic blood cells (Fig. 11.1). The bone marrow is housed in an inner space created in most bones by the opposing actions of osteoblasts and osteoclasts. This inner space or cavity consists of a labyrinth of communicating chambers formed by the crisscrossing of fine bony trabeculae. The bony framework is filled with a three-dimensional stromal cell network that forms the bedding for billions of blood-forming cells. The four main cell types of the bone marrow stroma are endothelial cells, fibroblasts, macrophages and energy-rich fat cells. From birth up to about 5 years the bone marrow cavity is fully occupied by proliferating haemopoietic cells. The haemopoietic cell mass consists of pluripotent stem cells, differentiated stem cells, precursor blood cells as well as the highly specialized and mature erythrocytes, neutrophils, monocytes, eosinophils, basophils, lymphocytes and platelets, which are continuously released into the peripheral circulation (Fig. 11.2). After the age of 5 years, bone growth exceeds that of the blood-forming elements and large parts of the bone marrow are replaced by fat. In adults about 75% of the marrow cavities are replaced by fat, so-called white marrow (in contrast to red marrow of blood-forming elements). By the age of 20 years, long bones house only 10% of haemopoietic cells, and by middle age it is the marrow of the truncal bones; that is, vertebrae, pelvis, ribs and sternum that is almost totally responsible for haemopoiesis.

Circulating cells

All cells of the haemopoietic and lymphoreticular systems are continuously being replaced and spend part of their lives in the bone marrow, part in the circulation and part in the tissues. Red blood cells and platelets only survive in the circulation and do not leave the vascular system at all during their 4-month lifespan. Neutrophils are predominantly intravascular cells where they survive for 6 h. They do leave the circulation in areas of inflammation where they survive for short periods of time, but do not return to recirculate. Monocytes circulate in small numbers, but the majority reside in the tissues as macrophages where they survive for 2–3 months. Macrophages do not re-enter the bloodstream for recirculation to other sites. Eosinophils and basophils circulate briefly before they leave the circulation to reside in the tissues for a short period of time. Lymphocytes circulate in small numbers, but spend most of their lifespan of 2–3 years in aggregates of lymphoid tissue, from where they frequently recirculate through the bloodstream to other sites (Fig. 11.3).

Red blood cells

The mature red blood cell or erythrocyte is a 7–8-μm cell with the shape of a biconcave disc and is highly specialized for carrying O_2. The cytoplasm is predominantly protein of which haemoglobin comprises 95%. The peculiar shape and deformability of erythrocytes are due to an integrated system of articulating proteins called the cytoskeleton. The cell is covered by a membrane that consists of 50% lipids arranged in a bilayer and 50% proteins. The thousands of membrane molecules create a multitude of antigens which

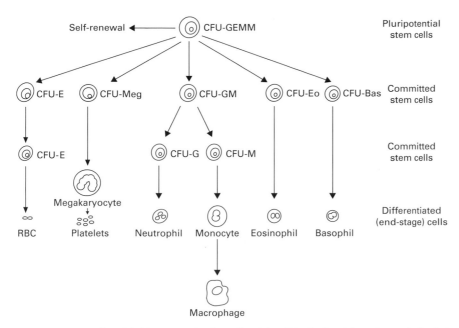

Figure 11.2. Proposed model of haemopoiesis where all peripheral blood cells originate from a single pluripotent stem cell. E: erythrocyte; Meg: megacaryocyte; Eo: eosinophil; Bas: basophil; (modified from Jandl, 1996).

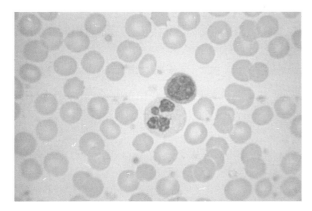

Figure 11.3. A peripheral blood smear showing normal red blood cells, platelets, a neutrophil and a lymphocyte.

make the surface of every individual's red cells quite unique. Some antigens are widely distributed in all humans and are even maintained across different species. Of particular importance to surgeons are the glycolipids which constitute the A and B antigens used for ABO blood typing. The cytoskeleton and membrane structure of erythrocytes serve as a prototype for all the other blood cells.

Neutrophils

Mature polymorphonuclear leucocytes or neutrophils circulate at a concentration of $2–7 \times 10^6$/ml of whole blood. The mature neutrophil is a round, but deformable cell of 13 μm that is characterized by two to five nuclear lobes connected by fine filamentous strands. The cytoplasm contains three types of granules: specific, azurophylic and gelatinase-containing granules. These granules harbours cytotoxic compounds such as myeloperoxide, elastase, lysozyme, components of the nicotinamide adenosine dinucleotide phosphate (NADPH) oxidase that generate toxic O_2 radicals, and various adhesion receptors. The receptor-rich plasma membrane is crucial for receiving signals and communication with the external world. The selectin and integrin groups of membrane receptors, respectively, regulate rolling along and tight adhesion to the endothelial cell lining of blood vessels, which are prerequisites for extravascular migration. Neutrophils are the circulating rapid response cells in host defense and within minutes of receiving signals can navigate and diapedese to areas of tissue injury where they respond to and release inflammatory mediators, interact with other cells, phagocytose foreign antigen and debris, and destroy unwanted material by both intra- and extracellular release of cytotoxic substances.

Monocytes

Monocytes constitute 3–8% of circulating white blood cells and their concentration in free-axial circulation is $0.2–0.8 \times 10^6$/ml of whole blood. At 16 μm across, mature monocytes are the largest blood cells in circulation. An indented nucleus occupies half the cell volume. The cytoplasm is granular due to cytotoxic granules. The monocyte is covered by a receptor-rich cell membrane which is connected by a cytoskeleton of actin filaments designed for locomotion. In addition to their phagocytic abilities and cytotoxic arsenal, monocytes have much more extensive resources than neutrophils for releasing

humoral mediators to control the local and systemic immunological response. Furthermore, monocytes can become transformed in the tissue spaces to become residential macrophages.
These specialized 'tissue monocytes' or macrophages can survive for 2–3 months and outnumber circulating monocytes by
100 : 1. Macrophages also have the capacity to present phagocytosed antigens to T- and B-lymphocytes, and thereby play
an important role in cell-mediated immunity and antibody
release.

Eosinophils

Mature eosinophils circulate at a concentration of 0.1×10^6/ml of whole blood and are the same size as mature neutrophils. Upon release from the bone marrow they leave the
bloodstream within one pass through the circulation and
diapedese through to patrol the epithelial surfaces of the
skin, gut and bronchial tree. They also accumulate in lymph
nodes where they interact with lymphocytes and take part in
early antigen recognition and phagocytosis of immune complexes. Their nuclei consists of two to three round or ovoid
lobes, and the cytoplasmic granules are larger than those of
neutrophils and of a single type. These brightly orange staining granules contain a mixture of basic and cationic proteins
which are highly toxic to parasites, tumour cells and antibody-
coated host cells.

Basophils

Mature basophils are the least common granulocyte (less
than 0.1% of leucocytes in whole blood) and similar to
eosinophils circulating numbers are subject to a circadian
rhythm with higher numbers at night. Also like eosinophils
they spend just a brief time in circulation before they migrate
to barrier tissues such as skin, mucosa and serosa. Their
nuclei are indistinctly lobulated, and the cytoplasm contains
large bluish granules which harbours a mixture of potent
inflammatory mediators including histamine. These mediators promote vasodilatation and increases endothelial permeability, both crucial components of an inflammatory
response to foreign antigen or injury.

Lymphocytes

Circulating lymphocytes amount to $1.5–4 \times 10^6$ cells/ml of
whole blood which is 30% of circulating leucocytes. However,
this is only a fraction of the mature lymphocyte pool since
99% of mature lymphocytes reside in the secondary lymphoid tissues such as the spleen and lymph nodes. Mature
lymphocytes contain a compact, rounded and sometimes
notched nucleus, and scant bluish cytoplasm lacking any
granules. Its cell contains quite unique receptors which
enable lymphocytes to recognize the universe of foreign antigens and create an immunity against them, thereby providing the opportunity for the host to develop and survive as a
unique or 'self'-identifiable individual. In addition to antibody secretion, activated lymphocytes release vast quantities

of mediators, particularly cytokines or interleukins (IL), for
interaction with and control over other cells.

B-lymphocytes

Mature B-lymphocytes released from the bone marrow
are virginal in that they have not yet undergone antigen-
dependent conversion. Antigen-dependent conversion occurs
in germinal centres of secondary lymphoid tissues and results
in two types of mature cells: that is, specialized end-stage
antibody-secreting B-cells called plasma cells, or alternatively, long-lived memory B-cells. These cells continuously
recirculate between different secondary lymphoid tissues.

T-lymphocytes

T-cell precursors are released from the bone marrow and are
concentrated in the thymus where they mature and from
where they are released to accumulate in the secondary lymphoid tissues. Mature T-cells only recognize antigen when it
is expressed on cell surface membranes in association with
major histocompatibility complex (MHC) antigens, and do not
respond to the self-components: that is, T-cells are self-tolerant.

Natural killer cells

These granular lymphocytic cells are released in mature form
from the bone marrow and circulate between the different
secondary lymphoid tissues. Their function lies somewhere
between granulocytes and lymphocytes. Natural killer (NK)
cells do not phagocytose, do not have the cell surface markers of mature lymphocytes, do not secrete antibodies, do not
develop immunological memory and do not use antibody-
dependent cell-mediated cytotoxicity (ADCC). They do recognize tumour cells, virus-infected cells, parasites, fungi and
bacteria. After recognition, they immediately discharge their
cytotoxic granules near the target cell, and move on. NK cell
function is locally enhanced by cytokines, particularly the
interferons (IFN).

Platelets

Mature platelets are released from the bone marrow by fragmentation of megacaryocytes. These anuclear cells of $2 \mu m$
in diameter circulate at a concentration of $200–400 \times 10^6$/ml
of whole blood. Some 30% of peripheral platelets are harboured in the red pulp of the spleen. The main function of
platelets are in haemostasis.

Stem cells

Stem cells for all the mature blood cells are released from the
bone marrow into the peripheral circulation in small quantities. They presumably recirculate to the bone marrow since
stem cell proliferation and maturation do not occur at any
other site in the normal adult. The physiological purpose of
stem cell recirculation is not clear, for they do not lodge in
peripheral tissues to become islands of haemopoiesis, but it
does provide the opportunity for peripheral stem cell harvesting for research and therapeutic purposes.

Tissue cells

As discussed earlier, lymphocytes and macrophages spend most of their relatively long lives in the tissue spaces, eosinophils and basophils spend most of their short lives in the tissues, whereas neutrophils leave the circulation only under inflammatory conditions. In the tissue spaces these cells of haemopoietic origin interact with each other as well as with stromal cells, endothelial cells, epithelial cells and all other cells. The elaborate system of intercellular communication is discussed later.

Endothelial cells

Although not a descendent of a haemopoietic stem cell, endothelial cells are integral components of both the haemopoietic and lymphoreticular systems. Until recently it was believed that endothelial cells have a phagocytic function in support of macrophages, and this presumed cooperation was called the reticuloendothelial system. Although this term is no longer used, we know that endothelial cells interact with blood cells to regulate haemostasis, control transfer of fluid and protein between blood and tissue spaces, regulate trafficking of all types of leucocytes between the circulation and tissue spaces and release mediators to communicate with other cells.

Fibroblasts

Fibroblasts are stromal cells that are important in creating the micro-environment in which blood cells can function. They have surface membrane receptors to communicate with the blood cells and also secretes several mediators including IL.

Reticular cells

Reticular cells are derived from fibroblasts and in conjunction with endothelial cells are responsible for creating the three-dimensional matrix that optimizes the interaction between macrophages, lymphocytes and antigen in tissues such as the bone marrow, liver sinuses, splenic red pulp, and subcapsular and paracortical regions of lymph glands.

Myofibroblasts

These fibroblast derivatives are found in the interstitial spaces of the pulmonary alveolar septa. They are attached to the epithelial basement membrane and their contraction effect the shape of both the alveoli and the interstitial space.

Macrophages

Monocytes that have become resident outside the circulation are called macrophages. They are continuously being replenished from the circulating monocytes. Macrophages are scattered throughout most tissues in the body, and in some tissues assume quite different morphological appearances and functions. These different looking macrophages have been given a variety of names that sometimes cause confusion.

Dendritic cells

These macrophages have a frilled surface membrane to enhance its capacity of antigen presentation to lymphocytes. Dendritic cells are found in all secondary lymphoid tissues as well as the thymus and are the most potent antigen-presenting cells (APC) of the immune system. After phagocytosis they can destroy antigen, but those foreign peptides that are presented on its surface membrane in association with MHC antigens, are recognized by T-lymphocytes, and result in a T-cell immune response.

Kupffer cells

Kupffer cells are macrophages that line the hepatic sinuses and develop tremendous phagocytic potential. It has been calculated that less than 1% of gut-derived bacteria and foreign antigen in the portal blood manages to pass through the liver into the systemic circulation due to the rapid phagocytosis and destruction by Kupffer cells. These cells have lost much of their antigen-presenting capabilities.

Pulmonary macrophages

The alveolar interstitial spaces are occupied by a mucopolysaccharide-containing gel and several resident cells including macrophages. Macrophages are also found within the alveolar spaces. These alveolar macrophages are 12–40 μm in diameter, have a lobulated nucleus, and have potent phagocytic and secretory capabilities. Macrophages are also found along the bronchial tree and pleura.

Langerhans cells

Langerhans cells are macrophages found in the epidermis and can be considered as dendritic cells since their strongest feature is antigen presentation. Their phagocytic capacity is secondary.

Peritoneal macrophages

The normal peritoneal cavity contains less than 100 ml of fluid and about 300 cells/mm^3, of which most are macrophages, but also some lymphocytes. These peritoneal macrophages are potent phagocytes and orchestrate peritoneal inflammation. They can also present antigen to lymphocytes to create an immune response.

Microglial cells

There are about 10–50 times more glial or support cells than neurones in the central nervous system (CNS). Oligodendrocytes, Schwann cells and astrocytes makeup the macroglia, whereas the microglia are macrophages. The function of these microglia is to remove foreign antigen and debris, as well as to present antigen to lymphocytes.

Mast cells

Mast cells contain pale round nuclei and a cytoplasm densely filled with bluish granules. They reside just below epithelial surfaces (skin, gut, respiratory tree, etc.) and around blood vessels. Although functionally akin to basophils, they are long living and thought to belong to the tissue macrophage family. They are not phagocytic and do not present antigen to lymphocytes. Upon binding of foreign antigen to its membrane receptors, degranulation occurs with release of histamine, heparin and other vasoactive peptides. Activation also results in the release of leukotrienes (LT) from the surface membrane. Mast cells are important effector cells of many of the manifestations of hypersensitivity or allergic reactions, such as urticaria, rhinitis and bronchospasm.

Lymphocytes

Although all lymphocytes originate from the pluripotent stem cells in the bone marrow, only B-lymphocytes reaches maturity in the bone marrow before release into the circulation. T-lymphocytes are released from the bone marrow in precursor forms and circulate to the thymus for further cell division and maturation. The bone marrow and thymus gland are called primary lymphoid organs. Mature T- and B-cells released from the thymus and bone marrow are concentrated in secondary lymphoid tissues. The major secondary lymphoid organs are the spleen and lymph nodes, but aggregates of secondary lymphoid tissue are also found below the mucosa of several organs (called mucosa-associated lymphoid tissue or MALT). MALT include Peyer's patches in the gut (also called gut-associated lymphoid tissue or GALT), the adenoids and tonsils (Waldeyer's ring), bronchus-associated lymphoid tissue (BALT), peritoneum-associated lymphoid tissue (PALT) and lymphoid aggregates in the genitourinary tract, conjunctiva and salivary glands. The functions of the secondary lymphoid tissue are to trap and concentrate foreign substances and antigens, and to allow division and differentiation of lymphocytes to produce antibodies, antigen-specific T-cells and secrete mediators that amplify the inflammatory and immune responses. In addition to these specialized aggregates of lymphocytes, scattered lymphocytes are also found in most tissue throughout the body. Lymphocytes frequently move and reside in many different tissues throughout their lifespans.

Thymus

The thymus lies partly in the neck anterior to the trachea and partly in the anterior mediastinum in the chest. The organ has a profuse blood supply and lymphatic drainage. It consists of two to three lobes subdivided in lobules by fibrous trabeculae. Each lobule has a cortex and a medulla containing epithelial cells and thymocytes, which are immature T-cells. The gland starts enlarging during foetal life and reaches its largest size at puberty after which it begins to regress. The main function of the thymus is a bed for T-lymphocyte maturation, which involves commitment of surface receptors to recognition of a specific antigen. Most of T-cell maturation occurs during foetal life and for a short time after birth. Removal of the thymus in the neonatal period therefore results in severe T-cell deficiencies, yet removal of the gland from an adult generally

has little effect since most T-cells have matured and populated the secondary lymphoid organs by this time. Adult thymectomy could result in T-cell deficiencies if T-lymphocytes are subsequently destroyed by chemotherapy or whole-body irradiation, for replenishment of secondary lymphoid tissue by new mature T-cells will not be possible.

Spleen

The spleen is a soft vascular organ of 150 g surrounded by a fibrous capsule and has a blood supply of 250 ml/min (i.e. 5% of the cardiac output). After entering the hilum the splenic artery divides into a latticework of arterioles. Each arteriole is surrounded by a cuff or peri-arteriolar lymphocytic sheath (PALS) forming the white pulp. The spongy reddish tissue in which the white pulp is embedded is called the red pulp. The red pulp consists of sinuses and splenic cords containing large quantities of red blood cells and macrophages. Since the spleen has an arterial supply but no afferent lymphatics it has been called the lymph gland or filter of the blood. By virtue of the unique vascular structure of the red pulp it is extremely proficient at monitoring blood cells passing through. Altered, imperfect or aging red cells are checked and then either remodelled or destroyed by the resident macrophages. The spleen also filters and removes foreign particles, antigens and defective white cells and platelets from the circulation. In addition to the large quantities of lymphocytes harboured in the spleen, up to 30% of the total platelet mass can be pooled in the spleen. The spleen also has an important immunological function. In addition to the liver and lung, the spleen is the third major macrophage-rich lymphoreticular organ, designed to filter blood borne organisms and antigen, both for antigen destruction and antigen presentation to the T- and B-lymphocytes.

Lymph glands

Lymph glands are small ovoid structures (usually less than 1-cm long) found in various regions of the body. Several afferent lymphatics enter a lymph gland and empty into a subcapsular sinus in which macrophages are found. The outer part of the gland is called the cortex where B-lymphocytes are organized in follicles. On exposure to antigen cortical follicles develop germinal centres containing dense populations of dividing B-cells. The interfollicular regions and the paracortex contain T-cells as well as macrophages. The macrophages trap, process and present the antigen to T-cells with specificity against that specific antigen. The central part of the gland is called the medulla and is predominantly made up of antibody-secreting plasma cells. The hilum of the lymph gland usually contains only one efferent lymphatic as well as a feeding artery and a vein. The efferent lymphatic contains lymph, antibodies and cells, and joins other lymphatics to form the thoracic duct that drains into the left subclavian vein. Lymph glands are highly efficient at trapping antigen and creating interactions between macrophages, B- and T-cells. These interactions result in destruction of the antigen and/or an immune response consisting of the production of antibodies and antigen-specific T-cells (Fig. 11.4).

Peyer's patches, adenoids, tonsils and other MALT

These are aggregates of lymphoid tissue found in and below the lining of various organs. The larger aggregates consist of an outer mantel zone of lymphocytes and macrophages, and an inner germinal centre. Their function is to trap antigen that passes directly through the mucosa and to destroy the antigen and/or generate an immune response similar to lymph glands.

Scattered lymphocytes

In addition to the aggregates of lymphocytes mentioned above, individual T- and B-lymphocytes, and NK cells are scattered throughout the body. These cells can recognize undesirable antigen or cells, and promote local inflammation or trigger an immune response.

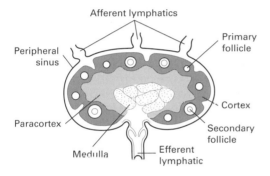

Figure 11.4. A diagrammatic illustration of the histology of a lymph node.

PHYSIOLOGY AND THE NORMAL RESPONSE TO SURGERY

Intercellular communication

Effective communication is crucial in a complex system of solid organs, tissue cells and different circulating cells all concerned with maintaining the integrity and defending the host against harmful antigens and intruders. The main components of intercellular communication are mediators (free-floating signals), membrane receptors (for receiving signals), intracellular signal transduction (interpreting the signals) and effector mechanisms (acting upon the signal) (Fig. 11.5).

Mediators

Mediators are defined as communication molecules derived from one cell type that act on another by virtue of specific receptors, and are intermediate in lifespan between the long-lived hormones and the short-lived and local acting neurotransmitters. These mediators are released by all blood and stromal cells of the haemopoietic and lymphoreticular systems, particularly macrophages, lymphocytes, endothelial cells and fibroblasts. Little is known about normal control mechanisms because under steady-state conditions mediators are released locally and act locally. Only when produced in excess are they detectable in the bloodstream. The terminology of mediators is confusing and the terms mediator, cytokine, growth factor, monokine, lymphokine and IL are often used interchangeably. In this chapter the term mediator will be used as the all-inclusive term for cellular

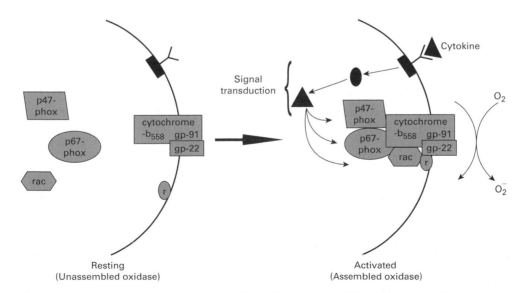

Figure 11.5. Cellular communication pathways illustrated in a neutrophil. In the resting neutrophil on the left the membrane oxidase complex responsible for producing toxic O_2 radicals is unassembled and therefore not active. On the right binding of a cytokine to its membrane receptor has resulted in signal transduction and assembly of the oxidase enzyme. The resultant effector response is a respiratory burst with VO_2 and production of free-O_2 radicals.

communication molecules, whereas cytokine will refer only to protein mediators, in contrast to lipid mediators and other cascade molecules. The list of cytokines continues to grow and many derive their names from the first function that was ascribed to them (i.e. colony-stimulating factors (CSFs), growth factors, IL, tumour necrosis factor (TNF) and IFN).

Growth factors

Several cytokines have been discovered that promote cellular proliferation; for example, platelet-derived growth factor (PDGF), endothelium-derived growth factor (EDGF), transforming growth factor beta (TGF-β), fibroblast-derived growth factor (FDGF) and epidermal growth factor (EGF).

Colony-stimulating factors

The five most important cytokines in this group are granulocyte-CSF (G-CSF), granulocyte–macrophage-CSF (GM-CSF), macrophage-CSF (M-CSF), multi-CSF and thrombopoietin. Receptors for the different CSFs are found on bone marrow stem cells, precursor cells as well as mature cells in circulation, and it is clear that they influence blood cells during all stages of their development, as well as the function of mature cells.

Interleukins

The IL group of cytokines are proteins that are produced throughout the body by macrophages, lymphocytes, endothelial cells, granulocytes and fibroblasts. They are numbered in order of discovery. IL-15, for example, is a recently discovered T-cell growth factor released by T-cells and endothelial cells.

Tumour necrosis factors α and β

TNF-α was originally described as a protein that could cause haemorrhagic necrosis in laboratory-induced sarcomas in mice. The TNF are potent pro-inflammatory cytokines that are released early during an inflammatory response and have a variety of effects on several different cell types.

Interferon-γ

These cytokines are released by activated helper T-cells and stimulate NK cells and macrophages for enhanced cell killing.

Lipid mediators

Activation of phospholipase A_2 (PLA$_2$) results in release of the plasma membrane phospholipids, lyso-platelet-activating factor (lyso-PAF) and arachidonic acid. These two membrane products are further metabolized into three classes of lipid mediators: PAF, LT and prostaglandins (PG). The latter two groups derived from arachidonic acid are collectively called eicosanoids. Examples of LT are LTA_4, LTB_4, LTC_4, etc. and examples of PG are PGA_2, PGE_2, PGI_2 and thromboxane A_2 (TXA_2). These lipid mediators possess variable and highly potent biological activities.

Circulating cascades

The complement, kinin, fibrinolytic and clotting cascades are systems of molecules circulating in the plasma. These plasma systems are not mediators in the strictest sense of the definition. However, under certain conditions, for example, exposure to foreign antigen, cellular injury or a break in the endothelial lining, these circulating molecules become activated and the different cascades produce compounds such as C3a, C5a, C567, bradykinin, kallikrein, plasmin, fibrinopeptides and others that have profound mediating effects on all the blood cells.

Receptors

The plasma membrane with its basic structure of a double layer of lipids and interspersed transmembrane glycoproteins is a biologically active structure. It is continually being renewed by endocytosis, which is a process whereby a part of the membrane is pinched off, internalized and recycled with the intracellular membranous structures such as lysosomes, Golgi apparatus or endoplasmic reticulum. Similarly, intracellular vesicles continuously fuse with the cell membrane to replenish membrane lipids and proteins. Thousands of membrane molecules are presented to the extracellular environment, and many are genetically coded for to be very specific receptors that bind particular ligands. A receptor's efficiency at binding its ligand can be increased either by increasing its affinity (usually by a conformational change) or by increasing the number of receptors. Receptor downregulation occurs by decreasing the affinity for its particular ligand or internalizing the receptor. Several types of receptors have been identified on the cells of the haemopoietic and lymphoreticular systems (e.g. immunoglobulin, IL and adhesion receptors).

Signal transduction

Binding of a ligand or mediator to its specific cell membrane receptor activates intracellular signal transduction pathways that modulate distinct, measurable effector responses. The key components via which G-protein-linked receptors, such as most of the cytokine receptors, transduce a signal are: the phospholipases C, D and A_2 (PLC, PLD and PLA$_2$), and second messengers such as diacylglycerol (DAG), inositol triphosphate (IP$_3$), phosphatidate and arachidonate. This signalling causes calcium mobilization, protein kinase C (PKC) activation and phosphorylation of serine/threonine or tyrosine residues. Although the direct causal links between ligand, phospholipases, second messengers, calcium, PKC, phosphorylated amino acids and effector function remain to be elucidated, much has already been learned. The expanding knowledge about the molecular mechanisms of signal transduction creates numerous therapeutic options for modifying cellular behaviour.

Effector response

Most mediators cause several effector responses in the same cell and also have effects on more than one cell type.

Furthermore, numerous different mediators are usually released simultaneously, some with opposing functions. The final response of a haemopoietic cell *in vivo* is therefore the result of very complex intracellular signalling indeed. The most important effector responses of haemopoietic cells are *haemopoiesis* (production of new blood cells from stem cells residing in the bone marrow), *chemotaxis* (one-directional movement of a blood cell along a chemical gradient), *adhesion* (firm adherence of longer than 30 s to an endothelial cell), *diapedesis* (movement of a blood cell through narrow tissue spaces by deforming itself), *phagocytosis* (ingestion of a particle by enveloping it in part of the surface membrane), *degranulation* (release of intracellular vesicles and their contents), *mediator release* (release of proteins from the cytoplasm or lipids from the surface membrane to influence the function of other cells), *antibody release* (release of immunoglobulin receptors from B-lymphocytes), *cytotoxicity* (killing of other cells by attaching to them and releasing toxic products in their proximity).

Haemopoiesis

Stem cells

All mature circulating blood cells originate from the same stem cells in the bone marrow. The pool of pluripotential ('master' or 'most senior') stem cells makeup less than 0.05% of the bone marrow mass and divides only about every 5 days. Yet with genetic pre-programming and appropriate stimulation with growth factors, these undifferentiated cells undergo differentiation through a series of cell divisions to form more committed stem cells. Committed stem cells are also called colony-forming units (CFUs) or colony-forming cells (CFCs). These CFUs differentiate further through a series of cell divisions to bring forth nine different fully functional and mature blood cells: that is, red cells, platelets, neutrophils, monocytes, eosinophils, basophils, B-lymphocytes, T-lymphocytes and NK cells. The lifespan of mature blood cells is variable, but brief; that is, 6 h for granulocytes, 10 days for platelets, 4 months for red blood cells and months to years for lymphocytes. It is calculated that under normal circumstances approximately 500 000 million blood cells are replaced each day (Fig. 11.2).

Colony-stimulating factors

The control of haemopoiesis is very complex indeed. CSFs and allied cytokines form complex signalling networks that act as positive and negative regulators of haemopoiesis. Under normal conditions haemopoiesis and the release of mature cells from the bone marrow occurs at a steady rate, and the numbers of circulating cells are maintained within narrow ranges. When secretion of mediators of haemopoiesis is increased as occurs during inflammation, bone marrow hyperplasia occurs and output of mature granulocytes can increase several folds. Erythropoiesis is stimulated by the renal hormone erythropoietin.

Erythropoietin

Erythropoietin, the glycoprotein hormone regulating red blood cell formation, is released by peritubular interstitial cells in the kidney. The kidney therefore has the dual function of controlling the blood volume as well as the red cell mass or haematocrit, which in turn determines blood viscosity. Viscosity is a crucial determinant of the speed of blood flow and thereby red cell and O_2 transport through the tissues. Tissue hypoxia results immediately in an increased cardiac output and blood flow, but prolonged hypoxia results in increased erythropoietin release and increased red cell production. The erythropoietin receptor (ER-R) on stem and precursor cells in the bone marrow is a G-protein-linked transmembrane peptide. The gene coding for erythropoietin is on the long arm of chromosome 7 and has been successfully transfected for commercial production of recombinant human erythropoietin (rEP). rEP is used clinically to stimulate erythropoiesis in patients wanting to donate blood pre-operatively for autotransfusion afterwards or post-operatively in patients in whom blood transfusion is prohibited (e.g. in Jehova's witnesses). It is also successfully used to treat the anaemia associated with chronic renal failure.

Oxygen carrying

The red blood cell

Red blood cells makeup 99% of the circulating cell mass. The normal venous haematocrit in men is 45% and in women 41%. The sole function of the red blood cell is to transport O_2. During the 1–2 s pass through capillary vessels, red blood cells (7–8 μm) have to deform and squeeze through 5 μm spaces in single file. This tight fit enhances gas exchange with the surrounding tissue cells. In circulation red blood cells form stacks or rouleaux, held together by large plasma proteins such as fibrinogen. At maturity red cells are cleared from the circulation by tissue macrophages, particularly those lining the sinuses of the liver, spleen and bone marrow. In the macrophage the cell membrane is rapidly degraded, the globin chains split into their constituent amino acids and the haem molecule split into its porphyrin ring and iron. The porphyrin ring is catabolized to bilirubin which is released into the circulation for recycling by the liver, and the iron molecule is transferred to transferrin for recycling. Most people have observed the colour changes from blue-black to purple-green to yellow as cutaneous macrophages degrade red cells and haem in a subcutaneous haematoma.

Haemoglobin

The normal adult haemoglobin molecule (Hb A) has a tetrameric structure and has a molecular weight of 64 458. It consists of four unbranched globin polypeptides: two identical α-chains and two identical β-chains (Fig. 11.6). Foetal haemoglobin (Hb F) has two α-chains and two γ-chains. Each globin chain has a haem group attached to it. The haem molecule

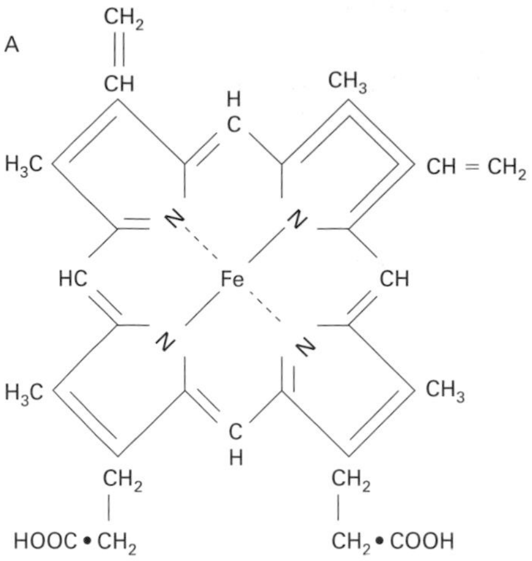

Figure 11.6. A haemoglobin molecule.

consists of a tetrapyrrole ring, protoporphyrin IX, surrounding a single ferrous ion. Free haemoglobin, that is haemoglobin not enveloped in a red cell plasma membrane are quickly bound to haptoglobin, a plasma transport protein, but large amounts can be toxic, causing vasospasm, endothelial cell leak and renal failure. Defects in globin synthesis in the cytoplasmic ribosomes of red cell precursors result in the haemoglobinopathies and thalassaemias. Defects in haem synthesis in the mitochondria of precursor cells result in the porphyrias.

Iron metabolism

Most cells harbour iron reserves in the centre of large cytoplasmic proteins called ferritin. About 60% of the body's excess iron is stored in the liver. Men loose about 1 mg of iron and females about 2 mg a day, mostly in faeces and menstrual fluid, and these amounts are absorbed from the diet by the mucosal cells of predominantly the jejunum. However, there is a daily re-cycling of 20 mg of iron in the normal adult. Free iron is toxic and as soon as it becomes available it is bound up by glycoproteins called transferrins. Each transferrin molecule can bind two ferric ions (Fe^{3+}) and transport them through the circulation. Receptors for transferrin (TfR) are found on the plasma membranes of all cells, but in cells with high iron requirements such as red blood cell precursors in the bone marrow, these receptors are greatly increased. Upon binding of an iron-laden transferrin molecule to a TfR, the receptor becomes internalized by endocytosis and the iron is released for haem synthesis or for storage in ferritin.

Oxygen delivery and consumption

The amount of O_2 delivered to tissues is a function of the quantity of blood flow, the amount of haemoglobin in the blood and the amount of O_2 bound to the haemoglobin.

The quantity of blood flow is determined by the pressure gradient, the radius of the vessel, the length of the vessel and the viscosity of the blood (haematocrit). Not surprisingly, at a normal blood pressure, optimal O_2 transport by whole blood occurs at a haematocrit of 40–45%. In a normal adult with a haemoglobin concentration of 15 g%, a temperature of 37°C, a pH of 7.4 and an O_2 tension (PO_2) in arterial blood of 90 mmHg, haemoglobin is 97% saturated. Under the same conditions and a venous PO_2 of 40 mmHg, haemoglobin is 75% saturated, indicating that 4.4 ml of O_2 is being released to the tissues per 100 ml of blood passing through. An essential feature of haemoglobin is that it has a strong affinity to bind O_2 at the high O_2 tensions in the alveolar capillaries, and a lower affinity for O_2 and thus release O_2 at the lower O_2 tensions in tissue capillaries. This is best explained by the sigmoidal O_2 dissociation curve. In intensive care patients with balloon-tipped pulmonary artery catheters in place, O_2 delivery (DO_2) can be calculated with the formula: DO_2 = cardiac output × haemoglobin concentration × O_2 saturation, and by comparing the O_2 content in arterial blood with that of the right ventricle, the consumption of O_2 (VO_2) can also be calculated. Interestingly, in septic patients, despite delivering large amounts of O_2 to the tissues, it is not consumed, presumably due to acquired errors of cellular metabolism.

Oxygen saturation

When O_2 is bound to the ferrous ion, oxyhaemoglobin turns bright red compared to the bluish colour of carboxyhaemoglobin. This fact is exploited by pulse oxymeters which determine haemoglobin colour transcutaneously as an index of the percentage of haemoglobin saturated with O_2. Pulse oxymeters are not accurate in patients with a haemoglobin less than 5 g%. Another caveat is that bound carbon monoxide (CO) also turns haemoglobin red which will therefore result in falsely high readings of O_2 saturation.

Haemostasis

The lining of blood vessels, consisting of a continuous layer of endothelial cells attached to a basement membrane, is essential for the normal laminar flow of blood. When this layer or the whole vessel wall is breached, the body employs a complex interplay of cells and circulating molecules to patch the hole and arrest the haemorrhage. The main components of a haemostatic response are endothelial cells, platelets, coagulation and fibrinolysis.

Endothelial cells

Endothelial cells lining arteries and capillary vessels are densely packed together, whereas in veins the arrangement is more loose in order that blood cells can diapedese into the tissues with ease. In normal laminar blood flow, neutrophils and platelets roll along the endothelial cells and no firm adhesion of neutrophils or aggregation of platelets takes place. During these steady-state conditions platelet aggregation is prevented by endothelial cell mediators released due to the shear force of flowing blood (e.g. nitric oxide (NO), tissue plasminogen activator (t-PA) and prostacyclin (prostaglandin I_2 or PGI_2)) (Fig. 11.7). Coagulation of plasma is prevented by thrombomodulin, a large endothelial cell membrane receptor, which binds thrombin and converts plasma protein C to activated protein C, a direct inhibitor of coagulation. Endothelial cells also release antithrombin III which is a polypeptide that neutralizes thrombin by binding to it. However, when the vascular tree is breached, endothelial cells can call several potent haemostatic mechanisms into play. It releases endothelin-1 (ET-1), a small peptide, which is one of the most potent vasoconstrictor substances known. Injured and activated endothelial cells upregulate the selectin, intercellular adhesion molecule (ICAM) and integrin groups of adhesion receptors on their cell membranes which all cause adhesion and activation of platelets. Retraction and loss of endothelial cells result in the exposure of platelets to the subendothelial basement membrane layer which contains von Willebrand factor (vWF), fibronectin and collagen, all potent binders and activators of platelets.

Platelets

Platelets are the most important circulating component responsible for haemostasis. The platelet cytoplasm contains numerous granules and is traversed by actin filaments that are connected to the plasma membrane and intracellular canalicular system. Free-rolling platelets become activated when they become adherent through specific surface membrane receptors to extracellular matrix molecules, fibronectin, collagen and vWF, or to endothelial cells. Activated platelets becomes 'sticky' by binding to fibrinogen, and sticky platelets clump or aggregate together. These activated platelets degranulate and also release eicosanoids and PAF from their surface membranes. Platelet granules contain numerous mediators and molecules including ADP, PDGF and coagulation factors. Through these molecules they effect the function of stationary as well as passing cells, particularly other platelets, and thereby propagate platelet aggregation and the formation of a haemostatic plug. Platelets contain numerous receptors for thrombin and the surface membranes of activated platelets become ideal platforms for plasma coagulation (Fig. 11.8).

Coagulation

Blood coagulation represents the conversion of the soluble plasma protein, fibrinogen, into an insoluble fibrillar polymer called fibrin, and plasma is thereby changed from a solution into a gel. Coagulation, that is conversion of fibrinogen to fibrin, is catalysed by the proteolytic enzyme thrombin; however, it is the end result of complex serial reactions involving circulating procoagulant proteins. These coagulation factors are named by Roman numerals in order of discovery from I to XIII. Traditionally coagulation has been described as following either an extrinsic (initiated by tissue thromboplastin) or

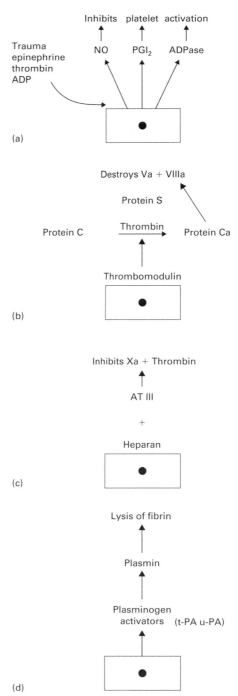

Figure 11.7. Mechanisms (a–d) whereby endothelial cells prevent inopportune platelet plug formation and coagulation. Endothelial cells synthesize NO, PGI_2 (prostacyclin), thrombomodulin, heparin and plasminogen activators, all of which prevent thrombosis and thereby help preserve vascular patency. AT III: antithrombin III (modified from Colman RW *et al.* Chapter 1, In: Colman RW *et al.* (eds), *Hemostasis and Thrombosis: Basic Principles and Clinical Practice*, 3rd edn. Philadelphia: JB Lippincott Company, 1994).

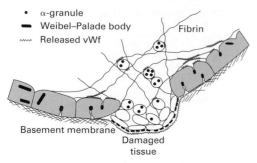

- α-granule
- Weibel–Palade body
- Released vWf

Fibrin

Basement membrane

Damaged tissue

Figure 11.8. A diagrammatic representation of the role of platelets in coagulation. After a breach in the endothelial cell lining, platelets in the presence of vWF, adhere to the exposed matrix. Activated platelets provide a template for activation of the coagulation cascades and thus formation of fibrin (modified from Jandl, 1996).

intrinsic (initiated by circulating factors) pathway, although it is now recognized that these two pathways are not the full story.

Fibrinolysis

Clot removal or fibrinolysis is mediated by the fibrin splitting protease called plasmin. Plasmin is formed from a precursor, plasminogen, by specialized plasminogen activators called t-PA and urokinase-type plasminogen activator (u-PA or urokinase). Streptokinase produced by several strains of haemolytic streptococci and produced commercially, indirectly activates plasminogen, and is therefore therapeutically used to lyse clots. Fibrin degradation products (FDPs) are potent inhibitors of coagulation, and when their plasma levels become elevated, for example, with disseminated intravascular clotting (DIC) and subsequent clot lysis, can cause a bleeding disorder.

Clinical assessment of haemostasis

History and physical examination

Ask about and look for petechia, purpura, echymoses, easy bruising or spontaneous bleeding from mucosal surfaces.

Platelet count

This test is automatically done as part of a full blood count. Platelet counts of less than 100 000 requires monitoring, but bleeding is rarely a problem with platelet counts between 50 and 100 000. Counts of less than 10 000, however, almost invariably leads to bleeding.

Bleeding time

The bleeding time after a small skin incision is a good indication of platelet function. Seepage of blood into filter paper normally stops after 7–8 min, but when platelet numbers are reduced below 10 000 or their function is impaired, bleeding can continue for up to 30 min.

Activated partial thromboplastin time

By adding an exogenous 'partial' thromboplastin such as soya phosphatide to whole blood, the intrinsic (particularly factors

XII, XI, IX and VIII) and final common pathways of coagulation are tested. This test is unaffected by factor VII deficiency. This test is frequently used to monitor heparin therapy, since heparin acts by enhancing antithrombin III and thereby inhibiting several coagulation factors, including factor X.

Prothrombin time

Adding a 'complete' tissue thromboplastin to whole blood tests the factor VII dependent part of the extrinsic (particularly factors VII, V and X) and final common pathways of coagulation. Results are usually given in terms of the international normalized ratio (INR). This test is frequently used to monitor warfarin therapy, since warfarin acts by inhibiting the vitamin K-dependent production of factors II, VII, IX and X by the liver.

Thrombin time

Adding thrombin to whole blood tests the conversion of fibrinogen to fibrin. When coagulation is prolonged by this test it suggests fibrinogen deficiency, or inhibition of thrombin by heparin or FDPs.

Immunity

Immunity means resistance or protection of the host (self) against foreign or environmental (non-self) agents. In the broadest sense the immune system refers to all the protective mechanisms used by the body. Traditionally, the non-specific protection mechanisms: for example, skin, mucous membranes, cough reflex, gastric acid and phagocytic cells such as neutrophils and macrophages have been referred to as innate immunity, whereas the specific protection mechanism based on the molecular recognition of self- and non-self-antigens by lymphocytes, have been referred to as acquired immunity.

Innate (natural/non-specific) immunity

The skin and mucous membranes provide highly efficient barriers against intrusion of foreign organisms or agents. Should either the skin or mucous membrane become breached, organisms and agents easily gain access to tissues, and tissues have to call upon cellular defense mechanisms for protection. The coordinated tissue response to foreign body intrusion or cellular injury is called inflammation.

Inflammation

The cellular injury resulting in inflammation may be caused by changes in temperature, ischaemia/reperfusion, infection or ionizing radiation, but the tissue response is very similar. Injured cells release mediators that are recognized by local stromal, endothelial and haemopoietic cells such as macrophages and lymphocytes. These response cells (sometimes referred to as the leucoendothelial system) in turn release inflammatory mediators. These mediators cause vasodilatation, increased capillary permeability with fluid and protein leak, and extravascular sequestration of large

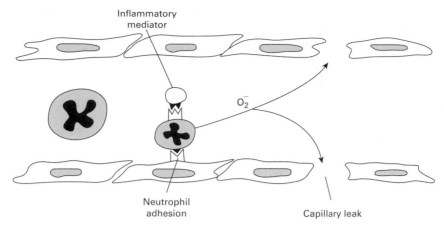

Figure 11.9. A schematic illustration of a capillary vessel during early inflammation. The endothelial cells express receptors which bind to neutrophil adhesion molecules. The firm adhesion results in neutrophil activation with release O_2 radicals and other mediators. The result will be endothelial cell activation and contraction with leakage of plasma into interstitial spaces.

numbers of neutrophils and macrophages in the injured area. The aim of inflammation is healing of injured tissues and host defense. Cellular debris and foreign antigen are phagocytosed and destroyed. Antigen may be presented to lymphocytes to produce memory cells for an enhanced response on a second exposure to the antigen. Inflammation can further be described as local and/or systemic (Fig. 11.9).

Local inflammation

The clinical signs of local inflammation have been described by Celsus (25 AD): 'Notae vero inflammationis sunt quattuor *rubor* et *tumor* cum *calore* et *dolore*', with Galen (AD 170) later adding '*Functio laesa*' to the definition. If the injurious agent is removed or overcome by the local inflammatory response, the inflammation will subside with complete restitution of the original architecture and function of the injured tissue (*resolution*), or when tissue had been destroyed, with the formation of *scar tissue*. Persistence of injury will result in *chronic inflammation* with gradual destruction to tissues caused by the inflammatory process. Should the body mount an *inadequate* inflammatory response, poor wound healing and uncontrolled infection may result. Under certain conditions a normal or *exaggerated* local inflammatory process can become deleterious; for example, intracranial inflammatory oedema after head injury, inflammatory bowel disease and laryngeal oedema in croup.

Systemic inflammation

In addition to local inflammation, tissue trauma and severe infection cause a systemic response expressed as tachycardia, fever or hypothermia, tachypnoea and evidence of inadequate organ perfusion or organ dysfunction. The systemic response to infection has traditionally been defined as sepsis. However, what was traditionally regarded as 'sepsis' is in fact a systemic

inflammatory response mounted by the host. In up to 50% of patients who appear 'septic' no source of infection can be found. This systemic inflammatory response can also result from several other insults such as acute pancreatitis, major trauma, burns, ischaemia/reperfusion (e.g. repair of abdominal aortic aneurysm) and haemorrhagic shock (e.g. massive gastrointestinal bleed). It is best to use the term systemic inflammatory response syndrome (SIRS) to describe the systemic inflammatory response common to a variety of clinical insults and to reserve the term sepsis for the systemic response to proven infection. The underlying mechanisms of SIRS are the same as those responsible for creating local inflammation (i.e. endothelial cells, circulating blood cells and inflammatory mediators). There is generalized vasodilatation, capillary leak with extravasation of fluid into extracellular spaces, and inflammatory cells can be found sequestered in virtually all organs. It is unclear whether this systemic inflammation is beneficial to the host. What is clear is that excessive systemic inflammation results in acute lung injury with pulmonary oedema and the adult respiratory distress syndrome (ARDS), as well as renal failure, liver failure and cardiac dysfunction; that is, so-called multiple organ failure (MOF).

Acquired (specific) immunity

This form of specialist host protection is only present in vertebrates. It is based on immunoglobulin and T-cell receptors (TcR+) recognizing specific antigens, with either acceptance of antigen as normal host (*self*) or activation of a response to destroy unacceptable or foreign (*non-self*) antigen. The main components responsible for antigen recognition are antibodies, APC, B- and T-lymphocytes. Tolerance of self-antigen, crucial to survival of the host, is thought to develop during early foetal life when potentially hostile lymphocytes are destroyed, and lymphocytes that can recognize self-antigen are allowed to proliferate. Exposure to non-self-antigen with the resultant secretion of specific antibodies and the development of memory lymphocytes begin soon after birth.

Antigens

Any molecule or agent capable of binding specifically to either lymphocytes or antibodies are called antigens. They are typically large molecules (>6000 Da) with chemical complexity. A hapten is an antigen that is too small to elicit an immune response on its own, but becomes immunogenic when bound to a carrier molecule. The part of the antigen recognized by a lymphocyte or antibody is called an epitope. Of the four major chemical classes, proteins are by far the most immunogenic. Carbohydrates are generally not immunogenic, but when bound to cell membrane proteins in the form of glycoproteins (e.g. ABO blood groups) become highly immunogenic. Lipids and nucleic acids are rarely immunogenic. Whereas antibodies and B-lymphocytes can bind to freely circulating antigen, T-cells can only recognize antigen that is presented on a cell surface membrane.

MHC molecules and antigen presentation

Several cell surface molecules are unique to a certain cell type, but constant in all individuals; for example, cluster determinant (CD) 4 on some lymphocytes in all humans, whereas others, for example, MHC class I and II molecules are present on the surface membranes of all cells in a specific individual, and are coded for by a set of unique MHC genes in that individual. The best-studied human MHC genes are the human leucocyte antigens (HLA) on chromosome 6. Whereas B-lymphocytes and antibodies can bind to freely circulating antigen, T-cell responses to antigen are MHC restricted; that is, T-cells can only recognize and respond to antigen when the antigen is presented together with MHC molecules on a cell surface membrane. Antigen presentation can occur on any cell type (e.g. virus-infected hepatocytes), but some cells such as macrophages are specialized APC. After antigen is phagocytosed by macrophages, the antigen is bound to MHC molecules on the endoplasmic reticulum and both are then recycled to the surface membrane for assessment by T-lymphocytes.

Lymphocytes

Specific antigen recognition by mature B-lymphocytes are via IgM and IgD immunoglobulin receptors (IgM$^+$ and IgD$^+$) which are pre-programmed to recognize specific antigens, whereas T-lymphocytes recognize specific antigen by a differently structured two-chain TcR$^+$. T- and B-lymphocytes interact closely in effecting an immune response. After the first encounter with an antigen, lymphocytes undergo transformation, proliferate and effect their immune functions such as antibody release, cytokine release, cell killing and destruction of antigen. These lymphocytes are considered primed and retain a memory of the event. Upon second exposure to the same antigen, the immune response is faster and much enhanced, the so-called memory response. Subpopulations of B- and T- lymphocytes are defined by serology using a series of cell surface antigens called CD antigens. CD4$^+$, CD8$^+$, CD19$^+$, CD34$^+$, CD44$^+$, etc. are numbered in sequence of their discovery and more than 130 have already been described. For example, B-lymphocytes also contain CD19, CD20, CD21, CD32, CD40 and CD79 antigens on their cell membrane. Mature T-lymphocytes are subdivided into two subpopulations, helper cells (CD4$^+$) and cytotoxic cells (CD8$^+$). When antigen expressed in association with MHC class II molecules bind their specific TcR on a CD4$^+$ T-cell, T-cell activation results in cytokine release. Cytokines affect the function of T-cells, B-cells and many other cell types. CD8$^+$ T-cells bind to antigen expressed on cell surfaces in association with MHC class I molecules, and activation of these T-cells results in killing of the infected cells.

Antibodies

An antibody is a soluble and circulating immunoglobulin receptor secreted by B-lymphocytes. Immunoglobulins belong to the class of proteins called globulins because of their globular structure.

Molecular structure

By using the enzyme papain, each immunoglobulin molecule can be split up into three fragments: two of which are the antigen-binding fragments (Fab) and one which is crystallizable fragment (Fc), and responsible for the biological activities of the molecule. Alternatively, mercaptoethanol, a reagent that breaks disulfide bonds, can be used to divide the immunoglobulin molecule up into four peptide chains: two identical heavy (H) chains and two identical light (L) chains (Fig. 11.10).

Antigen-binding (receptor) part

The receptor part of the immunoglobulin molecule resides in the variable region. It is quite amazing that this region is capable of enough variety to recognize probably all of the enormous number of antigenic substances in the universe, and may even create a response to antigen that have never been seen on earth. The variety results from a genetic mechanism unique to lymphocytes called rearrangement. A further result of genetic rearrangement is that the antigenic specificity of a single lymphocyte becomes fixed. Each B-lymphocyte therefore secretes antibodies of only one antigenic specificity, even though the antibodies may be of several different classes.

Classes (isotypes) of immunoglobulins

Immunoglobulins consist of five different classes based on the type of heavy chain: μ-chains in IgM, γ-chains in IgG, α-chains in IgA, δ-chains in IgD and ε-chains in IgE. These heavy chains are combined with one of the only two types of light chains: (k or λ. For example, the structure of an antibody of the IgG class can thus either be ($k2\gamma2$ or $\lambda2\gamma2$. Once bound to antigen, the biological functions of the immunoglobulin molecule is derived from the constant region, which is identical for all antibodies within a specific class.

Biological properties

Once bound to antigen, the biological effect of each class of immunoglobulin molecule depends on the constant region, which is identical for all antibodies within a specific class. For example:

IgG   IgG is the predominant immunogobulin in the intra- and extravascular fluid compartments, and makes up 15% of serum proteins. Its half-life of 23 days is the longest of all classes of antibodies. *Aggregation* of IgG molecules is an important prerequisite for several other biological functions. IgG molecules can cause *agglutination* or clumping of insoluble antigens such as micro-organisms, and *precipitation* of soluble antigens, thus promoting phagocytosis. IgG molecules is the only class of immunoglobulin that can pass through the *placenta* and transfer maternal immunity to the foetus. *Opsonization* is an IgG function whereby antibodies coat micro-organisms and thus prepare the organism for phagocytosis (Fig. 11.11).

In a process called *ADCC*, IgG molecules bind to micro-organism or tumour cells, and their Fc portions are in turn recognized by NK cells which kill by extracellular release of toxins. Other IgG functions are *complement activation, neutralization of toxin, immobilization of bacteria*, and *neutralization of viruses*.

IgM   IgM is the largest immunoglobulin molecule consisting of five subunits. It is found predominantly in the intravascular spaces and has a half-life of 5 days. It is the first antibody manufactured after immunization. IgMs are efficient at *agglutination* and are also the natural *isohaemagglutinins* against the ABO blood group antigens. IgM molecules are very efficient at initiating the *complement* sequence, it is not very efficient at other IgG functions.

IgA   IgA is a dimeric immunoglobulin with a half-life of 5 days found predominantly in *secretions* such as tears, saliva, colostrum, sweat and mucous. Due to its extensive secretion as part of MALT, it is often seen as the body's major antibody. It protects the host by preventing organisms attaching and penetrating epithelial cells. IgAs do not have complement receptors.

IgD   IgD molecules appear on the surface of *B-lymphocytes* at certain stages of development, but their biological function after antigen binding in the serum have not been defined.

IgE   IgE has the shortest half-life of all antibodies (2 days) and are also found in the lowest concentration in the serum. These molecules are predominantly found bound to basophils and mast cells, and are involved in hypersensitivity or *allergic* immune responses.

Serology

Serology is the *in vitro* study and clinical utilization of antigen–antibody interactions.

The *agglutination* reaction after antigen have bound to their specific antibodies, is widely used clinically; for example, for erythrocyte typing in blood banks, diagnosing auto-immune haemolytic disorders and detecting rheumatoid factor.

Immunoassays are used to quantify small amounts of antigen, antibody or antigen–antibody complexes. *Radioimmunoassays (RIA)*, in which antigen is labelled with a

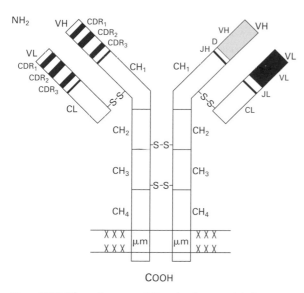

Figure 11.10. Schematic representation of an immunoglobulin molecule. Antigen is bound by the Fab regions whereas the Fc region mediates the biological activity such as opsonization.

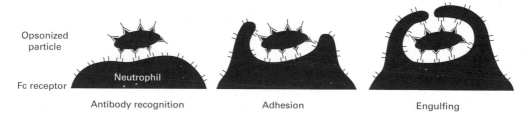

Figure 11.11. A diagrammatic representation of phagocytosis. The antigens on a particle is coated with antibodies. The phagocytic cell (macrophage or neutrophil) have receptors for the Fc portions of the immunoglobulin molecules on the particle. This aid with phagocytosis is called opsonization (from Benjamini *et al.*, 1996).

radioactive isotope, is sensitive for extremely small amounts of antigen and antibody. *Enzyme-linked immunosorbent assay (ELISA)*, a solid-phase immunoassay in which antigen is coated to a plastic surface and antibodies are labelled with a colour reagent, can be used for qualitative or quantitative determination of antigen or antibody.

Immunofluorescence is a method of detecting antigen by labelling antibody with fluorescent compounds. Fluorescein isothiocyanate (FITC), which fluoresces with a visible greenish colour, is one of the most commonly used fluorescent compounds in immunology.

Monoclonal antibodies are homogenous populations of antibody molecules, derived from a single lymphocyte, in which all antibodies are identical and of the same precise specificity for a given epitope. These monoclonal antibodies are used both for diagnostic purposes and as 'magic bullets' in immunotherapy of cancer. Most monoclonal antibodies are made in mouse cells, but with gene technology, *in vitro* production has become easier.

Response to surgery in normal patients

The insults to the patient

Tissue injury

Surgery cause *mechanical* tissue injury, which results in the release of humoral mediators to effect a local inflammatory response, but some mediators also spill over into the systemic circulation, causing a systemic inflammatory response. Resuscitation of surgical patients after variable periods of haemorrhagic shock may result in an *ischaemia/reperfusion* injury, particularly in the gut which undergoes disproportionate vasoconstriction during hypotension. Application of a tourniquet or vascular clamp during surgery (e.g. aortic aneurysm repair) results in distal ischaemia. During ischaemia, PLA_2 is activated which in turn results in the release of PAF. Reperfusion of ischaemic tissues leads to the generation of O_2 radicals and inflammatory mediators, and promotes neutrophil–endothelial cell interaction. Tissue injury sustained during ischaemia is thus much enhanced during the reperfusion period.

Bacterial load

When epithelial and mucosal barriers are broken during surgery, large amounts of bacteria and their products such as endotoxin can be introduced into the bloodstream, which will result in immediate inflammatory and immune responses to clear foreign antigen and prevent cellular injury.

Anaesthesia, invasive monitoring and blood transfusion

These also cause injury which may provide a cumulative insult of a significant proportion.

The patient's response

The body's normal response to a major surgical insult is a complex interaction of systems that can be strung together

as follows: *neuro-endocrine–metabolic–inflammatory–immunological.* The effects of this response are to cease bodily functions not essential to survival; to enhance functions crucial to survival; to mobilize reserves; to limit the injury size, destroy foreign and non-viable tissue, commence healing of the injury site and to retain a memory of the injurious agent for an enhanced response upon a second encounter. Healing and survival do not occur when the magnitude of the insult(s) overwhelm the body's normal response mechanisms, or when some of the defence mechanisms are deficient, such as occur under some pathological states.

PATHOLOGICAL STATES AND SURGICAL IMPLICATIONS

Disordered haemopoiesis/bone marrow failure

Aplastic anaemia

Aplastic anaemia is caused by depletion or dysfunction of the bone marrow pluripotential stem cell. The result is a reduction in the numbers of all blood cell precursors in the marrow as well as a circulating pancytopaenia. There are numerous causes of aplastic anaemia, but a surgeon is most likely to encounter primary (idiopathic) aplastic anaemia or aplastic anaemia secondary to chemotherapy, ionizing radiation, idiosyncratic drug reactions or infection. Bone marrow transplantation is the treatment of choice if no treatable underlying cause can be found.

Myelodysplastic syndromes

Myelodysplastic syndromes are a group of heterogeneous disorders characterized by defects in the production of one or more haemopoietic cell lines. The syndromes often occur in the elderly and may progress into acute leukaemia. Patients commonly present with anaemia, yet neutropaenia, thrombocytopaenia and monocytopaenia are also observed. The use of CSFs have met with some success in increasing blood counts as well as decreasing the number of infections.

Infiltrative myelopathies

When the bone marrow is infiltrated by non-haemopoietic cells, native haemopoietic cells are displaced, premature blood cells are released into the circulation, and anaemia and other cytopaenias result. The most common causes of infiltrative myelopathies are leukaemia, lymphoma, metastatic carcinoma and tuberculosis. The diagnosis is made by bone marrow aspiration and radionuclide scanning of the marrow. Treatment is that of the underlying condition.

Surgical implications

Surgery on patients with disordered haemopoiesis is fraught with potential complications. Anaemic patients have *hypoxic* tissues with deranged function, reduced numbers of granulocytes results in *impaired inflammation* and wound healing, reduced numbers of phagocytes and lymphocytes make the patients prone to bacterial, viral and parasitic *infections*, and thrombocytopaenia leads to a *bleeding* tendency. The outcome of surgery can be improved by transfusing the appropriate blood product peri-operatively. Transfusion of stem cells, bone marrow, fresh whole blood, packed red blood cells, neutrophil concentrates or platelet concentrates should be appropriately timed either pre-, intra- or post-operatively to achieve the optimal effect.

Transfusion of blood products

Preparation

A blood donation is taken by aseptic technique into bags containing an appropriate amount of anticoagulant – usually citrate, phosphate, dextrose (CPD). Before issue the following tests are carried out: ABO, RhD blood grouping, red cell antibody screen and serology tests to exclude syphilis, hepatitis B surface antigen (HbsAg), hepatitis C virus (HCV) and human immunodeficiency virus 1 and 2 (HIV-1 and 2). Currently HCV and HIV are excluded by detection of appropriate antiviral antibodies, and polymerase chain reaction (PCR)-based detection of viral nucleic acid. PCR testing has increased the sensitivity of screening of donors in the 'window period' prior to antibody formation.

Blood is stored at 4–6°C for up to 35 days. During the storage some changes may take place in the blood composition, there is a slow K^+ loss from the red cells into the plasma and a fall in the 2,3-diphosphoglycerate (2,3-DPG). The level of 2,3-DPG return to normal within 24 h after transfusion. Blood is usually processed and separated into its components before use. Whole blood is rarely used. Leucodepletion, the filtering of blood to remove the majority of white cells, is usually performed soon after collection and prior to processing. Leucodepletion reduces the risk of febrile transfusion reactions and alloimmunization. Its also effective at preventing the possible transmission of new variant Creutzfeldt–Jakob disease (nvCJD) and cytomegalovirus (CMV) transmission.

How safe is blood transfusions?

In the UK, most of the information about the safety of blood transfusions comes from the Serious Hazards of Transfusion (SHOT) scheme, which is a national reporting system for serious complications of blood transfusion. The Sixth Annual Report was published in July 2003. Data from SHOT provides great evidence about the risks of transfusions. In the UK each donated unit of blood is tested for HIV, Hepatitis B and C, syphilis, and red blood cell typing for ABO and RH(D) antigens is performed. A donated unit of blood can either be transfused whole (e.g. for babies) or split into several components that can be transfused to different patients. A request for *group and save* results in the patient's blood being typed for ABO and RH(A) antigens, and the plasma being tested for antibodies that could lyse red cells at 37°C. A request for a blood product results in a full *cross-match* between the patient's blood and the unit of blood product to be transfused (Fig. 11.12).

Administrative errors in blood transfusions

The most frequent adverse event of transfusion is 'wrong blood to patient', due to administrative errors. These errors arise from either taking the cross-match sample from wrong patient, wrong labelling, wrong collection from the hospital storage sites, and most importantly, failure of bedside checking before commencing the blood transfusion.

Red blood cells

Packed (plasma-depleted) red cells are the usual choice for most transfusions. Whole blood is used occasionally for treatment of acute blood loss or for exchange transfusions. The optimal pre-operative haemoglobin is unknown, but has arbitrarily been chosen as around 10 g%. However, surgery can very well be performed on asymptomatic patients with a haemoglobin of 7 g% and similar post-operative haemoglobin levels can result in a successful outcome without transfusion. Once taken out of cold storage, transfusion should be completed within 5 h. Infusion should be through a blood giving set. When infused rapidly red cells should be heated to body temperature in a specially designed blood warmer and not by any other means.

Autologous donation and transfusion

Fears over transmission of infections such as HIV has increased the demand for autotransfusions. There are three ways of administering autologous transfusions:
1. *Predeposit*: Blood is taken from patient who may potentially require a blood transfusion in the future elective surgery. Blood donation usually take place 2–3 weeks prior to surgery.
2. *Haemodilution*: Blood is taken from patient immediately before surgery starts and replaced with crystalloids and then re-infused at the end of surgery as needed.
3. *Salvage*: Blood loss during surgery is collected in special device and re-infused.

Platelets

Platelet concentrates can either be made from blood from a single donor or pooled from several donors. Once prepared platelets are kept at room temperature in a shaking rack and the shelf life is only 5 days. Once released from the laboratory infusion (through a blood giving set) should be rapid. Platelet transfusion is used in patients who are thrombocytopaenic or have disordered platelet function and whole are actively bleeding (therapeutic use) or at serious risk of bleeding (prophylactic use). For prophylaxis the platelet count should be kept above 5–10 × 10^9/l. For minor invasive procedures the platelet count should be kept above 50 × 10^9/l. Platelet transfusions should be avoided in auto-immune thrombocytopaenic purpura unless there is serious haemorrhage. They are contraindicated in heparin-induced thrombocytopaenia, thrombotic thrombocytopaenic purpura and haemolytic uraemic syndrome.

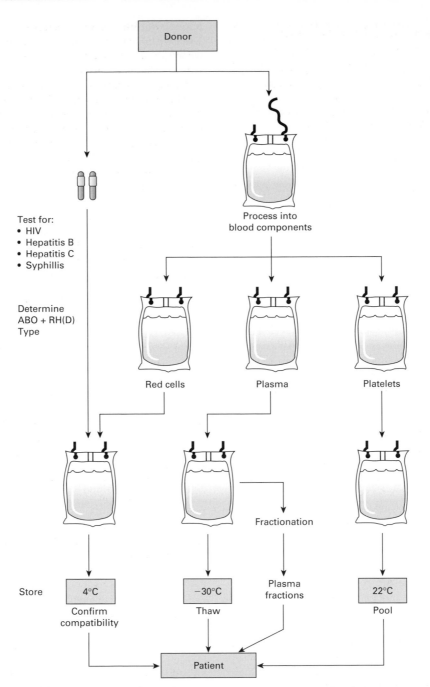

Figure 11.12. The blood transfusion process from donors to patients (from McLelland B. *Handbook of Transfusion Medicine*, 2nd edn. Norwich: HMSO, 1996).

Granulocyte concentrates

These are prepared from normal healthy donors or from patients with chronic myeloid leukaemia. They are used in patients with severe neutropaenia who do not respond to appropriate antibiotic therapy. It is often not possible to give sufficient amounts and carry the risk of transmitting CMV infection.

Stem cells

Stem cells can be harvested from the peripheral blood of a donor and transfusion into a recipient can be as efficient at restoring normal bone marrow as a bone marrow transplant. The technique has the advantage that contrary to bone marrow harvesting, it does not require a general anaesthetic. Harvesting and storage prior to planned high-dose

Table 11.1. Complications of blood transfusions.

Early	Late
Haemolytic reactions	Transmission of disease
• Immediate	*Virus*
• Delayed	• Hepatitis A, B, C and others
Reactions caused by infected blood	• HIV
	• CMV
Allergic reactions to white cells, platelets or proteins	*Bacteria*
	• *Treponema pallidum*
Pyrogenic reactions (to plasma proteins or caused by HLA antibodies)	• *Brucella*
	• *Salmonella*
	Parasites
TRALI	• Malaria
Clotting abnormalities after massive transfusion	• *Toxoplasma*
	• Microfilaria
Hyperkalemia	Transfusional iron overload
Citrate toxicity	Immune sensitization
Thrombophlebitis	Transfusion-associated graft-versus-host disease
Air embolism	
Circulatory overload	

chemotherapy with resultant bone marrow ablation, and subsequent intravenous autotransfusion of stem cells can result in complete reconstitution of all the bone marrow elements (Table 11.1).

Human plasma preparations

Fresh frozen plasma

Rapidly frozen plasma separated from fresh blood is stored at less than −30°C. Its main use is for the replacement of coagulation factors or with massive transfusion of packed cells, in liver disease and DIC, after cardiopulmonary bypass surgery, to rapidly reverse a warfarin effect and in thrombotic thrombocytopaenic purpura.

Cryoprecipitate

This is obtained by thawing fresh frozen plasma at 4°C and contains concentrated factor VIII and fibrinogen. It was widely used as replacement therapy in haemophilia A and von Willebrand's disease before more purified preparations became available. They are still being used to replace coagulation factors in patients that runs the risk of circulatory volume overload when fresh frozen plasma that is needed to replace significant coagulation deficits.

Freeze-dried factor VIII concentrates

They are used to treat haemophilia A and von Willebrand's disease. There small volume makes them ideal for patients at risk for circulatory volume overload. Their use is declining as recombinant forms of factor VIII become available.

Protein C concentrate

This is used in severe sepsis and with DIC to reduce thrombosis resulting from depletion of protein C.

Haemolytic transfusion reactions

Haemolytic transfusion reactions may be immediate or delayed. Immediate life-threatening reactions associated with massive intravascular haemolysis are the result of compliment-activating antibodies of IgM or IgG classes, usually with ABO specificity. Reactions associated with extravascular haemolysis (e.g. immune antibodies of the Rh system which are unable to activate complement) are generally less severe but may still be life threatening. The cells become coated with IgG and are removed in the reticuloendothelial system. Patients usually exhibit an unexplained anaemia with or without jaundice.

Clinical features of a major haemolytic reaction

Haemolytic shock phase – this may start within minutes after a few millilitres of blood have been transfused or may take 1–2 h after the end of the transfusion to develop. Symptoms include urticaria, lower backache, flushing, headache, shortness of breath, precordial pain and hypotension. These symptoms may be difficult to identify in the anaesthetized patient or the unconscious intensive therapy unit (ITU) patient. Laboratory examinations will reveal evidence of blood cell destruction, jaundice and disseminated intravascular coagulation. Urinalysis will demonstrate haemoglobinuria.

Due to the haemoglobinuria renal tubular necrosis may develop and progress to acute renal failure.

Management of immediate transfusion reaction

The transfusion should be stopped immediately. All compatibility blood labels and patient identification should be re-checked. The unit of donor blood and samples of the patient's blood should be send to the laboratory to be checked for grouping, direct antiglobulin test, plasma haemoglobinaemia, screening for DIC, bacterial contamination. Urine must be examined for haemoglobinuria. Further samples should be repeated after 6 and 24 h for a blood count, free haemoglobin and methaemalbumin estimations. The treatment is mainly supportive to maintain the blood pressure and renal perfusion. Aggressive fluid resuscitation should be started to establish diuresis. Frusemide are sometimes necessary. Hydrocortisone and antihistamine may help to alleviate shock, but in event of severe shock, intravenous adrenaline in small incremental doses may be required.

Febrile reactions because of white cell antibodies

HLA antibodies are usually the result of sensitization by pregnancy or previous transfusions. They produce rigors, pyrexia and in sever cases, pulmonary infiltrates. They are minimized by giving leucocyte-depleted packed cells.

Febrile or non-febrile non-haemolytic allergic reactions

These are usually caused by hypersensitivity to donor plasma proteins and if severe can result in anaphylaxis. Treatment is hydrocortisone and antihistamine. Washed red cells or frozen red cells may be needed for further transfusions.

Pro-inflammation/immunosuppression

A major blood transfusion (more than 6 units of red blood cells) is a potent inflammatory stimulus and is an independent risk factor for end organ injury (e.g. acute lung injury) and MOF after major trauma. It also causes prolonged immunosuppression which may adversely effect outcome after cancer surgery. The mechanisms of these immunological effects seem to be related to the leucocyte count and leucocyte release of mediators such as IL-8 and PAF in the stored blood products.

Transfusion-transmitted infections

The chance of receiving an infected unit from a British donor is now as low as 1 in 30 million for hepatitis C, 1 in 8 million for HIV and 1 in 260 000 for hepatitis B. Since 1995 only 16 cases of viral transmission was reported to SHOT, and no confirmed transmissions have been reported in the last 2 years. Reduction of the risk depends on exclusion of donors with lifestyle markers indicating a high risk for viral infection and serological testing (PCR-based detection of viral nucleic acid).

Transfusion-related acute lung injury

Transfusion-related acute lung injury (TRALI) is the clinical association of non-cardiogenic pulmonary oedema occurring within 6 h of transfusion. TRALI is emerging as possibly the most important cause of transfusion-associated mortality. It appears to be related to antibodies in the donor plasma against HLA or granulocyte antigens. The treatment of TRALI is supportive and most patients will require ventilation.

The future of blood transfusion

Bloodless medicine incorporates improved surgical techniques, careful pre-operative preparation and implementation of blood salvage and autologous transfusions to reduce transfusion requirement. There is also studies that indicate that lowering the haemoglobin trigger level for transfusion may improve the outcome in patients.

Blood substitutes

The ideal replacement for red cells should have equal clinical effectiveness, can be stored for long periods at room temperatures and is simple to use without the need for cross-matching. O_2 therapeutics encompass a range of red cell replacement, including haemoglobin-based products and perfluorocarbon emulsions, which serve to provide O_2-carrying capacity and volume restoration. The first haemoglobin-based O_2 carriers (HBOC) cause vasoconstriction, nephrotoxicity and had a short half-life. The first product to reach phase III trials (HemAssist, Baxter) was withdrawn after negative outcome in trauma and stroke patients compared to control patients.

Red blood cell/haemoglobin disorders

Anaemia with resultant tissue hypoxia can result in intra- and post-operative cardiovascular complications. Anaemia results from decreased red blood cell production (e.g. iron deficiency), production of abnormal red cells (e.g. thalassaemia) or increased haemolysis (e.g. sickle cell anaemia). Surgery may further precipitate haemolysis in patients with a sickling disorder. Causes of haemolytic anaemia are listed in Table 11.2.

Disordered haemostasis

Bleeding disorders

Vascular purpura

Vascular causes of bleeding are either due to congenital disorders of the vascular connective tissue (e.g. Marfan's disease) or acquired damage to blood vessel structure, function or support (e.g. corticosteroid use or vasculitides).

Platelet disorders

Deficiencies in either number or function of platelets can result in a bleeding tendency. Thrombocytopaenia follows either decreased production (e.g. bone marrow disease) or increased destruction (e.g. immune thrombocytopaenic purpura, drug-induced (heparin) thrombocytopaenia or hypersplenism. Circulating platelet numbers may be normal, but their function deranged in some congenital disorders of platelet metabolism (e.g. thrombasthenia). Acquired defects of

---

Table 11.2. Causes of haemolytic anaemia.

Primary defects of the red cell membrane
- Hereditary spherocytosis
- Hereditary elliptocytosis
- Paroxysmal nocturnal haemoglobinuria

Secondary defects of the red cell membrane
- Auto-immune haemolytic anaemia
- Burns
- Haemolysis caused by membrane lysins (e.g. venoms)

Haemolytic anaemia caused by infection of red cells
- Malaria
- Bacterial infections of red cells

Heinz body haemolytic anaemias
- Oxidative haemolysis
- Favism

Haemolytic anaemias caused by genetic aberrations of glycolysis
- G6PD deficiency
- Pyruvate kinase deficiency

Haemoglobinopathies
- Sickle cell disease (Haemoglobin S disorder)
- Haemoglobin C disorder

Haemolytic anaemias secondary to generalized disorders
- Chronic liver disease
- Acute or subacute infection
- Starvation/anorexia nervosa

Hypersplenism

G6PD: glucose-6-phosphate dehydrogenase.

platelet function include uraemia, and numerous drugs such as non-steroidal anti-inflammatory drugs including aspirin, antibiotics including penicillin and plasma expanders such as dextran.

Coagulation factor deficiencies

The most common congenital coagulation factor deficiencies are haemophilia A (factor VIII) and B (factor IX), and von Willebrand's disease, although deficiencies in most of the other factors have been described. Coagulation factor deficiencies can develop secondary to any one of the following:

(a) deranged production in the liver of the vitamin K-dependent factors II, VII, IX and X;
(b) plasma dilution after a massive blood transfusion;
(c) consumption as part of disseminated intravascular coagulation.

Thrombotic disorders

Surgery predisposes patients to thrombosis and thromboembolism which can result in significant post-operative morbidity and mortality.

Arterial thrombosis

It results at sites of damaged or breached endothelial cells such as with atherosclerosis, and can cause myocardial infarction, cerebrovascular accidents or mesenteric and limb ischaemia.

Venous thrombosis

It is the result of stasis, altered flow and an imbalance between the coagulation and fibrinolytic mechanisms. Several conditions increase the risk for venous thrombosis significantly.

Therapeutic options to prevent

The options to prevent arterial and venous thrombosis include: physical activity, graded compression stockings, electrical calf stimulation, external pneumatic calf compression, oral antiplatelet agents (such as low-dose aspirin), oral anticoagulation agents (such as low-dose warfarin) and subcutaneous anticoagulation agents (such as heparin).

Drug therapy to treat

Drug therapy to treat arterial and venous thrombosis include: oral anticoagulation agents (such as warfarin), intravenous anticoagulation agents (such as heparin) and intravenous thrombolytic agents (such as streptokinase).

Disseminated intravascular coagulation

DIC is characterized by widespread deposition of fibrin in small blood vessels; consumption and depletion of fibrin, coagulation factors and platelets; increase in FDPs and a bleeding tendency. This is induced by blood procoagulants either introduced into or produced in the bloodstream. These coagulant proteins overcome the normal physiological anti-coagulant mechanism (Table 11.3).

Clinical features

Patients may present with fulminant bleeding disorder (due to consumption of clotting factors, platelets and the production of breakdown products that further inhibit the coagulation pathway), or they may present with tissue ischaemia (due to clot formation and thrombi in the micro-circulation) or a combination of the two. They may also present with a less severe and more chronic form of DIC.

Pathogenesis

DIC may be triggered by the entry of procoagulant material into the blood circulation (e.g. amniotic fluid embolism, disseminated mucin-producing adenocarcinoma, acute monocytic leukaemia (AML), severe falciparum malaria, haemolytic transfusion and snakebites).

Table 11.3. Causes of disseminated intravascular coagulation.

Infections
- Gram-negative and meningococcal septicaemia
- Endotoxic shock
- *Clostridium welchii* septicaemia
- Severe falciparum malaria
- Viral infection: varicella, HIV, hepatitis, CMV

Obstetric
- Amniotic fluid embolism
- Septic abortion/postpartum sepsis
- Placental abruption
- Eclampsia
- Retained products of conception/intrauterine foetal death

Malignancy
- Disseminated adenocarcinoma
- Acute promyelocytic leukaemia

Widespread tissue damage
- Severe trauma, head injuries
- Extensive surgery
- Severe burns

Hypersensitivity reactions
- Anaphylaxis
- Incompatible blood transfusions

Vascular abnormalities
- Kasabach–Merritt syndrome
- Leaking prosthetic heart valves
- Cardiac bypass surgery
- Aortic aneurysms

Miscellaneous
- Liver failure
- Snakebites and invertebrate venoms
- Hypothermia/heatstroke
- Acute hypoxia

DIC may also be initiated by widespread endothelial damage and collagen exposure (severe sepsis, severe trauma, extensive surgery, severe burns).

In addition to its role in the deposition of fibrin in the micro-circulation, intravascular thrombin formation produces large amounts of circulating fibrin monomers which form complexes with fibrinogen. Fibrinolysis is stimulated by thrombi adhered to vascular walls and the release of split products interferes with fibrin polymerization, thus contributing to the coagulation defect. The combined action of thrombin and plasmin causes depletion of fibrinogen, prothrombin and factors V and VIII. Intravascular thrombin also causes widespread platelet aggregation and deposition in the vessels.

Laboratory findings

Tests of haemostasis
1. Low platelet count.
2. Low or deficient fibrinogen levels.
3. The thrombin time (TT) is prolonged.
4. High levels of fibrinogen and FDPs, such as D-dimers are found in the blood.
5. The prothrombin time (PT) and activated partial thromboplastin time (APTT) is prolonged.

Blood film examination
Picture of haemolytic anaemia/'micro-angiopathy' with prominent fragmentation of the red blood cells.

Treatment

1. The most important aspect of treating DIC is to treat or remove the underlying cause for DIC; for example eradication of sepsis, antibiotics, removal of foetus/products of conception.
2. Establishing intravenous access and restoration of circulating volume, while supporting respiratory, cardiovascular, renal and other systems appropriately.
3. Supportive therapy with fresh frozen plasma and platelet concentrates is indicated in cases where active bleeding takes place or where there is high risk of bleeding. Cryoprecipitate provides a more concentrated source of fibrinogen and packed red cell transfusion may be required. The use of heparin or antiplatelet drugs to inhibit the ongoing coagulation process may be indicated, although this may aggravate the bleeding tendency. The use of antithrombin and protein C concentrates to inhibit DIC appears promising.

Immune deficiency disorders

Immune deficiency disorders can be divided into five groups:
1. B-lymphocyte and antibody deficiencies;
2. T-lymphocyte deficiencies;
3. combined B- and T-cell deficiencies;
4. phagocyte and NK cell deficiencies;
5. complement deficiencies.

The causes of these deficiencies are either primary (congenital) or secondary.

Primary (congenital)

Congenital B-cell deficiency such as X-linked (Bruton's) agammaglobulinaemia in male babies is characterized by recurrent bacterial infections. The treatment is periodic injections of large amounts of IgG. Congenital thymic dysplasia (DiGeorge syndrome) results in a primary T-cell deficiency with recurrent and chronic infections. The treatment is transplantation of foetal thymus tissue. Severe combined immunodeficiency diseases (SCID) are a group of diseases resulting from a failure of lymphocyte stem cells to differentiate into B- and T-cells. These individuals are vulnerable to almost any type of infection, and unless treated by bone marrow transplantation will result in death within 1 year of birth. Chronic granulomatous disease (CGD) is a disease in which phagocytic cells have a defect in the NADPH oxidase responsible of generation of O_2 radicals. This results in inefficient bacterial killing and recurrent infections. Treatment is by antibiotic prophylaxis.

Secondary

The most common cause of secondary immunodeficiency in developed countries is the use of *chemotherapeutic drugs* in cancer therapy. Most of these agents are toxic to the bone marrow as well as T- and B-cell populations in the secondary lymphoid tissues. Deliberate *immunosuppression* in organ transplantation patients, or patients on *steroid treatment* for auto-immune or chronic inflammatory conditions, will also bring about immune dysfunction. In *leukaemia* normal lymphocytes are replaced by non-functioning cells and the haemopoietic elements in the bone marrow is displaced.

Acquired immune deficiency syndrome

Infection with HIV, a retrovirus of the lentivirus subgroup is these days one of the most frequent causes of immune deficiency. This syndrome give rise to a diverse range of symptoms and the development of opportunistic infections and malignancies. Most infections in the West result from the B clade of HIV-1, but different clades (HIV families, that can be distinguished on the basis of viral sequence) predominate in other parts of the world. In South Asia the E clade predominate and in sub-Saharan Africa the A and C clades are the most common. Infection with the related retrovirus, HIV-2, which is found predominantly in West Africa. This infection gives rise to a more protracted disease course. Patients infected with this virus have fewer signs of immune deficiency.

Epidemiology

The virus is transmitted in semen, blood and other body fluids, including breast milk. On a worldwide basis, the vast majority of transmissions occur during heterosexual intercourse. Other methods of transmission include homosexual intercourse, breastfeeding by infected mothers, sharing of contaminated needles by intravenous drug users. Infections from blood or blood products transfusions is rare now in countries where screening of donated blood is routine.

When performing a surgical procedure on an HIV-infected patient, it is crucial that the surgeon and allied health-care workers protect themselves against transmission of the virus by avoiding any direct contact with the patient's blood, tissues, semen, vaginal secretions, mucous membranes, skin lesions or any body fluid whatsoever. There is no evidence that the virus is transmitted by aerosol from the lungs. The risk of virus transmission by a needle stick injury from an infected patient is 0.4%. The most frequent causes of infection of health-care workers have been handling of needles, hand-to-hand transfer of sharp instruments, lengthy procedures associated with blood loss, emergencies, accidental trauma, and obstetric, gynaecological, orthopaedic, vascular and cardiothoracic procedures. Full precautionary measures include disqualifying any staff with defects in skin or immune barriers, impenetrable operating gowns, helmet head covering, protective eye wear, double gloving, needles handled by instruments only and no hand-to-hand passing of sharp instruments. In the event of contamination the area should be thoroughly cleaned with soap and water.

Pathogenesis

HIV causes its major effect through infection of the T-helper (CD4) cells and cells of the monocyte lineage. Entry into cells require both the presence of the CD4 molecule and a member of the chemokine receptor family (CCR-5, CXCR-4). Once inside the cell viral RNA is changed to DNA by a reverse transcriptase, incorporated into the host genome, and undergoes replication. The CD4$^+$ T-cells are destroyed as the new viral particles are released. An important feature of HIV infection is the rapid mutation rate of the virus in an infected individual. This rapid mutation rate is the result of both the error-prone nature of the enzyme reverse transcriptase and the high rate of viral replication. The significance of this is that the virus can readily adapt to become resistant to antiviral therapy and develop resistance against the bodies immune response directed against it.

Clinical features

After being infected with the virus, a prodromal period of about 6 weeks follows. This prodromal syndrome resembles infectious mononucleosis with transient lymphadenopathy, fever, malaise and occasionally meningoencephalitis. The viral load may be extremely high during acute infection. The majority of infected people then experience a protracted asymptomatic period. The virus however continues to replicate during this asymptomatic period and the CD4 T-cell count steadily falls. A number of HIV-related symptoms may develop, such as generalized lymphadenopathy, persistent

fever, weight loss, diarrhoea, skin changes, CNS manifestations. Haematological abnormalities include thrombocytopaenia, leucopaenia, neutropaenia, hypergammaglobulinaemia and anaemia. Infections may start to occur with organisms such as herpes simplex or zoster, *Pneumococcus* and *Salmonella*. When the CD4 count falls below $0.2 \times 10^9/l$, the patient becomes susceptible to a wide spectrum of opportunistic infections (*Streptococcus pneumoniae*, *Haemophilus influenzae*, *Pneumocystis carinii*, toxoplasmosis, *Mycobacterium tuberculosis*, atypical mycobacteria, histoplasmosis, *Cryptococcus*, cryptosporidiosis, fungal infections, Jamestown Canyon (JC) virus infection and CMV infections), malignancies (Kaposi's sarcoma and non-Hodgkin's lymphoma) and CNS disease such as dementia may develop. This stage of infection is classified by the Centre for Disease Control (CDC) as fully developed acquired immunodeficiency syndrome (AIDS). Many staging systems for HIV have been proposed and exist. Mostly clinicians determine the stage of infection according to the patients symptoms and the CD4 count. If available, the plasma viral load is progressively more being used to predict outcome and evaluate response to therapy (Fig. 11.13 and Table 11.4).

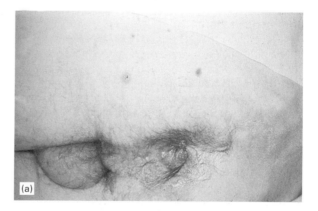

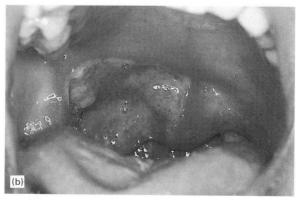

Figure 11.13. Photographs of a patient with AIDS: (a) shows perineal scarring after recurrent peri-anal infections and (b) a mouth ulcer on the hard palate, probably due to an opportunistic viral infection.

Table 11.4. Staging of HIV infection.

CD4 cell count ($\times 10^9$/l)	Stage	Clinical features
>0.5	Early	Low risk of disease
		Normal response to infection
0.2–0.5	Middle	Minor signs and symptoms
		Moderate risk of opportunistic infections
0.05–0.2	Late	High risk of opportunistic infections
		Benefit from prophylactic antibiotic and antiretrovirals
<0.05	Advanced	High risk of opportunistic diseases and death

Diagnosis

The diagnosis of HIV is confirmed by the presence of antibodies to HIV or the direct detection of HIV RNA in the plasma. Blood counts usually reveals a lymphopaenia and a fall of the CD4 : CD8 ratio from the normal value of 1.5–2.5 : 1 to less than 1 : 1.

Haematological aspects

Most often the blood picture will reveal a anaemia, thrombocytopaenia, neutropaenia and a lymphopaenia. Thrombocytopaenia may be immune based or secondary to bone marrow dysfunction. Bone marrow examination may also be valuable for the diagnosis of some opportunistic infections: for example tuberculosis, atypical mycobacterial infections, *Cryptococcus, Leishmaniasis and* histoplasmosis.

The drugs available in the treatment of HIV, especially azidothymidine (AZT), but also ganciclovir, pentamidine and trimethoprim, may also cause cytopaenias, especially in the presence of folate deficiency. Thrombocytopaenia may respond to steroid therapy or antiretroviral therapy.

Treatment

Treatment of HIV is both specific and supportive. Supportive treatment is aimed at preventing and treating opportunistic infections (e.g. with co-trimoxazole, isoniazid or antifungals). Lymphomas are treated the usual way with chemotherapy, although these have a tendency to be high grade and the prognosis is poor.

Specific treatment is aimed at suppressing viral replication. AZT was the first agent shown to be effective in suppressing viral replication. It has been followed by the development of a range of other reverse transcriptase inhibitors such as lamivudine and nevirapine. More recently protease inhibitors have been developed to reduce the viral load (e.g. indinavir, ritonavir and saquinavir). As the virus are likely to develop resistance against monotherapy, combination therapy with at least three drugs are widely recommended.

As these drugs have serious side effects and resistance may develop, the optimal time to start therapy is controversial. Most clinicians will start therapy if symptoms develop or if the CD4 count drops below 0.2×10^9/l.

The decision to operate as well as the performance of the surgery should be undertaken by an experienced surgeon. Post-operative complications such as wound and anastomotic dehiscence, and local as well as life-threatening systemic infections are common. When bowel is resected it may be prudent to avoid an anastomosis and bring both bowel ends to the surface. Anal fissures and superficial anal infections are best left well alone.

Auto-immune diseases

Auto-immune diseases result when the host loses tolerance to 'self-antigens' and mounts an immune response consisting of either auto-antibodies or auto-destructive T-cells, to one or more of its own constituent molecules. The triggers for loss of self-tolerance are usually a combination of genetic predisposition and environmental stimuli. The list of auto-immune diseases are continuously growing and only some of those that are frequently encountered by surgeons are mentioned here.

Auto-immune haemolytic anaemia

This results from antibodies formed against antigens on normal red cell surface membranes. It is often drug induced (e.g. penicillin), but under most circumstances the triggering stimulus is unknown. Antibodies are classified as 'warm' when they react optimally at 37°C or 'cold' when they attach to red cells only at temperatures below 37°C. Upon binding of the auto-antibodies to the surface membrane receptors, red cells are destroyed either by complement activation or phagocytosis by macrophages. The treatment of choice is steroids such as oral prednisolone. On occasion patients benefit from splenectomy.

Idiopathic thrombocytopaenic purpura

It is caused by auto-antibodies formed against surface membrane antigens on platelets. Binding of the antibodies result in platelet destruction, particularly in the spleen, and recurrent spontaneous haemorrhaging. Idiopathic thrombocytopaenic purpura often starts in childhood and treatment consists of steroids and repeated injections with immunoglobulin. Failure of medical treatment and recurrent spontaneous haemorrhaging are indications for splenectomy.

Graves' disease (auto-immune hyperthyroidism)

Graves' disease results from auto-antibodies that develop against the thyroid-stimulating hormone (TSH) receptor on thyroid cell membranes. Interestingly, binding of these antibodies with TSH receptors do not result in destruction of either the receptors or the cells, but instead cause long-term stimulation of the thyroid with the development of a goitre,

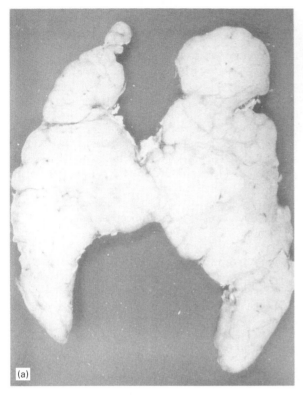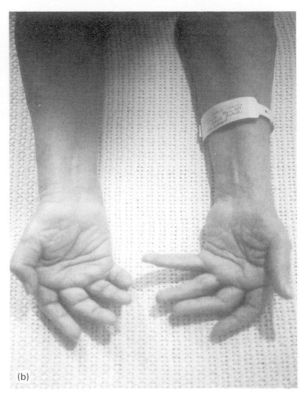

(a)   (b)

Figure 11.14. Auto-immune destruction of the thyroid gland and joints of the hands: (a) shows the characteristic woody appearance of a goitre removed from a patient with Hashimoto's disease and (b) the hands of a patient with rheumatoid arthritis.

excessive production of thyroxine hormones and the clinical syndrome of hyperthyroidism. The treatment is to suppress thyroid cell function by antithyroid drugs such as propylthiouracil and carbimazole, or destruction of thyroid cells by either radioactive iodine or a subtotal thyroidectomy.

Hashimoto's thyroiditis

Hashimoto's thyroiditis is a disease of middle-aged women that results from a B- and T-cell response to different components of the thyroid gland such as thyroglobulin and epithelial cell microsomes. There is an intense lymphocyte infiltration of the gland and the thyroid follicles are progressively destroyed. In an attempt to regenerate the gland becomes enlarged with a rubbery hard consistency, but patients are ultimately rendered hypothyroid. Treatment during the acute phase is with steroids and thyroxine. If pressure symptoms develop, a subtotal thyroidectomy should be performed (Fig. 11.14).

Rheumatoid arthritis

It is characterized by chronically inflamed synovial membranes which are densely infiltrated by B- and T-lymphocytes, as well granulocytes and macrophages. An abnormally produced IgM antibody called rheumatoid factor is detectable in the plasma. The persistent inflammation results in destruction of the cartilaginous joint surfaces with laying down of fibrous tissue, progressive restriction of movement and deformity. Medical treatment consists of analgesia, anti-inflammatory drugs (non-steroidal and steroidal) and immunosuppression. A range of surgical treatment options are available such as synovectomy, splintage, tendon repair, arthrodesis and joint replacement.

Myasthenia gravis

Myasthenia gravis results from auto-antibodies against the acetylcholine receptors at neuromuscular junctions. Binding of antibody blocks the receptor with resultant muscle weakness which is progressive until death ensues from respiratory failure. Treatment is by steroids, plasma electrophoresis and respiratory support. Occasionally thymectomy contributes to recovery.

Systemic lupus erythematous

Systemic lupus erythematous (SLE) is the consequence of auto-antibodies forming circulating complexes with DNA. The disease affects the skin, kidneys, joints, heart, CNS and peripheral arteries, and has protean manifestations, including Raynaud's phenomenon.

Cancer

Immune response to a cancer

There is some evidence that cancer cells have surface membrane antigens called tumour-specific antigens (TSA) or tumour-associated antigens (TAA) that are recognized by the immune system as non-self, and can elicit an immune response. Antibodies secreted by B-lymphocytes will coat tumour cells and with the help of complement and phagocytic cells can cause tumour cell destruction. CD8$^+$ T-lymphocytes and NK cells can cause direct tumour cell killing, whereas CD4$^+$ T-cells release cytokines to augment tumour cell killing by macrophages. The concept of immune surveillance as protection against cancer, whereby lymphocytes continuously check dividing cells for mutations and destroy unacceptable cells, has not been proved (Fig. 11.15).

Immune effects of a cancer

Part of the success of tumour cell growth may be due to their immunosuppressive capacities. Tumour cells release immunosuppressive mediators such as PG. In addition, T-lymphocytes residing in tumours may become antigen-specific suppressor T-cells; that is, they suppress proliferation and cytotoxicity of lymphocytes, NK cells and macrophages that are targeted against the tumour antigens. Tumour cells may also modify its cell surface antigens to escape an immune response, or by rapid growth simply overwhelm the immune defence mechanisms.

Immunodeficiency and cancer

Immunocompromised individuals such as patients after radiotherapy or chemotherapy, transplant patients on immunosuppressive drugs or those with an AIDS are at an increased risk of developing cancer. The risk is particularly for lymphoproliferative and cutaneous malignancies, which suggest that immune protection may be more important in some tumours than in others.

Immunodiagnosis of cancer

If tumour cells express surface membrane, cytoplasmic or secreted products of specific antigenicity and in sufficient quantities, it should be possible to detect these by developing monoclonal antibodies against them. Unfortunately these techniques have not yet reached widespread application in either screening for early cancer or follow-up of cancer. The three most commonly used antigens used for these purposes are: prostatic-specific antigen (PSA), used for screening and follow-up of prostate cancer; carcinoembryonic antigen (CEA), used for follow-up of colon cancer and α-fetoprotein, used for diagnosis and follow-up of liver cancer.

Immunotherapy of cancer

Numerous attempts have been made to employ immunological methods to treat cancer, but none have been very successful. The different techniques can be grouped together as active, passive and adoptive immunotherapy. *Active immunotherapy* refers to those techniques designed to enhance components of the immune system most likely responsible for antitumour activity. Bacillus Calmette–Guérin (BCG) has been used to enhance cellular immunity, particularly macrophage function, and various cytokines such as IFN, IL-1, IL-2, IL-4, IL-12 and TNF are being tested to enhance immune function. *Passive immunotherapy* usually refers to the use of monoclonal antibodies directed against TSA in an attempt to destroy the tumour cell. *Adoptive immunotherapy* refers to the transfer of immune components such as macrophages and NK cells from one individual to another. The most extensively studied in this group are known as lymphokine-activated killer (LAK) cells.

Lymph node surgery in malignant disease

Tumour cells invade the venules and lymphatics in and around the primary cancer and also float down the draining veins and lymphatics. Most of these circulating cancer cells are destroyed, but some can develop into metastatic tumour in either lymph glands or distant organs. Metastatic spread is not in a centrifugal manner and local lymph nodes are often bypassed with metastatic deposits developing in more distal nodes. Tumour deposits in local lymph nodes are a clear indication of the metastatic potential of the primary tumour and in general are associated with an unfavourable outcome. A curative operation for a primary cancer aims to remove the primary tumour, surrounding tissue infiltrated by tumour and regional lymph nodes with metastatic deposits. Block dissection of uninvolved nodes do not improve outcome and are infrequently performed. In breast and melanoma surgery, new techniques are being developed to diagnose lymph node deposits in order to prevent unnecessary block dissection.

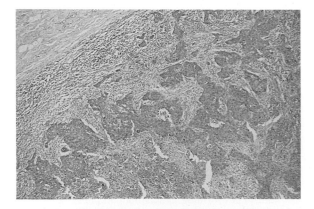

Figure 11.15. Histological slide of a patient with cancer of the breast. Note the infiltration of lymphocytes both into the connective tissue surrounding the cancer as well as directly into the cancer itself.

Approach and differential diagnosis of lymphadenopathy

The history and clinical examination is essential in the approach to the diagnosis of the cause of lymphadenopathy. The age of patient, duration of symptoms, associated symptoms of possible infective causes or malignant disease, whether the enlarged lymph nodes are painful or tender, consistency of the lymph nodes, their location and whether they are localized or generalized, are all important factors. Splenomegaly or hepatomegaly should be assessed. If the lymphadenopathy is localized, the appropriate lymphatic drainage area are particularly examined (Table 11.5).

Further investigations will depend on the initial history and clinical diagnosis but it frequently include a full blood count, blood film and erythrocyte sedimentation rate (ESR). Chest X-ray, monospot test, CMV, and *Toxoplasma* titres, and anti-HIV and Mantoux tests, are frequently suitable. In several cases it may be essential to make a cytohistological diagnosis, by either a fine needle aspirate or a lymph node biopsy. Computed tomography (CT) scanning is valuable in determining the cause or presence and extent of intra-abdominal or intrathoracic lymphadenopathy. In some cases of deep lymph node enlargement, where superficial lymph node enlargement are not available for biopsy, bone marrow biopsy, liver biopsies, CT or ultrasound guided fine or core needle biopsy may be needed. Occasionally laparoscopic or thoracoscopic lymph node biopsies is indicated and help to avoid the need for laparotomy or thoracotomy.

Splenic disorders

Splenic trauma

Trauma is the most common reason for operating on the spleen. The spleen is the most frequently injured solid organ in the abdomen and splenic injury can result in profuse bleeding that is often fatal. The degree of splenic trauma is graded as follows:

- *Grade I*: Subcapsular haematoma or capsular tear not actively bleeding.
- *Grade II*: Capsular and superficial parenchymal tear with minimal bleeding.
- *Grade III*: Deep parenchymal tears with active bleeding.
- *Grade IV*: Parenchymal tears extending to hilum, total disruption, hilar injuries.

Splenic injury can be caused by blunt or penetrating trauma to the torso. In patients with pre-existing splenomegaly or bleeding disorders: for example, leukaemia patients on chemotherapy, minimal trauma (sometimes not remembered by the patient) can result in splenic disruption. The spleen is frequently inadvertently or iatrogenic injured during abdominal surgery.

The diagnosis is made clinically or aided by diagnostic peritoneal lavage, ultrasound and CT scanning. Management

---

Table 11.5. Causes of lymphadenopathy.

Localized	Generalized
Local infection	*Infection*
• Pyogenic infection (e.g. pharyngitis, dental abscess, otitis media, actinomyces)	• Viral (e.g. infectious mononucleosis, measles, rubella, HIV, viral hepatitis)
• Viral infection	• Bacterial (e.g. syphilis, brucellosis, tuberculosis, *Salmonella*, bacterial endocarditis)
• Cat scratch fever	• Fungal (e.g. histoplasmosis)
• Lymphogranuloma venereum	• Protozoal (e.g. toxoplasmosis)
• Tuberculosis	*Non-infectious inflammatory disease* (e.g. sarcoidosis, rheumatoid arthritis, SLE, other connective disease, serum sickness)
Lymphoma	*Malignant*
• Hodgkin's disease	• Leukaemias, especially CLL, ALL
• Non-Hodgkin's lymphoma	• Lymphoma
Carcinoma	• Waldenström's macroglobulinaemia
	• Rarely secondary malignancy
	• Angioimmunoblastic lymphadenopathy
	Miscellaneous
	• Sinus histocytosis
	• Reaction to drugs and chemicals (e.g. hydantoins and related chemicals, beryllium)
	• Hyperthyroidism

All: acute lymphoblastic leukaemia.

of a splenic injury depends on the severity of the injury, the experience of the surgeon, and the facilities available. Grade I injuries may be treated by observation with regular follow-up haemoglobin checks (e.g. 4 hourly) and intermittent scanning (e.g. every 2–3 days). Splenic conservation surgery by fibrin glue, patching or packing with haemostatic material, suturing, partial resection or wrapping in absorbable sheets such as polyglycolic acid, may be considered for grade II and III injuries. Splenectomy should be performed for all grade IV injuries, and also for grade II and III injuries if facilities for close follow-up is not available and/or if the surgeon is inexperienced with dealing with splenic trauma.

Implantation of diced pieces of splenic tissue into the omentum after splenectomy, with the hope that these islands of splenic tissue will restore normal splenic function, have been tried for many years. Unfortunately, although successful implantation has been achieved, the ectopic splenic tissue has not been shown to be functional.

Hypersplenism

The syndrome of hypersplenism is caused by several different diseases, and is characterized by splenomegaly, reduced circulating numbers of one or more types of blood cells (e.g. red cells, platelets and neutrophils), and the release of immature cells by the bone marrow. The most common causes are lymphoma, leukaemia (particularly chronic lymphocytic leukaemia, CLL), B-thalassaemia, sickle cell disease, portal hypertension, rheumatoid arthritis, infection (e.g. malaria), infiltrative diseases (e.g. sarcoidosis) and lipid storage disease (e.g. Gaucher's disease). The decision to perform a splenectomy is based on the natural history of the disease and the severity of the cytopaenia (Fig. 11.16).

Other indications for splenectomy

Splenectomy is sometimes indicated as part of a cancer operation; for example, tumours near the greater curve of the stomach, near the tail of the pancreas, at the splenic flexure of the colon. On occasion a splenectomy is indicated as treatment for idiopathic thrombocytopaenic purpura and hereditary spherocytosis, or as a staging procedure for lymphoma. An abscess or hydatid cyst of the spleen are rare indications.

Haematological effects of splenectomy and hyposplenism
Red cell changes
The changes in red cell morphology include the presence of Howell–Jolly bodies and Pappenheimer (siderotic) granules in some cells. These red cell morphology may assist in the diagnosis of hyposplenism and evaluate residual or ectopic splenic function after splenectomy.

White cell changes
Postsplenectomy there is a mild permanent rise in both lymphocyte and monocyte count.

Platelet changes
The spleen normally pools up to a third of the circulating platelets. In the immediate period after a splenectomy, the platelet count rise steeply to levels of $600–1000 \times 10^9/l$. This thrombocytosis is usually temporary and fall to a level one-third higher than in normal subjects over the following 1–2 months. Occasional large and bizarre platelets can be seen in blood films.

Complications after splenectomy and asplenism
Bleeding
Bleeding may occur from the splenic bed, pedicle or short gastric vessels. Especially important where splenectomy was performed for thrombocytopaenia.

Atelectasis
Left lower lobe atelectasis is common after splenectomy. Active physiotherapy may prevent this complication.

Pancreatic tail injury
The tail of the pancreas is in close relation to the hilum of the spleen and may be injured during the surgical procedure. This may lead to a pancreatic leak and collection.

Fever
Postsplenectomy fever can occur in the absence of any source of infection.

Thrombocytosis
There is an immediate and progressive rise in the platelet count after splenectomy to levels of $600–1000 \times 10^9/l$. After a peak at days 7–12, platelet levels usually return to normal, but it may remain elevated for up to 3 months. If the platelet count is persistently elevated above $1000 \times 10^9/l$, prophylaxis against deep vein thrombosis should be instituted; for example, oral aspirin at 150 mg/day.

Overwhelming postsplenectomy infection
Following splenectomy, patients clear encapsulated bacteria less well from the bloodstream. This is particularly true for *S. pneumoniae*, but also for *Neisseria meningitidis*, *Escherichia coli* and *H. influenzae*. Overwhelming postsplenectomy infection occurs in 3–5% of patients, particularly in children, and has a mortality rate of 50%. Most serious infections occurs within the first 3 years of splenectomy.

Prophylactic vaccination
Prophylaxis is achieved by vaccination against pneumococci, meningococci and *H. influenzae*. Vaccines should preferably be given pre-operatively as soon as the decision is made to operate, because antibody titres are 50% greater than when vaccines are given in the post-operative period. The question of prolonged prophylactic antibiotics is still controversial. The standard recommended regimen is a daily

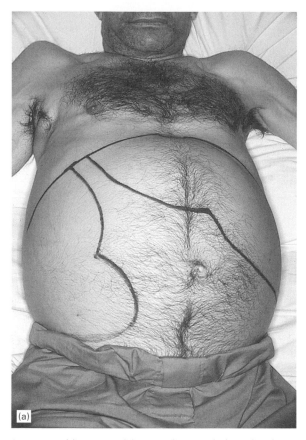
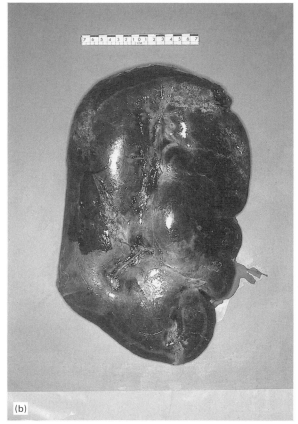

Figure 11.16. (a) Patient with hepato-splenomegaly due to lymphoma with the outlines of the liver and spleen marked on the skin. and (b) a spleen resected for hypersplenism in a patient with lymphoma. (photographs courtesy of Mr T Davidson, UCL Medical School).

dose of 250 mg penicillin VK orally for life, and to keep a supply of oral amoxicillin at home to start at the earliest sign of a fever or chest infection.

Recommendations for patients with no spleen or hypofunctioning spleen:

- Pneumococcal vaccine (Pneumovax II) 0.5 ml – 2 weeks before splenectomy or as soon as possible after splenectomy is performed in emergency situation.
- *H. influenzae* type B (Hib) vaccine 0.5 ml.
- Meningococcal polysaccharide vaccine for *N. meningitidis* type A and C 0.5 ml.
- Consider penicillin as prophylaxis (250 mg twice daily for life).

The three vaccines (subcutaneous or intramuscular) may be given at same time, but different sites should be used.

Organ transplantation

Transplanted non-self (allogeneic) cells have surface membrane antigens that stimulate a B- and T-cell immune response in the recipient that is intent on destroying the antigen and therefore the transplanted organ (graft rejection). Major advances have been made in both antigen matching between donor and recipient, and suppression of the immune response in the recipient.

The antigenic relationship between donor graft and recipient can be described as follows:

- *Autogeneic* when tissue is transplanted in the same individual to a different site in the body.
- *Syngeneic* when the transplant is between two individuals with identical genetic makeup (e.g. identical twins).
- *Allogeneic* when tissue is transplanted between two individuals with different antigenic makeups, and their tissues are therefore histo-incompatible.
- *Xenogeneic* when tissue is transplanted from one species to another (Fig. 11.17).

Transplantation/histocompatibility antigens
MHC antigens

These are the most important antigens (in humans called HLA) responsible for graft rejection. The surface molecules are divided into class I and class II MHC antigens. Each class of antigens are coded for by genes located at three different loci on chromosome 6; that is, loci A, B and C for class I, and

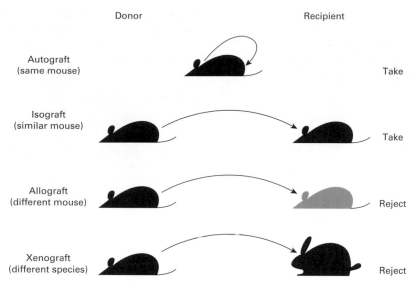

Figure 11.17. Different types of tissue transplantation (from Benjamini *et al.*, 1996.)

loci DR, DQ and DP for class II molecules and numerous different alleles, coding for different molecules, have been described for each locus. Although these antigens have been named and extensively studied in relation to transplantation surgery, they were not designed by nature for that purpose. The physiological role of the MHC antigens is that of antigen presentation in order that lymphocytes can determine whether it is self or non-self.

Minor histocompatibility antigens
These cell surface antigens are a mixed group that can also cause cell-mediated graft rejection, but induce a less potent immune response than the MHC molecules.

Blood group antigens
Blood transfusion was one of the first types of tissue transplantation. The major groups of antigens responsible for histocompatibility are designated as A, B and O. There are numerous other groups of blood cell antigens that are less likely to cause a significant haemolytic transfusion reaction (e.g. Kell, Duffy, Lewis, MN and Ss groups).

Tissue typing/antigen matching
Cross-match
During cross-matching, serum from the potential recipient is mixed with lymphocytes (organ transplant) or red blood cells (blood transfusion) to test whether the recipient has any antibodies that could be cytotoxic to the potential donor's cells. This is the only type of antigen matching performed before blood transfusion, and many organ transplant units propose that it is also a sufficient antigen-matching procedure before organ transplantation.

Serological tissue typing
The MHC antigen profile of both donor and recipient can be determined by using monoclonal antibodies and stored serum known to contain antibodies against specific MHC antigens. Usually only HLA-A, B, C and DR are tested for.

Mixed leucocyte reaction
In this procedure leucocytes from both donor and recipient are cultured together over a few days to test the parity (or disparity) between the cells.

Genotyping
In stead of typing the whole molecule, typing specific epitopes on HLA molecules have become possible by amplifying the DNA segment that codes for the epitope. Matching HLA at the genetic level is much more accurate than serological methods.

Graft rejection
Hyperacute rejection
Hyperacute rejection occurs within minutes of transplantation and is due to destruction of the transplanted organ by pre-existing antibodies in the recipient, similar to an ABO incompatible blood transfusion. There is no treatment to prevent or stop hyperacute rejection once it has started.

Acute rejection
Acute rejection is mediated by T-cells and is the common type of organ rejection seen in tissue mismatch after an allotransplant, or when insufficient immunosuppression is employed. This type of rejection begins within a few days after the transplant with a complete loss of function within 10–14 days.

Chronic rejection

Chronic rejection is mediated by both antibodies and T-cells, and occurs months after the transplanted organ had initially functioned normally. It is characterized by a slow and progressive organ failure, and little can be done to slow the process down.

Prevention

Over recent years it has become clear that graft survival is more dependent on adequate immunosuppression than on accurate tissue typing. The three most commonly used immunosuppressive drugs are azathioprine, steroids and cyclosporine. Newer drugs are being developed and the latest immunosuppressant to appear on the market is FK506. Other methods include antilymphocyte serum or globulin, monoclonal antibodies against lymphocytes, and total lymphoid irradiation. The price paid for effective immunosuppression and graft survival is the complications of immunosuppression as discussed earlier in this chapter.

FURTHER READING

Benjamini E, Sunshine G, Leskowitz S. *Immunology. A Short Course*, 3rd edn. New York: Wiley-Liss, Inc., 1996

Edwards SW. *Biochemistry and Physiology of the Neutrophil.* Cambridge: Cambridge University Press, 1994

Jandl JH. *Blood: Textbook of Hematology.* Boston: Little, Brown and Company, 1996

Provan D. *ABC of Clinical Haematology.* London: BMJ Books, 2003

12

Upper Gastrointestinal Surgery

TJ Wheatley

Consultant Upper GI Surgeon, Derriford Hospital, Plymouth, UK

CONTENTS

Anatomy	**230**
Stomach	230
Oesophagus	230
Duodenum, pancreas, hepatic, and biliary systems	231
Portal venous system	231
Investigations	**232**
Ultrasound	232
Computed tomography	233
Magnetic resonance imaging	233
Endoscopy	233
Endoscopic retrograde cholangio-pancreatography	233
Oesophageal function tests	233
Upper GI emergencies	**234**
Acute cholecystitis	234
Acute pancreatitis	235
Perforated viscus	236
Upper GI bleeding	237
Upper GI malignancy	**239**
Oesophageal carcinoma	239
Gastric carcinoma	240
Cancer of the GOJ	241
Pancreatic carcinoma	241
Hepatic tumours	243
Other upper GI conditions	**244**
Jaundice	244
Gallstones	245
Portal hypertension	246
Peptic ulcer	246
Gastro oesophageal reflux disease	247

ANATOMY

Stomach

The upper abdominal viscera can be related to the transpyloric plane. The normal stomach is impalpable with the fundus lying underneath the left diaphragm. The body of a stomach distended secondary to gastric outlet obstruction may be visible and palpable and a succussion splash may be heard within it. Gastric masses are rarely palpable and if at this stage they represent a malignant process, they will invariably be inoperable. The stomach has a rich blood supply which comprises the left gastric artery from the coeliac axis, the right gastric artery from the common hepatic artery, the right gastroepiploic artery from the gastroduodenal branch of the hepatic artery, the left gastroepiploic artery from the splenic artery and the short gastric arteries from the splenic artery. When the stomach is used as a conduit in the chest following oesophagectomy, the left gastric, left gastroepiploic, and short gastric arteries are divided and the organ suffers no ischaemic damage. Corresponding veins drain into the portal venous system and the lymphatic drainage follows perigastric glands and thence to groups around the spleen, aorta, retropancreatic, suprapancreatic, and subpyloric zones.

Oesophagus

The oesophagus is 25 cm long, extending from the pharynx to the cardia. It lies in the posterior mediastinum, and is traditionally divided into upper, middle, and lower thirds. The upper third is closely related anteriorly to the trachea, down to the carina. The middle third extends from the carina to approximately 7 cm above the diaphragmatic hiatus, and is related anteriorly to the pericardium. The lower third extends through the hiatus to include a short segment of intra-abdominal oesophagus, and is related (in the thorax) to the left atrium. The oesophagus receives its blood supply via direct branches from the aorta, and branches from other organs such as thyroid, trachea, and stomach. Venous drainage is via the azygos and hemiazygos veins. The vagus nerves lie closely applied to the surface of the oesophagus, and it must be remembered that the right recurrent laryngeal branch arises in the upper thorax, passing around the subclavian artery, and the left recurrent laryngeal branch passes around the ductus arteriosus. These branches can be injured during surgery on the upper oesophagus. The oesophageal hiatus is surrounded by the crura, pillars of diaphragmatic muscle that help contribute to the lower oesophageal sphincter. A hiatus hernia involves herniation of the proximal stomach through this area, and can predispose to gastro-oesophageal reflux. Massive hiatus hernia can occur where most, or all, of the stomach herniates into the thoracic cavity.

Duodenum, pancreas, hepatic, and biliary systems

Behind the stomach lies the lesser sac which separates the stomach from the pancreas, left kidney, left suprarenal, spleen, and splenic artery. The duodenum forms a 'C'-shape around the head of the pancreas, is 25 cm long and originates from the pylorus which is completely covered with peritoneum, following which it becomes a retroperitoneal organ. Thus, instrumental perforations of the second part of the duodenum during endoscopic retrograde cholangio-pancreatography (ERCP) present with non-specific abdominal symptoms since the duodenal and biliary secretions collect in the retroperitoneal space. The right and left hepatic ducts join in the porta hepatis to emerge as the common hepatic duct. The gallbladder drains through the cystic duct to join the common hepatic duct and form the common bile duct (CBD). The supraduodenal portion of the CBD is of variable length, depending on the length of the cystic duct, and the definition of this junction is of paramount importance during cholecystectomy and also to determine the type of biliary bypass required in inoperable obstructive jaundice due to periampullary carcinomas. The retropancreatic CBD joins the main pancreatic duct to form the ampulla of vater and this drains into the second part of the duodenum via the duodenal papilla (Fig. 12.1). A papillotomy or sphincterotomy performed either endoscopically or by open surgery deroofs the superior aspect of the ampulla of vater, thus enlarging the outlet of the CBD at its termination. In general terms this is a safe procedure because there are no major anatomical structures or blood vessels in the vicinity. The CBD is found at the free edge of the lesser omentum, to its left is the common hepatic artery and behind both these structures is the portal vein. Posterior to the free edge of the lesser omentum is the foramen of Winslow and behind this is the inferior vena cava. Thus, there is a short distance at this level between the portal vein and the inferior vena cava, which is utilised surgically in the construction of portacaval shunts.

Portal venous system

The portal venous system drains blood from all the abdominal viscera. The distal tributaries of this system correspond to the arterial blood supply to form, eventually, the inferior mesenteric vein and the superior mesenteric vein. The inferior mesenteric vein ascends to the left of the duodenojejunal flexure to join the splenic vein behind the pancreas. The superior mesenteric vein joins the splenic vein behind the neck of the pancreas at the transpyloric plane to form the portal vein which ascends behind the first part of the duodenum, behind the bile duct and hepatic artery into the porta hepatis. The portal vein divides into right and left branches which eventually drain into lobules of the liver and then reform as radicals of the hepatic vein through which they empty into the inferior vena cava (Fig. 12.2). Communications exist between the portal venous system and the systemic venous system at the oesophageal branches of the left gastric vein and the oesophageal veins of the azygos system in the thorax. A rise in

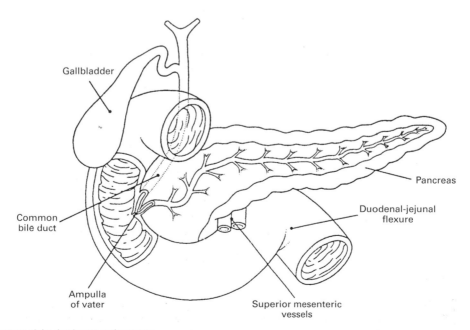

Figure 12.1. Anatomy of the duodenum and pancreas.

pressure in this system forms oesophageal varices. Communications also form between the superior haemorrhoidal branch of the inferior mesenteric vein and inferior haemorrhoidal veins, between tributaries in the mesentery and mesocolon and retroperitoneal veins, between portal branches in the liver and veins of the abdominal wall through veins passing along the falciform ligament to the umbilicus and between portal branches in the liver and veins of the diaphragm around the bare area of the liver.

INVESTIGATIONS

There are certain specialised investigations that can be used in the investigation of upper gastrointestinal (GI) conditions.

These do not replace a carefully taken history, but do provide a useful adjunct to clinical examination, and it is important to understand the uses and limitations of the various techniques.

Ultrasound

The use of high-frequency sound waves to image soft tissues is safe, effective, and widely available. The standard ultrasound examination involves a probe applied to the skin with a layer of conductive gel to provide a good interface for sound waves. These waves are produced in the probe at frequencies of 1–5 MHz and their reflections are collected and

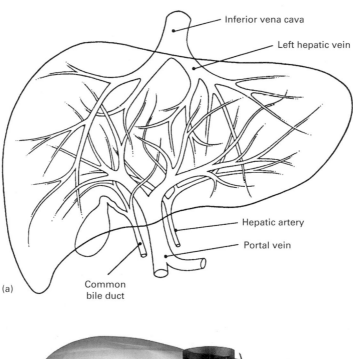

(a)

Inferior vena cava

Left hepatic vein

Hepatic artery

Portal vein

Common bile duct

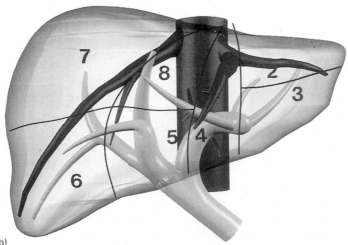

(b)

Figure 12.2. (a) Anatomy of the biliary system (b) Portal segmentation.

interpreted to produce a real time gray-scale image of the area under investigation. Generally, fluid-filled structures transmit ultrasound waves easily and appear black, whereas connective tissues reflect more waves and appear brighter on the screen. Interpretation of ultrasound images is much easier when seen at the time of scanning, while printed images are more difficult. The experience of the operator is a very important factor in the accuracy of information provided. Basic trans-abdominal scanning is a useful investigation for biliary, hepatic and pancreatic disease, and can be combined with Doppler scanning technology (so-called 'duplex' scans) to give information about blood flow. Biopsy of intra-abdominal structures, such as liver metastases, can be performed accurately under ultrasound guidance, as can the insertion of drains. Using ultrasound through the layers of the anterior abdominal wall limits the image quality, and probes have been developed to allow use within the peritoneal cavity (handheld and laparoscopic), and within endoscopes. Endoscopic ultrasound (EUS) is used to help stage upper GI malignancies, and investigate benign hepato-pancreato-biliary (HPB) conditions. Intra-operative ultrasound is also used for staging, and is helpful planning hepatic resections.

Computed tomography

Computed tomography (CT) scanning relies on multiple X-ray images taken as 'slices' and re-configured under computer control to display cross-sectional images of the body. Early scanners were slow and resolution was poor for structures measuring less than 1 cm, but newer scanners are much quicker using spiral scanning techniques, and provide greatly improved resolution. It is relatively straightforward with current technology to create computerised 3D images to allow easier appreciation of anatomy. CT scans of solid organs, such as the liver, spleen, and pancreas, are useful for both benign and malignant lesions; and staging of all upper GI cancers relies on CT scans of the chest and abdomen. CT scanning is much less operator dependant than ultrasound, and does not require real time images for accurate interpretation. As with ultrasound it is possible to perform interventional procedures (biopsy, drain insertion) under CT guidance.

Magnetic resonance imaging

Magnetic resonance imaging (MRI) scanning uses high-density magnetic fields to align hydrogen atoms within the body. Radio frequency (RF) pulses are then applied which make the atoms spin (or resonate) in a slightly different direction, and when the RF pulse ends the atoms return to their original orientation, releasing energy. This energy is detected by the scanner and interpreted to provide detailed images. These are similar to CT images in that they show cross-sectional views of the body, however MRI is better than CT for differentiating between certain soft tissues, and for imaging joints. For upper GI conditions it is useful for the liver

and pancreas, often in conjunction with CT. Increasingly the technique of magnetic resonance cholangio-pancreatography (MRCP) is being used to supplement and/or replace ERCP (see below), MRCP being non-invasive and avoiding the 0.1% mortality rate associated with ERCP.

Endoscopy

Upper GI endoscopy is a vital investigation for imaging the upper GI tract, and is sometimes referred to as OGD (oesophago-gastro-duodenoscopy). Using flexible endoscopes it is possible to directly visualise the oesophagus, stomach, and duodenum to check for mucosal abnormality and obtain biopsies. Modern video-endoscopes project the image onto a monitor allowing easier use, more accurate diagnosis, and the ability to record photographic and video images. Endoscopy is not only diagnostic, but also interventional, and has become first-line treatment for most cases of upper GI bleeding. Oesophageal strictures can be dilated, obstructing cancers can be stented, and polyps and early cancers can be resected. Most endoscopy can be performed using simple anaesthetic throat spray, but sedation is required for some patients and procedures. Morbidity and mortality are rare but include bleeding and perforation – which are more common with interventional techniques.

Endoscopic retrograde cholangio-pancreatography

ERCP is a variant of upper GI endoscopy, specifically used to visualise and instrument the CBD and pancreatic duct. Rather than the usual endoscope which views from the end, a 'side-viewing' scope is used which allows a view at 90° to the long axis of the scope. It is more difficult to manoeuvre this side-viewing scope through the stomach and pylorus, but once in the duodenum it allows an excellent view of the ampulla of Vater. ERCP is used to investigate and treat biliary and pancreatic pathology such as jaundice, acute pancreatitis, and chronic pancreatitis. MRCP provides good diagnostic images of the biliary and pancreatic tract, whereas ERCP has the advantage of allowing stent placement, or stone extraction, to deal with jaundice and cholangitis. The disadvantages are the risks of introducing infection, causing bleeding, inducing pancreatitis (1% of cases), and an overall mortality rate of 0.1%.

Oesophageal function tests

Oesophageal motility and acid exposure can be measured very accurately to provide useful information on oesophageal disorders. Most surgeons would insist on oesophageal function studies being performed before considering a patient for anti-reflux surgery. These investigations are performed by trained individuals and require careful interpretation by a specialist.

Manometry

Intra-oesophageal pressure readings are measured using catheters with multiple fluid-filled channels, or miniature pressure transducers. Manometry is commonly performed in a laboratory over a very short time period. It is possible to carry out 24-h ambulatory assessments, which may be combined with pH studies, for a more representative view of motility. Primary peristalsis is initiated by swallowing and progresses from the pharynx, terminating in relaxation of the lower oesophageal sphincter. Secondary peristalsis is initiated by distension of the oesophagus (e.g. by food bolus) and progresses in a similar fashion. Tertiary contractions do not result in peristaltic waves, and occur as isolated, sporadic events. Motility disorders include: achalasia, where failure of both normal peristaltic activity and relaxation of the lower oesophageal sphincter results in dysphagia and a dilated oesophagus proximal to the gastro-oesophageal junction (GOJ); and diffuse oesophageal spasm, where isolated high-pressure contractions cause chest pain. A low-pressure lower oesophageal sphincter is commonly seen in gastro-oesophageal reflux disease (GORD).

pH monitoring

Intra-oesophageal pH is measured with a transducer positioned 5 cm above the manometrically determined lower oesophageal sphincter. Ambulatory readings are taken over a 24- or 48-h period, and correlated with symptoms recorded by the patient. Normally, the pH is <4 for no more than 4% of a 24-h period, but with significant reflux the percentage is much higher. Some patients have a normal percentage of pH < 4, but very good correlation between reflux episodes and symptoms which often indicates significant reflux. Others have pH < 4 for more than 4% of the period measured, but no correlation with symptoms, suggesting reflux is an incidental finding. It is important that pH studies are interpreted carefully, and correlated with the patient's history.

UPPER GI EMERGENCIES

Acute cholecystitis

For more details see also the section Gallstones.

Acute cholecystitis is an inflammatory condition of the gallbladder, often, but not always, associated with the presence of gallstones. It is a common surgical cause of emergency admission to hospital, and is more common in women than men in keeping with the distribution of stone disease. The symptoms will initially resemble biliary colic, with right upper quadrant pain, and nausea, but symptoms persist and patients become systemically unwell. Fever, tachycardia, and mild jaundice may develop, and the pain may radiate to the scapula. An initial chemical inflammation is often superceded by bacterial infection with a deterioration in systemic symptoms. Clinical examination demonstrates localised tenderness in the right upper quadrant over the fundus of the gallbladder. Pain on inspiration while palpating in the right upper quadrant is called Murphy's sign, and is pathognomonic of cholecystitis.

Trans-abdominal ultrasound scanning is the investigation of choice for suspected acute cholecystitis, and should ideally be performed within 24 h of admission. The scan may confirm the presence of gallstones within the gallbladder, as well as a thickened gallbladder wall, and localised tenderness over the fundus ('sonographic Murphy's sign'). In severe conditions some pericholecystic fluid is present, and collections of fluid indicate a contained perforation. Varying degrees of dilatation of the biliary tree may be present, caused by inflammatory compression, bile duct stones, or Mirizzi's syndrome (see Gallstones). If the gallbladder is normal then the scan may help further the diagnosis, showing free fluid from a perforated viscus, or pancreatic oedema in acute pancreatitis.

The initial management of a suspected case of acute cholecystitis includes analgesia, antibiotics if bacterial infection is present, and intravenous fluids if dehydration and vomiting are present. Once the diagnosis is confirmed by ultrasound then definitive treatment should be planned. In patients fit enough for surgery, cholecystectomy is indicated, the timing of which is controversial. Standard treatment in the UK has been to allow the acute attack to settle with conservative treatment, and plan for an 'interval cholecystectomy' 6 weeks later. The practice in other countries, supported by clinical studies, is to perform an early cholecystectomy, within 3–4 days of the onset of symptoms. Proponents of the 'interval' approach claim that acute inflammation makes the early operation more difficult. However, 50% of people left to recover after an acute attack of cholecystitis will have further attacks before undergoing their interval cholecystectomy, and the early approach is not only more acceptable to most patients, but makes more efficient use of health care resources. Some patients treated conservatively do not settle and require surgery after a few days of treatment. A common scenario for this is a patient who develops an empyema of the gallbladder, where an obstructed cystic duct and undrained bacterial infection allows pus to collect within the lumen of the gallbladder. Cholecystectomy for acute cholecystitis is most commonly performed laparoscopically, but when performed in the acute setting may be more difficult, requiring an experienced surgeon, and resulting in a higher conversion rate to open surgery.

Some patients are unfit for surgery due to age, or co-morbidity, in which case conservative treatment may be their best, definitive option. There is a risk of further attacks though, and in such cases the risk of surgery must be carefully weighed against the risk of further episodes. Patients whose condition is so serious that surgery would be too dangerous during the acute attack may be treated by percutaneous cholecystostomy, where a drain is placed into the gallbladder lumen under ultrasound guidance and infected bile drained. This is usually a temporary procedure, until such time as the patient is fit for surgery.

On rare occasions acute cholecystitis develops in the absence of gallstones, so-called acalculous cholecystitis. This tends to happen in diabetic patients, and is often more serious than calculous attacks.

Acute pancreatitis

Acute pancreatitis is an acute inflammatory process of the pancreas, with variable involvement of other regional tissues or remote organ systems. It includes a spectrum of disease from a mild, self-limiting event, through to a severe, potentially fatal condition with associated multi-organ failure. There are 20–40 cases per 100 000 population per year in the UK, and the mortality rate remains unchanged at 10%. The majority of cases (80–90%) are caused by gallstones or alcohol ingestion; other rarer causes are listed in Table 12.1. The number of genuine idiopathic cases decreases as other possible causes are investigated.

The classic presentation is a sudden onset of severe epigastric pain, radiating to the back, associated with profuse vomiting. The patient will often be unable to keep still with the pain, in contrast to the immobile patient with peritonitis. A history of previously diagnosed gallstones, or alcohol consumption, is helpful, but not conclusive. Hypotension, tachycardia, tachypnoea, oliguria, and jaundice may be present, especially in severe cases. Biochemical tests are often crucial in the diagnosis, serum amylase measurement being the most widely recognised, with British Society of Gastroenterology guidelines suggesting a level four times above normal as diagnostic. It is important to remember that a raised amylase by itself is not diagnostic of acute pancreatitis, but has to be taken in context of the clinical picture. Also if the presentation is delayed then the peak level of amylase may be missed and the diagnosis may be more difficult. Serum lipase measurements are less widely available, but are more specific and remain elevated for longer than amylase – the diagnostic level is two times above normal. There is no correlation between amylase (or lipase) level and disease severity. Changes described on plain X-ray examinations include pleural effusions, localised ileus (sentinel loop), and radio-opaque gallstones, but these are non-specific. More specialised radiology can be helpful; ultrasound shows the presence of gallstones, as well as fluid collections, but is less good at visualising the pancreas, while CT scanning can be diagnostic in difficult cases. Rarely, acute pancreatitis is diagnosed at laparotomy when another intra-abdominal emergency is suspected.

Severity scoring is important in all cases of acute pancreatitis, and a variety of schemes are in use. The Glasgow scoring system is easily and widely used, and has been validated on UK patients. Scores ≥3 imply severe disease (Table 12.2). The APACHE II system is more complex, and relies on a wide selection of acute physiological readings, as well as attributing points for pre-existing chronic health problems. Scores ≥9 predict severe disease (Table 12.3). Whichever system is used it is important that severity scoring is performed within 48 h of onset to help identify those patients with predicted severe disease who will require more intensive management.

Patients with mild acute pancreatitis recover quickly with minimal supportive treatment. Adequate analgesia, careful fluid balance, and supplementary oxygen are usually all the measures that are required. Nasogastric drainage and urinary catheterisation are often unnecessary and within 3–5 days most patients are feeling better. It is important that such patients undergo ultrasound examination to look for gallstones, and if present these must be treated. The preferred management would be urgent cholecystectomy, if possible during that same admission, if not then within 2–4 weeks.

Table 12.2. Glasgow scoring system for acute pancreatitis.

Age	>55 years
White blood cell count	$>15 \times 10^9/l$
Glucose	>10 mmol/l
Urea	>16 mmol/l
PaO_2	<60 mmHg
Calcium	<2 mmol/l
Albumin	<32 g/l
Lactate dehydrogenase	>600 units/l
Aspartate or alanine aminotransferase	>100 units/l

Table 12.3. APACHE II scoring system parameters.

Acute physiology parameters	Chronic health parameters
Temperature	Age
Mean arterial pressure	Post-operative status
Heart rate	Liver disease
Respiratory rate	Cardiovascular disease
Oxygenation	Respiratory disease
Arterial pH	Renal disease
Na	Immunocompromised
K	states
Creatinine	
Packed cell volume	
White blood cell count	
Glasgow coma score	

Table 12.1. Rare causes of acute pancreatitis.

- Idiopathic
- Iatrogenic: ERCP, surgery
- Duct obstruction: cancer, adenoma
- Infective: mumps, coxsackie, HIV
- Metabolic: hypercalcaemia, hyperlipidaemia
- Drugs: loop diuretics, azathioprine
- Hypothermia
- Hereditary pancreatitis

The bile duct must be imaged to ensure absence of choledo-cholithiasis, either by ERCP, or on-table cholangiography.

Patients with predicted severe disease should be transferred to a high dependency or intensive care unit (ICU) for close monitoring and multi-system support as necessary. The overall mortality rate in this group is 20–30%, and supportive management in a critical care setting is essential to keep this as low as possible. No therapeutic agents have been found to significantly alter prognosis. These patients should all undergo CT scanning within the first 10 days of admission, to look for local complications. Acute fluid collections and necrosis seen on scans may require drainage, especially if infection is suspected. Drainage may be by percutaneous techniques for fluid collections which are accessible, or by laparotomy especially if infected necrosis is present. If gallstones are present ERCP and sphincterotomy may improve the condition if performed within 48 h of onset, though there is continuing controversy as to the role of urgent ERCP. If obstructive jaundice or cholangitis are present then ERCP is vital. After a severe attack cholecystectomy may be delayed until the patient is fit for surgery, or performed at the same time as surgery for local complications. Pseudocysts in the lesser sac may require formal drainage if they are symptomatic (pain, gastric compression) or persist for more than 6 weeks. Drainage may be endoscopic or surgical, and usually involves connection to the posterior wall of the stomach.

Nutrition is important in all patients with prolonged and severe illness, and the traditional management of acute pancreatitis involved 'resting the gut' by starvation to avoid unnecessary pancreatic stimulation. To counter this period of starvation, total parenteral nutrition (TPN) has been used to support patients in their acute phase. Recent work has shown that it is possible to use enteral nutrition without detriment, so long as the feed is supplied into the jejunum – either by a feeding jejunostomy, or by a naso-jejunal tube.

Perforated viscus

The oesophagus, stomach, and duodenum can all suffer from perforation, and by far the commonest cause of an upper GI perforation is a peptic ulcer in either the stomach or duodenum.

Perforated peptic ulcer

Complications of peptic ulcer disease are now much less common than 20 years ago due to improved medical management (see Peptic Ulcer, below), but perforations still imply a mortality of approximately 10% (higher in older patients). The well-recognised risk factors for developing a perforation are long-term non-steroidal anti-inflammatory drug (NSAID) use, and *Helicobacter pylori* infection.

The usual presentation is a sudden onset of severe epigastric pain, followed quickly by signs of peritonitis. Patients with perforated ulcers will lie still with a 'rigid abdomen', are often pale and clammy, and may show hypotension, tachycardia,

tachypnoea, and pyrexia. Breathing will be shallow as well as rapid because of peritonitis. Sometimes in elderly patients, and those taking steroids, the early symptoms may be mild, or absent. The initial peritonitis is chemical due to the presence of gastric and/or duodenal fluid in the peritoneal cavity, but within hours a bacterial peritonitis supervenes. Delays in appropriate treatment being started result in higher mortality and morbidity – after 24 h the mortality rate has increased by seven times.

The diagnosis is made on clinical grounds, and supported by the presence of free gas seen under the diaphragm on an erect chest X-ray, but it must be remembered that 20–30% of perforations do not show free gas. If the diagnosis is in doubt a left lateral, decubitus abdominal X-ray may show free gas more clearly against the liver, and contrast studies with water-soluble agents can confirm an ongoing leak from a perforation. Ultrasound and CT examinations may show free intraperitoneal fluid, and/or localised collections in late presentations, but are not part of the usual work-up of this condition.

The management of perforated ulcers includes initial resuscitation, treatment of the perforation and treatment of the ulcer. Resuscitation and optimisation requires intravenous fluids and antibiotics, urethral catheterisation to aid accurate fluid balance, naso-gastric drainage, oxygen by facemask, and prompt, adequate analgesia (usually opiates). A variety of options are available for treating the perforation, and are classified as conservative or surgical.

Conservative treatment relies on the fact that perforations have a tendency to seal themselves (up to 50% are sealed at time of presentation), and seeks to provide conditions for spontaneous healing to occur and persist, while also dealing with intra-abdominal sepsis. IV fluids, antibiotics, and acid anti-secretory drugs (H_2 blockers or proton pump inhibitors (PPI)) are given, and patients kept under close review. Contrast studies are helpful here to confirm sealed leaks, and ultrasound/CT scanning will show collections, which may then be drained percutaneously. A low threshold to revert to surgical management is important for those patients who deteriorate, or fail to improve.

Surgical treatment has two main aims: to close the perforation, and to deal with intra-abdominal sepsis. Surgery used also to include definitive treatment for the ulcer in the form of vagotomy and pyloroplasty, partial gastrectomy, or other anti-ulcer procedure. With current medical management being so effective, it is unusual to perform such procedures, unless the ulcer is too large to close adequately, or the ulcer has failed to respond to maximum medical treatment already. The majority of surgeons will deal with perforations at laparotomy, though it is possible to obtain similar results with a laparoscopic approach in certain cases. At laparotomy the perforation must first be identified, sometimes requiring exploration of the lesser sac to see the posterior wall of the stomach. Once the perforation has been found it may be closed by interrupted sutures, but if this is not possible a patch of omentum is sutured over the defect, taking care not to render the omentum ischaemic. Even after suture closure an omental patch should be performed as additional security. If the ulcer is in the stomach then a biopsy from its edge must be taken to exclude the possibility of malignancy. Thorough peritoneal lavage is performed, and there is no benefit in using solutions containing antibiotics or antiseptics compared to sterile water or normal saline. Whether to leave a drain in the abdomen is contentious, as it may be linked to increased morbidity, but many surgeons do drain the peritoneum after laparotomy.

Once the perforation has been successfully dealt with, the peptic ulcer must be treated with full medical management as described below. This will include eradication of *H. pylori* if present, stopping NSAIDs as appropriate (or switching to alternative analgesia), and a healing course of anti-secretory medication.

Perforated oesophagus

The oesophagus may rupture spontaneously during vomiting (Boerhaave syndrome), but by far the commonest cause of perforation is iatrogenic. Instrumentation of the oesophagus is increasingly common, both at diagnostic endoscopy, and therapeutic intervention for strictures, achalasia, and even endoscopic resections. The perforation rate varies from around 0.001% for diagnostic, flexible endoscopy, up to 5% for balloon dilatation for achalasia.

Patients complain of pain, which they can localise quite accurately to the level of the perforation. Surgical emphysema may develop within a few hours of perforation, as well as a high temperature. A history of recent oesophageal intubation, or vomiting raises suspicion, and a perforation confirmed by plain chest X-ray, contrast swallow, or sometimes repeat endoscopy. Prompt diagnosis and treatment are crucial to reducing mortality, which may be as high as 50%. Conservative management with antibiotics, parenteral nutrition and percutaneous drainage may be suitable for small perforations in an otherwise healthy oesophagus. Larger perforations, and those with associated oesophageal pathology (e.g. cancer), benefit from early surgery, to either repair or resect the affected oesophagus. If surgery is indicated it is best performed within the first 12 h following perforation, before mediastinal sepsis is established.

Upper GI bleeding

Bleeding from the upper GI tract places a high demand on medical services, because of both the number of admissions to hospital, and the often complex, multi-disciplinary approach required to treat those with significant bleeds. In the 1990's the incidence of upper GI bleeding was 103 cases per 100 000 population, and the in-patient mortality was 14%. One quarter of those presenting to hospital with a bleed are over 80 years old, which is a significant contributory factor to this high mortality rate. About a third of all

Table 12.4. Causes of upper GI bleeding and relative frequency.

- Peptic ulcer (35%)
- No cause found (25%)
- Oesophageal cause – oesophagitis, varices, Mallory–Weiss (19%)
- Gastric erosions (11%)
- Rare causes – vascular malformation, Dieulafoy lesion, haemobilia, aorto-duodenal fistula (6%)
- Malignancy (4%)

bleeds are due to peptic ulcers, with a variety of other causes listed in Table 12.4.

The majority of patients present with overt bleeding in the form of haematemesis and/or melaena, or more rarely with fresh bleeding per rectum. Haematemesis may produce fresh blood, as commonly seen with varices, or altered blood (coffee grounds) from a slowly bleeding ulcer. Melaena occurs when blood is partially digested during passage through the GI tract, resulting in a black, liquid stool with an unmistakable, foul smell. The passage of fresh blood per rectum from an upper GI source is a very worrying feature, as it implies a significant bleed causing rapid transit through the gut without time for melaena to form.

Some patients present with covert bleeding and are investigated for collapse or anaemia. In time it becomes obvious that they are bleeding, either by the appearance of overt bleeding, or as a result of endoscopic investigation.

The initial management of patients with bleeding is resuscitation appropriate to the severity of their condition. Most patients have a minor episode of bleeding and are never haemodynamically compromised by it, but others lose a lot of blood, relatively quickly and require prompt resuscitation. Patients who have lost a lot of blood will be tachycardic initially, and hypotensive as blood loss increases. Tachypnoea develops as oxygen delivery decreases, and at the same time conscious level is affected leading to restlessness, irritability, drowsiness, and even unconsciousness. Oxygen supplementation is often required, and intravenous fluid replacement must start immediately in patients who are compromised. It is important to remember that many patients take β-blockers regularly, so will not show a tachycardia, and that younger people can maintain their blood pressure well with significant blood loss so tachycardia is an important sign. Whether the intravenous fluid used is crystalloid or colloid is less important than the amount given, and it is important to have good venous access (two large bore cannulas). If a lot of blood has been lost the best resuscitation fluid is blood, even O-negative if there is no time for a cross-match. A clotting screen must always be performed on patients with bleeding, and those who require active resuscitation benefit from central venous pressure monitoring, and urethral catheterisation with hourly urine output measurement.

Table 12.5. Rockall scoring system for upper GI bleeding.

Age (in years)	<60	60–79	>80
	0	1	2
Shock	None	Systolic BP > 100 Pulse > 100	Systolic BP < 100
	0	1	2
Co-morbidity	None	Major co-morbidity (ischaemic heart disease etc.)	Renal or hepatic failure. Disseminated malignancy
	0	1	2
Endoscopic diagnosis	No lesion, or Mallory–Weiss	All other lesions	Upper GI cancer
	0	1	2
Stigmata of recent haemorrhage	None		Blood in upper GI tract, adherent clot, visible vessel, active bleeding
	0		2

Once patients have been stabilised the next step is diagnosing the cause of the bleeding, so that definitive treatment can be started. The single most important investigation for upper GI bleeding is endoscopy, and hospitals require 24-h access to endoscopy facilities. All patients with a bleed should have an endoscopy performed within 24 h of admission irrespective of the severity of the bleed and this needs to be done by an experienced endoscopist. Endoscopy should provide a diagnosis of the cause of the bleeding, and may allow treatment. Endoscopic findings, combined with clinical features, can be used in scoring systems to predict patients at high risk of both further bleeding, and poor prognosis (Table 12.5).

Endoscopic management of upper GI bleeding employs a variety of different techniques to arrest bleeding. Oesophageal varices have traditionally been injected with ethanolamine, or sodium tetradecyl sulphate (STD); more recently elastic bands have been used to ligate varices using devices attached to flexible endoscopes. Results from variceal banding are generally better than injection sclerotherapy, especially as design of banding devices improves, making them easier to use. Bleeding peptic ulcers can be treated by injection, coagulation, or clips. Injection therapy has been tried with many different agents: adrenaline, alcohol, STD, tissue glue, and fibrin are the commonly used ones. Coagulation can be achieved with diathermy (bipolar, monopolar, or argon beam), laser energy, or heat probe. All coagulation techniques rely on heating tissue, though they differ in how that heat is generated. Clipping devices are available that allow small metal clips to be delivered down the working channel of flexible endoscopes, as yet these are not widely used.

Endoscopic management of bleeding is accepted as first-line treatment in patients who are stable enough to tolerate it. It has been shown to decrease transfusion requirements, reduce the likelihood of re-bleeding, and decrease the need for surgery. Whether it decreases the mortality rate from bleeding is less certain. If endoscopic treatment fails the options for further treatment depend on the individual circumstances. If varices re-bleed after banding, then repeat banding should be performed. If primary control of variceal bleeding cannot be achieved then balloon tamponade with a Sengstaken–Blakemore, or Minnesota, tube should be attempted. These tubes have a large, distal balloon which is inflated in the stomach, and pulled back to lodge at the GOJ. The more proximal oesophageal ballon is then inflated, thus compressing the cardia and distal oesophagus to tamponade varices. If this fails then trans-jugular intra-hepatic portalsystemic shunting (TIPSS) will lower the portal venous pressure, and is very useful for preventing re-bleeding, and stopping primary bleeding. If TIPSS is unavailable, or unsuccessful then surgery with oesophageal transection using a circular staple gun is an option. For bleeding ulcers the choice is more straightforward: if bleeding cannot be controlled at the first endoscopy then surgery is necessary, and if the patient re-bleeds then it may be worth trying further endoscopic treatment, but surgery is usually more appropriate.

Surgery for bleeding ulcers has one main aim – to secure haemostasis. The bleeding point must first be displayed adequately, and a good pre-operative endoscopy is invaluable at identifying the anatomical location of the bleed. A gastrotomy, or duodenotomy is performed depending on where the lesion is, and the bleeding point is controlled by under-running the area with multiple sutures. If the lesion is a gastric ulcer then a biopsy must be taken, because of the risk of malignancy, and it may be possible to excise the ulcer and close the resulting gastric defect. It is usually unnecessary to perform a definitive anti-ulcer operation as an emergency, as medical management for peptic ulcers is currently preferable.

The successful management of upper GI bleeding requires close co-operation between physicians, endoscopists and surgeons, and benefits from clear, local guidelines outlining management pathways. Although the majority of patients presenting with bleeds will settle with minimal treatment, the 10–20% who do not need early, co-ordinated management to minimise mortality rates.

Table 12.6. **TNM staging classification for oesophageal cancer.**

Tx – Primary tumour not assessable	Nx – Regional nodes not assessable
T0 – No primary tumour	N0 – No regional nodes involved
Tis – Carcinoma in situ	N1 – Regional nodes involved
T1 – Tumour invading lamina propria/submucosa	
T2 – Tumour invading muscularis propria	Mx – Metastasis not assessable
T3 – Tumour invading adventitia	M0 – No distant metastasis
T4 – Tumour invading adjacent structures	M1 – Distant metastasis

UPPER GI MALIGNANCY

Oesophageal carcinoma

Cancer of the oesophagus has an incidence of 5–10 cases per 100 000 people in Western countries, but this varies widely throughout the rest of the world, and may get as high as 150–200 per 100 000 in parts of China and Iran. Worryingly, the incidence is increasing sharply, especially for tumours of the distal third of the oesophagus, and at the GOJ. Men are twice as likely to be affected than women, and people in their 60s and 70s are at highest risk. Aetiological factors are multiple, but oesophagitis is a common link, while smoking, alcohol ingestion, and nitrosamines in foodstuffs have all been implicated. Metaplasia of normal squamous epithelium to columnar (Barrett's oesophagus) is a significant risk factor for adenocarcinoma, and as Barrett's is linked to GORD the increasing incidence of GORD may partly explain the rise in number of oesophageal cancer cases.

The commonest presentation of oesophageal cancer is dysphagia, which is progressive. Initially patients notice that certain solid foods stick as they swallow, then they become unable to swallow solids and rely on soft, sloppy foods, then they can only tolerate liquids, until eventually complete dysphagia develops and they cannot even swallow their own saliva. Dysphagia is a very distressing symptom, and is invariably linked with weight loss, which worsens as dysphagia progresses. Tiredness and lethargy develop, linked both to the gradual starvation, and to anaemia from chronic low-grade blood loss. Occasionally, patients are diagnosed during investigation for anaemia, at endoscopy for other upper GI symptoms, and from screening programmes for Barrett's oesophagus.

Barium swallow may show features of a malignant stricture, or an irregular mucosa, but endoscopy is essential for visualisation of the tumour, and obtaining biopsies for histological diagnosis. Once a cancer has been confirmed further management depends on the patient's suitability for surgery, the stage of the cancer, and, of course, the patient's wishes. Surgical resection of oesophageal cancer is a major undertaking, and carries a mortality rate of 5–10% (lower in specialised centres), and significant co-morbidity, especially cardio-respiratory, increases this to unacceptable levels. If patients are fit enough for surgery then they will undergo staging investigations, otherwise they will require palliative care to control symptoms. Palliation of dysphagia can been relieved by physical methods such as dilatation, alcohol injection, laser re-canalisation, and stenting, the latter two being the commonest methods employed currently. Stenting has been revolutionised by the introduction of self-expanding metal stents (SEMS) that are introduced on a small diameter trocar over a guide-wire placed across the cancer, and then deployed to expand to a much larger diameter over a period of 12–24-h. SEMS are best used in patients with at least dysphagia to solids as they grip better in a relatively tight stricture, and are not without morbidity and mortality. They may block either with impacted food boluses, or with tumour overgrowth/ingrowth, and repeat endoscopic interventions are then required. Chemo- or radiotherapy has a role in palliating some patients' dysphagia, but can initially make symptoms worse before they improve due to tissue oedema.

Staging of oesophageal cancer must be performed pre-operatively to identify patients who have tumours that are suitable for resection. The current TNM (Tumour, Nodes, Metastases) staging classification for oesophageal cancer is shown in Table 12.6. A variety of investigations are required to produce an accurate pre-operative stage, these include CT scanning, EUS, and laparoscopy. CT scanning is good at detecting metastatic disease, particularly in the liver and lungs, but rarely detects peritoneal disease. It is not good at predicting T or N stage, but may show extension of a bulky tumour into adjacent structures (T4). EUS is much better at predicting T stage, and is now the investigation of choice for this aspect of staging. EUS is also better than CT at predicting lymph node involvement, and it is possible to perform fine needle aspiration of suspicious nodes with the right equipment. Laparoscopy is useful with distal oesophageal tumours to detect metastatic disease that would be missed at CT, such as peritoneal and omental seedlings, and small liver metastases.

Tumours are suitable for resection if pre-operative staging suggests no more than T3 disease, N0 or N1 lymph node status, and no distant metastases (i.e. T3, N1, M0, or better). Unfortunately, only 20% of patients who present with oesophageal cancer are suitable for resection, mainly because the presenting symptom, dysphagia, often occurs late in the disease process. Recent studies in the UK, Holland, and America have suggested survival benefits in certain patients receiving neo-adjuvant chemotherapy, and current practice in the UK is to offer this to patients with T2 and T3 tumours.

Patients with T1 tumours are offered surgery alone. A variety of operations are available, and a variety of different organs can be used to replace the resected oesophagus. The most commonly used organ for reconstruction is the stomach, which is mobilised at laparotomy by dividing the left and short gastric vessels, but preserving the gastro-epiploic arcade along its greater curve. Excising the lesser curve and GOJ provides a gastric tube that can be brought up to anastomose to the cervical oesophagus in most people. Colon and jejunum have been used instead if the stomach is not suitable, or fails. Mobilisation of the stomach may be combined with a right thoracotomy and resection of the mid/distal oesophagus (Ivor–Lewis procedure), a left sided thoraco-abdominal approach for tumours of the cardia, a right thoracotomy and cervical incision for resection of the majority of the oesophagus (three-stage, McKeown procedure), or just a cervical incision along with a trans-hiatal dissection to perform a subtotal oesophagectomy without need for a thoracotomy.

Significant complications from oesophagectomy include respiratory problems related to thoracotomy, myocardial infarction and arrhythmias, anastomotic leak, chylothorax from thoracic duct injury, anastomotic stricture, recurrent laryngeal nerve palsy, and death.

Survival rates from oesophageal cancer are low, due to the aggressive nature of the disease, and its tendency to present at an advanced stage. Of patients who undergo surgery, the 5-year survival rate is 20%, and the median survival is only 18 months. Those who are suitable only for palliation show a median survival of just 6 months.

Gastric carcinoma

Gastric carcinoma has an incidence of 10–20 cases per 100 000 people in the UK and USA, a rate that has fallen from 35 per 100 000 in the 1920s. As with oesophageal cancer, the site of cancers is changing, with a decrease in the number of distal tumours, and an increase in the number of proximal tumours. Men are 2.5 times more likely to develop gastric cancer than women, and over three-quarters of patients are 65 years or older. Chronic gastritis, leading to metaplasia, has been implicated in the aetiology, as seen in patients with pernicious anaemia. Recently the gastritis associated with *H. pylori* infection has been linked with gastric cancer, increasing the risk by up to 6 times. The exact role of *H. pylori* remains unclear though, as eradication treatment may increase the incidence of more proximal cancers. Other risk factors include smoking, a diet lacking in fresh fruit and vegetables, and having a first degree relative with gastric cancer.

The main, and often only, symptom of an early gastric cancer is dyspepsia. As the cancer becomes more advanced symptoms include anorexia, weight loss, vomiting, and anaemia. Unfortunately, dyspepsia is a very common symptom, and is often treated by patients and doctors alike with a variety of ant-acid therapies. Guidelines have been produced to encourage referral of patients with dyspepsia who

Table 12.7. Referral guidelines for suspected upper GI cancers (patients with dyspepsia).

Patient >55 years old, with dyspepsia
  – Continuous
  – Onset within 12 months

Dyspepsia with alarm symptoms
  – Weight loss
  – Anaemia
  – Anorexia

Dyspepsia with risk factors
  – Pernicious anaemia
  – Previous surgery for peptic ulcer
  – Atrophic gastritis
  – Intestinal metaplasia
  – First degree relative with gastric cancer

are at risk, and these are shown in Table 12.7. Even so, it is uncommon to see early gastric cancers and it is often the case that when advanced cancers are diagnosed patients have often had a long history of dyspepsia prior to diagnosis.

Although barium studies have been used to investigate dyspepsia, and diagnose gastric cancer, the investigation of choice is endoscopy, which allows visualisation of the mucosa, and diagnostic biopsy. Early cancers may be missed on barium examinations, and subtle changes are more easily seen at endoscopy, especially if dye-spraying techniques are used to accentuate mucosal abnormalities. Once a cancer has been diagnosed, staging investigations are required to enable an appropriate treatment plan to be discussed with the patient. The current TNM staging system is shown in Table 12.8. Staging investigations include CT scanning, EUS, and laparoscopy, in a similar fashion to oesophageal cancer. CT scanning provides good information about metastatic disease, detecting up to 80% of liver metastases, but is unreliable at predicting T stage (other than T4) and N stage. EUS is much better than CT at evaluating T stage and N stage, and fine needle aspiration cytology of suspicious nodes may increase sensitivity and specificity. Laparoscopy is advocated for all patients in whom a potentially curative gastric resection is contemplated, as it is highly accurate at detecting peritoneal disease and malignant ascites.

The mainstay of treatment for gastric cancer is surgery, which may be curative or palliative. Patients fit enough to withstand surgery, and who have localised disease on pre-operative staging, should undergo a potentially curative resection. Tumours in the distal 1/3 of the stomach can be resected with a subtotal gastrectomy, preserving a pouch of proximal stomach that is vascularised by the short gastric vessels. Intestinal continuity is restored with a gastro-jejunostomy, either as a loop, or as a Roux-en-Y reconstruction. Tumours of the proximal 2/3 require total gastrectomy, with a jejunal anastomosis onto the distal oesophagus. Some surgeons will

Table 12.8. TNM staging classification for gastric cancer.

Tx – Primary tumour not assessable	Nx – Regional nodes not assessable
T0 – No primary tumour	N0 – No regional nodes involved
Tis – Carcinoma in situ	N1 – 1–6 nodes involved
T1 – Tumour invading lamina propria/submucosa	N2 – 7–15 nodes involved
T2 – Tumour invading muscularis propria/subserosa	N3 – >15 nodes involved
T3 – Tumour penetrating serosa	
T4 – Tumour invading adjacent structures	Mx – Metastasis not assessable
	M0 – No distant metastasis
	M1 – Distant metastasis

create a pouch in the jejunum to act as a neo-stomach, but whether they improve nutrition significantly is unproven. Recently there has been much debate as to the extent of the lymphadenectomy that should be performed with a gastrectomy. The Japanese experience is that radical lymph node dissection to remove not only the lymph nodes immediately adjacent to the cancer (N1 nodes) but also those along the arterial supply to the stomach (N2 nodes) increases the survival rate. Such a radical resection (a D2 lymphadenectomy) has been compared in Western centres with the lesser procedure of just removing N1 nodes (D1 lymphadenectomy), and no survival benefit has been shown. However, as expertise in performing D2 resections has increased, so the mortality rate associated with surgery has decreased, and D2 resection is now recommended in specialist centres. Mortality rates from gastrectomy are 5–10%, with subtotal procedures being safer than total, and specialist centres achieving better results as with oesophageal resection. Specific complications include anastomotic leak, duodenal stump leak, and respiratory infections. Achieving adequate nutritional input can be difficult for many patients, and general advice to eat '*small amounts, more frequently*', may need to be combined with expert dietetic input. After total gastrectomy vitamin B12 is not absorbed due to lack of intrinsic factor, and parenteral supplementation must be given indefinitely.

Five-year survival after gastrectomy for cancer in Western centres has been 35–45%, some 20% worse than equivalent stage disease treated in Japan. The centralisation of cancer surgery to specialised centres has started to improve these figures, but there is still significant room for improvement.

Surgery may be required for palliation of gastric outlet obstruction caused by large cancers, or for persistent bleeding. Gastro-jejunostomy has been the operation of choice for obstructing tumours, and may be performed laparoscopically. Increasingly, SEMS have been used to stent such tumours, and may yet become as widely used as in oesophageal obstruction.

Adjuvant and neo-adjuvant chemo- and radiotherapy have been studied in gastric cancer with differing results. A recently published study from the UK has shown a definite survival benefit from neo-adjuvant chemotherapy, and this should be offered to patients.

Cancer of the GOJ

Cancer of the oesophagus and stomach is becoming more common at the GOJ, and this form of the disease presents its own particular problems. One issue is whether to treat such cancers as gastric or oesophageal, with important implications for chemotherapy and surgical approach. A classification is in use to help clarify the current situation:

Type I – cancer centered 1–5 cm above the GOJ.

Type II – cancer centered at the GOJ (from 1 cm above to 2 cm below).

Type III – cancer centered 2–5 cm below the GOJ.

For the purposes of resection, Type I should be managed by oesophago-gastrectomy, Type III by total gastrectomy, and Type II by whichever of the two approaches seems more appropriate.

Pancreatic carcinoma

Pancreatic carcinoma has an annual incidence in the UK of 10 per 100 000; this is now higher than it was 80 years ago. Men are more commonly affected than women by a factor of 1.5, and the age of presentation is usually 60–80. A diet rich in fats and meat is a risk factor, which reflects the high incidence in the Western world. Smoking is another well-established risk factor, as well as having a first degree relative with the disease. Chronic pancreatitis is linked with pancreatic cancer, but this link is probably casual rather than causal.

The majority of cases present with jaundice, which is classically painless, secondary to obstruction of the CBD by a tumour in the pancreatic head. In this situation the gallbladder is often palpable, in keeping with Courvoisier's law, which states that jaundice in a patient with a palpable gallbladder is unlikely to be due to gallstones. Pale stools, dark urine, and severe pruritus are common complaints, and as the tumour progresses pain may develop in the epigastrium, radiating to the back in advanced disease. Cachexia, nausea and vomiting are also seen in advanced disease, especially if gastric outlet obstruction occurs. Upper GI bleeding, acute pancreatitis, and thrombophlebitis are also recognised features of pancreatic cancer.

Liver function tests in a jaundiced patient will confirm an obstructed picture, with raised alkaline phosphatase, but the

Table 12.9. **TNM staging classification for pancreatic cancer.**

Tx – Primary tumour not assessable	Nx – Regional nodes not assessable
T0 – No primary tumour	N0 – No regional nodes involved
Tis – Carcinoma in situ	N1 – Regional nodes involved
T1 – Tumour confined to pancreas, <2 cm diameter	
T2 – Tumour confined to pancreas, <2 cm diameter	Mx – Metastasis not assessable
T3 – Tumour invading adjacent structures but not vessels	M0 – No distant metastasis
T4 – Tumour invading adjacent structures including vessels	M1 – Distant metastasis

definitive investigation is trans-abdominal ultrasound scanning. This will confirm obstruction of the biliary system, provide good views of the pancreas in 75% of cases and identify pancreatic masses, and may demonstrate metastatic disease in the liver if present. If a diagnosis of pancreatic cancer is suspected then a CT scan is the next step, and is part of the staging process. Modern CT scanning provides excellent cross-sectional imaging of the pancreas, and should be performed before any interventional procedure (such as ERCP) to relieve jaundice, as these may affect accurate interpretation of the scans. ERCP can be useful in the investigation of jaundiced patients with suspected pancreatic cancers, allowing imaging of both pancreatic and bile ducts, and the possibility of draining an obstructed biliary system with a stent. ERCP should only be used if the diagnosis is unconfirmed by other methods, and/or biliary drainage is required. Pre-operative drainage of the biliary tree with endoscopic, or percutaneous, stents or drains may increase the incidence of post-operative complications. Percutaneous biopsy of suspicious pancreatic masses is possible, but should only be performed if surgical resection is not suitable, as it may be complicated by seeding of tumour in the biopsy tract, pancreatitis, or visceral perforation.

There is overlap between diagnostic and staging investigations for pancreatic cancer, and the two may be completed together. CT scanning is the main staging investigation, and is useful in predicting tumour size and invasion of adjacent organs. The TNM staging system for pancreatic cancer is shown in Table 12.9. Involvement of the portal vein, superior mesenteric artery, or coeliac axis suggests irresectable disease, and is accurately shown by CT. Metastatic disease is shown well, other than small volume peritoneal lesions, but nodal disease is not easily assessed by CT. MRI scanning has not shown any significant advantage over CT, though MRCP images provide information previously obtained by ERCP, and may help to streamline the diagnostic/staging process. EUS is useful with small pancreatic lesions that are hard to assess on CT, and is more reliable than CT at predicting peripancreatic lymph node involvement, especially if combined with fine needle aspiration cytology via the EUS scope. Laparoscopy has been used increasingly in recent years to look for small volume metastatic disease in the peritoneal cavity, missed on CT scanning. It also allows sampling of

ascites, and can be combined with intra-operative ultrasound (via a laparoscopic probe) to provide direct ultrasonographic imaging of the primary lesion. The main advantage of a staging laparoscopy is in avoiding an unnecessary laparotomy, but if operative palliation of the tumour is suitable if resection is deemed impractical then laparoscopy itself is usually unnecessary.

Only 15–20% of patients will be suitable for resectional surgery. Tumours in the head of the pancreas require a Whipple's pancreaticoduodenectomy, those in the body/tail a distal pancreatectomy, and rarely a total pancreatectomy may be required. The Whipple's procedure involves removal of the head of the pancreas (divided at the level of the portal vein) along with the entire duodenum and distal stomach. The stomach, bile duct, and pancreatic duct are then anastomosed to the jejunum to restore continuity. A modification of the Whipple's is the pylorus preserving pancreaticoduodenectomy where no stomach is resected, and the duodenum divided just distal to the pylorus. This provides a better physiological result, but may compromise both tumour clearance at the duodenum, and lymphadenectomy. Distal pancreatectomy includes splenectomy, with ligation of the splenic vessels adjacent to the pancreas, but does not require any anastomosis. Total pancreatectomy may be required for diffuse involvement of the pancreas, and as a salvage procedure for post-operative complications from Whipple's including tumour involvement of the pancreatic transection margin. Complications after pancreatic resection include pancreatic leak, anastomotic leak, pancreatitis, and diabetes (after total pancreatectomy).

The majority of patients with pancreatic cancer require palliation, and the main symptoms are jaundice, pain, and vomiting. Jaundice can be relieved by placing a stent across the obstructed bile duct, either at ERCP, or by a percutaneous, transhepatic approach. Metal stents provide better palliation than plastic stents, as they are less prone to blocking and displacing. Pain can be relieved by analgesics, but coeliac plexus blocks are very effective treatment for pancreatic pain. Thoracoscopic division of splanchnic nerves can help reduce pain, but its role in pancreatic disease has not yet been established. Vomiting is often due to duodenal obstruction, and requires either stenting of the duodenum, or a surgical gastroenterostomy, which may be performed laparoscopically.

Palliation of all the above symptoms can be achieved at laparotomy, with a surgically fashioned hepatico-jejunostomy, gastro-enterostomy, and alcohol ablation of the coeliac plexus. While such a procedure provides good, durable palliation, it is at the expense of a laparotomy with inherent morbidity and mortality, and the choice between operative or non-operative palliation must be made carefully.

Neo-adjuvant chemo- or radiotherapy has no role currently in managing pancreatic cancer. Adjuvant chemotherapy with gemcitabine has been shown to improve post-operative survival, and to improve survival and quality of life in patients with inoperable disease. The prognosis from pancreatic cancer remains extremely poor however, with overall 5-year survival less than 5%, and in the region of 10% for those resected.

Hepatic tumours

Hepatocellular carcinoma (HCC) is the commonest malignant tumour seen in humans. Incidence varies widely from 5 per 100 000 in UK and USA, to 70–80 per 100 000 in parts of Asia and Africa. The main risk factor is chronic liver disease, and HCC often arises from cirrhosis due to chronic hepatitis B and C infection, as well as alcoholic liver disease and haemochromatosis. The majority of HCC are asymptomatic, until such time as they become large and/or multi-focal when they may cause a patient with cirrhosis to deteriorate with ascites, jaundice, and malaise. A palpable mass and pain from bleeding are other symptoms. While asymptomatic, HCC may be detected during ultrasonography for other reasons, or as part of a screening program. Measurement of α-fetoprotein will confirm the diagnosis if grossly elevated, but levels may be normal with small tumours, and mildly elevated in chronic liver disease. CT and MRI scanning provide further useful information over ultrasound, including detection of small tumours and differentiation from other liver tumours. Percutaneous biopsy of suspected HCC should not be performed, as tumour seeding in the needle tract is a well-recognised phenomenon, and jeopradises potentially curative resection.

Treatment options for HCC include surgical resection, tumour ablation, and chemotherapy. Surgery may involve partial hepatectomy, or total hepatectomy and transplantation. Liver resection in cirrhotic patients carries increased risk of morbidity and mortality, and this risk increases with the Childs grade (see Table 12.10). Childs C patients would not be offered surgery, and the risks in Childs A are still significant. Numerous methods of ablating liver tumours when surgery is not appropriate have been developed, including ethanol injection, cryotherapy, radio-frequency ablation, microwave, and electrolysis. Chemotherapy is only of value if given transarterially, and combined with embolisation of the feeding artery (chemo-embolisation).

The most common form of liver tumour seen in the UK is metastatic cancer, arising from primaries in the GI tract, breast, and lung. The majority of liver metastases are unsuitable for any form of surgical treatment, the exception being those that originate from colorectal cancers. Between 40% and 50% of patients with colorectal cancer will develop liver metastases, and without treatment these will prove fatal often within 1 year. If these metastases are suitable for surgery then 5-year survival rates of 20–30% have been demonstrated, with operative mortality rates of around 5%. Such results rely on patients with potentially resectable disease being identified and reviewed by specialist surgeons with experience of hepatic resection. Liver metastases are often asymptomatic, and their detection at a stage where surgery may be appropriate relies on imaging at 6–12 monthly intervals after a colorectal cancer resection. Ultrasound is the most appropriate screening technique, but should only be performed if a patient would be a suitable candidate for liver resection (fit enough and young enough for major surgery). If metastases are detected then further imaging with CT and/or MRI provides accurate information about the distribution of disease within the liver. The best results are obtained from small volume lesions in a single lobe (right or left); but multiple lesions, affecting both lobes can be resected. The presence of extra-hepatic metastases is a contra-indication to resection, and a clear margin of 10 mm from tumour is desirable. An accurate knowledge of the segmental anatomy of the liver is essential for safe resection, and as techniques have been refined, and anaesthetic and perioperative care improved, so too have the results from surgery. The liver is extremely quick to regenerate,

Table 12.10. **Childs classification of patients with chronic liver disease.**

	Points		
	1	2	3
Bilirubin (μmol/l)	>35	35–51	>51
Albumin (g/l)	>35	28–35	<28
INR (prothrombin ratio)	<1.4	1.4–2.0	>2.0
Ascites	None	Slight	Moderate to severe
Encephalopathy	None	Slight	Moderate to severe
Childs grade	A = 5–6 points	B = 7–9 points	C = 10–15 points

and if sufficient functioning tissue to avoid hepatic failure is left behind, within several weeks this will have re-grown. It is possible to perform repeat resection if further metastases develop, but this becomes increasingly more complex.

Metastases not suitable for surgery may be treated with ablative techniques as described for HCC, and there is increasing interest in using these techniques as an adjunct to resection; both pre- and intra-operatively. Chemotherapy has a role in palliation of metastatic disease, but may also prove useful in down-staging previously irresectable lesions. Resection has been used on metastases from primaries other than colorectal cancer, but cases must be carefully selected and the survival benefit is unclear.

OTHER UPPER GI CONDITIONS

Jaundice

Jaundice is the yellow appearance of sclera, skin, and other tissues, seen as the clinical manifestation of hyperbilirubi-naemia. The upper limit of normal for serum bilirubin is 17 μmol/l, and concentrations above this represent bio-chemical jaundice. Levels over 40–50 μmol/l present as clin-ical jaundice when the yellow discolouration appears obvious, initially seen at the sclera. Jaundice is classified into pre-hepatic, hepatic, and post-hepatic causes (see Table 12.11), and the latter (also called obstructive jaundice) is the one which surgeons are most familiar with.

Jaundiced patients are often presented to surgeons with a diagnosis of obstructive, post-hepatic jaundice, already made. It is important though to consider other causes of jaun-dice in the history and examination, and questions should cover recent foreign travel, alcohol intake, drug history, blood transfusions, and sexually transmitted diseases. Examination may reveal signs of chronic liver disease such as finger club-bing, palmar erythema, spider naevi, and caput medusa.

Obstructive jaundice implies partial or complete occlusion of the biliary tree, and this results in progressive jaundice which may be profound, with bilirubin >100 μmol/l. Bilirubin is conjugated in the liver to form a water-soluble compound, and if the flow of bile is obstructed this accumulates in the blood, and is excreted by the kidneys. The decreased flow of bile into the bowel results in fewer bile pigments in faeces, and

together this accounts for the pale stools and dark urine asso-ciated with obstructive jaundice. Bile acids become more con-centrated in the blood, and cause significant pruritus.

Patients with obstructive jaundice may give a history of pain in the epigastrium and right upper quadrant suggestive of symptomatic gallstones, or may have painless jaundice, which is always suspicious of malignant biliary obstruction. Inflammatory changes from stones in the gallbladder cause fibrosis, so the finding of a palpable, distended gallbladder on examination suggests that gallstones are not the cause (Courvoisier's law), raising the possibility of malignancy.

Liver function tests in obstructive jaundice tend to show grossly elevated alkaline phospatase, with minimal elevation of transaminases, whereas these changes are reversed in hepatic jaundice. The absence of bile in the bowel decreases fat absorption, which decreases absorption of fat-soluble vitamin K, which decreases production of prothrombin by the liver. Coagulation studies show an increased prothrom-bin time, which is commonly expressed as the International Normalised Ratio (INR).

Blood tests do not diagnose obstructive jaundice, and the definitive investigation is an ultrasound scan of the abdomen. This must document whether the bile ducts (intra- and extra-hepatic) are dilated or not, and if dilated a search for the cause attempted. Ultrasound is the best imaging for showing gallstones, but visualisation of the CBD, especially the distal portion, is difficult with overlying bowel, and stones here are often missed. Large tumours in the pancreatic head may be obvious on ultrasound, but smaller lesions, bile duct tumours and strictures may be impossible to detect. Further imaging is almost always required; the choice depends on the likely cause of obstruction and the patient's clinical condi-tion. If gallstones are seen on ultrasound then an ERCP is both diagnostic and therapeutic, allowing CBD stones to be removed via a sphincterotomy, or a biliary stent to be placed to drain the obstructed system and facilitate further endo-scopic or operative treatment. If cholangitis is present, irre-spective of cause, then the biliary system must be drained as a priority, either at ERCP, or via a percutaneous transhepatic approach. If the clinical situation is less urgent, and stones are not suspected, then CT and/or MRI scanning are essen-tial to determine the obstructing lesion and direct further management. These scans are best obtained before any

Table 12.11. **Classification of jaundice.**

Pre-hepatic	Hepatic	Post-hepatic
Haemolytic anaemia	Acute hepatitis	Gall stones
Mechanical heart valves	Drug induced liver failure	Biliary tumours
Hypersplenism	Alcoholic liver disease	Biliary strictures
Transfusion reaction (severe)	Cirrhosis	Pancreatic tumours
		External biliary compression

attempts at stenting if at all possible, as stents and the trauma caused by their insertion can affect the images produced, and make diagnosis more difficult.

Gallstones are a common cause of obstructive jaundice, usually through their presence in the CBD, and may pass spontaneously, or require removal at endoscopy or surgery. Rarely they cause jaundice by becoming impacted in Hartmann's pouch and exerting external pressure on the common hepatic duct (Mirizzi's syndrome). Cancer of the head of the pancreas is another common cause, and its management is discussed further (see Pancreatic Cancer). Bile duct tumours are rare, and occasionally are suitable for surgical resection depending on CT/MRI imaging. If irresectable they require stenting to palliate the jaundice. Biliary strictures may be the sequelae of gallstones, chronic pancreatitis, or operative trauma, and need stenting or operative repair. Extrinsic compression of the biliary tree is most commonly seen from portal lymphadenopathy as part of a systemic malignancy such as lymphoma, or metastatic carcinoma. Biliary stenting relieves jaundice while chemo- or radiotherapy is administered, if appropriate.

Jaundiced patients are prone to coagulation defects (see above), renal failure (hepato-renal syndrome), infectious complications, and poor wound healing. They need parenteral vitamin K and careful fluid balance while jaundiced, and if interventional procedures, including surgery, are performed antibiotic cover is essential. It must be remembered that they are high-risk patients, and the above factors are anticipated and managed proactively.

Gallstones

Gallstones are common, and are estimated to be present in 20–30% of people in developed countries. Only 20–30% of these people will develop problems related to their stones, and it is important to try and differentiate between symptomatic and asymptomatic stones. Gallstones contain cholesterol, bile pigments, or a mixture of these compounds, and it is clear that their aetiology is multi-factoral. Obesity, ileal resection, and haemolytic anaemia have all been linked to gallstone formation, the only certain factors about their formation is that they are twice as common in women as men, and become increasingly common with age.

Gallstones may cause a variety of symptoms depending on which part of the body they are in. The commonest problems arise from stones in the gallbladder, and present as biliary colic or cholecystitis. Biliary colic is a self-limiting condition characterised by right upper quadrant pain, often severe, caused by temporary cystic duct obstruction. The pain is associated with nausea, and occasional vomiting, and may radiate to the back. If the pain does not settle within a few hours, and a fever and raised white cell count develop, then a diagnosis of acute cholecystitis is more likely (see Acute Cholecystitis). Unrelieved obstruction of the cystic duct may lead to formation of a mucocele, as mucus secretions collect and produce a tense swollen

gallbladder. Infection within an obstructed gallbladder results in an empyema. Stones in the CBD may cause obstructive jaundice (see Jaundice), as may stones impacted in Hartmann's pouch (Mirizzi's syndrome). Infection can occur within an obstructed biliary system, giving rise to cholangitis, associated with the classic features of Charcot's triad (pain, fever, and jaundice). This may respond to antibiotic therapy, but occasionally requires prompt drainage of the infected system too, either by ERCP, or by a percutaneous, trans-hepatic route. Gallstones passing through the extra-hepatic biliary system are one of the commonest causes of acute pancreatitis (see Acute Pancreatitis). On rare occasions a biliary-enteric fistula may develop between an inflamed gallbladder and the duodenum, stomach, or colon, and may result in stones passing into the bowel directly. If a large stone passes into the small intestine in this manner then a 'gallstone ileus' can develop when the stone impacts at the ileo-colic junction, causing small bowel obstruction. The classic features of this condition seen on a plain abdominal film are dilated loops of small bowel, gas in the biliary tree, and a calcified stone in the right iliac fossa. Gallstones are associated with carcinoma of the gallbladder, which is fortunately extremely rare as it is a very aggressive cancer.

Trans-abdominal ultrasound scanning is the investigation of choice for investigation of suspected gallstones, as it not only demonstrates stones but can also identify the thickened gallbladder wall of cholecystitis, and the dilated bile ducts of obstructive jaundice. Trans-abdominal ultrasound is poor at detecting CBD stones, and ERCP, MRCP, CT, EUS, or operative cholangiography may be necessary.

The treatment of choice for symptomatic gallstones is surgery, and cholecystectomy is one of the commonest elective procedures performed by general surgeons. Over the last 15 years laparoscopic cholecystectomy has become the accepted approach for the majority of patients, with less postoperative pain, and shorter hospital stay. Five per cent of laparoscopic procedures have to be converted to open cholecystectomy for reasons such as technical failure, bleeding, and unclear anatomy, and this conversion rate decreases with the experience of the surgeon. Bile duct injury is the feared complication of cholecystectomy, and occurs in 0.1–0.2% of laparoscopic procedures – a figure which is not significantly different to historical data from open cholecystectomy.

One revolution that the laparoscopic era has brought to gallbladder surgery is the management of bile duct stones. In the days of open surgery 10% of patients were found to have CBD stones at operation, and these were managed by bile duct exploration as part of the same procedure. Laparoscopic exploration of the bile duct is a more complicated procedure, and management of duct stones has evolved accordingly, as has understanding of their natural history. Various systems have been proposed to predict patients who are at risk of having bile duct stones, and common indicators are: abnormal liver function tests, a history of obstructive jaundice, dilated CBD at ultrasound, a history of acute pancreatitis. Patients at risk of CBD stones should have imaging of their duct performed, either pre-operatively with one of the methods mentioned above, or during surgery by cholangiography or intra-operative ultrasound. Duct stones may be removed at ERCP or by operative duct exploration, both laparoscopically or open. It has become clear that the natural history of CBD stones is that the majority of small stones will pass spontaneously from a normal duct.

A variety of non-operative techniques have been tried in the management of gallstones, but none have become popular. Dissolution therapy with ursodeoxycholic acid was only suitable for limited patients, took up to 2 years to work, and stones recurred quickly once therapy was stopped. Extracorporeal shockwave lithotripsy (ESWL) has become very popular in the management of renal stones, but was associated with pain, pancreatitis, bile duct obstruction, and incomplete stone clearance when used on gallstones. Patients who are medically unfit for surgery may be stabilised by percutaneous drainage of the gallbladder (cholecystostomy), and stones may be extracted along the drainage tract – but recur rapidly as with dissolution therapy, and definitive surgical treatment is often preferable once their condition improves.

It is important to remember that 70–80% of gallstones are asymptomatic, and there is little evidence currently that intervention for asymptomatic stones is necessary or desirable. Gallstones found incidentally during investigations for other symptoms should be treated with caution. The fact that at least 5% of patients who undergo cholecystectomy have persistent symptoms post-operatively should serve as a warning that the presence of gallstones on ultrasound and vague abdominal symptoms does not necessarily mean that the two are connected.

Portal hypertension

If the pressure in the portal venous system is greater than 12 mmHg then portal hypertension exists. The commonest cause of this in Western countries is alcoholic cirrhosis causing obstruction to portal venous flow, but numerous other causes are recognised and are classified (as for jaundice) into pre-hepatic, hepatic, and post-hepatic (Table 12.12). The portal venous system has been described (see Anatomy), and in portal hypertension the sites of portal-systemic communication open up, commonly resulting in oesophageal and gastric varices that can bleed profusely. The other major complication of portal hypertension is ascites. The management of variceal bleeding has been described (see Upper GI Bleeding), and includes injection sclerotherapy, endoscopic banding, TIPSS, and oesophageal transection. Rarely, splenic vein thrombosis results in left-sided portal hypertension, leading to splenomegaly and gastric varices. Splenectomy with division of the short gastric vessels is an effective treatment for this situation.

Ascites is mostly managed medically, with a low-sodium diet and diuretics, though paracentesis is used to ease the discomfort of tense ascites, and may be used repeatedly if

Table 12.12. **Classification of portal hypertension.**

Pre-hepatic	Hepatic	Post-hepatic
Portal vein thrombosis	Cirrhosis	Budd–Chiari syndrome
Splenic vein thrombosis	Hepatitis	Pericarditis
Extrinsic compression	Schistosomiasis	
	Sarcoid	

medical measures are ineffective. Portal-systemic shunting has been helpful at controlling ascites, and is now usually performed as a TIPSS procedure. Shunts between the peritoneal cavity and the systemic venous system have been created surgically for over 30 years, and can provide excellent relief from ascites refractory to other treatment, but complications are multiple, including infection, blockage of shunt, and disseminated intravascular coagulation, and such shunts are now performed rarely.

Operating on patients with portal hypertension is technically challenging, as multiple dilated veins are found within the abdomen, making surgery difficult, bloody and slow. These dilated veins do not seal well with diathermy, and suturing of bleeding points is often the best course of action.

Peptic ulcer

The management of peptic ulcer disease has changed dramatically in the last 20 years as the aetiology of peptic ulceration has become more clearly understood, and more powerful and effective medical treatment has evolved. At the same time there has been a dramatic decrease in both elective and emergency surgery for peptic ulceration. Aetiological factors in peptic ulceration include *H. pylori* infection, NSAID ingestion, smoking, renal failure, liver disease, and Zollinger–Ellison (ZE) syndrome. *H. pylori* is by far the most important, and adequate management of *H. pylori* is the mainstay of modern ulcer therapy. *H. pylori* is a spiral, gram-negative bacteria which is spread by direct contact, and infects up to 60% of the population, though only 5–10% of those infected develop ulceration. *H. pylori* causes increased gastrin levels, a rise in gastric acid production, and also has a direct effect on gastric and duodenal mucosa. NSAIDs have both a localised and systemic effect on gastric and duodenal mucosa, which seems to be through their inhibition of cyclo-oxygenase enzyme (particularly COX-1).

Patients with ulcers have a variety of symptoms, including epigastric pain, anorexia, vomiting, and weight loss. Epigastric pain may be relieved by food, or associated with anorexia, and radiates through to the back. Some patients are asymptomatic. Examination is often unremarkable, except for melaena when there has been bleeding, or a succussion splash with gastric outlet obstruction. The diagnostic investigation is upper GI endoscopy, which allows visualisation of ulcers as well as gastric biopsy. All patients with peptic ulceration must be investigated for *H. pylori* by, serology, breath testing, CLO test, or histology. The last two are performed on biopsies taken at endoscopy and are the most accurate. All gastric ulcers must be biopsied from their margin to exclude the possibility of malignancy.

Treatment depends on the presumed causal factor. If *H. pylori* is identified it must be eradicated. If NSAIDs are being used they should be stopped if at all possible and alternative analgesia used. If neither *H. pylori* is identified or NSAIDs are being used then the initial presumption should be a false-negative result from the *H. pylori* test, and eradication prescribed – other causes of ulceration are extremely rare. Eradication of *H. pylori* is achieved by a combination of antibiotics in conjunction with an anti-secretory agent – a common combination would be a PPI, with clarithromycin and amoxycillin, or metronidazole. This 'triple therapy' would be given for one week, and followed by continuing anti-secretory therapy for 8–12 weeks to heal the ulcer, which must also be prescribed for NSAID induced ulcers.

If ulcers fail to heal then repeat testing for *H. pylori* must be performed, and this is most effective by CLO test and histology at repeat endoscopy. Persistent infection must be treated before alternative diagnoses are sought, and a different combination of antibiotics over a 2-week period is recommended. NSAID ingestion must be re-assessed, and malignancy excluded with endoscopic biopsies. In the absence of other causes ZE syndrome must be considered, where gastrin-secreting tumours result in high-gastric acidity and resistant peptic ulceration. Serum gastrin levels must be measured to diagnose ZE syndrome, and the possibility of multiple endocrine neoplasia (MEN) considered.

Surgery for peptic ulcer disease is now much less common than it used to be. Elective surgery is extremely rare, and consisted of acid-reducing procedures (vagotomy, selective vagotomy, antrectomy), and gastric resections. Complications from these operations were common, and recurrent ulceration well recognised. It is still occasionally necessary to perform elective surgery for resistant ulcer disease, but only after all medical treatment has been tried thoroughly. Emergency surgery for complications is still common, but less common than 20 years ago. The treatment of bleeding ulcers and perforations has been described already (see Upper GI Bleeding and Perforated Viscus). Gastric outlet obstruction may result from scarring and fibrosis secondary to ulceration in the pyloric region and duodenum, and this often requires surgical intervention. Balloon dilatation at endoscopy is a good first-line treatment, but may result in perforation requiring surgery. Operative treatment of gastric outlet obstruction includes pyloroplasty, gastro-enterostomy, and distal gastrectomy.

Gastro-oesophageal reflux disease

Gastro-oesophageal reflux occurs when gastric contents pass retrograde through the GOJ into the oesophagus. Everybody experiences episodes of reflux, but in 10–40% of the population of the UK this occurs frequently enough to significantly impair their quality of life. The incidence of this problem seems to be increasing, though it is hard to accurately measure just how many people are affected. What is clear is that it is a highly significant problem accounting for a large number of attendances at both primary and secondary care, and requiring a large amount of money for therapeutic measures (mainly anti-secretory agent prescriptions). There are a number of mechanisms which help to prevent GORD, including a lower oesophageal 'sphincter', the diaphragmatic crura at the hiatus, and the presence of a short segment of distal oesophagus within the abdominal compartment. Some patients with GORD have a hiatus hernia, but it must be realised that the presence of a hiatus hernia does not imply reflux (most hernias are asymptomatic for GORD), and that having reflux does not imply the presence of a hiatus hernia (30–90% of reflux patients have a hernia).

Symptoms are variable; 'heartburn' is common with retrosternal burning and discomfort, regurgitation of food and acid into the mouth is unpleasant, and dysphagia to both solids and liquids can occur. Symptoms are worse when lying down, or bending over, and waking at night choking is described. Respiratory disease may be worsened by nocturnal aspiration, and teeth may be eroded by gastric acid. Clinical examination is unremarkable, and the diagnosis is most often obtained from history alone.

The majority of reflux responds to lifestyle adjustments and medical treatment. Losing weight, stopping smoking, avoiding spicy foods and alcohol help some people, but most require some form of acid reduction therapy with either H_2 antagonists, or PPIs. Surgical intervention is only considered in cases that do not respond to medical therapy, and sometimes when patients request surgery as an alternative to life-long medication. Some patients have only a partial response to high doses of PPIs, and others have relief of the acid-related problems, but still have a large volume of gastric fluid regurgitating into their oro-pharynx.

Before considering surgery the oesophagus must be investigated to prove the diagnosis of GORD, and show motility disorders and anatomical variants. Endoscopy with distal oesophageal biopsies should be performed, as well as manometry and 24-h pH studies (see Oesophageal Function Tests).

There are many types of anti-reflux operations, but most include some form of fundoplication. The principles of a fundoplication procedure include reducing hiatus hernia if present, restoring a length of intra-abdominal oesophagus, and repairing the diaphragmatic hiatus. The commonest anti-reflux procedure is the Nissen fundoplication that involves a 360° wrap of the gastric fundus around the distal oesophagus. Various partial fundoplications exist with either anterior or posterior wrapping of the fundus over 180° or 270°. The development of laparoscopic surgery has renewed enthusiasm for anti-reflux surgery, as it can be performed without the need for a painful laparotomy or thoracotomy. The results from well-selected patients are good, with 85–95% reporting cure or significant improvement of reflux. Patients must know that certain complications occur with anti-reflux surgery: dysphagia affects at least 30% immediately post-operatively, but this resolves over the first 3 months; gas-bloat affects up to 30% where inability to belch air from the stomach causes gastric distension. Persistent dysphagia can be treated with endoscopic balloon dilatation.

There is a well-described link between GORD and Barrett's oesophagus, and between Barrett's and oesophageal cancer (see Oesophageal Cancer). It would seem logical that a mechanical solution to reflux as provided by surgery would help prevent progression of Barrett's, but so far there is no evidence to support this theory. Anti-reflux surgery is not indicated as treatment for Barrett's oesophagus alone.

13

Lower Gastrointestinal Surgery

Douglas M Bowley and Christopher Cunningham

Department of Colorectal Surgery, John Radcliffe Hospital, Headley Way, Headington, Oxford, UK

CONTENTS

Surgical anatomy	249
Colorectal investigations	250
Radiology	250
Anorectal physiology	250
Endoscopy	250
Colorectal emergencies	250
Obstruction	250
Diverticulosis	252
Lower GI haemorrhage	252
Anorectal sepsis	253
Colorectal injury	254
Foreign body	254
Inflammatory bowel disease	254
Ulcerative colitis	254
Crohn's disease	255
Colorectal cancer	255
Background and aetiology	255
Preoperative staging of colorectal cancer	256
Management of early cancer	256
The management of advanced cancer	257
Metastatic cancer	257
Pathology	258
Non-surgical treatment of colorectal cancer	258
Adjuvant therapy	258
Neoadjuvant therapy	258
Palliative therapy	259
Screening and surveillance for colorectal cancer	259
Population screening	259
Anal cancer	260
Minor anorectal conditions	260
Fistula-in-ano	260
Anal fissure	260
Haemorrhoids	261
Prolapse	261
Functional anorectal disorders	262
Constipation	262
Anal incontinence	262
Minimally invasive colorectal surgery	263
Further reading	263

SURGICAL ANATOMY

Accurate understanding of the pelvic anatomy is critical to achieving good oncological and functional outcomes after rectal excision. Heald et al. (1998) in Basingstoke introduced the concept of total mesorectal excision during the 1980s. Total Mesorectal Excision (TME) consists of separate high ligation of the inferior mesenteric vessels to define the proximal limits of the lymphatic clearance, followed by rectal mobilisation with sharp dissection under direct vision in the avascular plane outside the mesorectum excising the entire mesorectum and leaving the autonomic nerve plexuses intact. This surgical innovation has been shown to reduce local recurrence dramatically, while maximising the chances of sphincter-preserving surgery.

Permanent impotence in men has been reported to be almost universal in some series of abdominoperineal excisions of rectum and occurs in up to half of all men after anterior resection of the rectum for rectal cancer. The incidence of permanent bladder denervation after rectal excisional surgery has been reported to be up to 19% in some series. The presumed mechanism for sexual and urinary dysfunction is damage to the pelvic autonomic parasympathetic and/or sympathetic nerves during surgery.

The risk of sympathetic nerve damage occurs in the abdomen during ligation of the inferior mesenteric artery pedicle, and high in the pelvis during initial posterior rectal dissection adjacent to the large hypogastric nerves. Lower down, risk to the parasympathetic nerves occurs while dissecting laterally near the pelvic plexus, and during deep dissection of the anterior aspect of the rectum away from the seminal vesicles and prostate near the cavernous nerves. The anterior dissection is thought to be the point of highest risk to the nerves governing erectile function.

COLORECTAL INVESTIGATIONS

Radiology

Barium enema

Barium enema is usually 'double contrast' with air and liquid barium insufflated into the colon. Barium enema is able to show detail of the mucosa and gives a permanent record of the bowel examination; it remains the gold standard for demonstrating the extent and severity of colonic diverticular disease.

Abdominal and pelvic computed tomography

Computed tomography (CT) is used in the staging of colorectal cancer and is also especially helpful in complicated diverticular disease.

CT colonography

CT colonography uses computer programming to combine helical CT scans in order to create two- or three-dimensional images of the interior of a patient's colon acquired after bowel preparation and insufflation of air into the colon. These images can be rotated for different views and even combined for a complete view of the colon that is known as 'virtual colonoscopy'. For the detection of frank colon cancers and polyps greater than 10 mm, the accuracy of CT colonography appears to be comparable to conventional colonoscopy with few false positives or negatives.

Magnetic resonance imaging

The overall accuracy of magnetic resonance imaging (MRI) for preoperative staging of rectal cancer in studies using a body coil ranges from 59% to 95%, with that for nodal staging ranging between 39% and 95%. Many centres now use MRI to predict which rectal cancers should undergo neoadjuvant chemoradiation therapy prior to rectal excision.

Endoanal MRI is particularly useful in imaging fistula-in-ano. MRI of primary fistulas may change the surgical approach in 10% of patients, but for recurrent fistula-in-ano surgery guided by MRI reduces further recurrence of fistula-in-ano by 75% and should be done in all patients with recurrent fistula.

Anorectal ultrasound

Anal ultrasound is the definitive way to image the anal sphincters, in addition ultrasound is used to stage rectal cancer. Ultrasound examination of the normal rectum demonstrates five distinct layers; this enables accurate assessment of depth of penetration of tumour through the bowel. Endoanal ultrasonography is effective for T staging, although it is least accurate for T2 and T4 tumours. It has been recommended as the investigation of choice in the selection of patients for potentially curative local excision of rectal cancer.

Anorectal physiology

Anorectal physiology can provide helpful information in the management of patients with constipation and anal incontinence. Anal manometry provides objective measurement of the resting and squeeze pressure within the anal canal. Resting pressure is largely due to the internal anal sphincter; squeeze pressure is a reflection of the voluntary muscles of the anal canal (external sphincter and puborectalis). Normal resting canal pressure is 50–70 mmHg and the resting pressure in the anal canal increases from cranial to caudal, creating a 'high-pressure zone' 1 or 2 cm from the anal verge. In normal individuals, the maximum squeeze pressure is an additional 50–100% of the resting tone. The anal canal is rich in sensory receptors and when rectal distension is detected, the internal sphincter reflexely relaxes and the external sphincter contracts. This rectoanal inhibitory reflex enables rectal contents to be 'sampled' by the anal canal mucosa and facilitates discrimination between gaseous and non-gaseous contents of the rectum.

Endoscopy

Colonoscopy provides detailed views of the colon and rectum, and enables interventions such as biopsy and polypectomy. However, it is an invasive technique, requiring bowel preparation, skilled practitioners and exposes the patient to the risks of perforation (0.06–2%) and bleeding after polypectomy (0.4–2.7%). Most colorectal cancers are assumed to have a premalignant adenomatous polyp phase; therefore colonoscopy provides the opportunity for cancer screening and prevention. The USA National Polyp Study observed a 70–90% lower than expected incidence of colorectal cancer in patients undergoing colonoscopy compared to three reference populations. Indications for colonoscopy are given in Table 13.1.

Wireless capsule endoscopy represents a major advance in the imaging of the small intestine. It is able to capture video-images of the mucosal surface of the entire length of the intestine, which can then be interpreted by an observer.

COLORECTAL EMERGENCIES

Obstruction

Volvulus

Although the incidence of sigmoid volvulus is rare in Western countries, it is one of the most common causes of emergency large-bowel surgery in other countries, particularly in Africa. In the UK, sigmoid volvulus often occurs in elderly and frail patients. The clinical symptoms and signs are those of colonic obstruction, often the abdomen is hugely distended and 'drum-like' and the rectum is empty on digital examination. The diagnosis is supported by a typical X-ray appearance. In the absence of signs of peritonitis, detorsion of the volvulus can be attempted by use of a rigid sigmoidoscope and a flatus tube; however, flexible sigmoidoscopy may be more effective. If colonic ischaemia is suspected, then prompt laparotomy is indicated. Recurrence rates after

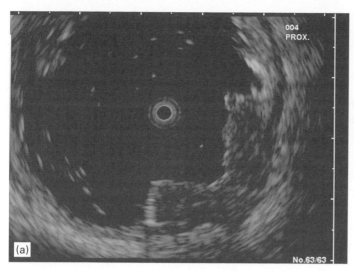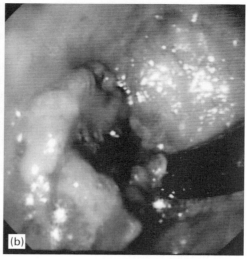

Figure 13.1. (a) Rectal cancer viewed at endoscopy and (b) transrectal ultrasound. Cancer (labelled A) arising at anorectal junction seen at endoscopy (retroflex manoeuvre) and same cancer at endorectal ultrasound. The muscularis propria lesion is seen within the bowel wall. This layer is lost at C indicating local invasion and the tumour was staged as T3.

Table 13.1. Indications for lower GI endoscopy.

Colonoscopy	Flexible sigmoidoscopy
Dark red rectal bleeding	Bright red rectal bleeding
Iron deficiency anaemia	Left-sided abnormalities on other imaging
Change in bowel habit	Left-sided mass
Suspected inflammatory bowel disease	Population screening
Further assessment of abnormalities suspected on other imaging	
Population screening	

endoscopic detorsion are high and an operative procedure is usually recommended. The options are fixing the colon without resection (colopexy) or a resection with either a colostomy or an anastomosis. Simply fixing the colon without resecting the volvulus is associated with high recurrence rates and a resection is usually undertaken. The decision to anastomose or not will be taken according to the state of the patient and the skills of the operator. Volvulus may also occur in the caecum or transverse colon, but is much less common.

Malignancy

About 15–20% of patients with primary colorectal cancer present with intestinal obstruction. Preoperative staging of the disease is valuable; if there are extensive liver metastases then a palliative stenting procedure is justified.

Single-stage surgery is considered the preferred option for an obstructing lesion of the right colon. However, in the management of malignant left-sided colonic obstruction, staged procedures are usually advocated because of the risk of anastomotic complications. The options for surgery include proximal diversion, resection without anastomosis and resection with primary anastomosis. Resecting the entire distended proximal colon and forming an ileo-sigmoid anastomosis is an attractive option, but postoperative bowel function can be relatively poor. If it is decided to perform a segmental colectomy, then an on-table colonic lavage is usually undertaken.

With the development of self-expanding metallic stents (SEMS), colonic obstruction can be relieved rapidly and effectively. SEMS may be used as a temporary measure to decompress the obstructed bowel so that surgical resection can subsequently be performed in an elective setting with proper bowel preparation, a so-called 'bridge to surgery'. SEMS may also serve as a definitive palliative treatment for patients with advanced or disseminated disease.

Pseudo-obstruction

Colonic pseudo-obstruction is also called Ogilvie's syndrome, and mimics the appearances of obstruction (with colonic distension) although mechanical obstruction is absent. It typically occurs in patients hospitalised for other reasons, such as recent surgery, trauma or infection. It is thought to occur due to an imbalance in the autonomic supply of the colon, with over exaggerated effects of the sympathetic nervous system.

The diagnosis rests on the exclusion of mechanical obstruction by contrast enema or flexible endoscopy. Treatment is initially conservative, with attempts to correct underlying causes if possible, correction of electrolyte abnormality and stopping of drugs that affect colonic motility, such as opiates and anti-cholinergics. Nasogastric decompression and intravenous fluids are likely to be required. Plain X-ray of the abdomen is essential to monitor the diameter of the colon, particularly the caecum. Gross distension (>12 cm) suggests imminent perforation. Colonoscopy can be therapeutical and some authorities recommend intravenous neostigmine (2.5 mg in 100 ml of saline over 60 min) to hasten colonic decompression. This must be given in a 'high care' nursing setting with cardiac monitoring to detect bradycardia. Surgery can be indicated in Ogilvie's Syndrome, if there are signs of colonic ischaemia or perforation.

Diverticulosis

Diverticulosis coli is a common colonic condition of the elderly in Western societies, up to two-thirds of people aged over 80 years are affected; however, most are asymptomatic. Diverticulosis has been labelled a disease of Western societies, as the disorder is rare in rural Africa and Asia and highly prevalent in Europe, USA and Australia.

Colonic diverticula typically form in parallel rows between the taenia coli because of weakness of the muscle wall at site of penetration of the vasa recta supplying the mucosa. It is thought that increased intraluminal pressure causes the mucosa to herniate through the muscle wall to create the diverticula. The underlying problem is thought to be dietary deficiency of fibre.

Complications of diverticular disease

Diverticulitis has been likened to appendicitis, with a diverticulum becoming obstructed by inspissated stool in its neck. The inflammatory process varies in severity from inflammation alone to pericolic abscess to free perforation of the colon with faecal peritonitis. Most patients present with symptoms of pain and signs of tenderness or a mass accompanied by varying degrees of systemic inflammatory response. CT scanning is regarded as the diagnostic modality of choice. Endoscopy is generally avoided due to the increased risk of perforation.

Pericolic abscess may result from the perforation of a diverticulum; when identified an abscess should be drained percutaneously if possible. Diverticular disease may lead to fistulas into adjacent organs; the most common is colovesical fistula. Colovaginal fistula may also occur and are more common if the patient has had a previous hysterectomy. Diverticular disease is the commonest cause of major lower gastrointestinal (GI) bleeding (see following section).

Treatment is based on confirming the diagnosis (exclusion of co-existing colonic carcinoma is sometimes difficult as the features of both conditions can appear to overlap on colonic imaging) and conservatism is generally advised for mild attacks. Treatment with antibiotics usually settles mild attacks and dietary advice is given to increase both fibre and fluid in the diet. Pericolic abscess should be treated by percutaneous drainage and patients with peritonitis or colonic fistulas are usually submitted to laparotomy and colonic resection. Whether to reconstruct intestinal continuity or leave the patient with a Hartmann's operation is dependant on the patient's general condition, the state of the bowel (presence of infection usually precludes anastomosis) and the skill, and experience of the surgeon.

Lower GI haemorrhage

Lower GI hemorrhage is defined as the abnormal loss of blood from the GI tract distal to the ligament of Treitz. Bleeding can be occult, slow, moderate, or life-threatening.

Diverticular disease

Diverticular disease is the most likely cause of lower GI hemorrhage in adults and accounts for between 30% and 40% of all cases. The severity of bleeding caused by diverticular disease ranges from mild to life-threatening. Approximately 80% of bleeding episodes caused by diverticular disease stop spontaneously.

Inflammatory bowel disease

Inflammatory bowel disease (ulcerative colitis (UC) and Crohn's disease (CD)) is a common source of lower GI hemorrhage, usually manifesting as bloody diarrhoea. Although the risk of life-threatening GI hemorrhage is reported to be low in these disorders, it does occur and occasionally mandates emergent operation. Ischaemic colitis should also be considered in the differential diagnosis.

Arteriovenous malformations

Arteriovenous malformations, also known as vascular ectasias, angiomas and angiodysplasias, are degenerative lesions of the GI tract that occur with increasing frequency as patients age. It is estimated that up to 30% of the population greater than 50 years of age have arteriovenous malformations. It is thought that colonic muscle wall contraction leads to intermittent partial obstruction of the submucosal veins and these veins become dilated and tortuous, resulting in incompetence of the precapillary sphincters, which results in arteriovenous communications. Arteriovenous malformations are usually multiple and occur most frequently in the ascending colon, particularly in the caecum. The caecum is the single most likely location of arteriovenous malformations because, according to Laplace's law (tension in wall α internal pressure × radius), it has the greatest wall tension. Bleeding caused by arteriovenous malformations is characteristically chronic, slow, intermittent and recurrent. Endoscopic coagulation is the treatment of choice.

Neoplasia

Although bleeding commonly occurs with both benign adenomatous polyps and adenocarcinomas of the colon and rectum, large-volume bleeding is an unusual presenting sign.

Benign anorectal conditions

Colonic, anorectal and peristomal varices arise as a complication of portal hypertension and can cause painless, massive lower GI hemorrhage. Nevertheless, it is the more humble anorectal conditions that present more typically with lower GI bleeding. In a review of nearly 18 000 patients with lower GI bleeding, haemorrhoids, fissure and fistula-in-ano were the cause in 11% of patients. It is, therefore, important to thoroughly examine the anorectum early in the evaluation before proceeding to more invasive and complex diagnostic methods. Digital rectal examination, proctoscopy and sigmoidoscopy should be performed in all patients with rectal bleeding. Discovery of benign anorectal disease does not eliminate the possibility of a more proximal bleeding source, and complete colonic evaluation is recommended.

Upper GI bleeding

Approximately 10% of cases of bright red rectal blood loss actually occurs as a result of massive, continuous, life-threatening bleeding from an upper GI source (i.e. proximal to the ligament of Treitz). Normally upper GI bleeding presents as melaena due to digestive alteration of the blood in the small intestine. When the upper GI blood loss is massive, with rapid transit of blood down the intestine, this digestive process does not have time to take place.

Management of lower GI bleeding

Resuscitation of the patient is the priority, with airway control and provision of oxygen plus large bore intravenous access. Blood should be taken for estimation of haemoglobin, urea, electrolytes, liver function and coagulation profile. Blood should be cross-matched and blood, and products given as required. Urinary and nasogastric catheters are helpful and arterial blood gas analysis will also help to guide the resuscitative effort. The history is important and evidence should be sought of previous GI bleeding, peptic ulcer or inflammatory bowel disease, liver disease, non-steroidal or warfarin usage. The abdomen and anorectum must be carefully examined and bedside examination of the anal canal and rectum are mandatory. If there is any suspicion of an upper GI source, this should be ruled out by upper GI endoscopy.

Colonoscopy is the diagnostic procedure of choice because of its diagnostic accuracy and therapeutical capability. As many lower GI bleeds subside spontaneously, the traditional management has been to wait, then to prep the bowel and undertake endoscopy. Recent evidence supports the use of early colonoscopy after mechanical bowel preparation. Colonoscopy must only be performed in a stable patient. Endoscopic haemostasis either by adrenaline injection or bipolar coagulation has been shown to reduce the requirement for surgery.

If upper and lower GI tract endoscopy fail to identify a source of bleeding, nuclear scintigraphy may be indicated. The role of technetium-labelled red blood cell scintigraphy in lower GI hemorrhage is controversial because its accuracy in locating the precise site of hemorrhage is variable, with reports of false localisation ranging from 3% to 59%.

Angiography can detect hemorrhage at a rate of 0.5–1 ml/min. The technique is performed via transfemoral placement of an arterial catheter. The hallmark of a positive examination is extravasation of contrast material into the lumen of the bowel. Angiography requires the availability of a skilled radiologist and the overall sensitivity of angiography is variable, and may be as low as 40%. If a bleeding source is identified then vasopressin may be infused down the angiography catheter. Vasopressin is a pituitary extract that causes arteriolar vasoconstriction and bowel wall contraction. Another angiographic option for control of hemorrhage is selective transcatheter embolisation of the bleeding site.

Emergency operations for acute lower GI bleeding may be required in approximately 15% of patients. The indications for an operation are persistent or recurrent haemorrhage leading to haemodynamic instability despite resuscitation or a high transfusion requirement. In general, patients with ongoing bleeding who have required transfusion of six or more units of blood should undergo an operation. If the bleeding site has been successfully localised, segmental resection is the treatment of choice because of its low morbidity, mortality and rebleed rate. If operation is required before accurate localisation of the bleeding site has been possible, then attempts should be made intraoperatively to identify the precise cause. Blind segmental colectomy should not be performed because of its high risk of rebleeding and associated mortality. Intraoperative colonoscopy should be undertaken; if diagnostic confusion still exists, oesophogastrodueodonoscopy (OGD) should be repeated and a paediatric colonoscope used to perform on-table small-bowel enteroscopy as small intestinal sources such as arteriovenous malformations, diverticula and neoplasia account for up to 5% of all cases of severe lower GI bleeding. If the bleeding site remains unidentified, then subtotal colectomy with ileorectal anastomosis or ileostomy should be undertaken.

Anorectal sepsis

Anorectal sepsis is a common feature of acute surgical takes all over the world. Presenting features are usually pain with fever and malaise. Perianal abscess is usually obvious, but intersphincteric abscesses may cause pain without obvious pointing of an abscess at the anal margin and examination under anaesthetic may be necessary to achieve a diagnosis. Perianal abscess is thought to arise through infection of an anal gland and anal fistula may result. Treatment of the acute infection is to relieve the abscess. Examination of the anal canal with a bi-valved speculum (Eisenhammer) with gentle pressure on the abscess may reveal evidence of an internal opening, and some surgeons routinely lay open such fistulas acutely. However, there is some evidence that simple drainage of the abscess will allow resolution of the infection without subsequent fistula formation. Pus should be sent routinely for microbiology and the abscess drained with an incision circumferential to the anal canal over the fluctuant part. Pus must be drained and the cavity irrigated. Packing with gauze should be avoided, as it is very painful to remove on the ward. The patient must be followed up carefully to identify those who require further treatment of anal fistula (see below).

Anorectal sepsis may progress to become the disease eponymously credited to Prof. Jean-Alfred Fournier, a Parisian dermatologist and venereologist. Fournier's gangrene is a rapidly progressive infection of the perineal soft tissue and polymicrobial cultures of anaerobes and aerobes are the rule rather than the exception. Anorectal sepsis is a common precursor for Fournier's gangrene and early aggressive treatment is associated with a reduced mortality rate. King Herod the Great of Judaea is suspected to have succumbed to Fournier's gangrene in association with diabetes mellitus, a common co-factor in the condition.

Colorectal injury

Rectal injuries usually occur in association with pelvic fractures, although impalement injuries and penetrating injuries of the abdomen or perineum from knives or gunshots can also damage the rectum. A high index of suspicion is required as these injuries can be subtle and are easily missed. In stable trauma patients were clinical suspicion exists, careful clinical examination aided by flexible endoscopic examination is vital. Initial experience with rectal injury was obtained in warfare where wounds can be severe with gross destruction and contamination plus delay from point of wounding to definitive surgical care. Experience with such wounds led to a policy of treatment based on faecal diversion with exposure, debridement and repair of the rectal wound, distal washout of the rectum and pre-sacral drainage. There is evidence that the majority of rectal injuries encountered in civilian practice do not require such an aggressive surgical approach and can be treated with simple faecal diversion alone. In impalement injuries, careful perineal debridement is necessary and sphincteric damage should ideally be assessed and managed by an expert.

Defunctioning colostomy was the standard management of penetrating colonic injury from the time of World War II until 1979 when the first randomised trial was undertaken which showed that primary repair of colonic injuries was appropriate for selected patients. A *Cochrane Database Review* from 2003 demonstrated that mortality was not significantly different between patients with penetrating colonic injury treated by primary repair or faecal diversion. However, total complications were significantly less in the primary repair group. While

primary repair is appropriate for non-destructive (involvement of <50% of the bowel wall without devascularisation) colon wounds in the absence of peritonitis, patients with penetrating intraperitoneal colon wounds that are destructive (involvement of >50% of the bowel wall or devascularisation of a bowel segment) should undergo resection and primary anastomosis. However, if there are significant associated injuries, there has been haemodynamically instability, or the patient has serious underlying co-morbidity, serious consideration should still be given to the use of colostomy.

Colonic injury after blunt trauma is rare and difficult to diagnose. There is little guidance in the literature to know what is the best way to manage these injuries; however, experience of treating patients with penetrating colonic injury suggests that primary repair (or resection and anastomosis) is appropriate in the absence of delay to diagnosis, severe associated injury or haemodynamic instability.

Foreign body

Human beings appear to have an inexhaustible fascination for inserting objects into their rectums. Retained rectal foreign bodies can present a challenge in management. Digital rectal examination, proctoscopy and abdominal radiography are helpful and soft or low-lying objects can be grasped and removed safely in the emergency department. However, simply grasping objects may result in upward migration toward the sigmoid. Insufflation of air with a rigid or flexible sigmoidoscope proximal to the object can break the apparent 'vacuum seal' and aid retrieval. Many innovative approaches (such as obstetrical forceps) have been used, but occasionally general anaesthesia with transrectal manipulation and bimanual palpation is necessary to withdraw the foreign body. Laparoscopy may help to retrieve objects, but laparotomy and colotomy may ultimately be required.

INFLAMMATORY BOWEL DISEASE

Ulcerative colitis

UC is characterised by ulcerative inflammation of all or part of the colonic mucosa, at presentation half of patients have inflammation confined to the rectum. UC is characterised by exacerbation and remission and may be associated with extraintestinal manifestation such as arthropathy or sclerosing cholangitis.

Symptoms of UC include rectal bleeding and urgency, tenesmus and diarrhoea. Medical therapy is the mainstay of treatment and the goal is first to induce and then maintain remission of the colitis. UC can be either distal or extensive; in distal UC, the inflammation is limited to the area below the splenic flexure and is amenable to oral or topical treatment. In extensive UC, inflammation extends proximal to the splenic flexure and requires oral therapy with or without topical therapy. Disease severity is classified as mild (<4 stools/day, with or without blood, and no systemic signs of toxicity), moderate 4–6 stools/day with minimal signs of toxicity), or severe (>6 bloody stools a day accompanied by signs of toxicity, including fever, tachycardia, anaemia or elevated erythrocyte sedimentation rate).

The 5-aminosalicylic acid (5-ASA) agents are the treatment of choice for mild to moderate disease. Corticosteroids are useful agents to help induce remission in severe colitis; intravenous cyclosporine can be used in refractory disease but if remission does not occur, then colectomy is indicated.

Once remission has been initiated, maintenance should be achieved with aminosalicylates, orally, topically (by enemas) or in combination. In some patients, immunomodulation may be required with azathioprine or 6-mercaptopurine.

Crohn's disease

CD is a chronic transmural inflammation that may affect any part of the GI tract, from the mouth to the anus. In approximately one-third of cases, the disease is confined to the small intestine, whereas approximately one-half of patients will have involvement of both the small intestine and the colon (ileocolitis). In approximately 20% of cases, only the colon is involved. Most patients present with symptoms of abdominal pain and tenderness, chronic or nocturnal diarrhea, rectal bleeding, weight loss and fever. Perianal disease is occasionally the dominant feature of CD.

CD evolves over time from a primarily inflammatory disease into one of two clinical patterns: stricturing (obstructive) or penetrating (fistulising). The 5-ASA compounds are effective for establishing remission of mild to moderate CD. Budesonide, a newer corticosteroid with a lower systemic bioavailability than the older corticosteroids, is indicated for mild to moderate CD involving the ileocaecal area. Corticosteroids are used in order to induce remission and azathioprine or 6-mercaptopurine can be used in conjunction with steroids for establishing remission in patients with refractory, moderate to severe CD and as corticosteroid sparing maintenance agents. Surveillance full blood counts must be undertaken, every 3 months, as long as patients continue azathioprine, in view of the risk of agranulocytosis. The novel agent, infliximab, which is an antagonist of tumour necrosis factor α, has shown it is effective in fistulous CD but must be used with care as there is a risk of anaphylaxis (it contains non-human protein) and there are reports of reactivation of latent tuberculosis in patients after treatment.

Surgical therapy

Between 30% and 40% of patients with UC will eventually require surgery. Surgical removal of the entire colonic and rectal mucosa in UC can be curative. Surgery is required for emergency presentations, such as toxic colitis, bleeding or perforation, or for colitis refractory to optimal medical therapy. Longstanding total colitis increases the risk of carcinoma and surgery is required if there is dysplasia in the colon or rectum. Restoration of intestinal continuity after removal

of the colon and rectum is by creation of a neorectum fashioned from the terminal ileum and anastomosed to the anal canal; the so-called ileal pouch operation.

The primary indications for surgery in patients with CD are intestinal obstruction and septic complications, such as internal fistula or abscess. Other indications include perforation, hemorrhage, failure to thrive despite optimal medical therapy and carcinoma. One of the main principles of operating for CD is to maintain as much small bowel length as possible. Microscopic disease may be present at resection margins without compromising results and strictureplasty is preferred over resection when possible. Smoking after a surgical resection doubles the risk of recurrence and use of 5-ASA drugs also reduces the risk of recurrence after surgery.

Perianal disease in CD

CD has a well-recognised association with perianal lesions, which may be primary Crohn's associated fissures or ulcers, or secondary lesions such as tags, fistulas or rectal stricture. The perianal manifestations range from mild to severe (so-called watering can perineum) and are usually amenable to surgical therapy. In some cases proctectomy may be required.

COLORECTAL CANCER
Background and aetiology

Each year colorectal cancer affects 32 000 people in the UK and is responsible for around 22 000 deaths. In males it is second only to lung cancer and in females it falls third behind lung and breast cancer. In the developed world, life-time risk of colorectal cancer is around 1 : 25 and this is increased by genetic predisposition and certain conditions such as chronic colitis. Colorectal cancer is mainly a disease of the elderly with a marked rise in incidence after age 70 years, however, 10% of individuals are under age 55 years at diagnosis.

In 1972, Burkitt described the relationship between diet and incidence of bowel cancer; he hypothesised that a diet rich in fibre was associated with regular bulky stools and reduced bowel carcinogenesis, perhaps by reducing exposure of colonic mucosa to dietary carcinogens. It does seem likely that the combination of high fibre and low fat may be protective against bowel cancer. Protection against colorectal carcinogenesis is also derived from dietary supplements of calcium and folate and evidence from the Nurses Health Study (North America) suggested that oestrogen in the form of hormone replacement therapy (HRT) lowers the incidence of colorectal neoplasia. There has been interest in the potential influence of non-steroidal anti-inflammatory drugs in colorectal carcinogenesis. Cyclooxygenase (COX)-2 inhibition appears to have potent effects on the colonic mucosa, increasing apoptosis and reducing cellular proliferation. It is also likely that these drugs function through COX-independent mechanisms. Impressive effects on the growth on adenomas have been described in certain polyposis syndromes and uncontrolled population studies suggest a reduction in colorectal cancer associated mortality. However, these effects may be subject to many confounding factors and the exact influence on colorectal cancer incidence has yet to be determined.

Chronic inflammatory conditions often predispose to carcinogenesis and in the colon and rectum this is best demonstrated by chronic UC. The risk of developing malignancy is related to the duration and extent of colitis. An approximate incidence of 10% per annum after a decade of extensive colitis is often cited. However, careful surveillance for dysplasia and precursor lesions followed by colectomy can reduce this risk. Similar risks and surveillance strategies apply to Crohn's colitis.

Vogelstein has proposed a model for colorectal carcinogenesis; with cancer resulting from an accumulation of somatic genetic defects manifested in the progression from small adenoma to larger adenoma and ultimately cancer. The time course to this endpoint is around 10 years but typically, conditions which lead to familial predisposition hasten this pathway to carcinogenesis with inherited mutations in the critical cancer genes or systems which maintain the integrity of DNA replication and repair. Examples of this are seen in familial adenomatous polyposis where an inheritable inactivating mutation in the antigen presenting cells (APC) gene occurs and hereditary non-polyposis colorectal cancer (HNPCC) where defects in DNA mismatch repair genes result in a high frequency of mutation.

Clinical presentation

Clinical presentation is determined by the site of tumour within the bowel (Table 13.2). Transient changes in bowel function are common as a result of GI infection and functional bowel disease such as irritable bowel syndrome. However, persistence of bowel symptoms for more than 6 weeks is of concern, particularly in those over 40 years of age; malignant disease should be excluded in this group. As a generalisation, cancers of the left colon and rectum present with change in bowel habit and/or bleeding whereas right colon cancers cause anaemia and small bowel obstruction. General malaise, anorexia and weight loss, and uncommon features of bowel cancer generally reflect the presence of metastatic disease.

The majority of patients with colorectal cancer are detected through out patient investigation, but as many as 25–30% are diagnosed as emergencies with obstruction and perforation being common features. Most patients presenting to outpatients have no abnormality detected on clinical examination. However, an abdominal mass may be detected, of which a caecal tumour in the right iliac fossa is the most common. Rectal examination and rigid sigmodoscopy may detect a distal sigmoid colon or rectal lesion; however, normal clinical examination does not exclude significant bowel pathology.

Bowel symptoms suggestive of malignant disease are usually best investigated by direct visualisation of the mucosa by means of colonoscopy. However, limited endoscopy resources coupled with increased complications from colonoscopy mean that double-contrast barium enema is often undertaken as an alternative. The disadvantage is reduced sensitivity and specificity. When the presenting symptom is rectal bleeding alone, flexible sigmoidoscopy may be sufficient.

In an emergency setting, patients present with the consequences of obstruction, perforation or bleeding. It may be impossible to distinguish bowel cancer from other pathology particularly diverticular disease. Plain abdominal X-ray may confirm the diagnosis with dilated large bowel, and second stage investigation with water-soluble contrast enema and CT scan should provide a definitive diagnosis and help plan appropriate management through disease staging.

Preoperative staging of colorectal cancer

Following the diagnosis of bowel cancer staging is important in determining the optimum management plan and in providing prognostic information. Three areas need to be considered.

Local invasion

This is particularly important in rectal cancer where proximity of tumour to the circumferential margin of resection can determine the need for neoadjuvant chemoradiotherapy. In the rectum this information is obtained by specialist assessment by MRI and/or endoluminal ultrasound to clearly define the layers of the bowel wall, surrounding mesorectal fat and the enveloping mesorectal fascia. In colon cancer, local assessment by CT scan is adequate, and can provide information on invasion of adjacent structures, such as ureter or duodenum, which can assist surgical planning.

Metastatic disease

Bowel cancer most commonly spreads to liver and lung, and these organs should be assessed routinely before surgery. CT scan of abdomen and chest offers the most accurate and convenient means and also provides a baseline for subsequent routine examinations.

Synchronous lesions

Adenomas are found in 20% of patients with colorectal cancer and around 3% have multiple cancers. Identifying these lesions preoperatively can dramatically alter surgical planning. Colonoscopy or barium enema should be undertaken. Occasionally, obstructing cancers can preclude examination of the proximal bowel.

Management of early cancer

Some cancers are diagnosed at an early stage and this is best demonstrated by the finding of invasive cancer in a polyp. Endoscopic removal of the polyp is adequate treatment in many cases and this should be balanced against the risk of

Table 13.2. Presentation of colorectal cancer.

Site	Bleeding	Constipation or obstruction	Diarrhoea
Rectum	Bright or dark	Disturbance of bowel function common with frequent defaecation and tenesmus. Locally advanced cancers may obstruct	May be spurious due to obstruction or result from mucus production
Left colon	Dark and mixed with stool	Tendency to constipation and erratic bowel habit leading to obstruction	May be spurious due to obstruction or result from mucus production
Right colon	Usually occult resulting in anaemic	Liquid stool makes obstruction a late symptom. Advanced caecal lesions cause small bowl obstruction	Large mucin producing cancers may cause loose stools

colonic resection. The presence of poorly differentiated cancer, lymphovascular invasion and involvement of the excised margin would suggest that resection should be undertaken.

Small rectal cancers can be removed by full-thickness local excision. This is best achieved with transanal endoscopic microsurgery (TEM) using sophisticated instrumentation offering a magnified view and precise surgical technique. This is an area of increasing experience as early cancers are likely to be asymptomatic and therefore diagnosed in screening programmes.

The management of advanced cancer

The majority of bowel cancers are managed by surgical resection. The principle of surgery is to remove the primary tumour with draining lymph nodes while preserving anatomical planes around the mesentery. This is best demonstrated in the rectum where the application of this principle, termed 'total mesorectal excision' has resulted in a reduction in local recurrence of cancer. The main arterial supply and venous drainage are identified and divided. The bowel ends are then divided at appropriate points determined by the need to achieve an adequate margin around the cancer and leave healthy, well vascularised normal bowel that can be sutured or approximated by stapling devices. The resulting anastomosis is critical and problems in healing lead to dehiscence or 'leak'. This commonly results in re-operation and is associated with high morbidity and mortality. In some cases where the cancer is immediately above or invading the sphincter muscle it is not possible to form an anastomosis and an abdominoperineal excision is performed. This involves the complete removal of the anus and rectum with formation of a permanent colostomy. Segmental colonic resections are usually described in a logical fashion according to the involved segment: right hemicolectomy, left hemicolectomy, sigmoid colectomy. Removal of the rectum with formation of an anastomosis is often abbreviated to 'anterior resection' indicating that the rectum surgery is performed through the anterior or abdominal route rather than perineal or posterior approach.

Under some circumstances the surgeon may regard formation of an anastomosis as unsafe. This situation most often arises in emergency surgery where bowel perforation or obstruction has led to contamination of the peritoneal cavity. An anastomosis is avoided by forming a stoma, where the proximal end of bowel is brought to the skin through a separate trephine in the abdominal wall. The resulting stoma is known as a colostomy or ileostomy depending on the origin. The most common procedure at which a colostomy is formed is a Hartmann's resection, where sigmoid pathology is removed with the formation of an end colostomy. This colostomy can be reversed at a later date but in this generally elderly population up to 40% of patients choose not to have further surgery. If a high-risk anastomosis is formed, for example, deep in the pelvis after a low anterior resection a temporary ileostomy or colostomy may be formed to protect the downstream join in the bowel should it fail to heal. The use of a defunctioning stoma in this fashion tends to reduce the sequelae of a failed anastomosis. This type of stoma is usually a 'loop' and can be closed when the primary anastomosis has been confirmed to have healed adequately, usually after 3–4 months.

Metastatic cancer

Twenty-five per cent of patients with bowel cancer present with metastatic disease, most commonly affecting the liver. There are several treatment options depending on the extent of metastatic disease and the patient's symptoms and wishes. In those patients with advanced metastatic disease treatment is aimed at optimising palliation. Early use of chemotherapy has been shown to increase quality and length of survival in metastatic colorectal cancer. However, some patients choose not to have treatment until symptoms develop. If significant symptoms can be attributed to the primary cancer within the bowel then a range of surgical options can be explored. Surgical resection as described above for localised disease can provide effective treatment for bowel symptoms, arising from bleeding or obstruction of the lumen. If patients are unfit for surgery, cancers causing obstruction can be treated with endoluminal stenting where an expandable metallic stent is deployed across the stricturing tumour opening the lumen to relieve the obstruction. Rectal cancer symptoms such as tenesmus, bleeding, discharge or obstruction can be improved by transanal resection, radiotherapy, stoma formation or combination treatment.

Localised metastatic disease, either at time of initial presentation or following primary surgery may be amenable to potentially curative treatment. Surgical resection of liver secondaries is associated with a 5-year survival of 20–25% in experienced centres. The population with advanced disease who may benefit from liver resection is increased by a multimodal approach using neoadjuvant chemotherapy and local treatments such as high-intensity focussed ultrasound, radio frequency and cryo-ablation, which induce tumour necrosis. Poor prognostic factors for failure of hepatic resection include large or multiple metastases, surgical clearance margin of less than 1 cm, metastases appearing within 6 months of surgery and the presence of involved lymph nodes in the primary colonic resection.

Pathology

Three gross morphological forms of colorectal cancer exist: polypoid, ulcerative and stricturing. The vast majority are adenocarcinomas. Carcinoid tumours, lymphoma, sarcoma and adenosquamous cancers are also described. The histology of adenocarcinomas is characterised further on the basis of differentiation and mucin production: well differentiated cancers (where cells show a propensity to form glandular structures from which there were derived) and those without mucin production are associated with an improved prognosis. Histological factors such as vascular and lymphatic invasion within the tumour are also associated with poorer prognosis.

Pathological staging systems are important in determining appropriate treatment as well as standardising populations for research and audit. For these reasons, accurate staging in colorectal cancer is vital. Pathological staging offers the definitive report but as noted above radiological staging in rectal cancer is an important determinant of treatment.

Pathological staging

Dukes' stage is the most widely employed staging system. It lacks detail on local tumour invasion but overall provides a robust if rather crude predictor of prognosis. Dukes' classification has been largely abandoned in favour of the internationally agreed Union Internationale Contre Cancer (UICC) tumour, nodes, metastases (TNM) system of classification, the principles of which are shared with many cancers. In North America, The American Joint Committee on Cancer (AJCC) system is employed. Table 13.3 summarises these systems.

TNM classification offers more detail and flexibility without becoming unduly complex. The modification to Dukes stage detailing apical lymph node involvement is a useful prognosticator: C2 is associated with a 5-year survival of 35% compared to 55% associated with C1 disease. In the TNM system, N1 or N2 may or may not involve the apical lymph node and accordingly this useful prognostic factor is lost.

The TNM staging system is also employed in preoperative clinical and radiological assessment. This is identified by prefixing a report with 'c', for example, cT3N2M0. Pathological stage is prefixed by 'p' and if neoadjuvant treatments may have changed the pathological stage the report is prefixed by 'yp'.

NON-SURGICAL TREATMENT OF COLORECTAL CANCER

Chemotherapy and radiotherapy have well-defined roles in the treatment of colorectal cancer. They can be considered in three forms: adjuvant, neoadjuvant and palliative.

Adjuvant therapy

Chemotherapy in the form of 5-fluorouracil (5-FU) and folinic acid increases survival in patients following potentially curative surgery. This effect is through eradication of occult metastases and offers an overall improvement in survival by approximately 5%. However, in those patients at higher risk of metastatic disease (those with lymph node involvement) this benefit may increase to 20%. Therefore, it is generally advised that adjuvant chemotherapy with 5-FU is reserved for patients with lymph node involvement. In practice, adjuvant therapy is frequently extended to younger patients with no lymph node involvement where the primary tumour shows vascular invasion, peritoneal (T4) disease or poor differentiation. However, in all patients the potential benefits of adjuvant therapy must be balanced against the risk of side effects and accordingly it tends to be employed less often in elderly patients with comorbidity, especially ischaemic heart disease.

Short course preoperative radiotherapy given over 1 week and followed immediately by surgical resection has been shown to reduce local recurrence in rectal cancer. However, it is probable that only a subset of rectal cancers may benefit and ideally these can be identified by accurate preoperative staging. Radiotherapy in this context does not offer any reduction in tumour size as surgery is undertaken before tumour regression occurs.

Postoperative radiotherapy is of benefit in rectal cancer patients where the cancer is shown to have threatened the resection margin. This has some disadvantages compared to preoperative treatment in that the surgical field including the neorectum is irradiated causing deterioration in function and increased side effects form collateral damage to other structures such as small bowel.

Neoadjuvant therapy

Neoadjuvant treatment is employed with the aim of reducing tumour size, thereby improving the chances of curative resection. It is employed in the treatment of rectal cancers where preoperative staging suggest the circumferential margin of the mesorectum may be threatened or involved with tumour. This group of patients receive radiotherapy as a long course: 45 Gy over 5 weeks combined with 5-FU. A complete pathological response with no cancer present in the resected specimen is occurs in 10–15% of patients.

Neoadjuvant chemotherapy is also used in the treatment of liver metastases, potentially reducing tumour size to improve the chances of successful surgical resection.

Palliative therapy

In patients with metastatic disease not suitable for surgical resection, chemotherapy in the form of 5-FU may be employed. In this setting increased survival can be achieved but the benefits need to be balanced against the potential side effects. More recently, Irinotecan and Oxaliplatin have been used at earlier stages of palliative treatment. They are generally more efficacious than 5-FU, but more expensive and with an increased incidence of adverse effects. Palliative radiotherapy can be targeted for symptom relief in locally advanced rectal cancer. It is also valuable in the treatment of painful bone metastases from colorectal cancer.

Screening and surveillance for colorectal cancer

Colorectal cancer presents an ideal opportunity for asymptomatic population screening. There is a protracted premalignant phase (adenoma), which can be identified and removed endoscopically halting the development of invasive disease. Several methods of population-based screening and surveillance of high-risk groups exist.

Population screening

Faecal occult blood testing

Cancers and large adenomas bleed into the bowel lumen and this can be detected by simple stool analysis. Various forms of faecal occult blood testing (FOBT) exist and these vary in sensitivity and specificity. Three large randomised trials in England, Denmark and the USA have demonstrated a reduction in colorectal cancer deaths with FOBT. Healthy individuals over age 45 years are invited to perform FOBT every 2 years. Those with positive FOBT undergo colonoscopy. This approach leads to the earlier diagnosis of colorectal cancer and in the Nottingham (UK) trial colorectal cancer mortality was reduced by 17%.

Flexible sigmoidoscopy

Seventy per cent of cancers and adenomas occur in the rectum and sigmoid colon within reach of a flexible sigmoidoscope. A single flexible sigmoidoscopy examination between 55 and 65 years is likely to reduce the incidence of colorectal

Table 13.3. **Pathological staging of colorectal cancer.**

Stage	Degree of invasion	Lymph node status	Metastasis
Dukes A	Confined to bowel wall	Not involved	Absent
Dukes B	Through muscularis propria	Not involved	Absent
Dukes C1	Any	Local lymph node(s) involved	Absent
Dukes C2	Any	Apical lymph node ± others involved	Absent
Dukes D	Any	Any	Present
Tis	*In situ* cancer, basement membrane intact	Any	Any
T1	Into submucosa	Any	Any
T2	Into muscularis propria	Any	Any
T3	Through muscularis propria	Any	Any
T4	Breaches peritoneal surface. Includes free perforation, abscess and invasion of adjacent organ	Any	Any
Nx	Any	Lymph nodes not assessed	Any
N0	Any	None	Any
N1	Any	1–3 lymph nodes	Any
N2	Any	>3 lymph nodes	Any
Mx	Any	Any	Not assessed
MO	Any	Any	Absent
M1	Any	Any	Present
AJCC I	Submucosal or into muscularis propria	Not involved	Absent
AJCC II	Though muscularis propria	Not involved	Absent
AJCC III	Any	Involved	Absent
AJCC IV	Any	Any	Present

cancer through two means. Firstly, all polyps identified at this examination are removed and with them the risk of developing into invasive disease. Secondly, those individuals with large, multiple or severely dysplastic adenomas undergo colonoscopy to exclude more proximal lesions. Although this screening method will detect some early cancers, the main thrust is to remove adenomas and identify the subgroup of patients at high risk who are likely to benefit from more intensive follow up.

Colonoscopy

This provides a sensitive and specific means of examining the bowel but it is expensive and associated with a relatively high incidence of complications which makes it unsuitable for population-based screening. However, it is the method of choice in the surveillance of high-risk individuals such as those with a genetical predisposition or chronic colitis.

Faecal DNA analysis

Extraction of DNA from stool is now feasible and some genetic abnormalities commonly found in colorectal cancer can be detected, including mutations in k-ras, APC, p53 and BAT26. This approach is likely to become more sensitive with improved techniques and ultimately may be used in combination with flexible sigmoidoscopy or non-invasive approaches such as virtual colonoscopy.

ANAL CANCER

Anal cancer is rare, accounting for less 5% of large-bowel tumours. Over 80% of anal cancers are squamous cell in origin, however, malignant melanoma may occur in the anal canal. The recognition of a high incidence of squamous cell carcinoma of the anus amongst some homosexual men led to the search for an infective aetiological agent. Risk factors for anal cancer include a history of genital warts and evidence now suggests an association between human papilloma virus types 16, 18, 30, 31 and 33, and anal cancer. It is believed that anal cancer may occur due to progression of anal intraepithelial neoplasia in a manner analogous to intraepithelial carcinoma of the cervix, vulva or vagina.

Anal cancer typically presents with pain and bleeding, and these symptoms are often initially disregarded or misdiagnosed. Clinicians must be most suspicious of a patient with an indolent anal ulcer or rectal bleeding who complains of persistent or severe pain.

Treatment is usually by combination chemo and radiation therapy using 5-FU and mitomycin C combined with high-dose external beam irradiation. Surgery is reserved for those who relapse despite oncological therapy; however, small lesions at the anal margin may still be treated by local excision only.

Anal cancer spreads to inguinal lymph nodes which should always be assessed by the clinician. Typically, inguinal nodes are included in the radiation field.

MINOR ANORECTAL CONDITIONS

Fistula-in-ano

The so-called 'cryptoglandular hypothesis' ascribes the aetiology of fistula-in-ano to the glands that sit in the intersphincteric space around the anal canal. Spread of sepsis from an infected gland leads to perianal abscess which usually presents acutely (see above). Epithelialisation of the track leads to establishment of a fistula-in-ano. A classification of fistulas by the late Sir Alan Parks in 1976, described four main groups; intersphincteric, transsphincteric, suprasphincteric and extrasphincteric. A full assessment of a fistula-in-ano requires the identification of the internal and external openings, the primary track, any secondary extension and any diseases complicating the situation. Extensions occur in approximately 10–15% of patients, and are more prevalent in recurrent or Crohn's fistulas.

The goal of treatment of fistula-in-ano is to eradicate the fistula while maintaining continence.

Up to 25% of fistulas recur, and recurrence is usually due to sepsis missed at surgery and left untreated. MRI is effective at identifying the cause for recurrent sepsis and surgery guided by MRI can reduce further episodes of recurrence by up to 75%.

The best way to cure fistula is to lay open the track and allow it to heal by secondary intention, thus obliterating the fistula; however, in order to achieve this, a varying amount of sphincter muscle must be divided. The majority of fistulas will be amenable to this technique, but laying open of high or transphincteric fistulas may result in incontinence. There are various options for the treatment of high or complex fistulas, from the use of permanent seton sutures, to mucosal advancement flaps or the use of tissue glues.

Anal fissure

Anal fissure is a linear split in the lining of the lower half of the anal canal and may be primary, or related to other pathology, such as CD.

The cause of anal fissure is unclear, but the initiating event is usually thought to be the difficult passage of a constipated stool that traumatises the anal canal. Patients with anal fissure are likely to have high resting pressures in the anal canal and it is thought that high resting pressures in the canal lead to relative hypoperfusion and reduced tissue oxygen tensions, impairing healing. This understanding underpins the therapeutical strategy, which is based on interventions that reduce the resting pressures in the canal. However, an important subgroup of patients develop anal fissure despite normal or low pressures (e.g. it is common postpartum).

Patients usually present with pain at defaecation and there may be some associated bright red bleeding. Visual inspection of the anus while gently everting the perianal skin is usually sufficient to make the diagnosis and further examination may be too painful in a conscious patient. Always bear in mind the possibility of other diagnoses; CD, sexually transmitted disease (e.g. syphilis and herpes simplex) and anal carcinoma.

Management is based on altering two factors; the stool consistency and the resting muscle tone in the anal canal. Dietary advice to increase fluid and fibre in the diet helps and stool-softening agents such as isphagula can be useful. In the past, resting tone in the anal canal was reduced surgically by submitting the patient to an anaesthetic and dilating the anal canal. This caused an injury to the internal sphincter and reliably reduced the resting tone, but in an uncontrolled manner with an unacceptably high rate of anal incontinence. Controlled surgical spincterotomy is still considered by many to be the 'gold standard' against which other therapies must be judged.

Haemorrhoids

Haemorrhoids, or piles, are a common complaint which patients tend to use as a 'catch-all' diagnosis to encompass a variety of anal conditions. To the colorectal surgeon, haemorrhoids refer to the symptoms that arise from the anal cushions. These cushions are three submucosal spaces filled with arteriovenous communications, which lie in the upper half of the anal canal and help to keep it 'airtight' at rest. Haemorrhoids are said to have occurred when the cushions bleed or prolapse, or both.

Haemorrhoids have been arbitrarily classified as:
- *First degree*: bleeding alone.
- *Second degree*: prolapse on defaecation with spontaneous reduction.
- *Third degree*: prolapse on defaecation requiring manual reduction.
- *Fourth degree*: prolapse on defaecation, unable to replace.

The bleeding of haemorrhoids is classically bright red in colour and seen on the toilet paper or in the toilet pan. A rectal neoplasm can produce similar bleeding and steps must be taken to exclude such a lesion. Flexible sigmoidoscopy is the investigation of choice in bright red rectal bleeding. Advice about dietary changes (to include more fibre and fluid) may be sufficient to manage some haemorrhoidal symptoms. Other interventions may be in the outpatient setting or surgical.

Outpatient treatment for haemorrhoids is usually by the application of rubber bands or by injection of 5% phenol in almond or arachis oil as a sclerosant. A recent meta-analysis suggested that rubber-band ligation was better than sclerotherapy.

Surgical haemorrhoidectomy is usually described as the Milligan–Morgan technique, with excision of the three cushions to leave a 'clover leaf' type wound in the anal canal. This is a painful operation and careful attention should be paid to the perioperative regime. Pre- and postoperative aperients, intraoperative local anaesthetic with postoperative balanced analgesia and antibiotics is thought to be the optimal regime.

Skin bridges need to be preserved between the pile excision wounds to prevent anal stenosis.

In 1998, Longo introduced a new surgical approach to haemorrhoids, stapled haemorrhoidectomy or **p**rocedure for **p**rolapsed **h**aemorrhoids (PPH). In this technique, a circumferential strip of mucosa is excised from above the dentate line by use of a stapling device. Pain is less compared to conventional surgical haemorrhoidectomy, with earlier return to the activities of daily living. Initial enthusiasm for this procedure has been tempered by reports of rare, but very serious, complications such as sepsis and anovaginal fistulation and the technique is clearly operator dependant.

Prolapse

Rectal prolapse is a distressing condition for the patient. Approximately 50–75% of rectal prolapse patients suffer from associated anal incontinence, and the prolapse itself is socially embarrassing. Although the majority of patients are elderly women, prolapse can occur at all ages and is not infrequent in infants under the age of 2 years. Prolapse in infancy is usually precipitated by acute diarrhoeal illness or severe coughing; however, the association of rectal prolapse in infancy and cystic fibrosis makes a sweat test mandatory.

The cause of rectal prolapse in adulthood is unknown; however, rectal prolapse is thought to begin as an internal intussusception. A typical patient will have a lax pelvic floor and a floppy, redundant sigmoid colon. Patients usually present with complaint of a lump that prolapses at defaecation and either reduces spontaneously or has to be manually replaced. Incontinence and evacuatory difficulties are commonly associated. Occasionally, prolapse presents as an emergency and prolonged difficulty replacing the prolapse can lead to its strangulation. The best way to reduce an apparently irreducible prolapse is to raise the foot of the bed and coat the prolapse liberally with sugar; the osmotic effect reduces oedema and the prolapse can then be replaced.

The best way to confirm the diagnosis in the outpatient setting is to ask the patient to go to the clinic toilet and demonstrate the prolapse. Colonic investigation is recommended, although very elderly patients are unsuitable for colonoscopy and either CT colonography or flexible sigmoidoscopy is all that is required.

There have been many surgical approaches described for rectal prolapse, but they can be broken down into two main types: abdominal or perineal. Initial surgical attempts were perineal; Thiersch's anal encirclement operation was described in 1891 and Delorme's mucosal sleeve resection was described in 1900. The perineal approach may also involve rectosigmoidectomy (Altemeier operation). Abdominal approaches can be open or laparoscopic and surgeons may elect to remove redundant colon or not.

Abdominal approaches have lower recurrence rates than the perineal approaches, (in a major retrospective series from the University of Minnesota, the recurrence rate after abdominal procedures was 5% and 16% after perineal rectosigmoidectomy) but as the patients are often elderly and very frail; a perineal operation, which avoids the morbidity of abdominal surgery is attractive.

Solitary rectal ulcer syndrome (SRUS) is frequently, but not universally, associated with internal intussusception or full-thickness rectal prolapse. SRUS without full-thickness prolapse usually responds to dietary and biofeedback treatment; however, an abdominal procedure is usually indicated if there is associated full-thickness prolapse.

FUNCTIONAL ANORECTAL DISORDERS

Constipation

There is a large variation in stool frequency between individuals and infrequent bowel actions in the absence of symptoms can be regarded as part of the normal spectrum of bowel function. However, constipation is a symptom that may affect a quarter of the population at some time and patients with decreased bowel frequency or impaired rectal evacuation have impaired quality of life and consume a large amount of healthcare resources. Many different processes can result in the final common symptoms of constipation and no single treatment will be effective across the board. The multidisciplinary team approach is valuable in the management of difficult constipation.

For people with mild longstanding constipation investigations are not required, and dietary management is usually sufficient to relieve symptoms. When chronic constipation is more severe, detailed consideration of likely causes and other treatments is warranted. Psychological morbidity, such as depression is commonly associated with severe constipation and should be considered as part of the overall evaluation of the patient.

Many patients with mild constipation can be managed with simple bulking agents or laxatives. In elderly patients with resistant constipation, a stimulant such as senna, possibly combined with a bulking agent, is more effective and cheaper than lactulose. Polyethylene glycol-based laxatives (such as Movicol) may be effective in patients with idiopathic constipation and faecal impaction.

For many patients, however, laxatives do not provide sustained relief of symptoms. In addition increasing dietary fibre has been shown to worsen symptoms in many patients by causing increased bloating without improvement in bowel function.

Severe intractable constipation with resistance to laxatives in the presence of an apparently normal (non-dilated) colon is seen most commonly in women of reproductive age. Appropriate investigation include transit studies and anorectal physiology. Defaecating proctography may also be helpful. Behavioural therapy has become established as the most effective form of treatment for patients with either slow transit or impaired evacuation, when traditional treatments

have failed. These behavioural treatments must be provided by experts and comprise a multimodal approach, consisting of habit training, biofeedback (teaching the patient to normalise pelvic floor function while watching real time feedback of sphincter function) help in decreasing the use of laxatives and psychological support. Such treatment will be effective in about two-thirds of patients.

Patients with a dilated rectum and faecal impaction (idiopathic megarectum) are usually teenagers or young adults of either sex. They have often soiled since childhood. In some the problem has a behavioural basis, whereas in others there may be subtle neuromuscular abnormalities of the gut. Constipation with faecal impaction is also seen in elderly patients, especially those in care. Poor general health, impaired mobility, inadequate toilet facilities, endocrine abnormalities (such as hypothyroidism) and drugs may all contribute. Patients with idiopathic megarectum should have their bowel emptied completely before titrating an osmotic laxative. Such a laxative may be required in the long term, although behavioural treatment seems also to help some of these patients. Hirschsprung's disease should always be considered in the differential diagnosis for patients with severe intractable constipation as, although usually diagnosed and treated in infancy, the diagnosis may have been missed. Anorectal physiology is diagnostic for Hirschsprung's as the anorectal inhibitory reflex is absent.

If conservative treatment of intractable idiopathic constipation fails, then subtotal colectomy with ileorectal anastomosis may be considered; however, this has a high failure rate and is associated with significant morbidity. A colostomy may relieve symptoms but it is an unattractive option for most patients, and abdominal pain and bloating may persist. Sacral nerve stimulation has been shown to produce a clinical benefit for patients with idiopathic constipation with improvements in symptoms of abdominal pain and bloating, plus improvement in overall quality of life scores. Almost all patients with spinal injury experience constipation and, along with bladder control, bowel control is the function that individuals with spinal-cord injury would most like to regain. All spinal-injured patients should have dedicated bowel continence regimes initiated by their carers but sacral nerve stimulation has also been shown to be of benefit in this group of patients.

Anal incontinence

Anal incontinence affects approximately 2% of the adult population of both sexes and all age groups. The commonest overall causes of faecal leakage are probably idiopathic degeneration of the internal anal sphincter and faecal impaction with overflow. Faecal impaction typically occurs in children or institutionalised elderly patients. The commonest cause of anal incontinence in young women is obstetrical damage to the anal sphincter. Approximately a third of first vaginal deliveries result in sphincter damage, although two-thirds of these will be asymptomatic. An estimated 1% of vaginal deliveries results in a third degree tear into the anal sphincter complex. Sphincter damage can also result from surgery, such as haemorrhoidectomy or internal sphinctertomy for anal fissure. Anal endosonography enables identification of structural damage to the sphincter muscles and anorectal physiology complements this investigation and gives valuable additional information.

Continence depends on a number of factors, notably normal anatomy and function of the internal–external anal sphincters and of the pelvic floor muscles, and normal anal–rectal sensation. Other variables that play a part in preserving continence are stool volume and consistency, intestinal transit and normal mental function. A complete history, examination for inflammatory bowel disease, sphincter damage or faecal impaction, and correction of predisposing factors can lead to successful treatment in many patients.

Loperamide reduces the force of bowel contractions and enhances absorption of water from the stool. It may also increase the resting pressure in the anal canal. It can be effective in patients with faecal urgency or leakage and the dose should be titrated to achieve control of symptoms. Dietary modification may also be helpful. Additional behavioural interventions, with bowel focused counselling (biofeedback), including advice on resisting urgency and titrating loperamide can lead to marked improvement in the symptom sometimes even when there is structural damage to the sphincter.

In patients with structural defects in the external anal sphincter, an overlapping repair of the sphincter will improve continence in the majority of patients, but the long-term results are less reliable. Silicone biomaterial may be injected to augment a weak internal anal sphincter and sacral nerve stimulation can be a useful therapy for a patient with a structurally intact sphincteric complex.

The final surgical options are reconstruction of the sphincter or permanent faecal diversion. An electronically stimulated gracilis muscle flap can be used to create a neosphincter around the anal canal and some centres implant artificial neosphincters. Both of these operations have been associated with implant-related infection and impaired evacuation.

MINIMALLY INVASIVE COLORECTAL SURGERY

Laparoscopic techniques have been shown to reduce the physical impact of surgery on patients. Benefits include lesser cosmetic insults, less pain, earlier mobilisation and earlier return to normal functioning. In a randomised trial, laparoscopic colorectal surgery resulted in a significant reduction of 30-day postoperative morbidity compared to open surgery. Concerns over the oncological effectiveness appear to be unfounded. In a randomised trial from Spain cancer outcomes were at least as good in the laparoscopic group compared with the open group. Laparoscopic colorectal surgery is technically very demanding and also requires increased resources. Its growth in the UK has been slow. Robotic surgical techniques are also showing promise in facilitating laparoscopic colorectal surgery.

TEM is a minimally invasive technique that facilitates the resection of rectal lesions that would otherwise be too high in the rectum for conventional per anal excision. The technique involves inserting a large operating endoscope through the anus. TEM is suitable for benign rectal lesions and is also used for resection of early (T1 and T2) rectal cancers, thus avoiding the morbidity of abdominal surgery. The local recurrence rate after TEM (5–9%) is lower than traditional transanal resection (12–25%), but concerns remain about the oncological effectiveness of the technique for all but the earliest cancers.

FURTHER READING

Atkin WS, Saunders BP. Surveillance guidelines after removal of colorectal adenomatous polyps. *Gut* 2002; **51**(Suppl 5): V6–V9

Vernava 3rd AM, Moore BA, Longo WE, Johnson FE. Lower gastrointestinal bleeding. *Dis Colon Rectum* 1997; **40**(7): 846–858

Stollman N, Raskin JB. Diverticular disease of the colon. *Lancet* 2004; **363**(9409): 631–639

Heald RJ, Moran BJ, Ryall RD, Sexton R, MacFarlane JK. Rectal cancer: the Basingstoke experience of total mesorectal excision, 1978–1997. *Arch Surg* 1998; **133**(8): 894–899

Eke N. Fournier's gangrene: a review of 1726 cases. *Br J Surg* 2000; **87**(6): 718–728

Braga M, Vignali A, Gianotti L, Zuliani W, Radaelli G, Gruarin P, Dellabona P, Di Carlo V. Laparoscopic versus open colorectal surgery: a randomized trial on short-term outcome. *Ann Surg* 2002; **236**(6): 759–766

Lacy AM, Garcia-Valdecasas JC, Delgado S, Castells A, Taura P, Pique JM, Visa J. Laparoscopy-assisted colectomy versus open colectomy for treatment of non-metastatic colon cancer: a randomised trial. *Lancet* 2002; **359**(9325): 2224–2229

Kamm MA. Faecal incontinence. *Br Med J* 2003a; **327**(7427): 1299–1300

Kamm MA. Constipation and its management. *Br Med J* 2003b; **327**(7413): 459–460

14

Hernia Management

Andrew N Kingsnorth

Department of Surgery, Level 7 Derriford Hospital, Plymouth, UK

CONTENTS

A brief history	**264**
Tension-free hernia repair	267
Laparoscopic repair	267
Essential anatomy of the abdominal wall	**267**
External anatomy – the surface markings	267
The subcutaneous layer	268
Superficial nerves	268
The external oblique aponeurosis	269
The conjoint tendon	270
The fascia transversalis – the space of Bogros	270
The peritoneum – the view from within	270
Aetiology	**271**
Exertion and herniation	272
Economics	**272**
Economics of hernia repair	272
Return to normal activity and work	273
Economics of laparoscopic surgery	273
Principles in hernia surgery	**274**
Prosthetic biomaterials	**274**
Anaesthesia	**275**
Technique for local anaesthesia	275
Complications of hernia in general	**276**
Incarceration, obstruction and strangulation	276
Richter's hernia	277
Littre's hernia – hernia of Meckel's diverticulum	277
Groin hernias in children	**277**
Incarceration and strangulation	277
Clinical diagnosis of inguinal hernia in a child	278
The operation	278
Diagnosis of a lump in the groin in the adult	**278**
Inguinal hernia – the adolescent and the adult	278
Femoral hernia	279
Other groin swellings	279
Clinical examination	280
Anterior open repair of inguinal hernia in adults	**280**
The Lichtenstein technique	280
Strangulated hernia	281
Postoperative care	281
Laparoscopic groin hernia repair	**281**
Disadvantages of laparoscopic hernia repair	282
Femoral hernia	**282**
The three open approaches	282
Open prosthetic repair	282
Laparoscopic repair	282
Umbilical hernia in adults	**283**
Incisional hernia	**284**
Incidence	284
Aetiological factors	284
Principles of open repair	284
Further reading	**285**

A BRIEF HISTORY

An appreciation of the history of hernia surgery may prevent us repeating the mistakes of the past and put in perspective the knowledge that has been accumulated in order to allow development of the successful techniques used today.

The high prevalence of hernia, for which the lifetime risk is 27% for men and 3% for women has resulted in this condition inheriting one of the longest traditions of surgical management. The Egyptians (1500 BC), the Phoenicians (900 BC) and the Ancient Greeks (Hippocrates, 400 BC) diagnosed hernia. During this period a number of devices and operative techniques have been recorded. Attempted repair was usually accompanied by castration, and strangulation was usually a death sentence.

Greek and Phoenician terracottas (Fig. 14.1) illustrate general awareness of hernias at this time (900–600 BC) but the condition appeared to be a social stigma and other than bandaging, treatments are not recorded. The Greek physician Galen (129–201 AD) was a prolific writer and one of his treatises was

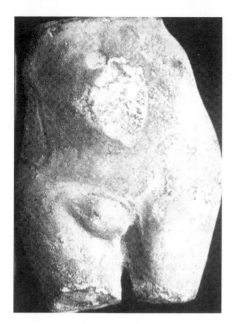

Figure 14.1. Greek terracotta illustrates general awareness of hernias around 900 BC.

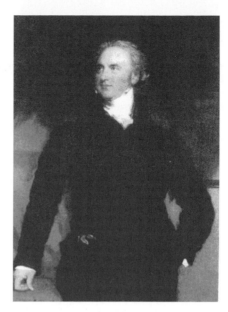

Figure 14.2. Sir Astley Paston Cooper (1768–1841). Surgical Anatomist, London, England.

a detailed description of the musculature of the lower abdominal wall in which he also describes the deficiency of inguinal hernia. He described the peritoneal sac and the concept of reducible contents of the sac.

During the dark time of the Middle Ages there was a decline of medicine in the civilized world and the use of the knife was largely abandoned and few contributions were made to the art of surgery, which was now practised, by itinerants and quacks. With the rise of the universities such as the appearance of the school of Salerno in the 13th century, there was some revival of surgical practice. At this time three important advances in herniology were made: Guy de Chauliac, in 1363, distinguished femoral from inguinal hernia. He developed taxis for incarceration, recommending the head-down, Trendelenburg position. Guy was French and studied in Toulouse and Montpelier and later learned anatomy in Bologna from Nicole Bertuccio. Guy wrote extensively about hernia in his book Chirurgia principally about diagnosis and methods of treatment. He described four surgical interventions one of which was a herniotomy without castration, another consisting of cauterization of the hernia down to the os pubis and third consisting of transfixion of the sac to a piece of wood by a strong ligature. His fourth method however was conservative treatment with bandaging and several weeks bed rest accompanied by enemas, bloodletting and special diet. At the time he was the authorative expert on hernia:

- Hernia surgery has a 3500-year history.
- Castration was an essential part of the earliest operations for hernia, which carried with it an obvious stigma.
- The Dark Ages until the 16th century halted further progress in effective treatment.

- Femoral hernia was distinguished from inguinal hernia in the 14th century.

The renaissance brought burgeoning anatomic knowledge, now based on careful cadaver dissection. William Cheselden successfully operated on a strangulated right inguinal hernia on the Tuesday morning after Easter 1721. The intestines were easily reduced and adherent omentum was ligated and divided. The patient survived and went back to work. Without adequate interventional surgery some patients survived hernia strangulation when spontaneous, preternatural fistula occasionally followed infarction and sloughing of a strangulated hernia. Cheselden's Margaret White survived for many years 'voiding the excrements through the intestine at the navel' after simple local surgery for a strangulated umbilical hernia. The closure of such a fistula in the absence of distal bowel pathology was described by Le Dran, who had noted that it was quite common for poor people with incarcerated hernias to mistake the tender painful groin lump for an abscess and incise it themselves. He found that these painful wounds with faecal fistulas required no more than cleaning and dressing.

The great contribution of the surgical anatomists was between the years 1750 and 1865 and was called the age of dissection. The main contributors were Antonio Scarpa and Sir Astley Cooper and few major advances in our knowledge of the anatomy of the groin have been made since this time. The names of these great anatomists are Pieter, Camper, Antonio Scarpa, Percival Pott, Sir Astley Cooper, John Hunter, Thomas Morton, Germaine Cloquet, Franz Hesselbach, Friedrich Henle and Don Antonio Gimbernat.

Astley Cooper's seminal monograph was written in 1804 (Fig. 14.2). Sir Astley Cooper (1768–1841) trained at St Thomas's hospital, London and became a surgeon at Guy's Hospital and from 1813 to 1815 was Professor of Comparative Anatomy of the Royal College of Surgeons. Cooper published six magnificent books, two of which covered the subject of hernia, which were liberally illustrated by his own hand from dissections he had performed personally. Cooper was a charismatic lecturer and socialite and had an extensive surgical practice, which included being Sergeant Surgeon to King George IV. Cooper's recognition of the transversalis fascia positions him as one of the most important contributors to present day surgery which emphasizes this layer as being the first layer to be breached in groin hernias.

The first accurate description of the ilio-pubic tract, an important structure utilized in many sutured repairs for inguinal hernia, was made by Jules Cloquet (1790–1883). Cloquet was Professor of Anatomy and Surgery in Paris and Surgeon to the Emperor. Cloquet researched the pathological anatomy of the groin in numerous autopsy dissections and their reconstruction in wax models. He was the first to observe the frequency of patency of the processus vaginalis after birth and its role in the production of a hernia sac later in life. Franz Hesselbach was an anatomist at the University of Wurzburg who described the triangle now so important in laparoscopic surgery which originally defined the pathway of direct and external and supravesical hernias. The triangle as defined today is somewhat smaller.

As so often in surgery a new concept was needed before further progress could be made in herniology. Two pioneers – the American Marcy (Marcy, 1887) and the Italian Bassini (1884) – vie for priority for the critical breakthrough. Both appreciated the physiology of the inguinal canal and both correctly understood how each anatomic plane, transversalis fascia, transverse and oblique muscles and the external oblique aponeurosis, contributed to the canal's stability. Bassini made another important advance when he subjected his technique to the scrutiny of the prospective follow-up. Bassini's 1890 paper is truly a quantum leap in surgery. He decided to open the inguinal canal and approach the posterior wall of the canal which he achieved by reconstruction of the inguinal canal into the physiological condition, a canal with two openings one abdominal the other subcutaneous and with two walls, one anterior and one posterior through the middle of which the spermatic cord would pass. Bassini dissected the indirect sac and closed it off flush with the parietal peritoneum. He then isolated and lifted up the spermatic cord and dissected the posterior wall of the canal, dividing the fascia transversalis down to the pubic tubercle. He then sutured the dissected conjoint tendon consisting of the internal oblique, the transversus muscle and the 'vertical fascia of Cooper', the fascia transversalis, to the posterior rim of Poupart's ligament, including the lower lateral divided margin of the fascia transversalis. Bassini stresses that this suture line must be approximated without difficulty; hence the early dissection separating the external oblique from the internal oblique must be adequate and allow good development and mobilization of the conjoint tendon.

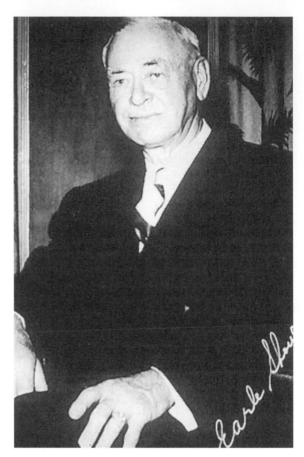

Figure 14.3. Earle E Shouldice (1890–1965). Lecturer in Anatomy, University of Toronto, Canada.

The Bassini operation re-emerged as the Shouldice repair in 1950s (Fig. 14.3). Earl Shouldice (1890–1965) also promulgated the benefits of early ambulation and opened the Shouldice clinic, a hospital dedicated to the repair of hernias to the abdominal wall. A huge experience accumulated with an annual throughput of 7000 herniorrhaphies per year, enabled the surgeons at the Shouldice clinic to study the pathology in primary and recurrent hernias and to emphasize adjuncts to successful outcomes. Continuous monofilament wire was used in preference to other suture materials and the hernioplasty incorporated repair of the internal ring, the posterior wall of the inguinal canal and the femoral region. The cremaster muscle and fascia with vessels and genital branch of genitofemoral nerve were removed and the posterior wall after division was repaired by a four-layer imbrication method using the ilio-pubic tract as its main anchor point. Until the introduction of mesh, the Shouldice operation became the gold-standard for inguinal hernia repair:

- The surgical anatomy of the groin, on which modern hernia surgery is based, was defined between 1750 and 1865.
- Bassini described his revolutionary operation in 1890.

- The Shouldice Clinic revived the Bassini operation in the latter half of the 20th century.

Tension-free hernia repair

Irving Lichtenstein is the revolutionary thinker who introduced tension-free prosthetic repair of groin hernias into everyday, commonplace, outpatient practices. As well as being an office procedure under local anaesthetic, Lichtenstein pioneered the idea that hernia surgery is special, that it must be performed by an experienced surgeon and cannot be relegated to the unsupervised trainee doing 'minor' surgery. The key feature of Lichtenstein's technique is the 'tensionless' operation. With his co-workers Shulman and Amid, he has developed a simple prosthetic operation, which can be performed on outpatients. As a pioneer, Lichtenstein worked hard to promulgate his ideas but even so the first edition of his book '*Hernia Repair Without Disability*' written in 1970 sold rather poorly and never went beyond the first printing. Subsequent additions however, required numerous reprints to meet demand paralleling the increase in popularity and worldwide success of the mesh-patch repair devised by Lichtenstein:

- Irving Lichtenstein had faith in his new operation in spite of opposition from the surgical establishment.
- Mesh has contributed more to improvements in hernia surgery outcomes in the 20th century than any other factor.

Laparoscopic repair

Laparoscopic repair continues to develop its place in the surgical armamentarium of inguinal hernia. The use of the laparoscope has been extended to repair incisional, ventral, lumbar and paracolostomy hernias. This latter technique is rapidly gaining in popularity.

The first attempt to treat an inguinal hernia with the laparoscope was made by P. Fletcher of the University of the West Indies in 1979. He closed the neck of the hernia sac. The first report of the use of a clip (Michel) placed laparoscopically to close the neck of the sac was made by Ger in 1982, who reported a series of 13 patients: all the patients in this series were repaired through an open incision except the 13th patient who was repaired under laparoscopic guidance with a special stapling device. The 3-year follow-up of that patient revealed him to be free of an identifiable recurrence. Ger continued his efforts to repair these hernias laparoscopically. He reported the closure of the neck of the hernia sac using a prototypical instrument called the 'Herniostat' in beagle dogs. The results in these models appeared to be promising. In that same article, he reported the potential benefits of the laparoscopic approach to groin hernia repair as:

1. Creation of puncture wounds rather than formal incisions.
2. Need for minimal dissection.
3. Less danger of spermatic cord injury and less risk of ischaemic orchitis.

4. Minimal risk of bladder injury.
5. Decreased incidence of neuralgias.
6. Possibility of an outpatient procedure.
7. Ability to achieve the highest possible ligation of the hernial sac.
8. Minimal postoperative discomfort and a faster recovery time.
9. Ability to perform simultaneous diagnostic laparoscopy.
10. Ability to diagnose and treat bilateral inguinal hernias.

These potential advantages and advances in the laparoscopic repair of hernias continue to be the recognized goals that each method is attempting to achieve:

- Laparoscopic repair of an inguinal hernia was first performed in 1982.
- Laparoscopic hernia repair requires greater skills than laparoscopic cholecystectomy or fundoplication.
- The learning curve for laparoscopic hernia repair may be as high as 250 hernias, before recurrence rates reach an acceptable level.
- Incisional hernia may be an area for the development of laparoscopic techniques.

ESSENTIAL ANATOMY OF THE ABDOMINAL WALL

The anatomy of the abdominal wall is well documented in several standard texts on anatomy, which contain accurate and detailed information that is readily available. The lined drawings in this chapter have been adapted from published reports for anatomists and surgeons with particular attention to applied surgical anatomy and anatomical variance of the normal. Pathological processes further disorganize the underlying anatomy and the surgeon who seeks to make a success of hernia repairs should fully understand these anatomic variations. Today the surgeon should individualize the operation for the anatomy encountered.

Under normal circumstances the musculo-aponeurotic layers of the abdominal wall are designed to retain the contents of the peritoneal cavity. There are certain limited areas however where the underlying anatomical structure is deficient and where hernias develop. This deficiency is most notable in the groin area in relation to the inguinal and femoral canals but there are several other sites notably the umbilicus, epigastrium, lumbar triangle, obturator canal, sciatic foramina, perineum, pelvic sidewall and the spigelian line. The list is quite long and the clinician may or may not encounter one of the rarer types of abdominal wall hernias in a lifetime.

External anatomy – the surface markings

The abdominal wall, bounded by the lower margin of the thorax above, and by the pubes, the iliac crests and the inguinal ligaments below, is easily recognized in the upright man. Vertically down the centre of the abdomen the depression of

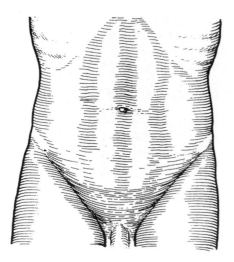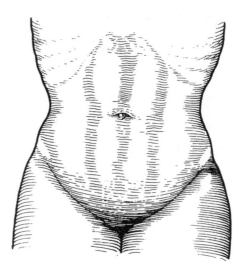

Figure 14.4. Topographical anatomy of the abdomen shows the distinctly different male and female characteristics.

the linea alba is obvious and is usually more apparent above the umbilicus. The umbilicus lies at the junction of the upper three-fifths and lower two-fifths of the linea alba. In the healthy young adult the rectus muscle is prominent on either side of the linea alba. The rectus muscle is particularly prominent inferolaterally to the umbilicus: this infra-umbilical rectus mound is of surgical importance. With ageing and obesity, the lower abdomen sags but the infra-umbilical rectus mound remains obvious and visible to the subject, even into old age.

The outer margin of each rectus is indicated by a convex vertically directed furrow, the semilunar line (linea semilunaris), which is most distinct in the upper abdomen where it commences at the tip of the ninth costal cartilage. At first it descends almost vertically, but inferior to the umbilicus it gently curves medially to terminate at the pubic tubercle. It is along this line that the internal oblique aponeurosis bands and splits to enclose the rectus muscle in the upper two-thirds of the abdomen. The broad furrow of the inferior semilunar line is also described as the Spigelian fascia and is the site of herniation. In the lower abdomen the configuration varies, a wider pelvis and greater pubic prominence being important female characteristics (Fig. 14.4).

The surgeon must be aware of the elastic and connective tissue lines in the skin (Langer's lines) if optimum healing is to be obtained. Incisions made at right angles to Langer's lines gape and tend to splay out when they heal. The longitudinal contraction of the healing wound, particularly when the wound crosses a skin delve or body crease, can make healing very unsightly with contracture and for these reasons vertical incisions over the groin should be avoided. However, rapid abdominal access requires adequate vertical incisions and they continue to remain in everyday general surgical and gynaecological practice particularly in emergency surgery.

The subcutaneous layer

Beneath the skin there is the subcutaneous areolar tissue and fascia. Superiorly over the lower chest and epigastrium, this layer is generally thin and less organized than in the lower abdomen where it becomes bilaminar – a superficial fatty stratum (Camper's fascia) and a deeper, stronger and more elastic layer (Scarpa's fascia). Scarpa's fascia is well developed in infancy, forming a distinct layer which must be separately incised when the superficial inguinal ring is approached in childhood herniotomy.

In the lower abdomen the deeper fascia (Scarpa's) is more membranous with much elastic tissue and almost devoid of fat. This fascia does not pass down uninterrupted to the thigh and perineum as the superficial fatty fascia does; instead, the deep fascia is attached to the inner half of the inguinal ligament, to the anterior fascia lata of the thigh and to the iliac crest laterally. Medially it forms a distinct structure containing much elastic tissue and descends, almost as a band, from the pubis to envelop the penis as the suspensory ligament. Internally it can be traced as a thin layer over the penis and scrotum. Behind the scrotum it becomes continuous with the deep layer of the superficial fascia of the perineum (Colles' fascia).

Superficial nerves

The most caudal of the abdominal wall nerves are derived from the first lumbar nerve; they are the ilio-hypogastric and ilio-inguinal nerves. The ilio-inguinal nerve is generally smaller than the ilio-hypogastric nerve – if one is large the other is smaller and vice versa. Occasionally the ilio-inguinal nerve is very small and may be absent. The anterior cutaneous branch of the ilio-hypogastric nerve emerges through the aponeurosis of the external oblique just above the superficial inguinal ring and innervates the skin in the suprapubic region. The ilio-inguinal nerve passes through the lower inguinal canal and becomes superficial by emerging from the superficial inguinal ring to supply the skin of the scrotum and a small area of the medial upper thigh.

The genitofemoral nerve arises from the first and second lumbar nerves and completes the innervation of the abdominal wall and groin areas. At first it passes obliquely forwards and downwards through the substance of the psoas major. It emerges from the muscle and crosses its anterior surface deep to the peritoneum, going behind, posterior to, the ureter. It divides a variable distance from the deep inguinal ring into a genital and a femoral branch. The genital branch, a mixed motor and sensory nerve, crosses the femoral vessels and enters the inguinal canal at or just medial to the deep ring. The nerve penetrates the fascia transversalis of the posterior wall of the inguinal ligament either through the deep ring or separately medially to the deep ring. The nerve traverses the inguinal canal lying between the spermatic cord above and the upturned edge of the inguinal ligament inferiorly; the nerve is vulnerable to surgical trauma as it progresses along the floor of the canal (the gutter produced by the upturned internal edge of the inguinal ligament). The genital nerve supplies the motor function to the cremaster muscle and the sensory function to the skin of the scrotum. The femoral branch enters the femoral sheath lying lateral to the femoral artery and supplies the skin of the upper part of the femoral triangle.

The external oblique aponeurosis

The aponeurosis of the external oblique muscle fuses with the aponeurosis of the internal oblique in the anterior rectus sheath. This line of fusion is considerably medial to the semilunar line – the fusion line is oblique and somewhat semilunar, being more lateral above and more medial below. In fact, the external oblique aponeurosis contributes very little to the lower portion of the anterior rectus sheath. This latter point is of considerable importance in inguinal hernioplasty (Fig. 14.5).

There is a defect in the external – oblique aponeurosis just above the pubis. This aperture – the superficial inguinal ring – is triangular in shape and in the male allows passage of the spermatic cord from the abdomen to the scrotum. In the female the round ligament of the uterus passes through this opening. The superficial inguinal ring is not a 'ring'; it is a triangular cleft with its long axis oblique in the same direction but not quite parallel to the inguinal ligament. The base of the triangle is formed by the crest of the pubis and the apex is lateral towards the anterior superior iliac spine. The superficial inguinal ring represents that interval between the aponeurosis of the external oblique which inserts into the pubic bone superiorly and, as the inguinal ligament, inserts into the pubic tubercle inferiorly. The aponeurotic margins of the ring are described as the superior and inferior crura. The spermatic

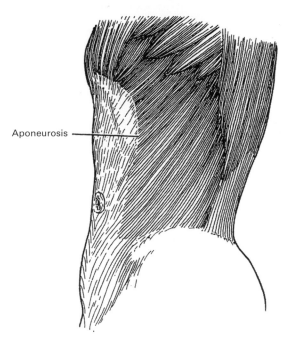

Aponeurosis

Figure 14.5. The external oblique muscle and its aponeurosis invests the abdomen.

cord, as it comes through the superficial ring, rests on the inferior crus which is a continuation of the floor of the inguinal canal (the upturned internal margin of the inguinal ligament).

The crura of the superficial ring are joined together by intercrural fibres derived from the outer investing fascia of the external oblique aponeurosis. The size and strength of these intercrural fibres vary.

The external oblique aponeurosis in the region of the groin forms a free border known as or the inguinal ligament, which is simply the lower margin of this aponeurosis; it is not a condensed thickened ligamentous structure. The ligament presents a rounded surface towards the thigh where the aponeurosis is rolled inwards back on itself to make a groove on its deep surface. Laterally the ligament is attached to the anterior superior iliac spine and medially to the pubic tubercle and via the lacunar and reflected inguinal ligaments to the iliopectineal line on the superior ramus of the pubis. The inguinal ligament is not straight; it is concave, with the concavity directed medially and upward towards the abdomen.

The medial attachment, or continuation, of the inguinal ligament as the lacunar (Gimbernat's) and the pectineal (Cooper's) ligament gives a fan-like expansion of the inguinal ligament at its medial end, which curves posteriorly to the iliopectineal ligament. This expansion has important surgical implications.

The lacunar ligament is a triangular continuation of the medial end of the inguinal ligament. Its apex is at the pubic tubercle, its superior margin continuous with the inguinal ligament and its medial margin is attached to the iliopectineal

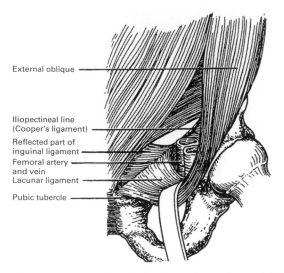

External oblique

Iliopectineal line
(Cooper's ligament)

Reflected part of
inguinal ligament
Femoral artery
and vein
Lacunar ligament

Pubic tubercle

Figure 14.6. The upper abdominal surface of the attachment of the inguinal ligament to the pubic tubercle is the floor of the inguinal canal.

line on the superior ramus of the pubis. Its lateral crescentic edge is free and directed laterally, where it is an important rigid structure in the medial margin of the femoral canal. The ligament lies in an oblique plane, with its upper (abdominal) surface facing superomedially and being crossed by the spermatic cord, and its lower (femoral) surface looking anterolaterally. With the external oblique aponeurosis and the inguinal ligament, the superior surface forms a groove for the cord as it emerges from the inguinal canal (Fig. 14.6).

The conjoint tendon

The conjoint tendon has a very variable structure and in 20% of subjects it does not exist as a discrete anatomic structure. It may be absent or only slightly developed, it may be replaced by a lateral extension of the tendon of origin of the rectus muscle or it may extend laterally to the deep inguinal ring so that no interval is present between the lower border of the transversus and the inguinal ligament. A shutter mechanism for the conjoint tendon can only be demonstrated when the lateral side of the tendon, that is the transversus and internal oblique muscles, extend onto and are attached to the iliopectineal line. The extent of this insertion is very variable.

The fascia transversalis – the space of Bogros

The fascia transversalis lies deep to the transverse abdominal muscle plane. It is continuous from side to side and extends from the rib cage above to the pelvis inferiorly.

In the upper abdominal wall the fascia transversalis is thin, but in the lower abdomen and especially in the inguinofemoral region the fascia is thicker and has specialized bands and folds within it. In the groin region, where the fascia transversalis is an

important constituent of the posterior wall of the inguinal canal and where it forms the femoral sheath inferiorly to the inguinal ligament, the anatomy and function of the fascia transversalis is of particular importance to the surgeon. As originally described by Sir Astley Cooper in 1807 the fascia transversalis, in the groin, consists of two layers. The anterior strong layer covers the internal aspect of the transversalis muscle where it is intimately blended with the tendon of the transversus muscle. It then extends across the posterior wall of the inguinal canal medial to the deep ring aperture and is attached to the inner margin of the inguinal ligament. The deeper layer of fascia transversalis, a membranous layer, lies between the anterior substantial layer of fascia transversalis and the peritoneum. The extraperitoneal fat lies behind this layer between it and the peritoneum (Fig. 14.7). The deep epigastric vessels run between the two layers of fascia transversalis. Defects in it, congenital or acquired, are the aetiology of all groin hernias.

The peritoneum – the view from within

Hernia sacs are composed of peritoneum and they may contain intra-abdominal viscera. From within they consist of the peritoneum, then a loose layer of extraperitoneal fat, then the deep membranous lamina of fascia transversalis, then the vessels such as the epigastric vessels in the space of Bogros, then the stout anterior lamina of fascia transversalis, then the muscles and aponeuroses of the abdominal wall. The preperitoneal space lies in the abdominal cavity between the peritoneum internally and transversalis fascia externally. Within this space lies a variable quantity of adipose tissue, loose connective tissue and membraneous tissue, and other anatomical entities such as arteries, veins, nerves and various organs such as the kidneys and ureters. The clinically significant parts of the preperitoneal space include the space associated with the structural elements related to the myopectoneal orifice of Fruchaud, the prevesical space of Retzius, the space of Bogros and retroperitoneal periurinary space. The myopectineal orifice of Fruchaud represents the potentially weak area in the abdominal wall, which permits inguinal and femoral hernias. The preperitoneal space lies deep to the supra-vesical fossa and the medial inguinal fossa is the prevesical space of Retzius. The space of Retzius contains loose connective tissue and fat but more importantly vascular elements such as an abnormal obturator artery and vein. Bogros' space, which is a triangular area between the abdominal wall and peritoneum, can be entered by means of an incision through the roof and floor of the inguinal canal through which the posterior preperitoneal approach for hernia repair can be achieved. In the groin these muscles and aponeuroses are variously absent over the inguinal and crural canals. The myopectineal orifice of Fruchaud, which is divided into two parts by the inguinal ligament (Fig. 14.8). This concept of one groin aperture is relevant for mesh repairs, whether anterior open operation or posterior laparoscopic operation. The boundaries of the myopectineal

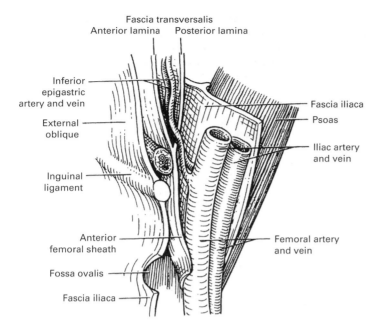

Fascia transversalis
Anterior lamina   Posterior lamina

Inferior
epigastric
artery and vein

External
oblique

Inguinal
ligament

Anterior
femoral sheath

Fossa ovalis

Fascia iliaca

Fascia iliaca

Psoas

Iliac artery
and vein

Femoral artery
and vein

Figure 14.7. The bilaminar fascia transversalis in
the groin.

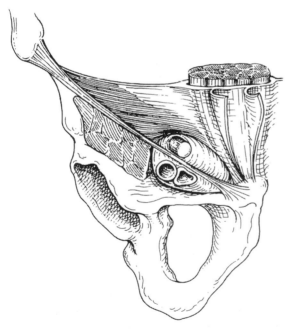

Figure 14.8. The myopectineal orifice of Fruchaud: the area of the
groin closed by fascia transversalis with the inguinal canal above and
femoral canal below the rigid inguinal canal.

orifice of Fruchaud are superiorly the 'arch' of the transversus
muscle, laterally the iliopsoas muscle, medially the rectus
muscle and inferiorly the pecten of the pubis. The space is utilized in both the trans-abdominal preperitoneal (TAPP) and
the totally extraperitoneal (TEP) laparoscopic approaches to

the repair of inguinal and femoral repairs. A thorough understanding of the limits of this myopectineal orifice is necessary
to accomplish an effective repair of the inguinal floor with the
laparoscopic methodology.

AETIOLOGY

The pathogenesis of groin hernia is multifactorial. As indirect
inguinal hernias are so common in infancy the first surgical
speculation was that they were due to a developmental defect.
Indirect inguinal hernia arises from incomplete obliteration of
the processus vaginalis, the embryological out pocketing of
peritoneum that precedes testicular descent into the scrotum.
The testes originate along the urogenital line in the retroperitoneum and migrate caudally during the second trimester
of pregnancy to arrive at the internal inguinal ring at about
6 months of intrauterine life. During the last trimester they proceed through the abdominal wall via the inguinal canal and
descend into the scrotum, the right slightly later than the left.
The processus vaginalis then normally obliterates postnatally
except for the portion surrounding and serving as a covering
for the testes. Failure of this obliterative process results in congenital indirect inguinal hernia. Additional support for the congenital theory of indirect inguinal herniation is the finding at
autopsy that 15–30% of adult males without clinically apparent
inguinal hernias have a patent processus vaginalis at death.
A Bedouin mother and her four daughters with indirect
inguinal hernia in whom there was no evidence of collagen diseases, normal hormone profile and normal pelvic anatomy
suggests that in adult females as well, there is genetic hetero-
geneity.

Read made the crucial clinical observation which next advanced our understanding of the aetiology of inguinal hernia. In 1970 he noted, when using the preperitoneal approach to the inguinal region, that the rectus sheath is thinner and has a 'greasy' feel in those patients who turned out to have direct defects. This observation was confirmed by weighing samples of constant area; specimens from controls weighed significantly more than those from patients with indirect, pantaloon and direct hernias (in that order). Bilateral hernias were associated with more severe atrophy. Adjustment for age and muscle mass confirmed the validity of the primary observation. And, if surgical technical failure can be excluded, the logical treatment of recurrent herniation is prosthetic repair. This concept was enthusiastically promulgated by Irving Lichtenstein, one of the earliest protagonists of prosthetic repair for primary inguinal hernia:

- The aetiology of inguinal hernia is multifactorial.
- Genetic inheritance has a role.
- Indirect hernias originate from a patent processus vaginalis.
- A weakening of the transversalis fascia is the major factor contributing to the development of direct hernia, and also indirect hernia (20% of males at autopsy have an intact transversalis fascia, a patent processus and no hernia).
- Smoking weakens collagen tissue including the transversalis fascia.

Exertion and herniation

There is no evidence that strong muscular or athletic exertion causes inguinal hernia in the absence of a fascial and/or muscular abnormality – either acquired connective tissue disease or congenital anomaly of the abdominal wall. Indeed, inguinal hernia is rare in weightlifters. However, in a study of inguinal hernia and a single strenuous event, in 7% of patients the hernia subjectively was attributable to a single muscular strain. At the moment the relative importance of genetic, anatomic and environmental (smoking and heavy manual work) factors cannot be construed in each case. Manual work or strain is never, or very rarely, the sole cause of inguinal hernia.

The aetiology of groin hernia has an importance in terms of prevention; smoking is a causal agent.

ECONOMICS

Economic evaluations of new and existing healthcare interventions are an essential input into decision-making. Healthcare systems around the world face steady increases in expenditure resulting from demographic change and improvements in medical technology. Increasingly, payors must choose which interventions will be provided and which will not be reimbursed from limited public or private funds. This creates difficult choices. In the UK the National Institute for Clinical Excellence (NICE) synthesizes evidence and reaches a judgement as to whether on balance the intervention can be

recommended as a cost-effective use of National Health Service (NHS) resources. In 2000, NICE published recommendations for the use of laparoscopic hernia surgery and recommended its use, outside centres of expertise only in cases of bilateral inguinal hernia or recurrent inguinal hernia.

It is no longer sufficient to consider the clinical or therapeutic effects of healthcare interventions: purchasing choices will be predicated on studies which identify, measure and value what is given up when an intervention is used (the cost) and what is gained (improved patient health outcomes). This requires explicit economic evaluation of healthcare interventions. Purchasers have a fixed budget and are aware of the opportunity costs of interventions. Increasingly they are likely to require evidence of effectiveness and cost effectiveness, and they may develop contracts and enforce protocols to ensure this:

- In a socialized system of healthcare (NHS), healthcare interventions must be cost-effective.
- Laparoscopic repair for inguinal hernia is at least £350 more expensive than open repair.

The type of economic evaluation depends upon the outcome measure chosen:

1. *Cost-minimization analysis* is appropriate only when the outcomes of two or more interventions have been demonstrated to be equivalent, in which case the least costly alternative is the most efficient, and only cost analysis is required.
2. *Cost-effectiveness analysis* includes both costs and outcomes using a single outcome measure, usually a natural unit. This allows comparisons between treatments in a particular therapeutic area where effectiveness is unequal, but not between therapeutic areas where natural outcome measures differ.
3. *Cost-utility analysis* combines multiple outcomes into a single measure of utility (e.g. a quality adjusted life year, or QALY). This allows comparisons between alternatives in different therapeutic categories with different natural outcomes.
4. *Cost-benefit analysis* links costs and outcomes by expressing both in monetary units, forcing an explicit decision about whether an intervention is worth its cost. Various techniques have been used to attach monetary values to health outcomes, but the technique remains rare in health economics.

Economics of hernia repair

Hernia repair is an established and effective procedure and its relatively fixed cost and high volume amongst surgical procedures means that economic evaluation of the procedure itself has become a priority. Hernias create pain and discomfort for patients and limit ability to work or carry out other productive activities. While the increased risk of surgical procedures in elderly people means that repair of some small direct hernias may not be mandatory, there would seem to be clear clinical and economic arguments in favour of carrying out hernia repairs amongst the majority of the working population.

The experience from the Shouldice clinic in Canada and the results from the US support the use of limited hospitalization for the repair of hernias. Laparoscopic inguinal hernia surgery has not been proven to represent an economic benefit for the unilateral primary hernia. There may be some benefit for the patient with bilateral and/or recurrent herniation:

- Hernia repair is common (20 million world wide, 100 000 in the UK annually).
- Hernia surgery is carried out most efficiently in dedicated units.
- Ambulatory care is the most cost-effective means of care.
- Local anaesthesia reduces complexity, time and money utilized (see below).

Return to normal activity and work

There is enormous variation in reported times for return to normal activity and work. For instance, in a socialized system of healthcare where patients' expectations and the insurance system still favour hospitalization, length of hospital stay after hernia surgery may be in excess of 8 days. Even in the USA, where a headlong rush for day-care surgery in ambulatory units has taken place, length of stay may be several days in institutions where reimbursement is not as strictly controlled as the private sector.

Advice concerning return to normal activity has been poorly managed by surgeons. Recent studies indicate that factors limiting a patient's return to activity and work are governed principally by perceived amount of postoperative pain. Socioeconomic factors strongly influence this perception over and above the actual procedure performed or the anatomy involved. In patients having National Insurance compared with patients having private insurance, the duration of postoperative pain and the days off work have been compared. The differences between the two groups were striking: the median duration of postoperative pain in the National insurance group was 27 days, with 36.5 days off work. In the private insurance patients the duration of postoperative pain was 7.5 days and they went back to work after only 8.5 days. Personal motivation, therefore, appears to be the most important factor affecting clinical outcome and return to activities. Callesen from Copenhagen has demonstrated that well-defined recommendations and improved pain management can shorten convalescence. One hundred patients having elective herniorraphy under local anaesthetic and managed analgesia were recommended to have 1 day of convalescence for light/moderate work and 3 weeks for strenuous physical activity. The overall median absence from work was 6 days; the unemployed returning to activities in just 1 day, those in light/moderate work in 6 days and those in heavy jobs by 25 days. A more detailed prospective study of return to work after inguinal hernia repair has been undertaken by Jones and colleagues: data was collected by personal interviews, written surveys and medical record reviews in 235 patients, the main outcome measures being actual and expected return to work. Age, educational level, income level, occupation, symptoms of depression and the expected day of return to work (10 days) accounted for 61% of the variation in actual (12 days) return to work:

- Length of hospital stay is controlled overwhelmingly by the surgeon.
- In the majority of cases local anaesthesia and a 1–2 h recovery in hospital is sufficient.
- Most patients can return to normal activities within 7–10 days of an uncomplicated, primary inguinal hernia repair.

Economics of laparoscopic surgery

The majority of laparoscopic adaptations of the general surgical operations have proven to be cost effective due to the diminution in the length of hospital stay. The great exception is that of the laparoscopic repair of inguinal hernias, which are always more costly.

Some 'economic' arguments have been used to support the rapid diffusion of laparoscopic surgery. Studies often quote reductions in the length of in-patient hospital stay in comparison with standard surgical procedures and imply that this will necessarily save hospitals money. This is, however, not necessarily the case, and hospital managers are increasingly questioning the appropriateness of procedures which involve purchase of sophisticated and expensive capital equipment and considerably increased theatre time, resulting in lower patient throughput for surgical procedures. Available time in the operating theatre is a scarce resource, and although operating time in laparoscopic surgery declines as experience increases, Cushieri estimated that on average it will continue to take about one-third longer than the corresponding conventional operation, with the excess of time over open surgery the higher the more complicated the basic operation. Time, however, has proven that once past the 'learning curve' many of these operations are as long or shorter than that of the open method.

The data comparing the open versus laparoscopic repair of inguinal hernias is now voluminous. Suffice to say that the vast majority of reports have identified the same findings that are commonly known. That is, in general, the operation is more expensive but the postoperative pain is diminished and the return to work notably shorter. The learning curve and the payors of these operations will force this procedure into the hands of a few skilled surgeons with excellent outcomes. Even in this instance, this will be for the bilateral and recurrent hernias.

Unlike the data of the laparoscopic inguinal herniorraphy, the clinical and economic benefits are rather clearer with the laparoscopic repair of incisional and ventral hernias. A shorter period of hospitalization is seen with this approach and is associated with fewer complications than that of the open methods. In the hands of experts, the laparoscopic method is associated with less cost than the open repair. This fact is primarily based upon the decreased length of stay of the laparoscopically repaired patients:

- For inguinal hernia the UK NICE recommends the laparoscopic approach for recurrent and bilateral hernias (and not primary hernia).
- Laparoscopic repair should be carried out by experienced surgeons in well-equipped units.
- Laparoscopic techniques continue to evolve.

PRINCIPLES IN HERNIA SURGERY

There are three principles which dictate the management of all abdominal wall hernia patients.

1. The patient must be adequately prepared for surgery. The mortality from hernia operations, particularly the mortality and morbidity of strangulated femoral hernias in older women, is almost entirely due to operating when the patient is in a less than optimal physiological condition. Hernias almost never require emergency surgery, although they may require urgent surgery as soon as the patient is rendered fit. To operate before adequate rehydration and renal function is restored, or before the cardiorespiratory status is assessed and stabilized, is to court disaster. Even in the very elderly, mortality can be reduced to a minimum; death is usually a result of complications of the strangulated hernia rather than associated diseases which should have been adequately treated before the urgent operation. For elective hernia repair the same golden principle applies – do not operate until the patient has been fully assessed and is in an optimum physiological state.

2. The contents must be reduced after inspection at open operation and following careful inspection for viability. If strangulation has occurred infarcted contents must be resected. The dangers of forcible reduction of contents into an inadequate cavity when there is 'lack of storage capacity of the abdominal cavity' or when organs have lost the right of domain must be appreciated.

3. The defect must be repaired. When repairing abdominal wall hernias with the pure tissue repair the principle is to repair each layer of the defect discreetly. One may also reinforce weak layers with mesh to restore the patient's anatomy so that it resembles the normal unoperated condition. The process of repair in aponeurosis is slow. Only tendinous/ aponeurotic/fascial structures can be successfully sutured together: suturing red fleshy muscle to tendon or fascia will not contribute to permanent union of these structures. Nor will it reconstruct anything resembling the normal anatomy!

Frequently, particularly with the repair of the larger incisional and ventral hernias, the reconstruction of the patient's anatomy is not feasible. The use of a prosthetic biomaterial is the only option for these individuals. When this is the case, the surgeon must assure that a large overlap of the prosthetic is used so that the resulting repair will be sound and permanent.

Table 14.1. The main indications for the use of prosthetic materials.

Absorbable prosthetic materials	Temporary replacement of absent tissue (e.g. smaller infected wounds)
Collagen based products	Form a 'neo-fascia' to repair defects in the abdominal wall
Flat prosthetic biomaterials	Differ in weight, porosity and thickness and utilized for fascial reinforcement
Dual sided mesh products	The smooth surface is designed for use in the intra-peritoneal space

PROSTHETIC BIOMATERIALS

The use of prosthetic biomaterials in the repair of hernias of the abdominal wall is now routine practice in many countries. In the USA and Europe over 90% of all inguinal and ventral hernias are repaired with a prosthetic material or device. In other parts of the world, this is not the case. Limitations on the use of these products include a natural reluctance to place a biomaterial into a primary hernia or the cost of these products.

Incisional hernias will develop in approximately 13% of laparotomy incisions. The risk of herniation is increased by fivefold if a postoperative wound infection occurs. Other factors that predispose to the development of a fascial defect include obesity, poor nutritional status, steroid usage, etc. While some of these may be avoided, those patients that are found to have such a hernia can present difficult management problems due to the high potential for recurrence. Without the use of a prosthetic biomaterial, the recurrence rate is as high as 51%. The use of a synthetic material will reduce this rate to 10–24%.

The 'ideal' prosthetic product has yet to be found. There are at least eighty different products that can be used in the repair of inguinal, ventral, incisional and other hernias of the abdominal wall. In many of the products there is a paucity of published literature that verifies the claims that are made by the manufacturers. Surgeons recognize that the main purpose in the use of these materials will be the repair of a fascial defect in the abdominal wall. The main indications of use of the materials are listed in Table 14.1.

Synthetic prosthetic biomaterials can be divided into the absorbable and non-absorbable products. The absorbable biomaterials (polyglycolic or polyglactic acid) have been used to cover polypropylene prosthetics used to repair a fascial defect in an effort to protect the viscera from that product or as a temporary closure of the abdominal wall for intra-abdominal sepsis. While these materials may appear to have a role in the prevention of adhesions, they may, in fact, enhance their development because of the inflammatory response that develops as a natural consequence of the use of these materials. There is no clinical data to support this type of usage of the absorbable biomaterials. Recent laboratory studies have shown that this technique may not achieve its intended result.

Non-synthetic biomaterials are based on either the use of porcine tissues to produce a collagen matrix or on cadaveric skin. All of the products are not truly absorbable as they are intended to provide a scaffold for the native fibroblasts to incorporate natural collagen to repair a fascial defect.

Synthetic non-absorbable biomaterials are of many types, sizes and shapes. The use of these products is common in the repair of inguinal hernias. The current use of a prosthesis in the tension-free concept of a repair of the incisional hernias has gained widespread acceptance. The detailed description of the available prosthetic materials is beyond the scope of this chapter:

- Mesh utilization has become routine in countries where it is affordable.
- Careful consideration should be given to the use of mesh in younger patients.
- With meticulous technique mesh reduces recurrence rates by a factor of three in inguinal and incisional hernia.
- Mesh design and mesh materials are undergoing continuous development.
- A small proportion of patients may react adversely to prosthetic mesh.

ANAESTHESIA

Even though local anaesthesia with sedation (so called monitored anaesthesia care) is a more cost-effective anaesthetic technique for inguinal hernia repair, general and regional anaesthesia remain the most popular techniques in most district general hospitals. Interestingly, specialized hernia centres use local infiltration anaesthesia in more than 90% of these cases. The few audit data that exists indicate that on a national and regional scale, general anaesthesia is used in 60–70% of cases, regional anaesthesia in 10–20% and local infiltration anaesthesia in only 5–10% of cases.

General, regional or local anaesthesia is suitable for the repair of most hernias and the type of anaesthesia employed may depend on the preferences and skills of the surgical team rather than the wishes of the patient. In socialized systems of healthcare there are no effective incentives for the widespread adoption of cost-effective techniques and for this reason in Europe general anaesthesia and regional anaesthesia predominate. In contrast in the USA where market forces prevail and the payor can demand that the less expensive local anaesthesia is utilized for herniorrhaphy, local anaesthesia is employed on a much larger scale.

Local anaesthesia for hernia repair does have particular advantages – organizational and economic as well as clinical. Local anaesthesia can be administered by the operator, thus no medical anaesthetist is required; the patient does require shared care during an operation performed under local anaesthetic and local practice, and clinical governance guidelines

will dictate whether the monitoring of the local anaesthetic with sedation is undertaken by a medical anaesthetist, a nurse anaesthetist, an operating department assistant or even in some healthcare environments no specialist monitor. Peripheral oxygen saturation must be monitored with a pulse oximeter, especially if intravenous sedation is being used. In addition intravenous access should be established in order that the complications of inadvertent intravascular injection of local anaesthetic agents, which may result in cerebral and cardiovascular side effects can be counteracted. Blood pressure should be recorded on arrival in the operating theatre and after the injection of local anaesthetic, and preferably monitored throughout the procedure. This may be done by connecting the patient to a cardiac monitor supervised by the anaesthetic nurse throughout the operation and regularly recording pulse, blood pressure and respiratory rate. Emergency resuscitation equipment, including the requirements for endotracheal intubation, must be available in the event of severe respiratory depression needing intubation.

Modern general anaesthesia makes it possible for safe operations to be performed on patients who are to go home 2 h or so later. The need for tracheal intubation is no longer a contraindication to day surgery. The speed of recovery from general anaesthesia is paramount to facilitate full and rapid recovery to consciousness and a degree of physical performance commensurate with returning home by private car or taxi.

While the advantages and disadvantages of local or general anaesthesia must be considered for each and every patient, for open operations the patient's views should not be overruled by the surgeon's personal preference:

- The use of local anaesthesia in inguinal hernia surgery requires the acquisition of additional skills.
- Patients having surgery under local anaesthesia should be carefully monitored.
- A rate of 90% of patients having inguinal hernia repair under local anaesthesia is achievable.

Technique for local anaesthesia

The recommended local anaesthetic agent is a mixture of bupivacaine and lignocaine with the addition of adrenaline 1 : 200 000. The benefits of this mixture are the rapid onset of action of the lignocaine solution, the prolonged action of the bupivacaine and the possibility of reduced local haemorrhage with the addition of adrenaline. In practice 3×10 ml ampoules of bupivacaine 0.25% solution with adrenaline 1 : 200 000 are admixed with 3×10 ml ampoules of 1% lignocaine to produce 3×20 ml anaesthetic solutions. This 60 ml volume of local anaesthetic is suitable for most patients except the excessively lean or excessively obese patient where the volume may be reduced or increased by up to 10 ml. The technique of application of the inguinal block can be achieved by a variety of techniques including the one described in the foregoing section of this chapter. If a preoperative inguinal block is applied, the surgeon should have handy on the scrub nurses trolley a 5 ml supplement of 1% lignocaine which can be used intraoperatively should the need arise. Many experienced operators will use this supplementary local anaesthetic around the pubic tubercle before attempting dissection of the spermatic cord in this area. Amid from the Lichtenstein clinic has given an account of the step-by-step, infiltrate-as-you-go procedure of local anaesthesia for inguinal hernia repair. Care must be taken to avoid direct intravascular injection during the infiltration, which is a very rare event since the only major vein in the region is the femoral vein, which should be far from the wandering tip of the infiltrator's needle.

Although pre-anaesthetic drugs are unnecessary, patient morale is improved by giving midazolam intravenously just before the start of the procedure. In most patients the dose should be no more than 2 mg midazolam, except for young anxious patients where the dose required may be up to 4 mg, and in elderly patients with comorbid cardiorespiratory disease when sedation is contraindicated or unnecessary:

- A detailed knowledge of groin anatomy is required to achieve effective administration of local anaesthesia for hernia surgery.
- Improved local anaesthetic agents have increased their effectiveness.
- Surgical technique must be adapted to the local anaesthetic situation.

COMPLICATIONS OF HERNIA IN GENERAL

Includes the following:

1. Rupture of the hernia – spontaneous or traumatic.
2. Involvement of the hernial sac in the disease process: (a) mesothelial hyperplasia; (b) carcinoma; (c) endometriosis and leiomyomatosis; (d) inflammation – peritonitis, acute appendicitis.
3. Incarceration, obstruction and strangulation. *Reductio-en-masse.*
4. Maydl's hernia and afferent loop strangulation. Strangulation of the appendix in a hernial sac. Richter's hernia. Littre's hernia.
5. Herniation of female genitalia. Pregnancy in a hernial sac.
6. Urinary tract complications, hernia of the bladder, the ureter and of a urinary ileal conduit.
7. Sliding hernia.
8. Testicular strangulation in: (a) infants; (b) adults with large giant inguinoscrotal hernias.

Incarceration, obstruction and strangulation

Incarceration is the state of an external hernia, which cannot be reduced into the abdomen. Incarceration is important because it implies an increased risk of obstruction and strangulation. Incarceration is caused by (a) a tight hernial sac neck; (b) adhesions between the hernial contents and the sac lining – these adhesions are sometimes a manifestation of previous ischaemia and inflammation; (c) development of

pathology in the incarcerated viscus, e.g. a carcinoma or diverticulitis in incarcerated colon; (d) impaction of faeces in an incarcerated colon.

Incarceration is an important finding. It should urge the surgeon to undertake operation sooner rather than later. If reduction of a hernia is performed it should be gentle; forcible reduction of an incarcerated hernia may precipitate *reductio-en-masse* (see below). If bowel with a compromised blood supply is reduced, stricturing and adhesions between gut loops will follow. This will lead to intestinal obstruction some weeks or months later. The best policy is to operate on incarcerated hernias and check the viability of the gut at operation.

Incarceration in an inguinal hernia is the commonest cause of acute intestinal obstruction in infants and children in the UK. In adults, postoperative adhesions account for 40% of cases of obstruction, external hernias for 30% and malignancy for 25% of cases. In tropical Africa, strangulated external hernia is the commonest cause of intestinal obstruction in all age groups.

Patients presenting with symptoms of intestinal obstruction should have all the potential hernial sites very carefully examined. The sites of obstruction are inguinal, femoral, umbilical, incisional, Spigelian, and obturator and perineal hernial orifices in that order. A partial enterocoele (Richter's hernia) is a particularly treacherous variety of hernia, especially in infancy. Partial enterocoele is a potentially lethal and easily overlooked complication of 'port site' hernia following laparoscopy.

Strangulation is the major life-threatening complication of abdominal hernias. In strangulation the blood supply to the hernial contents is compromised. At first there is angulation and distortion of the neck of the sac; this leads to lymphatic and venous engorgement. The herniated contents become oedematous. Capillary vascular permeability develops. The arterial supply is occluded by the developing oedema and now the scene is set for ischaemic changes in the bowel wall.

The gut mucosal defenses are breached and intestinal bacteria multiply and penetrate through to infect the hernial sac contents. Necrobiosis and gangrene complete a sad and lethal cycle unless surgery or preternatural fistula formation save the patient. Hypovolaemia and septic shock predicate vigorous resuscitation if surgery is to be successful.

Forty per cent of patients with femoral hernia are admitted as emergency cases with strangulation or incarceration, whereas only 3% of patients with direct inguinal hernias present with strangulation. A groin hernia is at its greatest risk of strangulation within 3 months of its onset. The general public, especially the elderly, should be aware of the potential dangers of a lump in the groin. The most easily missed of these lumps in the groin is a femoral hernia in an obese patient in whom the consequences of a missed diagnosis carry a high morbidity and mortality.

Obturator hernias are very prone to strangulation; however, their elective repair is rarely feasible and a high index of suspicion particularly in elderly, emaciated female patients with symptoms of intestinal obstruction is required. Clinical

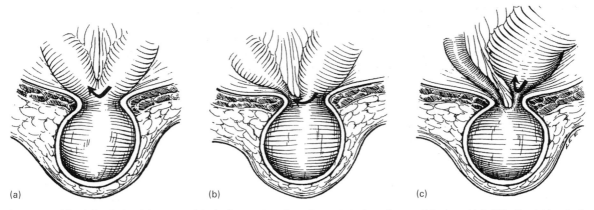

Figure 14.9. Richter's hernia (partial enterocoele). The figures show the antimesenteric circumference of the bowel is held by the rigid neck of the hernial sac.

suspicion combined with preoperative ultrasonography or computed tomographic (CT) scan can correctly diagnose obturator hernia preoperatively and result in successful surgery:

- Incarceration should be treated urgently.
- External hernias are one of the commonest causes of intestinal obstruction.
- Strangulation should be treated emergently after adequate resuscitation.
- Femoral and obturator hernias frequently present with strangulation and should be considered in a patient with an unidentified cause for intestinal obstruction.

Richter's hernia

Partial enterocoele, the eponymous Richter's hernia, occurs when the antimesenteric circumference of the intestine becomes constricted in the neck of a hernial sac without causing complete intestinal luminal occlusion (Fig. 14.9).

Richter's hernia is most frequently found in femoral or obturator hernias, although the condition has been described at other sites and there is an increasing incidence at laparoscope insertion sites, therefore awareness of this special type of hernia with its misleading clinical appearance is important.

According to localization and the mode of herniation and entrapment, the clinical picture and course can vary considerably. There are four main groups:

1. The obstructive group, in which early diagnosis and therapy leads to an excellent prognosis.
2. The danger group, in which symptomatology is vague and subsequent delay in surgery is responsible for a high death rate.
3. The postnecrotic group in which local strangulation and perforation leads to formation of an enterocutaneous fistula; the fistula may close spontaneously ('the miracle cure') or remain chronic.
4. The 'unlucky' perforation group, in which the postnecrotic abscess, as a result of unlucky anatomical constellations,

accidentally finds its way into another compartment, resulting either in a large abscess with severe septic/toxic load or in peritonitis; both of these would lead to a high death rate.

Littre's hernia – hernia of Meckel's diverticulum

Meckel's diverticulum is the most common congenital anomaly of the gastrointestinal tract arising as a result of incomplete dissolution of the vitello-intestinal duct. Approximately 4% of patients with Meckel's diverticulum develop complications, Littre's hernia being one of the least common. A Meckel's diverticulum may be a chance finding in an inguinal hernia. It has been described in incarcerated inguinal hernia in infants: in infants the diverticulum frequently becomes adherent to the sac and as a consequence the hernia becomes irreducible. This can be diagnosed when after taxis of a right inguinal hernia in an infant, part of the hernia remains unreduced.

GROIN HERNIAS IN CHILDREN

Some 3–5% of full-term babies are born with clinically apparent inguinal hernias, in preterm babies this incidence is substantially increased up to 30%. Inguinal hernia is the commonest indication for surgery in early life. Approximately 20–25 live births per 1000 require operation for inguinal hernia of which some 10% require emergency admission for incarceration and strangulation. The ratio of boys to girls is 9 : 1, which yields an incidence in male children of 4.2%.

Incarceration and strangulation

Ten per cent of children with inguinal hernias present as emergencies with incarceration or strangulation. Incarceration or strangulation has its highest frequency in the first 3 months of life; thereafter the incidence falls off so that incarceration is very rare after the sixth birthday. The incidence of incarceration is higher in premature and low birthweight children. Incarceration or strangulation is 10 times more frequent in male than in female children. While incarceration is not infrequent, strangulation (an irreducible hernia containing viscera with a critically compromised blood supply) is very rare.

Treatment by sedation and gallows traction (Solomon position) is recommended initially. Eighty per cent of incarcerated hernias reduce spontaneously if the child is adequately sedated.

Prompt elective operation for inguinal hernia in infants is recommended, the probability of incarceration being 1 : 4 for hernias in male children diagnosed under 12 months of age:
- Groin hernia incarceration and strangulation is common in premature infants.
- Resuscitation and preparation for surgery must take place in the environment of a paediatric unit.
- Infant groin hernia is a specialist operation.

Clinical diagnosis of inguinal hernia in a child

A lump in the groin of a child is a common condition that presents to surgeons. In making a diagnosis, the sex and age of the patient and the history of the onset of the lump are critical determinants. Physical diagnosis usually only confirms what can be discovered by careful history-taking.

Sixty per cent of inguinal hernias are apparent within the first 3 months of life; the remainder are discovered in well baby clinics or at school medical examinations. Few inguinal hernias are first noticed after 5 years of age.

Inguinal hernias may present at birth or at any date after that, and they are more frequent on the right side than the left side. Their early history often distinguishes them from other lumps. In the infant or child the lump is most often noticed by the mother. The lump is more prominent when the child screams or moves about vigorously, whereas it often disappears in the relaxed child; indeed when the child is brought to be examined in the clinic it may not be apparent. The mother's word alone is enough to make a diagnosis. The lump appears initially as a 'bulge' at the medial end of the groin. It increases in size and may progress down into the scrotum. Episodes of irreducibility are frequent.

The inguinal hernia in the male child should be distinguished from the hydrocoele. The symptoms are similar, except that with hydrocoele the mother will have noticed the swelling in the scrotum before there was a swelling in the groin. She may notice that the swelling is only in the scrotum.

On clinical examination the hernia extends from the superficial ring to the scrotum. The hydrocoele extends from scrotum towards the superficial ring; it may not extend as far as the groin crease and external ring. The hernia is reducible and if it contains gut it will reduce with a gurgle. The hydrocoele is readily transilluminable:
- The diagnosis of groin hernia in an infant can be accepted on the basis of the history from the mother.

- Hydrocoele and hernia should be distinguished.
- Planned, elective surgery is the norm for infant hernia.

Burd and colleagues have suggested a strategy for the optimal management of metachronous hernias in children. A decision analysis tree was constructed with three approaches:
1. Observation and repair of a contralateral hernia only if it later becomes apparent.
2. Routine contralateral groin exploration.
3. Laparoscopy to evaluate the contralateral groin for a potential hernia.

The results indicated that observation was favoured over laparoscopy, and laparoscopy over routine exploration, with respect to preventing spermatic cord injury and preserving future fertility. Although observation was the favoured approach with respect to cost, laparoscopy was less expensive when the expected incidence of metachronous hernias was high. It was concluded that observation is the preferred approach to metachronous hernia repair because it results in the lowest incidence of injury and costs, and in most patients and is associated with a minimal increase in anaesthesia related morbidity and mortality. Laparoscopy may be advantageous for patients of high risk for development of a contralateral hernia.

The operation

In babies and young children, the inguinal canal has not yet developed its oblique adult anatomy. The superficial ring is directly anterior to the deep ring and the sac is indirect. There is no acquired deformity of the canal. In these cases the fascia transversalis is normal and a simple herniotomy is all that is necessary. Straightforward inguinal herniotomy should give a 100% cure rate.

DIAGNOSIS OF A LUMP IN THE GROIN IN THE ADULT

Although the distinction between femoral and inguinal hernias is difficult enough for practising surgeons, the clinical distinction between indirect and direct inguinal hernia is correct in little more than 50% of cases even in experienced hands. Even the position of fixed landmarks such as the midpoint of the inguinal ligament and the mid inguinal point cannot be accurately distinguished. Every groin lump should be carefully evaluated and hernias must be distinguished from other lesions.

Inguinal hernia – the adolescent and the adult

In the male adolescent or young adult the lump is most likely to be an indirect inguinal hernia. The story then is that when the lump first appeared there was acute, quite severe pain in the groin that passed off and after a day or two went away altogether. The pain may have been related to straining or lifting or playing some violent game. Overall however, it has been estimated that only 7% of patients can attribute the presence of a hernia to a single muscular strain. At first the lump comes and goes, disappearing when the sufferer goes to bed at night and not being present in the morning until he gets out of bed and stands up. The lump comes in the groin and goes obliquely down into the scrotum. The patient usually describes the sequence well. This is the classic description of an indirect (oblique) inguinal hernia in the young adult.

In the older man an indirect hernia can occur, but a direct inguinal hernia is more likely. The story here is usually of some associated strain, often at work, the lump then appearing 1 or 2 days after the initial pain in the groin has gone away. Such a hernia may not reduce spontaneously. In the older male the lump may be associated with coughing, straining to micturate or disturbances in bowel habit. In these circumstances other predisposing conditions, respiratory disease or urinary tract obstruction or colonic disease that results in constriction of the lumen must be excluded as potentiating factors.

A varicocoele cannot easily be confused with an inguinal hernia in the male. The varicocoele is invariably in the left inguinoscrotal line – it is like a mass of worms and disappears spontaneously if the subject lies down. It has no cough impulse.

Inguinal hernias are more common in adult males than adult females in a ratio of 10 : 1. However, inguinal hernias do occur in women; indeed, indirect inguinal hernias in women are as common as femoral hernias in women, a fact that is often forgotten in the differential diagnosis. Direct inguinal hernias are very rare in women:

- Direct and indirect inguinal hernias cannot be reliably distinguished.
- Straining and coughing potentiate and are not a cause of groin hernia.
- Beware the femoral hernia in a fat female with intestinal hernia.

Femoral hernia

A femoral hernia accounts for approximately 5–10% of all groin hernias in adults. Most femoral hernias occur in women aged over 50 years. Atrophy and weight loss are common in patients with femoral hernias. The incidence of femoral hernias, male to female, is generally reported to be about 1 : 4. The different pelvic shape and additional fat in women render them more prone to femoral hernias than are men. Women with femoral hernias are usually multiparous – multiple pregnancy is said to predispose to femoral herniation. Femoral hernias are as common in men as in nulliparous women.

Groin pain with a recent onset irreducible groin lump is the presentation in 27%, a painless reducible groin lump occurs in 10%, a painful and reducible groin lump in 7%. Groin pain with no other symptoms and no complaint of a groin lump is the presentation in 3% of patients. Six per cent of patients present with recurrent obstructive symptoms. Missing the diagnosis of femoral hernia has dire consequences. Such patients are often frail and elderly with severe coexisting diseases and late hospitalization is one of the main causes of unfavourable outcome.

Other groin swellings

Other structures in the groin each contribute to the harvest of swellings, pains and discomforts patients complain of. These include:

1. *Vascular disease*: (a) Arterial – aneurysms of the iliac and femoral vessels; these may be complicated by distal embolization or vascular insufficiency which will make the diagnosis easy. Femoral aneurysm as a complication of cardiac catheterization or transluminal angioplasty is a recent arrival in the diagnostic arena. (b) Venous – a saphenavarix could be confused with a femoral hernia. Its anatomical site is the same, but its characteristic blue colour, soft feel, fluid thrill, disappearance when the patient is laid flat and the giveaway associated varicose veins should prevent misdiagnosis. (c) Inguinal venous dilatation secondary to portosystemtic shunting can result in a painful inguinal bulge that can even become incarcerated. Preoperative Doppler ultrasound in cirrhotic patients with suspected inguinal hernias is advised.

2. *Lymphadenopathy*: Chronic painless lymphadenopathy may occur in lymphoma and a spectrum of infective diseases. Acute painful lymphadenitis can be confused with a tiny strangulated femoral hernia. A lesion in the watershed area, the lower abdomen, inguinoscrotal or perineal region, the distal anal canal or the ipsilateral lower limb quickly resolves the argument.

3. *Tumours*: Lipomas are very common tumours. The common 'lipoma of the cord', which in reality is an extension of preperitoneal fat is frequently associated with an indirect or direct inguinal hernia. Fawcett and Rooney examined 140 inguinal hernias in 129 patients to study the problem of lipoma. A fatty swelling was deemed significant if it was possible to separate it from the fat accompanying the testicular vessels. The fatty swelling was designated as being a lipoma if there was no connection with extraperitoneal fat and was designated as being a preperitoneal protrusion if it was continuous through the deep ring with extraperitoneal fat. Protrusions of extraperitoneal fat were found in 33% of patients and occurred in association with all varieties of hernia. There was a true lipoma of the cord in only one patient. It was concluded that the forces causing the hernia were also responsible for causing the protrusion of extraperitoneal fat. Read has commented that occasionally extraperitoneal protrusions of fat may be the only herniation and therefore inguinal hernia classifications need to include not only fatty hernias but sac-less, fatty protrusions. Lipomas also occur in the upper thigh to cause confusion with femoral hernias. A lipoma is rarely tender; it is soft with scalloped edges and can be lifted 'free' of the subjacent fat.

4. *Secondary tumours*: A lymph node enlarged with metastatic tumour usually lies in a more superficial layer than a

femoral hernia. Such lymph nodes are more mobile in every direction than a femoral hernia and are often multiple. A metastatic deposit of a tumour arising from the abdominal cavity such as adenocarcinoma can present as a rock-hard immobile mass that can be confused as either a primary incarcerated inguinal hernia or a postoperative fibrotic reaction following an inguinal hernia repair.

5. *Genital anomalies*: (a) Ectopic testis in the male – there is no testicle in the scrotum on the same side. Torsion of an ectopic testicle can be confused with a strangulated hernia. (b) Cyst of the canal of Nuck – these cysts extend towards, or into, the labium majorum and are transilluminable.

6. *Obturator hernia*: An obturator hernia, especially in a female lies in the thigh lateral to the adductor longus muscle. Vaginal examination will resolve the diagnosis. Elective diagnosis is rarely entertained.

7. *Rarities*: (a) A cystic hygroma is a rare swelling; it is loculated and very soft. Usually the fluid can be pressed from one part of it to another. (b) A psoas abscess is a soft swelling frequently associated with backache. It loses its tension if the patient is laid flat. It is classically lateral to the femoral artery. (c) A hydrocoele of the femoral canal is a rarity reported from West Africa. In reality it is the end stage of an untreated strangulated femoral epiplocoele. The strangulated portion of omentum is slowly reabsorbed, the neck of the femoral sac remains occluded by viable omentum, while the distal sac becomes progressively more and more distended by protein-rich transudate.

Clinical examination

The groin should be examined with the patient standing erect and again with the patient lying flat. Hernias are sometimes only apparent when the patient stands up or only when the patient strains or coughs (Fig. 14.10).

When the patient is examined a rapid decision should be made as to whether the lump is a hernia or not a hernia – this is the crucial initial decision to make. A hernia has a cough impulse, changes in size when the patient strains or lies down and may be reducible. The other lumps in the groin do not change their disposition when the patient stands or lies down.

Reducing the hernia and then using one finger to hold it reduced while the patient coughs is a useful test which will enable the inguinal canal or the femoral ring to be identified, almost with certainty. Scrotal hernias must be separated from other scrotal lumps – hydrocoele, varicocoele, testicular tumours, epididymal cysts, etc. If the hernia is reducible, the diagnosis is obvious. A cough impulse is a characteristic of hernias, but not of other scrotal masses.

The advent of sophisticated radiological investigation has enabled small and occult hernias to be more easily diagnosed. The chief utility of ultrasound is to enable scrotal and other swellings to be clearly differentiated:

- In the absence of a clinical hernia, do not rely on radiological examination to make the diagnosis.

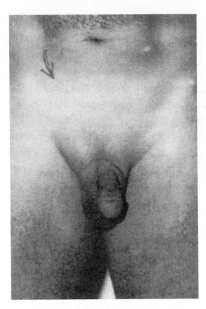

Figure 14.10. An inguinal hernia in the adult is above and medial to the inguinal ligament and pubic tubercle as the hernia emerges from the superficial inguinal ring.

- Radiological assessment helps identify the origin of unusual lumps in the groin and scrotum.
- Expertise is required to interpret radiological images of the groin.

ANTERIOR OPEN REPAIR OF INGUINAL HERNIA IN ADULTS

The Shouldice operation is the gold standard for sutured repair. The most essential part of the Shouldice operation is the repair of the fascia transversalis which is divided along the length of the canal, beginning at the deep inguinal ring and continuing down to the pubic tubercle. The fascia transversalis is repaired in four layers and the deep ring is carefully reconstituted using a 'double-breasting' technique (Fig. 14.11).

The Lichtenstein technique

The true tension-free hernioplasty using mesh and no suture closure of the hernial defect was introduced in 1984 by Irving Lichtenstein in Los Angeles. Repair of the posterior wall with a suture line is abandoned, except for a simple imbrication suture for large sacs that aided flattening of the posterior wall before placement of the mesh. In the UK, the Lichtenstein technique was first reported by Kingsnorth and colleagues, and subsequently by a private hernia clinic, The British Hernia Centre. Mesh repair is associated with three times fewer recurrences than non-mesh, in the repair of inguinal hernia. The incision, exposure, dissection of the canal and cord, and the dealing with indirect hernial sacs are identical to that described for the Shouldice operation. Polypropylene mesh precut to

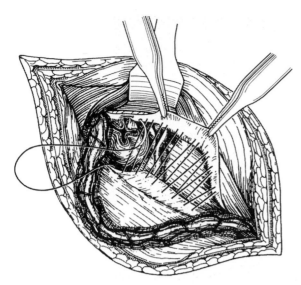

Figure 14.11. The second layer of suturing in the multi-layered Shouldice repair: the lower lateral flap of fascia transversalis is sutured to the undersurface of the upper medial flap along the 'white line' or 'arch'.

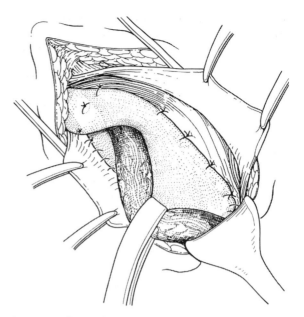

Figure 14.12. The completed Lichtenstein operation showing coverage of the posterior inguinal wall and overlap of 1–2 cm medially, laterally and superiorly.

8 cm × 16 cm is tailored to the individual patient's requirements. This will involve trimming 1–2 cm of the patch's width and the upper medial corner so that it will tuck itself between the external oblique and internal oblique muscles without wrinkles. After tailoring the mesh is sutured to the inguinal ligament and conjoint tendon and closed around the spermatic cord to recreate the internal ring. (Fig. 14.12)

Strangulated hernia

The use of mesh is not absolutely contraindicated if the amount of contamination is kept to a minimum and broad-spectrum antibiotics are used during and after the operation for several days. The Shouldice operative technique is recommended to treat a strangulated inguinal hernia, where there is gross contamination following bowel perforation due to necrosis. The additional risk of infection in this situation militates against the use of mesh, infection of which may cause morbidity.

Postoperative care

Immediate active mobilization is the key to rapid convalescence. The 'patient with a hernia' must not be allowed to become institutionalized into the 'postoperative patient'. If the operation has been performed under local anaesthesia, the patient should be helped to walk as soon as he is returned to the ward. If general anaesthesia has been used, the patient must be made to get up and walk as soon as he is conscious. There may be slight pain after surgery and a suitable mild analgesic should be prescribed. Analgesics with narcotic properties are never needed.

If social circumstances allow, patients should be discharged within a few hours of operation with minimal discomfort for which mild analgesics are prescribed. Unrestricted activity is encouraged, and indeed most patients should resume normal activity in 2–10 days. 'Take it easy' is the wrong advice.

Integrity of the hernia repair depends on good surgical technique, rather than any supposedly deleterious, premature physical activity undertaken by the patient. Return to full activity does not increase recurrences and indeed caution will engender anxiety and perhaps justify the patient's decision to remain off work for up to 6 weeks. It is contradictory and counterproductive to warn against strenuous activity and is a recipe for long-term disability. Troublesome wound soreness is rare 7–10 days after the operation.

The recurrence rate after inguinal hernia repair is operator dependent: the choice of operator is as important as the choice of operation:

- Mobilization and return to activity must be actively encouraged by verbal and written information to patients and their carers.
- Inadequate home support can compromise recovery.
- Properly fixated mesh is stronger than inate tissues, allowing early return to normal activity.

LAPAROSCOPIC GROIN HERNIA REPAIR

Laparoscopic repair involves placement of a preperitoneal prosthetic biomaterial. The repair follows the same principles as the open preperitoneal (Stoppa) repair. After reducing the

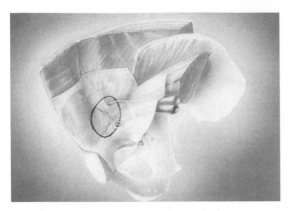

Figure 14.13. Mesh in the preperitoneal space overlying the myopectineal orifice.

hernia sac a large piece of mesh is placed in the preperitoneal space covering all potential hernia sites in the inguinal region (Fig. 14.13). The mesh becomes sandwiched between the preperitoneal tissues and the abdominal wall and, provided it is large enough, is held there by intra-abdominal pressure until such time as it becomes incorporated by fibrous tissue.

The choice between the TAPP and the TEP repair is merely a matter of personal preference. There is no clinical difference between the conversions to open, the complications seen, or the recurrence rates between these two operations in experienced hands. The TEP may be the more expeditious and less costly procedure based upon operating room expenses.

Disadvantages of laparoscopic hernia repair

It is estimated that it may take as many as 100 laparoscopic hernia repairs before an inexperienced laparoscopic surgeon can bring the operating time for laparoscopic hernia repair into a range similar to that for open hernia repair. On the other hand, the surgeon that is experienced with other advanced laparoscopic operations will take approximately 30–50 cases to build an adequate experience and a decreased operative time. Since operating time is expensive this has significant cost implications. Added to this, laparoscopic hernia repair is already more costly than open repair, principally because of the use of disposable instruments. These costs, however, can be brought into a range similar to that of open repair by using reusable rather than disposable instruments and by suturing rather than stapling or tacking when indicated. A hidden cost, often not considered, is use of the laparoscopic equipment itself, which is currently less durable and more expensive than conventional instruments. These costs can be minimized by frequent use and extra care by nursing and medical staff during their use.

Laparoscopic hernia repair is technically more demanding than open anterior approaches. This, combined with a poor knowledge of the preperitoneal anatomy by many, will limit its use to surgeons with a special interest in laparoscopic or

hernia surgery. Nevertheless, it has advantages in terms of reduced postoperative pain, lower wound morbidity, a more rapid return to normal activity, and less chronic pain and numbness than open repair. The benefits that are realized to the individual patients can be expanded into the societal advantages because these patients are returned to the work force more rapidly. Many surgeons are finding this technique more beneficial for the patients with bilateral and/or recurrent hernias. These advantages need to be balanced against increased costs and a high recurrence rate in the learning curve period.

FEMORAL HERNIA

A femoral hernia is a variety of groin hernia – a defect in the fascia transversalis which occurs when the femoral sheath, a funnel of fascia transversalis enclosing the femoral vessels beneath the inguinal ligament, becomes dilated. A peritoneal sac enters the femoral funnel and then, as a plunger, causes it to dilate. As the lacunar ligament medially and the pectineal ligament posteriorly are unyielding, strangulation is common at the neck of the sac.

The three open approaches

1. The low approach is recommended for the easily reducible uncomplicated femoral hernia especially in the thin patient, and in the frail American Society of Anesthesiologists (ASA) class 3 or 4 patient, when it can be undertaken electively using local anaesthesia.
2. The inguinal approach is best used when there is a concomitant primary inguinal hernia on the same side which can be repaired simultaneously.
3. The extraperitoneal approach is used when obstruction or strangulation are present, in patients who have undergone previous groin surgery, when inguinal and femoral hernias occur together, and in bilateral cases where both sides can be repaired simultaneously.

Open prosthetic repair

The use of prosthetic biomaterials is becoming the preferred method. This is especially true for recurrent repairs in which the recurrence rate is at least 25%. The concept of the plug-and-patch repair for femoral hernia is based upon the 'umbrella plug' and 'dart' repairs for inguinal hernia. The plug is fixed in position in the defect with non-absorbable sutures (Fig. 14.14). This will prevent the migration of the plug.

Laparoscopic repair

The repair of femoral hernia with the laparoscopic placement of a preperitoneal mesh is identical to the TAPP or the TEP inguinal operations. There is no difference in technique

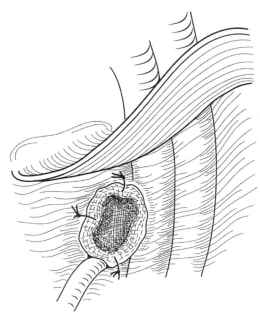

Figure 14.14. Insertion of a plug to repair a femoral hernia.

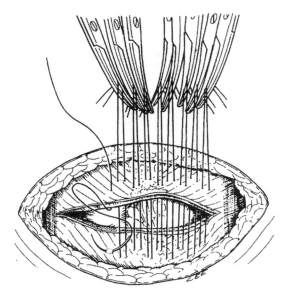

Figure 14.15. The first layer of sutures placed in the Mayo repair: the sutures are left lax and held in haemostats.

because the exposure of the myopectineal orifice by these two procedures will provide an excellent visualization of the femoral hernia.

UMBILICAL HERNIA IN ADULTS

Umbilical hernias in adults can be a cause of considerable morbidity and if complications supervene they can lead to death. Umbilical hernias are much less frequent in the adult population than inguinal hernias and account for 0.03% of the hernia operations performed in the UK. Of the patients with umbilical hernias, 90% are women, invariably women who are overweight and multiparous. Umbilical hernias have a high risk of incarceration. When these hernias incarcerate and strangulate, they frequently contain transverse colon and/or stomach. Strangulated umbilical hernias have a considerable morbidity dictated by the age of the patient and concomitant disease, atherosclerosis, obesity and diabetes mellitus.

Most patients with umbilical hernias complain of a painful protrusion at the umbilicus. This discomfort is indication enough for operation. In many patients, this protrusion may be asymptomatic but will be discovered by the primary physician or general practitioner on routine physical examination. Frequently, it is found in association of an inguinal hernia by the surgeon. Absolute indications for surgery include obstruction and strangulation. Irreducibility is not an absolute indication for surgery: many long-standing umbilical hernias have many adhesions in a loculated hernia and are thus irreducible. In larger hernias the overlying skin may become damaged and ulcerated. Skin complications may dictate the need for

operation after the skin sepsis has been controlled. Surgery is advised for all umbilical hernias unless there are strong contraindications, which include obesity, chronic cardiovascular or respiratory disease, or ascites (umbilical hernias can be manifestations of cirrhotic or malignant peritoneal effusions). In even these situations, however, the need for surgery may dictate that the procedure be performed after adequate preoperative preparation of the patient.

Umbilical hernias are an important complication of cirrhosis and ascites; the ascites should be controlled either medically or with a shunt before hernia repair is undertaken. Umbilical herniation is sometimes a consequence of chronic ambulatory peritoneal dialysis (CAPD). In all patients that are to initiate CAPD, any hernia that is found prior to the insertion of the catheter must be repaired.

The overlapping fascial operation as described by Mayo can be used successfully in patients where there are no risk factors (Fig. 14.15). However, the use of a prosthetic biomaterial for the repair of the larger defects has been associated with a lowered rate of recurrence. There are few reports in the literature of the results of the repair of this type of hernia.

The use of the laparoscopic repair of these hernias has also been reported with acceptable results and may become a viable alternative to the repair of this hernia:

- Early diagnosis and repair represents optimal management for umbilical hernia.
- A large incarcerated umbilical hernia in an obese patient represents a considerable operative risk.
- An asymptomatic umbilical protrusion in a patient with ascites does not warrant surgical intervention.

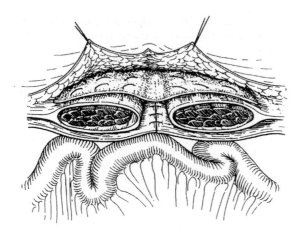

Figure 14.16. Incisional hernia repair using a mesh onlay.

INCISIONAL HERNIA

An incisional hernia is a bulge visible and palpable when the patient is standing and often requiring support or repair. Sixty per cent of patients with incisional hernias do not experience any symptoms; however, symptoms that predicate medical advice include difficulty in bending, cosmetic deformity, discomfort from the size of the hernia, persistent abdominal pain and episodic subacute intestinal obstruction. Incarceration persisting to acute intestinal obstruction and strangulation necessitate emergency surgery.

It is sometimes difficult to differentiate between a hernia and subcutaneous fat or small bowel in the hernia versus in close proximity to a weakened anterior fascia. In most situations and particularly for massive complex incisional hernias a CT scan may be much more efficient and accurate in defining the defect and planning the preoperative preparation of the patient and the operation chosen (Fig. 14.16).

Incidence

The overall incidence of incisional hernias is difficult to estimate, but at least 10–15% of abdominal operations are followed by incisional hernia. Certainly the reported incidence of this complication has fallen in the past 10 years, during which major sepsis has diminished, non-irritant, non-absorbable sutures have been introduced and the technique of wound closure has been emphasized. Incisional hernias are slightly more frequent in males than females.

Long-term prospective studies of laparotomy wound has revealed a high incidence of late wound failure in patients who have undergone laparotomy but who had sound wounds without herniation when examined at 1 year. More than half the incisional hernias first appeared more than 1 year after the initial operation. These 10-year results confirm that there is a continued attrition of the healed laparotomy wound, with incisional hernias developing up to and after 10 years.

Abdominal fascial closure of midline laparotomy wounds with a continuous, non-absorbable suture results in a significantly lower rate of incisional hernia than using either non-absorbable or interrupted techniques. The recent adoption of the laparoscopic techniques for the treatment of intra-abdominal pathology will undoubtedly decrease the occurrence of the midline incisional hernias. However, this change will probably require a new generation of surgeons to emerge from the training programmes.

Aetiological factors

The important causative factors include sepsis, steroid and other immunosuppressant therapy, and inflammatory bowel disease. Obesity is an important risk factor both for the occurrence of the original incisional hernia and for the likelihood of recurrence of the hernia after repair. Less significant factors include age and sex, anaemia, malnutrition, hypoproteinaemia, diabetes, type of incision, postoperative intestinal obstruction and postoperative chest infection.

Midline incisions are at greater risk than paramedian incisions. Lower midline incisions seem to be at greater risk than upper midline incisions:

- Incisional hernias are common and are largely a consequence of faulty surgical techniques used in closure of laparotomy wounds.
- All fit patients with incisional hernias should be offered surgery to improve quality of life and reduce complications.
- Experienced surgeons should repair complex hernias.

Principles of open repair

The following principles should be followed:

1. Whenever possible the normal anatomy should be reconstituted. In midline hernias this means the linea alba must be firmly reconstructed; in more lateral hernias there should be layer-by-layer closure as far as possible. However, the use of sutures with the repair of these hernias is associated with a rate of recurrence. For this reason, the ability of the reconstitution of the linea alba may not be feasible or advisable. This is not always possible with the larger hernias and certainly not done with the laparoscopic repair.
2. Only tendinous/aponeurotic/fascial structures should be brought together. *In situ* darning over the defect without adequate mobilization and apposition of the aponeurotic defect gives a 100% recurrence rate.
3. The suture material must retain its strength for long enough to maintain tissue apposition and allow sound union of tissues to occur. A non-absorbable material must, therefore, be used.
4. The length of suture material is related to the geometry of the wound and to its healing. Using deep bites at not more than 0.5 cm intervals, the ratio of suture length to wound length must be 4 : 1 or more.

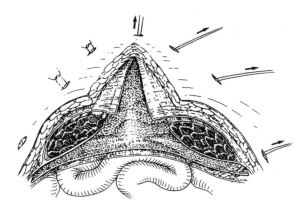

Figure 14.17. Incisional hernia repair using a mesh sublay with fixation by through-and-through sutures.

5. Repair of an incisional hernia inevitably involves returning viscera to the confines of the abdominal cavity with a resultant rise in intra-abdominal pressure. It is important to minimize this. Preoperative weight reduction is the first precaution. This, unfortunately, is generally not possible. Therefore the surgeon will usually be forced to repair these hernias with little consideration for the increase in the intra-abdominal pressure. In the majority of situations, this is not a clinical issue as few patients will not experience this increase in the intra-abdominal pressure that is clinically significant.

6. A tension-free repair with prosthetic reinforcement is recommended, for which there are several different approaches:

   • The mesh is placed over the defect (onlay) and sutured in position (Fig. 14.16).

   • The mesh is placed in the preperitoneal (and retro-muscular) space (Fig. 14.17) so that it does not contact the bowel (sublay). Each rectus sheath is incised along its medial border and opened in the midline to expose the anterior and posterior aspects of the rectus muscle, which by blunt dissection is mobilized to its entire width along the length of the defect. The mesh is then placed posterior (retro-) to the rectus muscles, after first closing the posterior leaf of the sheath/peritoneum with monofilament nylon. The mesh is secured with interrupted absorbable sutures between the edges of the mesh and the underlying posterior rectus sheath/peritoneum. The layered closure is completed by approximation of the anterior rectus sheath over the prosthesis.

   • The mesh is placed between the unapproximated fascial edges (inlay). This exposes the bowel to the undersurface of the mesh and should only be used in the exceptional circumstance of inability to close the fascial layers without hernioplasty techniques (less than 5% cases).

Whichever technique is employed, the mesh must overlap each margin of the aponeurotic defect by some 3–4 cm and must be well fixed to the aponeurosis.

Studies have shown a rate of recurrence that is consistently improved with the use of a synthetic biomaterial as an element to the open repair of incisional and ventral hernias. If there is any tissue loss, a defect greater than 4 cm or any risk factors prosthetic mesh reinforcement is mandatory.

FURTHER READING

Kingsnorth AN, LeBlanc KA. *Management of Abdominal Wall Hernias*. London and New York: Arnold, 2003

15

Vascular Surgery

JR Barwell[1] and ZH Khan[2]

[1]Consultant Vascular and Renal Transplant Surgeon, Derriford Hospital, Plymouth, UK [2]Locum Consultant Vascular Surgeon, Derriford Hospital, Plymouth, UK

CONTENTS

Disorders of the arterial system	**286**
Anatomy	286
Physiology	286
Pathology	287
Risk factors for atherosclerosis	287
Epidemiology, clinical features and management of arterial disease	287
Investigation of arterial disease	288
Arterial surgical techniques	289
Atherosclerotic occlusive disease	292
Degenerative aneurysmal disease	295
Abdominal aortic aneurysms	296
Diabetic foot	296
Arterial trauma	297
Complications of arterial surgery	297
Disorders of veins of the lower limb	**298**
Anatomy	298
Pathophysiology	298
Classification	299
Varicose veins	299
Venous ulceration	301
Deep venous thrombosis	302
Venous malformations	303
Further reading	**303**

Vascular surgery is concerned with the investigation and treatment of arterial diseases affecting the aorta and its branches and the arteries in the limbs and the neck, but excluding the coronary arteries. It is also concerned with the management of diseases of the venous system.

DISORDERS OF THE ARTERIAL SYSTEM

Arterial surgery has evolved rapidly over the last 50 years with the development of bypass techniques, prosthetic materials, sutures, percutaneous procedures and imaging. The number of patients treated annually continues to increase in parallel with the increasing age of the population.

A comprehensive review of the basic sciences in relation to the specialty of vascular surgery is beyond the scope of this book; however, some significant features are covered below.

Anatomy

The heart pumps blood into the aorta, a large diameter vessel. With repeated branching the total cross-sectional area of the vessels increases in size until that of the capillaries is approximately 1000 times that of the aorta.

Collateral circulation

The development of collateral circulation is an important concept in arterial disease. In acute ischaemia the rapidity of onset prevents adequate collateral development; however, with slowly progressive chronic ischaemia, the collateral development may be so extensive as to fully compensate for major arterial occlusions (Fig. 15.1).

Physiology

Blood flow in an artery is related to:
- pressure gradient across the segment;
- diameter of the vessel;
- viscosity of the blood.

In patients with occlusive arterial disease, stenoses or occlusions proximal or distal to the area being assessed reduce the pressure gradient either by reducing the perfusion pressure or increasing the peripheral resistance. Low-pressure gradients across a graft or diseased arterial segment reduce the flow and therefore predispose to thrombosis.

Inflow pressure will also be reduced in patients with a reduced cardiac output and therefore patients who have stenotic arterial disease are particularly at risk of acute thrombosis during periods of reduced cardiac output from whatever cause.

Increased blood viscosity due to polycythaemia or dehydration can reduce blood flow. Malignancy or chemotherapy

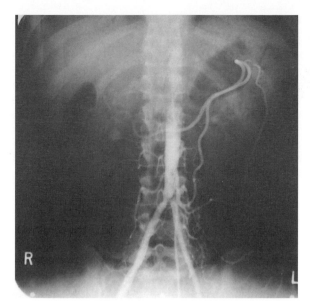

Figure 15.1. Marginal artery of the colon demonstrating the collateral circulation in a patient with superior mesenteric artery occlusion.

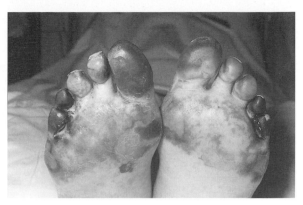

Figure 15.2. Cold injury.

can induce hypercoagulability. Both can increase risk of thrombosis in the arterial or venous circulation.

Pathology

The arterial system may be affected by various pathological processes:

- *Embolism* lodging at arterial branching points. They may result from:
  - thrombus or material from aneurysms or atheromatous plaques;
  - intracardiac thrombus in relation to myocardial infarction or arrhythmias;
  - cardiac tumour.
- *Occlusive disease* which may result from:
  - atherosclerosis;
  - vasculitis, often associated with an underlying systemic illness or connective tissue disorder.
- *Aneurysm*:
  - degenerative;
  - false, due to trauma or breakdown of an arterial anastomosis;
  - infective;
  - inflammatory.
- *Thoracic aortic dissection*:
  - possibly leading to distal ischaemic complications of limbs or organs. Not to be confused with thoracic aortic *aneurysm*, although this may be a late complication.
- *Fistulas*:
  - arterio-venous, secondary to trauma or aneurysm;
  - aorto-enteric, usually following aortic surgery.

- *Trauma*:
  - penetrating or blunt, leading to haemorrhage and/or distal ischaemia;
  - may be iatrogenic.
- *Vasospastic disorders*
  - Raynaud's phenomenon;
  - vibration white finger.
- *Cold injury* (Fig. 15.2)

Risk factors for atherosclerosis:

- smoking,
- hypercholesterolaemia,
- hypertension,
- diabetes mellitus,
- homocysteinaemia.

Patients with any atherosclerosis should be considered as having a systemic disease. They carry an increased risk of ischaemic stroke, coronary artery disease and reno-vascular disease. Risk factor management therefore plays an important part in such patients. They should be encouraged and helped to stop smoking. Blood pressure should be monitored and controlled. Anti-platelet therapy should be instigated: low-dose aspirin if tolerated or clopidogrel (and rarely a combination of the two). Hypercholesterolaemia should be sought and treated; there is evidence that all patients with arterial disease below the age of 75 benefit from low-dose statin therapy even if they have a normal baseline plasma cholesterol concentration.

Epidemiology, clinical features and management of arterial disease

These will be dealt with separately under the following headings concerning manifestations of most common arterial disorders:

- atherosclerotic occlusive disease,
- degenerative aneurysmal disease,
- diabetic foot.

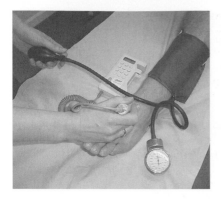

Figure 15.3. Ankle/brachial pressure index measurement.

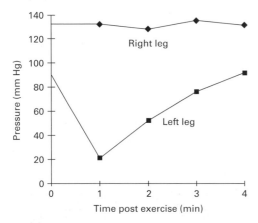

Figure 15.4. Exercise test result showing a normal pressure response in the right leg and an abnormal response (the pressure drops suddenly on exercise as perfusion is inadequate to meet demand) in the left where there is a femero-popliteal occlusion.

Investigation of arterial disease

Ankle/brachial pressure index (ABPI)

The ankle and brachial pressures are measured using a sphygmomanometer cuff to externally occlude the vessel at the lower calf and a Doppler ultrasound probe to detect blood flow at the ankle and ante-cubital fossa (Fig. 15.3). The pressure at which flow can be just detected at the ankle should be the same or higher than a similar measurement at the brachial artery (index 0.9–1.2). Some patients with occlusive disease may have normal resting pressures and others who have rigid arteries due to calcification may have spuriously high pressures detected at the ankle (e.g. diabetics). An index of about 0.7 indicates moderate ischaemia and if it falls below 0.5 the ischaemia is severe and often associated with rest pain.

Exercise testing

The patient is exercised at a set speed and gradient on a treadmill (Fig. 15.4) for a specified time or until the onset of claudication. The ankle pressures are measured before and at 1-min intervals after completion of exercise until the pressure returns to the pre-exercise level. Normal patients show a rise after exercise due to the increase in systolic pressure and the peripheral vasodilation. In patients with occlusive disease, the pressure falls after exercise and the extent and duration of the fall crudely correlates with the severity of the arterial disease. This is a useful test for distinguishing between arterial and non-arterial claudication.

B-mode ultrasound

This is an effective screening tool for the presence of an abdominal aortic aneurysm.

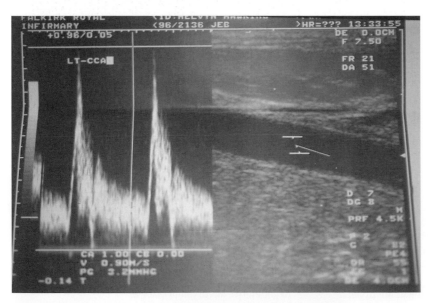

Figure 15.5. Duplex scan of common carotid artery showing normal flow velocities.

Duplex ultrasonography

A duplex scan combines the imaging of B-mode ultrasound scanning with Doppler flow measurements and therefore gives both anatomical and haemodynamic information (Fig. 15.5). This non-invasive test is now the procedure of choice in the investigation of peripheral and carotid artery disease. High-flow velocities and turbulence across a lesion can be used to accurately assess and map arterial stenoses and occlusions. Wave pattern analysis also detects upstream disease.

Computed tomography angiography

A bolus of contrast is given via a peripheral vein. Advances in the speed and resolution of modern computed tomography (CT) scanners make this the investigation of choice for assessment of the thoracic and abdominal aorta and all its major branches (Fig. 15.6).

Magnetic resonance angiography

Advances in technology and the introduction of gadolinium as a contrast medium has increased the role of magnetic resonance angiography (MRA) in the investigation of arterial disease and it is likely to become increasingly relevant in the future.

Angiography

Trans-femoral angiography is an invasive procedure involving the direct puncture of the common femoral artery, passage of a catheter into the distal aorta and injection of a contrast medium (Fig. 15.7). The images are stored digitally and processed to eliminate the images of everything except the contrast-filled arteries (digital subtraction angiography). Angiography is not without complications: haemorrhage, false aneurysm formation, arterial thrombosis and peripheral embolisation. With the increased diagnostic accuracy of duplex ultrasonography and CT angiography, direct arterial puncture is usually now reserved for when a synchronous intervention (e.g. angioplasty) is planned.

Arterial surgical techniques

Heparin therapy

- Intravenous (i.v.) systemic heparinisation: give 5000 units as a bolus i.v. followed by 350 units/kg/24 h adjusted accordingly to the partial thromboplastin time and maintaining a ratio of 2.0–2.5;
- intra-operative heparinisation: give 5000 units i.v. 2 min prior to clamping;
- intra-operative irrigation solution: usually used in a concentration of 10 units/ml saline;
- DVT prophylaxis: unfractionated heparin in a dose of 5000 units subcutaneously two or three daily or fractionated heparin 2500 units subcutaneous daily.

The half-life of unfractionated heparin in the plasma is about 1.5 h. Its effects may be immediately reversed by giving protamine sulphate i.v. in a dose of 10 mg/1000 units of heparin. The dose is reduced as the time interval from injection of heparin increases.

Seldinger technique

This is the technique for inserting catheters transcutaneously into the arterial circulation for endovascular procedures. The artery, usually the common femoral, is cannulated with a needle and a flexible wire is inserted through the

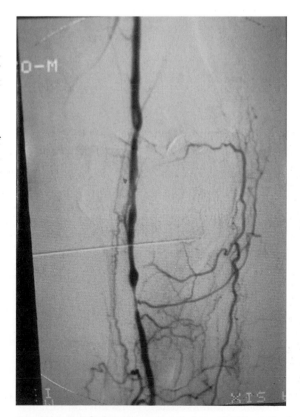

Figure 15.7. Digital subtraction angiogram of superficial femoral artery.

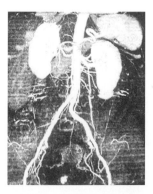

Figure 15.6. CT angiography of abdominal aorta.

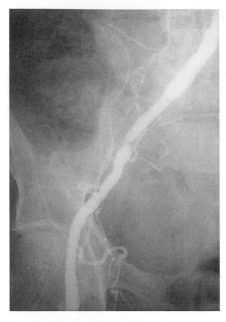

Figure 15.8. External iliac stenosis.

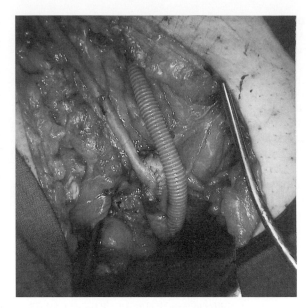

Figure 15.10. Saphenous vein graft and Dacron graft.

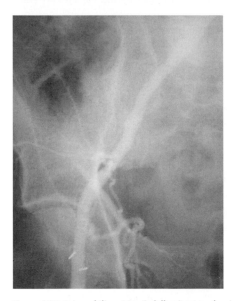

Figure 15.9. External iliac stenosis following transluminal angioplasty.

needle. This wire is then used to position the catheter in the appropriate place in the arterial circulation.

Angioplasty

This technique involves the passage of an especially strong balloon catheter into the artery under radiological control, followed by the dilatation of a localised stenosis or the recanalisation of a short occlusion (Figs 15.8 and 15.9). It is most successful in the iliac arteries and least successful

below the popliteal. It is not of value in calcified stenoses or those that are asymmetrical (the normal area of wall dilates without compressing the plaque). Longer occlusions may be more successfully treated with subintimal passage of the balloon. Complications include acute thrombosis of the dilated segment, rupture of the artery and peripheral embolisation.

Suture materials

Suture materials for vascular anastomoses which fulfil the requirements of non-thrombogenicity, a low coefficient of friction and maintaining strength indefinitely (for prosthetic graft anastomoses) are:

- polypropylene (monofilament),
- polytetrafluoroethylene (PTFE) (monofilament).

Arterial grafts

The type of graft used depends on the diameter of the vessel required and on the availability of an autograft.

Autologous vein

The long saphenous vein is usually used, providing its diameter on duplex scanning is 3.5 mm or above (Fig. 15.10). Arm veins are less robust and tend to dilate with time but are a good option if no leg veins are available. They should be marked pre-operatively, under duplex control if necessary. The vein may be prepared by removing and reversing it before reinsertion. It may also be used in the '*in situ*' mode, whereby it is not removed but simply anastomosed at both ends after destroying the valves with a valvulotome. All the side branches have to be ligated.

Expanded PTFE

This has a lower long-term patency and much higher infection rate than autogenous vein.

Dacron

These grafts have a well-established place in large arterial reconstruction and they have yet to be surpassed for long-term patency and strength. They may be impregnated with rifampicin to render them more resistant to infection or heparin to lower their thrombogenicity.

Endarterectomy

This is a technique used to deal with short occlusions or stenoses due to atheroma in large diameter or high-flow arteries and has the advantage of not using a prosthesis. It is the procedure of choice for disease at the common carotid or common femoral artery bifurcations.

The artery is exposed and clamped and then opened longitudinally and a plane of cleavage developed between the inner two-thirds and the outer third of the media. Distally the edge of the intimal flap must be sutured down to prevent it being dissected by the flowing blood. The arteriotomy is then closed. A vein or prosthetic patch is used if the artery is likely to be narrowed.

Bypass procedures

Blockages or a narrowed area may be bypassed using the materials and techniques described above. There are a few conditions which must be satisfied for success:

- there must be a high-pressure inflow and a low-resistance outflow;
- there must be no narrowing of the anastomosis or kinking, twisting or compression of the graft;
- there should be a minimum of turbulence at the anastomoses;
- the materials used should be non-thrombogenic;
- the diameter of the graft should approximate to the diameter of the vessel being bypassed.

Fasciotomy

Fasciotomy is indicated for:

- acute compartment syndrome following trauma or successful revascularisation in patients with acute ischaemia;
- exercise related compartment syndrome.

Vertical incisions are made on the medial and lateral aspects of the leg. The superficial anterior, lateral and posterior compartments can be decompressed and by retraction of the gastrocnemius and soleus posteriorly the deep compartment can be entered. The skin should not be closed, as even this can cause compression in the grossly swollen limb, but a subcuticular prolene suture can be placed for later skin closure by simple traction on the suture ends.

Occasionally fasciotomy is required in the upper limb following revascularisation in acute ischaemia.

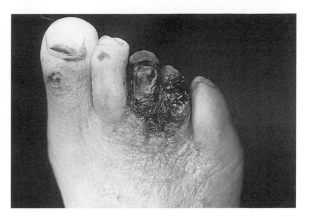

Figure 15.11. Diabetic digital gangrene.

Amputation

Absolute indications for amputation in vascular disease include:

- rest pain not relieved by any other technique;
- infected diabetic gangrene not responding to conservative measures;
- extensive gangrene with loss of function.

Relative indications are:

- intractable ischaemic ulceration;
- critical ischaemia with severe deformity, paralysis or major venous occlusion.

The amputation should be carried out at as distal a level as is compatible with primary healing. Many investigative techniques have been tried to assess the level of the amputation but none has been uniformly successful.

Partial foot amputations

This level of amputation is usually only of value in the diabetic patient. It is usually carried out for diabetic gangrene with sepsis. Individual toes may be amputated or if the infection has spread to the centre of the foot a metatarsal may be removed with the toe (ray amputation) to encourage drainage (Fig. 15.11). If several toes are involved and the gangrene has spread to the forefoot, an amputation through the metatarsals using a plantar flap may be appropriate. All these procedures give good functional results and the patient may walk without a prosthesis, but note the comments in the section on the diabetic foot below.

Below knee amputation

The flaps used should be either a long posterior flap or the 'skew flap' technique with anteromedial and posterolateral flaps. This tibia should be divided 10–15 cm below the tibial plateau and the anterior border of the tibia should be bevelled. The fibula should be cut at least 2 cm above the tibial bone section.

Amputations in the region of the knee have been advocated but in patients with vascular disease but are difficult to attach a prosthetic limb to.

Above knee amputations

The flaps used are usually equal anterior and posterior. The level of bone section is the junction between the proximal two-thirds and distal one-third of the femur. The bone end should be rounded and the muscle flaps sutured across it to give protection to the bone.

Rehabilitation

The immediate goals are:
- obtain primary healing,
- minimise swelling,
- prevent flexion contractures.

After the first week, the goals are:
- strengthen remaining muscles;
- train patient in crutch walking;
- start walking in temporary prosthesis in the form of a pneumatic bag in a frame the personal aid for mobility and health monitoring (PAMM aid).

After 6 weeks the stump should be suitable for casting and fitting with a definitive limb. However, the stump will continue to shrink and will require refitting on several occasions in the first year. Later, 70% of below knee amputees and 30% of above knee amputees should be able to walk independently with a prosthesis.

Atherosclerotic occlusive disease

Atheromatous plaques

These lesions tend to occur at areas of high turbulence such as arterial bifurcations, suggesting that endothelial damage is an important early factor. Endothelial damage results in deposition of fibrin, platelets and 'foamy' macrophages containing progressively large volumes of cholesterol. Substances released from platelets or the vessel wall cause smooth muscle proliferation and fibrosis.

Atheromatous plaques contain three major components:
- cholesterol – mainly in the form of cholesterol esters;
- cells – mainly smooth muscle cells and macrophages;
- proteins – mainly collagen, elastin and glycosaminoglycans.

Plaques vary enormously in their relative content of these components and in advanced lesions, fibrin, blood cells and calcium may also be found. They cause progressive narrowing of the lumen of the artery and lead to chronic occlusion. A tight stenosis can induce an acute arterial thrombosis.

Patterns of occlusive disease

Legs

Chronic leg ischaemia

Intermittent claudication

In the male general population aged 40–49 years the prevalence of intermittent claudication is approximately 0.5–1%. By 60–69 years this rises approximately four-fold. The prevalence in women is roughly half that in men.

Typically the pain is described as 'cramp like' and felt after walking for a certain distance commencing more rapidly

when walking rapidly or uphill. The pain is most often felt in the calf but may develop in the foot, thigh or buttock. It is usually relieved by resting for 2–3 min after which the patient may walk further. This must be differentiated from other causes of intermittent leg pain such as:

- *Arthritis*: Pain is typically felt as soon as the patient starts to walk, tends to be worse in the mornings and is often partially relieved by exercise. It is often present at rest.
- *Neurogenic*: Pain usually arises from cauda equina or nerve root compression. It commences after walking a short distance and is only slowly relieved at rest and often only after sitting down. It is commonly associated with back pain or sciatica.
- *Venous claudication*: There is always a clear history of ileofemoral venous thrombosis. The pain characteristically is described as 'bursting' and is only slowly relieved by resting with the limb elevated.
- *Compartment syndrome*: This usually affects the anterior compartment of the leg in young athletic individuals and is associated with 'tightness' and swelling of the anterior compartment.

About 75% of patients presenting with claudication will show improvement or maintenance of symptoms. At most only about 10% will ever need amputation or limb salvage procedures. The risk of amputation is increased five-fold in diabetics. However, the mortality from all causes in claudicants at 5, 10 and 15 years is approximately 30, 50 and 70%, respectively, which is about twice the rate in the control population. Patients with claudication are therefore up to seven-times more likely to die than to lose a leg.

The aims of treatment are therefore to reduce the rate of deterioration by risk factor management (see above) and exercise to stimulate development of the collateral circulation, possibly as part of a supervised programme.

There is no evidence that vasodilating drugs have any effect on claudicants but metabolically active drugs such as naftidrofuryl or viscosity-reducing drugs like oxpentifylline may have a marginal effect.

Disease causing isolated calf symptoms is often limited to the superficial femoral or popliteal artery and balloon angioplasty of these lesions tends to be technically feasible. However there is no level one evidence that angioplasty is superior to conservative management. Supra-inguinal disease often causes thigh and/or buttock symptoms and may have a poorer response to conservative management. It would seem sensible to offer balloon angioplasty, with a complication risk of 1–4%, to patients with short lesions (<10 cm) not responding to a trial of conservative management.

Critical ischaemia

This is defined as rest pain most nights in spite of adequate analgesia, tissue loss or an ankle Doppler pressure <50 mmHg. Rest pain is an unremitting pain felt in the toes or the forefoot. It tends to be worse in bed and may be partially relieved by hanging it out of the bed or walking round. It is a particularly debilitating form of pain. Pain felt only in the leg or thigh at night is *not* ischaemic rest pain. Tissue loss in this context implies gangrene or ulceration of the non-diabetic foot with an ABPI < 0.5.

Critical ischaemia usually requires intervention, often a combination of open surgery and endovascular procedures, to salvage the leg or primary amputation.

Re-vascularisation of the leg requires that three factors be addressed:
1. *Inflow*: Haemodynamically significant stenoses (>50%) or occlusions in the aorto-iliac segment must be treated, either by angioplasty ± stenting of short iliac lesions or aorto-bi-femoral, axillo-bi-femoral or femero–femoral cross-over grafting if the lesion is too long. If the common femoral and profunda femoris arteries are patent this will usually be sufficient to salvage a leg with rest pain but more distal reconstruction is usually required if there is tissue loss. Endarterectomy may be used for localised stenoses or occlusions of the aorta, common iliac or common femoral arteries.
2. *Conduit*: For long occlusions of the femero–popliteal and crural vessels the preferred conduit is long saphenous vein (Fig. 15.12). If this is not available and vein cannot be harvested from the contra-lateral leg or arms then a prosthetic graft may be necessary. A cuff of vein interposed between the prosthesis and the artery at the distal anastomosis improves patency. Subintimal angioplasty is a technique whereby balloon angioplasty is deliberately performed in the space between the intima and media, rather than the lumen of the artery. Much longer lesions (>10 cm) can now be treated in this way. There is much debate regarding the relative long-term patency of infra-inguinal bypass grafts or subintimal angioplasty and clinical trials are underway. As long as the conduit remains patent for sufficient time to allow healing of distal tissue loss and a collateral circulation to develop then limb salvage is usually achieved if the inflow and profunda vessels remain open.
3. *Run-off*: There must be a patent crural vessel in continuity with the arch vessels of the foot. This is necessary either for a bypass graft to be anastomosed onto or for a subintimal angioplasty tract to re-enter an arterial lumen. Any re-vascularisation procedure will fail if this condition is not met.

Acute leg ischaemia

An acutely ischaemic leg is either due to an embolus lodging in a previously healthy artery (Fig. 15.13) or thrombosis in an artery which virtually always has underlying disease or has been damaged by a traumatic event. The occlusion has been too sudden for an effective collateral system to develop and this is a surgical emergency. The diagnosis and management of an acutely ischaemic leg is challenging but can be extremely rewarding.

The history is of sudden onset coldness, weakness, pain and numbness of the affected limb. On examination pulses are absent and diagnosis is obvious if the foot is white. However the foot may appear pink, especially if dependant, by the time the patient arrives in hospital. Clues to the urgency of the situation are neuromuscular deficit and/or tender muscle compartments. The former may be quite a subtle altered sensation and weakness of extension of the great toe compared to the other side, the latter signifies

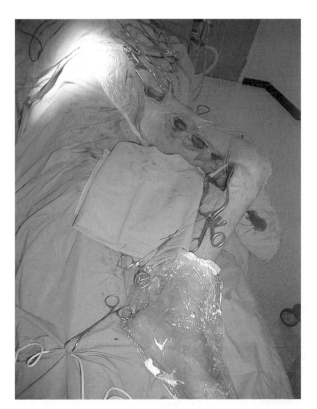

Figure 15.12. Reversed vein arterial bypass surgery.

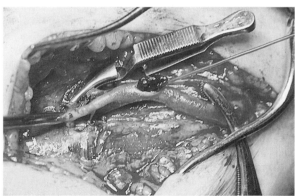

Figure 15.13. Brachial embolectomy.

severe muscular ischaemia which will progress to muscle death over a few hours. Extensive fixed mottling of the skin suggests that the limb is unsalvageable.

An embolus should be strongly suspected if there is no previous history suggestive of peripheral vascular disease, no signs of chronic ischaemia (hair loss, nail disruption, muscle wasting), palpable pulses in the other foot and the patient is in atrial fibrillation. If all the above conditions are met an embolectomy under local anaesthetic can be limb and life saving in even the most elderly patients.

Acute intra-arterial thrombosis may occur in a tightly stenosed atherosclerotic vessel, a stenosed bypass graft, a peripheral aneurysm or following trauma (blunt, penetrating or iatrogenic). Rarely intra-arterial thrombosis may occur in previously healthy vessels when there is a severe systemic illness (e.g. malignancy, HIV, anti-phospholipid syndrome). Stasis and thrombosis in diseased vessels may be induced by dehydration, immobility, low cardiac output or polycythaemia. The mortality associated with acute ischaemia remains high as thrombosis or embolism is not infrequently a pre-terminal event in patients dying from other causes such as cardiac failure. In these cases aggressive treatment may be contraindicated.

Management of the acutely ischaemic leg involves:
- if irreversibly ischaemic, amputate when demarcated;
- immediately heparinise (may double limb-salvage rate);
- after successful embolectomy, anticoagulate, if not contraindicated, to prevent recurrence;
- if thrombotic, investigate acutely with a view to immediate limb salvage surgery as above;
- following successful re-vascularisation, the limb must be checked for evidence of compartment syndrome and fasciotomy should be performed if in any doubt.

Intra-arterial thrombolysis: (Fig. 15.14)
This technique is now less commonly used in the acutely ischaemic leg for the following reasons:
- it was expensive, not always successful, had a high re-occlusion rate and carried a significant morbidity especially in the elderly (haemorrhage, haemorrhagic stroke and distal embolisation);
- there was usually an underlying problem that required surgery anyway;
- if neuromuscular deficit was present the technique could be too slow to prevent permanent tissue damage.

Arms

Very few patients present with symptoms related to major occlusive arterial disease of the arms but symptoms of claudication and rest pain do occur. Brachial emboli are relatively common and the presentation is nearly always with numbness and weakness rather than a white hand. Management involves local anaesthetic embolectomy followed by long-term anti-coagulation.

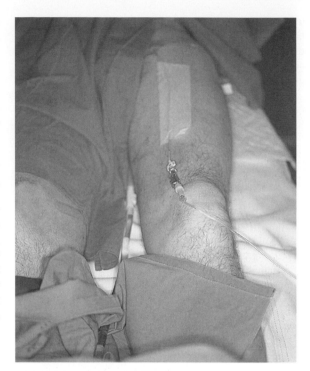

Figure 15.14. Intra-arterial thrombolysis.

Raynaud's disease is common in younger patients. Vasospasm causes coldness and pallor in relation to certain stimuli (usually cold) followed by blue then red discoloration and pain as the arterial circulation dilates again. Occasionally, the disease is severe enough to produce digital ulceration or gangrene. The majority of patients can be managed by avoidance of cold stimuli and the use of heated gloves if needed. Nifedipine can give short-term relief but headache often limits its use in the long term. Episodes of ulceration or gangrene may require guanethidine blockade or hospital admission for prostacyclin infusion or trans-thoracic endoscopic sympathectomy.

Mesentery

In the chronic situation the patient usually presents with severe cramp-like abdominal pain occurring 20–30 min after food and lasting up to 2 h. This is associated with fear of eating, marked weight loss and diarrhoea. Acute mesenteric ischaemia often leads to irreversible gut ischaemia requiring resection.

Renal

The presentation is with hypertension or chronic renal failure often exacerbated by treatment with angiotensin-converting enzyme (ACE) inhibitors. Endovascular intervention is usually successful but open surgery is occasionally required.

Cerebral

Internal Carotid artery (Fig. 15.15)

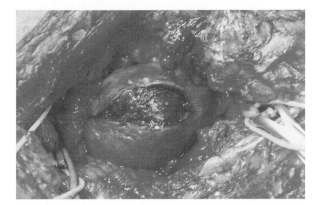

Figure 15.16. Thrombosed popliteal aneurysm.

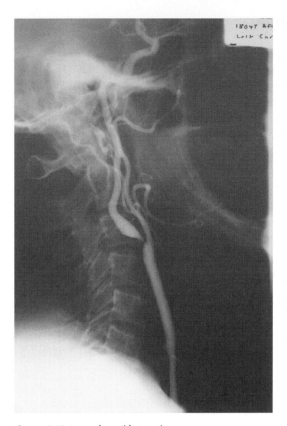

Figure 15.15. Internal carotid stenosis.

Patients present in three principal ways:
1. ischaemic stroke without full recovery;
2. stroke with recovery taking >24 h;
3. transient ischaemic attack (TIA) in which the neurological deficit lasts <24 h. This may affect the cerebral hemisphere producing contralateral symptoms or amaurosis fugax giving ipsilateral blindness due to retinal artery embolisation.

Patients with symptomatic carotid disease have an increased risk of debilitating ischaemic stroke; management strategies are aimed at reducing this risk. Large studies from Europe and America have indicated that patients with stenoses >70% who have had symptoms within the past 6 months do better with surgical plus best medical management than medical management alone, provided the surgical team are experienced. The benefit from surgery appears to be greatest within the first few weeks following symptoms.

Patients with asymptomatic carotid disease have a lower risk of stroke but recent evidence shows that this risk is further reduced with surgical intervention. Patients with asymptomatic carotid disease undergoing major cardiac surgery are at high risk of peri-operative stroke; surgical correction prior to cardiac surgery reduces this risk considerably.

The operation of choice for a stenosis of the origin of the internal carotid artery (the commonest lesion) is endarterectomy with or without a patch. Clamping of the carotid artery during surgery naturally puts the patient at risk of intra-operative stroke. Insertion of a temporary bypass shunt may reduce this risk but carries morbidity itself. Many units are now performing the operation under local anaesthetic; a shunt can be inserted if there is any indication of cerebral ischaemia. Stroke rate from the operation should now be >2–3%. Endovascular management of carotid disease is being evaluated as an alternative in clinical trials.

Vertebral artery

Symptoms arising from vertebral artery disease are often ill defined. The usual symptoms are related to positional or rotational vertigo and occasionally to cortical visual disturbances. An occlusion of the proximal subclavian artery can result in the subclavian steal syndrome when the arm is exercised as blood is diverted from the posterior cerebral circulation by reverse flow in the vertebral artery. This can be treated by an endovascular procedure to the subclavian stenosis or a carotid to subclavian artery bypass at the root of the neck.

Degenerative aneurysmal disease

An aneurysm is defined as an artery that has expanded by 50% of its normal diameter. It should be remembered that the vessel also expands in length and therefore becomes tortuous. The nature of the pathological process is not fully understood. The arterial media has an increased protein content and reduced elastin and smooth muscle with resulting expansion of the collagenous adventitia. Atherosclerotic changes to the intima are probably secondary to damage due to flow disturbances within the aneurysmal vessel. An inflammatory infiltrate is seen in all vessel layers.

Although virtually any artery may be involved, the common sites in order of frequency are:
- aorta;
- iliac artery;
- popliteal artery; (Fig. 15.16)
- femoral artery;
- rarely visceral arteries.

Abdominal aortic aneurysms

90% of aortic aneurysms affect the infra-renal abdominal aorta, 8% the thoracic aorta and 2% both (thoraco-abdominal). If the aneurysm is operated on before rupture, the mortality should be 5% or less. Following rupture, it is thought that well over 50% of patients die, frequently undiagnosed, before arrival in hospital and the mortality of those receiving an operation approaches 50%.

Asymptomatic AAA

Ultrasound screening studies have shown an incidence of 5% in males aged 65–74, four times > that in females. A single ultrasound scan at the age of 65 in males is a cost effective tool for detecting asymptomatic AAA and arrangements are underway for a national screening programme.

Large studies have concluded that small infra-renal AAAs, less than 5.5 cm in antero-posterior diameter as measured on ultrasound, can safely be entered into a surveillance programme of 6-monthly repeat ultrasounds. As long as they remain asymptomatic and expand slowly (<0.5 cm in 6 months) they carry an annual rupture rate of 1%. Aneurysms >5.5 cm carry an annual rupture rate of about 10% which increases with aneurysm size and this is an indication for aneurysm repair if the patient is fit for surgery.

Symptomatic AAA

Symptoms of abdominal or back pain, which may radiate to the groin, or tenderness on palpating an aneurysm should be taken as a predictor of imminent rupture and repair should be undertaken as soon as possible.

The differential diagnosis includes:

- sciatica,
- osteoporotic vertebral collapse,
- renal or ureteric pain,
- pancreatitis,
- perforated duodenal ulcer,
- myocardial infarction.

Ruptured AAA

This surgical emergency should be suspected in anyone with abdominal or back pain and collapse. A pulsatile mass can usually, but not always, be palpated. If the diagnosis is obvious then immediate surgical repair is indicated. CT should only be performed if there is doubt about the diagnosis and the patient is well compensated.

Open repair

The aneurysm is replaced by inserting a prosthetic graft inside the aneurysm after appropriate mobilisation and clamping of the arteries (Fig. 15.17). The graft may be a simple tube graft to above the aortic bifurcation or may extend as a 'trouser' graft distally to one or both iliac or femoral arteries. The operation carries a mortality of around 5% but returns the patient to a life expectancy equal to their age matched peers.

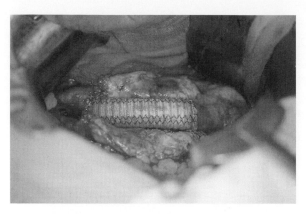

Figure 15.17. Gelatin-impregnated Dacron graft replacing aortic aneurysm.

Endovascular aneurysm repair (EVAR)

A covered stent graft is deployed under X-ray control via an open approach to the femoral arteries avoiding the need for aortic cross-clamping. The procedure carries a lower operative mortality but a cumulative annual 10% re-intervention rate for device failure or slippage or continued aneurysm expansion is required. Patients require annual CT surveillance. Long team outcomes for EVAR are as yet unknown. EVAR confers to survival benefit over conservative management in patients unfit for open surgery.

Aneurysm at other sites

Femoral and popliteal aneurysms are treated by simple graft replacement. A thrombosed femoral or popliteal aneurysm is a surgical emergency which carries a 25% risk of limb loss.

Diabetic foot

Diabetes mellitus is becoming more prevalent especially in the developed nations. Tissue loss and sepsis in the feet of diabetic patients is common and is due to a combination of the following:

- Atherosclerotic occlusive peripheral vascular disease.
  - Diabetes mellitus is a potent risk factor; the vessels are characteristically very calcified and often confined to the calf vessels, indeed the popliteal pulse is frequently present.
- 'Small vessel' occlusive disease in the vessels distal to the arterial arches of the foot.
- Peripheral neuropathy, leading to pressure areas or sepsis due to unnoticed foreign bodies in the foot.
- Charcot's changes in the joints between the bones of the foot, leading to deformity and ulceration at resulting pressure points.

Management

- Preventative:
  - Good glycaemic control.

- Risk factor management for peripheral vascular disease.
- Fanatical foot care; podiatrist, chiropidist, well-fitted shoes.
- Re-vascularisation:
  - Concept of 'supercharging' the arterial supply to encourage healing may be beneficial with calf vessel angioplasty or vein graft to the dorsalis pedis artery.
- Debridement:
  - Surgical to bleeding tissue, larval or chemical (de-sloughing dressings with anti-septic properties).
- Antibiotics:
  - For systemic sepsis or frank cellulitis; systemic antibiotics will not enter dead tissue so are not a substitute for debridement.
- Hyperbaric oxygen:
  - There is some evidence that this enhances healing.
- Primary amputation:
  - Digital if blood supply to foot adequate, that is, foot pulse or biphasic signal on hand-held Doppler assessment.
  - 'Salami slicing' amputations over a period of months can be very counter-productive, slowing the patient's rehabilitation and may well lead to a higher eventual level of amputation.
  - Otherwise active diabetics who suffer significant foot sepsis at a young age may be better served with a primary below knee amputation.
  - The combination of peripheral vascular disease chronic renal failure and diabetes invariably results in a major amputation once tissue loss occurs.

Arterial trauma

(See also Chapter 7)

Arterial injury may occur as a result of penetrating injury from missiles or sharp instruments, blunt injury in relation to fractures, injury in relation to acute deceleration (thoracic aorta) or as a result of invasive surgical or radiological procedures.

The types of arterial injury are:
- penetration or laceration of the artery,
- transection of the artery with retraction of the ends,
- transection of intima with intact adventitia,
- contusion and thrombosis,
- distal embolisation.

The signs of arterial injury are:
- absent or diminished peripheral pulses with or without peripheral ischaemia;
- major haemorrhage;
- large or expanding haematoma;
- bruit at or near the site of injury;
- pulsatile mass at the site of injury.

Management

In patients with penetrating injury the site of injury to the artery is usually obvious and preliminary arteriography is

unnecessary. If there is major haemorrhage, immediate exploration is required. In those with penetrating injuries in the root of the neck or the chest or in those with major soft tissue or bony injuries, arteriography is of value if the patient is clinically stable. If in doubt, explore.

Complications of arterial surgery

Patients undergoing vascular surgery suffer the same complications as those undergoing any major surgical procedure but in addition there are some complications to which they are particularly prone and these are discussed below.

Cardiac

Patients with arterial disease all have a degree of coronary artery disease and any hypotensive episode, common during major surgery, enhances the risk of myocardial infarction. The peak incidence of cardiac ischaemia occurs on post-operative day 2–3.

The following co-morbidities predispose to myocardial infarction:
- Previous myocardial infarction: If the patient has suffered a previous myocardial infarction either within 3 months, 4–6 months or more than 6 months previously then the re-infarction risk is 37%, 16% and 6%, respectively.
- Angina pectoris; unstable > stable.
- Uncontrolled moderate to severe hypertension.
- Left ventricular failure.
- Arrhythmias.

Respiratory

Most patients with arterial disease have a compromised respiratory system due to chronic smoking. Chronic obstructive pulmonary disease, poor nutrition, emergency surgery, duration and type of anaesthesia, site of incision and prolonged post-operative ileus or immobility are all risk factors for post-operative respiratory complications. These include acute respiratory failure, atelectasis, and bacterial pneumonitis.

Cerebral

Due to concomitant carotid artery and cerebrovascular disease any hypotensive episode may result in an ischaemic stroke.

Renal

Interference with renal arteries during aortic surgery, episodes of hypotension or myoglobinuria following re-vascularisation all contribute to the development of renal failure. This may be reduced by maintaining a satisfactory blood volume and maintaining a high urine output.

Reperfusion injury

When tissue that has been ischaemic for an extended period (>6 h) is re-vascularised various vasoactive substances enter the blood stream causing severe hypotension often requiring inotropic support. Inflammatory mediators are also released which can cause a systemic inflammatory response syndrome (SIRS) and end organ damage. Coagulation cascades may be triggered and large quantities of myoglobin spill over from the dead muscle cells into the circulation.

Haemorrhage

The use of heparin will increase the risk of haemorrhage but it is essential to prevent thrombosis during arterial cross-clamping. In patients requiring major transfusion, coagulopathy is common and should be anticipated by early correction with clotting factors. Meticulous anastomotic technique is required to minimise bleeding.

Limb ischaemia

This may take the form of distal embolisation resulting in minor digital ischaemia (trash foot) or major ischaemia due to graft thrombosis. Distal embolisation should be prevented by suitable techniques such as preliminary iliac clamping before mobilisation of the aorta in patients with aortic aneurysms. Early major graft occlusion requires early re-exploration and usually indicates a defective technique, poor conduit or inappropriate patient selection. Late graft occlusion is usually due to disease progression or neo-intimal hyperplasia.

Compartment syndrome

This complication is commonest after successful treatment of acute ischaemia. It must be expected and looked for so that early decompression may be undertaken before irreversible ischaemic damage has occurred.

Graft infection

This complication is a major disaster. In the early post-operative period it should be prevented by the use of prophylactic antibiotics (usually given at the time of surgery and continued for 1–2 days), the avoidance of haematoma, careful wound closure to prevent ischaemic necrosis of the wound, meticulous attention to aseptic techniques and the use of rifampicin-bonded grafts. Late infections result from bacteraemia and therefore patients with prosthetic grafts should receive antibiotic prophylaxis during any invasive procedure.

Methicillin-resistant *staphylococcus aureus* (MRSA) graft infection is becoming a major problem in many vascular units in the UK. Risk can be reduced by pre-operative eradication of MRSA from the patient, the use of autologous vein as a conduit whenever feasible, meticulous wound care and hygiene post-operatively and the avoidance of injudicious use of antibiotics on the unit. Management of these patients is very challenging once this infection has set in.

Lymphatic leak

This is common in the groin following reconstruction. A lateral approach to the femoral artery and layered closure reduces the incidence but there is no foolproof method of avoiding this complication. It usually ceases spontaneously in 7–10 days. Care must be taken to avoid secondary infection as this is a major source of graft infection.

DISORDERS OF VEINS OF THE LOWER LIMB

Anatomy

The venous system in the leg is anatomically divided into two main components, deep and superficial. The deep veins are in close proximity to the arteries supplying the lower limb, from which their names are derived. In the calf these tend to be paired, on either side of the artery, and are termed venae comitantes. The superficial veins lie superficial to the deep facia and are unaccompanied by arteries. There is much overlap in the distribution of the territories drained, but tributaries from the medial aspect of the leg mostly join the long saphenous system while those from the lateral aspect of the calf join the short saphenous system. Perforating veins connect the deep and superficial venous systems by passing through the deep fascia; the normal direction of flow in these veins is from superficial to deep.

Pathophysiology

The major venous plexuses in the lower leg and foot are anatomically positioned so that they are compressed during normal ambulation, thus pumping venous blood towards the heart. Their position, between the soleus and gastrocnemius muscles in the calf and between the first and second muscle layers of the sole of the foot, is such that even muscle contractions while stationary are sufficient to pump blood proximally. The investing deep fascia surrounding the calf muscles ensures that much of the pressure generated by the muscular contractions, in excess of 200 mmHg, is transmitted directly to the deep calf veins. This force is also transmitted to the superficial veins via the connective tissue.

The muscle pumps are at their most efficient during normal ambulation, any deviation from this reducing their activity. Such gait abnormalities may be caused by:
- Localised or generalised muscle weakness;
- Localised or generalised neurological disorders;
- Ankle joint stiffness, due to an arthropathy, the effect of trauma or under-use;
- Knee, hip or spinal pathology;
- Frailty in elderly patients;
- Pain.

Bicuspid valves throughout the venous system maintain the unidirectional flow of blood towards the heart. These counteract the effect of gravity on the column of blood from the head to the foot. The term venous reflux describes the flow of blood, towards the feet and occurs to a minor degree in normal subjects, as the valves are closing. When prolonged, due to valve malfunction, it is termed venous insufficiency and

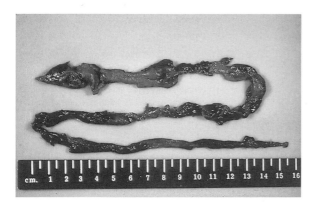

Figure 15.18. Thrombectomy specimen showing foci of white thrombus from within the value cusps and dark consecutive thrombosis between.

leads to venous hypertension. Valve damage is usually primary (i.e. of unknown aetiology), but may be secondary to previous thrombus formation and subsequent recanalisation and scarring within the vein (Fig. 15.18).

The walls of varicose veins have been shown to be deficient in elastin and collagen and are dilated and tortuous. It is not known whether these changes are primary, leading to valve failure and venous hypertension, or if these changes are secondary to the effect of high venous pressure following valvular insufficiency.

Venous hypertension is responsible for the symptoms and skin complications of varicose veins. Many of the early symptoms may be related to venous congestion but as the hypertension becomes established microcirculatory changes occur. There has been much debate as to the exact mechanism by which they lead to tissue damage and poor tissue healing. Perivascular fibrin cuffs, seen in tissue biopsies from lipodermatosclerotic skin, might provide a barrier to the diffusion of oxygen, causing local necrosis. White cell trapping within tissues exposed to high venous pressures is well documented, causing neutrophil degranulation and activation of various inflammatory cascades leading to tissue damage.

Classification

In order to standardise descriptions of venous disorders the CEAP-Classification was presented by the American Venous Forum in 1995 and takes into account clinical signs (C), aetiology (E), anatomical distribution (A) and pathophysiological dysfunction (P). The clinical signs considered by this classification are summarised below:
- Class 0: No visible or palpable signs of venous disease.
- Class 1: Telangiectases (intradermal vein ectasias) or reticular veins (impalpable, dilated, tortuous subcutaneous veins, not belonging to saphenous veins or their major branches).
- Class 2: Varicose veins (palpable).
- Class 3: Oedema.

- Class 4: Skin changes ascribed to venous disease (e.g. pigmentation, venous eczema, lipodermatosclerosis).
- Class 5: Skin changes as defined above with healed ulceration.
- Class 6: Skin changes as defined above with active ulceration.

The aetiology part of the assessment recognises congenital (E_C), primary (E_P) and secondary (E_S) venous disease. The anatomic part describes disease as in superficial (A_S), deep (A_D) or perforating (A_P) veins. The physiology of the venous disease is described as refluxing (P_R), obstructive (P_O) or combined (P_{RO}).

Varicose veins

Epidemiology

Varicose veins are extremely prevalent; 10–25% of the adult population in the Western world. It was thought that the incidence of varicose veins was lower in males and outside the western world, but this has recently been disputed. However it appears that even if the prevalence of varicose veins, and perhaps venous insufficiency, is similar in developing countries, the number of symptoms and complications they cause is almost certainly lower. Classical teaching is that the incidence of varicose veins is higher in occupations involving prolonged periods of standing or sitting and in pregnancy. While this has been supported by some but by no means all studies, it is likely that their symptoms are worse.

Clinical features

Patients with varicose veins complain of a rather nebulous set of symptoms namely leg aches, swelling, restlessness and pain or itching over specific veins. These are difficult to quantify and correlate poorly with the visible extent and size of the varicosities, which causes a problem for health care providers who are increasingly encouraged to only intervene surgically for symptoms rather than for pure cosmesis. From the epidemiological data outlined above, it would appear that female caucasian legs are more susceptible to the skin changes brought on by venous hypertension; it would be reasonable to assume that they are also likely to genuinely suffer more symptoms from their varicose veins.

The skin changes occur in the gaiter region, between the knee and the malleoli, and may consist of venous eczema and/or lipodermatosclerosis. These are often a prelude to venous ulceration and are an indication for intervention.

Assessment

The sites of venous reflux can be estimated from the anatomical distribution and hand-held Doppler assessment. The Trendelenberg tourniquet test is less often employed now but may be a useful examination of venous reflux. The patient lies supine and the examiner raises the leg and massages the dilated veins towards the trunk until they are empty. A tourniquet is then applied around the upper third of the thigh and the patient is asked to stand. Filling below the tourniquet

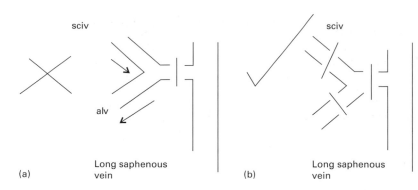

Figure 15.19. Ligating branches of the long saphenous vein. (a) Only the common stem of the superficial iliac vein (sciv) and the anterolateral vein (alv) are ligated resulting in continued reflux down the thig and 'recurrent' varicose veins. (b) Correct procedure where all three veins are ligated.

indicates incompetence between the deep and superficial systems (i.e. short saphenous or perforator(s)). Release of the tourniquet will show whether there is reflux from above (i.e. sapheno-femoral or a perforator depending on the position of the tourniquet). Repeating this test by applying the tourniquet at different levels will give added information.

Hand-held Doppler assessment with the patient standing can diagnose reflux in the popliteal fossa or at the sapheno-femoral junction. Flow is augmented by manually squeezing the calf. Reflux is present if reverse flow of more than 1 s is detected on releasing the calf. Popliteal fossa reflux may be in the deep veins or the sapheno–popliteal junction and requires confirmation with venous duplex imaging. This is also required for the pre-operative assessment of recurrent varicose veins, where there is any suggestion of deep venous thrombosis (DVT) now or in the past or if the distribution of veins is unusual.

Management
Graduated compression hosiery

Compression stockings worn by the patient during the day controls many of the symptoms from varicose veins. They may be helpful in distinguishing symptoms from the varicose veins from other pathologies. They may reduce the chance of ulceration in patients with significant skin changes awaiting surgery.

Compression sclerotherapy

This technique requires no anaesthetic. The needle is placed in the filled vein as the patient stands but the injection should be made with the patient supine and the leg held above the heart. This partly empties the vein and the blood remaining adjacent to the needle tip is swept away with the index finger and thumb of the other hand before the sclerosant is injected into the empty vein. Direct pressure is maintained over the point of injection as graduated compression is applied over the leg from the base of the toes upwards. Extravasation of sclerosant outside the venous lumen may cause cutaneous ulceration. Most units reserve this therapy for varicosities or thread veins not associated with main stem (long or short saphenous) reflux.

Open surgery

Immediately before surgery the varicosities of the leg are marked while the patient stands. Surgery is then undertaken guided by the pre-operative assessment:

Sapheno-femoral junction disconnection ('Trendeleberg's operation' or 'high tie')

The sapheno-femoral junction should be exposed by an incision in the groin crease immediately medial to the femoral pulse. Care must be taken to identify positively the long saphenous vein before dividing it. Careful ligation and division of the tributaries should be carried out (Fig. 15.19).

Long saphenous stripping

Sapheno-femoral junction disconnection may be carried out under local anaesthetic but this procedure requires general or regional anaesthesia. New venous tributaries tend to re-connect the junction with the long saphenous remnant (neovascularisation); long saphenous vein stripping significantly reduces the recurrence rate compared to junction disconnection alone. Damage to the saphenous nerve trip in the lower leg can be reduced by only stripping as far as the knee and towards the foot.

Sapheno–popliteal junction disconnection

The position of the sapheno–popliteal junction is very variable and occasionally the short saphenous vein will have a major connection with the medial thigh vein. The junction should be marked pre-operatively either by hand-held Doppler or preferably with venous duplex. It is then approached through a transverse incision with the patient prone. Evidence is emerging that the junction is missed in a proportion of cases even by experienced surgeons using these techniques. The upper 10 cm of the vein should be avulsed rather than a longer section stripped as the latter may damage the sural nerve, rendering the heel anaesthetic. Sensory nerve damage is common after a dissection of the popliteal fossa and occasional damage of a motor nerve can be devastating. Serious neurological sequelae occur in about 1% of cases and are probably much higher in redo surgery.

Calf phlebectomy

Calf phlebectomy is necessary to remove the varicose tributaries in the leg and thigh, which will otherwise remain even if the saphenous reflux is dealt with. Local areas of cutaneous neuropraxia are common.

Straightforward varicose vein surgery in otherwise fit patients can conveniently be done on a day basis. The aim should be to return the patient to full activity within 2 weeks following operation.

Complications of surgery include:
- damage to the common femoral or popliteal vein;
- DVT or pulmonary embolism;
- damage to sural, saphenous, femoral, tibial or common peroneal nerves;
- haematoma, wound infection and wound edge necrosis;
- recurrence of varicose veins; about 15% at 5 years.

Endovascular treatment of varicose veins

These techniques aim to oblitrate the lumen of the long saphenous vein and its tributaries by percutaneous methods. A catheter with a specialised tip is advanced from the knee or ankle under ultrasound control as far as the sapheno-femoral junction. Heat is generated at the catheter tip either by pulsed laser or radiofrequency energy whilst external pressure closes the vein.

Foam sclerotherapy is similar to injection sclerotherapy but the sclerosant is mixed with carbon dioxide or air under pressure, spreading the sclerosant throughout the veins under ultrasound control.

Early results for these techniques are promising and they appear to be safe. The longer term outcomes are currently being assessed in randomised controlled trials.

Venous ulceration

Epidemiology

It is estimated that 0.3% of the population has an active leg ulcer at any one time. For one patient with an open ulcer there are about three with a healed ulcer who should be considered at risk due to the natural history of high ulcer recurrence rates, so the overall prevalence of healed and open ulcers is around 1%. The prevalence of open leg ulceration rises exponentially with age, being rare below the age of 40 but >2% over the age of 80; a huge drain on community nursing resources. The incidence of ulcers in females is 2–3 that in males.

Studies into the natural history of varicose veins showed that the late incidence of venous ulcers is related to the severity of the varicose veins earlier in the study and the development of ulceration is related to the severity of venous incompetence. A history of DVT is a common finding in patients with leg ulceration but surprisingly few patients suffer ulceration following DVT.

Assessment

The key to the management of leg ulcers is to understand their aetiology. 70% of leg ulcers are purely venous, 10%

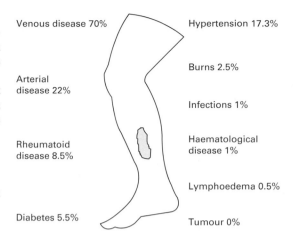

Figure 15.20. Conditions associated with leg ulceration.

purely arterial and 10% mixed arterial and venous. Diabetes mellitus and rheumatoid disease are important co-factors in some patients. In 10% no arterial or venous insufficiency is found on investigation and these probably represent postural problems or insufficiency in the lymphatic system; they are managed in the same way as venous ulcers (Fig. 15.20).

The appearance of the ulcer is of little value but clinical examination may reveal other signs of arterial or venous insufficiency.

The ABPI is a very useful guide with the following arbitrary cut off points (beware in diabetics):
- >0.8 = 'pure venous' ulcer,
- between 0.8 and 0.5 = 'mixed arterial/venous' ulcer,
- <0.5 = 'pure arterial' ulcer; manage as a critically ischaemic limb.

Venous duplex should be carried out to map the pattern of reflux in all patients with leg ulcers. In 60% the reflux is confined to the superficial (saphenous) veins, in 5% the deep veins alone and in 35% both deep and superficial veins are involved. In the latter group the reflux may be in all the deep venous segments or just in certain segments (segmental deep reflux).

It should be remembered that visible varicosities are only present in 40% of patients with superficial venous reflux.

1% of leg ulcers are due to a cutaneous malignancy (usually a squamous or basal cell carcinoma). Any ulcer failing to heal at 3 months or having an unusual clinical appearance should be biopsied.

Management of pure venous ulcers

The management is primarily aimed at treating the underlying venous hypertension. Much of it can be achieved successfully in specialist nurse led clinics, on a shared care basis with community nurses, with easy access to the vascular services.

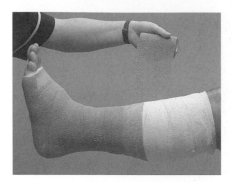

Figure 15.21. Multilayer compression therapy.

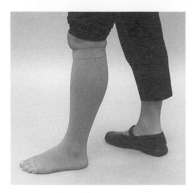

Figure 15.22. Graduated compression hosiery.

Elevation

The patient must be encouraged to regularly spend periods during the day lying down with the leg elevated on pillows so that the foot is above the heart. They should avoid sitting or standing for long periods with their legs fully dependant.

Exercise

Too often patients are told to rest. Walking activates the venous muscle pumps as does regularly moving the ankles and toes. Ankle flexion is possible within multilayer compression and it should be encouraged. The degree of ankle mobility is directly proportional to the leg ulcer healing rate.

Graduated compression

For the treatment of open ulceration multilayer elastic systems are superior to single bandages and should allow a pressure of 40 mmHg or more at the ankle, reducing to about half that below the knee. The first layer should be a generous one of wool roll followed by a bandage to compress the wool such as a white crepe bandage. On this foundation the elastic compression bandages should be applied (Fig. 15.21).

Healing rates of 60% or more at 6 months should be possible, but 20% remain unhealed at 1 year.

Healed legs should be fitted with compression hosiery aiming for an ankle pressure of 18 mmHg (Fig. 15.22). These should be worn during the day indefinitely and be renewed once in 3 months.

Superficial venous surgery

This does not improve ulcer healing rates but there is now level one evidence that it is very important in reducing ulcer recurrence. In patients with isolated superficial reflux or mixed superficial and segmental deep reflux, representing 85% of patients with venous leg ulcers, simple varicose vein surgery reduces the ulcer recurrence rate at 3 years from 50% to 20%. In the elderly a sapheno-femoral or sapheno–popliteal junction ligation can be carried out under local anaesthetic.

Perforator surgery

There has been a recent resurgence in the popularity of perforator ligation due to the advantages of the endoscopic subfascial approach, without the difficulties relating to a large wound, by the development of endoscopic techniques through a more proximal, smaller incision ('SEPS'). In fact this technique is usually combined with open saphenous vein surgery and it is probably the latter that has the greater effect on venous hypertension.

Local treatment of the ulcer

Usually a simple non-adherent dressing is all that is required as a primary dressing under the compression. Chemical or larval debridement can be employed if there is excessive slough. Systemic antibiotics are only useful if there is frank cellulitus, only then should ulcers be swabbed for bacteriology as they will always share the patient's normal skin flora. Split or pinch skin grafts are often used on large ulcers and can be placed under compression bandages; there is no level one evidence regarding their effect on healing rate.

Nutrition

Obese patients should be advised that weight loss will help their ulceration and undernourished patients will have slow healing. Any underlying anaemia should be addressed.

Management of mixed arterial/venous ulcers

The conservative measures are as for pure venous ulceration. A reduced level of compression should be employed, aiming for 23 mmHg at the ankle, under close supervision. If the ulcer fails to heal or gets worse then the patient should be investigated with a view to re-vascularisation.

Deep venous thrombosis

See also Chapter 1.

Deep venous thrombosis (DVT) is the process by which thrombus forms in the deep veins of the calf, thigh or pelvis – or any combination of these.

Presentation

The thrombosis may be occlusive or non-occlusive and the process may start at any level, usually in the valve sinuses. It may start in the lower leg and progress proximally, but equally may start in the pelvis, or synchronously at several levels. Since many of the underlying factors are systemic, there are often bilateral thromboses. DVT commonly follows major surgery or serious illness, it is common in patients suffering from cancer and may be the initial presentation; invariably so if the thrombosis is extensive enough to cause venous gangrene.

Any DVT may embolize, the larger life-threatening emboli usually coming from the pelvic veins. Commonly, the patient who has sustained a fatal pulmonary embolism has no leg swelling, suggesting that the thrombus was large, pelvic, non-occlusive and so poorly attached to the vein wall. About 50% of major, life-threatening pulmonary emboli are preceded by a small herald embolus.

Investigation

Duplex ultrasound is the best way to look at the deep veins of the leg, the critical areas to scan being the popliteal, femoral and pelvic veins of the suspected and the other leg. Young patients with no obvious predisposing factors for thromboembolic disease should be investigated early for hypercoagulability syndromes. Blood samples should be taken prior to starting the heparin infusion.

Management

Anticoagulation should be started on suspicion of a DVT pending confirmation by investigation. Warfarin should be continued for 3 months (6 months for a pulmonary embolus).

Thrombolysis or thrombectomy may have to be considered in *phlegmasia cerulea dolens* when there is sudden massive swelling and impending venous gangrene, but in less desperate situations the advantage of these treatments is outweighed by the potential complications of bleeding, re-thrombosis or embolisation.

The swollen leg must be elevated well above the level of the heart until the swelling subsides. Elevation, if it is high enough, will always reduce the leg swelling, when graduated compression hosiery may be safely applied.

Vena-caval filters are reserved for patients having recurrent pulmonary emboli in spite of full anticoagulation.

Longer-term sequelae

In 90% of cases of DVT the occlusion resolves as the clot contracts and recanalises. However, valvular function is lost more

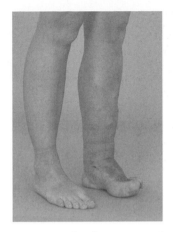

Figure 15.23. Klippel–Trenaunay syndrome.

often than not and persistent swelling and venous hypertension usually follow. Late ulceration rates are reduced by prescribing long-term graduated compression hosiery to all patients following a DVT.

Venous malformations

The commonest congenital venous anomalies are:
• Klippel–Trenaunay syndrome (Fig. 15.23);
• arterio-venous anomalies;
• phlebangiomas.
The Klippel–Trenaunay syndrome is associated with congenital varicose veins, haemangiomas and limb overgrowth. The distribution in the leg is almost invariably posterolateral. The pelvis is the commonest site for arterio-venous abnormalities and they are best managed by a combination of embolisation by selective catheterisation and graduated compression. Following fusion of the epiphyses, bone shortening may be undertaken. Capillary and cavernous haemangiomas should not normally be operated on, the mainstay of treatment being graduated compression and foam sclerotherapy.

FURTHER READING

Earnshaw JJ, Murie JA. *The Evidence for Vascular Surgery.* Shropshire: TFM Publishing Ltd

16

Endocrine Surgery

David Lee and Robert G Hardy

Department of General Surgery, Royal Infirmary, Edinburgh, UK

CONTENTS

Thyroid glands	**304**
Embryology	304
Anatomy	304
Blood supply	305
Histology	306
Physiology	306
Clinical examination	306
Investigations	306
Thyroid disorders	307
Parathyroid glands	**310**
Embryology	310
Anatomy	310
Physiology	311
Parathyroid disorders	312
Adrenal glands	**313**
Anatomy	313
Histology	313
Physiology	313
Glucocorticoids	314
Mineralocorticoids	314
Disorders of the adrenal glands	315
Hypothalamus/pituitary gland	**317**
Anatomy	317
Physiology	317
Pituitary tumours	318
Tumours of the gastro-intestinal tract and pancreas	**318**
Multiple endocrine neoplasia	**320**
Further reading	**320**

THYROID GLAND

Embryology

The thyroid gland is formed from an ectodermal down-growth from the first and second pharyngeal pouches and descends to its final level just below the cricoid cartilage. The line of descent is known as the thyroglossal tract and, by the time of birth, this has normally involuted and disappeared. During descent, the thyroid gland comes in contact with the ultimobranchial bodies from the fourth pharyngeal pouches and cells from these are thought to form the parafollicular, calcitonin producing or 'C-cells' of the thyroid. On reaching its final position, the thyroid divides into two lobes with a central bridge or isthmus. The site of origin forms the foramen caecum of the tongue.

Embryological abnormalities are:
- failure of descent – this may result in a lingual thyroid, an upper midline neck swelling, or a pyramidal lobe.
- cell nests in a persisting thyroglossal tract – these may result in a thyroglossal cyst.
- over descent resulting in a retrosternal goitre.
- agensis of one lobe – this may cause confusion on an isotope scan with a solitary nodule in one lobe and a cold area on the contralateral side.

Anatomy

The normal thyroid gland consists of two lateral lobes joined in the midline by a bridge of thyroid tissue or isthmus. The lobes extend from the level of the thyroid cartilage superiorly to the 5th or 6th tracheal rings inferiorly. The isthmus is variable in width and rests on the 2nd to 4th tracheal rings. Occasionally a pyramidal lobe extends from the isthmus superiorly and may reach as high as the hyoid bone (Figs 16.1 and 16.2).

The gland is encased in a sheath of pre-tracheal fascia which is attached to the arch of the cricoid cartilage and the oblique line of the thyroid cartilage. The thyroid therefore moves upwards on closure of the larynx on swallowing.

The *anatomical relations* of the thyroid are as follows:
- *Medially* (from below upwards)
  - trachea, oesophagus, and recurrent laryngeal nerve;
  - cricoid cartilage;
  - thyroid cartilage;
  - cricothyroid and inferior constrictor muscles;
  - external branch of the superior laryngeal nerve.

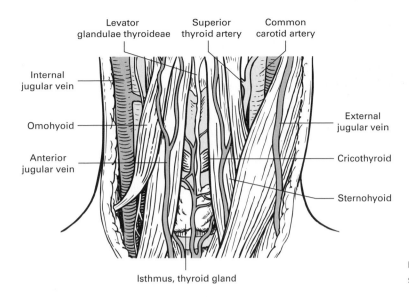

Figure 16.1. Dissection of the front of the neck showing the position of the thyroid gland.

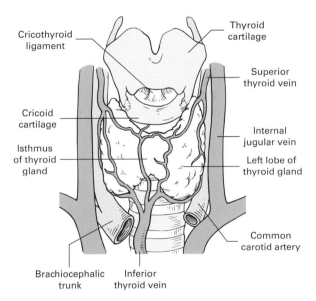

Figure 16.2. Anterior surface of the thyroid gland.

- *Anteriorly*
  - sternohyoid and sternothyroid;
  - anterior border of sternocleidomastoid.
- *Postero-laterally*
  - the carotid sheath containing the common carotid artery, internal jugular vein and vagus nerve.
- *Posteriorly*
  - cervical pre-vertebral muscles.

The relation to the parathyroid glands is very variable. The superior glands most commonly are adjacent to the intersection of the recurrent laryngeal nerve and the inferior thyroid artery, and the inferior glands are at the lower pole of the lobe or inferior to this.

Blood supply

At rest, the thyroid gland has the highest rate of blood flow of any organ in the body.

Thyroid arteries

The *superior thyroid artery* arises at the origin of the external carotid artery, runs downwards to the superior pole of the thyroid lobe, divides into 2–3 branches and enters the lobe on its posterior aspect.

The *inferior thyroid artery* arises from the thyro-cervical trunk which originates from the first part of the subclavian artery. It ascends initially, then turns medially at the level of the cricoid cartilage. From here it passes posterior to the internal jugular vein, the common carotid artery and the vagus nerve in the carotid sheath, and also behind the sympathetic trunk. It enters the posterior aspect of the thyroid at about the middle of the lobe.

The *thyroid ima artery* is rare and enters the thyroid isthmus inferiorly. It may arise from the brachiocephalic trunk, the left common carotid artery or even the aortic arch.

Venous drainage

The *superior thyroid vein* arises from the posterior aspect of the superior pole of thyroid and turns to immediately enter the internal jugular vein.

The *middle thyroid vein* runs laterally from the antero-lateral aspect of the thyroid lobe to enter the internal jugular vein.

The *inferior thyroid vein* arises as a leash of small vessels from the inferior aspect of the lower pole of each thyroid lobe to form a single vein. The veins from each side run in parallel inferiorly to enter the brachiocephalic veins immediately before they unite to form the superior vena cava.

An accessory vein may also run upwards from the isthmus, particularly if a pyramidal lobe is present.

Histology

The thyroid gland is formed of multiple follicles. These are spherical and encased by a single layer of cubicle follicular cells. The content of each follicle is known as 'colloid' and stains pink on haematoxylin-and-eosin (H & E) staining.

Between the follicles are clusters of cells – lymphocytes, macrophages and 'C-cells' or parafollicular cells.

Physiology

Over 90% of absorbed iodine (approximately 75 μg daily) is taken up by the thyroid gland as iodide. This is actively transported from the circulation into the colloid of the follicles where it is rapidly oxidised, bound to tyrosine, forming mono-iodotyrosine. It then becomes attached to thyroglobulin molecules. The mono-iodotyrosine is further iodinated to form di-iodotyrosine. Linkage of two di-iodotyrosine molecules with liberation of alanine results in thyroxine (T_4) while linkage of one mono-iodotyrosine molecule with one molecule of di-iodotyrosine, results in tri-iodothyronine (T_3). The condensation of di-iodotyrosine and mono-iodotyrosine results in the formation of 'reverse T_3' which is physiologically inactive. A normal thyroid gland produces approximately 80 μg/day of free thyroxine. In the follicles, T_3 and T_4 remain bound to thyroglobulin.

Thyroid secretion is controlled by a negative feedback mechanism involving the anterior pituitary gland. Thyroid stimulating hormone (TSH) from the anterior pituitary circulates to the thyroid where it binds to receptors on the cell membrane increasing thyroid cellular activity. This results in hydrolysis of thyroglobulin, releasing T_3 and T_4 into the plasma. Thyroxine is carried in the serum, mostly bound to thyroxine-binding globulin (TBG), although some is also carried to thyroxine-binding pre-albumin (TBPA) and to albumin itself. A small amount of thyroxine circulates free in the plasma and this is thought to be the physiologically active component which exerts negative feedback to the pituitary release of TSH. The biological half-life of T_4 is 6–7 days and of T_3 is only a few hours. It is thought that T_3 may be the active molecule and that the majority of T_4 may be converted to T_3 at a cellular level.

Thyrotrophin releasing hormone (TRH), a tri-peptide amide, is formed in the hypothalamus and passes down in the hypothalamic-pituitary portal venous system to stimulate the release of TSH, over-riding the negative feedback of T_4 and regulating the system.

The main effects of thyroxine are:
• increase in oxygen consumption in the tissues (calorogenic action),
• influences growth and maturation,
• helps to regulate body basal metabolic rate,
• increases absorption of carbohydrate from the intestine.

Clinical examination

The following points should be noted on history taking:
• any swelling – duration, progression, regression, fluctuation,
• pain,
• obstructive features – swallowing, breathing,
• voice change,
• difficulty coughing,
• symptoms to suggest hypo- or hyper-function,
• family history of thyroid or other endocrine disease,
• past medical history,
• drug history.

Rapid onset of a painful swelling usually suggests a cyst. A fluctuant swelling may suggest cyst or multinodular goitre. Compressive symptoms are most commonly associated with retrosternal goitre but may also suggest thyroiditis or malignancy. Voice change should be checked for vocal cord palsy and if confirmed is very suggestive of malignancy. A strong family history of thyroid disorders should alert the clinician to the possibility of auto-immune thyroiditis but a strong history of associated other endocrine disorders may suggest a multiple endocrine neoplasia (MEN) syndrome.

Toxic features with a diffuse goitre may be noted in either primary or pituitary-stimulated thyrotoxicosis. However toxicity with a nodular goitre may suggest a solitary toxic nodule or an advanced multinodular goitre.

Clinical examination should look for systemic features of thyroid disease, especially toxicity. Local examination should differentiate between diffuse or nodular goitre. Any nodule should be inspected for size, shape, fluctuance, whether solitary or part of a multinodular goitre, any retrosternal extension, and any associated cervical lymphadenopathy.

Investigations

The investigations for a patient with goitre are:
• thyroid function tests, *
• serum calcium,**
• thyroid antibodies (anti-peroxidase),
• X-rays of neck, thoracic inlet, chest,**
• ultrasound scan,
• isotope scan (essential in a thyrotoxic patient with a solitary thyroid nodule – differentiates a hot nodule in a normal gland from a cold nodule in a toxic gland),**
• computerised tomography (CT)/magnetic resonance imaging (MRI) scan (especially for suspected retrosternal gland),
• respiratory function tests (especially in a patient with stridor),
• fine-needle aspiration cytology (FNAC) (for a solitary nodule),**
• indirect laryngoscopy (especially for a re-do thyroidectomy, suspected malignancy or significant voice change).**

* = essential in all cases of goitre
** = essential pre-operative investigation

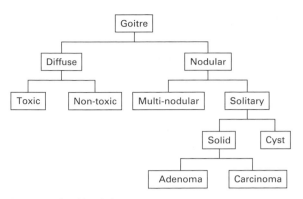

Figure 16.3. Thyroid pathology.

Thyroid disorders

Goitre is defined as enlargement of the thyroid and may be either diffuse or nodular. Diffuse forms may be toxic or non-toxic and nodular forms may be either multinodular or solitary (Fig. 16.3).

Diffuse goitre
Primary thyrotoxicosis

Primary thyrotoxicosis is an auto-immune disorder associated with a marked lymphocytic infiltrate into the gland. At least 90% of cases have associated positive thyroid auto-antibodies. The majority of patients have elevated T_4 levels, pure T_3 thyrotoxicosis being exceedingly rare. In both cases TSH is totally suppressed and this differentiates from pituitary-stimulated thyrotoxicosis where the TSH is markedly elevated. Clinical features are identical in all types and all forms can be associated with eye signs.

• lid retraction;
• lid lag;
• exophthalmos;
• ophthalmoplegia;
• diverging squint;
• corneal ulceration and blindness.

The earliest eye signs are lid retraction and lid lag. Examination for exophthalmos is best carried out from above, looking down. Ophthalmoplegia can affect any of the extra-ocular eye muscles, but most commonly the lateral rectus. Severe proptosis can result in a fixed diverging squint and inability to close the eye-lid, but this is extremely rare. Treatment is by orbital decompression possibly supplemented by lateral tarsorrhaphy.

Treatment of primary thyrotoxicosis may be either medical, surgical, or by use of radioiodine.

Medical treatment is by administration of oral medication, either carbimazole or propylthiouracil. Treatment should not be continued beyond 18 months because of risk of marrow suppression. However, about 40% of patients will remain euthyroid on cessation of treatment at this time and require no further therapy. There is some evidence to suggest that this group of patients may have a tendency to hypothyroidism in later life.

Radioiodine, administered as a single oral dose, may be given as a tailored dose to try to render the patient euthyroid. Such patients have a tendency to become more and more hypothyroid in time, even up to 10 years after treatment, and therefore require prolonged follow-up. Alternatively the radioiodine can be given as an ablating dose to produce hypothyroidism, followed by thyroxine therapy, without need for prolonged review. Because of early anxiety about possible risks of thyroid malignancy and potential teratogenic effects, radioiodine was only administered to patients aged 45 and over. However initial worries do not seem to have been confirmed and many centres now administer radioiodine to young patients as primary treatment for thyrotoxicosis.

Surgery was previously by bilateral sub-total thyroidectomy. However, because of the problems associated with treating the occasional patient who develops recurrent hyperthyroidism after surgery, many centres now perform total thyroidectomy accepting the need for life-long thyroxine and the possibility of permanent hypoparathyroidism. Certainly a thyroid remnant of over 6 g in weight has an unacceptable rate of recurrence of approximately 1%. The patient must be rendered euthyroid before surgery either with anti-thyroid drugs or iodide. The use of β-blockers alone is not advised but may be used to complement pre-operative management.

Initial post-operative hypothyroidism should not be treated if the patient is asymptomatic but the patient should be closely observed by regular thyroid function tests for 6 months at which time the ultimate thyroid function will have stabilised and a decision can be made about replacement therapy. Obviously if the patient becomes symptomatic during this time, then replacement therapy with thyroxine should be instituted.

Any eye signs may be exacerbated especially after radioiodine, but also occasionally after surgery. There is some evidence that immediate replacement therapy with thyroxine may reduce this problem. Other post-operative problems associated with thyroidectomy are:

• reactionary haemorrhage;
• hypocalcaemia;
• delayed hypothyroidism;
• hypoparathyroidism;
• recurrent laryngeal nerve palsy;
• external laryngeal nerve palsy.

Diffuse non-toxic goitre
The commonest causes are:
• physiological;
• colloid;
• iodine deficiency;
• dyshormonogenetic;
• thyroiditis;
• myxoedema.

Physiological goitre is usually a minimal diffuse swelling occurring at puberty, in pregnancy or at the menopause and reverses totally. Colloid goitre can result in a very large goitre and may require cosmetic surgery. Numerous syndromes may be associated with dyshormonogenetic goitre for example Pendred's syndrome with congenital deafness, and again many of these require surgery for cosmetic reasons.

Thyroiditis can occur in various forms including viral, Riedel's and Hashimoto's auto-immune thyroiditis. Auto-immune thyroiditis results in a marked lymphocytic infiltrate into the gland with ultimate destruction of thyroid function. Such patients require long-term follow-up of thyroid function to determine the timing and amount of thyroxine replacement. Hashimoto's thyroiditis can usually be diagnosed by serum auto-antibody estimation of peroxidase. Although auto-immune thyroiditis does not require surgery per se, it does predispose to malignancy for example lymphoma, and therefore a discrete nodule appearing in the gland may require surgery. Fine needle aspiration (FNA) can be exceedingly difficult to differentiate between lymphoma cells and the lymphocytes of thyroiditis and formal resection for histology is frequently necessary.

Nodular goitre
Multinodular goitre
Multinodular goitre is exceedingly common world-wide, occurring in about 4% of the world's population. The aetiology is unknown. The natural history is a progressive enlargement of the goitre with an increase in the size and number of the nodules, with a tendency to hyperthyroidism in later life. Multinodular goitre is associated with a low incidence of malignancy. Since this malignancy may not affect the largest nodules in the goitre, FNA cannot be relied on for the definitive exclusion of malignancy.

Multinodular goitre alone is not an indication for treatment. Medial therapy by suppression of TSH using thyroxine, has failed to have any impact on the progression of the disease and seems inappropriate in view of the tendency of the gland to become hyperthyroid. Radioiodine has also been tried without marked success. Treatment is therefore by surgery which will also afford the opportunity to examine the gland histologically.

Surgical treatment of multinodular goitre should be by total lobectomy or total thyroidectomy. Sub-total resection results in a reported 15% recurrence rate requiring further surgery. Re-resection of a lobe which has previously had a sub-total resection is associated with a 2–4% incidence of permanent recurrent laryngeal nerve damage.

The indications for surgery are:
- cosmetic;
- large dominant nodule;
- increasing gland size;
- increasing size of one nodule;
- retrosternal extension;
- hyperthyroidism;
- symptomatic airway or oesophageal compression.

Massive cervical enlargement may not be associated with any compression symptoms. Any patient presenting with dysphagia, dyspnoea, or venous compression should be suspected of having a retrosternal goitre, malignancy or thyroiditis.

In those patients not treated surgically, long-term follow-up is recommended by serial ultrasound scanning and thyroid function tests.

Solitary thyroid nodule
Solitary thyroid nodules may be either:
- cysts (10%);
- adenoma (70%);
- malignancy (20%).

Cysts. The aetiology is unknown. Histology consists of a thin-walled cyst with a fibrous capsule. In an uncomplicated cyst the fluid is clear. Clinically the patient may present with sudden appearance of a painful swelling indicating haemorrhage into the cyst and, although this may be frightening to the patient, it is rarely associated with any significant compression problems. Where ultrasound scan confirms a thin-walled cyst, treatment is by simple aspiration. However, if any of the following are present:
- scan suggests a thick-walled cyst;
- scan suggests a solid component to the cyst;
- scan suggests any irregularity in the line of the cyst wall;
- fluid aspirate is blood stained;
- swelling does not disappear completely on aspiration;
- swelling recurs rapidly after aspiration

then treatment should be by surgical removal. The incidence of malignancy in apparently simple thyroid cysts referred to a surgical clinic has been reported to be as high as 10% and is usually associated with a small papillary carcinoma in the wall of the cyst. The cytology of the fluid is unreliable in excluding malignancy.

Solitary thyroid adenoma. The aetiology is unknown. The histology is of a follicular lesion with a thin capsule and no cell infiltrate into or through the capsule. The natural history of follicular adenoma is of progressive enlargement. It is unclear whether follicular adenoma progresses to micro-invasion into the capsule and ultimately to frank carcinoma in a step wise fashion.

Investigation is by:
- thyroid function tests to exclude a toxic hot nodule;
- ultrasound scan to exclude a cyst;
- FNAC.

Since the cytology of follicular adenoma and carcinoma is identical, it is impossible to exclude malignancy by FNAC of a follicular lesion. The treatment of a solitary thyroid nodule which shows follicular cells on FNAC is by thyroid lobectomy. If the lesion is an adenoma, lobectomy is curative since these lesions are not multifocal. Frozen section histology to try to confirm the diagnosis of malignancy or adenoma can be technically very difficult and is not always accurate, even in the most expert hands.

In a patient who is biochemically thyrotoxic with a solitary nodule, an isotope scan is useful to confirm whether the nodule is a 'hot' hyperfunctioning adenoma with a surrounding suppressed gland or whether the patient has primary thyrotoxicosis and has a cold nodule present. This differentiation is vital if surgery is contemplated.

Malignancy. Despite its vascularity, the thyroid is rarely the site of secondary malignancy. Patients with spread from bronchogenic and breast carcinoma have been described but are very rare and kidney tumour (hypernephroma) is responsible for most cases. Since the thyroid is an ectodermal tissue, the commonest primary malignancy is an adenocarcinoma. In the elderly patient however, a primary non-Hodgkin's lymphoma may develop and this is particularly common in patients with known Hashimoto's thyroiditis.

1. *Thyroid lymphoma* is a non-Hodgkin B cell lymphoma. Diagnosis by FNAC may be difficult, particularly in the presence of thyroiditis, and therefore open biopsy may be necessary. Surgery is usually not possible and therefore most patients are treated by external radiotherapy. The tumour tends to occur in the elderly and the 5 year survival figure is very low.

2. *Adenocarcinoma* can be sub-classified according to the cell of origin into tumours arising from follicular cells or from the parafollicular or C-cells (produce calcitonin).

   • *Medullary carcinomas* arise from C-cells and can be subdivided into two types:

     The sporadic tumour with no family history presents as a solitary nodule and is treated by total thyroidectomy, node dissection and thyroxine replacement. There is no indication to suppress TSH with this tumour as it is not TSH dependent. Patients should be followed by regular calcitonin assays to detect early recurrence. The 5 year survival figure is 50%.

     The familial form is usually multifocal in origin and is associated with MEN (MEN) II syndrome (see below). The treatment is as for sporadic medullary carcinoma but it has a less favourable prognosis, especially in the MEN IIB subtype. In patients who are known to belong to MEN II families, it may be possible to detect and treat those members of the family who will develop medullary carcinoma before they actually develop the disease (see below).

   • *Adenocarcinoma* arising from follicular cells can be subdivided into differentiated and undifferentiated forms. The former are papillary and follicular carcinomas and it is likely that the undifferentiated form, which occurs in elderly patients, may represent a progression from one of the differentiated forms.

     Papillary carcinoma is the commonest thyroid malignancy, accounting for over 60% of cases. It tends to occur under the age of 40, is particularly common in teenagers, but can arise at any age. The younger the patient, the more pure is the histological form and the better the life expectancy, with teenagers having a normal life expectancy in almost all cases. In older patients, variant forms of papillary carcinoma are encountered, such as 'follicular variant' and 'tall columnar cell variant', and these have a poorer prognosis.

The patient usually presents with a solitary thyroid nodule and is euthyroid. Metastases are present on approximately 50% of cases to ipsilateral cervical nodes. Distant metastases are exceedingly rare. Diagnosis is made by FNAC confirming papillary cells with optically clear nuclei and nuclear clefts. Since the tumour is usually multifocal in site in the thyroid, total thyroidectomy is recommended. Where enlarged nodes are present, these should be removed. Block neck dissection affords no clear benefit over simple node excision. Patients with micro-papillary carcinoma (<1 cm) with no nodal involvement should receive thyroxine at a dose to suppress TSH. For all other cases, radioiodine should also be administered about 6 weeks post-surgery.

It is important that these patients are followed up to ensure that their TSH remains suppressed. Thyroglobulin should also be assayed regularly and may give an indication of early tumour recurrence.

Follicular carcinoma can also occur at any age but is most common in the middle-aged female. It is not associated with the good prognosis of papillary carcinoma, 5 year survival rates being about 50%. Histologically the tumour exists in two forms: micro-invasive follicular carcinoma and frankly invasive follicular carcinoma.

The micro-invasive form has a thick capsule with tumour cells penetrating into the capsule but not through into the thyroid substance. There is no vascular or lymphatic invasion. This tumour presents as a solitary nodule and is not multifocal in the thyroid. Treatment is therefore by thyroid lobectomy and thyroxine at a dose to suppress TSH. This results in a good long-term remission.

Invasive follicular carcinoma tends to spread by the vascular as well as the lymphatic route. The patient's presentation may therefore be by metastatic disease, especially if spread is to bone. The majority of patients present with a solitary thyroid nodule and the tumour is diagnosed histologically by tumour capsule penetration into the surrounding thyroid and/or by lymphatic and vascular invasion. Since the cell structure of follicular adenomas, micro-invasive carcinomas, and invasive carcinomas is identical, FNAC is unable to differentiate between these, and formal excision by lobectomy is necessary for accurate diagnosis.

Treatment of invasive carcinoma is by total thyroidectomy, central neck node clearance to the carotid sheaths laterally, radioiodine ablation at 6 weeks and thyroxine to suppress TSH. Bone metastases may require local therapy with external radiotherapy and tend to be radiosensitive.

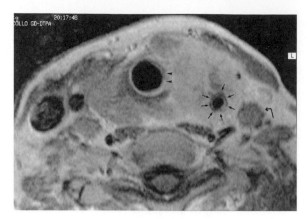

Figure 16.4. MRI of undifferentiated carcinoma of the thyroid gland showing invasion of the tracheal wall and common carotid artery.

Undifferentiated carcinoma is a highly aggressive and unpleasant tumour. It is difficult to diagnose by FNAC, is not amenable to surgical resection, and progresses rapidly in the neck producing obstructive problems (Fig. 16.4). It responds poorly to radiotherapy and patients rarely survive beyond 1 year. Tracheostomy for respiratory obstruction is not recommended. This usually has a very short-term effect with the patient progressing to further respiratory obstruction due to tumour fungating at the tracheostomy opening.

Retrosternal goitre

This may be sub-classified into two types:
1. *Congenital*, which is due to overdescent of the thyroid into the superior mediastinum. This is rare, non-progressive and usually asymptomatic requiring no treatment.
2. *Acquired* which is usually secondary to multinodular goitre with nodule formation occurring retrosternally. Such nodules tend to progressively enlarge with time and will ultimately produce compressive symptoms such as dysphagia, dyspnoea or venous obstruction.

Retrosternal goitre has a higher incidence of malignancy than cervical multinodular goitre, the incidence in some series being as high as 17%.

Over 80% of patients with retrosternal goitre are detected clinically. Dullness to percussion over the upper sternum, and head and neck congestion on arm elevation are classical signs, but inability to feel the lower border of a goitre on swallowing should alert the clinician. A chest X-ray may confirm a superior mediastinal mass. Respiratory function tests may suggest airway compression. Ultrasound scan may fail to delineate the lower border of a goitre suggesting the presence of a retrosternal component but cannot visualise the mediastinal component. The preferred mode of investigation is CT or MRI scan which will confirm the diagnosis and demonstrate the extent of the mediastinal goitre. This should be performed in all cases prior to surgery.

If the patient is fit for surgery, retrosternal goitre is an absolute indication for surgery. Even if it is not causing compression symptoms, it will tend to enlarge and ultimately cause problems. The smaller the nodule, the easier it is to remove through the cervical route and over 95% of mediastinal goitres should be removable through a cervical incision. It is unacceptable to treat mediastinal goitre by sternotomy and excision without first attempting removal through a cervical incision and without treating the cervical goitre as well.

Thyroglossal cyst

Along its line of embryological descent from the foramen caecum of the tongue to its position in the neck, the thyroid gland may leave behind a tract of ectodermal cells, and in later life these may form a *thyroglossal cyst*. These cysts can be either supra- or infra-hyoid and on clinical examination move on swallowing and on tongue protrusion. To demonstrate this clearly it is important that the patient's jaw is fixed open while she/he protrudes and retracts her/his tongue.

The treatment for thyroglossal cyst is excision together with the thyroglossal tract from the isthmus of thyroid to base of tongue, including excision of the central portion of the hyoid bone. Simple cyst excision has a high incidence of recurrent cyst formation.

Occasionally a thyroglossal cyst may become infected to form a thyroglossal abscess. These are best treated by simple needle aspiration and antibiotics rather than formal incision and drainage which usually results in a thyroglossal sinus.

A patient may occasionally present with a papillary carcinoma either arising in a thyroglossal cyst or arising apparently from thyroid cells left on the line of descent.

PARATHYROID GLANDS

Embryology

There are normally four parathyroid glands in the neck, two arising from the third and two from the fourth pharyngeal pouches. The superior glands arise from the fourth pharyngeal pouch in a position adjacent to the upper-central part of the thyroid gland. The inferior parathyroids arise from the third pharyngeal pouch and normally descend past the superior glands with the descent of the thymus to end in a position adjacent to the lower pole of thyroid or upper cornua of thymus.

Anatomy

Although, classically, there are four parathyroid glands, two superior and two inferior (Fig. 16.5), this is variable and up to 10 glands have been identified in one patient. In addition, parathyroid rests of cells may be found along the line of descent of the parathyroids, especially into the thymus gland. These probably account for the lack of need for vitamin D or calcium replacement in some patients who undergo total parathyroidectomy.

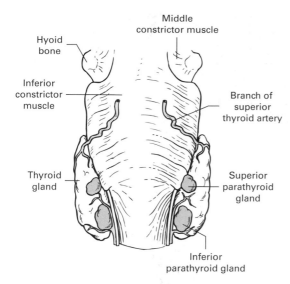

Figure 16.5. Posterior surface of the thyroid gland showing the parathyroid glands.

The superior parathyroid glands tend to be constant in their position, in the vicinity of the site where the inferior thyroid artery crosses the recurrent laryngeal nerve.

The inferior parathyroid glands are more variable in position but in almost 90% of people, they are situated in the region of the lower pole of thyroid, upper cornua of thymus, or in the tract between.

However, the inferior glands may be situated some considerable distance from this area. The glands may not descend fully with the thymus, or may over-descend. They may be found therefore in the normal line of descent from above the upper pole of thyroid, anywhere to the lower pole of thyroid, down into the upper cornua of thymus and may even descend into the superior mediastinum. If arrested on descent behind the thyroid, they may take up a position within a cleft in the thyroid gland and become intra-thyroid.

A gland may deviate from its normal line of descent ending up in an ectopic position. Glands have been described in the neck between trachea and oesophagus, retro-oesophagus, laterally in the neck and within the carotid sheath. A gland may descend into the thorax and may be intra-thymic, or in the superior or anterior mediastinum and be extra-thymic. Individual reports have described glands found in the middle mediastinum, intrapericardium, subpleural, in the posterior mediastinum and even intra-pulmonary.

Physiology

Parathormone (PTH) is an 84 amino acid polypeptide of molecular weight 9500. Although the parathyroid gland has two populations of cells (chief cells and oxyphil cells), both of which produce PTH, there is no evidence that they produce different types of PTH. The active part of the molecule is the 34 amino acid amino-terminal but only the intact molecule is effective biologically; 98% of circulating PTH is as inert fragments. Previous radio-immunoassays for PTH measured only the carboxyl part of the molecule but it is now possible to assay the entire molecule giving accurate values for PTH levels in the circulation.

The main actions of PTH are:

- increases serum calcium;
- depresses serum phosphate;
- increases phosphate excretion in the urine;
- direct effect on bone by stimulating osteoclastic activity;
- increases calcium absorption from the kidney;
- in the presence of vitamin D, enhances intestinal absorption of calcium.

Secretion of PTH is inhibited by a negative feedback effect of ionised calcium on the parathyroid glands. Prolonged hypomagnesaemia inhibits PTH secretion and may be associated with hypocalcaemia.

Total body calcium is approximately 1.5% of body weight and most is skeletal. Serum calcium (2.2–2.5 mmol/l) is carried mainly bound to protein, predominantly albumin, but also exists in a partially ionised state. It is the ionised component which is essential for coagulation, cardiac and skeletal muscle contraction and nerve function. Calcium absorption from the gastro-intestinal tract is decreased by substances which form insoluble calcium salts for example phosphates and oxalates, or by alkalis which form insoluble calcium soaps. High protein diet increases the absorption of calcium. Excess calcium is excreted in the stool but excess absorbed calcium is excreted by the kidneys.

Vitamin D is a term applied to a group of closely related sterols produced by the action of ultraviolet light on provitamins, predominantly in the skin by the action of sunlight. Vitamin D_3 (cholecalciferol) is converted in the liver to 25-hydroxy-cholecalciferol and is hydroxylated in the kidney to 1-25-dihydroxy cholecalciferol by the enzyme α-1-hydroxylase. The formation of 1-25-dihydroxy vitamin D_3 is enhanced by the presence of PTH. Patients with chronic renal failure lack α-1-hydroxylase and therefore fail to produce 1-25-dihydroxy vitamin D_3. With PTH, 1-25-dihydroxy vitamin D_3 increases intestinal absorption of calcium and phosphate and increases phosphorus absorption from the proximal tubule of the kidney. It is also involved in bone demineralisation.

Calcitonin produced from the parafollicular cells of the thyroid acts to lower elevated serum calcium but does not appear to play a major role in calcium haemostasis in man.

Hypocalcaemia thus results in an elevated PTH by a reduced negative feedback on the parathyroid glands. This stimulates the formation of 1-25-dihydroxy vitamin D_3 and together these act to return serum calcium levels to normal.

Hypercalcaemia results in a decreased PTH secretion, reduction in 1-25-dihydroxy vitamin D_3 and formation of 24-25-dihydroxy vitamin D_3 instead which is much less biologically active and results in a lowering of serum calcium levels.

Parathyroid disorders

Hypoparathyroidism almost always occurs following parathyroid surgery or post-thyroidectomy by inadvertent removal or ischaemic damage to the glands (see below – 'post-operative hypocalcaemia').

Hyperparathyroidism may be primary, secondary, or tertiary.

Primary hyperparathyroidism

Primary hyperparathyroidism results from over-activity of one or more of the parathyroid glands, resulting in elevation of detectable PTH and hypercalcaemia, where there has been no pre-existing condition which has stimulated parathyroid activity. Over 90% of cases are related to a solitary parathyroid adenoma. In approximately 1% of cases, adenomata may exist in two or more glands. The remainder of cases are associated with four gland hyperplasia and where this occurs, especially if the glands are large and the patient is young, the clinician should be alerted to the possibility of MEN syndrome (see below).

Studies on the prevalence of the disease suggest that this is constant world-wide at 1/1000 population. The majority of cases are now detected from routine blood testing using multiphasic automated biochemistry machines and the detection rate is approximately 25 new cases/100 000 patients assayed.

Although it is now less common to see patients with overt symptoms or signs associated with primary hyperparathyroidism, cases still present. The commonest clinical presentations are in patients who present with fractures, especially if through a bone cyst, or with renal calculi. Occasional patients are detected with hypercalcaemia associated with hypertension.

Despite the fact that 50% of patients are classified as 'asymptomatic', following treatment and cure of the hypercalcaemia, many of these patients realise an improvement in their well-being with improved concentration, less depression, improved grip strength and an improvement in their Quality of Life scores. The elderly apparently mildly demented patient may suddenly recover mental function, and mild 'dementia' is therefore not a contraindication to parathyroidectomy, but rather an indication for treatment.

Three complications which tend to arise in the untreated case, may be irreversible and have a effect on the patient's long-term morbidity and mortality rates:

- *Bone*: It is estimated that patient presenting with primary hyperparathyroidism have bone mineral density only approximately 60–70% of the average population. Some patients have values much below this. Following parathyroidectomy, only a small proportion of this is re-couped. Since the majority of patients are middle-aged to elderly females, this aspect exacerbates any tendency to osteoporosis and predisposes to fractures.
- *Cardiovascular system*: Hypertension associated with hyperparathyroidism is irreversible once established.
- *Kidney*: Renal failure once established is irreversible.

Diagnosis

After confirmation of hypercalcaemia (either total calcium balanced against serum albumin or ionised calcium), other causes of hypercalcaemia must be excluded for example disseminated malignancy. The diagnosis of hyperparathyroidism is confirmed by elevated intact PTH in the presence of hypercalcaemia.

In the past 5–10 years, major advances have been made in the pre-operative detection of the site of the abnormal parathyroid gland. Increasing expertise in ultrasound scanning, isotope studies using Sestamibi, and MRI scanning have all resulted in accurate localisation in over 90% of cases. Concordance between two of these modalities has a very high accuracy rate. Such accuracy has allowed mini- and laparoscopic exploration of the neck targeted to the affected gland alone with a high degree of success. Some experienced endocrine surgeons still advocate a full neck exploration with four glands visualisation but many surgeons are now changing to local targeted exploration as the primary procedure.

Management

Parathyroidectomy is the accepted treatment for primary hyperparathyroidism. Increasingly 'asymptomatic' patients being picked up incidentally by biochemical analysis are being offered surgery before the development of any long-term complications.

Four gland exploration and removal of the diseased gland is successful in curing the disease. Mini- or laparoscopic exploration with a single gland visualisation and removal, may afford the possibility that a second gland may rarely be missed. In this situation, many surgeons advocate a 'rapid PTH assay' to be performed within 20 min of surgery. A drop of 50% from a pre-operative value confirms that the disease has been cured.

The post-operative drop in serum calcium can take several hours to days to stabilise. Approximately 50% of patients become hypocalcaemic post-operatively and may require calcium and even vitamin D supplementation. Full bone re-mineralisation does not occur and the hypertension and abnormal renal function, if present, do not recover.

Secondary/tertiary hyperparathyroidism

Secondary hyperparathyroidism is a physiological response from the parathyroid glands to a chronically low calcium state, which in the UK is most commonly due to chronic renal failure.

Tertiary hyperparathyroidism results from secondary hyperparathyroidism where the glands have been stimulated for so long they become autonomous and hyperfunctional.

Unlike primary hyperparathyroidism, secondary and tertiary hyperparathyroidism may be managed medically or surgically.

It is estimated that 40% of patients maintained on haemodialysis for >3 years develop significant hyperparathyroidism. The main indications for surgical treatment are marked progression of bone disease with osteoporosis, sub-periostial erosions and non-healing fractures, soft tissue and vascular calcification, and intractable pruritus. This is associated with marked elevation of serum bone alkaline phosphatase and intact serum PTH.

Surgical treatment depends on whether the patient is on a waiting list for renal transplantation. In that case, some residual parathyroid tissue should be preserved. Either a sub-total parathyroidectomy can be performed excising 3½ glands leaving approximately 30 mg of parathyroid tissue at a site carefully marked, or alternatively total parathyroidectomy and muscle implantation of $15–20 \times 1\,mm^3$ cubes of parathyroid tissue. The usual site for implantation is the brachioradialis of the forearm not being used for haemodialysis. If a successful renal transplant is not performed, approximately 20% of patients will develop hyperfunction of the remaining piece of tissue requiring further surgery to this. Patients who are not for renal transplant should have a total parathyroidectomy performed. With either situation, it is recommended that tissue is cryopreserved and available for implantation should the need arise. In many patients this will not be necessary, either no treatment being required or a small dose of vitamin D to maintain calcium stasis.

Following successful renal transplantation, patients with secondary hyperparathyroidism should revert to normal PTH levels in 1–4 months. This is because the α-1-hydroxylase in the renal graft will result in active formation of 1-25-dihydroxy vitamin D_3 and therefore an increased absorption of calcium and regression of the hyperplastic glands.

Approximately 20% of patients with successful renal grafts will have developed tertiary hyperparathyroidism prior to surgery and this will persist with hyperplastic parathyroid glands or tissue. In this situation parathyroid surgery is commonly necessary. If the renal graft is rejected at some future date, further hyperparathyroidism is likely to develop in any parathyroid remnant or graft.

Post-operative hypocalcaemia

Hypocalcaemia is exceedingly common following both thyroidectomy and parathyroidectomy and if transient and minimal, requires no treatment.

Despite clearly identifying all adjacent parathyroid glands or identifying all parathyroid glands at thyroid surgery, permanent hypoparathyroidism can still occur. Most experienced endocrine surgeons do not advocate ligation of the inferior thyroid artery laterally because of the risk of devascularising the parathyroid glands. Instead they recommend ligating the branches of the inferior artery medially on the thyroid capsule medial to the nerve, having identified the parathyroid glands clearly.

However, isotope studies have shown no difference in the activity of the parathyroid glands whether the vessels are ligated laterally or medially and cases of hypoparathyroidism do still occur despite extreme care with the blood supply to the parathyroid glands. Also, the incidence of permanent hypocalcaemia is similar.

Permanent hypoparathyroidism requires permanent vitamin D therapy, possibly supplemented with oral calcium.

ADRENAL GLANDS

Anatomy

There are two adrenal glands, one situated above each kidney. Both glands have a rich arterial blood supply, mainly from the suprarenal arteries from the aorta, branches from the renal arteries, and branches from the phrenic vessels. The venous drainage is normally by a single vein, on the right side draining directly into the inferior vena cava, and on the left side into the left renal vein.

Each gland consists of two parts, an inner medulla which secretes catecholamines, mainly epinephrine and norepinephrine, and an outer cortex which secretes steroids, particularly glucocorticoids, mineralocorticoids and sex hormones. The medulla and cortex function as two separate endocrine glands, each independent of the other, under a different method of regulation and control, and with different functions.

The adrenal medulla can be regarded as a sympathetic ganglion in which the post-ganglionic neurones have no axons but merely secrete directly into the circulation. Cell nests, paraganglia, can frequently be found near the thoracic and abdominal sympathetic ganglia which resemble cells from the adrenal medulla and may be the site of extra-adrenal type tumours (phaeochromocytoma).

Histology

Histologically the adrenal cortex is divided into three zones – zona glomerulosa, zona fasciculata and zona reticularis – from the outside in. All three zones produce glucocorticoids and sex hormones, but mineralocorticoids, especially aldosterone, are only produced by the zona glomerulosa.

Physiology

Adrenal cortex

Glucocorticoid release is controlled by secretion of adrenocorticotrophic hormone (ACTH) from the anterior pituitary gland into the circulation. Mineralocorticoid secretion is stimulated by the renin–angiotensin mechanism.

Hormones produced from the adrenal cortex are all derived from cortisone and are based on the cyclopentanoperhydrophenanthrene nucleus. This nucleus contains 19 carbon atoms. At the C-17 position there is a side chain. Those with two carbon atoms in the side chain are known as C-21 steroids and those with no carbon atoms are known as C-19 steroids. C-19 steroids with an oxygen atom at the side chain are 17-ketosteroids and those with a hydroxyl group are 17-hydroxy corticosteroids. C-19 steroids are androgenic.

C-21 steroids have either a mineralocorticoid or glucocorticoid effect depending on whether their primary effect is on sodium–potassium excretion or predominantly on glucose and protein metabolism respectively.

The predominant steroids produced by the adrenal cortex are as follows:

- *Glucocorticoids*: cortisol and corticosterone.
- *Mineralocorticoid*: aldosterone.
- *Androgens*: predominatly androstenedione, 11-hydroxy-androstenedione, testosterone, and the inactive precursor dehydroepiandrostenedione sulphate(DHA-S)

Small amounts of progesterone and oestrogens are also synthesised.

Individual tumours may arise which produce an excess of each of these hormones:

- Cushing's syndrome or Cushing's disease – glucocorticoids;
- Conn's syndrome – mineralocorticoids;
- adrenogenital syndrome – sex hormones.

Glucocorticoids

Approximately 15–20 mg of cortisol is secreted daily. Corticotrophin releasing hormone (CRF) from the hypothalamus is carried to the anterior pituitary gland in a portal venous system and stimulates release of ACTH. The ACTH circulates to the adrenal cortex where it stimulates synthesis and release of cortisol (very little cortisol is actually stored in the adrenal gland). Approximately 95% of glucocorticoid circulates bound to an α-globulin and the remainder is free steroid. A negative feedback effect from the free cortisol inhibits release of both CRF from the hypothalamus and ACTH from the anterior pituitary gland. There is a normal diurnal variation in glucocorticoid levels in 24 h with a trough at approximately 4 a.m.

The main actions of glucocorticoids are:

- *Metabolic*: glucocorticoids increase protein metabolism, hepatic glycogenesis and gluconeogenesis causing a rise in blood sugar. They therefore have an anti-insulin action in the peripheral tissues and exacerbate diabetes.
- *Negative feedback* on ACTH secretion, either directly in the anterior pituitary gland or via corticotrophin releasing hormone (CRH) inhibition from the hypothalamus.
- *Stress reaction*: 'Stress' results in an increase in ACTH and glucocorticoids. This response is essential for life and appears to have vital intracellular functions, especially the maintenance of blood pressure.
- *Increased tendency to peptic ulceration* by lowering gastric mucosal resistance and increasing acid secretion.
- *Slight mineralocorticoid effect* resulting in sodium retention and potassium excretion with water retention.
- *Increased fat metabolism.*
- *Effect on vascular smooth muscle* being essential for the normal response to epinephrine and norepinephrine. Corticoid insufficiency results in capillary dilatation and increased permeability.

- *Anti-inflammatory action* by reducing lymphocyte and eosinophil counts in the peripheral blood and inhibiting normal antibody response.

Mineralocorticoids

Approximately 100–200 μg of aldosterone is produced daily. Normal blood levels are 5–6 ng/100 ml. Aldosterone circulates unbound and has a half-life of approximately 20 min.

Aldosterone production is normally controlled by the renin–angiotensin mechanism but can be released by direct stimulation of high levels of ACTH. Decreased renal perfusion causes release of renin from the juxtaglomerular apparatus of the kidney. This converts angiotensinogen to angiotensin-1 in the circulation and then to angiotensin-2 in the lungs. Angiotensin-2 acts on the zona glomerulosa of the adrenal cortex to release aldosterone.

Aldosterone now acts on the distal renal tubule exchanging sodium for potassium and hydrogen ions. This results in sodium retention and a potassium diuresis with an acid urine. The sodium ions retain water in the circulation resulting in an increased plasma volume with an aim to restore renal perfusion. Aldosterone acts on sweat glands, salivary glands and the gastro-intestinal tract to increase sodium resorption at these sites also.

Adrenal medulla

The adrenal medulla produces both the catecholamines, epinephrine (adrenaline) and norepinephrine (noradrenaline). Norepinephrine is also formed at adrenergic nerve endings. Norepinephrine is formed from the essential amino acid phenylalanine and epinephrine is formed by methylation of norepinephrine. The enzyme for this only exists in the adrenal medulla. Catecholamines are broken down in the circulation to metanephrines which are then oxidised to form 4-hydroxy-3-methoxy mandelic acid (VMA). The catecholamines and their breakdown products are excreted through the kidney, half as metanephrines, one third as VMA and the remainder as free hormone.

Catecholamines are not essential for life but are essential for reaction to acute stress (preparation for 'flight or fight'). The sympathetic nervous system stimulates the adrenal medulla to release catecholamines directly into the circulation. In view of the anatomical position of the adrenal glands, this is directly into the upper inferior vena cava and directly to the heart for immediate effect.

The main actions of catecholamines are:

- increase the heart rate;
- raise blood pressure;
- raise blood sugar;
- stimulate the metabolic rate;
- lower the threshold in the reticular formation of the brain re-inforcing the state of arousal;
- dilate the pupils;
- increase hepatic and skeletal muscle glycogenesis;
- mobilise free fatty acids.

Epinephrine and norepinephrine have different actions. Norepinephrine produces peripheral vasoconstriction in all peripheral vessels while epinephrine produces vasodilatation in liver and skeletal muscle resulting in a drop in total peripheral resistance. Norepinephrine therefore produces a rise in systolic and diastolic blood pressure while epinephrine causes an increase in pulse pressure.

Disorders of the adrenal glands

Cushing's disease/Cushing's syndrome

Cushing's disease is the excess production of glucocorticoids secondary to over-stimulation of the adrenal cortex by a pituitary tumour producing excess ACTH. Cushing's syndrome is the excess presence of glucocorticoids secondary to an autonomous glucocorticoid adenoma, adrenal carcinoma, ectopic ACTH production or the administration of large doses of steroids as medical therapy.

Clinically the patient presents with truncal obesity, moon face, hypertension, diabetes, abdominal striae, acne and a buffalo hump, and experiences profound weakness. Pituitary ACTH-producing tumours tend also to produce skin pigmentation as ACTH has a similar molecular structure to melanocyte-stimulating hormone (MSH). Because patients have a tendency to bruise easily with delicate skin which is easily damaged, and have an increased risk of infection, post-operative problems are increased.

Diagnosis

Diagnosis is by detection of an elevated plasma cortisol with lack of diurnal variation. Because other conditions can produce a similar pattern (e.g. excess alcohol production), a low dose Dexamethasone suppression test should be performed to confirm the diagnosis. Dexamethasone suppresses ACTH production but does not interfere with cortisol assay. Therefore, in a patient who does not have Cushing's syndrome, Dexamethasone, by suppressing ACTH, will suppress cortisol.

If cortisol levels are not suppressed, the next step is to measure plasma ACTH (by a radio-immunoassay) and to perform a high dose Dexamethasone suppression test to determine suppression of urinary 17-hydroxy-corticosteroids.
- *Undetectable ACTH* indicates a primary adrenal tumour.
- *Elevated ACTH* may be due to either pituitary or ectopic ACTH production.
  - Pituitary ACTH hypersecretion (Cushing's disease) is partially suppressed by a high dose Dexamethsone suppression test with 17-hydroxy corticosteroids being reduced to <50% of baseline.
  - Ectopic ACTH production is unaffected by a high dose Dexamethasone suppression test in which case 17-hydroxycorticosteroids will not be suppressed.

If the diagnosis is adrenal Cushing's syndrome, the tumour can normally be localised by a CT scan or an iodo-cholesterol scan. Failure to localise with the isotope scan raises the suspicion of malignancy. Adrenal tumours <5 cm in diameter are usually benign but tumours >8 cm have a high incidence of malignancy.

Management

Symptoms of Cushing's syndrome can be reduced by metyrapone or aminoglutethamide but effects are usually temporary. However the use of these drugs may reduce the incidence of post-operative complications outlined above, especially risk of sepsis.

Most centres would now accept that a unilateral adrenalectomy for a tumour <5 cm should be performed by laparoscopy in all cases. The long-term side effects and complications of a large incision which would otherwise be necessary are unacceptable. The technique is not easy and patients should be referred into a main centre where the expertise for this exists. As experience is obtained, larger tumours and bilateral surgery is now being carried out by more centres.

Because of suppression of the contralateral gland, unilateral adrenalectomy will result in hypo-adrenalism which may last for several months before the contralateral gland regains function. Glucocorticoids will be necessary throughout this time. Bilateral adrenalectomy will require not only glucocorticoid replacement but also life-long mineralocorticoid.

Patients with bilateral adrenal hyperplasia due to Cushing's disease may be treated by excision of the pituitary adenoma or by bilateral adrenalectomy. In those cases treated by adrenalectomy, the pituitary tumour will tend to enlarge and in 20% of patients will cause symptoms (*Nelson's syndrome*). This causes hyperpigmentation, headache, increased levels of sex hormones and optic chiasma compression resulting in bi-temporal hemianopia and ultimate blindness. To prevent this, the pituitary should therefore be irradiated.

Primary hyperaldosteronism (Conn's syndrome)

Hyperaldosteronism may be either primary or secondary.

Primary disease (Conn's syndrome) is due to excess production of aldosterone, most commonly due to an adrenal adenoma. This results in excess sodium and water retention with loss of potassium and hydrogen ions. Patients therefore become hypertensive with hypokalaemic alkalosis. In this situation, the juxtaglomerular apparatus is not stimulated and renin levels are therefore low.

Secondary disease is due to impaired renal perfusion most commonly associated with renal vascular disease or malignant hypertension. This results in excess production of renin from the juxta-glomerular apparatus, ultimately causing excess aldosterone production. Renin levels are therefore high.

Diagnosis

The diagnosis of Conn's syndrome rests on having a high index of suspicion. The diagnosis may not be obvious because many patients with hypertension are prescribed diuretics which cause hypokalaemia. Initially, hypertension and hypokalaemia may therefore simply be mistaken for effects of therapy. Renin levels may aid in making the diagnosis. A CT scan showing a small adrenal mass in a patient suspected of having Conn's syndrome, may aid in confirming the diagnosis.

An adenoma may be detected by iodo-cholesterol scanning. Carcinomata tend not to show with isotope scans. Only two cases of ectopic aldosterone producing adenomas have been described, one in the kidney and one in the ovary. Bilateral adenomata are exceedingly rare.

Management

Patients may be controlled medically, initially by spironolactone. If the patient is elderly and the dose is small, this may be the preferred treatment. Otherwise it is most cost-effective to treat surgically.

In patients who are on a large dose or who experience side effects of the drug, such as impotence, gynaecomastia, hypotension and weakness due to hypokalaemia, surgery is indicated. Since these tumours are normally unilateral and small, laparoscopic adrenalectomy is the treatment of choice. Total adrenalectomy is normally performed rather than simple extirpation of the tumour from the gland.

Since there is no glucocorticoid suppression of the contralateral gland, post-operative steroids are not necessary. However, the occasional patient may experience problems with mineralocorticoid suppression of the opposite gland and this may not recover instantly. Weight loss, hyperkalaemia and hypotension within 1 week of surgery indicate a need for mineralocorticoid replacement by fludrocortisone. This rarely requires to continue beyond 1 month.

Phaeochromocytoma

Phaeochromocytoma is a tumour which produces excess of epinephrine or norepinephrine and is situated either in the adrenal medulla or in related chromaffin cells. It results in hypertension, initially episodic then sustained. A family history of phaeochromocytoma, bilateral disease, associated medullary carcinoma of thyroid, hyperparathyroidism, neurofibromatosis or ganglioneuromatosis should alert one to the possibility of MEN II (see below).

Clinically the patient presents with hypertension, episodic flushing, palpitations, headaches and anxiety. There may be associated persistent tachycardia, weight loss, and a tendency to diabetes. Malignancy is rare but multiple tumours occur in about 10% of patients.

The hypertension during an attack can be profound and may be lethal, causing cerebral vascular accident (CVA), myocardial infarction or sudden cardiac arrythmias. Cardiomyopathy is a major complication of phaeochromocytoma.

Diagnosis

Urinary assay of VMA or metanephrines is the main first investigation. Excitation and suppression tests are dangerous and should be avoided. It is essential that the hypertension

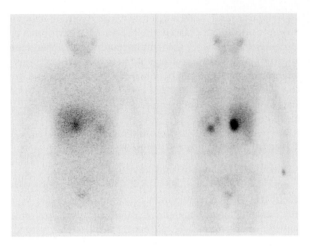

Figure 16.6. MIBG scan in patient with bilateral phaeochromocytomas.

is treated early and the patient completely adrenergic blocked as soon as the diagnosis is made and before further tests are performed.

The main differential diagnoses to exclude are hyperthyroidism, carcinoid syndrome, labile hypertension and pre-eclampsia.

Localisation is vital before any surgery is contemplated. Over 90% of phaeochromocytomas are within the adrenal area. Tumours producing epinephrine are rarely extra-adrenal and therefore extensive localising tests are not indicated for these.

However, primarily norepinephrine producing tumours can occur remotely from the adrenal and tests to localise must be performed. Extra-adrenal tumours are usually found along the line of the aorta, occasionally along the thoracic aorta. Tumours have been identified in the genital organs, hernial sacs, bladder wall, mediastinum and up into the neck.

CT or MRI scanning may demonstrate a mass. Meta-iodobenzylguanidine labelled with I[131] (MIBG) concentrates in chromaffin tissue and may therefore demonstrate phaeochromocytomas (Fig. 16.6). Angiography may demonstrate the tumour clearly as it is frequently very vascular. Selective venous sampling from adrenal veins may localise the side.

Management

Treatment with α-blockers, for example phenoxybenzamine, should be started immediately the diagnosis is made. The use of β-blockers should only be started after the patient is α-blocked to avoid a hypertensive crisis. When medical treated is established, localising studies can be conducted.

Treatment is by surgery which must only be performed in the safely blocked patient. Initial concerns about laparoscopic resection have been overcome by several studies and this is now the approach of choice in the smaller tumours (<5 cm). Even bilateral phaeochromocytomas are now dealt with laparoscopically. Of equal importance is the skill and experience of the anaesthetist who must be prepared to deal with the wild fluctuations of blood pressure which can occur during this procedure. The use of intravenous magnesium is now more widely advocated as a means of stabilising the blood pressure throughout surgery but separate infusions of phentolamine or nitroprusside to control hypertensive episodes, and norepinephrine to control hypotension, must still be in place.

The majority of patients will have an adrenal adenoma or a solitary tumour and will be cured by excision. There is a recurrence rate of 5% in the contralateral gland, even years later. Adrenal carcinomas are rare and have usually metastasised by the time of presentation.

Congenital adrenal hyperplasia

Congenital adrenal hyperplasia is the commonest form of virilisation and is due to a genetic enzyme defect which results in deficient secretion of cortisol. This results in reduced negative feedback to the pituitary resulting in a very high ACTH. This produces adrenal hyperplasia and excess androgen production, especially androsterone which is converted to testosterone peripherally. Androsterone is a 17-ketosteroid and testosterone is not. Therefore, virilisation with an elevated urinary 17-keto steroid level suggest adrenal origin, while a normal or only slightly elevated 17-ketosteroid suggests excess testosterone from ovary or testis.

Congenital adrenal hyperplasia is treated by glucocorticoids which supply cortisol requirements and suppress the ACTH. Cosmetic surgery may be required.

Virilism due to an adrenal tumour is usually secondary to a large malignant tumour. Surgical resection is still indicated despite the size, to control symptoms and to treat the tumour. Occasionally a good long-term remission may be obtained.

Asymptomatic adrenal tumours

The finding of an adrenal mass which is non-functional (an 'incidentaloma') requires investigation. Many are picked up on abdominal CT scanning being used for investigation of other intra-abdominal problems. CT should always be performed to accurately localise the tumour, its site and its attachments. Tests of function must always be performed. A previous history of malignancy, especially bronchus or breast, should alert one to the possibility of a secondary deposit.

In a truly non-functioning tumour, FNA should be performed. If the tumour is adrenal in origin and not a metastasis, a decision regarding surgery must be made. If the tumour is <4 cm it is acceptable to simply follow the patient with regular scanning to ensure there is no enlargement occurring. Tumours larger than this, or where steady enlargement is seen on sequential scans, should be removed. A high percentage of tumours >8 cm will be malignant.

Neuroblastoma

For more details refer to Chapter 21.

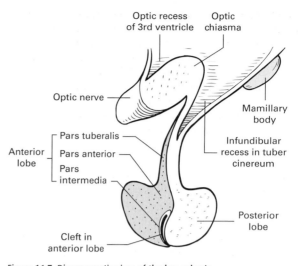

Figure 16.7. Diagrammatic view of the hypophysis.

Adrenal cysts

There have been about 200 cases of adrenal cysts described in the world literature. Many are large but are rarely malignant and are usually removed after initial needle decompression.

HYPOTHALAMUS/PITUITARY GLAND

Anatomy

The hypothalamus is situated at the anterior end of the diencephalon. It contains clearly defined nuclei such as the supraoptic and paraventricular nuclei, and other nuclear areas which are less well defined. The hypothalamus is connected to the pituitary gland by both neural and vascular connections.

The pituitary gland is situated in the pituitary fossa or sella turcica under the diaphragma sella. The posterior pituitary gland, or neurohypophysis, arises from an evagination of the floor of the third ventricle and is therefore primarily neural (Fig. 16.7). It receives fibres from both the supraoptic and paraventricular nuclei. The anterior lobe, or adenohypophysis, and the intermediate lobe of the pituitary, arise from Rathke's pouch which is an evagination of the roof of the pharynx. The anterior pituitary receives very few nerve fibres from the hypothalamus but there is a portal system of vessels from the hypothalamus to the anterior pituitary via the pituitary stalk.

Anatomical relations of the pituitary gland are:
- inferiorly and anteriorly – sphenoidal air sinuses;
- superiorly – optic chiasma;
- posteriorly – dorsum sella, vestibular artery and pons;
- laterally – cavernous sinuses.

Physiology

As well as its endocrine functions, the hypothalamus is involved in temperature regulation, appetite, and defensive reactions such as fear and rage. This latter action is probably related to the neuroendocrine control of catecholamine release, mainly via the adrenal medulla.

The hypothalamus releases hormones which travel down the hypothalamic-pituitary portal venous system and are known as 'messenger hormones'. These are:
- thyrotrophin releasing hormone (TRH);
- corticotrophin releasing hormone (CRH);
- luteinising hormone releasing hormone (LHRH);
- prolactin inhibiting factor (PIF);
- growth hormone releasing and inhibiting factor.

The supraoptic nuclei, via the neural connections to the posterior pituitary gland, are responsible for release of vasopressin or antidiuretic hormone(ADH) and the paraventricular nuclei stimulate release of oxytocin.

Six hormones are released by the anterior pituitary gland:
- thyroid stimulating hormone (TSH);
- adrenocorticotrophic hormone (ACTH);
- follicle stimulating hormone (FSH);
- luteinising hormone (LH);
- prolactin;
- growth hormone.

The intermediate lobe of the pituitary produces α- and β-melanocytic stimulating hormones (MSH).

LH, FSH and TSH and glycoproteins. Each has an α- and β-subunit, the α- part being identical between the hormones. ACTH is a 39 amino acid polypeptide. The 4–10 part carboxy terminus of the amino acid sequence is identical to that of melanocyte-stimulating hormones and accounts for the pigmentation associated with excess ACTH secretion. Prolactin is an amino acid polypeptide with a molecular weight of 21 500. Its release increases markedly during pregnancy to act on the breasts where it is essential for initiation of lactation. Growth hormone is a 191 amino acid polypeptide with a molecular weight of 22 000.

Growth hormone and prolactin are not subject to feedback loop control and all, except growth hormone, are trophic hormones that regulate function in other endocrine organs.

Pituitary tumours

Pituitary tumours can be subdivided into adenomas and microadenomas. Microadenomas are tumours with a diameter of <1 cm and are further subdivided into endocrine-active or endocrine-inactive tumours, the former producing characteristic syndromes:
- pituitary-stimulated hyperthyroidism (excess TSH);
- Cushing's disease (excess ACTH). This may also produce Nelson's syndrome following treatment by bilateral adrenalectomy;
- acromegaly or gigantism (excess growth hormone);
- amenorrhoea/galactorrhoea (excess prolactin).

Large adenomas of the pituitary may extend into the suprasellar region and produce pressure on the optic nerves and optic chiasma. This results in bitemporal hemianopia.

Diagnosis of endocrine-active tumours is by hormonal analysis and assays are available for all trophic hormones. Skull X-rays may demonstrate expansion of the pituitary fossa but CT and MRI scanning allow visualisation of macro- and micro-adenomata.

TUMOURS OF THE GASTRO-INTESTINAL TRACT AND PANCREAS

The upper gastro-intestinal tract and pancreas produce many hormones. Overproduction produces many specific clinical syndromes especially of insulin, gastrin, glucagon, pancreatic polypeptide, vasoactive intestinal polypeptide (VIP), secretion and somatostatin. Some of these may be associated with MEN syndromes.

Insulinoma

Insulin is produced by the β-cells of the islets of Langerhans of the pancreas. These tumours are usually solitary, <3 cm in diameter, and may be situated in any part of the gland. Over 90% are benign. Multiple insulinomata should alert to the possibility of MEN I.

Clinically, patients usually present with psychiatric symptoms with bizarre behaviour, sweating and tremulousness. Whipple's triad is present in most cases:
- symptoms precipitated by fasting;
- significant hypoglycaemia during symptomatic episodes;
- relief of symptoms by glucose.

Most patients are obese due to associated hunger. The diagnosis can be difficult and only one-third of patients are diagnosed within 1 year of onset of symptoms.

Diagnosis

Diagnosis is confirmed by hypoglycaemia on fasting (up to 72 h) during which time the patient should have an attack. This can be confirmed by measurement of elevated insulin and lowered blood sugar. Failure to provoke an attack during this time precludes the diagnosis. Provocation tests are unreliable, can be dangerous and are no longer used.

Localisation of the tumour can be difficult. CT scanning is unreliable. Angiography is only accurate in about 50% of cases. Percutaneous transhepatic catheterisation of the splenic vein with serial venous sampling along the line of the vein may help to indicate which end of the pancreas is the problem.

Management

Urgent surgery is required. Careful palpation of the pancreas will delineate the tumour in 90% of patients and if it superficial, the tumour can be enucleated. If deep seated, partial pancreatectomy is required. Where the tumour cannot be palpated, proximal or distal pancreatectomy should be performed depending on the results of the serial venous sampling. If the patient has metastatic disease, removal of as much tumour as possible is justified in order to try to relieve symptoms.

Gastrinoma (Zollinger–Ellison syndrome)

Zollinger–Ellison (ZE) syndrome is a disease of fulminant peptic ulceration associated with high gastric acid secretion secondary to excess gastrin production. Tumours usually arise from the G-cells of the islets of the pancreas but about 5% of patients have solitary submucosal gastrinomas in the first or second part of the duodenum. Approximately two-thirds are malignant and 75% of patients have multiple tumours. About one-third of patients have MEN I syndrome. G-cell hyperplasia of the gastric antrum is very rare.

Clinically, patients present with fulminant peptic ulceration. Any patient who presents with more than one ulcer, or who has ulceration in the second part of the duodenum or more distally, should be suspected of having ZE syndrome. The excess acid in the duodenum destroys pancreatic lipase in one-third of patients resulting in steatorrhoea and loose stools.

Diagnosis

Diagnosis no longer depends on studies of gastric acid secretion. Gastrin assays are available (normal <200 pg/ml) and a level of over 500 pg/ml to several thousands may be obtained in ZE syndrome. Very high levels suggest malignancy, especially with liver secondaries. The diagnosis may be confirmed in patients with borderline levels by performing provocation tests using calcium or secretin, following which gastrin levels will rise. The main differential diagnoses are of other conditions producing hypergastrin secretion (pernicious anaemia, hypochlorhydric gastritis, gastric outlet obstruction, short bowel syndrome, and renal insufficiency).

Localisation is difficult. CT scanning and angiography may be misleading. Serial splenic vein sampling for gastrin may indicate the site of tumour deposits. Selective angiography may demonstrate hepatic metastases. Endoscopic ultrasound should help to define any submucosal lesions and may also assist with lesions in the head of pancreas.

Management

Initial treatment should be with proton pump inhibitor (PPI) to reduce acid concentration and bring the disease under control.

Pancreatectomy and duodenal submucosal resection is only successful in a small minority of cases. The tumour is usually multifocal and frequently malignant. Laparotomy is justified however to treat the 20% who can be cured by tumour excision.

Failure of medical treatment may therefore dictate total gastrectomy. It is of note that after total gastrectomy, many gastrinomas appear to remain dormant and occasionally regress. In intractable malignant disease, streptozotosin may be of some value. The 5 year survival figure is about 60%.

Glucagonoma

Glucagonoma is produced from the α-cells in the pancreatic islets. It is a rare tumour, usually affecting middle-aged women and is normally benign.

Glucagon is a polypeptide of molecular weight 3500. In the liver it stimulates adenosine-3-5-monophosphate to activate phosphorylase which breaks down glycogen and stimulates gluconeogenesis resulting in a rise in blood sugar.

Patients present with a symptom complex of necrotising migratory dermatitis, stomatitis, weight loss, mild diabetes and anaemia. Diagnosis is confirmed by an elevated serum glucagon level. Pancreatic arteriography usually localises the tumour and treatment by pancreatic resection is curative. Rarely, irresectable tumours can be treated by streptozotosin.

Vipoma

It is thought that these tumours may arise form the non-β-cells of the pancreatic islets. A variety of polypeptides result, the most active of which is VIP. Classically, these tumours produce 'pancreatic cholera' with profuse watery diarrhoea, hypokalaemia, and achlorhydria (WDHA) with extreme weakness syndrome. VIP is structurally very similar to secretin and Prostaglandin E which both increase intestinal motility and cause diarrhoea.

Diagnosis is confirmed by profuse diarrhoea (>30 times/day) with the passage of over 5 l of fluid, profound hypokalaemia, achlorhydria and high levels of serum VIP; 80% are solitary in the body or tail of pancreas and can be easily removed. CT scanning and angiography should be used to localise the tumour prior to surgery.

Approximately 50% are malignant and of these, 75% have metastasised by the time of presentation. If the tumour cannot be located, distal pancreatectomy should be performed. If symptoms persist, steroids or indomethacin may be of value in controlling symptoms. In addition, selective arterial administration of streptozotosin to the tumour or selective embolisation may improve symptoms. Following successful treatment there may be a rebound of gastric hypersecretion which may need treatment.

Carcinoid tumours/carcinoid syndrome

Carcinoid tumours arise from Amine Precursor Uptake Decarboxylase (APUD) cells and can be found anywhere in the gastro-intestinal tract. They produce an excess of serotonin (5-hydroxytryptamine). The most common site is the appendix or distal small bowel but they have been described to arise anywhere in the gastrointestinal (GI) tract, in the lungs and intra-ovarian. Tumours are usually asymptomatic secretion wise, the serotonin being broken down in the liver, and they normally present with local problems for example appendicitis, small bowel obstruction. Appendix carcinoids rarely metastasise.

Metastatic spread occurs in 10% of cases and is mainly from small bowel carcinoids to the liver. Once in the liver, tumour can now liberate serotonin directly into the systemic circulation which will cause the classic symptoms of carcinoid syndrome (flushing, diarrhoea, bronchoconstriction, and right sided cardiac valve disease). Ovarian and bronchial carcinoids can obviously cause carcinoid syndrome without hepatic metastases because of venous drainage directly into the systemic circulation. Various hormones in addition to serotonin have been implicated in the production of symptoms: catecholamines, histamine, kallikrein, prostaglandins, ACTH and calcitonin.

Carcinoid syndrome can usually be confirmed by the detection of the breakdown product of serotonin on the urine (5-hydroxy-indole-acetic acid – 5-HIAA). Low levels however do not absolutely exclude the diagnosis.

Treatment is by resection of the primary tumour. Hepatic metastases may be treated by hepatic arterial embolisation since these tumours seem to be dependent on the hepatic arterial circulation and not on the portal venous flow. Multiple liver metastases can also be simply enucleated from the liver parenchyma to good effect. Streptocintocinon may also be infused through the hepatic artery and be of value.

Carcinoid tumours of the foregut and lung usually belong to MEN I syndrome.

These tumours grow slowly and prognosis depends on the primary site:

- appendix carcinoids are usually small and solitary. They rarely metastasise and are usually cured by appendicectomy.
- Small bowel tumours are associated with a 70% 5 year survival rate. Only 40% of patients with inoperable metastases and 20% with liver secondaries will survive 5 years.

MULTIPLE ENDOCRINE NEOPLASIA (MEN)

Cells which secrete amine and polypeptide hormones, APUD cells, have many common characteristics:

- ability to store amines (A);
- ability to take up amine precursors such as dopamine (PU);
- possession of a decarboxylating enzyme, α-1-decarboxylase, which is necessary for amine synthesis (D).

APUD cells have specific chemical and immunofluorescent properties. They are derived from the neuroectoderm and migrate from the neural crest to their specific endocrine tissues where they secrete specific substances. Cells exist in the anterior pituitary, adrenal medulla, thyroid, gastrointestinal tract and pancreas.

Tumours and hyperplasia of these cells may result in specific endocrine syndromes and may be cross-related, occurring in one individual or one family with association of different but related endocrine syndromes. These syndromes of multiple tumours from APUD cells are known as MEN syndromes.

The commonest tumours arise from the anterior pituitary, adrenal medulla, pancreas and C-cells of the thyroid gland. In described syndromes, parathyroid hyperplasia is also found but it is unclear why this is involved since PTH is not formed by APUD cells.

Two main groups of associated tumours have been described, MEN I and MEN II.

MEN I

MEN I is an association of hormone over-production from the parathyroid, pancreatic, islets of Langerhans of the pancreas and anterior pituitary. There is quite a variation of described syndromes in MEN I and individual families may have a tendency to have only specific tumours in that family unit. Some members of MEN I families have also been described with thyroid, adrenal and soft tissue tumours such as lipomata. Any patient presenting with a foregut or lung carcinoid tumour should immediately alert the clinician to the possibility of MEN I.

The commonest abnormality is hyperparathyroidism due to parathyroid hyperplasia(95%). Gastrinomas occur in about 40% and insulinomas in about 10%. Pituitary tumours causing acromegaly or prolactinomas are rare.

Tumours tend to be transmitted as an autosomal dominant trait and therefore screening of close family members should be performed.

MEN II

MEN II, also known as Sipple's syndrome, consists of a triad of hormonal tumours – parathyroid hyperplasia, medullary carcinoma of thyroid, and phaeochromocytoma. MEN II is divided into two types: MEN IIA in which the predominant lesion is medullary carcinoma of thyroid: and MEN IIB in which there is associated multiple neuromas, ganglioneuromas and a Marfan type habitus.

All patients presenting with medullary carcinoma of thyroid should be screened for MEN II and if any associated tumours are detected, close family screening should be performed. The medullary carcinoma of MEN II is more aggressive than the sporadic form, especially in MEN IIB. In known MEN II families, chromosomal analysis of neonates will detect inheritance of the gene. In these children, calcitonin assay following pentagastrin stimulation will detect a premalignant phase of medullary carcinoma, and a total thyroidectomy should be performed. Since the youngest age described of established medullary carcinoma in MEN is 3 years, surgery is recommended before this age. Such surgery will result in marked improvement in life expectancy.

Urinary catecholamines and VMA estimations must be carried out and if a phaeochromocytoma is detected, this requires treatment prior to treatment of any of the other lesions of the syndrome.

FURTHER READING

Buchanan MA, Lee D. Thyroid auto-antibodies, lymphocyte infiltration and the development of post-operative hypothyroidism following hemi-thyroidectomy for non-toxic nodular goitre, *J Roy Coll Surg Edinb* 2001, Apr; 46(2): 86–90

Lee D and Marson LP. "Surgical Management of Thyroid Diseases" in *Advanced Surgical Practice* (2002) ed: Aljafri and Kingsnorth Chapter 32, pages 481–498

Wheeler MH. Thyroid surgery and the recurrent laryngeal nerve. *Br J Surg* 1999; **86**: 291–292

Dralle H. Lymph node dissection and medullary thyroid carcinoma. *Br J Surg* 2002; **89**: 1073–1075

Wheeler MH. Retrosternal goitre. *Br J Surg* 1999; **86**: 1235–1236

Mehrotra P. et al. Ultrasound scan-guided core sampling for diagnosis versus freehand FNAC of the thyroid gland. *The Surgeon* 2005; **3**(1): 1–5

Berti et al. Limits and drawbacks of video-assisted parathyroidectomy. *Br J Surg* 2003; **90**: 743–747

Ganger M. Endoscopic subtotal parathyroidectomy in patients with primary hyperparathyroidism. *Br J Surg* 1996; **83**: 875

Kaplan EL. Endocrine surgery. *J Am Coll Surg* 1999; **188**: 118–126

Biertho L. et al. Image-directed parathyroidectomy under local anaesthesia in the elderly. *Br J Surg* 2003 ; **90** : 738–742

Duh Q-Y. Adrenal incidentalomas. *Br J Surg* 2002; **89**: 1347–1349

Miccoli P. et al. Adrenal surgery before and after the introduction of laparoscopic adrenalectomy. *Br J Surg* 2002; **89**: 779–782

Dudley NE & Harrison BJ. Comparison of open posterior *versus* transperitoneal laparoscopic adrenalectomy. *Br J Surg* 1999; **86**: 656–660

Assalia A & Ganger M. Laparoscopic adrenalectomy. *Br J Surg* 2004; **91**: 1259–1274

Skogseid B. Multiple Endocrine Neoplasia type 1. *Br J Surg* 2003; **90**: 383–385

Eriksson B & Oberg K. Neuroendocrine tumours of the pancreas. *Br J Surg* 2000; **87**: 129–131

17

The Breast

Steven D Heys

Department of Surgery, University of Aberdeen, Foresterhill, Aberdeen, UK

CONTENTS

Basic biology 322
Anatomy of the breast 322
Anatomy of the axilla 324
Congenital abnormalities of the breast 325
Physiological changes in the female breast 325

Diagnostic modalities used in the assessment of breast disease 325
Clinical assessment 325
Imaging 325
Fine needle aspiration cytology 327
Breast biopsy 328

Benign breast disorders 329
Infections 329
Mammary duct fistula 330
Mammary duct ectasia 330
Nipple discharge 330
Nipple retraction (inversion) 331
Nipple and areola skin disorders 332
Mastalgia 332
Fibroadenomas 333
Breast cysts 334
Mammary dysplasia 334
Fat necrosis 335
Mondor's disease 335
Gynaecomastia 336

Carcinoma of the breast 336
Introduction 336
Epidemiology and risk factors 336
Breast cancer: pathological types 338
Prognostic factors in breast cancer 340
Staging of breast cancer 341
Clinical features 342
Diagnosis 343
Treatment 343
Breast reconstruction 345
Adjuvant therapy 346

Metastatic breast cancer 347
Paget's disease of the nipple 348
Phylloides tumour of the breast 348
Breast cancer in the elderly 348
Bilateral breast cancers 348
Breast cancer during pregnancy and lactation 349
Breast cancer in the male 349
Screening for breast cancer 349

BASIC BIOLOGY

Anatomy of the breast

Embryology

The breast is a modified sweat gland which originates from the ectodermal layer of the embryo between the fifth and sixth week of gestation. It arises from the 'milk lines', which are two ridges of ectodermal thickening, running from the axilla to the groin. Although most of the 'milk line' eventually disappears, a prominent ridge remains in the pectoral area to form the breast. The ectoderm in this area subsequently grows into the underlying mesoderm as a series (15–20) of buds. These ectodermal buds, which are initially solid, eventually form the lactiferous ducts and their associated alveoli. The adjacent mesenchyme develops into the surrounding adipose and connective tissues. During the final 2 months of gestation, the ducts become canalised and a 'mammary pit' is formed in the ectoderm. The lactiferous ducts subsequently communicate with the mammary pit.

Gross anatomy
Morphological features

The breast is situated within the subcutaneous tissue of the anterolateral chest wall. It extends from the second to the sixth rib and from the edge of the sternum to the mid-axillary line, overlying the pectoralis major, serratus anterior, upper part of the rectus sheath and external oblique muscles. The breast extends in a supero-lateral direction along the border of the pectoralis major muscle, through the foramen of Langer in the deep fascia of the axilla, to lie close to the pectoral group

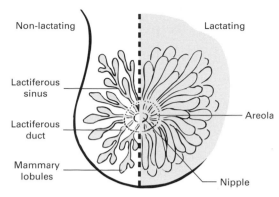

Figure 17.1. Anatomy of the breast and- chest wall. Permission from *Essential Clinical Anatomy*, Williams & Wilkins, Baltimore.

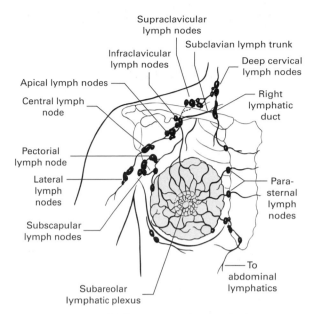

Figure 17.2. Anatomy of axilla. Permission from *Gray's Anatomy*, 35th edn., Churchill Livingston, p. 648, 1973.

of axillary lymph nodes. This is termed the axillary tail of Spence. The breast is separated from the muscles it overlies by the deep fascia. However, between the breast and the deep fascia is the retromammary space which contains loose areolar tissue. Supporting connective tissue strands pass between the dermal layer of the skin and the underlying breast. They are well developed in the upper aspect of the breast and are referred to as the suspensory ligaments of Cooper.

The nipple usually lies at the level of the fourth intercostal space and 15–20 lactiferous ducts open onto its surface through small openings. Surrounding the nipple is the areola which is made up of pigmented skin and subcutaneous tissue in which lie smooth muscle fibres. The epithelium contains sweat glands, sebaceous glands and accessory mammary glandular tissue (Figs 17.1 and 17.2).

Arterial supply and venous drainage
The blood supply to the breast is from the perforating branches of the internal thoracic artery (lateral edge of the sternum), the lateral thoracic artery and the pectoral branch of the acromiothoracic artery (the latter two derived from the axillary artery). In addition, there is also a variable blood supply from perforating branches of the intercostal arteries and from the subscapular artery. The venous drainage is through veins corresponding to the arterial supply.

Lymphatic drainage
The lymphatic drainage of the breast is predominantly through lymph vessels which are located in the interlobular connective tissues. These lymph vessels communicate with the cutaneous and subcutaneous lymphatic plexuses, the subareolar plexus of Sappey, and a plexus lying beneath the breast on the deep fascia covering the pectoralis major muscle. It has been estimated that approximately 75% of the lymph drainage of the breast is to the axillary groups of lymph nodes. These are the anterior (or pectoral nodes) which are situated along the lateral thoracic vessels, the posterior (or subscapular nodes) which are on the subscapular vessels, the central group of lymph nodes lying within the axilla, and the apical group sited at the apex of the axilla (Fig. 17.3).

These lymph nodes can be subdivided anatomically, depending on their relationship to the pectoralis minor muscle: level 1: nodes lying below the muscle; level 2: nodes lying behind the muscle and level 3: nodes above the muscle in the apex of the axilla. The lymphatic drainage from the apical nodes is to the supraclavicular and lower cervical groups of nodes. However, it is also recognised that 25% of the lymph drainage of the breast (medial aspect) is to the internal thoracic nodes and, in addition, some lymphatic drainage is through the lymphatics of the anterior abdominal wall.

Microscopic anatomy
The breast is composed of glandular elements, fibrous and fat tissues. The glandular part of the breast consists of between 15 and 20 lobes. A lobe has approximately 30 lobules, which terminate in the acini (10–100). The acini are separated from each other by the intralobular connective tissue and the lobules are separated from each other by fine connective tissue. Light microscopic examination of an acinus demonstrates that it is composed of two cell types: the secretory epithelial cell and the contractile myoepithelial cell. The terminal duct and the acini of a lobule are termed the 'terminal duct lobular unit'. These ducts unite to form subsegmental and segmental ducts, which in turn drain into the lactiferous ducts and sinuses. The lactiferous ducts (15–20) pass towards the nipple and areola, where they undergo dilatation to form the

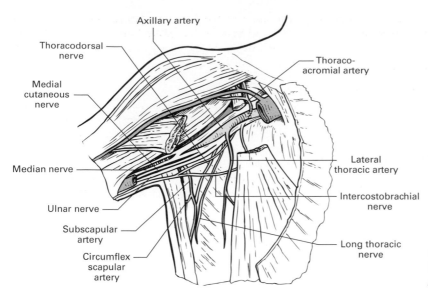

Figure 17.3. Lymphatic drainage of the breast. Permission from *Essential Clinical Anatomy*, Williams & Wilkins, Baltimore.

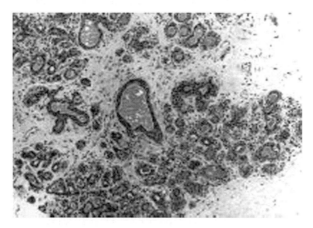

Figure 17.4. Microscopic anatomy of the breast. Permission from *Atlas of Human Histology*, di Fiore MSH (ed.), Lea and Febiger, Philadelphia, p. 245.

lactiferous sinuses. The sinuses open onto the surface of the nipple through separate ductular orifices (Fig. 17.4).

Anatomy of the axilla

Structure

The axilla is a pyramidal space with an apex, base (or floor) and four walls – anterior, posterior, medial and lateral. The apex is bordered by the outer border of the first rib, the posterior surface of the middle third of the clavicle and the upper border of the scapula. The base of the axilla is formed by skin and deep fascia, the axillary fascia. The anterior wall is made up of the pectoralis major, the pectoralis minor and subclavius muscles, and the clavipectoral fascia (lying between the lower border of subclavius and upper border of pectoralis minor). The extension of the clavipectoral fascia, running from the lower border of the pectoralis minor muscle to the floor of the axilla, is termed the suspensory ligament of the axilla. The posterior wall of the axilla comprises the subscapularis, teres major and latissimus dorsi muscles. The medial wall is formed by the first five ribs, the intercostal muscles and the overlying serratus anterior muscle. The lateral wall is the intertubercular sulcus of the humerus, the coracobrachialis and biceps muscles. The structures passing through the axilla are important and include blood vessels, nerves, lymphatic vessels and lymph nodes (see above), areolar tissue and fat.

Neurovascular contents

The axillary artery and vein, together with the brachial plexus of nerves, run from the apex of the axilla along its lateral wall into the upper arm. Two important nerves running through the axilla are the long thoracic and the thoracodorsal nerves. The former lies along the posterior aspect of the medial wall of the axilla and supplies the serratus anterior muscle. The latter is joined by the thoracodorsal vessels on the anterior surface of subscapularis and supplies motor fibres to the latissimus dorsi muscle. The intercostobrachial nerve (lateral cutaneous branch of the second intercostal nerve) traverses the axilla and supplies the skin of the floor of the axilla and inner aspect of the upper arm, communicating with the posterior brachial cutaneous branch of the radial nerve. A second intercostobrachial nerve, also supplying the axilla and medial aspect of the arm, is commonly given off from the lateral cutaneous branch of the third intercostal nerve.

Congenital abnormalities of the breast

A variety of congenital anomalies of the breast may occur.

Types of abnormalities
Supernumery nipples and breasts
Accessory nipples can be found anywhere along the 'milk line', from the axilla to the groin, but most often are found below the normal breast. Accessory breasts (with or without nipples) may also occur along the 'milk line' but are usually found in the axilla.

Congenital inversion of the nipple
This arises because the mammary pit fails to become evaginated to form the nipple. This may spontaneously correct itself during pregnancy or by traction on the nipple.

Other abnormalities
These include amastia (congenital absence of a breast) or breast hypoplasia, both with a variable degree of underdevelopment of the pectoral muscles. Less commonly, this may be found in association with defects of the upper limb and this is known as Poland's syndrome.

Physiological changes in the female breast

Menstrual cycle
Changes occur in the breast in a cyclical fashion during the menstrual cycle. After cessation of menstruation there is proliferation of ductal and ductular cells. Subsequently, in the second phase of the menstrual cycle, there is proliferation of the terminal duct structures, in association with increased mitosis in the basal epithelial cells and stromal cell proliferation. In addition, the stroma of the lobules becomes oedematous during this phase. However, towards the end of the cycle there is a reduction in cell numbers through the process of apoptosis. These changes are dependent on the stimulatory effects of oestrogens and progestogens.

Pregnancy and lactation
Marked changes occur in the breast during pregnancy under the influence of a variety of hormones (e.g. oestrogens, progestogens, prolactin, insulin, growth hormone and chorionic gonadotrophins). There is an increase in the number and size of lobules, and an increase in the number of acini within each lobule. During the third trimester, secretory vacuoles of lipid material appear in the epithelial cells, and is the precursor of milk production. Following birth, milk is secreted by the epithelial cells into the ductules, mainly under the influence of prolactin. Once breast feeding has ceased, these changes regress with atrophy of the gland, hyalinisation of the lobules and reduction in the size of the ducts, occurring over approximately 3 months.

Involution changes
From the age of 35 onwards, progressive involutional changes occur in the female breast. There is a gradual involution of breast glandular elements, especially lobules, a thickening of the basal lamina of the acini, a reduction in the amount of inter- and intralobular connective tissue but with an increase in the amount of fat within the breast. In some women there may be almost total disappearance of the lobules as ageing progresses.

DIAGNOSTIC MODALITIES USED IN THE ASSESSMENT OF BREAST DISEASE
Clinical assessment

A thorough history is necessary in all women presenting with breast disease. Careful details about the presenting breast complaint (lump, pain, nipple discharge, etc.) should be taken and, in addition, the following points should be carefully noted:
1. *Past history*: This should include menopausal status, age at menarche, parity, age at first full-term pregnancy, breast feeding, usage of oral contraceptives and/or hormone replacement therapy (HRT), previous history of breast disease.
2. *Family history*: Relatives (in particular first degree) with breast cancer, ovarian cancer or family members with any type of cancers (ages of onset and relationship).

Clinical examination of the breast should be carried out. In particular, inspection of the breast is carried out with the patient sitting and with their arms elevated and on their hips. With the patient reclining (arms behind head) both the breasts (quadrants and tail) are palpated using the flat of the hand. The axilla is examined and lymph node status ascertained; the supraclavicular area is palpated for lymphadenopathy (examiner standing behind the patient). Although clinical examination is crucial it does have some limitations. For example, an experienced clinician will only diagnose 8 out of 10 cancers presenting to a symptomatic breast clinic. Therefore, other modalities are necessary to confirm or establish the nature of breast symptoms and/or lesions.

Imaging

Mammography
Mammography (soft tissue radiography) involves having two radiographs taken of the breast: cranio-caudal and oblique views of each breast. The total X-ray dose is usually less than 1 mGy. This technique is most useful when the breasts contain little of dense glandular tissues and are

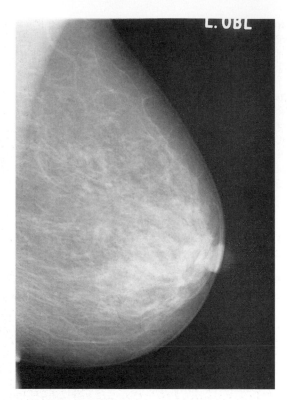

Figure 17.5. Normal mammogram.

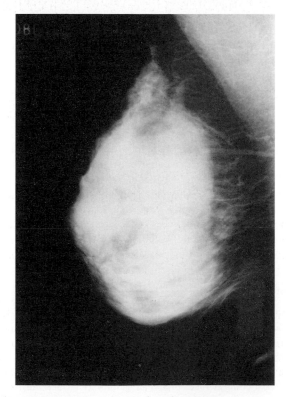

Figure 17.6. Mammogram showing dense breast tissue.

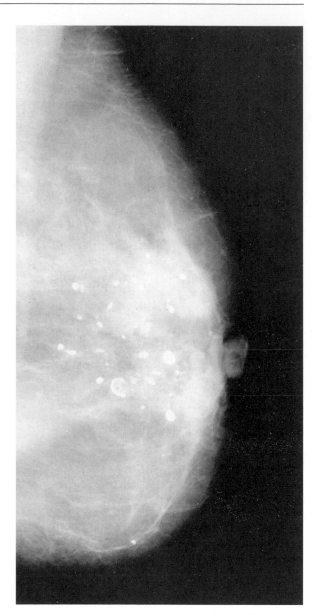

Figure 17.7. Mammogram demonstrating benign microcalcification.

composed predominantly of fat (Fig. 17.5). Therefore, in younger women (with dense glandular elements in the breasts) it is less accurate and reliable (Fig. 17.6). In general, mammography is reserved for women over the age of 35 years but should be carried out in younger women if there is a good clinical indication (e.g. suspicion of cancer).

The mammographic features of malignancy include: (i) microcalcification, comprising multiple particles of irregular size and density (see Figs 17.7 and 17.8 for examples of benign and malignant microcalcification); (ii) an opacity with characteristically irregular or spiculated margins (Fig. 17.9) and (iii) an area of distortion of the normal breast architecture

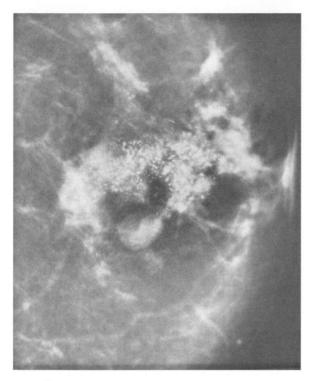

Figure 17.8. Mammographic appearances of microcalcification associated with malignancy.

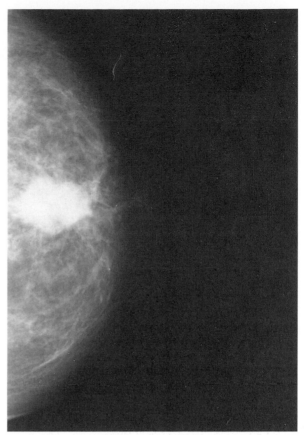

Figure 17.9. Characteristic appearances of a breast cancer on mammography.

(Fig. 17.10). These can be compared with the appearances of a breast cyst shown in Fig. 17.11. In some patients, axillary lymph nodes may also be visible, whilst in others thickening (oedema) and retraction of the skin of the breast can be seen. The sensitivity of mammography ranges from 75% to 90%, whilst its specificity varies from 70% to 85%.

Ultrasonography

Breast ultrasound is being used with increasing frequency in clinical practice. It is most useful in distinguishing solid from cystic lesions (Fig. 17.11), in imaging the dense breast tissue in young women; it may also be helpful when mammography has been performed and has not been diagnostic. As with most ultrasound investigations, breast ultrasound is operator dependent and the sensitivity varies from 70% to 90%, with a specificity of approximately 80–95%.

Magnetic resonance mammography

Preliminary studies have shown that magnetic resonance mammography (MRM) can have a sensitivity of between 88% and 100% but with a specificity ranging from as low as 37–97%. This does limit the widespread clinical use of MRM. However, in patients with suspected local recurrence it can be very useful in identifying this and MRM also can allow the detection of multifocal disease within the breast. Other potential uses for MRM include assessing the response to

primary chemotherapy and there are trials which are evaluating its use as a screening technique, particularly in its role in younger women.

Fine needle aspiration cytology

After clinical examination and imaging procedures have been carried out and a 'lump' has been documented, a definitive diagnosis is required. The latter can be established by carrying out fine needle aspiration cytology (FNAC) obviating the need for a formal biopsy (requiring surgery) or a core or TruCut biopsy (which can be uncomfortable for the patient).

FNAC is performed using a standard (10 ml) syringe and needle (21G); a special gun containing the syringe may be used. The needle is inserted into the palpable lump and suction is applied to the syringe in order to aspirate material into the needle. Multiple passes are made into the lump, in a range of directions, in order to obtain as representative an aspirate as possible. The needle is then withdrawn from the lump and the contents of the needle spread out onto

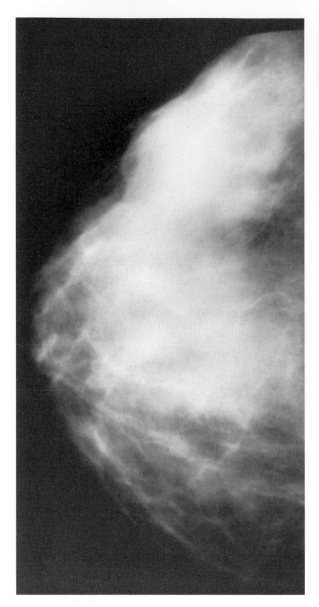

Figure 17.10. Mammographic appearances of a breast cancer showing increased density and architectural changes.

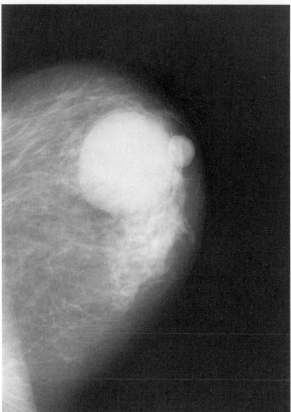

Figure 17.11. (a) Mammographic appearances of a breast cyst.

microscope slides, with some being dried in air and others put into a fixative solution. The cells can then be stained (e.g. Giemsa, Papanicolaou, haematoxylin and oesin) prior to microscopic examination. Many major centres have a cytologist present at the breast clinic who will examine and report on the breast aspirates whilst the patient is at the clinic and an immediate report is provided. The scoring system used for reporting the results of FNAC is shown in Table 17.1. The sensitivity of FNAC is approximately 95% (ranging from 80% to 99%), with a specificity of 98% (ranging from 95% to 99%) (Figs 17.12 and 17.13).

If a lesion in the breast has been detected on either mammography or ultrasonography (but is not clinically detectable) then cytological examination of the lesion can still be made. This is carried out either stereotactically using mammographic-guided fine needle aspiration (FNA) or by ultrasound-guided FNA. Established centres using triple assessment (clinical examination, imaging (mammography, ultrasonography) and FNAC) report a sensitivity of more than 95%, specificity of more than 96% and a predictive value of more than 97%, with this approach. However, in some patients it is still not possible to make a definitive diagnosis despite use of triple assessment and in these cases a biopsy will be required for histological examination.

Breast biopsy

Needle biopsy
Breast biopsy can be performed under local anaesthesia by using a 'TruCut' needle or a 'drill'-type needle which removes a core of tissue. Both of these techniques can be uncomfortable and lead to bruising. However, they allow an assessment of tumour type and grade of tumour to be determined.

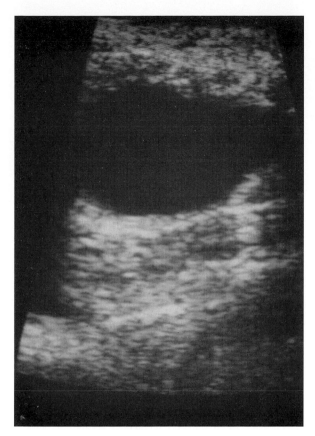

Figure 17.11. (b) Ultrasonographic appearances of a breast cyst.

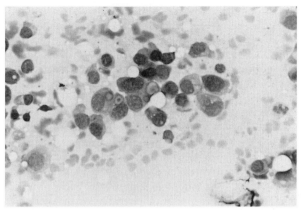

Figure 17.13. Malignant cells obtained using FNAC.

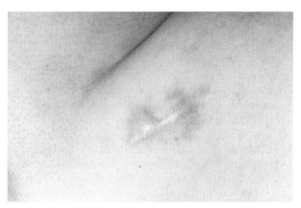

Figure 17.14. Example of a thickened scar in a radial skin incision following biopsy for benign breast disease.

Table 17.1. **Fine needle aspiration cytology scoring system.**

C0	No epithelial cells present
C1	Scanty benign epithelial cells
C2	Benign epithelial cells
C3	Atypical cells
C4	Cells which are highly suspicious of cancer
C5	Definitely malignant cells

Operative biopsy

Operative biopsy (incisional or excisional) can be performed under a local or general anaesthetic. The skin incision should be made circumferentially (Langer's lines) and not radially as this can result in hypertrophic scarring (Fig. 17.14).

BENIGN BREAST DISORDERS

Infections

Non-lactating breast

Infections in non-lactating breasts usually occur in the peri-areolar region as periductal mastitis, typically in pre-meno-pausal women. The precise aetiology is unknown but smoking is thought to play a role in the pathogenesis of this condition. Various bacteria, such as staphylococcus pyogenes, strep-tococci, enterococci and anaerobic organisms, have been implicated. Less commonly, infections can occur in the more peripheral parts of the breast.

Periductal mastitis usually presents as a tender swelling in the periareolar region. There may be erythema of the overlying

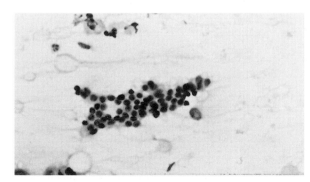

Figure 17.12. Benign cells obtained using FNAC.

and surrounding skin, and features of abscess formation. These changes tend to be localised to a segment of the breast but the infection may spread to involve most of the breast. In addition, there may also be a discharge from the nipple and/or nipple retraction. Systemic manifestations of sepsis (fever, leucocytosis, systemic upset) may be present.

With localised infection, and in the absence of an obvious abscess, the treatment is systemic antibiotic therapy. If a small collection of pus is present (confirmed clinically, ultrasonographically) this should be aspirated with a fine bore needle; this can be repeated. However, if this is unsuccessful or the abscess is large then incision and drainage of the abscess under general anaesthesia is required. Although the infective episode resolves with treatment recurrent infections/abscesses occur in many patients. A mammary duct fistula may develop (usually as a result of surgical intervention) and will require definitive treatment (see later). It should also be noted that inflammatory cancers of the breast can present in a similar way, and biopsies of the abscess cavity may be required for definitive histological examination.

Lactating breast

Infections may occur during lactation. The organisms most commonly involved are staphylococcus pyogenes and epidermidis. The bacteria may originate from the mother or the child and access to the breast parenchyma through a break in the skin of the nipple is believed to occur. Engorgement of the breast with milk and delay in ductal clearance are additional important factors. The clinical features and treatment of these infections are as already described above. The baby may still be fed from the uninfected breast if the patient wishes.

Other infections

Other, uncommon acute and chronic infections and inflammatory processes can also affect the breast and axilla. These include, tuberculosis, actinomycosis, fungal infections, pilonidal sinus disease, and the spread of infections from the chest wall.

Mammary duct fistula

A mammary duct fistula is an abnormal connection between the skin (usually periareolar) and a major breast duct (usually subareolar). As already discussed, the commonest cause is periductal mastitis, with the fistula typically arising as a result of surgical intervention.

Clinically, the condition usually presents as a discharging area(s) in the breast in the vicinity of the areola; recurrent episodes of infection involving the fistula is not uncommon (Fig. 17.15). Treatment of this condition requires excision of the whole fistula tract, and adjacent area of scar tissue, with healing either by secondary intention or by primary closure under antibiotic cover. However, in some patients the fistula can recur and more radical surgery (subareolar duct excision) is required.

Mammary duct ectasia

There has been much debate as to the relationship between periductal mastitis and mammary duct ectasia. Although it has often been held that these are variants of the same pathological process, with the former possibly resulting in the latter, the two conditions are probably different. Periductal mastitis occurs in young pre-menopausal women whilst mammary duct ectasia occurs more commonly in peri- and post-menopausal females. Histological examination shows there is dilatation of ducts filled with inspissated breast secretions and lipid-filled macrophages. In some patients, there may be squamous metaplasia of the lactiferous ducts and fibrous tissue formation. However, duct dilatation is common and occurs in approximately 50% of women over the age of 60 years.

Clinically, mammary duct ectasia presents as nipple discharge, often affecting multiple ducts. The discharge varies in colour from clear to black, and in many of the cases it contains blood (microscopic or macroscopic). It is often thick and white. The patients may also have varying degrees of nipple retraction. If treatment is required (for symptomatic control or diagnostic uncertainty), and as multiple ducts are likely to be involved, subareolar duct excision should be carried out.

Nipple discharge

Nipple discharge is relatively common in the female population and is the third commonest cause of referral to a specialist breast clinic. However, it has been estimated that less than 10% of cancers are associated with breast discharge.

Nipple discharge can be categorised into several types: clear or watery, milky, serous, multicoloured or blood stained. In addition, the discharge may come from a single or from multiple ducts. The most common causes of the different types of nipple discharge are shown in Table 17.2. However, in a very small number of cases of watery or serous discharge coming from a single duct, an underlying cancer may be found. In a small number of women with prolonged,

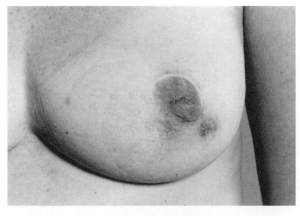

Figure 17.15. Example of a mammary duct fistula.

profuse, bilateral milky discharge abnormal serum prolactin levels may suggest a prolactinoma of the pituitary gland.

After clinical examination of the breast various investigations are undertaken. The discharge should be tested for the presence of blood (e.g. Labstix testing) and examined microscopically for the presence of malignant cells. All patients over the age of 35 years should also have mammography; ultrasound examination of the breast may reveal the presence of dilated lactiferous ducts, particularly those close to the nipple and areola. In some patients, if there is discharge from a single duct, a ductogram (injection of contrast material into the duct) may demonstrate an intraduct papilloma, carcinoma or duct ectasia. In many women in whom no underlying cause for the discharge has been found, the discharge may resolve, be intermittent and/or of small amount which does not concern the patient (see Fig. 17.16 for management). However, if there is a large amount of discharge, if it comes from a single duct or

tests suggest underlying pathology (e.g. prominent red blood cell content, atypical or malignant cells), then the duct should be removed surgically (microdochectomy). In older women or those not intending to conceive and breast feed, if the duct cannot be identified or the discharge comes from several ducts, then subareolar central duct excision is undertaken through a circumareolar incision.

Nipple retraction (inversion)

The terms nipple retraction and inversion have come to be used interchangeably. However, nipple inversion is most often used when the whole of the nipple is permanently pulled inwards, whilst nipple retraction is used to describe variable degrees (usually intermittent) of the nipple being pulled inwards.

Congenital nipple inversion (of variable degree) occurs in up to one-fifth of all women. This is usually of no clinical significance unless it interferes with breast feeding. The woman may present because of the cosmetic deformity. However, two of the most common causes of nipple retraction are mammary duct ectasia and periductal mastitis. Clinically, this manifests as a transverse depression in the nipple which progresses to complete retraction (there may also be an associated nipple discharge). This process may be intermittent in its early stages and can be present in both breasts. Nipple retraction may also occur in patients with breast cancer. In the latter this is unilateral and there may be an associated breast lump, with or without a nipple discharge (often blood stained).

Table 17.2. **The risk of breast cancer occurring in patients with certain types of benign breast disease.**

Type of benign breast disease	Risk of developing breast cancer
Sclerosing adenosis	1.5–2
Papilloma (one)	1.5–2
Moderate hyperplasia but there is no cellular atypia	1.5–2
Atypical ductal hyperplasia	4–5
Atypical lobular hyperplasia	4–5

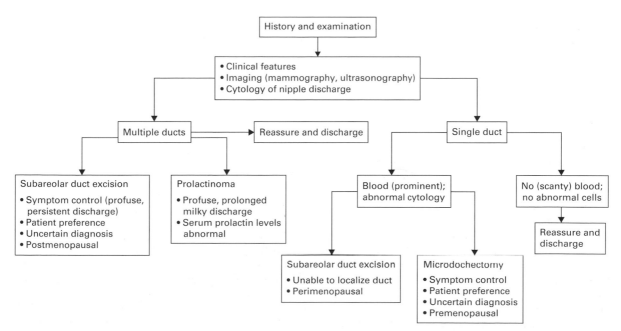

Figure 17.16. Scheme of management for patients with nipple discharge.

Investigations of patients with nipple retraction include mammography and, if appropriate, ultrasonography to determine if there is an underlying tumour present. However, in the absence of malignancy, and in the majority of women, reassurance only is required. In young women and in those seeking cosmesis, surgical correction with eversion of the nipple may be carried out. However, this may cause damage to the underlying ducts and can interfere with attempts at breast feeding subsequently.

Nipple and areola skin disorders

The skin of the nipples may become involved with dermatitis and/or eczematous skin disorders. These often affect both nipples; the typical skin changes being erythema and scaliness. However, these must be differentiated from Paget's disease of the breast (see later).

The glands of Montgomery (large sebaceous glands opening onto the areola) may become blocked with the formation of a lump in the areola. This can be removed if necessary.

Mastalgia

Breast pain is one of the commonest symptoms in patients attending a specialist breast clinic, occurring in up to 50% of the patients. Furthermore, up to two-thirds of women will experience breast pain during their life-time. In some women, this may be of a minor nature occurring infrequently, but in others this may be severe pain which can interfere with their life-style.

Breast pain is commonly categorised into two main types: cyclical and non-cyclical. Whilst breast pain is considered as a benign condition, it has been estimated that breast pain may be the presenting symptom in up to 10 of patients with breast cancer.

Cyclical mastalgia

Cyclical mastalgia usually affects younger women, with the median age being 35 years. The mastalgia is related to the menstrual cycle and is commonly described as a fullness, heaviness, discomfort or pain (of varying degrees of severity), felt particularly for the few days prior to the onset of menstruation. The mastalgia is often described as occurring in the upper and outer quadrant of the breast, and may be bilateral. In some cases the pain/discomfort may be referred to the upper arm or axilla. The mastalgia usually abates after the onset of menstruation, only to return as the menstrual cycle progresses. Physical examination may reveal no overt clinical abnormality apart from some tenderness. Examination, on the other hand, may demonstrate associated breast nodularity (localised, diffuse, uni- or bilateral).

Non-cyclical mastalgia

Non-cyclical mastalgia occurs in an older age group of women and is not related to the menstrual cycle. It may occur intermittently, although in some patients it can be continuous. This type of pain is usually felt in the medial aspect of the breast and also in the periareolar regions; it may resolve spontaneously. In addition to pain and discomfort arising in the breast, non-cyclical mastalgia may also arise from the musculoskeletal system, for example Tietz's syndrome (pain arising from the costochondral areas).

Pathogenesis

The relationship of cyclical mastalgia to the menstrual cycle has suggested that there may be a hormonal basis for the symptom complex; for example, abnormal levels of gonadotrophins, oestrogens or prolactin. However, to date, no consistent abnormalities in circulating levels of these hormones have been demonstrated. An alternative explanation, therefore, is that there is an increased sensitivity to circulating hormones, possibly at the level of the hormone receptors within the breast tissues. Other suggestions for the cause of mastalgia have included an increased water retention within the breast tissues, an increased dietary intake of saturated fats or deficiencies of vitamins (e.g. B1, B6 and E). In addition, the intake of methylxanthines has been suggested to be an important 'trigger' mechanism, although the precise reasons for this remain unclear.

More recently, interest has focused on alterations in essential fatty acids, in particular, gammalinolenic acid, in patients with mastalgia. For example, some studies have shown that patients with mastalgia have low circulating levels of gammalinolenic acid. Furthermore, women with severe cyclical breast pain appear to have low plasma levels of the metabolites of gammalinolenic acid, although it is unclear whether this represents a dietary deficiency or some abnormality in metabolism. The possible reasons why there changes in essential fatty acids may be important are as follows: (i) steroid hormones may become esterified to fatty acids in their target tissues and the resultant esters (e.g. with saturated fats) are more potent; (ii) saturated fatty acids have a higher affinity for hormone receptors than unsaturated fats and an excess of saturated fats in the cell membranes will enhance receptor expression; (iii) the prostaglandins (PGE_1), synthesised from gammalinolenic acid metabolites, can reduce the trophic effects of prolactin on breast tissue. Although some of these mechanisms may also be important in the aetiology of non-cyclical mastalgia, this is less well understood.

Management
Investigations
A careful history should be taken from patients with mastalgia (a pain diary will help to differentiate cyclical from the non-cyclical variety) and a careful examination carried out (in up to 10% of patients with breast cancer, pain is the presenting symptom). Investigations that may be required are breast imaging (mammography and/or breast ultrasound) and FNAC.

Treatment

One of the most important aspects of therapy in patients with mastalgia is reassurance; approximately two-thirds of patients requiring no other forms of therapy. However, when treatment is required then a variety of substances are available, not all of which have been shown to be effective in randomised-controlled trials. These are each discussed in more detail below.

Dietary alteration

One small study has shown that reducing substantially the dietary fat intake resulted in a significant improvement in breast tenderness. Certain foods (e.g. caffeine) may trigger episodes of mastalgia.

Gammalinolenic acid

Trials have shown that gammalinolenic acid can be effective in reducing breast pain and tenderness. In patients with cyclical mastalgia up to 60% appear to benefit, whereas only approximately 40% of those with non-cyclical mastalgia will have relief of pain. Patient compliance is excellent and side effects are minimal (occasionally patients may experience mild gastrointestinal symptoms). It is recommended that up to 320 mg/day should be given for at least 4 months as it may take this long to achieve the maximum benefit.

Danazol

Danazol is a synthetic steroid derived from ethisterone. It binds with a marked affinity to androgen receptors, with less affinity for progesterone and oestrogen receptors (OR). Randomised-controlled studies have also shown that danazol can significantly reduce breast pain and tenderness if given in doses of 100–200 mg twice daily for 3–6 months. However, although this is an effective therapy (80% with cyclical and 40% with non-cyclical mastalgia experience relief of symptoms), androgenic side effects (e.g. hirsutism, acne, deepening of the voice), weight gain, headache and nausea are relatively common. These side effects may occur in up to 30% of patients.

Bromocriptine

Bromocriptine is a dopamine agonist which stimulates dopamine receptors and lowers circulating levels of prolactin (by inhibiting pituitary secretion). Randomised-controlled studies have demonstrated that bromocriptine (5 mg/day) is beneficial, with up to 55% with cyclical and 30% of patients with non-cyclical mastalgia gaining significant relief. Unfortunately, side effects (e.g. nausea, headache, postural hypotension, constipation) occur in up to one-third of patients and can be treatment limiting.

Tamoxifen

The anti-oestrogen tamoxifen also reduces breast pain and tenderness. However, its product licence does not include the treatment of mastalgia.

Goserelin

Goserelin is a synthetic analogue of naturally occurring luteinising hormone releasing hormone (LHRH). When given over a long period it causes an inhibition of pituitary luteinising hormone (LH) secretion leading to falls in serum testosterone levels in men and serum oestradiol in women. Although it may result in significant improvements in breast symptoms in up to 90% of women with cyclical mastalgia, the side effects (headaches, hot flushes, loss of libido, vaginal dryness) are treatment limiting.

Other drug treatments

A variety of other agents have been used in the treatment of mastalgia, including antibiotics, pyridoxine, diuretics and progestogens. However, none of these has been proven to be effective in randomised-controlled trials.

Surgery

Surgical treatment for mastalgia is rarely indicated. However, very occasionally the mastalgia may be refractory to all forms of therapy and may be very incapacitating for the patient. In these rare instances, and with assistance from a psychologist, mastectomy (with or without breast reconstruction) may be indicated.

Fibroadenomas

Fibroadenomas are the commonest benign tumours to arise in the breast and are most often seen in women under the age of 35 years. They comprise approximately 10% of symptomatic breast lumps. In older women, particularly after the menopause, they are quite uncommon. In the latter age group they can undergo involution and become calcified. Large, rapidly growing fibroadenomas may occur in girls and young women.

Clinically, fibroadenomas are smooth, well-circumscribed, mobile lumps and in a few patients they can be multiple. Their size can vary, ranging from less than 1 cm to more than 10 cm in diameter. Those greater than 5 cm in diameter are termed 'giant fibroadenomas' (which are more common in non-caucasions).

Fibroadenomas are derived from the intralobular stroma and are composed of both fibrous and glandular elements. Histologically, there is an abundant fibroblastic stroma which surrounds glandular and cystic cavities lined by an epithelium (pericanalicular type) or there is a more active proliferation of the connective tissue stroma with a resultant compression of the glandular spaces (intracanalicular type). The epithelium in a fibroadenoma may be hormonally sensitive and result in an increase in size during the menstrual cycle, pregnancy and lactation.

The diagnosis is confirmed by imaging (ultrasound and/or mammography) and FNAC. It has been recommended that fibroadenomas of greater than 4 cm in size should be removed. This is carried out through a circumferential incision, under general (or local) anaesthesia. However, if triple assessment confirms the diagnosis the fibroadenoma may be left alone (approximately 20% of fibroadenomas will regress with time) depending on patient preference. However, if it enlarges in size or causes symptoms, it should be removed.

Breast cysts

Breast cysts are a common cause of referral to a specialised breast clinic, with up to 7% of all women presenting with a palpable cyst at some time during their life. The true incidence of cysts amongst the general population has been estimated to be as high as 20%. Cysts most commonly present in the 35–50-year age group as a lump (circumscribed, smooth, mobile) with a variable degree of discomfort or pain; up to 30% of such women will have multiple cysts. The aetiology of breast cysts is poorly understood. Although hormones have been implicated no consistent differences in hormonal levels in women with cysts have been identified.

A breast cyst arises from a breast lobule and on microscopy it is found to be lined by either a flattened epithelium (simple cysts) or by columnar secretory epithelium (apocrine cysts). Biochemically the contents of these two types of cysts are different. For example, simple cysts have high sodium and low potassium concentrations, with a sodium : potassium ratio of greater than 4 and a pH of less than 7.4. However, apocrine cysts have low sodium and high potassium concentrations, with a sodium : potassium ratio of less than 4 and a pH of greater than 7.4. The fluid from these cysts also contains a range of hormones, enzymes and growth factors.

The diagnosis of a cyst is confirmed by triple assessment. Mammography typically shows a well-defined opacity, although this may be difficult to demonstrate in dense breasts (Fig. 17.11(a)). Ultrasound examination, however, usually confirms that the lesion is a cyst (Fig. 17.11(b)). FNAC usually reveals straw-coloured fluid (sometimes bluish-green or brown). The fluid normally is not sent for cytological assessment. However, if the cyst is blood stained the fluid should be sent for cytological examination to exclude malignant cells and the presence of an intracystic growth. Following aspiration of a cyst the breast must be carefully examined to ensure that there has been complete resolution of the lump. If there is a residual palpable lump then this should undergo FNAC in case there is an underlying cancer.

Many surgeons will re-examine the breast 6–8 weeks later to determine if the cyst has re-accumulated. If so, it may be aspirated on a second and possibly third occasion. Although the management of cysts which repeatedly re-fill is debatable, it is probably best to excise them for therapeutic reasons as well as to exclude an underlying malignancy. Some authors have reported an increased tendency for cysts to repeatedly re-fill when associated with an underlying malignancy. The management of patients with multiple cysts also poses problems, as they may require repeated aspirations. A 3-month course of danazol may reduce the number and subsequent rate of cyst

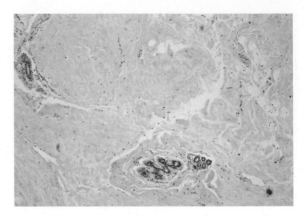

Figure 17.17. Histological appearances seen in fibrocystic disease – fibrous obliteration of the normal breast parenchyma (×50).

formation. However, the side effects of danazol (see section on Treatment) must be taken into account when prescribing this form of therapy.

There is a continuing debate as to whether breast cysts are associated with an increased risk of developing breast cancer. Some studies have suggested that those with multiple, bilateral and apocrine cysts are at most risk. Other long-term studies have failed to demonstrate any link to subsequent development of malignancy.

Galactocole
This is a benign lesion which usually occurs under the areola in women who are pregnant or lactating. Clinically, the lesion is a smooth, well-defined lump and can become quite large. FNAC will result in the aspiration of milky fluid (can be inspissated) with resolution of the lump.

Mammary dysplasia

General
The aetiology of mammary dysplasia (also termed fibrocystic disease, fibroadenosis, cystic mastopathy) is poorly defined but is thought to arise as a result of a disordered proliferation and involution of breast tissues that occurs as part of the normal cyclical physiological process during the reproductive years (see section on Physiological changes in the female breast). Thus, it tends to occur in women in the 25–45-year age group and presents clinically as mastalgia, breast lump or nodularity, particularly in the second part of the menstrual cycle. Microscopy of breast tissues reveals a variety of pathophysiological changes (Figs 17.17 and 17.18); these are discussed in more detail below.

Microarchitectural changes
Adenosis
Adenosis is associated with an increase in acini and glandular tissue. There may be an increase in the myoepithelial component and in the connective tissue of the lobule.

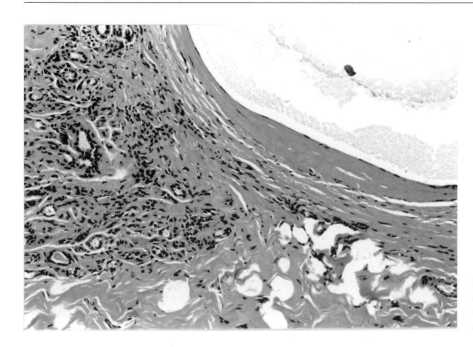

Figure 17.18. Histological appearances of fibrocystic disease – cyst formation, fibrosis and sclerosing adenosis (×150).

Sclerosing adenosis

This is characterised by prominent intralobular fibrosis and proliferation of small ductules or acini. The fibrosis may be extensive resulting in dense spiculated strands with prominent architectural distortion of the normal breast pattern. Complex sclerosing lesions are variants of this but are associated with prominent epithelial hyperplasia. In addition, there may be an increase in the myoepithelial component. As a result of the accumulation of dense fibrous tissue these lesions may be difficult to differentiate clinically and mammographically from breast cancers.

Epitheliosis

This is characterised by hyperplasia of the epithelium lining the terminal ducts and acini. The proliferation of epithelium may result in a solid mass with obliteration of the ducts or it may take the form of epithelial projections which grow into the ducts (ductal papillomatosis). The morphological appearance of the epithelial cells can vary and different degrees of atypia may be seen. A variant is atypical lobular hyperplasia which is characterised by hyperplasia of the terminal duct and acini; this has some of the features of lobular carcinoma *in situ* (LCIS). The importance of this lies in the increased risk of the subsequent development of breast cancer (see later).

Fibrosis (sclerosis)

There is a substantial increase in the content of dense fibrous tissue, with loss of elastic tissue, fat and epithelial elements.

Cyst formation

Numerous cysts (macro or micro) may also develop and this is discussed in more detail in the appropriate section above.

Fat necrosis

Fat necrosis of the breast occurs most commonly in obese and post-menopausal women. Frequently, patients give a history of trauma to the breast and complain of a subsequent breast lump. The lump may be difficult to differentiate (clinically and mammographically) from a breast cancer as it can be hard, be associated with skin tethering and show varying inflammatory changes in the overlying skin of the breast. Macroscopically, the tissue is yellow in colour and haemorrhagic; microscopically there is necrosis of fat, scar formation and infiltration with polymorphs, macrophages and giant cells. Although FNAC may be helpful, biopsy may sometimes be necessary to obtain a definitive diagnosis.

Mondor's disease

This is characterised by thrombophlebitis of the superficial veins of the breast but the aetiology is unknown. Clinically, this presents as taught, firm, subcutaneous bands with associated skin dimpling and retraction. The clinical features usually resolve spontaneously but if there is associated discomfort, non-steroidal anti-inflammatory drugs may be helpful.

Gynaecomastia

Gynaecomastia is defined as enlargement of the male breast. This can occur unilaterally or bilaterally and can range from a minimal increase of the breastplate beneath the areola to resembling the female breast. Microscopically, there is proliferation in the dense connective tissue and hyperplasia of the ductal lining cells resulting in the formation of a multi-layered epithelium.

The aetiology is unknown, but some studies have shown an alteration in the ratio of the circulating levels of androgens and oestrogens. It is also postulated that there is an alteration in the sensitivity of hormonal receptors in the breast tissue. Conditions in which gynaecomastia can occur include certain cancers (testicular, lung, adrenal), testicular absence or maldevelopment (congenital, acquired), liver disease, testicular damage (viral orchitis, torsion, chemotherapy, etc.), chronic renal disease and hyperprolactinaemia. Drugs may also cause gynaecomastia and include diuretics (e.g. spironolactone), anti-androgens, oestrogens, cardiac drugs (e.g. digoxin), metoclopramide, anti-hypertensive agents (e.g. methyldopa) and tricyclic anti-depressants and some proton pump inhibitors. However, 25% of cases of gynaecomastia occur at the time of puberty and a further 25% are idiopathic, with no underlying cause being demonstrated.

A thorough history and examination of the breasts and axillae, chest, testes and abdomen should be performed in all patients. Mammography and FNAC may also be performed. Further investigations may include liver function tests and measurement of serum androgen, oestrogen and prolactin levels and a chest radiograph. Abdominal and testicular ultrasound examinations may also be required.

If there is an underlying cause for the gynaecomastia treatment of this will usually result in resolution of the gynaecomastia. However, in the absence of any demonstrable cause, and particularly in young patients, reassurance is frequently all that is required as the condition tends to be self-limiting. If the gynaecomastia persists and/or the patient is concerned by the appearances then surgical excision may be indicated.

CARCINOMA OF THE BREAST

Introduction

Breast cancer accounts for approximately 24% of all malignancies occurring in the female population in industrialised western societies and 18% of deaths in women due to malignant disease. In the UK there are approximately 117 cases per 100 000 women (34 000 new cases per annum). Thus, 1 at least 12 women will develop breast cancer during their lifetime and the incidence is rising by approximately 2% per annum. Breast cancer rarely occurs in women under the age of 25 years. Thereafter, the incidence increases steadily until at the time of the menopause, where the incidence plateaus out. After the menopause there is again a steady increase in

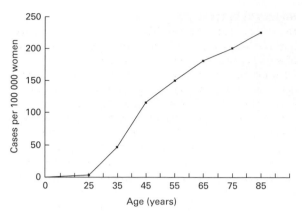

Figure 17.19. Incidence of breast cancer and age of diagnosis.

Table 17.3. Age-standardised incidence of breast cancer amongst different countries.

Country	Incidence
England	54.0
Scotland	59.6
USA	77.8
Sweden	60.7
Yugoslavia	37.7
Japan	19.7

Data are for 100 000 of the population, taken from 1980s.

the incidence of breast cancer, although this is less rapid than before (Fig. 17.19).

Epidemiology and risk factors

Benign breast disease

The relationship between benign breast disease and the subsequent development of breast cancer has been a matter of debate for some time. It appears that most benign conditions of the breast do not increase the risk of developing breast cancer (e.g. fibrocystic disease, cysts, fibroadenomas). However, there are some benign conditions which do increase the risk, in some instances substantially; these are listed in Table 17.2.

Geographical factors

There is a difference in the incidence in breast cancer between different countries and these are illustrated in Table 17.3. The reasons for these differences are unclear. However, although genetic aspects are important, environmental factors play a key role. For example, the incidence of breast cancer in the daughters of immigrants who arrive from countries with a low-prevalence approaches the high level found in the established indigenous population.

Hormonal factors

Data has accumulated from different epidemiological studies that a prolonged exposure to oestrogens may increase the risk of subsequently developing breast cancer. Therefore, the following have been shown to increase the relative risks of developing breast cancer: early menarche, delayed menopause, late age of birth of first child and nulliparity.

The possible relationship of the oral contraceptive pill to breast cancer has also been considered and discussed in detail. A recent large study (involving >150 000 women) found that there was a small increase in the number of cancers diagnosed in women when taking the contraceptive pill and during the 10 years after stopping its usage. However, after this 10-year period there was no increased risk of developing breast cancer. Other studies have found that it is the prolonged use of the oral contraceptive pill prior to the first pregnancy which is most likely to predispose to breast cancer.

Recent studies have demonstrated that HRT may possibly predispose to breast cancer. For example, it has been shown in a recent meta-analysis from the USA that an exposure of 5–10 years to HRT was associated with an increased risk of breast cancer in those women with a family history of breast cancer. Furthermore, an analysis from the UK also suggested that 5 years of HRT resulted in an increase in an individuals' risk of developing breast cancer.

Furthermore, a recent study from the UK (the million women study) has suggested that the risk of developing breast cancer was dependent on the type of preparation used. For example, after 10 years of combined oestrogen/progesterone HRT there would be expected to be an excess of 19 cases of breast cancer per 1000 women who had not used HRT, and for oestrogen-only HRT there would be only five extra cases per 1000 women not taking HRT.

Ionising radiation

An increased risk of breast cancer occurs as a result of exposure to ionising radiation. For example, in survivors of atomic bomb explosions, in patients who have received multiple and high-dosage chest radiographs, and in women who have received radiotherapy which has included the breast, there is an increased risk of breast cancer. This risk is most apparent if the exposure to the radiation occurred in those under 30 years of age.

Of particular concern has been the risks that might be associated with the use of radiation (mammography) in screening populations for breast cancer. However, it has been estimated that if 2 million women above the age of 50 years received a low-dose mammogram (mean radiation dose of 0.15 cGy), there would be one excess breast cancer per year in the population after a latent period of 10 years.

Genetic factors

It has been estimated that approximately 5% of patients under the age of 50 years with breast cancer have a genetic predisposition to developing breast cancer. For example, breast cancer

(BRCA1) gene, which is found on the long arm of chromosome 17 and is implicated in approximately 4% of all breast cancers, has been cloned. It has been found that mutations of this gene are associated with a high risk (up to 85%) of developing breast cancer before the age of 80 years. Furthermore, approximately one-half of these cases will occur before the age of 50. A second breast cancer gene (BRCA2) has been identified on the long arm of chromosome 13. A range of mutations of these genes has been described which alter the estimated risk. These mutations can also occur in the sporadic form of breast cancers. In the inherited type of breast cancer other genetic defects have been established.

For example, there is either a mutation or loss of heterozygosity of the p53 tumour-suppressor gene on the short arm of chromosome 17. This occurs in the Li–Fraumeni syndrome; soft tissue sarcomas and other types of epithelial tumours occur in members of these families. Another type of genetically determined breast cancer is the Lynch type II syndrome (autosomal dominant with high penetrance), where there is a high incidence of breast and ovarian cancers. The earlier the age of onset of the breast cancer, the more likely it is that there is a genetic susceptibility to the disease.

The relatives of some patients are also at increased risk of developing breast cancer and most familial types of breast cancer is due to mutations in more common genes but which have a lower penetrance. The magnitude of this is dependent on several factors. For example, the relative risk if the mother had the disease is 1.8, whilst with a sister it is 2.5. If both first-degree relatives were affected, the risk rises to 5.6 (approximately 40%). Further studies have shown that the relative risk for sisters of patients with bilateral disease is approximately 5.3. However, if the age of presentation of the cancer is less than 40 years of age then the relative risk increases to approximately 9 (i.e. approaches 80%).

A variety of guidelines have been developed for following-up patients who have been identified as being at increased risk of breast cancer (e.g. those of the Association of Breast Surgery, Scottish Intercollegiate Guidelines Network, etc.). However, the following would indicate patients considered to be at 'high risk' (i.e. three times that of the general population). It should be remembered that there may be variations and these criteria frequently change as this field progresses:

1. One first-degree male relative with breast cancer diagnosed at less than 40 years of age.
2. Two first- or second-degree relatives with breast cancer and who have been diagnosed at less than 60 years of age, or ovarian cancer at any age.
3. Three first- or second-degree relatives with breast or ovarian cancer which has been diagnosed at any age.
4. A first-degree relative with bilateral breast cancer under the age of 60 years.
5. A first-degree male relative with breast cancer at any age.

Having identified these patients a possible follow-up programme is as below:

- *If less than 30 years of age*: no mammography and annual clinical examination.

• *If aged 35–49*: annual mammography from when the patient is 5 years prior to the age of diagnosis of the relative.
• *Over the age of 50*: mammography every 18 months.

Other alternative strategies for the management of patients at high risk include chemoprophylaxis or prophylactic mastectomy and in some patients the latter will be discussed with the patient.

Healthy life-style

Obesity

Obesity is associated with an increased risk of breast cancer in post-menopausal women, the mechanisms of which may be hormonal. It has been demonstrated that obese women metabolise androstenedione (from the adrenal gland) into oestrogen in the adipocytes. The circulating levels of oestrone are higher in obese post-menopausal women than non-obese individuals. In pre-menopausal women obesity may be associated with a reduced risk of breast cancer, although the reasons for this difference are unclear.

Diet

Attention has focused on the role of dietary fat in the pathogenesis of breast cancer. Animal studies have shown that the total fat consumption, and more importantly, the composition of fats in the diet are important in the development of breast cancer. In studies in man, close correlations between the *per capita* consumption of fat and breast cancer mortality rates have been demonstrated. However, when individuals are considered the association is lacking. There is no well-established relationship between dietary fat consumption and an individual persons risk of developing breast cancer.

Anti-oxidant nutrients (e.g. fruit, greens) may be important in protecting against the development of breast cancer. These molecules protect against reactive oxygen species which can damage DNA within the cell. Examples of these substances are vitamins A, C and E, and selenium. Other dietary substances which may be important in causing breast cancer are the heterocyclic amines (found in char-broiled foods) and plant oestrogens (soy products).

Exercise

Physical activity, especially in the teenage and young adult years, may protect against breast cancer in both pre- and post-menopausal women. One explanation for this has been the exercise-induced delay in the onset of the menarche and the reduction in the number of menstrual cycles.

Alcohol

Alcohol consumption increases the risk of breast cancer. An intake of more than 15 g of alcohol per day has been found to be associated with a significant increase in the risk of breast cancer, when compared with people who do not consume alcohol. This may be because of a hormonal effect – alcohol consumption results in increased circulating levels of oestrone and oestradiol.

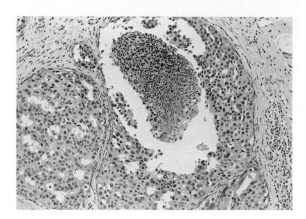

Figure 17.20. An example of DCIS: high-grade DCIS with comedo necrosis distending and filling terminal ducts. Note the cellular pleomorphism and well-defined cell borders (×150).

Cigarette smoking

There is controversy regarding the role of smoking in the aetiology of breast cancer. Although some studies have suggested there is an increased risk (possibly due to carcinogens in smoke) others have shown a reduced risk (possibly due to decreased circulating levels of oestrogens). There is no convincing evidence that smoking causes breast cancer although a small number of studies have indicated there may be a very weak link.

Breast cancer: pathological types

Non-invasive breast cancer

There are two main types of non-invasive breast carcinoma: ductal carcinoma *in situ* (DCIS) and LCIS. Of these, DCIS is the more common histological type.

Ductal carcinoma *in situ*

DCIS is characterised by an abnormal proliferation of breast epithelial cells lying within the duct but not penetrating the basement membrane (Fig. 17.20). Different types of DCIS can be recognised histologically: (i) comedo (characteristic central necrosis); (ii) cribriform (sieve-like appearance); (iii) papillary or micropapillary (the epithelium forms projections into the ducts) and (iv) solid (sheets of cells fill the duct system). Different types of DCIS may be found in the same breast, but the comedo type is recognised as the most aggressive biologically. DCIS may also arise in several areas of the breast and the risk of this occurring is related to the size of the detected DCIS. For example, one study reported that if the area of DCIS was less than 2.5 cm, DCIS was found in other areas of the same breast in less than 15% of cases and there was no evidence of microinvasion by tumour cells.

However, if the DCIS was greater than 2.5 cm, then almost one-half of these patients had other areas of DCIS within the same breast and, furthermore, in over 40% of these cases there was evidence of microinvasion, with 4% having lymph node metastases. In addition, there is also a risk of patients with DCIS subsequently developing invasive cancer. Although different estimates of this risk have been reported, approximately 2% of these patients are likely to develop invasive breast cancer each year.

Clinically, DCIS may present as an incidental finding on a mammogram (localised, widespread, or multifocal microcalcifications, of variable density and branching pattern (Fig. 17.8), or a soft tissue mass), as a blood-stained (or less commonly serous) nipple discharge, a palpable mass or it may occur in association with Paget's disease of the nipple. The treatment of DCIS is controversial, with trials currently evaluating several treatment regimens. If mastectomy is performed, there is a 98% 5-year survival rate. However, this is probably excessive treatment in many cases and more conservative surgery for the treatment of a circumscribed area of DCIS (excising the area of DCIS only) has also been carried out. This approach, however, is associated with a recurrence of DCIS in up to 30% of cases, particularly with the comedo-type DCIS. The role of radiotherapy and/or tamoxifen treatment in preventing local recurrence following conservative surgery remains unclear and is currently being evaluated. It is recommended that, if the area of DCIS is extensive (>2.5 cm), or if there are multiple sites of DCIS within the same breast, mastectomy should be performed.

Lobular carcinoma *in situ*

LCIS is less common than DCIS and has no characteristic clinical or radiological features. It is not associated with microcalcification (although very rarely microcalcification has been reported). Pathological examination is characterised by a proliferation of cells in the terminal ducts and/or acini. LCIS can be both multicentric and bilateral (30%). It has been estimated that up to 1% of patients per annum will develop invasive cancer, but this may be in either breast (in contrast with DCIS) and histologically this may be either lobular or ductular carcinoma.

Following the diagnosis of LCIS in a breast biopsy the treatment is contentious. Small incidental findings (pathological assessment) are of doubtful clinical relevance. However, most commonly the patients are monitored by regular clinical examination and mammography (e.g. at yearly intervals). However, very anxious patients and especially those with evidence of multicentricity may wish to consider the option of bilateral mastectomy with or without reconstruction.

Invasive breast cancer

The commonly occurring invasive cancers and their relative frequencies are listed in Table 17.4 and are discussed in more detail below.

Invasive ductal carcinoma

The most commonly occurring type of breast cancer is the invasive ductal carcinoma of no special type (75–80% of all

Table 17.4. **Frequency of invasive breast cancers.**

Type	Frequency (% of total)
Invasive ductal carcinoma	75–80
Invasive lobular carcinoma	<5
Tubular carcinomas	<5
Medullary carcinomas	<5
Mucinous carcinomas	<5
Inflammatory breast cancer	2–5

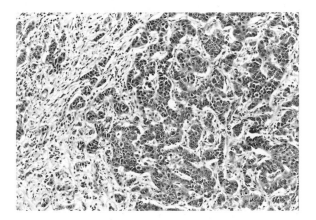

Figure 17.21. Invasive ductal carcinoma of no special type (×250).

cases). Histologically, the tumour cells can be arranged in groups, cords and can also form gland-like structures set in a dense fibrous stroma, which gives the tumour a hard consistency (scirrhous tumour) (Fig. 17.21).

The degree of aggressiveness of these tumours is variable and can be determined from the cytological and histological appearances of the tumour cells. Bloom and Richardson developed a grading system (1–3) for these tumours which was based on three characteristics: (i) the formation of tubules; (ii) the degree of nuclear pleomorphism and (iii) the mitotic rate. Grade 3 tumours have the worst prognosis, with grade 1 tumours having the best outcome.

Invasive lobular carcinoma

Invasive lobular carcinoma occurs much less frequently, comprising less than 5% of all breast cancers. Histologically, there are strands of tumour cells which infiltrate into the surrounding stromal tissues; typically these are one cell in width ('Indian filing'). Tumour cells may also be found in concentric rings around normal ducts (Fig. 17.22). However, in some cases it can be difficult to differentiate between an invasive ductal and an invasive lobular cancer. Furthermore, both of these types may co-exist in the same tumour. This tumour can be multicentric within the same breast and is bilateral in up to 20% of patients.

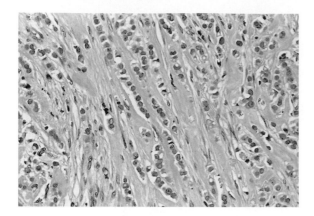

Figure 17.22. Invasive lobular carcinoma, with 'Indian filing' (×125).

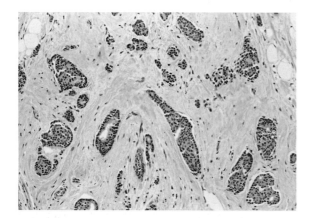

Figure 17.23. Tubular carcinoma (×150).

Tubular carcinoma

Tubular carcinomas are usually small and well-differentiated tumours. Histologically, they are characterised by the tumour cells being arranged into well-differentiated tubular structures.

The tumour cells have a low mitotic rate and there is little nuclear pleomorphism. The stromal tissue is also very dense and can be found within the tubular structures (Fig. 17.23). Patients with this type of tumour generally have an excellent prognosis as it usually remains confined to the breast and rarely metastasises, either regionally or more distally.

Medullary carcinoma

Medullary carcinomas constitute less than 5% of all breast cancers. They have a well-defined margin and are soft. Histologically, they are characterised by a marked lymphocytic infiltration, high cellularity and have less fibrous tissue than is seen in other histological types of breast cancer. They are less commonly associated with axillary gland metastases than are invasive ductal cancers. Even if the axillary lymph glands do contain tumour the prognosis is still better than for the invasive ductal tumour type.

Mucinous carcinoma

Mucinous tumours comprise less than 5% of all breast cancers. They tend to occur in the older population and are believed to be more slowly growing than other types, rarely metastasising to the regional lymph nodes. Histologically, there are large areas of mucin in the tumour. The tumour cells themselves can be seen to lie within pools of mucin forming small islands of cells or gland-like structures. This type of tumour is also associated with a good prognosis.

Inflammatory breast cancer

Inflammatory breast cancer occurs in approximately 2–5% of patients with malignant lesions in the breast. It is recognised clinically by redness of the skin and signs of inflammation of the breast, often with peau d'orange of the skin. The histological findings may be non-specific, but the characteristic feature is invasion of the dermal lymphatics by malignant cells and tissue oedema, and a variable degree of infiltration of the breast by inflammatory cells. It is biologically more aggressive than the other tumour types and is associated with a worse prognosis.

Prognostic factors in breast cancer

Prognostic factors relating to the degree of tumour spread and its biological behaviour have been identified. These factors determine the outcome (disease recurrence) and survival for the patient and are discussed in more detail below.

Tumour size

This is an important prognostic indicator. Generally, the larger the tumour clinically the worse the prognosis, with tumours less than 0.5 cm having an excellent prognosis and those greater than 4 cm a poor outcome. Tumours less than 1 cm have a good prognosis but in 15% of these patients there is histological evidence of lymph node involvement with tumour.

Tumour type

Invasive ductal carcinomas of no special type have a worse prognosis than certain tumours of a special type (e.g. tubular, lobular, mucinous or medullary cancers).

Tumour grade

Tumours can be graded (1–3) using the Bloom and Richardson classification (tubule formation, mitotic rate and nuclear pleomorphism). Grade 3 tumours have the worse prognosis.

Cell kinetics

Cell proliferation has been shown to be a prognostic indicator. Those tumours with enhanced rates of mitosis, increased percentage of cells in the S-phase of the cell cycle and with tumour cells showing the greatest expression of the Ki67 nuclear antigen (expressed by proliferating cells) have a poorer prognosis.

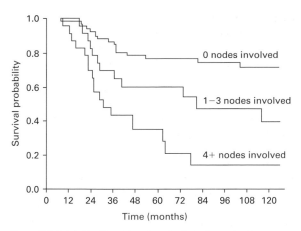

Figure 17.24. Relationship of lymph node status to survival in patients with breast cancer.

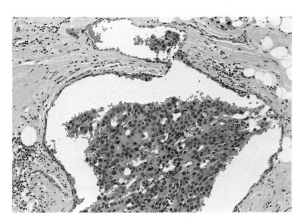

Figure 17.26. Invasive ductal carcinoma invading into vascular lymphatic spaces (×250).

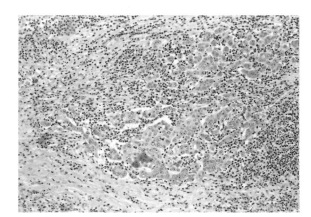

Figure 17.25. Ductal carcinoma infiltrating into a lymph node, pleomorphic cells in a lymphoid background (×150).

Table 17.5. The Nottingham Prognostic Index (NPI).

- NPI = 0.2 × tumour size (cm) + lymph node status (1–3 according to stage A–C) + tumour grade (I–III).
- An NPI of less than or equal to 3.4 is good prognosis, 3.41–5.4 is moderate prognosis, and greater than 5.4 is a poor prognosis. Patients in the good prognostic group have a 15-year survival of 85%, but patients with an NPI of equal to or less than 2.4 have a 15-year survival of 94%.

Lymph node status
This has been shown to be the single most important prognostic indicator (Fig. 17.24). If there is no lymph node involvement by tumour patients have an 85% 5-year survival. However, if there is lymph node involvement then the 5-year survival is reduced to 65%. Furthermore, this reduction in survival is related to the number of lymph nodes being involved – the greater the number the poorer the survival (Fig. 17.25).

Lymphatic or vascular invasion
Invasion of the lymphatic system or blood vessels (Fig. 17.26) has also been shown to be a poor prognostic indicator.

Hormone receptor status
OR status has been shown to be a prognostic indicator, with approximately 60% of tumours being OR positive. Those patients whose tumours strongly express OR receptors have a survival advantage, when compared with patients who have no OR expression. Progesterone receptors (PR) depend on a

satisfactory OR pathway for their presence, which correlates, therefore, with OR status. However, there is some evidence to suggest that the presence of both OR and PR expression is associated with a better prognosis than OR expression alone.

Other prognostic indicators
A variety of other possible prognostic indicators are currently being evaluated. These include the expression of growth factor receptors (e.g. epidermal growth factor and its receptor, EGFR), expression of cell adhesion molecules, expression of oncogenes and products (e.g. c-erbB-2) and mutations of wild-type-suppressor genes (e.g. p53).

Prognostic indices
Combinations of these prognostic indicators have been developed using statistical modelling techniques in an attempt to improve prognostic information. One such example is the NPI which takes into account the tumour size, tumour grade and lymph node staging. This allows the identification of the likelihood of survival of patients with breast cancer (Table 17.5).

Staging of breast cancer

Several staging systems have been developed for use in patients with breast cancer. However, the TNM system is the one which is most frequently used and is given in Table 17.6.

Table 17.6. Staging of breast cancer.

TNM system

Primary tumour – (T)

TX	Primary tumour cannot be assessed
T0	No evidence of primary tumour
TIS	Carcinoma *in situ*, Paget's disease
T1	Tumour <2 cm in greatest dimension
T1a	<0.5 cm in greatest dimension
T1b	>0.5 cm but <1.0 cm in greatest dimension
T1c	>1 cm but ≤2.0 cm in greatest dimension
T2	Tumour >2 cm but <5 cm in greatest dimension
T3	Tumour >5 cm in greatest dimension
T4	Tumour of any size with direct extension to the skin or chest wall
T4a	Extension to chest wall
T4b	Oedema, or ulceration of the skin of the breast or satellite skin nodules confined to the same breast
T4c	Both T4a and T4b
T4d	Inflammatory carcinoma (diffuse browny induration of the skin, with an erysipeloid edge, often with no underlying palpable mass)

Regional lymph nodes – (N)

NX	Regional lymph nodes cannot be assessed
N0	No regional node metastases
N1	Mobile homolateral axillary nodes
N1a	Nodes not considered to contain tumour
N1b	Nodes considered to contain tumour
N2	Homolateral axillary nodes fixed to each other or to adjacent structures
N3	Metastases to ipsilateral internal mammary nodes

Distant metastases – (M)

MX	Presence of distant metastases cannot be assessed
M0	No distant metastases
M1	Distant metastases (includes metastases to supraclavicular lymph nodes)

Table 17.7. Staging of breast cancer UICC staging.

Stage	Corresponding TNM
0	Tis, N0, M0
I	T1, N0, M0
II	T1, N1, M0; T2, N0–1, M0
III	Any T, N2–3, M0; T3 any N, M0
IV	Any T, any N, M1

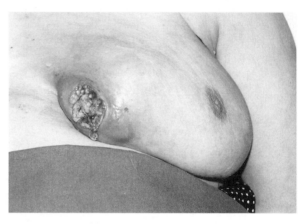

Figure 17.27. Locally advanced carcinoma of the breast with associated skin ulceration.

This is a clinical staging system and the measurements of tumour size and lymph node status are established on clinical examination. In pathological staging, the prefix 'p' must be added in front of the T or N. Another commonly used staging system is that advocated by the Union Internationale Contre Cancer (UICC) in 1987. The correlation of this with the TNM system is shown in Table 17.7.

Clinical features

The majority of women present with a breast lump, which is confirmed on examination. In two-thirds of patients it is in the upper outer quadrant of the breast and characteristically is well defined, hard and with an irregular surface. The lump may be fixed to the skin or to the underlying chest wall and retraction or dimpling of the skin may be seen. The skin of the breast must be carefully examined for the presence of erythema which may indicate an inflammatory cancer (see

above). Locally advanced cancers are characterised by oedema, skin infiltration, satellite skin nodules, ulceration, fixity to the chest wall and/or large fixed axillary nodes (N2) (Fig. 17.27). Some patients may also have oedema of the ipsilateral arm. However, not all cancers have these features and occasionally some may be difficult to differentiate clinically from benign tumours such as fibroadenomas. Other breast cancers may present as a diffuse nodularity, with no localised lump being found, and up to 10% of patients with breast cancer may present with pain as the predominant complaint.

The nipple should also be carefully examined for the presence of distortion or inversion. A nipple discharge may be present. This often contains blood and emanates from one duct. However, a variety of other nipple discharges (clear, coloured) may be present (see section on Nipple discharge). The presence of a scaly, erythematous nipple should raise the suspicion of Paget's disease of the nipple (see later).

Less commonly, patients may present with features of regional tumour spread (e.g. involved and enlarged axillary lymph nodes). Alternatively, metastatic disease in distant sites may be responsible for symptoms; for example, breathlessness (intra-thoracic metastases), bone pain and pathological fractures, jaundice and abdominal pain (liver metastases), ascites (intra-abdominal metastases), neurological symptoms (intracerebral metastases), difficulty in walking (spinal cord compression), etc.

Diagnosis

Triple assessment

The investigations that are used to establish the diagnosis of breast cancer include mammography, ultrasonography of the breast, FNAC and biopsy. These have all been discussed earlier in this chapter.

Staging investigations

All patients should have a full blood count, urea and electrolytes (including serum calcium), liver function tests (bilirubin, transaminase, alkaline phosphatase and gamma glutamyl peptidase) and a chest radiograph performed. In patients with small tumours (T1, N0), and in the absence of suggestive clinical features, further imaging to detect metastatic disease (bone scans, abdominal ultrasound) has been shown to be unnecessary, as they have a very low incidence of detecting metastases. However, in patients with larger or more advanced tumours or if abnormalities have been detected on the basic staging investigations then further appropriate imaging investigations should be undertaken (e.g. isotope bone scans, abdominal ultrasound, CT scans of thorax and/or brain).

Treatment

General

Treatment of breast cancer requires a multidisciplinary approach with input from the surgeon, radiotherapist and medical oncologist, cytologist and pathologist, radiographer and radiologist, and nurse counsellor and psychologist. The patient and partner should also be given the opportunity to participate and make informed choices (if they wish) in the decision-making processes, following full discussion and provision of appropriate information.

The treatment of a patient with a palpable breast cancer comprises the management of the lesion in the breast (to achieve local control of disease) and treatment of possible regional metastases in the tumour-draining lymph nodes (to obtain regional control of disease and to determine prognostic outcome) and possible adjuvant therapy. In addition, patients who are considered to be at a high risk of having occult micrometastatic disease (e.g. grade 3 tumours, nodal invasion) may also require adjuvant chemotherapy and/or hormonal therapy.

Primary breast tumour

Treatment of the primary breast tumour

The treatments initially advocated for breast cancer were based on the belief that cancer cells spread in a centrifugal pattern – from the tumour to the regional-draining lymph nodes and then sequentially to the vascular system and distant metastatic sites. Thus, it was recommended that a radical mastectomy (which includes removing the pectoralis major muscle) should be undertaken. However, in the 1920s and 1930s this approach was challenged and surgeons

began to realise that less radical surgery was associated with good results. Indeed, Geoffrey Keynes in the UK had treated early breast cancers by local excision of the tumour and implantation of a radioactive source (radium seeds) at the site of the excised tumour 'bed'.

Randomised-controlled trials (both Europe and the USA) evaluated more precisely the role of breast conservation surgery versus mastectomy in the treatment of patients with breast cancer. It was demonstrated that if the clinical size of the tumour was 2 cm or less (T1) then wide local excision of the tumour or a 'quadrantectomy' (for tumours 2–4 cm (T2)), in conjunction with radiotherapy given to the breast in the post-operative period, could be carried out safely. When this approach was compared with patients undergoing mastectomy there were no differences in survival between the two groups of patients. It has been documented, however, that there is a small increased risk of local recurrence of disease following breast conservation, when compared with mastectomy – up to 1% ('recurrent disease') of patients per annum on a cumulative basis for the first 10 years; 0.5%, thereafter, will have local recurrence of disease.

However, a number of clinical and pathological features have been identified which are considered to be contraindications to breast conservation because they are associated with a much higher risk of local recurrence of disease; for example, tumours with a clinical size of greater than 4 cm, incomplete excision of tumour, extensive associated DCIS, lymphatic or vascular invasion, high histological tumour grade. Of course, the patients' own wishes must also be taken into consideration when planning the treatment. If breast conservation is undertaken then radiotherapy is also given to the breast (4500–5000 cGy) and the patient should be seen by the radiotherapist pre-operatively to make sure that the patient is suitable for radiotherapy (e.g. severe disease of the lungs and heart may preclude the use of radiotherapy because of the risks of radiation-induced damage to these structures).

Locally advanced breast cancers

Locally advanced breast cancers (LABC) occurs in up to 15% of patients presenting with breast cancer (Fig. 17.27). LABC can be defined as:

1. presence of a large tumour (>5 cm: T3);
2. fixation of the tumour to the chest wall, skin oedema (peau d'orange) or infiltration, with or without ulceration (T4);
3. large, fixed or matted axillary lymph nodes (N2);
4. inflammatory carcinoma (localised or generalised induration of the breast, oedema and erythema of the skin, especially in the lower half of the breast (T4d)).

If these patients undergo surgical resection of the tumour, approximately 50% of patients will develop a local recurrence of disease and the 5-year survival is very low (<10%) with most patients dying from metastatic disease. Therefore, combination chemotherapy is given primarily (neo-adjuvant chemotherapy) with the aim of destroying micrometastatic disease and destaging the primary tumour. This may enable breast-conserving surgery to be undertaken subsequently. Although different regimens have been used, most of these contain doxorubicin or other anthracyclins, which have been shown to be the most active chemotherapeutic agents against breast cancer cells. More recently the taxanes group of agents, in particular docetaxel, has been shown to be at least as active as doxorubicin and to be active even against tumours which are resistant to doxorubicin.

Using this approach, complete and partial clinical responses (UICC criteria) can be usually obtained in approximately 70–80% of all patients – the smaller the initial tumour the higher the clinical and pathological response rates. Following neo-adjuvant chemotherapy surgery is undertaken (usually quadrantectomy or mastectomy). Complete destruction of all tumour cells in the breast occurs in up to 15% of cases, the remaining patients have varying numbers of residual tumour cells.

Radiotherapy is given to the breast (or chest wall) and lymph-draining areas approximately 4 weeks after surgery. Using this approach, survival rates have ranged from 35% to 65% at 5 years. However, recent studies have suggested that there may be a slightly higher risk of local disease recurrence in patients with large tumours which have been successfully downstaged with chemotherapy and then in whom breast conservation surgery has been carried out.

Impalpable lesions

If an impalpable abnormality is detected in the breast, which is shown to be malignant on FNAC (stereotactically, ultrasound guided) further treatment is necessary. In the first instance, the lesion is removed in order to obtain a histological diagnosis and assessment, in particular whether this is an *in-situ* or an invasive cancer. Pre-operative localisation of the abnormality is carried out by inserting a wire into the lesion under mammographic or ultrasound control. This will enable the lesion to be accurately found and removed at operation. The excised tissue is orientated and is then X-rayed to ensure that the abnormality (e.g. opacity, microcalcification) has been removed. The breast specimen is inked and sent fresh to the pathology department, where 3-mm thick slices are cut which are then X-rayed again so that paraffin sections can be cut of abnormal areas for histopathological examination.

The extent of, or need for, further surgery will depend on whether this is an *in-situ* cancer or an invasive tumour. Small invasive lesions, particularly if of low grade, carry a very good prognosis and a local excision may be all that is required. However, if the lesion is larger or there is multifocal disease then consideration should be given to mastectomy because of the increased risk of recurrent malignancy or the subsequent development of further invasive cancers in the residual breast.

Axillary lymph nodes

Treatment of the axillary lymph nodes

The lymphatic drainage of the breast has already been described in some detail (see previous section). It is essential to have an accurate histological assessment of the lymph nodes in the axilla because this will provide prognostic information about the disease (and determine the need for adjuvant therapies) and is also required to achieve adequate 'regional' control of disease. Clinical assessment of the axillary node status is most unreliable, in some studies less than 60% of involved nodes are clinically detectable. Radiological imaging procedures (mammography and ultrasound) do not reliably detect tumour-involved lymph nodes. Although magnetic resonance imaging and positron-emission tomography have shown some promise they are not used in routine pre-operative assessment of the axilla. Therefore, some form of axillary surgery to remove the lymph nodes and examine them histologically is the only way, at present, of accurately determining if they are involved with tumour. There are various surgical approaches (i.e. axillary sample, dissection and clearance).

Axillary sample

This involves the removal of four or more lymph nodes (confirmed at operation) from the proximal anterior/pectoral and central group of draining lymph nodes in the axilla. This has been shown to provide an accurate assessment of the nodal status of the axilla. Some surgeons, however, have had difficulty in identifying the required number of lymph nodes and have questioned whether sampling is an adequate procedure to stage the axilla. If the sampled nodes contain malignant cells, then radiotherapy to the axilla and supraclavicular areas (4500 cGy) is given. The internal thoracic group of lymph nodes should also be considered. It has been estimated that approximately 90% of women with internal thoracic node involvement also have axillary nodes involved with tumour. If there is a strong possibility of tumour spread to the internal mammary group of lymph nodes (e.g. from tumours in the medial aspect of the breast), these nodes can also be irradiated.

Axillary dissection

An alternative approach to axillary node sample is dissection of the axilla to various anatomical levels, as outlined below:

Level 1: removal of lymph nodes lateral to the inferior border of the pectoralis minor muscle.

Level 2: removal of level 1 lymph nodes and those behind and in front of pectoralis minor muscle.

Neither a level 1 nor 2 dissection of the axilla is an adequate therapeutic manoeuvre on its own. For example, if level 1 nodes are involved there is a 10% chance of further nodal involvement at level 2 or 3; if level 2 nodes are involved there is a 50% chance of level 3 nodes being involved with tumour. Radiotherapy to the axilla, therefore, is also required in patients with involved lymph nodes and who have undergone level 1 or 2 dissections. The likelihood of lymphoedema is significantly increased with irradiation of the axilla following axillary dissection.

Axillary clearance

This is the removal of all the axillary lymphatic tissue (also termed a level 3 axillary dissection). In order to achieve this, division or removal of the pectoralis minor muscle allows better access to the upper aspect of the axilla. The axillary contents (fat, fascia, lymphatic tissue) are cleared, starting from the apex (outer border of the first rib), below and medial to the axillary vein. The brachial plexus, the major axillary vessels, the long thoracic nerve and the thoracodorsal vessels and nerve are preserved during dissection. With a thorough axillary clearance no further treatment of the axilla is required, irrespective of whether there is involvement of the lymph nodes by tumour. Radiotherapy to the axilla following a clearance is associated with up to 30% incidence of lymphoedema. However, this does not result in a substantial improvement in regional disease control. Axillary surgery is not recommended for DCIS or minimal cancers.

Sentinal lymph node biopsy

Recently, the use of sentinal node biopsy has been advocated for patients with invasive breast cancer. The theoretical basis of this technique is that the malignant cells will desiminate in an orderly fashion to the axillary nodes, spreading firstly to the 'sentinal' lymph node. Therefore, by removing this lymph node for histological examination a representative view of the state of axillary nodal involvement can be achieved with the minimum of disruption to the axilla itself.

There are different techniques which are available to localise the sentinal node, but basically either an injection of a radio-colloid and/or a vital blue dye is given to the patient either peritumourally or subdermally (usually in the periareolar region).

At the time of surgery, the sentinal node can then be localised using a probe to detect the radioactively labelled colloid which has accumulated in it and the site marked. Through a small incision the sentinal node(s) are located and if the blue dye has also used, this will give a further visual identification of the sentinal node.

A recent meta-analysis of more than 60 studies of sentinal node biopsy has suggested that there is a false negative rate of approximately 8% with this procedure, and in studies of smaller numbers of patients it was even higher at up to 25%. In some centres sentinal nodes are examined using 'frozen sections', or by imprint cytology and if there is evidence of metastatic tumour in the node, an axillary clearance can be carried out immediately. This removes the requirement for a patient to undergo a second operative procedure.

However, whilst the technique has been adopted widely in surgical practice the evidence from a randomised-controlled trial that it is as effective and efficient as axillary sampling is still awaited.

Morbidity of axillary treatment

Axillary surgery and radiotherapy are associated with a recognised morbidity. During surgery, there is the risk of damage to nerves, most commonly the intercostobrachial nerve, not

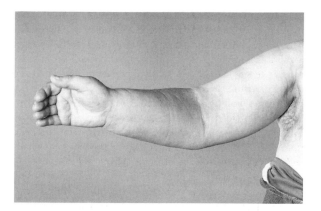

Figure 17.28. An example of lymphoedema of the arm following axillary clearance (level 3).

infrequently cut and resulting in anaesthesia and/or paraesthesia of axilla and inner aspect of upper arm. The long thoracic and thoracodorsal nerves may also be damaged on occasions. Furthermore, wound seromas or infections may occur in up to 5% of patients. Radiotherapy may also be associated with nerve damage, and more rarely a brachial plexopathy. Both radiotherapy and surgery are associated with some reduction in the range of movements at the shoulder joint (particularly in elderly patients). Less than 10% of patients will develop lymphocdema (variable degree) following radiotherapy or a level 2 or 3 axillary dissection (Fig. 17.28).

Breast reconstruction

Breast reconstruction aims to reverse the deformity of the breast and chest wall following breast surgery for cancer. This requires a team approach with the breast surgeon (and/or a plastic and reconstructive surgeon), the radiotherapist and medical oncologist and nurse counsellors being involved. The reconstructive surgery may be undertaken immediately at the time of the mastectomy or delayed for a short period until adjuvant therapies have been completed. There does not appear to be any detrimental effects of immediate reconstruction in terms of subsequent local or systemic relapse of disease. There are several approaches currently used in reconstruction. The choice will depend on the surgeon, the available skin on the chest wall (quality and quantity), the amount of skin, fat and muscle in other areas (back, abdomen) and the patients' own wishes. The various procedures used include:

Breast implants

These can be inserted at the time of the mastectomy or after the use of a tissue expander to produce an increase in chest wall skin.

Tissue expansion

Tissue expansion involves the insertion of a breast-shaped 'bag' which has a filling port (usually sited in axilla). This is gradually (over weeks) filled with saline and results in an expansion of the overlying area of skin. The expander can then be removed and replaced with a silicone breast prosthesis. Alternatively, the expander may also be a breast prosthesis and can then be left *in situ* once the required degree of skin expansion and shape of the breast mound has been achieved. Concern has been expressed because of the silicone content of the prosthesis and the expander, and its possible association with connective tissue disorders. However, this association has not been definitively established. Complications occurring with the use of these implants include infection of the prosthesis, formation and contraction of a fibrous capsule around the prosthesis, rupture and leakage of silicone from the prosthesis.

Myocutaneous transposition flaps

If the simpler forms of breast reconstruction discussed above are not suitable then myocutaneous flaps (e.g. latissimus dorsi, transverse rectus abdominis) may be employed. For example, myocutaneous flaps are used if the skin of the chest wall is of poor quality (e.g. has been damaged by radiotherapy), if a large amount of skin was removed at the time of mastectomy or if the patient's breasts are very large. One such flap is the latissimus dorsi flap which involves the transfer of an ellipse of skin and latissimus muscle from the back; this receives its blood supply from the thoracodorsal neurovascular pedicle. More recently an 'extended' latissimus flap procedure can be undertaken where much more muscle and subcutaneous fat is taken and used to reconstruct the breast. An alternative is the transverse rectus abdominis muscle (TRAM) flap in which an ellipse of skin, fat and rectus muscle from the lower abdominal wall are utilised. This may remain attached to its vascular pedicle, but if this is not possible the TRAM flap can be a free flap (based on the deep inferior epigastric vessels) and requires a microvascular anastomosis. Newer techniques involve not removing the muscle but this is more complicated and is not yet used widespread. Complications associated with this procedure include flap necrosis, infection and abdominal wall herniation.

Reconstruction of the nipple and areola can be achieved using a variety of techniques (e.g. tissue from the other nipple, skin from the labia minora or upper thigh). Also, techniques using skin from the breast mound can also be used to create a nipple and this can be carried out under local anaesthetic. The areola colour can be developed and modified by using tattooing techniques. An alternative to this, which gives excellent cosmesis, is to use a prosthetic nipple which 'sticks' to the skin and is removable. In patients with a ptotic remaining breast, surgery to correct this and thus achieve symmetry may also be required in order to provide a 'match' for the reconstructed breast.

Adjuvant therapy

Following definitive surgical therapy of the primary breast cancer adjuvant therapy may be considered necessary to deal with suspected occult micrometastases. This may take the form of either chemotherapy or hormonal therapy; in some patients both forms of treatment may be used.

Adjuvant chemotherapy

There is well-documented evidence that the administration of chemotherapy (two or more agents) will improve survival (overall and disease free), albeit in a small group of women. These effects are greatest in women who are younger than 50 years of age and particularly in patients who have lymph node involvement by tumour.

Initially, combination chemotherapy comprising cyclophosphamide, methotrexate and 5-fluorouracil (CMF) was given at monthly intervals for 6 months and this was shown to be beneficial in reducing disease recurrence and increasing overall survival. In recent years, the Early Breast Cancer Trialists Collaborative group has carried out an overview to examine all the studies. The key points to emerge from this overview are that:

(a) Patients aged under 50 years benefit more than those who are older than this in terms of reduction in the risk of death.

(b) Patients with tumour involving lymph nodes in the axilla gain more benefit than those whose axillary nodes are not involved by tumour. However, there is still a significant but smaller benefit in the latter category of patients.

(c) A doxorubicin-containing regimen also reduces the risk of death when compared with combination chemotherapy regimens which do not contain an anthracycline such as doxorubicin.

Whilst there are different combination chemotherapy regimens in usage throughout the world, one which is commonly used is four cycles of doxorubicin and cyclophosphamide given to patients at 21-day intervals. There are several trials which are evaluating other combinations of chemotherapeutic agents, particularly the taxanes (paclitaxel and docetaxel), but their role in adjuvant chemotherapy requires further clarification.

Recent studies have indicated that the use of monoclonal antibodies, Trastuzumab (Herceptin®) can improve the survival if given in the adjuvant setting and after surgery to those patients whose tumours overexpress the Her-2 receptor.

Hormone therapy

Drug treatment

Adjuvant hormonal therapy with tamoxifen (20 mg/day) has also been shown to improve time to disease recurrence and overall survival. The greatest effect is seen in post-menopausal women and in those in whom the tumours are OR positive. However, beneficial effects are seen in younger women and those with OR-poor tumours. In addition, those patients whose tumours are OR negative, but PR positive, will also benefit from tamoxifen therapy.

It has been estimated that the annual odds of death in women taking tamoxifen is reduced by approximately 17% (a 6% absolute improvement in survival at 10 years). The duration of taking tamoxifen is also important. There appears to be a better effect if it is taken for more than 2 years; there does not appear to be any advantages in taking tamoxifen for longer than 5 years. There is some preliminary evidence to suggest that by then taking an aromatase inhibitor (which prevents the synthesis of oestrogens in peripheral tissues) for a further 5 years, the risk of disease relapse can be halved. However, further studies are required to confirm these benefits.

Of concern have been the possible side effects of long-term tamoxifen use, in particular the risk of endometrial cancer. However, this must be balanced against the protective effect of tamoxifen in post-menopausal women in reducing cardiovascular-associated disorders (e.g. strokes). In addition, tamoxifen may reduce the risks of the development of a contralateral breast cancer by up to 30% although this benefit is less pronounced with time. Other side effects of tamoxifen include vaginal dryness, loss of libido and hot flushes. Weight gain is often attributed to tamoxifen but in placebo-controlled trials this did not appear to be confirmed. A small number of patients may develop retinal damage.

Recent studies have suggested that another aromatase inhibitor (anastrozole) is also effective when used in the adjuvant setting. However, at the present time it is indicated for use if patients have the thrombotic or uterine side effects of tamoxifen. A recent update of the clinical trials has given further evidence to indicate that anastozole is more effective and increasing numbers of patients are being treated with this as first-line treatment. As an alternative, however, there is also evidence to suggest that changing a patients hormonal treatment to aromatase inhibitor, after two or three years. Tamoxifen treatment, reduces the risk of disease recurrence more than by simply taking five years of tamoxifen treatment.

Ovarian ablation

Ovarian ablation has also been shown to improve survival in pre-menopausal women. The reduction in the annual odds of death is 25% (a 10% reduction in the risk of death after 5 years), which is comparable to that demonstrated from the use of chemotherapy. Ovarian ablation may be achieved by radiotherapy, surgery and more recently by using LHRH agonists.

Metastatic breast cancer

Patients with metastatic disease may present because of symptoms caused by the metastatic deposits. However, up to one-half of patients who present with a loco-regional recurrence of disease either have demonstrable metastatic disease at the time of presentation or shortly thereafter. Once metastatic breast cancer has been diagnosed the mean survival of these patients is approximately 18–24 months. Thus, the primary aim of any treatment is to palliate and improve the quality of life.

Treatment for such patients can be divided into (i) those aimed primarily at control of symptoms (e.g. general supportive care; relief of debilitating, disabling and distressing symptoms; management of pathological fractures; correction of disorders of body functions, etc.) and (ii) treatment to retard the growth of the tumour. These latter treatments are either chemotherapy or hormonal therapy.

Chemotherapy

Chemotherapy is associated with side effects which can impair the patients' quality of life and a considered decision must be made as to which patients are most likely to gain benefit (and what these benefits are) from chemotherapy. Patients who are most likely to benefit are those with a good performance status, metastatic disease in one or only a few sites and previous beneficial response to hormonal therapy. Combination chemotherapeutic regimens are used, most often containing one of the anthracyclin group of drugs. The response rates to these regimens vary but may be as high as 60%. However, the median time to disease relapse is only 6–10 months. Following further relapse of disease, other chemotherapeutic regimens may be tried but the response rates are usually less than 25%. More recent chemotherapeutic approaches to the treatment of metastatic disease have included the administration of docetaxel (50% of patients resistant to anthracyclins may respond) and high-dose intensification regimens. However, further studies are required to clearly define the place of these latter treatments in patients with metastatic disease. A small group of women (up to 20% in some series) have a prolonged (5 year) survival benefit with palliative chemotherapy.

Hormonal therapy

Hormone therapy has the advantage of less severe side effects than chemotherapy. Hormone therapy would be indicated in patients who were unfit for chemotherapy and also in those with disease present in multiple sites and with bone metastases. Responses to hormonal therapy have been reported in up to 60% of patients whose tumours have a high level of OR. Response rates are unlikely in OR negative tumours or in patients with hepatic metastases. If patients have been taking tamoxifen as adjuvant therapy before the development of metastatic disease then only 20–30% will respond to second-line hormonal manipulation, for example using medroxyprogesterone or aromatase inhibitors. It is also important to remember that even if patients demonstrate no response to first-line hormonal therapy, 20% will respond to second-line hormonal treatment. A further 10–15% may show a response to third-line hormonal treatment. In pre-menopausal women ovarian ablation (e.g. oophorectomy or radiation-induced menopause, LHRH agonists) is tried initially. Following relapse, aromatase inhibitors (e.g. aminoglutethamide, 4-hydroxyandrostenedione) or progestogens (e.g. medroxyprogesterone acetate) can be tried. Post-menopausal women are treated with anti-oestrogens or other hormonal treatments (see above).

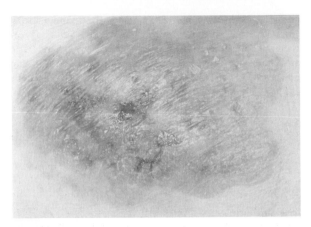

Figure 17.29. Paget's disease of the nipple.

Paget's disease of the nipple

Paget's disease of the nipple was first described over 200 years ago by Sir James Paget. Clinically, this is recognised by reddening, excoriation and/or scaling of the skin of the nipple with or without a nipple discharge (Fig. 17.29). These appearances may resemble eczema or dermatitis but are unilateral. This is associated with an underlying intraduct carcinoma and up to one-half of the patients have a palpable lump. If there is a palpable lump present then up to 90% of this group of patients will have an invasive cancer present. In the absence of a palpable lump up to one-third of patients will have an invasive cancer.

Histologically, Paget's cells are located in the epidermis of the nipple. Morphologically, these cells are large and rounded, with vacuolated cytoplasm and pleomorphic hyperchromatic nuclei. Their origin is unclear but it is believed that they have migrated from the underlying cancer through the mammary ducts or, alternatively, they are malignant cells that have arisen in the skin of the nipple.

The treatment of Paget's disease has been controversial. If local excision and breast-conserving surgery only is carried out, then tumour recurrence may occur in up to 40% of patients. Therefore, some surgeons advocate mastectomy and axillary surgery.

Phylloides tumour of the breast

Phylloides tumours (previously called 'cystosarcoma phylloides') account for up to 1% of all breast neoplasms. Although they can be found in any age group the median age is 45 years and they present clinically as a discrete lump in the breast. Macroscopically, they range in size from a few millimetres to up to several centimetres in diameter; when cut they demonstrate cystic cavities associated with fronds of tissue projecting into them. Microscopically, they have two distinct components: an epithelial component which covers the fronds of tissue and a stromal component. The stromal component is more cellular than that seen in a fibroadenoma. Furthermore, the cells may show mitoses have marked nuclear pleomorphism and may have an infiltrative border. The histological appearances may resemble a sarcoma and biologically the tumour may behave either as a benign lesion (85%) or a malignant growth (15%). In the latter situation, they metastasise via the blood stream to lungs and bone. Spread to regional tumour-draining lymph nodes rarely occurs with phylloides tumours.

It may be difficult to determine the likely behaviour of a phylloides tumour. However, factors which are considered to be important are the number of mitoses per 10 high-power microscopic fields ($\times$400); 0–4 mitoses being benign, 5–9 potentially malignant and 10 or more malignant. Benign lesions are treated conservatively whilst those with features of a sarcoma are treated by a mastectomy. Treatment of the lesion is usually wide local excision with careful follow-up for local recurrence of disease. If the tumour recurs further local excision or mastectomy will be required. Unfortunately, when the tumour recurs it tends to be biologically more aggressive, with the tumour cells having a higher mitotic rate. The tumours are not radio- or chemo-sensitive.

Breast cancer in the elderly

The incidence of breast cancer continues to rise through life with 40% of all cases occurring in patients older than 70 years. A small number of these patients, because of concurrent disease, will be unfit for any form of loco-regional therapy other than tamoxifen (20–40 mg/day). With tamoxifen as the sole therapy it has been shown that approximately one-half of the tumours will show a reduction in size and of these, up to 50% will be complete responses (6–12 months of treatment may be required). However, approximately 50% of those tumours which initially responded to tamoxifen will relapse within 2 years, with tumour growth then occurring. It should also be noted that if the tumours are OR negative they are unlikely to respond to tamoxifen and OR status should be established before commencing therapy. In general, therefore, it is recommended that older patients should be treated along the same principles as outlined previously. Stage for stage the results of therapy in women over 65 years are comparable to younger women. However, population-based audit shows that the prognosis in women over 80 years is worse than younger age groups.

Bilateral breast cancers

A second primary cancer in the opposite breast may be found either at the time of the initial presentation (synchronous tumour, 0.5–2%) or more commonly at a subsequent date (metachronous cancer, 3–9%). A woman who has a primary breast cancer has a four- to sixfold risk of developing a cancer in the opposite breast. Other risk factors for the development of a cancer in the opposite breast include LCIS and multifocal disease.

The prognosis for patients with bilateral breast cancers depends on the staging of the tumours and treatment should be appropriate for the disease stage. Patients who have a genetic predisposition (mutations of the putative breast cancer gene(s) and associated genomic abnormalities (e.g. loss of heterozygosity of the p53-suppressor gene)) are at very high risk of developing bilateral breast cancers. In these patients, consideration may be given as to whether prophylactic mastectomy (with or without reconstruction) should be undertaken.

Breast cancer during pregnancy and lactation

Breast cancer presenting during pregnancy or lactation occurs in up to 3 in 10 000 pregnancies, and comprises less than 2% of all breast cancer cases. The median age of these patients is 34 years or less, depending on the series. Earlier studies had suggested that the prognosis was worse in pregnant women with breast cancer, when compared with those who were not pregnant. This is partly due to the fact that presentation tends to be delayed and up to 70% of pregnant women with operable breast cancer have involved axillary nodes. When compared stage for stage with non-pregnant women there appears to be no difference in prognosis. However, in general young women with breast cancer, aged 30 years or less, tend to have a worse prognosis than those aged 35 years or more.

The treatment of the breast cancer should be as for the general population. For example, mastectomy can be safely undertaken. Lumpectomy and axillary surgery, if deemed appropriate, may be carried out in the third trimester. However, radiation treatment should be delayed until after the birth of the baby. If the patient requires adjuvant therapy then this should be delayed until after the first trimester (the most likely time for teratogenic effects). The risks to the foetus of chemotherapy in the second and third trimesters are unclear. The foetus tends to be small and premature labour is a risk, thus some clinicians would delay chemotherapy until after delivery.

Patients presenting with LABC and who would normally be treated with neo-adjuvant chemotherapy pose a particularly difficult problem. If the pregnancy is in the third trimester a decision may be taken to delay treatment until after the delivery. If the pregnancy is in the first or second trimester consideration has to be given to terminating the pregnancy prior to starting such therapy. However, this is a complex problem and requires a multidisciplinary approach between the surgeon, obstetrician, medical oncologist, psychologist, and the patient and her partner.

Breast cancer in the male

Cancer of the male breast accounts for 0.5–1% of all breast cancers and less than 1% of all male malignancies. Only 5% of male breast cancers occur before the age of 40 years and the median age of presentation is 68 years (older than that of the female population who develop breast cancer). The aetiology of male breast cancer has not been elucidated but there are risk factors which may predispose to the development of breast cancer. These include increased levels of oestrogens either in the circulation or in the breast tissue (Kleinfelters syndrome, treatment with oestrogens for prostatic cancer), increased prolactin levels, exposure to ionising radiation, genetic predisposition and occupational risk factors (steel and news printing workers).

The clinical presentation is usually a lump, most commonly centrally placed or in the upper outer quadrant. Up to 20% of patients may have nipple discharge which can be either serous or sero-sanguineous. Histologically, invasive ductal carcinomas of no special type comprise the majority of cancers, as in the female population. All histological types of cancer may be found with the exception of lobular cancer which occurs less frequently. In approximately 80% of tumours, there are oestrogen or PR present. The reported 5-year survival for male patients with breast cancer has ranged from 36% to 75%, but when the patients age, tumour stage, lymph node and hormonal status are taken into account the survival is comparable with that of female patients.

Treatment is as described for female breast cancer. Control of loco-regional disease (with surgery and radiotherapy) is important. In addition, systemic therapy is required for overt or occult micrometastatic disease and this may involve either hormone or chemotherapy.

Screening for breast cancer

Clinical studies have demonstrated that mammographic screening of women can reduce the number of deaths from breast cancer. In particular, studies (USA, Europe) have demonstrated that if women aged 40–74 years of age underwent regular screening there was a decrease in mortality from breast cancer of approximately 25% over 15 years, with the most benefit being found in those women over 50 years of age.

In 1988 a UK National Health Service Breast Screening Programme was introduced. The aim of this programme was to reduce deaths from breast cancer by approximately 25% by the year 2000, provided that at least 70% of women in the population being screened attend for mammography. Women aged 50–64 years were invited to attend a screening centre for a single, high-quality mediolateral oblique view mammogram, every 3 years. However, there was concern that a single view mammogram could miss abnormalities that would have been detected if two mammographic views had been taken. Therefore, two views are now usually taken at the first screen.

If any abnormality is detected it is assessed to determine if any other diagnostic investigations are required. For example, clinical examination, further mammographic examinations, ultrasound assessment and FNAC may all be carried out. Further diagnostic procedures may be required after these assessments to establish the nature of the abnormality detected in the breast. This process requires a multidisciplinary team composed of radiologists, surgeons, cytologists and pathologists, who are specifically trained and experienced in the diagnosis and treatment of breast disease. The results of the screening programme are constantly being audited and evaluated. Findings, to date, suggest that the cancers detected through breast screening are smaller and at an earlier stage (*in-situ* disease, absence of nodal spread) than the tumours of those patients who attend symptomatic breast clinics.

18

Thoracic Surgery

C Peter Clarke

Austin & Repatriation Medical Centre, Heidelberg, Victoria, Australia and
Department of Surgery, University of Melbourne, Victoria, Australia

CONTENTS

Surgical anatomy	351
Tracheobronchial tree	351
Pleural space	352
Mediastinum	353
Oesophagus	353
Vagal and phrenic nerves	353
Diaphragm	353
Symptoms of respiratory disease	354
Investigation	354
Investigative procedures	354
Lobar and pulmonary collapse	356
Thoracotomy	357
Techniques	357
Management of intercostal catheters	358
Complications	358
Pulmonary operations	360
Thoracic trauma	361
Thoracic diseases and their treatment	361
Congenital lesions	361
Empyema	362
Mediastinitis	363
Bronchiectasis	363
Lung abscess	363
Spontaneous pneumothorax	363
Lung cancer	364
Malignant pleural effusion	366
Bronchial obstruction	366
Surgical emphysema	366
Oesophageal diseases	366
Further reading	368

SURGICAL ANATOMY

Tracheobronchial tree

The larynx is the gateway to the tracheobronchial tree and is guarded by the false and true vocal cords. The true vocal cords are important in phonation and also participate in the protection of the airway from fluid and food during deglutition. They are largely controlled by the recurrent laryngeal nerves which both originate in the chest from the vagus nerve and thus are liable to be compromised by any intrathoracic disease.

The main body of the larynx is protected by the hyoid bone and the trachea is suspended from the cricoid bone. There is a membrane in between and this is a useful landmark for emergency cricothyroidotomy or insertion of a minitracheostomy (Fig. 18.1). The trachea and main bronchi are held open by cartilaginous rings. In the former, the rings are incomplete with a posterior membrane and immediately behind the membrane lies the cervical oesophagus. The recurrent laryngeal nerves ascend in this groove. The tracheobronchial tree is lined with ciliated epithelium containing glands secreting mucus and mucus is passed upwards after trapping inhaled particles of foreign material. When the

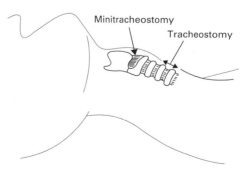

Figure 18.1. Pharynx showing cricothyroid membrane for minitracheostomy.

lining is damaged, such as by chronic smoking, the mucus becomes tenacious, the cilia are deficient and the patient has to cough to clear mucus adequately. This is particularly noticeable first thing in the morning and an early morning cough is the hallmark of chronic smokers.

The lungs are divided into lobes, three on the right and two on the left, and each lobe has two or more segments each served by an independent bronchus. A knowledge of the bronchial anatomy is important for bronchoscopy so that the correct segment can be readily identified (Fig. 18.2). The lungs receive their blood supply from bronchial arteries and are not dependent on the pulmonary circulation. The lymphatic drainage of the segments is first to segmental then hilar lymph nodes and ultimately up to the scalene node on either side. There is, however, a significant cross over of lymphatic drainage from one side to the other, particularly from the left lower lobe to the subcarinal and right-sided glands (Fig. 18.3).

Pleural space

The pleural space is a potential space between the lungs and chest wall and normally only contains a few millilitres of fluid but it both secretes and absorbs approximately 600 ml

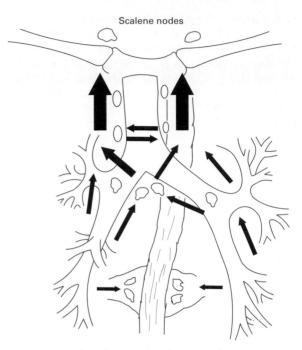

Figure 18.3. Lymohatic drainage of the lungs. Note there is more crossover from the left to right than right to left side.

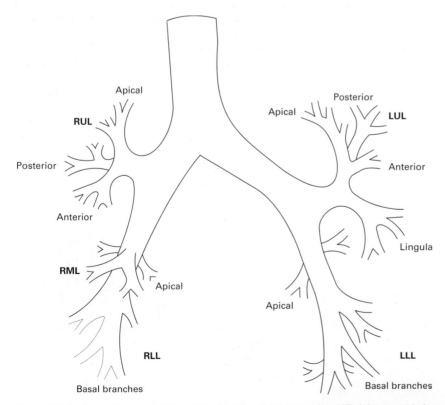

Figure 18.2. Anatomy of the bronchial tree. RUL: right upper lobe; RML: right middle lobe; RLL: right lower lobe; LUL: left upper lobe; LLL: left lower lobe.

of fluid each day. When there is increased fluid production or a decreased ability to reabsorb the fluid, such as may occur with lymphatic blockage, then a pleural effusion results. Generally, if this is secondary to heart failure, the effusion is a transudate, but if it is secondary to infection or tumour it is an exudate. The pleural space is much deeper posteriorly than anteriorly and this needs to be taken into account when planning a thoracentesis.

Mediastinum

The mediastinum is the space between the two pleural cavities and is divided into an anterior, middle and posterior mediastinum (Fig. 18.4). Certain tumours are characteristically found in one or other space–thymomas occur in the anterior mediastinum and neurofibromas in the posterior mediastinum.

Oesophagus

The oesophagus runs from the pharynx to the cardia and has a short cervical part, a longer intrathoracic part and a short upper abdominal part. It runs behind and is closely approximated to the trachea as far as the bifurcation, and the arch of the aorta crosses it. The least protected part of the oesophagus is the lower intrathoracic section and this is where spontaneous rupture generally occurs. The entrance to the abdomen is controlled by slips of the diaphragm called crurae and if these become lax then a sliding or paraoesophageal hernia may occur. Sliding hernias are associated with dysfunction of the natural valve occurring at the cardia and are often associated with acid reflux leading to reflux oesophagitis and sometimes stricture formation.

Vagal and phrenic nerves

The vagal and phrenic nerves have complex passages through the thoracic cavity. On the right-hand side the vagus nerve gives off the recurrent laryngeal nerve quite early which passes around the subclavian artery before ascending to the larynx; it then passes to the back of the hilum of the lung where it breaks into a plexus only to reform and run down to the stomach along the oesophagus. The anatomy of the left vagal nerve is similar excepting that the recurrent laryngeal nerve has a longer course as it passes around the ductus arteriosus before ascending to the neck. Both phrenic nerves lie in a more anterior position and run down on the pericardium to the diaphragm. The left phrenic nerve tends to run somewhat more anteriorly than the right phrenic nerve.

Diaphragm

The diaphragm is a large muscle separating the thoracic and abdominal cavities and has an important function in normal respiration. The bulk of the diaphragm is innervated by the phrenic nerve but the peripheral part gets its nerve supply from the adjoining intercostal nerves. As the intra-abdominal pressure is greater than that in the chest, a paralytic diaphragm will appear to be higher than a normal diaphragm and does not move appropriately with respiration. In the condition known as eventration of the diaphragm there is deficient muscle and the fibrous part is stretched with poor but normal movement. Large diaphragmatic hernias associated with agenesis of the relevant lung and malrotation of the bowel are a neonatal emergency (see Chapter 21). Smaller hernias characteristically occur anteriorly (Morgagni hernia) and posteriorly (Bochdalek hernia) and are less of a problem unless bowel becomes trapped in them (Fig. 18.5).

The chest is built like a bellows with 12 ribs on each side; the upper ones are articulated at the costotransverse angle

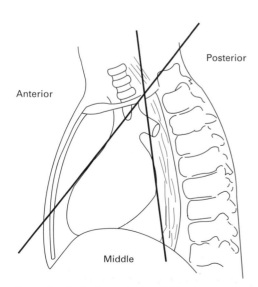

Figure 18.4. Mediastinum showing divisions.

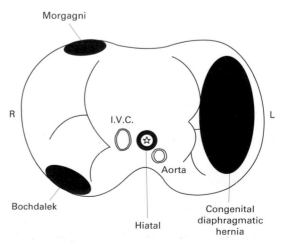

Figure 18.5. Sites if hernia. IVC: inferior vena cava.

and expand the chest as they rise and fall in a bucket-handle motion. This along with the rise and fall of the diaphragm allows air to be taken in and blown out from the lungs. The lungs have a natural elastic recoil which lessens with age. The normal intrathoracic pressure varies between -5 and $+20\,cm\,H_2O$.

SYMPTOMS OF RESPIRATORY DISEASE

The main symptoms are:
- *Cough*: particularly a persistent cough in a person who does not normally cough, or increased cough in smokers.
- *Sputum production*: normal sputum is clear; a yellow or green colour implies infection. An increasing amount of sputum is also a sign of infection.
- *Haemoptysis*: bleeding from the lung is generally bright and usually presents as streaks in the sputum, particularly first thing in the morning. Haemoptysis is rarely confused with a haematemesis as the blood is dark and altered blood in the latter. Bright blood coming from the upper airways can be confused with haemoptysis. A large haemoptysis is characterized by coughing up of clots and the patient often notices a preceding gurgle in the throat which brings on the cough.
- *Breathlessness*: implies loss of pulmonary function. A reasonable assessment of pulmonary function can be obtained from a careful history of the distance a patient can walk before becoming breathless and their normal level of activity.
- *Wheeze*: implies airway obstruction and is particularly significant if it is unilateral or occurs only in certain positions.
- *Chest pain*: lateral constant aching pain or pleuritic pain may indicate chest wall involvement by the underlying disease process. Central chest discomfort may be a sign of mediastinal adenopathy.

The signs to look for are:
- Use of accessory muscles in breathing and the shape of the chest which is barrel shaped in emphysema.
- Central cyanosis.
- Finger clubbing and hypertrophic osteoarthropathy is found in carcinoma of the lung and chronic suppurative chest disease, but can also be found in other conditions such as liver disease and congenital cardiac disease.
- The chest should be resonant to percussion and dullness implies solid lungs or pleural fluid. On auscultation bronchial breathing may be heard above the pleural fluid and rhonchi and crepitations may be detected.

INVESTIGATION

All patients with chest disease should have a chest radiograph and this needs to be inspected in a routine manner, carefully examining the bony skeleton, diaphragm and mediastinum before assessing the lung fields on each side. If a routine is

developed then such things as cervical ribs or bony metastases will not be overlooked by focusing on the obvious abnormality in a chest radiograph. Both anteroposterior and lateral views should be carefully examined.

Other routine tests are full blood count, serum urea and electrolytes and sputum examination both for cytology and culture, including acid-fast bacilli. The best sputum for examination is that produced first thing in the morning and a good routine is to get samples of 3 consecutive days' early morning sputum for examination. If an effusion is detected, this should be aspirated, an estimate made as to whether it is an exudate or a transudate and a specimen sent for cytology and culture (Table 18.1).

Most patients with an abnormality on the chest X-ray will also need a computed tomographic (CT) scan for precise localization of the lesion and to show the mediastinal structures and in particular, enlarged lymph nodes. This scan should also include the thoracic inlet and upper abdomen.

Magnetic radiation imaging (MRI) scans do not usually add further information than is available on a CT scan but are useful for vascular anomalies and when there is a question of neurological involvement.

More recently positron emission tomography (PET) scans (Fig. 18.6) have become available and are particularly useful in staging lung cancer and in the diagnosis of solitary pulmonary nodules. A labeled sugar (FDG 18) is given which is taken up preferentially by active tissues giving rise to a hot area on the scan.

Investigative procedures

Bronchoscopy

Rigid bronchoscopy was popularized by Chevalier Jackson in the 1920s and flexible bronchoscopy introduced by Ikeda in 1964. Flexible bronchoscopy using the fibreoptic bronchoscope can be performed as a day procedure under local anaesthetic and light sedation and is most useful for diagnosis. Investigative procedures include obtaining bronchial washings, bronchial lavage whereby a lobe is washed out and the cells obtained examined, cup biopsy and needle aspiration biopsy. Coagulation abnormalities should be excluded before biopsies are taken.

Table 18.1. **Differences between exudative effusion and transudate.**

	Exudate	Transudate
Colour	Dark yellow	Pale yellow
Pleural fluid/serum protein ratio	>0.5	<0.5
Pleural fluid/serum LDH ratio	>0.6	<0.6
LDH	>200 U	<200 U

Note: LDH – Lactic dehydrogenase.

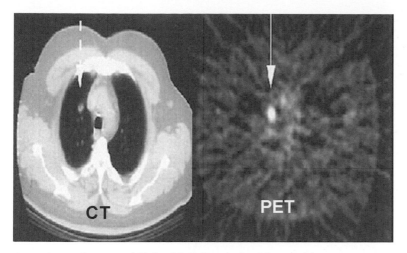

Figure 18.6. A solitary non-calcified nodule is shown in the Right upper lobe. It is active on a PET scan which makes it likely to be malignant.

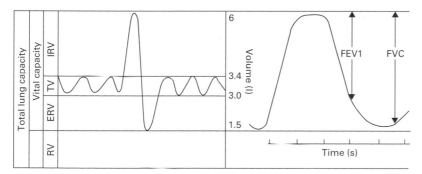

Figure 18.7. Basic spirometry. RV: residual volume; ERV: expiratory reserve volume; TV: tidal volume; IRV: inspiratory reserve volume; FEV1: forced expiratory capacity in 1 s; FVC: forced vital capacity.

For therapeutic purposes a rigid bronchoscopy gives better access to the airways but is uncomfortable and best done under a general anaesthetic. Respiration is maintained by a Venturi jet insufflator. It is the procedure of choice in the investigation of patients with massive haemoptysis, for the removal of inhaled foreign bodies and laser resection of endobronchial lesions or insertion of stents. Larger biopsies of tissue can be obtained through the rigid bronchoscope and if significant bleeding occurs this can usually be controlled with a pledget soaked in adrenaline.

Mediastinoscopy

The scalene lymph gland guards the gateway of the lymphatic channels draining the lungs into the subclavian veins and has long been biopsied as a diagnostic procedure in lung disease. Carlins extended the usefulness of scalene gland biopsy by introducing the mediastinoscope in 1959 to allow for direct biopsy of the mediastinal glands. An incision is made transversely just above the xiphisternal notch, the pretracheal fascia opened and the paratracheal fascia explored by blunt dissection. The mediastinoscope allows careful inspection of

the tissues and identification and biopsy of the paratracheal glands. The procedure has been extended by anterior mediastinotomy (Chamberlain procedure) through the bed of the second or third costal cartilage which allows a more direct approach to subaortic and subcarinal glands (see below).

These procedures are widely used for the staging of lung cancer, particularly when a CT scan shows enlarged mediastinal glands.

Video-assisted thoracoscopic surgery

A minimally invasive inspection of the pleural space allows sampling of effusions and pleural biopsy along with biopsy of all the mediastinal nodes on the same side but does not allow biopsy of the contralateral nodes.

Thoracocentesis

Thoracocentesis for pleural effusion is usually done for diagnostic purposes. The actual tap can be done with a needle, venous cannula or trochar and catheter and, unless the chest radiograph shows a loculated effusion, it is done posteriorly over the seventh or eighth rib where the pleural space is

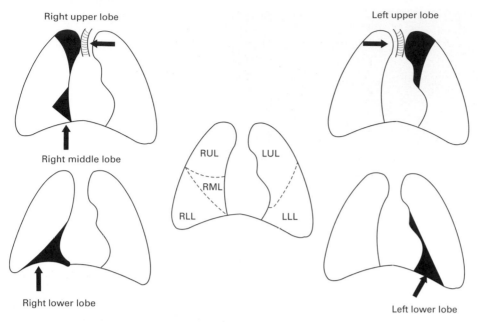

Figure 18.8. Radiographic appearance in lobar collapse.

deepest. The patient sits up and leans forward on a support and the procedure is done under a local anaesthetic. Fluid is sent for biochemistry, culture, cell count and cytology. Transudates have a low protein count and are likely to be due to cardiac failure, whilst exudates have a high protein count and are generally secondary to infection or malignancy. Large effusions are best managed by insertion of an inter-costal catheter, which is preferably placed in the mid-axillary line at the sixth or seventh intercostal space as this is an area devoid of overlying muscles. The pleural space should be emptied completely but the drainage may need to be inter-rupted if the patient experiences chest pain as the lung re-expands. On rare occasions, re-expansion pulmonary oedema can occur if the effusion is drained too quickly.

Pulmonary function

Pulmonary function should be measured before contem-plating lung resection. In a fit patient, this need be no more than basic spirometry (Fig. 18.7). Smoking, which causes lung cancer, may also lead to a degree of emphysema, and these patients require full bronchospirometry with and without bronchodilators and an estimate of pulmonary dif-fusion. In marginal cases, a pulmonary exercise test measur-ing the oxygen uptake during exercise is also helpful and a ventilation–perfusion scan, particularly if it is quantified, gives an estimate of the relative contribution of each area of the lung to the overall function. This information is helpful in estimating the likely respiratory function after pulmonary resection. Clinical evidence of pulmonary hypertension is a contraindication to major pulmonary resection and if suspected can be confirmed by non-invasive means.

Patients who have marginal pulmonary function improve if they cease smoking and are given an intensive regimen of bronchodilators and corticosteroids, and should be reassessed after 2 weeks of treatment to see if pulmonary function has improved sufficiently to allow surgery.

LOBAR AND PULMONARY COLLAPSE

When a bronchus is blocked, the area of the lung beyond it loses its aeration and collapses. This gives a characteristic appearance on the chest radiograph (Fig. 18.8). If the whole lung collapses there is an associated mediastinal shift to that side and hyperexpansion of the other lung.

In young patients, the cause is most likely to be an inhaled foreign body or postinfective stricture, but in older patients the most likely cause is bronchogenic carcinoma. Patients with severe asthma may get plugs of tenacious sputum which block the bronchus.

A collapsed area of lung leads to breathlessness as there is continued pulmonary blood flow in that part without any corresponding aeration and it is also liable to become infected. A patient with a collapsed lobe should have a bron-choscopy, both as a diagnostic and a possible therapeutic procedure.

The best management of lung cancer is to resect it but if this is not feasible intrinsic endobronchial cancers can be resected with a laser or removed manually with biopsy forceps. Sometimes these blockages are due to extrinsic compression in which cases, if there is a useful distal lumen, a stent can be inserted.

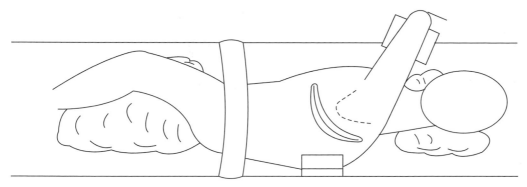

Figure 18.9. Posterolateral thoracotomy.

THORACOTOMY

Techniques

Posterolateral thoracotomy

The standard approach to the lung is through a posterolateral thoracotomy with the patient in a full lateral position and anaesthetized with a double-lumen tube so that the upper lung can be isolated and collapsed (Fig. 18.9). The incision curves around the tip of the scapula and the latissimus dorsi and serratus muscles are divided as far as possible distally to preserve their nerve supply. The ribs are counted from above, remembering that the top rib which is easily palpable is the second because of the insertion of the major fascicle of the serratus anterior muscle into that rib. The chest is then opened through the fifth or sixth interspace, depending on the site of pathology. This is usually done through the bed of the periosteum stripped from the upper surface of the rib. The posterior end of the rib is either divided or the costotransverse joint disarticulated to allow easy spreading. In older patients with brittle ribs, the whole rib should be resected. Perichondral sutures are used to hold the ribs together during closure and each layer then repaired with absorbable sutures.

Although this incision gives superb access, it is associated with considerable postoperative discomfort and a long recovery period. When the proposed procedure is straightforward, adequate access can be achieved through a *muscle-sparing incision* by mobilizing the muscles and pulling them to one or other side with retractors. There is no early benefit from this approach given the excellent analgesia that can be obtained using an epidural or extrapleural catheter and local anaesthetic, but there is a significant improvement in early mobilization.

Anterior thoracotomy

An anterior thoracotomy, curving the incision beneath the breast, gives access to the anterior mediastinum and is also useful for lung biopsy in patients on ventilators who do not tolerate collapsing a lung or being placed in the lateral position.

Axillary thoracotomy

An axillary thoracotomy is also a muscle-sparing technique which gives good access to the apex of the lung or the sympathetic chain posteriorly. The arm must be held in a vertical position with the patient leaning slightly backwards and care must be taken not to injure the long thoracic nerve.

Mediastinotomy

An anterior mediastinotomy dividing the sternum in the midline is a standard approach for cardiac surgery but is also useful in thoracic surgery for lesions in the anterior mediastinum or where both lungs need to be approached at the same time such as when there are multiple metastases. The sternum is reconstituted with wire sutures either passing through the sternum itself or around the sternum taking care not to injure the internal mammary vessels. This incision is usually better tolerated by patients than a lateral thoracotomy.

Video-assisted thorascopic surgery

Video-assisted thorascopic surgery (VATS) has the advantage of avoiding the necessity to spread the ribs, which reduces postoperative neuralgia and muscle damage. The patient is placed in the lateral position with a double-lumen tube and two or more ports introduced after collapsing the lung. The first port is generally introduced in the mid-axillary line at the sixth or lower interspace after carefully passing a finger into the chest to make sure there are no pleural adhesions. The other ports are then introduced under vision and placed in an arc pointing to the expected pathology so that the surgeon is working forwards and instrument clash is prevented (Fig. 18.10).

Vision is obtained using a telescope to which a video camera is attached and this allows everyone in the operating theatre to observe the operation. Although a superb view of the intrathoracic organs is obtained, the downside is that tactile ability is lost. Practically every intrathoracic procedure can be done using a video-assisted thoracoscopic approach.

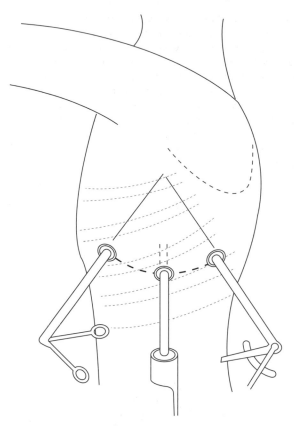

Figure 18.10. Placement of ports in an arc for video-assisted thoracoscopic.

There are some procedures for which this approach is the method of choice and these include management of:
• spontaneous pneumothorax,
• malignant pleural effusion,
• pleural biopsies,
• pleural-based lesions,
• excisional biopsy of peripheral nodules in the lung.
This approach can also be used for pulmonary resections particularly if the mass lesion in the lobe is less than 3 cm in diameter. Quite apart from patient satisfaction with faster recovery and less post operative neuralgia, there have been studies to show that the immune response for malignancy is better preserved in these patients because of the lessened trauma of operation.

One drawback of a VATS approach is the inability to palpate the lung either to localize the lesions or for detection of all lesions when secondary tumours are being resected. Ultrasound probes are helpful but can be difficult to interpret. A simple approach is to pass the hand up from below through the diaphragm from a subcostal incision, hand-assisted thoracoscopic surgery (HATS). The fingers pass between the radial fibres of the diaphragm with minimal effect on diaphragmatic function (Figure 18.11b,i&ii). The necessary

abdominal excision is much better tolerated than the alternative of performing a thoracotomy and spreading the ribs. This technique can also be adapted for minimally invasive oesophageal surgery; however, in this instance a special port is required in order to retain the intra-abdominal gases.

Management of intercostal catheters

After a thoracotomy, intercostal catheters are generally placed to lie at the apex and base of the chest with the intention of keeping the pleural space empty. If an intercostal catheter has to be inserted without an operation, then the area of choice is in the axilla where there are no muscles covering the chest wall and the scar is cosmetically acceptable. This can be done under local anaesthetic remembering that the most painful layers are the skin and pleura.

The catheter is introduced across the top of the rib as the intercostal vessels lie in the groove below a rib and, unless it is clear there is a large effusion or pneumothorax, then a finger should be carefully inserted first to ensure that there is a patent pleural space (Figure 18.11a). Many of the catheters come with a trocar which stiffens the catheter and aids its placement in the desired position after insertion.

The catheters are connected by tubing to an underwater seal which acts as a one-way valve and also allows for visual estimation of the intrathoracic pressure. The classic three-bottle system (Fig. 18.12) incorporates a bottle to collect fluid from the chest, a bottle to regulate the suction pressure and a bottle to act as a safety valve between the system and the suction source. There are several varieties of disposable receptacle which incorporate this three-bottle system into one unit.

Generally, gentle suction is applied to keep the pleural space empty and this is set at 20 cmH$_2$O, which is just above the normal range of pressure found in the pleural space.

There are some instances, however, where suction is not used and the most important is after a pneumonectomy when it is important to keep the mediastinum centrally placed. The tube is left in the post-pneumonectomy space to allow detection of postoperative bleeding and also as a means either of adding air or removing fluid or air in order to keep the mediastinum in a median position. Generally, the tube is clamped and only released for a minute or so each hour, during which time the patient is asked not to cough, and it is removed as soon as it is clear that there is no post-operative bleeding.

Complications

Apart from the usual complications after any surgery, such as wound infection, deep vein thrombosis and pulmonary embolism, particular complications after pulmonary surgery are:
• sputum retention,
• bronchopleural fistula,
• cardiac arrhythmias.

The key to avoiding *sputum retention* is good postoperative analgesia. There are some situations where coughing postoperatively is particularly difficult, such as if there has been damage to the recurrent laryngeal nerve during the course of a pulmonary resection. This may have been deliberate when glands from the aortopulmonary area have been involved and are removed. Patients with increased or tenacious sputum need either repeat nasolaryngeal suction or minitracheostomy. The latter can be inserted using a Seldinger technique through the cricothyroid membrane which is the most comfortable procedure for the patient.

A *bronchopleural fistula* may occur because of faulty technique, infection or because the suture line has become involved with tumour. The most important bronchopleural fistula occurs after a pneumonectomy when the postpneumonectomy space will become infected. The patient characteristically coughs up serosanguineous fluid and a chest

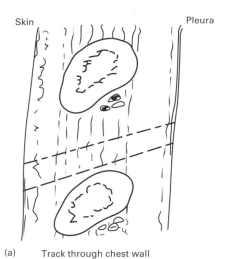

Skin   Pleura

(a)   Track through chest wall

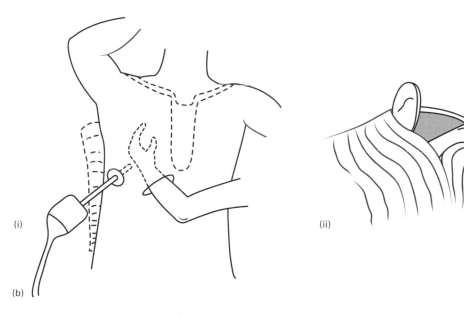

(i)

(ii)

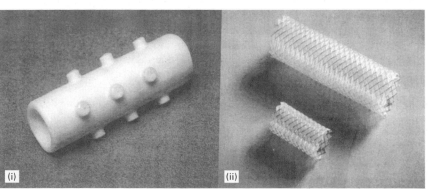

(c)   (i)   (ii)

Figure 18.11. (a) Track for insertion of Intercostal catheter. (b) (i) Approach for HATS and (ii) Passing fingers thru diaphragm. (c) (i) Dumon stent and (ii) Wallstent.

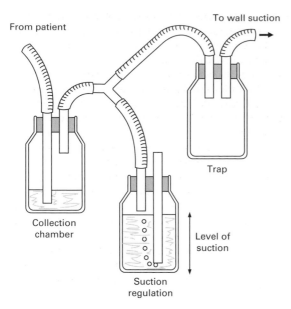

From patient

To wall suction

Trap

Collection chamber

Level of suction

Suction regulation

Figure 18.12. Three-bottle system of underwater sealed drainage.

radiograph shows a drop in the fluid level. In an emergency situation, the patient should be placed with the pneumonectomy space dependent and an intercostal catheter introduced to empty the space. When there is an early breakdown of the stump, then it may be possible to resuture it; however, in the presence of significant sepsis, formal drainage of the pneumonectomy space, either with rib resection and tube or a skin flap, is necessary with later closure of the stump and space once the situation has been stabilized. This may be done by means of a muscle or omental flap or by a thoracoplasty or even a combination of these manoeuvres.

Arrhythmias are common after thoracic surgery, particularly in elderly patients, after a pneumonectomy and especially when the pericardium has been opened. If digitalization is carried out this must be done slowly and even so may not eliminate arrhythmias. As arrhythmias can be brought under control quickly with modern drugs, it is reasonable to closely monitor them and treat arrhythmias as and when they occur, rather than performing preoperative digitalization.

PULMONARY OPERATIONS

Pulmonary operations vary from pneumonectomy to small-wedge biopsies for diagnostic purposes. A pneumonectomy used to be the standard operation for lung cancer but is not suitable for many elderly patients and can lead to long-term problems as the patient ages and the residual lung becomes emphysematous. It has been demonstrated that a lobectomy gives just as good results in most cases. The right lung accounts for some 55% of overall ventilation as against the left lung which accounts for 45%. Before planning a pneumonectomy

it is generally wise to have a ventilation–perfusion scan to ensure that the remaining lung is normal and get an assessment as to the effectiveness of the remaining lung.

Lesser procedures include segmental resection of an anatomical segment of a lobe of lung and wedge resections. Persistent air-leaks used to be a problem with them but the use of staplers and tissue glues has improved their safety.

Transplantation of the lung

Transplantation of the lungs may be performed as single-lung transplant, double-lung transplant or combined with heart transplantation. The main indications are end-stage pulmonary fibrosis, cystic fibrosis and emphysema. Limiting factors are the difficulty in obtaining suitable donor lungs and problems with the need for immunosuppression after the operation. At present, lung transplants do not do as well in the long-term as heart transplants as a significant number develop obliterative bronchiolitis.

The current 5-year survival in most series is only the order of 50% with upto 20% of patients developing a tumour during the same time of which the most common on is a lympho proliferative disorder.

Lung volume reduction

Although lung transplantation can be performed for emphysema, the large number of patients with emphysema precludes this being a useful overall modality, and this has sparked a renewal of interest in lung volume reduction surgery. This was originally performed in the 1950s by Brantigan who put forward the idea that the hyperinflated lungs work better if reduced in size, mainly because of the improved breathing dynamics. Difficulty with controlling air leaks led the procedure to fall into disfavour but modern techniques, such as use of buttresses of bovine pericardium and the use of tissue glues, has made it a feasible proposition.

The aim is to remove approximately 25–30% of the lung, selecting those areas which are poorly ventilated and perfused. This removes the stenting from the thoracic cage, allows the diaphragm to work properly as it is no longer flattened all the time, and reduces the tendency of the smaller bronchioles which are not held open by cartilaginous rings to collapse.

Patients likely to benefit from lung volume reduction surgery have relatively pure emphysema of a heterogenous nature. This means that they have a minimum of sputum production and easily controlled bronchospasm not requiring systemic steroids and that a ventilation–perfusion scan shows areas of mismatch between the lung being perfused and ventilated. These areas are usually at the lung apices and can be safely resected without reducing pulmonary function yet reducing the overall size of the lungs. Well selected patients should get several years of functional improvement before they once again deteriorate as their underlying loss of elasticity degenerates with age.

The procedure however carries a significant mortality and morbidity related to the patient's poor pulmonary function with associated lack of pulmonary reserve and is usually done after a course of pulmonary rehabilitation. There has been recent interest in attempting to achieve the same result but insertion of endobronchial valves to isolate the dysfunctional areas and lead to their collapse; however, these procedures are still experimental.

THORACIC TRAUMA

For more details refer Chapter 7.

Amongst trauma fatalities, 50% have significant thoracic trauma.

Several complications of thoracic trauma can be rapidly fatal:

- *Obstruction of the airways.* Re-establishing an adequate airway, by intubating the patient if necessary, should be the top priority.
- *Tension pneumothorax* results in pulmonary collapse and a shift of the mediastinum to the contralateral side with severe haemodynamic compromise. Successful treatment depends on early recognition and evacuation of the air.
- *Open pneumothorax* is easily recognized and requires control by whatever means are to hand in the first instance.
- A *massive haemothorax* presents with shock and hypoxia. Intercostal catheters are inserted and if there is continuing drainage, then an exploratory thoracotomy is necessary. The bleeding is generally from a torn intercostal artery or major pulmonary vessel.
- A *flail chest* leads to inefficient respiration. If it is placed posteriorly, it can be stabilized by lying the patient against pillows, but an anterior flail requires fixation of the flail or splinting by positive pressure ventilation.
- A *cardiac tamponade* should be suspected in any patient if severe shock fails to respond to resuscitation. The usual signs of tamponade are masked in the acute situation and cannot be relied on. If an echocardiogram is available, a quick diagnosis can be made, but otherwise a trial paracentesis should be performed.

Other serious complications include:

- *Pulmonary contusion* which can lead to respiratory failure requiring respiratory assistance.
- A *traumatic aortic rupture* which can be instantaneously fatal and generally occurs at the junction of the transverse aorta with the descending aorta. In survivors, the only part of the aorta which remains intact is the adventitia, leading to a localized false aneurysm which can rupture at a later time. Generally, it is the result of a deceleration injury in a younger person and the cardinal sign is widening of the mediastinum on a plain chest radiograph. If suspected, an aortogram should be performed and early repair undertaken.
- *Tracheobronchial rupture* which occurs in the lower main trachea or the origin of the major bronchi and is also the result of a deceleration injury. If complete rupture occurs, there is a pneumothorax with massive air leak on the side involved which necessitates early exploration. A partial

rupture may cause haemoptysis and when suspected a bronchoscopy should be performed. If neglected the rupture heals with excessive granulation tissue, leading to subsequent collapse of the lung.

- *Oesophageal rupture* which is comparatively rare as the oesophagus is a mobile organ. It can be involved in penetrating injuries, but the commonest form of rupture is when there is sudden compression of the chest with a closed glottis.
- *Ruptures of the diaphragm* which are generally secondary to abdominal compression and occur most commonly on the left-hand side. They are best repaired from below in view of the associated abdominal injuries. Occasionally, they present late when they are hard to differentiate from an eventration of the diaphragm. The issue can be solved by thoracoscopy and direct examination of the diaphragm.
- *Myocardial contusion* which commonly affects the right ventricle as it lies directly behind the sternum. There is subsequent splinting of the ventricle with resultant poor cardiac output requiring a high venous filling pressure and treatment with cardiac stimulants.
- *Fractures of the sternum* which indicate significant injury, especially in the elderly, and associated myocardial injury needs to be excluded. They take some 6 weeks to heal but are generally impacted and rarely need fixation.
- Similarly *fractures of the first rib* which are indicative of significant injury as it is a short thick rib. Because of the adjacent vessels and brachial plexus, a careful examination for the integrity of nerves needs to be made and, if necessary, a CT scan with contrast performed to rule out injury to the vessels.

To keep the matter of chest injuries in perspective, however, it should be kept in mind that of all chest injuries that require admission to hospital, most will require observation and pain relief and some will also require insertion of intercostal catheters in order to keep the pleural space empty and a number may require ventilatory assistance only 5% will require open operative intervention.

THORACIC DISEASES AND THEIR TREATMENT

Congenital lesions

For more details refer Chapter 21.

Congenital lesions of the respiratory tract are relatively rare and often associated with cardiac abnormalities. Both agenesis and hyperplasia of the lung and areas of tracheal hypoplasia may occur. The trachea can also be constricted if there is a vascular aortic ring, with respiratory difficulties requiring urgent division of the ring.

Congenital cysts

Congenital cysts of the lung may require attention if they compress normal lung tissue. Sometimes a whole lobe may be emphysematous and enlarged, causing significant respiratory embarrassment in the first 6 months of life, and needs to be resected. Bronchogenic cysts are rarely a problem unless they cause compression of a bronchus or pulmonary artery or become infected. They are most likely to be found as an incidental finding on a chest radiograph and are easily managed by unroofing the lesion by a video-assisted thoracoscopic approach (see above). They are lined with ciliated respiratory epithelium. Duplication cysts are remnants left over during the maturation of the original paired intestinal tracts into one and are recognized both from their position and simpler lining. Pericardial cysts are often called 'springwater cysts' because of the clear contents and are found adjacent to the heart.

Hamartomas

Hamartomas are chondromatous malformations within the lung and present as non-calcified coin lesions. In older patients they are a particular problem if no earlier chest radiographs are available and usually need to be resected to rule out the possibility of an early bronchogenic carcinoma. The PET scan is useful in sorting out which ones can be safely watched.

Pulmonary sequestration

A pulmonary sequestration is a part of the lung that gets an abnormal blood supply directly from the aorta. They can be extralobar having no communication with the bronchial tree or intralobar when the bronchial anatomy is normal. They rarely cause any problem unless they become infected when recurrent infection is the rule. They are commoner in the lower lobes than the upper lobes and are commonest on the left-hand side. The blood supply from the aorta may arise from below the diaphragm, and this needs to be kept in mind when they are being explored.

Chest wall deformities

A variety of chest wall deformities usually present in early childhood and often become more pronounced during later growth. The common ones are:

- pectus excavatum when there is an indrawing of the lower sternum;
- pectus carinatum when the sternum is pushed forward in a beak-like manner;
- Poland's anomaly which consists of agenesis of the pectoral muscles on one or other side in association with poor development of the ribs in that area.

Correction of the deformity is rarely required for physiological reasons but is commonly done for cosmetic reasons.

Some severe pectus deformities can compress the right ventricle with impaired cardiac output but this is only present in extreme cases. Most of the patients have normal pulmonary function before surgery which is reduced following repair of the pectus because of the splinting of the chest wall.

The classical repair of pectus excavatum deformity is the Ravitch repair which consists of a transverse sternotomy and mobilization of the lower sternum dividing the costal cartilages on each side and holding the freed sternum forwards with a transverse bar. More recently the Nuss bar has become popular for younger patients with compliant chest walls. The curved bar is placed by a minimally invasive approach to lye behind the sternum and then flipped to exert pressure pushing the sternum forwards.

Empyema

Empyema denotes the accumulation of pus in a natural cavity and if the location is not specified it is taken as an intrapleural collection as this is the commonest site. An empyema generally evolves in three phases:

1. Exudative: thin fluid-containing polymorphonuclear cells and bacteria.
2. Fibropurulent: thicker fluid-containing fibrin with a turbid appearance.
3. Organizing: thick pus with a rind of fibroblasts sealing off the cavity.

An untreated empyema may eventually point through the chest wall as an 'empyema necessitans'.

The aetiology may be:

- effusion following pneumonia,
- ruptured lung abscess,
- secondary to a subphrenic abscess,
- post-traumatic infected haemothorax,
- oesophageal perforation,
- postoperative.

A plain radiograph demonstrates the presence of fluid and an empyema is then confirmed by the associated physical signs (fever, sweats) and the presence of pus at thoracentesis. When detected, empyema requires cover with appropriate antibiotics and early drainage.

In the exudate phase, the pleural space can be drained by insertion of an intercostal tube, but when the empyema has progressed to the fibropurulent stage the space needs to be cleaned out either at VATS or minithoracotomy.

Once the empyema has become organized, the underlying lung is trapped by the fibrin shell and the alternative treatments are either a full decortication, which restores mobility of the chest wall and allows the underlying lung to re-expand but does necessitate a major operation, or the alternative of rib resection and tube thoracostomy. A variant of the latter procedure is to turn in a skin flap (the Elloesser procedure originally described for tuberculous empyema), which can then be fitted with a colostomy bag, and may be a more comfortable alternative for the patient.

When there is a large residual space, such as an infected post-pneumonectomy space, and the patient's condition has stabilized, then the space can be filled and closed using a muscle or omental flap or a combination of these. Another approach is to perform a thoracoplasty whereby the chest wall is allowed to sink in after removal of the ribs but this leads to chest deformity and often chronic back pain and is best avoided.

Mediastinitis

Mediastinitis is usually due to perforation of a viscus and this is generally the oesophagus. The commonest forms of perforation are iatrogenic during the course of an endoscopic examination and spontaneous (Boarehaave) rupture. It is brought on by vomiting with a closed glottis and characteristically occurs low down on the left-hand side of the oesophagus, which is the least supported area. When a Boarehaave rupture occurs, there is sudden onset of chest pain and breathlessness, and a chest radiograph will show evidence of air in the mediastinum and pleural fluid on the side of rupture if there has been a rupture into the pleural space. Aspiration shows gastric contents.

The principles of treatment are appropriate broad-spectrum antibiotic cover and urgent repair of the split if it has occurred within the last 24 h with drainage of the mediastinum. A gastrograffin swallow is necessary to show the exact site of the rupture unless it has already been identified at endoscopy.

After 24 hours, primary repair of the perforated oesophagus becomes a problem and if there is extensive mediastinitis, then immediate oesophagectomy with secondary reconstruction may be considered. If the rupture has occurred at the site of a stricture or malignancy, this needs to be attended to at the same time.

Bronchiectasis

Bronchiectasis is a condition where there is chronic inflammation of the lobar bronchi which become dilated and chronically infected. It generally follows a childhood infection of which whooping cough used to be the commonest cause. It can be circular or cylindrical depending on the length of bronchus involved. These may be localized or generalized. Characteristically, patients have a persistent cough bringing up large amounts of purulent sputum each morning and are liable to intermittent haemoptysis.

Treatment consists of keeping the airways free of pus by postural drainage each morning and in severe cases later in the day as well and managing episodes of active infection. The main investigation used to be bronchography but this has been supplanted by high-resolution CT scans with 3D reconstruction, which is much better tolerated by the patient. Localized areas of bronchiectasis can be treated by surgical excision but widespread bronchiectasis is a medical condition requiring life-long management.

Lung abscess

A lung abscess is a necrotic and often cavitated mass of infected lung tissue. The causes are:

- *Aspiration*: this may occur in alcoholics or under general anaesthesia.
- *Post-pneumonic*: commoner in alcoholics, patients who are immunosuppressed and diabetics.

- Secondary to *regional or distal sepsis, bronchostenotic lesion* or *foreign body*.

The clinical presentation is with foul sputum and a radiologically localized opacity proceeding to cavitation. If a lung abscess bursts into the pleural space, then a pyopneumothorax will occur.

Management is based on appropriate antibiotic cover and ensuring there is free drainage through the bronchial tree. An early bronchoscopy is mandatory to rule out an underlying bronchostenotic lesion, obtain a sample for culture and ensure that there is free drainage.

Lung abscesses in older patients that do not show strong evidence of healing within 4 weeks should be regarded with some suspicion and resected if the patient's condition allows.

Spontaneous pneumothorax

Spontaneous pneumothorax in its commonest form is a disease of young adults, occurring more frequently amongst males than females, and is due to rupture of a bleb. These are usually found at the apex of the upper lobes and, although their origin is still obscure, they probably follow minor infection with patchy fibrosis and contraction of areas on the surface of the lung creating blebs in between. Rarely, they may occur in women at the time of menses and may be associated with Marfan's syndrome, *Pneumocystis carinii* infection, particularly in patients with AIDS, granulomas and lymphangioleiomyomatosis. It is commoner amongst smokers and seems particularly prevalent at times of sharp barometric change.

In adults with emphysema, the cause is a ruptured bulla and continuing air leaks are often a significant problem. The bullae are distinguished from blebs in that they are surrounded by lung tissue (Fig. 18.13).

The clinical presentation of spontaneous pneumothorax is a sudden onset of pleuritic chest pain and breathlessness. It is often confused with a myocardial infarction but the diagnosis becomes apparent by the absence of breath sounds on one side and is confirmed with a chest X-ray.

If the pneumothorax is shallow, it may be aspirated and the patient observed; otherwise an intercostal catheter should be inserted. Of patients having their first episode, 80% will not have any further problems, but if a recurrence occurs then the likelihood of further episodes is of the order of 50% and increases with subsequent recurrences. Whilst spontaneous pneumothorax is rarely fatal, excepting in the rare event of a tension pneumothorax or simultaneous bilateral pneumothoraces, it accounts for significant use of hospital beds and loss of time from work. Early definitive treatment can save much subsequent morbidity and the introduction of VATS has allowed for aggressive early management leading to minimal periods of hospitalization and reduction in the likelihood of troublesome postoperative neuralgia. The management of the apical blebs by ligation or excision alone is insufficient as they may recur and a pleurodesis should also be performed. In young patients, this is best done either by a

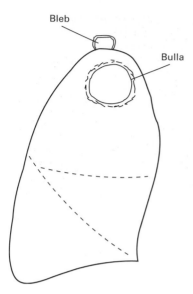

Figure 18.13. Blebs versus bullae.

formal pleurectomy or abrasion, but in older patients talc can be used as an irritant, as the possibility of long-term induction of tumour caused by the irritant is not relevant.

A plan for the management of spontaneous pneumothorax is:
- pneumothorax <15% – aspirate and observe,
- pneumothorax >15% – intercostal catheter with suction.

Indications for surgery are:
- *Definite*:
  - tension pneumothorax,
  - bilateral pneumothorax,
  - recurrent pneumothorax,
  - haemopneumothorax,
  - continuing air leak >5 days.
- *Relative*:
  - occupation,
  - availability of medical care.

A rare variant that is best operated on at the time of diagnosis is *spontaneous haemopneumothorax*. This occurs when an adhesion which is usually apical is torn as the lung deflates and there is continuing bleeding with consequent hidden blood loss. The blood needs to be evacuated and the adhesion fulgurated.

Lung cancer

Cancer of the lung is the leading cause of cancer-related death in males and the incidence is rising in females. Regrettably it is closely related to tobacco smoking and control in the future depends largely on government measures to reduce tobacco consumption.

From a practical point of view, lung cancers are categorized as small or non-small cell cancers.

Table 18.2. World Health Organization histologic classification of lung cancer.

Dysplasia/carcinoma *in situ*

Squamous cell carcinoma

Small cell carcinoma
1. Oat cell carcinoma
2. Intermediastinal cell type
3. Combined oat cell carcinoma

Adenocarcinoma
1. Acinar adenocarcinoma
2. Papillary adenocarcinoma
3. Bronchioalveolar carcinoma
4. Solid carcinoma with mucus formation

Large cell carcinoma variations
1. Giant cell carcinoma
2. Clear cell carcinoma

Adenosquamous carcinoma
Carcinoid tumours
Bronchial gland carcinoma
1. Adenoid cystic carcinoma
2. Mucoepidermal carcinoma
3. Others

Small cell cancers

Small cell cancers tend to occur centrally and grow rapidly, spreading widely through the blood stream at an early stage and are rarely amenable to surgical resection. If detected early and resected, then adjuvant chemotherapy should be given postoperatively because of the likelihood of distal metastases. In most large series, small cell cancers account for approximately 20% of cases overall.

Non-small cell cancers

The commoner tumours are non-small cell cancers and these fall into two main groups:
- *squamous cell cancers*, which tend to occur centrally but metastasize through the blood stream relatively late;
- *adenocarcinomas*, which generally occur more peripherally but have a greater tendency to metastasize distally early in the course of the disease.

Both varieties initially spread via the lymphatic drainage system. The World Health Organization histological classification of all lung cancers is shown in Table 18.2.

Staging of lung cancer involves an assessment of the primary lesion (T) and whether draining lymph nodes are involved (N) and the presence or absence of distal metastases (M) (Table 18.3).

Surgical removal is the preferred treatment for patients with non-small cell lung cancer but this is only possible if the patient can withstand a pulmonary resection and the tumour is confined to the lung. Only 15% of potential candidates turn out to have resectable lesions overall; 85% do not

Table 18.3. **TNM staging system for lung cancer (abridged from UICC).**

Primary tumours (T)

TX	Occult carcinoma
TIS	Carcinoma *in situ*
T1	Tumour <3 cm not abutting pleura or involving a main bronchus
T2	Tumour >3 cm extending to invade pleura or up to 2 cm from main carina
T3	Tumour with direct extension into chest wall, diaphragm, mediastinum but not involving mediastinal structures directly or with 2 cm but not involving carcina
T4	Tumour with direct invasion of mediastinal structures or with presence of a malignant pleural effusion

Nodal involvement (N)

N0	No evidence of regional node metastases
N1	Metastases to hilar regional nodes
N2	Metastases to ipsilateral mediastinal or subcarinal nodes
N3	Metastases to contralateral mediastinal nodes or supraclavicular nodes

Distal metastases (M)

M0	No known distal metastases
M1	Distal metastases present

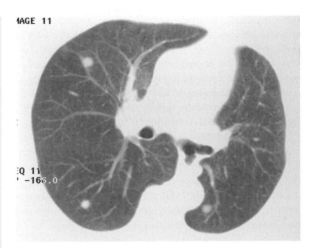

Figure 18.14. Metastatic tumour to the lung, demonstrated on CT.

because of age, poor pulmonary function, associated cardio-vascular disease and early spread of the cancer.

Staging procedures include:

- chest radiograph;
- CT scan of the chest and upper abdomen (Fig. 18.14);
- bronchoscopy;
- mediastinoscopy;
- anterior mediastinotomy and VATS exploration of the pleural space.

MRI has only a limited role and is generally no better than CT scanning. In the future, PET scanning may limit the necessity for more invasive procedures by showing whether the lymph glands are involved. Patients with adenocarcinomas should have skeletal radionuclide scans and CT scans of the head because of the increased likelihood of occult distal metastases.

Some younger and fitter patients with locally advanced non-small cell lung cancer, while not resectable in an ortho-dox sense, may benefit from neo-adjuvant chemotherapy and radiotherapy given with the object of downstaging the tumour and allowing subsequent resection but this must still be regarded as a largely experimental programme.

Secondary tumours

The lung is a common site for secondary tumours as it acts as a large filter. These are commonly multiple rather than solitary and affect both lungs. Occasionally, a secondary lesion in the lung, when resected, is so characteristic that the primary site is obvious but more commonly, although it is considered to be a secondary tumour, the primary site remains occult. An exhaustive search for a hidden primary may often be unrewarding but in males it is important to rule out carcinoma of the prostate and in females carcinoma of the breast and ovaries as these are amenable to hormone or cytotoxic chemotherapy.

When the primary site has been well controlled and there is a significant interval between the original operation and development of a pulmonary metastasis, it is worthwhile resecting the pulmonary lesion if there is no evidence of metastases elsewhere. Some tumours, particularly sarco-mas, have a predilection to metastasize to the lung, which is often the only site of metastasis, and particularly as they tend to occur in younger patients, should be treated aggres-sively resecting all the lesions but sparing as much lung tissue as possible.

Pleural-based tumours

Benign pleural-based tumours such as fibromas are rela-tively uncommon and cause only local symptoms as they increase in size. They are cured by surgical excision.

The pleura is a common site for metastatic tumours which are generally manifested by the development of an effusion. An insidious pleural effusion occurring in a patient over 50 years of age is very likely to be secondary to malignancy. Useful palliation can be afforded by removing the pleural fluid and performing a pleurodesis with an irritant such as talc.

A primary malignancy arising in the pleura, *malignant mesothelioma*, is uncommon except where there has been previous asbestos exposure. Once asbestos has been inhaled it cannot be removed from the lung and may cause asbesto-sis or fibrosis of the lung along with characteristic pleural plaques. After a lag period of some 20–30 years, a malignant mesothelioma may develop. This type of cancer is found in areas where there has been industrial use of asbestos such as in ship building. The tumour often causes a pleural effusion and local pain, is difficult to cure and the management is largely palliative.

The commonest *benign* tumour of the chest wall is a neurogenic tumour such as a neurofibroma or schwannoma developing on an intercostal nerve or a ganglioneuroma developing on the sympathetic system. These are usually within the chest and located posteriorly. They may be associated with multiple neurofibromatoses along with *cafe-au-lait* skin lesions in von Recklinhausen's disease but most commonly they occur as isolated tumours. There is a tendency for them to slowly increase in size when they are liable to undergo malignant change. They also tend to infiltrate along the nerve sheath and this can be a problem if the tumour infiltrates through the intervertebral foramen and presses on the spinal cord.

Tumours of the ribs manifest themselves by the presence of a palpable lump and are often painful as the weakened rib fractures. They may be primary lesions such as chondromas or secondary tumours from elsewhere. If they are localized, they are best removed by an *en bloc* incision.

MALIGNANT PLEURAL EFFUSION

This often appears insidiously and manifests itself by increasing dyspnoea with or without an unproductive cough. Aspiration of the effusion will show an exudate with malignant cells detected in approximately 50% of patients. If the patient has only a few weeks to live then they should be aspirated for comfort as required.

Patients with recurrent effusions in whom no diagnosis has been made and those with known malignancy but who are expected to at least 3 months and have a reasonable level of activity beforehand should have a video-assisted thoracoscopic inspection with biopsy and insulation of talc in order to obtain a pleurodesis, if necessary. An alternative in patients with known malignant effusion is to insert an intercostal catheter and attempt a chemical pleurodesis using an agent which will spread over the surface of the lung and promote a pleural reaction such as Bleomycin.

Occasionally a patient will have a trapped lung which cannot re-expand yet when the effusion recurs they get a mediastinal shift with increasing dyspnoea. If there is no intra-abdominal spread of the malignancy then this can be controlled by a pleuroperitoneal shunt. As the abdominal cavity has a higher natural pressure than the thoracic cavity the shunt is fitted with a valve which is placed under the skin over the costal margin. The patient pumps this fluid from the chest into the peritoneal cavity on a regular basis where it is reabsorbed.

BRONCHIAL OBSTRUCTION

In patients with lung cancer the bronchus can be obstructed by tumour growing directly in the lumen or by compression from surrounding masses. This leads to collapse of the lung beyond with dyspnoea and pulmonary infection.

Intraluminal tumour can be resected using an electric resectoscope, a laser or a cryoprobe. Whichever technique is used the rigid bronchoscope is preferred in order to allow for a thorough bronchial toilet and for maintenance of an airway if there is significant bleeding. Commonly a fibre-optic bronchoscope will be used in conjunction with the rigid bronchoscope in order to direct the probe.

When the bronchus is compressed but there is a patent bronchus beyond the obstruction then it can be dilated and a stent inserted. There are a variety of plastic and metal expandable stents available (Figure 18.11c,i&ii). The plastic stents are easier to remove but the metal stents have thinner walls and generate a better residual force to prevent recompression. Some of these are also covered with plastic and they are particularly useful for the management of oesophagobronchial fistulae. Malignant oesophagobronchial fistulae may require the insertion of stents in both the oesophagus and tracheobronchial tree for adequate control.

SURGICAL EMPHYSEMA

Surgical emphysema occurs when air is driven out into the tissues. The usual mechanism follows injury or surgery when this is a space with an air leak into it and an opening in the chest wall from within. When the patient coughs air is driven out into the tissues.

A small amount of surgical emphysema is not a problem but if it continues it can track up into the head and neck and around the eye lids causing the patient to become blind and paic-stricken and also has the potential to track around the larynx and can cause a change of voice and respiratory obstruction.

The appropriate management is to insert a chest tube with suction and if this fails to control the surgical emphysema and it becomes a significant problem then it can be controlled by a tracheostomy. This prevents the patient from raising the intrapressure by coughing but still allows toilet of the airways.

OESOPHAGEAL DISEASES

For more details refer Chapter 12.

Investigation of oesophageal disease is primarily by oesophagoscopy, which can be rigid or flexible. The rigid oesophagoscope is particularly useful for examination of the cervical oesophagus and when removing difficult foreign bodies such as bones, whereas the flexible oesophagoscope (generally a gastroscope is used) allows full examination of the oesophagus, even in patients with other problems such as kyphoscoliosis, and also examination of the stomach and duodenum for associated disease.

A *barium swallow* will show whether there is any hold up or abnormality in the oesophagus and if this is performed as a cine barium swallow, then a good idea of oesophageal motility is also obtained.

Oesophageal pressures may be measured using a perforated catheter with side holes and an electronic probe with microtransducers. The upper sphincter pressure is of the order of 70–108 mmHg and the lower sphincter pressure is 15–30 mmHg. Abnormal propulsion may be detected.

Measurements of oesophageal pH are useful in sorting out whether central chest pain is oesophageal or cardiac. If the pain is associated with episodes of low pH, this is a good indication that the pain is due to reflux oesophagitis.

Patients with oesophageal carcinoma should have a CT scan, which demonstrates if the tumour is infiltrating the adjacent structures and may also show paraoesophageal lymphadenopathy or distant metastases, particularly those in the liver. An intraoesophageal ultrasound examination is also a good way of estimating the depth of tumour in the wall of the oesophagus and the presence of paraoesophageal adenopathy. Special ultrasound probes are available which allow direct biopsy of the paraoesophageal glands.

If there is obstruction to swallowing it is called dysphagia, but if there is just pain on swallowing it is known as odonyphagia. Oesophageal pain may be characteristic such as heartburn associated with acid reflux and associated hiatal hernia, but can also be quite obscure and mimic cardiac disease.

Oesophageal atresia

The most important congenital disorder of the oesophagus is oesophageal atresia which presents as an emergency in a neonate (see also Chapter 21). The commonest form is when there is a blind oesophageal upper pouch and the lower oesophagus communicates with the trachea. If the baby is allowed to feed, inhalation and pneumonia occurs. All newborn babies should be tested by the passage of a catheter as a routine. When detected, early surgical repair is performed with an end-to-end anastomosis possible in most cases.

Achalasia

Another congenital disorder is achalasia of the oesophagus in which there is a deficiency in the neural control of the lower oesophagus leading to a failure of this area to relax during swallowing and eventually the formation of a megaoesophagus. Simple balloon dilatation rarely provides long-term relief and the best management is a Heller's myotomy which can be done through a video-assisted thoracoscopic or laparoscopic approach.

Other motility problems

Apart from achalasia of the oesophagus, other oesophageal motility problems include cricopharyngeal spasm and pulsion diverticulum. Traction diverticulum of the oesophagus follows infection and is rarely a problem as the mouth of the diverticulum is usually quite wide. In the case of pulsion diverticulum, however, the diverticulum forms proximal to an area of spasm and can be a cause of dysphagia. Treatment consists of removing the diverticulum but also performing a myotomy of the oesophagus below the level of the diverticulum.

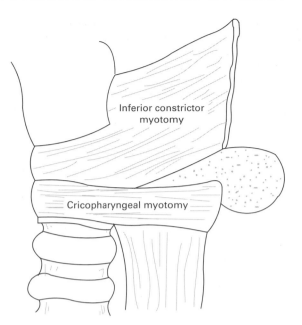

Figure 18.15. Pharyngeal pouch through Killia's dehiscence.

A similar condition occurs with cricopharyngeal spasm when a pharyngeal pouch occurs through Killian's dehiscence of the pharynx, generally on the left-hand side (Fig. 18.15). Treatment similarly consists of removing the pouch and dividing the cricopharyngeal muscle. This disorder most commonly occurs in elderly patients and is often associated with reflux oesophagitis which also requires attention. As there is a higher than average instance of secondary carcinoma formation at the level of the cricopharyngeal spasm, an oesophagoscopy is always required and care needs to be taken to identify the true passage which lies anteriorly; otherwise the pouch can be ruptured. In frail patients an endoscopic approach can be used to divide the cricopharyngeus muscle and widen the neck of the pouch so it drains into the oesophagus.

Cysts

Paraoesophageal developmental or duplication cysts are rarely a problem unless they become infected but can cause concern when detected at routine chest radiograph.

Strictures

Strictures of the oesophagus may be congenital due to failure of the lumen to canalize properly, but are most commonly secondary to reflux oesophagitis or ingestion of sclerosing agents such as caustic soda. Tumours may also present as strictures or they may occur following radiotherapy for oesophageal carcinoma.

They can be managed by dilatation passing a series of bougies over a guide wire or by balloon dilatation. Bulky tumours can be re-canalized with the aid of a laser passing the beam down a fibreoptic cable to vaporize the exophytic tumour. If there is a rapid recurrence of symptoms then a stent can be placed across the stricture. These have no intrinsic motility and the patients are only able to tolerate soft diets. The metal-expandable stents are particularly useful for malignant strictures but should be avoided in benign conditions as they are prone to erode into surrounding structures in the long term.

Oesophageal tumours

Benign tumours of the oesophagus are rare. The most common are leiomyomas which are usually asymptomatic but can cause dysphagia. If suspected they can be managed by a thoracoscopic approach.

Carcinoma

Oesophageal carcinoma has widespread epidemiological variation with an incidence varying markedly in different parts of the world which may be partly related to dietary habits. In the upper two-thirds of the oesophagus, squamous cell carcinoma is the commonest variety but in the lower third approximately half the cases are adenocarcinoma. When an adenocarcinoma is found in the oesophagus it generally arises in Barrett's mucosa which is columnar epithelium found in patients who have had severe reflux. As this is a premalignant condition patients with Barrett's changes should be kept under regular gastroscopic surveillance and consideration given to resection if severely dysplastic changes are found.

The location of the oesophagus immediately adjacent to vital structures and the inability to resect part of it and pull the ends together makes any attempt at surgical removal a much greater technical challenge than removing carcinomas in other parts of the intestinal tract. A large proportion of patients presenting are elderly and have poor pulmonary function from associated smoking or present with metastatic disease and are unsuitable for surgery. It is important, however, to keep the patient swallowing, particularly as inability to cope with saliva production is particularly distressing and palliation can be afforded by judicious dilatation, resection of exophytic endoluminal tumours with a laser or insertion of a stent.

There has been a great deal of interest in neo-adjuvant therapy attempting to reduce the bulk of the tumour prior to surgery. This appears to be much more effective for squamous cell carcinomas than adenocarcinomas.

If the tumour is in the lower oesophagus or cardia, then an Ivor Lewis type of resection is the preferable operation mobilizing the stomach and performing a high anastomosis in the right chest. This is better than a left thoracoabdominal approach as there is significant disability from disrupting the costochondral junction and a high anastomosis is associated with fewer problems from secondary reflux oesophagitis.

In tumours of the upper two-thirds of the oesophagus, a total oesophagectomy is preferable, performing an anastomosis in the neck. In this situation it is useful to bring the stomach up anteriorly behind the sternum which allows subsequent radiotherapy to the bed of the oesophagus if necessary without fear of an oesophagobronchial fistula. Some surgeons prefer to regard oesophageal tumours as essentially incurable and perform palliation by means of a transhiatal oesophagectomy, pulling the stomach up into the neck but not attempting to dissect out the associated glands.

In patients who have had previous gastric surgery or if, for some reason the stomach is unsuitable then the colon is a useful alternative. The small bowel is difficult to handle as a conduit but a free graft of small bowel taken with its pedicle and implanting the arteries and veins into vessels in the neck allows for repair of local problems in the cervical oesophagus, such as if part of a major conduit is lost because of inadequate perfusion.

The main complications after an oesophagectomy are breakdown of the anastomosis or bronchopneumonia due to inhalation of food from stasis in the conduit.

FURTHER READING

Pearson FG, Deslavriers J, Ginsberg R. *Esophageal Surgery*, 1st edn. Edinburgh: Churchill Livingstone, 1995

Pearson FG, Cooper JD, Deslauriers J, Ginsberg RJ, Herbert CA, Patterson GA, Urschel HC. *Thoracic Surgery*, 1st edn. Edinburgh: Churchill Livingstone, 2002

Kaiser LR, Singhal S. *Surgical Foundations: Essentials of Thoracic Surgery*, 1st edn. London, UK: Elsevier, 2004

Walker WS, *Video Assisted Thoracic Surgery*, 1st edn. London, UK: T&F STM, 1999

19

Genitourinary System

Neil Harris[1] and Andrew Dickinson[2]

[1]Department of Urology, Derriford Hospital, Plymouth, UK [2]Consultant Urological Surgeon, Derriford Hospital, Plymouth, UK

CONTENTS

Anatomy and developmental anomalies	**369**
Kidney	369
Ureter	370
Bladder	370
Prostate	371
Testis	371
Penis and urethra	371
Urological symptoms	**372**
Functional urinary symptoms	372
Haematuria	373
Pain	373
Urological history and examination	**374**
History	374
Examination	375
Investigations	**375**
Urine tests	375
Blood tests	375
Imaging	376
Investigation of common urological conditions	379
Common diseases and their treatment	**380**
Kidney	380
Ureter	383
Bladder	385
Prostate gland	387
Testis and scrotum	388
Penis and urethra	389
Aspects of general surgery and gynaecology that may cause urological problems	**390**
General surgery	390
Gynaecology	390
Further reading	**390**

Urology is the study of diseases of the urinary tract and the male reproductive system. Some of the earliest operations described are urological procedures and the ancient Egyptians are known to have performed surgical castration and cystolithotomy (open removal of bladder stones).

Functional disorders of micturition may lead to urine incontinence or urine retention. Metabolic abnormalities result in renal stone disease. Developmental abnormalities are seen in the neonate and the developing child (see also Chapter 21). Urological cancers are common and their management can affect continence, fertility and, of course, quality of life (QoL).

Despite the numerous diseases that can affect the urinary tract, the presenting symptoms are few, making accurate diagnosis dependent on the careful imaging of structural abnormalities as well as a functional assessment of voiding and renal function.

ANATOMY AND DEVELOPMENTAL ANOMALIES

Kidney

Gross anatomy

The adult kidney, a paired organ, is 11-cm long, weighs 150 g and lies in the retroperitoneum. Posteriorly, the upper half lies on the diaphragm with the psoas, quadratus lumborum and transversus abdominis muscles from medial to lateral on the lower half.

Anteriorly, the right kidney is covered on its medial aspect by the second part of the duodenum and the liver overlying the upper pole and hepatic flexure of the colon covering the lower part of the anterolateral aspect. The left kidney has the tail of the pancreas together with the edge of the greater curve of the stomach separated by the lesser sac on its medial aspect, the spleen lateral to this and the lower half of the kidney related to the splenic flexure of the colon.

Both kidneys have the adrenal glands superomedially.

Surgical anatomy

The 11th and 12th ribs are floating ribs and related to the upper half of the kidney. They provide useful surface markings for loin incisions, which divide skin, latissimus dorsi muscle, external and then internal oblique muscles. The pleura lies in the upper part of the incision and can be punctured, causing a pneumothorax. The transversus abdominis muscle is then divided and the kidney, surrounded by the

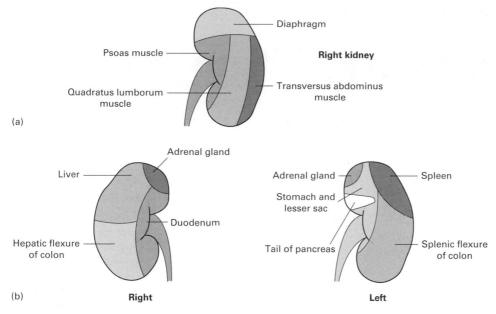

Figure 19.1. (a) Posterior and (b) anterior relations of the kidney.

perinephric fat contained within the Gerota's fascia, lies in the retroperitoneal space (Fig. 19.1). It should be noted that the pleural cavity may be deliberately opened during surgery to improve access to the upper pole of the kidney.

Other common approaches to the kidney include the transabdominal route (e.g. via a subcostal incision) and also laparoscopic approaches which can be either transabdominal or retroperitoneal.

Developmental anomalies

For more details refer also to Chapter 21.

The kidney can fail to develop from its primitive precursor, the metanephros, giving rise to a small dysplastic often cystic remnant. The ureter and trigone are normal. If renal dysplasia is bilateral, the neonate will be in renal failure (Potter's syndrome) and will die *in utero*.

The kidneys may fuse during embryological development. If one shifts to the other side (crossed renal ectopia), the ureter crosses the midline on its route to the bladder.

If fusion occurs at the lower pole of each kidney, ascent into the upper retroperitoneum is impaired by the inferior mesenteric artery. Due to its shape, such a kidney is called a horseshoe kidney. It has an anomalous blood supply which makes renal or aortic surgery difficult. Similarly, if the developing kidney remains within the pelvis and fails to ascend correctly, a *pelvic kidney* will result.

Ureter

Surgical anatomy

The ureter is a 25-cm long muscular tube; the upper half lies in the retroperitoneum and the lower half in the pelvis.

Three areas are narrow and are particularly prone to obstruction by ureteric stones:

1. The upper part at its junction with the pelvis (the pelvi-ureteric junction, PUJ).
2. The lower part as it passes through the bladder detrusor muscle (vesico-ureteric junction, VUJ).
3. At the junction of the upper and lower half as it passes over the bifurcation of the common iliac artery.

Urine is propelled down the ureter by peristalsis and this worm-like motion (vermiculation) can be demonstrated at operation by pinching the ureter gently with forceps. This can be used to distinguish the ureter from the nearby iliac vessels. The ureter passes through the bladder wall obliquely. This acts as a flutter valve so when the bladder contracts during voiding the intravesical ureter is compressed, thereby preventing reflux of urine.

Developmental anomalies

The renal pelvis divides inside the kidney to form the major and minor calyces. This division may occur early giving rise to two ureters draining the kidney and joining at a variable distance to form a common ureter. Occasionally, such duplex ureters fail to join and each drains separately into the bladder. The ureter draining the upper part (or moiety) of the kidney passes into the lowest and medial most aspect of the bladder. The ureters therefore cross, as they pass down to the bladder.

Bladder

Surgical anatomy

The normal adult bladder is a hollow muscular organ with a capacity of about 500 ml and lies in the bony pelvis. In the child, the shallow pelvis allows the bladder to rise up into the abdomen making suprapubic puncture relatively easy.

Developmental anomalies

In utero urine drains from the bladder to the placenta via the urachus along the umbilical cord. At birth the urachus closes to form a fibrous cord connecting the dome of the bladder to the umbilicus. Occasionally, it can remain patent or develop cysts that become inflamed. Occasionally, the urachal remnant can undergo malignant change.

As part of a major congenital abnormality of the lower abdominal wall musculature the bladder may open directly onto an incompletely formed abdominal wall; so-called ectopia vesicae. Previously the bladder was excised and the ureters diverted into the rectum (uretero-sigmoidostomy). With modern surgical reconstructive techniques it is now possible to close the bladder and repair the abdominal wall a few days after birth.

Prostate

Surgical anatomy

The prostate gland is rudimentary until adolescence when it grows to about the size of a large grape and weighs about 15 g. It lies at the exit of the bladder with the urethra passing through it. Proximally lies the bladder neck, distally the external urethral sphincter. In the prostatic urethra, the ejaculatory ducts drain out at the verumontanum. This is a surgical landmark for the proximal limit of the external sphincter. Super-posteriorly lie the seminal vesicles and together with the prostate they rest on the posterior condensation of pelvic fascia (Denonvilliers fascia). Digital rectal examination allows the posterior aspect of the prostate to be palpated.

Continence mechanisms

The bladder neck or internal urinary sphincter is automatic and unlike the external urinary sphincter are not under voluntary control (Fig. 19.2). For normal voiding, both these sphincters must relax. If the external sphincter is damaged it is possible to remain continent with the internal sphincter alone. The operation of transurethral resection of the prostate (TURP) removes the prostatic adenoma obstructing the prostate urethra, and it is common for the bladder neck and the internal sphincter to be resected as well. This leads to retrograde ejaculation following TURP.

Testis

Surgical anatomy

The normal adult testis is an ovoid sphere measuring $5 \times 4 \times 3$ cm. Posterolaterally lies the epididymis, which is continued superiorly as the vas deferens. This lies in the spermatic cord together with the testicular artery, pampiniform plexus of veins, nerves and lymphatics. Around the

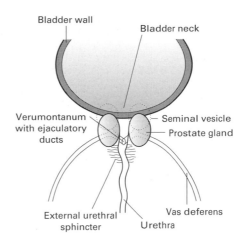

Figure 19.2. Male continence mechanism.

testis lies the tunica vaginalis, a double layer of peritoneum brought down as the testis descends during embryological development from its abdominal position in the foetus.

Developmental anomalies

The testis may fail to descend completely into the scrotum, but remain either intra-abdominal or within in the inguinal canal. A testis may have a strong cremasteric reflex and be retractile but such a testis can usually be brought down into the child's scrotum by gentle massage. If it cannot be brought down, it requires surgical mobilization and fixation in the scrotum (orchidopexy) (refer to Chapter 21).

The testis lies surrounded by the tunica vaginalis. In some cases the testis is so mobile that the free movement allows it to twist and obstruct its blood supply. Testicular torsion is acutely painful and requires surgical exploration. The testis is untwisted and if viable returned to the scrotum and anchored with sutures to prevent a recurrence. As the testicular mobility is bilateral, the other testis should be fixed prophylactically at the same time (refer to Chapter 21).

Penis and urethra

Surgical anatomy

The urethra is about 20-cm long in the adult male and comprises the prostatic urethra, the membranous urethra and the penile urethra, which passes from the bulb of the penis along the shaft to the meatus. The female urethra is much shorter and is surrounded by the sphincter muscle.

Developmental anomalies

During development, the male urethra may fail to form a complete tube to the end of glans and open onto the ventral surface of the penis. This is termed hypospadias. The foreskin is often deficient ventrally and has the appearance of a dorsal hood. As the foreskin may be used in the reconstructive surgical repair of a hypospadias, circumcision under these circumstances is contraindicated (refer to Chapter 21).

UROLOGICAL SYMPTOMS

The three main urological symptoms are:
1. functional urinary symptoms,
2. haematuria,
3. pain.

Functional urinary symptoms

The micturition cycle involves two relatively discrete processes:
1. bladder filling and urine storage,
2. bladder emptying.

Therefore, for descriptive purposes symptoms affecting the lower urinary tract (LUTS) can be divided into 'storage' and/or 'voiding'. The term 'prostatism' should be abandoned and terms such as bladder outflow obstruction (BOO) due to benign prostatic enlargement (BPE) should only be used when an appropriate diagnosis has been made:

Storage symptoms	Voiding symptoms
Frequency	Hesitancy
Urgency	Reduced stream
Nocturia	Straining
Incontinence	Terminal dribble
	Prolonged voiding times
	Post-micturition dribble

Voiding symptoms

The longer urethra and the prostate gland in men makes them more likely to complain of 'voiding' symptoms, whereas the shorter urethra and changes in pelvic floor musculature following childbirth means that 'storage' symptoms are more common in women.

However, men with BOO due to BPE will often complain of both storage and voiding symptoms. The symptoms typically have a slow, gradual onset with periods of apparent improvement due to compensatory increases in detrusor contractions develop to overcome the obstruction. The patient will find he has to pass urine more frequently during the day. Eventually he will reduce fluid intake to try and limit the need to pass urine at night. This may lead to a life dominated by having to know the location of all public conveniences since the bladder will be incompletely emptied at voiding and thereby refill quickly, reducing its effective capacity.

As the obstruction increases the bladder detrusor muscle may decompensate and *acute urine retention* be precipitated. This can occur secondary to constipation, a urine infection or simply delaying passing urine, for example waiting until the end of the after-dinner speeches! The pain of acute retention of urine is intense and felt suprapubically.

The patient is agitated and restless and will seek urgent medical help.

In contrast, *chronic urine retention* is painless. Over a long period of time the bladder is incompletely emptied at each void and the residual volume of urine gradually increases, leading to a reduced effective storage capacity and a chronically distended bladder. The bladder becomes full more quickly and the frequency of voiding increases. Eventually the bladder never completely empties. The post-micturition dribble increases and eventually becomes continuous. This is chronic retention with overflow incontinence. Occasionally, high pressure in the chronically overfilled bladder results in damage to the kidneys. This is known as an obstructive uropathy and must be treated with catheterization of the bladder and eventually outflow surgery (usually a TURP) to relieve the high-pressure retention. A post-obstructive diuresis may occur when this pressure is relieved.

As stated above, these symptoms are most commonly due to obstruction from enlargement of the prostate gland or, rarely, failure of the bladder neck sphincter to relax and open during normal voiding. In malignant enlargement of the prostate gland, urinary symptoms may develop more quickly without episodes of remission. A urethral stricture will produce a poor urine stream, but usually the bladder empties completely, and hesitancy and nocturia are not characteristic.

LUTS are a feature in women with urethral stenosis or obstruction of the urethra by a gravid uterus or severe genital organ prolapse. Failure of the normal sphincter mechanisms to relax and open during voiding will lead to voiding symptoms. This is seen after spinal trauma and in some patients with multiple sclerosis.

Storage/filling symptoms

The normal detrusor muscle undergoes receptive relaxation to allow urine storage, without causing a rise in intravesical pressure. When the bladder capacity is reached, sensory stimuli generate a desire to void and, when socially appropriate, the detrusor muscle contracts and voiding takes place due to the rise in intravesical pressure. If the ability for receptive relaxation is lost, the sensory stimuli are produced before the bladder is full and an intense urge to void is experienced. This recurs again as the bladder refills. The urge to void can be so intense that the patient becomes incontinent. This is known as *urge incontinence* and often includes the triad of symptoms:
1. urgency of micturition,
2. frequency of micturition,
3. urge incontinence.

These symptoms are seen in detrusor overactivity, formerly called detrusor instability, which can be proven with urodynamics (UDS). This condition may be secondary to increased stimulation of the trigone, for example bladder stone, urine infection, malignant cystitis or a neurological cause such as stroke. Alternatively, if no cause for the detrusor overactivity is identified, it is termed primary detrusor overactivity.

The term *overactive bladder* (OAB) is also used and can be defined from either UDS findings (e.g. detrusor overactivity) or symptoms (e.g. urgency).

Symptoms due to detrusor underactivity

If the bladder is chronically distended, it can lose the ability to contract during normal voiding. The sensory stimuli of the over-stretched bladder are lost and the bladder becomes a flaccid, painless storage bag. Voiding may be achieved by abdominal straining or direct suprapubic pressure. Overflow incontinence of urine may occur. This is seen in the end stages of outflow obstruction due to prostate disease or as part of an autonomic neuropathy (e.g. in a diabetic patient).

The diagnosis of detrusor underactivity (DUA) is made following formal UDS assessment, although its presence may be suspected with an appropriate history and simple flow rate measurement. It often coexists with other symptoms of BOO.

Symptoms of pelvic floor dysfunction weakness

Urine incontinence may occur when there is a sudden rise in intra-abdominal pressure (classically coughing or sneezing), so-called *stress incontinence*. If this is demonstrated by objective measurement (UDS), it is called urodynamic stress incontinence (USI). Although occasionally seen in men following traumatic or iatrogenic damage to the urinary sphincter, this is a symptom most commonly seen in women with damage to the muscles and/or nerves and/or connective tissue within the pelvic floor following childbirth.

Often the women will wear sanitary towels to avoid wetting their clothes, thereby coping with, but hiding the problem. The number of times the pads become wet and need changing is a good estimate of the severity of the incontinence.

Haematuria

Haematuria is the presence of blood in the urine. If it is visible, it is called frank, or macroscopic, haematuria. Whether the blood appears at the beginning, during or the end of the urine stream gives little useful information as to the likely cause and all forms of haematuria require a full evaluation.

Classically, glomerulonephritis produces a smoky brown haematuria and at microscopy (using phase contrast) cells may be misshapen (dysmorphic).

Haematuria identified at urine microscopy is as important a sign as frank haematuria and requires an equally full investigation. Dipstick testing of urine, often performed as a screening test in asymptomatic patients, may be the first indication of haematuria, but can give false-positive results and therefore confirmation by urine microscopy may be appropriate.

Pain associated with haematuria, either when passing urine or over the renal or bladder area, suggests an inflammatory cause, for example infection or mechanical trauma from a stone. Painless macroscopic haematuria may be the first sign of a bladder or kidney cancer. Associated symptoms such as malaise, anorexia and weight loss may be present, due to disseminated disease or paraneoplastic syndrome. Haematuria following direct trauma to the renal tract will be evident from the history, but bleeding following minimal trauma should be investigated carefully as there may be some underlying pathology. Patients on anticoagulants who develop haematuria also require full investigation, as a lesion in the urinary tract may be unmasked by the anticoagulants.

Blood found in the urine of a menstruating woman may be a contaminant, but the urine should be tested again after the period has finished.

Haemospermia

Blood in the ejaculate (haemospermia) is usually non-sinister up to the age of 40 or 50 years. Occasionally, a cancer of the prostate or bladder may present with haemospermia.

Red coloured urine may be caused by drugs (e.g. rifampicin) and some food stuffs (e.g. beetroot). Microscopy, however, will fail to demonstrate red cells.

Pain

Pain in the urinary system relates to the anatomical site fairly accurately.

Kidney and ureter

Pain and tenderness in the kidney, because of their retroperitoneal location, are felt posteriorly in the loin and renal angle. Pain from a stone passing from the renal pelvis down the ureter may be felt initially posteriorly. The pain then radiates around the loin into the iliac fossa and scrotum. Renal colic produces an intense, severe colicky type pain where the patient can find no relief by either movement or rest. In contrast, pain from a renal tumour or pyelonephritis is likely to be constant, but less intense.

Bladder and prostate gland

Acute retention of urine results in an intense pain suprapubically, with an unremitting desire to void. A similar pain can be experienced in a urinary infection, although more commonly there is severe suprapubic pain unrelieved by voiding which itself is painful. Irritation of the trigone, either by inflammation or mechanical trauma from a stone or catheter, can cause pain referred to the urethral meatus.

Inflammation of the prostate causes a variety of urinary symptoms, which can include perineal and penile pain, as well as and a dull suprapubic or ill-defined rectal discomfort. These symptoms form part of the *chronic pelvic pain syndrome*. This syndrome can also affect women. In a minority of cases a diagnosis of *interstitial cystitis* can be made (*see below*).

Scrotum and penis

Sudden onset of severe testicular pain associated with a dull abdominal ache is classically seen with torsion of the testis.

Such pain will persist for many hours until untwisting the testis relieves the ischaemia. Inflammation of the epididymis and testis (epididymo-orchitis) has a more gradual onset, often developing over several days. The pain can become intense but signs of inflammation, swelling and redness of the scrotum are also present.

A malignant testicular tumour may cause mild pain or discomfort, but most commonly it is painless. Similarly, cystic swelling such as hydrocoele or epididymal cysts are usually painless, although once noticed by the patient they can become a constant worry and source of discomfort. The dilated pampiniform plexus of veins in a varicocoele is usually asymptomatic, but can cause discomfort.

Penile pain is relatively uncommon. Pain on erection occurs in Peyronie's disease (a fibrosis of the corpora cavernosum, resulting in a curved erection), but this is usually self-limiting.

UROLOGICAL HISTORY AND EXAMINATION

History

The presenting symptoms should be assessed in context. The age of the patient, any past surgery or present medication will often direct the doctor towards the most likely pathologies to consider. For example, urinary infections in a child will have a different list of likely causes from those in an elderly man, a pregnant woman or an immunosuppressed transplant patient.

Presenting complaint

For most of the major symptoms ask about:
- onset,
- duration,
- severity.

The sudden onset of pain in renal colic or acute urine retention contrasts with the gradual build up of pain from a renal tumour or the slow development of LUTS due to outflow obstruction. The duration of pain from renal colic will be a few hours and will recur, whereas pain from a urine infection will be persistent. Other features such as pain, haematuria or incontinence should also be established.

The severity and inconvenience to the patient of their LUTS can be best assessed by direct questions or examples:
- How many times does the patient get up at night to pass urine?
- How many times is the patient incontinent or have to change their pads?
- Does the patient take longer to pass urine than their friends of the same age?
- Are trips out of the house or holidays limited by access to a toilet?

Frequency–volume charts can be filled in by patient's, to allow an objective and recordable assessment of their voiding pattern throughout the day and night.

Special questionnaires

Various useful and internationally validated scoring questionnaires have been developed to assess and monitor a patient's symptoms. They also provide a measure of QoL and can be used to assess the results of treatment. Such questionnaires exist for LUTS due to BPE (the International Prostate Symptom Score, IPSS), various aspects of continence (International Continence Society, ICS) and International Index of Erectile Function (IIEF).

Social and occupational history
Occupation or past occupation

Exposure to chemical carcinogens such as 2-naphthylamine or benzidine in the chemical or rubber industries may take 20 years to induce bladder cancer. Smoking is now the commonest aetiological factor in patients with transitional cell carcinoma (TCC).

Foreign travel

A trip to Egypt or Central Africa may result in exposure to *Schistosomiasis haematobium* (a trematode parasite fluke that lives in fresh water snails and parasitically in the human bladder and pelvic blood vessels) causing haematuria. Dehydration during a holiday to a hot climate may be the start of renal stone formation.

Family history

A family history of renal failure or polycystic kidney disease may reveal anxieties about kidney failure. A recent diagnosis or death from cancer of a family member or friend may provoke anxiety about non-specific symptoms. A family history of prostate cancer may be important.

Medical history
- *Neurological diseases*: For example Parkinson's disease, multiple sclerosis, diabetes, a stroke or back injury may cause abnormal bladder function and lead to various LUTS.
- *Past infections (either venereal or urinary)*: It may indicate underlying urinary tract pathology.
- *Medication*: Diuretics may explain mild LUTS. Antihypertensives may indicate intrinsic kidney disease.

Surgical history
- *Childhood problems* should be asked about specifically, as the patient may forget to mention them. Recurrent urine infections as a child may suggest reflux treated by surgical re-implantation of the ureters.
- *Undescended testes* that have been either excised or placed in the scrotum (orchidopexy).
- *Abdominal or pelvic surgery* can cause denervation injury to the bladder (e.g. abdomino-perineal resection of the rectum).
- *Ureteric injury* may occur in abdominal or gynaecological operations. Previous pelvic surgery may also result

in fistulas, which can present with incontinence and/or abnormal discharge.

Obstetric history

Damage to the pelvic floor during pregnancy can lead to stress incontinence. Problems with vaginal delivery or a forceps delivery may also damage the perineum causing various LUTS.

Examination

- All patients with urological symptoms must have their *blood pressure* measured.
- Signs of *dehydration* such as a dry mouth and tongue may indicate renal failure or the polyuria of diabetes.
- *Cervical lymph nodes* may be enlarged due to metastatic spread from any urological cancer.
- Sit the patient up to look at the *back* and *loins*. A forgotten laminectomy scar may be seen or the vesicles of shingles identified that would explain the loin pain.
- *Tenderness over the kidney* should be tested by gentle pressure over the renal angle.
- *Abdominal examination* allows palpation for the kidneys and bladder – the kidneys by bimanual examination with a hand posteriorly lifting up the kidney towards the examining abdominally placed hand; the bladder by percussion over the suprapubic region. A suprapubic mass can be shown to be a bladder if it disappears when the patient is catheterized. Occasionally, an enlarged liver or spleen will be detected as an incidental finding.
- Examine the *foreskin* to exclude a phimosis and signs of hypospadias. Palpate the *scrotal contents* to feel the normal features of the testis and epididymis. A cystic mass such as a hydrocoele or epididymal cyst will transilluminate, whereas a testicular mass will not. Stand the patient up to exclude an inguinal hernia and palpate the cord while the patient coughs for an impulse in a varicocoele.
- *Rectal examination* is performed to palpate the prostate gland and identify any malignant changes in the gland. A hard lump in either or both lobes suggests a cancer and a biopsy is needed to obtain histological proof.

INVESTIGATIONS

Urine tests

Dipstick testing

This is a valuable test as it gives an immediate result. Urine is tested for glucose to exclude diabetes mellitus and the presence of red blood cells. The latter test is based on the peroxidase-like activity of haemoglobin and is very sensitive, although false positives are seen. Protein in the urine can also be detected and its presence suggests an inflammatory process such as infection or protein loss from a glomerular or tubular lesion (e.g. glomerulonephritis).

Microscopy and culture

A mid-stream specimen of urine (MSSU) is collected, taking precautions to minimize contamination. Microscopy also allows red blood cells to be identified. If a urine infection is present, pus cells will be seen and bacteria will grow on the culture plates. If pus cells are present without evidence of infection (sterile pyuria), tuberculosis should be considered and special stains and culture medium used. Any bacterial cultured is tested for antibiotic sensitivities, according to local protocols.

Phase contrast microscopy allows the shape of the red blood cells to be assessed. They may be abnormal (dysmorphic) in glomerular bleeding.

Urine cytology

The urine specimen is fixed in formaldehyde, centrifuged to collect the cellular sediment and this is examined microscopically after Papanicolaou staining. Neoplastic cells can be identified by their characteristic features, which include abnormal nuclear : cytoplasm ratios and ploidy status.

Molecular markers

Several new molecular markers have been developed as a means to detect bladder cancer non-invasively, using exfoliated cells from patient's voided urine and bladder washings. They generally exhibit greater sensitivity but lower specificity than urine cytology. These markers are based on the pathogenesis of bladder cancer and include telomerase, survivin, bladder tumour antigen (BTA) and nuclear matrix protein (NMP-22). They are not yet in routine clinical use, but as refinements continue, their utilization is likely to become increasingly widespread.

24-h urine collection
Creatinine measurement

The urinary excretion of creatinine over 24 h (u) together with the urine volume (v) and plasma creatinine concentration (p) can be used to calculate the creatinine clearance (uv/p). This gives a working guide to the glomerular filtration rate (GFR), which is a surrogate for renal function. Alternatively, the renal clearance of radioisotopes can be used as a quicker, but less physiological measure of GFR.

Stone metabolites

24-h urinary calcium, uric acid and oxalate can be measured in recurrent stone formers.

Blood tests

General tests

Malignant disease and chronic inflammation in the urinary tract may alter haemopoiesis. A measurement of haemoglobin and red blood cell parameters is essential. Renal function is estimated by serum urea and creatinine concentrations. Electrolyte concentrations, especially potassium, may be abnormal in renal failure. In metabolic or malignant bone disease, serum calcium and alkaline phosphatase will be abnormal, with high serum calcium also found in hyper-parathyroidism.

Special tests

Prostate-specific antigen (PSA) is a glycoprotein, responsible for liquefying semen *in vivo*. As a tumour marker it is used to aid in the diagnosis and also monitor treatment of prostate cancer. It should be remembered that the 'normal range' for PSA varies with age and that PSA levels can also be effected by other conditions, such as urinary tract infection (UTI). The widespread use of PSA testing as part of a process of prostate cancer screening (particularly in the USA) has significantly reduced the proportion of patients diagnosed with advanced stage prostate cancer. In the UK, however, the use of PSA for screening remains controversial.

The tumour markers alpha-fetoprotein (AFP), lactic dehydrogenase (LDH) and beta-human chorionic gonadotrophin (β-HCG) are used to monitor treatment of testicular germ cell tumours. An elevated AFP implies the presence of non-seminomatous elements in the tumour.

Imaging

Ultrasound scan

This versatile, non-invasive and safe technique is used widely in the investigation of the urological patient. The kidneys are scanned via the loin and the bladder assessed transabdominally. A transrectal probe is used for prostate scanning and facilitates accurate guiding of the prostate biopsy needle. A smaller probe with higher frequency (and better image resolution) is available for very precise scanning of the testes.

Kidney

- Accurate assessment of the renal outline will identify a renal mass and distinguish between a fluid-filled cyst (probably benign) and a solid mass (possibly malignant).
- Shows the renal pelvis and any hydronephrosis or mucosal lesion (e.g. upper tract TCC).
- Shows parenchymal changes such as scarring from pyelonephritis or reflux.
- Renal stones will cast an acoustic shadow. This is especially useful for radiolucent stones.
- Guides percutaneous biopsy or placement of percutaneous drainage catheters.
- Identifying tumour thrombus in the renal vein or the inferior vena cava (IVC), especially when used in duplex mode to detect blood flow.
- May detect radiolucent stones.

Bladder

- Accurate measurement of bladder volume pre- and post-micturition. Can be used to assess post-void residual volume.

- Measures bladder wall thickness. Bladder wall hypertrophy is seen secondary to outflow obstruction and in other chronic inflammatory conditions, such as schistosomiasis.
- Bladder mucosal lesions, such as tumour, may be clearly shown although muscle invasion by bladder cancer can not be accurately assessed.
- Dilated lower ureter often visible. Obstruction from a stone or tumour can usually be seen.

Prostate

- Transrectal ultrasound scanning of the prostate can reveal abnormal echoic areas that can indicate malignancy. A channel down the probe allows ultrasound-guided biopsy.

Testes

- Accurately identifies testicular masses. These are invariably malignant.
- Cysts are well demonstrated (e.g. hydrocoele and epididymal cyst).
- Varicocoeles can be shown to fill when the patient coughs.
- A swollen inflamed epididymis due to epididymitis may be difficult to differentiate from a testicular torsion clinically, but may be distinguished by ultrasound, especially if duplex (combined Doppler) mode is used to assess blood flow.

Limitations of ultrasound

- Fails to show the ureter throughout its length. Ultrasound can miss ureteric stones and tumours.
- Does not assess renal function. An obstructed but non-dilated kidney may look normal on an ultrasound scan.
- Will not detect all stones. For this reason a plain abdominal radiograph (kidney, ureter and bladder, KUB) is performed as part of a renal tract ultrasound scan to look for renal stones and bone abnormalities.

Intravenous urogram

This invasive technique, also referred to as the intravenous pyelogram (IVP), involves injection of an intravenous bolus of an iodine-based radio-opaque solution (Conray or Hypaque) and taking sequential radiographs using ionizing radiation. To obtain the best concentration of the contrast in the kidneys, the patient may be dehydrated for a few hours before the test.

A plain abdominal radiograph or 'scout' film is taken initially to identify any renal stones that may be later obscured by contrast and to assess the bony skeleton for abnormalities.

Following the injection of intravenous contrast, radiographs are taken at 5 and 15 min. After a further 20 min, a further film is taken to demonstrate the KUB. Further films may be taken if particular features need to be assessed, for example oblique films or delayed films. Finally, the patient is asked to void and a post-micturition film is taken. If there is delayed renal function due to an obstructive hydronephrosis, films at 12 or 24 h can be taken to demonstrate contrast at the level of obstruction.

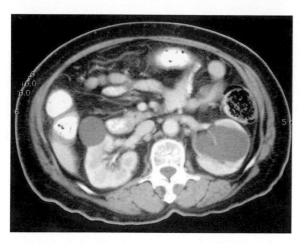

Figure 19.3. CT scan demonstrating bilateral renal cysts.

Uses

- Crude assessment of renal function can demonstrate a non-functioning kidney.
- Anatomical demonstration of renal pelvis and calyces. Distortion may indicate a renal mass.
- Demonstration of hydronephrosis and the level of any obstruction.

Disadvantages

- Invasive and uses ionizing radiation.
- Can miss renal masses and does not differentiate between solid and cystic lesions.
- Limited use in renal failure, due to poor renal function or perfusion.

Computed tomography scan

In computed tomography (CT) scanning, a thin, collimated X-ray beam is directed through the patient and images detected via a series of X-ray detectors arranged circumferentially. It provides an excellent method of staging renal, ureteric and bladder cancers. Although also used to stage prostate cancer, it remains relatively inaccurate.

Intravenous contrast can be administered to demonstrate functioning renal tissue. The timing of image acquisition, relative to the contrast injection can be used to determine whether renal masses enhance and by measuring the relative tissue densities on the scan (*Hounsfield units*), fat, fluid and blood can be accurately differentiated (Fig. 19.3). This allows renal lesions such as angiomyolipoma and haemangioma to be identified. CT scanning is the ideal way of demonstrating a retroperitoneal or pelvic collection of pus and oral contrast agents can be used to opacify small bowel and differentiate it from lymph nodes.

In some hospitals, CT scanning is also beginning to replace conventional intravenous urogram (IVU) in the initial diagnosis of acute loin pain, in patients with suspected renal or ureteric stones. The scan is usually performed without contrast and will detect a greater proportion of calculi than plain X-rays. It involves a similar radiation exposure as a standard IVU series and is considered to be the best investigation for detecting renal and ureteric stones.

Magnetic resonance scan

By employing a strong electromagnetic field, small magnetic changes can be stimulated in body tissues and the signal generated when the dipole is lost can be detected and measured. This non-invasive method of imaging is excellent at staging certain urological tumours, including prostate cancer. Lymph nodes can also be well demonstrated.

Using catheters

Micturating cystoureterogram

A catheter is passed into the bladder and the urine drained out. Contrast is used to fill the bladder. The catheter is removed and the patient positioned to allow radiographical screening of the KUB during voiding. This allows an assessment of ureteric reflux to be made.

Retrograde ureterogram

This is usually performed under general anaesthesia in the operating theatre. A ureteric catheter is passed, via a cystoscope, into the ureteric orifice and contrast injected directly up the ureter. Using radiographical screening the flow of contrast into the ureter is demonstrated and any obstruction or filling defects shown.

Antegrade uretogram

Contrast is injected, via a percutaneous nephrostomy tube while radiographical screening, to demonstrate any hold up to the free flow of contrast down the ureter.

Urethrogram

This is performed to assess a urethral stricture or, in cases of trauma, to the urethra, to assess rupture. Contrast is injected down a metal probe or catheter passed into the meatus and radiographs are taken.

Vasogram

This test demonstrates vasal obstruction in an infertile (azoospermic) male. Under a general anaesthetic the vas is identified either percutaneously or after a scrotal incision. A fine needle is passed into the lumen and contrast is injected antegradely. A radiograph will demonstrate contrast in the seminal vesicles if there is no obstruction.

Functional tests

Nuclear isotope renography

Mercaptoacetyltriglycine renogram

The compound mercaptoacetyltriglycine (MAG 3) labelled with an isotope of technetium is now the most commonly used agent for renography. An intravenous bolus is given

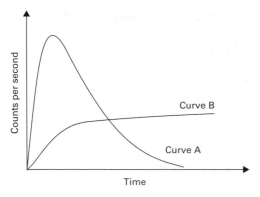

Figure 19.4. Renogram curve.

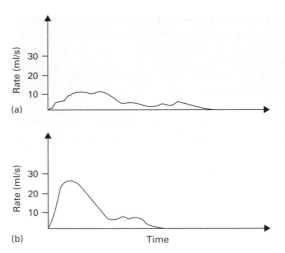

Figure 19.5. Urine flowmetry: (a) obstructed flow or poor detrusor muscle contraction and (b) non-obstructed flow.

and the uptake and rate of excretion by the kidneys is measured, by the rise and fall of radioactive activity, using a gamma camera placed posteriorly against the patient's back. In Fig. 19.4, curve A shows a rapid uptake by the kidney to a maximum with a smooth decay as the isotope is excreted with the urine. Curve B shows a reduced uptake suggesting reduced renal function. However, no fall in the curve is seen. This is characteristic of an obstructed kidney, where the urine containing the isotope is not excreted. Classically, this pattern is seen in a PUJ obstruction. Occasionally, urine production is poor and the isotope is excreted slowly or the calyces and renal pelvis are dilated and baggy and take a long time to fill. An intravenous diuretic is routinely given to increase urine (and isotope) excretion and determine whether the delay in excretion is due to an obstruction. The relative differential function of the kidneys can be assessed from the renogram (e.g. 60% right and 40% left). However, to assess absolute function of each kidney, the GFR must be measured and this is not usually assessed using MAG 3.

Chromium ethylenediaminetetraacetic acid clearance
Ethylenediaminetetraacetic acid (EDTA) labelled with a radioactive an isotope of chromium is given intravenously and measurement of blood and urine concentration gives a close approximation to the GFR. The agent is filtered at the glomerulus only, with little or no tubular secretion occurring. It therefore provides a quick and convenient test of GFR.

Dimercaptosuccinic acid renogram
This agent is both filtered and resorbed by the kidney. It has high cortical fixation and is therefore the agent of choice for renal cortical imaging in cases of acute pyelonephritis and renal scarring. A non-functioning obstructed kidney can also have its tubular function assessed by a static renogram using technetium-labelled dimercaptosuccinic acid (DMSA).

Bone scan
Radioisotope bone scanning, using technetium-99m tracer, is the standard method for assessing potential bone metastases

from prostate cancer. With widespread bone metastases, a so-called *superscan* image may be seen. This superscan demonstrates high uptake throughout the skeleton, with poor or absent renal excretion of the isotope. Although used particularly for patients with prostatic cancer, bladder and renal cancer can also metastasize to bone.

Urodynamics
The purpose of a UDS evaluation is to provide a pathophysiological diagnosis for a patient's voiding symptoms. In addition, it is often possible to reproduce their symptoms at the time of performing UDS. There are various aspects to a UDS assessment, but not every patient will require all the tests.

Urine flow test
This is the simplest form of UDS assessment and provides an objective measurement of urine flow. A reduced flow may indicate outflow obstruction or poor detrusor muscle contraction. Urine is voided directly onto a motor-driven rotating disc. The change in electrical impedance induced by the stream of urine is plotted by a pen recorder previously calibrated to give a curve of rate of voiding in ml/s against time. (Fig. 19.5) Flow testing is usually combined with an ultrasound measurement of residual urinary volume, which is frequently elevated when flow rates are reduced.

Cystometrogram
Cystometry is used to evaluate the storage and voiding phases of micturition and to determine the pressure–volume relationship of bladder function. The *filling* phase allows diagnosis of detrusor overactivity and reduced compliance, whereas the *voiding* phase looks at flow and detrusor pressures (p_{det}). The poor flow rate curve (Fig. 19.5(a)) is most commonly seen in men with BOO due to prostatic disease. However, a poorly contracting detrusor muscle can result in a similar flow pattern.

The difference between the two is the intravesical pressure generated by the contracting bladder and this parameter is displayed on the cystometrogram. A thin catheter is passed into the bladder and is attached to a fluid pressure transducer. A simultaneous measurement of the flow rate plotted against intravesical pressure will demonstrate the cause of the poor flow. To record abdominal pressure, a similar catheter attached to a second transducer is placed in the rectum and the two signals are subtracted electronically to give a pure reading of the detrusor pressure.

Videourodynamics cystometrogram
This combines the pressure and flow measurements of a videourodynamics (VUDS) cystometrogram together with radiographical screening of contrast in the bladder during filling and voiding. The images are recorded on videotape and can be analysed after the test. The technique allows additional useful information to be obtained such as degree of bladder neck opening and descent, the presence of any vesico-ureteric reflux (VUR) and the shape/caliber of the urethra.

Endoscopic examination
Cystourethroscopy
By direct visualization of the urethra and bladder, stones or tumour can be identified directly. This may be done under a local anaesthesia, but with a general anaesthesia therapeutic procedures can also be carried out, for example fragmentation of bladder stones or transurethral resection of bladder tumours (TURBT).

Ureteroscopy and renoscopy
Ureteroscopy is defined as upper urinary tract endoscopy (ureteroscopy) and is performed most commonly with an endoscope passed through the urethra, bladder and then directly into the ureter. Indications for ureteroscopy have broadened from diagnostic endoscopy and now include a variety of additional minimally invasive therapies. Flexible ureteroscopes are a recent development, allowing improved access to the upper ureter and kidney, but more limited therapeutic options due to their smaller size.

Endoscopic stone fragmentation, treatment of upper urinary tract urothelial malignancies, division of strictures and repair of PUJ obstructions (PUJO) all are current treatments facilitated by contemporary ureteroscopic techniques. To achieve stone fragmentation and tissue fulguration, it is possible to use standard monopolar diathermy, various types of laser and other lithoclastic modalities. With this progression of ureteroscopic procedures from diagnostic to more complex therapeutic interventions, one would expect a proportional increase in the rate and severity of complications. However, with improved instrumentation and an evolution of surgical technique, the complication rate from most procedures has decreased significantly.

Investigation of common urological conditions
Haematuria
Macroscopic haematuria always requires investigation. However, the evaluation of patients with microscopic (or *dipstick*) haematuria is more controversial, but in general should be investigated in individuals >40 years of age. A typical haematuria evaluation will include the following investigations:

- An MSSU is sent for microscopy, culture and sensitivities to demonstrate any urinary infection.
- Urine may be sent for cytology where TCC is suspected. A positive result is helpful, but malignancy is not excluded by a negative result.
- All patients must have a cystoscopy. With modern flexible cystoscopes, this can performed under a local anaesthesia and with open access haematuria clinics it is often done at the time the patient is first seen, along with the additional imaging investigations.
- Imaging the upper tract presents some difficulties. An ultrasound scan is non-invasive and excellent at identifying a renal mass. However, urothelial lesions may be missed. An IVU will show the collecting system and ureter but is not as reliable at demonstrating a renal mass. If in doubt both tests should be performed.
- Blood tests to demonstrate a normal haemoglobin and renal function are necessary and in certain patients the PSA will be measured.

Urine outflow obstruction
- An MSSU is sent and the urine examined with a *dipstick* to exclude microscopic haematuria or urine tract infection.
- Flow rate testing to determine maximum flow rate and voided volume.
- An ultrasound scan of the bladder to measure the post-micturition residual urine. The upper tracts should also be scanned for hydronephrosis if there is any evidence of renal failure.
- Blood tests for haemoglobin and renal function.
- Plain abdominal radiograph may be taken if bladder or renal tract stones are suspected.
- A *frequency–volume chart* and/or *IPSS questionnaire* is completed.

Urinary incontinence
- A urine culture should be performed to exclude a UTI.
- Stress incontinence in women can often be demonstrated at physical examination by getting the patient to cough whilst observing the urethral meatus. This test can be quantified using the *pad test*: the female patient is fitted with a dry, weighed sanitary towel and then given fluid to drink and standardized exercises to perform. The pad is weighed at the end of the test to measure the urine lost.
- An ultrasound scan of the bladder will demonstrate if the bladder fails to empty on voiding.

- If the incontinence is associated with urgency, then detrusor overactivity is likely and UDS should be performed.

Urinary stones
- Ideally send the stone for biochemical analysis.
- Serum calcium to identify hyperparathyroidism.
- 24-h urine collection for calcium, uric acid and oxalate should be performed in recurrent stone formers. Cystinuria should also be excluded, but is very uncommon.

Loin pain
- A plain abdominal radiograph may identify a possible stone and this should be confirmed by an IVU or CT urogram.
- Urinalysis for blood. This will usually be present if a stone is passing down the ureter.
- If the loin pain is less acute, or exposure to ionizing radiation contraindicated, an ultrasound scan of the kidney will demonstrate any hydronephrosis or renal masses.

Urinary infection
- Urine should be sent for microscopy and culture and the infection treated with appropriate antibiotics.
- It is usually appropriate to establish the likely cause of an infection. A haematuria evaluation should be performed if indicated (see above). In young girls, reflux may be a cause of recurrent UTI and a micturating cystoureterogram (MCUG) may be required.

A number of conditions that were hitherto diagnosed when patient's developed symptoms are now detected as incidental findings, or during routine (or selective) screening. The two main urological conditions to which this applies are detection of early prostate cancer and the detection of asymptomatic renal tumours as incidental findings during the investigation of other conditions. The significance of this change is that the conditions are now being diagnosed at an earlier *stage*, which has implications for both treatment and prognosis.

COMMON DISEASES AND THEIR TREATMENT

Kidney

Inflammation

Pyelonephritis
This is a urine infection leading to inflammation of the kidney. Clinically it is associated with a high temperature, rigors and vomiting. In recurrent cases renal scarring may occur, particularly if the infections occur in childhood.

Glomerulonephritis
Acute glomerulonephritis is the term applied to a wide range of renal disease, in which an immunological mechanism triggers inflammation and proliferation of glomerular tissue. The condition can occur following a streptococcal throat infection and may present as a sudden onset of haematuria

and proteinuria. This clinical picture often is accompanied by hypertension, oedema and impaired renal function. Other types of glomerulonephritis have an unknown aetiology and are usually more gradual in onset, with slowly developing renal impairment. Microscopic haematuria can be a feature. These conditions all require expert management by nephrologists.

Stones
Stone formation occurs as a result of an imbalance between the solubility of salts and their crystallization. In the Western world, 70–80% of stones are composed of calcium oxalate. Ureteric stones form initially in a renal papilla from a small submucosal concretion. As the crystallization increases, it separates from the papilla and passes into the collecting system with the urine. Before they pass into the calyces, such stones are seldom symptomatic although they can be associated with recurrent urinary infections. Conversely, a staghorn renal calculus that fills the renal pelvis and calyces is formed within the collecting system. Such stones are often seen with urine chronically infected with *Proteus mirabilis*. This bacterium splits urea to ammonia, alkalinizes the urine and precipitates magnesium ammonia phosphate. This becomes calcified and the stone may form a complete cast of the collecting system.

Treatment
- Small kidney stones can be fragmented by extracorporeal shock wave lithotripsy (ESWL). The technique uses a machine to generate shock waves, which are focussed through the skin and body tissues onto the dense stones, leading to fragmentation. It requires analgesia and careful monitoring afterwards to ensure the stone fragments pass down the ureter satisfactorily.
- Direct access to the renal collecting system via a percutaneous tract can allow larger stones to be removed endoscopically – known as percutaneous nephrolithotomy (PCNL).
- Staghorn stones represent a surgical challenge. If there is minimal renal function, then a nephrectomy may be the best way of eradicating the stone and the recurring urine infections. If renal function is good, percutaneous removal of the stone (PCNL) can be attempted. Sometimes fragments remain and these can be removed using ureteroscopy and appropriate fragmentation techniques, such as the laser (see above), or ESWL. Any remaining fragments may act as a nucleus for new stone formation and will act as a reservoir for continuing infection.
- Patients with stones in the ureter usually present acutely, with severe loin pain ('renal colic'). The majority of these stones are <5 mm in diameter and will pass spontaneously. However, larger ureteric stones often require surgical intervention. Various techniques can be utilized, but ureteroscopy and fragmentation (using a laser) is the most widely used, along with ESWL in certain situations.

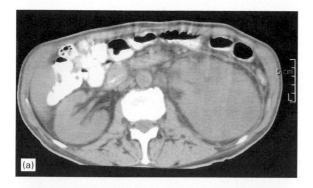

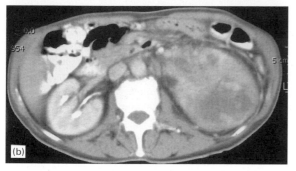

Figure 19.6. CT: renal cell carcinoma of the left kidney showing (a) pre- and (b) post-contrast images.

• The management of patients with a ureteric stone causing obstruction and in whom the urine becomes infected, represents a urological emergency. Urgent decompression of the infected and obstructed kidney is required by insertion of a percutaneous nephrostomy, or placement of a ureteric stent to 'bypass' the obstruction and allow drainage of the infected urine.

Tumour

Adenocarcinoma

Adenocarcinoma of the kidney (also known as renal cell carcinoma) is the most common type of renal tumour. It can occur at any age, but is commonest in the sixth and seventh decade. About 60% of cases occur in men. Presenting symptoms can include haematuria, loin pain or a palpable mass. However, an increasing number of renal tumours are now diagnosed as incidental findings on CT or ultrasound scan, following investigation for other conditions (Fig. 19.6). Occasionally, a tumour will present with a paraneoplastic phenomena, such as thromboembolism, polycythaemia or anaemia. The primary tumour may metastasize directly to adjacent lymph nodes and the adrenal gland or distantly to the lungs and occasionally bone.

Treatment of renal cell carcinoma depends on its stage, at presentation. If the tumour is confined to the kidney, radical nephrectomy (removing the kidney, perinephric fat and adrenal gland) is frequently curative. The operation can be performed using the traditional open approach, or via a minimally invasive laparoscopic approach. In addition, small, peripherally placed tumours may be amenable to removal by partial nephrectomy or enucleation. If the cancer has spread beyond the capsule of the kidney, or has metastasized, the disease is usually incurable. The cancer does not respond to radiotherapy, although palliation from painful bony metastases can sometimes be achieved with localized irradiation. Immunotherapy, using agents such as alpha-interferon and interleukin-2, has been shown to increase median survival, but is not curative.

Transitional cell carcinoma

This uncommon tumour may be associated with an existing bladder TCC. The condition may present as haematuria, 'clot colic' or be found incidentally, or during surveillance of a patient with known bladder cancer. Treatment for a localized tumour is nephroureterectomy. Metastatic disease is incurable and treated symptomatically.

Wilms' tumour

For more details refer to Chapter 21.

Wilms' tumour (malignant nephroblastoma) is an uncommon tumour of young children. It usually presents as an abdominal mass in a child under the age of 5 years. The majority cases are curable with a combination of surgery, chemotherapy and radiotherapy and it requires expert management in a paediatric oncology unit.

Trauma

For more details refer to Chapter 7.

Blunt trauma

Renal trauma is often associated with multiple injuries, particularly blunt trauma. Management should initially be aimed at resuscitation, using Advanced Trauma Life Support (ATLS) algorithms. The vast majority of patients with *isolated* renal trauma can be managed conservatively and do not require surgery. All patients with suspected renal injury should undergo CT scanning after resuscitation to confirm the diagnosis and assess the severity of the injury, along with any other associated injuries. In haemodynamically unstable patients, a 'single-shot' IVU may be performed prior to laparotomy to demonstrate a normal functioning kidney on the undamaged side. Management of a damaged solitary kidney requires greater effort to preserve it. Although surgical exploration of a bleeding kidney is occasionally necessary, it is not uncommon to find the bleeding impossible to stop and nephrectomy is then required. Complications following renal trauma are rare, but include urinoma, delayed haemorrhage, arteriovenous (A-V) fistula formation and occasionally hypertension.

Penetrating trauma

A loin injury from a knife or bullet wound is more likely to require surgical exploration. Again, a CT scan should be obtained, following resuscitation using ATLS protocols.

Renal failure

For more details, see Chapter 8.

Acute renal failure

This may be caused by:

- pre-renal factors (e.g. hypotension),
- renal factors (e.g. glomerulonephritis),
- post-renal factors (the clinical situation most commonly presenting to the urologist) (e.g. bilateral obstructive uropathy).

An obstruction causing a sudden complete blockage of two previously normal kidneys is uncommon (e.g. bilateral ureteric stones). The sudden presentation of anuria, dehydration and abnormal biochemistry is more often due to a chronic condition causing the long-term partial obstruction of the kidneys. For example, backpressure from a chronically distended bladder, or malignant obstruction from a carcinoma of the prostate in men, or carcinoma of the cervix in women.

Clinically, the patient is often confused and disorientated. Fluid balance is abnormal either with oedema and heart failure due to overload or dehydration from vomiting. The serum urea and creatinine will be raised and when the obstruction is released, a dramatic osmotic diuresis can occur, placing the patient in danger of dehydration unless careful fluid balance is maintained. The serum potassium may be raised and this can cause cardiac dysrhythmias and death. The potassium level must be treated urgently, either by dialysis or short-term measures such as shifting the potassium from the serum back into the cells using glucose and insulin intravenously, or calcium resonium to absorb it directly from the gut.

Patients with an obstructive cause of anuria should be catheterized to allow any urine in the bladder to be drained and any potential backpressure on the kidneys to be released. Any urine that is then produced can be measured accurately. A renal ultrasound scan will demonstrate a hydronephrosis and percutaneous placement of a nephrostomy tube will bypass the obstruction and allow the renal function to recover. Once the renal function is stable, the management of the cause of the obstruction can be planned.

Chronic renal failure

Renal damage from such causes as diabetic nephropathy, glomerulonephritis, polycystic renal disease or poor recovery from a treated obstructive uropathy can lead to permanent loss of renal function. The remaining renal tissue may then be inadequate for normal biochemical and fluid homoeostasis. A diet low in protein to reduce nitrogen products (urea) for excretion, along with fluid restriction will help limit the need for dialysis. Secondary effects of chronic renal failure, including anaemia, hypertension and osteoporosis, must also be controlled with drugs such as erythropoietin (to stimulate erythropoiesis) and angiotensin-converting enzyme (ACE) inhibitors. Nephrotoxic drugs including gentamicin and non-steroidal anti-inflammatory drugs (NSAIDS)

should also be avoided. With end-stage renal failure (ESRF) the renal function eventually becomes inadequate to maintain haemostasis and the patient requires dialysis or renal transplantation.

Dialysis

The principle of dialysis is to allow diffusion of water, electrolytes and waste products in the blood across a semi-permeable membrane into a solution that can then be discarded.

In *peritoneal dialysis*, the solution is run into the peritoneal cavity via an abdominally placed catheter. Diffusion takes place across the peritoneum, which acts as the membrane. The fluid is then drained out via the catheter and the process repeated until the biochemical status of the patient is satisfactory. This may take several hours and must be performed daily.

In *haemodialysis*, blood is circulated through filters. The blood flows across a semi-permeable membrane (the dialyzer or filter), along with solutions that help remove toxins. Haemodialysis requires a blood flow of 400–500 ml/min and a standard intravenous line in an arm or leg cannot support that amount of flow. Therefore, in long-term haemodialysis, an A-V fistula is surgically formed for example between the radial artery and cephalic vein at the wrist. Dilated veins with fast-flowing blood open up in the arm and by direct puncture blood can be drawn off into the dialysis machine and then run back into an adjacent puncture site. Anticoagulation is required to prevent clotting during dialysis.

Transplantation

The natural response of the body to foreign tissue is to reject it, by way of an immune response. In kidney transplantation, the best immunologically matched kidney to the patient's own tissues is selected to reduce rejection and immunosuppressor drugs are used to 'damp down' the normal immune response. A pre-transfusion with donor-specific blood may reduce immunorejection and can be used routinely.

The kidney donor's blood and tissue are matched as closely as possible with the recipient's blood ABO and major histocompatibility complex (MHC) antigens to reduce the risk of subsequent graft rejection.

The donor kidney is placed in the right or left iliac fossa and the renal vessels anastomosed end-to-side to the external iliac vessels or end-to-end to the internal iliac vessels. The ureter is implanted directly into the bladder. Immunosuppression is achieved using a combination of drugs, including cyclosporin/tacrolimus, OKT3® (monoclonal antibody), azathioprine and prednisolone. Despite these precautions, *acute* rejection is frequently seen in the months following transplantation and the transplanted kidney occasionally has to be removed. Some patients also suffer from *chronic* rejection where the initially good renal function deteriorates over several years until the patient develops chronic renal failure again and must return to dialysis.

Ureter

Reflux

If the anti-reflux valve mechanism at the VUJ is ineffective, urine will reflux up the ureter when the bladder contracts during voiding. When the bladder is empty and relaxes, the refluxed urine in the ureters refills the bladder so giving an effective residual volume that can become infected and lead to recurrent urine infections. Refluxing urine can lead to pressure damage in the kidney and infected urine can lead to pyelonephritis, both of which may lead to renal scarring and renal tubular damage, particularly if it occurs in childhood. This condition is a developmental anomaly and is seen in children when the kidneys are still growing and are most susceptible to damage (see Chapter 21).

Reflux can be demonstrated by a MCUG. Most cases may be managed by prophylactic antibiotics to prevent the complications of infections and as the child grows the anti-reflux valve mechanism may improve. For those with severe or persistent reflux, a surgical operation to re-implant the ureter obliquely in the bladder wall or endoscopic injection of bulking agents into the area of the ureteric orifice can be employed.

For children with severe reflux, renal damage can be irreversible and chronic renal failure may develop.

Hydronephrosis

This term is used to describe a dilated renal pelvis. It is also used to describe a dilated pelvis and ureter, although technically this is hydronephroureterosis. A hydronephrosis may be obstructive or non-obstructive.

Obstructive hydronephrosis

A ureter may be obstructed in four different ways (Fig. 19.7):

1. *A mass within the lumen*: A ureteric stone, blood clot or sloughed necrotic papilla may all get stuck within the ureter and cause obstruction.
2. *Narrowing of the wall*: A stricture may result from previous surgery such as ureteroscopy or damage at open surgery (e.g. anterior resection). Fibrotic narrowing is seen as a result of chronic inflammatory conditions, such as renal tuberculosis and schistosomiasis. A tumour is a cause of "mass within the lumen" and failure of normal ureteric peristalsis in the region of the PUJ leads to classical PUJ obstruction.
3. *Pressure from outside compressing the ureter*: Metastatic lymph nodes or retroperitoneal fibrosis (RPF) can result in ureteric obstruction.
4. *A mass at the end of the ureter obstructing outflow of urine*: A bladder carcinoma or prostate carcinoma infiltrating the trigone of the bladder can occlude the ureteric orifice. In women, carcinoma of the cervix can cause a similar effect. A chronically distended bladder (due to benign prostatic hypertrophy (BPH) or urethral stricture) can cause backpressure and hydronephrosis.

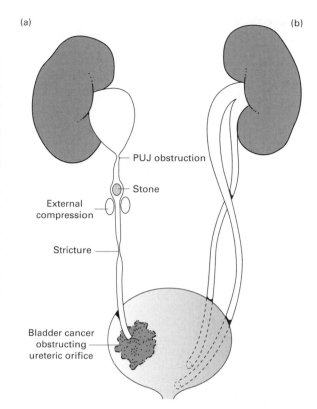

(a)   (b)

- PUJ obstruction

- Stone

External compression

Stricture

Bladder cancer obstructing ureteric orifice

Figure 19.7. (a) Kidney showing sites of possible ureteric obstruction and (b) kidney with duplex ureters.

Non-obstructive hydronephrosis

A dilated renal pelvis and ureter may be chronically distended rather than obstructed (e.g. VUR may produce a distended system). Following corrective surgery for a PUJ obstruction the hydronephrosis may seem unchanged, but prompt drainage will be demonstrated by renography. The congenital megaureter is another example of a dilated, but not obstructed ureter.

Ultrasonography will confirm the presence of a dilated system and an IVU may reveal the level of the obstruction. Isotope renography, using MAG 3, gives a functional measure of renal excretion and drainage and is an accurate way of quantifying obstruction, but will not show the anatomical level of obstruction.

If an obstructive cause is suspected, a cystoscopy and retrograde ureteropyelogram (RGPG) will confirm the site of obstruction and often gives an indication as to the cause of the obstruction. If an RGPG fails, percutaneous nephrostomy and antegrade ureterography usually demonstrates the level and cause of obstruction reliably.

At the time of imaging it is possible to place an indwelling ureteric stent. This is a hollow plastic tube with a draining hole along its length and ends that curl up, hence the name double pigtail or double J® stent. This may be placed retrogradely or antegradely along the ureter from the renal pelvis to the bladder, effectively bypassing the obstruction. Further treatment will depend on the cause of the hydronephrosis.

Alternatively, in some circumstances CT and magnetic resonance imaging (MRI) scanning may be used to diagnose the site and cause of an obstruction, particularly for conditions in and around the kidney.

Tumour

A TCC occasionally develops in the ureter or renal pelvis, and the tumour may cause haematuria and ureteric obstruction. Invasion can occur early because of the thin ureteric wall, resulting in lymph node metastases. Surgical treatment in the form of a nephroureterectomy is the usual treatment, but low-grade upper tract TCCs are increasingly being treated with endoscopic ablation and regular surveillance.

Stones

Ureteric colic due to a stone passing down the ureter is one of the commonest urological emergencies. The severe pain must be distinguished from the pain of biliary colic or a ruptured abdominal aortic aneurysm (AAA) and therefore an IVU, or CT urogram, is needed to confirm the diagnosis and establish the level the stone has reached. Pain relief using NSAIDS or opiates is usually effective.

Around 70% of ureteric stones of 5 mm or less in size will pass spontaneously. However, ureteric obstruction is not uncommon. Urgent relief of this obstruction is essential if the system becomes infected and this is achieved with percutaneous nephrostomy or retrograde placement of a ureteric stent. If the stone is far enough down the ureter, direct ureteroscopic manipulation and fragmentation (using a laser or lithoclast) is possible. Direct treatment of a ureteric stone by ESWL, although possible, has variable success.

Trauma

Injury to the ureter is most commonly the result of surgical intervention. Damage during ureteroscopy, bowel or gynaecological surgery is well recognized. End-to-end re-anastomosis of the ureter is possible if little or no length has been lost. If the ureter is damaged close to the bladder, re-implantation is usually preferred. If the damage is higher with significant loss or ureter, a Boari flap, using a flap of bladder or direct anastomosis to the normal ureter on the other side (a transuretero-ureterostomy) will deal with the problem. The anastomosis should be stented with a ureteric stent until it has healed (Fig. 19.8).

PUJ obstruction (PUJO)

Classical PUJO is due to abnormal ureteric peristalsis at the PUJ, or to external compression by vessel adjacent to the PUJ. This obstruction may be intermittent, precipitated by drinking large volumes of fluid. Surgery to widen the drainage through the PUJ and excise the redundant dilated portion of

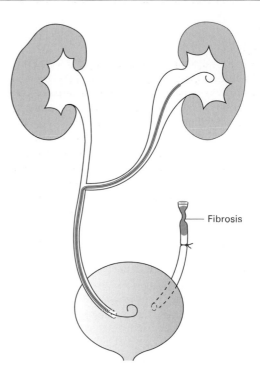

Figure 19.8. Transuretero-ureterostomy with an indwelling double J® ureteric stent across the anastomosis from the bladder to the pelvis of the affected kidney.

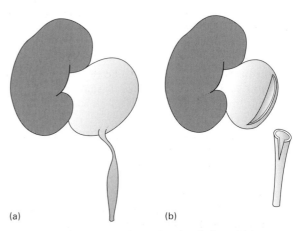

(a)   (b)

Figure 19.9. Anderson–Hynes dismembered pyeloplasty: (a) PUJ obstruction with hydronephrosis and (b) a contractile segment of ureter is excised and the ureter spatulated to anastomose to the trimmed renal pelvis.

renal pelvis (pyeloplasty) is generally effective at relieving the symptoms (Fig. 19.9). Surgery can be carried out through a standard loin incision, or laparoscopically. Various minimally invasive endoscopic techniques are also used, but these tend to have lower success rates.

Bladder

Inflammation

Cystitis (inflammation of the bladder) may be caused by infection, mechanical trauma (e.g. stone or catheter), malignant disease (e.g. carcinoma *in situ* of the bladder), radiotherapy or intravesical chemotherapy. The symptoms are pain and frequency of voiding. An uncommon inflammatory condition is interstitial cystitis, which may form part of a *chronic pelvic pain syndrome*. In this condition, which is commoner in women, none of the above causes are demonstrated, but histologically the bladder biopsy shows an excess of mast cells, thought to release histamine so causing inflammation. Treatment is symptomatic, although agents such as intravesical dimethyl sulphoxide (DMSO), pentosan polysulphate (Elmiron) and regular cystodistension are used with some success.

The symptoms of cystitis are also seen in young women who have recently become sexually active. Some of the discomfort probably arises as a result of mild trauma to the urethra, giving the sensation of a constant urge to void ('honeymoon cystitis').

Stones

Bladder stones are seen most commonly in developing countries and this may be linked to diet and increased prevalence of UTI. In more affluent countries, most bladder stones develop as a result of urinary stasis, due to BOO, or in neurogenic bladders (e.g. following spinal injury).

Like all stones, those in the bladder may give rise to haematuria, urinary infections, pain and sepsis. Many stones can be fragmented and removed endoscopically, although large stones may have to be removed at open surgery (cystolithotomy). In men with outflow obstruction, it is often necessary to improve voiding and reduce subsequent urinary stasis, by performing a TURP.

Tumour

The commonest bladder cancer type is a TCC. In countries where schistosomiasis is endemic, squamous carcinoma of the bladder is common. Adenocarcinoma is rare.

Transitional cell carcinoma

Classically, a TCC presents with painless haematuria, although urine infection is also commonly seen. Cystoscopy allows a biopsy to confirm the diagnosis and a resection biopsy of the base of the tumour will allow the pathologist to stage the tumour, by determining whether muscle invasion has occurred.

Treatment depends on the tumour stage and the general fitness of the patient. If the tumour is superficial (i.e. has not invaded muscle), simple endoscopic resection may be sufficient. This may be combined with adjuvant intravesical instillation of mitomycin C or epirubicin to reduce recurrence rates. Nevertheless, recurrence of new tumours in the bladder is common and so repeat check cystoscopies are

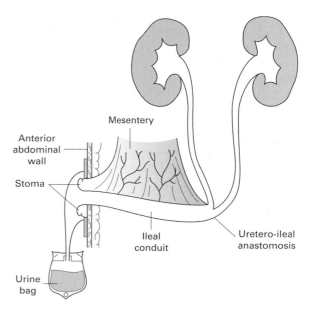

Figure 19.10. Ileal conduit urine diversion.

necessary. The majority of superficial bladder cancers (>80%) will not progress to muscle invasion. However, they do have a tendency to recur over a period of many years. If a superficial bladder cancer is poorly differentiated and invasion of the *lamina propria* is demonstrated histologically (G3 pT1), the disease may be treated as though it were muscle invasive, as the disease tends to run a more aggressive course with an increased likelihood of progression to muscle-invasive disease.

If the tumour has invaded the muscle of the bladder wall (>pT2), it is termed invasive. Local resection is unlikely to remove the entire tumour and the options for cure are radical radiotherapy or total removal of the bladder by surgery (cystectomy) and a urinary diversion procedure. If staging by CT or MRI scans reveal the disease has spread to lymph glands or beyond, the tumour is incurable and it is managed symptomatically. Adjuvant chemotherapy may be used in an attempt to improve long-term survival following cystectomy.

Adenocarcinoma

Adenocarcinoma of the bladder and squamous carcinoma of the bladder are both treated by cystectomy, if they are not metastatic, as they are both resistant to radiotherapy.

Urine diversion

In the UK, the most commonly performed urine diversion is an ileal conduit (Fig. 19.10). A segment of small bowel is isolated, along with its blood supply. The divided ends of the remaining ileum are anastomosed to maintain bowel continuity. The cut ends of the ureters are implanted into one end of the *ileal conduit* and the other end brought out as a stoma (urostomy) on the right side of the abdomen. A stoma bag is then applied to collect the urine (Fig. 19.10).

Alternatively, it is possible to use bowel to create a new reservoir, or *neobladder*. This 'orthotopic bladder' can be anastomosed to the urethra and if the sphincter mechanism is preserved, controlled voiding in the normal way is usually possible. Alternatively, the bowel urine reservoir can be drained onto the abdominal wall via a narrow lumen tube such as the appendix. Its closing pressure is such that the urine storage reservoir is continent and it is drained by the patient catheterizing the reservoir, via the stoma.

Trauma

For more details, see also Chapter 7.

Blunt abdominal trauma will produce the most dramatic effect if the bladder is full at the time. Rupture of the bladder frequently results and this will usually require surgical repair. Pelvic fractures may also rupture the bladder. Resuscitation of the patient and careful assessment of the bony injuries are required before the bladder is repaired. Catheterization, via a suprapubic cystotomy if necessary, will be required in the interim.

Functional abnormalities

Detrusor overactivity

An OAB may be seen in patients with intravesical inflammation (e.g. due to UTI or bladder stones) or as a result of neurological pathology causing overactivity of the detrusor muscle. The condition also occurs secondary to BOO. A third group has primary detrusor overactivity. They are neurologically intact, have a normal bladder capacity, but have symptoms of urine frequency, urgency and sometimes urge incontinence. A UDS demonstrate high detrusor pressure contractions at small bladder volumes.

Medical treatment aims to 'paralyse' the detrusor by blocking cholinergic receptors using anticholinergic drugs. Commonly used drugs include oxybutynin, tolterodine and trospium. As a result of generalized anticholinergic activity, side effects of these drugs are common and include dizziness, blurred vision and a dry mouth. Experimental drugs being used to treat OAB include resiniferatoxin, botulinum toxin and capsaicin.

Occasionally, surgical treatment may be necessary if medical treatments fail or are not tolerated. Surgical treatment also aims to paralyse part of the detrusor muscle, as well as improve bladder compliance and capacity. This is achieved by cutting the bladder in half and then resuturing it with an interposing opened length of ileum in the opened bladder (clam ileocystoplasty). As a last resort, urinary diversion with an ileal conduit may be successful.

Sacral nerve neuromodulation is also emerging as a potential treatment for cases refractory to drug therapy.

DUA and failure

Chronic retention of urine or the end stage of neurological diseases, such as diabetic neuropathy or multiple sclerosis,

may result in the bladder becoming a flaccid, acontractile bag able to store urine, but unable to contract to expel it. Occasionally, long-term indwelling catheter drainage will allow the contracted bladder to regain some muscular tone. However, intermittent self-catheterization (ISC) is probably the best treatment, if this can be tolerated.

Bladder neck pathology

The internal or bladder neck sphincter is found only in men. Its primary function is to close during ejaculation to prevent the semen passing retrogradely into the bladder. The physiological function of this smooth muscle sphincter is usually compromised following TURP or bladder neck incision (BNI), leading to retrograde ejaculation.

The external sphincter mechanism is involved in maintaining continence. During normal micturition this sphincter relaxes as the detrusor muscle contracts. If this does not take place in a coordinated manner, for example following interruption of spinal micturition pathways after spinal cord injury, the sphincter remains closed, causing detrusor–sphincter dyssynergia (DSD). This can result in high-pressure chronic retention and irreversible obstructive nephropathy. Medical treatment aims to block the adrenergic receptors, using uroselective alpha-blockers (e.g. tamsulosin) to reduce sphincter tone. Surgical treatment consists of endoscopic division of the sphincter, but the patient must be warned about irreversible retrograde ejaculation, following division of the internal sphincter.

Spinal pathology

Spina bifida

Children born with a spinal defect often have neurological problems affecting the lower limbs, bladder and rectum. Many patients have neuropathic bladders and may require surgery because of severe voiding dysfunction. Options include management by either an indwelling catheter, ISC or urinary diversion. Due to immobility and chronically poor voiding, renal stone formation and recurrent UTIs are common.

Spinal trauma

Traumatic spinal injury may result in paraplegia and an abnormally functioning bladder. Initially, during spinal shock, there is suppression of autonomic and somatic activity and the bladder becomes acontractile, areflexic and painlessly distended. It must therefore be drained, to prevent overdistention injury. As the neurological lesion stabilizes, reflex voiding may return, but this depends on the level of injury. Detrusor hyper-reflexia and DSD may also be present. Self-catheterization, a permanent indwelling catheter or urinary diversion are all options. Renal stone disease is common due to immobility and urinary stasis.

Incontinence

The various causes of urinary incontinence have been described above.

Stress incontinence, more correctly known as *USI*, is a common problem seen both by urologists and gynaecologists. Risk factors for the condition include female sex, advancing age, childbirth and obesity. Initial treatment is aimed at strengthening the pelvic floor, reducing unnecessary intra-abdominal pressure and trying to elevate the prolapsed urethra. Physiotherapy, in the form of intensive pelvic floor training, to strengthen the pelvic floor structures, together with weight loss and cessation of smoking improve symptoms in at least half of patients. Contemporary surgical treatment options aim to support the urethra and/or elevate the bladder neck and include colposuspension and the use of tension-free mid-urethral slings. Potential complications of these procedures include voiding and sexual dysfunction. In frail patients, a vaginal pessary may be used to support the urethra and bladder neck.

Prostate gland

Inflammation

Prostatitis may be acute or chronic. Symptoms of perineal or rectal discomfort with non-specific urinary symptoms are common. Occasionally, the prostatitis is bacterial and is treated effectively with a fluoroquinolone antibiotic. More often the condition is abacterial and may be a feature of the *chronic pelvic pain syndrome*. This form of prostatitis tends to run a chronic course and is refractory to antibiotic treatment. Symptomatic treatment using NSAIDS and alpha-blockers may be helpful.

Tumour

Benign prostatic enlargement

Although BPE does not necessarily cause BOO, the two are frequently linked and it is common for elderly men with troublesome urinary symptoms to present to the doctor complaining about 'their prostate gland'. Conversely, a patient with classical symptoms of BOO may still have an obstructive prostate, even if the gland feels small on rectal examination.

Many patients reach retirement before they complain of troublesome LUTS, although on direct questioning, they may admit to having had LUTS for some years beforehand. A full history and examination, along with appropriate tests to confirm the diagnosis is essential. Diagnosis is usually confirmed following exclusion of other conditions (e.g. prostate cancer, urethral strictures) and when flow rate measurement has revealed an obstructed pattern, characteristic of the condition.

The following options are available for the management of BPE.

General supportive advice

A reduction of fluid intake, particularly in the evening, will reduce urine production at night. Voiding twice before going to bed may help to empty the bladder and reduce troublesome nocturia. Reassurance that the patient's symptoms are not due to prostate cancer is usually greeted with relief.

Medical treatment

Alpha-blockers The uroselective alpha-1-blockers (e.g. tamsulosin, alfuzosin) now form the mainstay of medical management of BPE. They work by relaxing the smooth muscle around the bladder neck and prostate and so help increase urine flow. They have a rapid onset in alleviating some of the symptoms, but do not cure BPE. The drugs are usually well tolerated, but side effects include lethargy and postural hypotension.

5-alpha-reductase inhibitors These drugs block the enzyme 5-alpha-reductase, which converts testosterone to the active metabolite, dihydrotestosterone, which promotes BPE. Finasteride, taken orally, may take upto 4 months before any reduction in size of the prostate, or improvement in symptoms, is noted. A newer drug in this class is dutasteride, which is said to have a more rapid onset. The drugs are also well tolerated, but the prostate will regrow if treatment is stopped. Side effects include a reduced libido.

Surgical treatment

The commonest operation is TURP, in which the enlarged and obstructing adenoma is excised, using an endoscope and cutting diathermy loop. A laser can also be used to vaporize the tissue, but long-term results are still unproven. Open operations to remove the prostatic adenoma are less commonly performed, but may occasionally be required for very large adenomas. A BNI or transurethral incision of the prostate gland (TUIP) can be performed to release any bladder neck constriction, without removing any prostatic tissue.

Several other methods exist to shrink the prostate, using different types of energy. These include thermotherapy and microwave therapy, where the prostate is heated to shrink it.

Cancer

There is a wide range of incidence of adenocarcinoma of the prostate worldwide, but in the West it is the commonest cancer diagnosed in men over 65 years. Symptoms from the primary tumour may be indistinguishable from BPE, hence the importance of palpating the prostate and measuring the PSA in men with LUTS.

When the diagnosis is in doubt, a biopsy (ideally guided by a transrectal ultrasound scanner) is required. The PSA level may be normal in localized prostate cancer, but its level is important to monitor the response of the disease to treatment. It is invariably raised in metastatic prostate cancer.

The cancer most commonly metastasizes to bone and a bone scan is ideal for staging the disease. MRI scanning gives a satisfactory assessment of enlarged lymph nodes and may confirm extension of the tumour beyond the capsule of the prostate.

If the tumour is confined to the prostate, curative treatment can be offered in the form of radical external beam radiotherapy, localized implantation of radioactive seeds (brachytherapy) or the surgical removal of the prostate gland

and its capsule at open operation (radical prostatectomy). This technically demanding procedure can be performed via a standard open lower abdominal approach, a perineal approach or laparoscopically. It requires the urethra and bladder neck to be joined together when the gland has been removed. Side effects are significant and include erectile dysfunction (ED), urinary incontinence, bladder neck stricturing and damage to the rectum.

Metastatic prostate cancer is incurable, but significant improvements in survival, as well as relief of local and systemic symptoms of the disease are seen with androgen deprivation. This may be achieved by bilateral orchidectomy or, more commonly, by the use of drugs. These include gonadotropin-releasing hormone (GnRH) agonists (e.g. ®Zoladex), which block the release of gonadotropins from the pituitary gland and thereby inhibit production of testicular testosterone. These drugs are administered by monthly or 3-monthly depot injection. Antiandrogen tablets (e.g. bicalutamide, cyproterone acetate, flutamide) exist but may not represent a satisfactory monotherapy. However, GnRH agonists can be used in combination with antiandrogens to achieve maximum androgen blockade (MAB). Stilboestrol, which blocks the action of testosterone, is less widely used because of side effects, including thromboembolic events, but often gives a useful second line response when luteinizing hormone-releasing hormone (LHRH) analogue treatment has failed. The use of chemotherapy, using mitoxantrone, for advanced prostate cancer is currently being investigated, as is the use of GnRH receptor *antagonists*.

A variable time after introducing hormonal treatment, the cancer will become refractory to this androgen deprivation and it is said to be *hormone relapsed*. Painful bone secondaries can then be treated by local radiotherapy or analgesics. Treatment is generally symptomatic, although changing the hormonal treatment can sometimes achieve a useful secondary response.

Asymptomatic prostate cancer is a common finding at autopsy in men over 75 years. Elderly or frail men diagnosed with the disease may be best treated conservatively with active monitoring of their disease and treatment of symptoms as they occur.

Testis and scrotum

Inflammation

Orchitis is an acute inflammatory reaction of the testis secondary to infection. Most cases are associated with a viral mumps infection; however, other viruses and bacteria can cause orchitis. Inflammation and swelling of the epididymis is relatively common and there may associated orchitis – epididymo-orchitis. Usually, a specific organism is not identified, but the swelling and redness gradually resolve. This can be a painful and incapacitating condition, which requires bed rest, analgesics and antibiotic treatment. The symptoms usually develop more slowly than in testicular torsion and the men affected are usually older than the adolescents and young men affected by torsion. However, epididymo-orchitis can mimic a testicular tumour. If there is any doubt, an ultrasound scan may help to differentiate these conditions, but if the diagnosis is still in doubt, urgent scrotal exploration is necessary.

Fournier's gangrene is a rare necrotizing, inflammatory condition of the scrotum seen most commonly in elderly debilitated patients. The condition is also associated with diabetes and may occur following trauma or surgery. Initially a small black necrotic area develops in the scrotum. The inflammation spreads rapidly, due to synergism between aerobic and anaerobic organisms. The subcutaneous tissue becomes necrotic and gas-forming organisms may produce crepitus in the tissues. Urgent high-dose antibiotic treatment and radical surgical debridement of the affected tissues are required.

Swellings

These include:
- hydrocoele,
- epididymal cyst,
- tumour,
- varicocoele,
- inguinal hernia,
- testicular torsion.

A hydrocoele lies anterior to the testis and will transilluminate. With a large hydrocoele, the testis itself may be difficult to palpate. An epididymal cyst may have multiple septa and lies posterior and superior to the testis, within the epididymis. It may transilluminate.

A hydrocoele can be drained percutaneously with a needle, but commonly recurs. Otherwise all these cystic swellings can be excised surgically, or treated conservatively if the symptoms are minimal. Although they are usually painless, once a patient has noticed them, anxiety may make individuals conscious of them. If any doubt exists about whether the underlying testis is malignant, an ultrasound scan is a reliable way of excluding a testicular tumour.

A varicocoele results from the dilated pampiniform veins in the scrotum and cord. These veins can be ligated and divided in the inguinal canal, if they are symptomatic. Alternatively, embolization of the gonadal veins, using metallic coils, can be performed via the femoral vein.

In testicular torsion, the testis twists spontaneously on its spermatic cord, causing venous occlusion and subsequent arterial ischaemia. The majority of testes can be salvaged if scrotal exploration and untwisting of the cord is undertaken within 6 h. The peak age is 14 years, although a smaller peak also occurs in the neonatal period. The hydatid of Morgagni is a small embryological remnant located at the upper pole of the testis, which can occasionally twist and cause pain. The symptoms can mimic those of true testicular torsion.

Tumours

A solid swelling of the testis is assumed to be malignant until proved otherwise. Often the swelling is painless, but trauma may produce a pain or haemorrhage into the tumour, which can produce a painful inflamed scrotum, mimicking epididymo-orchitis. Diagnosis is greatly helped by testicular ultrasound scanning and the presence of raised tumour markers (AFP, β-HCG).

Occasionally, the tumour spreads to para-aortic lymph nodes, lungs, liver and brain. These may present with backache, haemoptysis, jaundice or neurological events. Testicular tumours occur in relatively young men, late teens to early 30s. Teratoma tends to occur in the younger age range and seminoma in the slightly older group.

Treatment consists of a radical orchidectomy via a groin incision. If tumour markers return to normal following surgery, it is likely there are no metastases. A complete staging, using chest and abdominal CT scanning, is required. Metastatic disease requires cisplatin-based chemotherapy. Post-chemotherapy residual metastatic teratoma masses require surgical excision.

Seminoma is extremely radiosensitive and if the tumour is confined to the testis, abdominal lymph nodes may be irradiated to treat undetected micrometastases. Following orchidectomy, localized (stage 1) teratoma can be monitored by a surveillance programme (withholding adjuvant treatments), utilizing regular CT scanning and blood tests for tumour markers. In the good prognosis group, only about 30% will relapse and require salvage chemotherapy, which is still curative in the majority of patients. With effective chemotherapy, over 90% of patients with a testicular tumour will be cured.

Rare testicular tumours include lymphoma in older men and rhabdomyosarcoma in infants.

Trauma

Direct trauma can cause testicular rupture, which requires surgical exploration and repair. Late presentation of trauma is not uncommon and a haematoma within the tunica vaginalis may form. This usually reabsorbs, but surgical exploration and drainage are occasionally necessary.

Fertility

Vasectomy is one of the commonest forms of contraception. Popularly regarded as a minor procedure, it is the urological procedure most likely to result in litigation. Post-operative haematoma or pain may be difficult to treat and sterility cannot be guaranteed until azoospermia has been confirmed on semen analysis. Even then, late recanalization of the vas is a rare but well-recognized complication.

Reversal of vasectomy may be attempted if the patient decides he wishes to have further children. Re-anastomosis of the vas is relatively straightforward. However, the longer it is since the vasectomy the greater the likelihood that sperm production and transport through the epididymis will be impaired.

Primary infertility is investigated initially with semen analysis to assess the number, motility and percentage of normal sperm. A hormonal screen is necessary to assess the

hypothalamic–pituitary–testicular axis and testicular biopsy may be performed to assess spermatogenesis.

Penis and urethra

Inflammation

Inflammation of the foreskin and glans (balanitis) can result in a phimosis. In recurrent cases, this is best treated by circumcision. If the foreskin is drawn back over the glans, a paraphimosis results. Although this can usually be reduced, a dorsal slit may be necessary in the acute situation.

Stricture

Trauma to the urethra, by a catheter or surgical instrument, or inflammation from an infection such as *Neisseria gonorrhoeae* may produce fibrosis resulting in a urethral stricture. This may be divided under direct vision using an optical urethrotome, but recurrence is common. Urethroplasty using buccal mucosal grafts or penile foreskin allows the stricture to be excised and replaced with healthier tissue.

Tumour

The male distal urethra is lined mainly by transitional cells and in the female, squamous epithelium. Carcinomas can occur but they are rare.

Squamous carcinoma of the penis usually presents as an ulcerated lesion beneath the foreskin. The tumour may be in the coronal groove. Biopsy is essential for histological confirmation and staging is by CT scanning to assess the inguinal lymph nodes. A localized tumour can be treated by amputation (partial or complete), local excision or external beam radiotherapy. Very small, localized penile cancers can be treated successfully with topical 5-fluorouracil preparations. Although metastatic squamous carcinoma is usually incurable its rate of growth may be quite slow. Often the patient is elderly and frail, and careful surveillance may be the best option.

Trauma

A degloving injury to the penis results in the loss of skin from the penile shaft. The shaft can be buried with scrotal skin to allow healing and then removed, thereby preserving the scrotal skin covering.

Fracture of an erect penis involves rupture of one or both of the corpora cavernosa. These should be repaired at open operation.

Erectile dysfunction

Failure of normal erections occurs with advancing age and it is estimated that around 20% of men between 50 and 70 years of age have moderate or severe ED. The cause of this impotence may be psychogenic, but organic causes (such as diabetes, smoking and peripheral vascular disease) are more likely with increasing age. The mainstays of treatment are the phosphodiesterase type 5 (PDE 5) inhibitors, such as sildenafil, vardenafil and tadalafil. These drugs inhibit breakdown of cyclic guanosine monophosphate (cGMP), thereby enhancing the normal erectile response. They are effective in psychogenic and organic ED. Other modalities of treatment are occasionally necessary including *intracavernosal* prostaglandin E1 and *intraurethral* vasoactive drug therapy, and vacuum constriction devices. An uncommon side effect of drug therapy for ED is a prolonged erection lasting several hours (priapism), which may lead to ischaemic injury to the erectile tissue in the corporeal bodies. If priapism does occur, the blood must be drained from the corpora cavernosa by direct aspiration, or by surgical formation of a shunt with the corpus spongiosum, or a saphenous vein. Priapism may also occur as part of a sickle cell crisis or in a patient with leukaemia.

ASPECTS OF GENERAL SURGERY AND GYNAECOLOGY THAT MAY CAUSE UROLOGICAL PROBLEMS

General surgery

Diverticular disease of the sigmoid colon may cause abscess formation that perforates into the bladder producing a colovesical fistula. Symptoms include recurrent urine infections and air bubbles in the urine passed down from flatus in the colon (pneumaturia). It is uncommon for a carcinoma of either the bladder or colon to cause a similar fistula.

A leaking AAA is occasionally misdiagnosed as ureteric colic. Any patient over the age of 50 years with sudden onset of abdominal/loin pain must *not* be diagnosed as having a symptomatic renal stone until radiological confirmation has been obtained, or an AAA excluded by ultrasonography.

Gynaecology

An *ectopic pregnancy* may cause lower abdominal pain and eventually an acute abdomen with shock. Establishing the date of a patient's last menstrual period is an important part of any history in a woman of childbearing age. *Ovarian cysts* may cause low abdominal pain and pelvic pain but these are easily identified by ultrasonography. A monthly cycle of lower abdominal pain and, more rarely, haematuria may result from *endometriosis*. Abdominal endometriosis can cause local fibrosis and ureteric obstruction.

Vaginal bleeding may present as 'haematuria'. A vaginal examination should always be performed at the time of cystoscopy to exclude a carcinoma of the cervix, or other pelvic mass. Locally advanced carcinoma of the cervix may present with hydronephrosis and renal failure due to local invasion, causing ureteric obstruction.

Following *hysterectomy*, unrecognized damage to a ureter may present as loin pain from an obstructive hydronephrosis, or a vaginal leakage of urine from a vesico-vaginal fistula.

FURTHER READING

Bullock, Sibley, Whittaker. *Essential Urology*. Livingstone: Churchill

Tanagho EA & McAninch JW. *Smith's General Urology*, 14th edn. Lang Publishing, Norwalk Connecticut, USA

Lloyd-Davies W, Parkhouse H, Gow J, Davies D. *Colour Atlas of Urology*, 2nd edn. London: Wolfe Publishing, 1994

Walsh P, Retik A, Vaughan E, Wein A (eds). *Campbell's Urology*, 7th edn. Philadelphia: Saunders, 1998

20

Head and Neck

Walter WK King[1], John KS Woo[2] and Dennis SC Lam[3]

[1]Centre Director, Plastic & Reconstructive Surgery Centre, Hong Kong Sanatorium & Hospital, Hong Kong; Honorary Clinical Professor, Department of Surgery, The Chinese University of Hong Kong [2]Consultant in Otorhionolaryngology, Department of Surgery, Prince of Wales Hospital, The Chinese University of Hong Kong; Honorary Clinical Associate Professor, The Chinese University of Hong Kong [3]Professor and Chairman, Department of Ophthalmology & Visual Sciences, The Chinese University of Hong Kong, Hong Kong

CONTENTS

Ocular injury	**391**
Ocular infection	**392**
Eyelid	392
Orbit	393
Conjunctiva	393
Cornea	393
Inflammatory disorders of the ear, nose, sinuses and throat	**394**
The ear	394
The nose and sinuses	396
The throat	397
Foreign bodies in the ENT	**398**
Aural foreign bodies	398
Nasal foreign bodies	399
Ingested foreign bodies	399
Epistaxis	**401**
Identification of the bleeding source	401
Surgery for local control of bleeding	401
Arterial ligation	401
Transnasal endoscopic ligation	402
Hereditary haemorrhagic telangiectasia	402
Endoscopy of the ENT	**402**
Otoscopy	402
Nasendoscopy	402
Pharyngolaryngoscopy	403
Head and neck tumours	**403**
Skin	403
Scalp	405
Oral cavity and oropharynx	405
Nasopharynx	407
Larynx and hypopharynx	408
Paranasal sinuses	410
Neck masses	410
Salivary gland disease	413
Further reading	**413**

OCULAR INJURY

Ocular injuries may occur as a result of thermal, radiation, chemical or physical insults. If the eye or periorbital region is involved in the injury, proper assessment, including a detailed history, visual acuity testing, pupillary responses, external eye surface inspection and the inner eye structures examination, must be carried out.

If retained intraocular foreign body is suspected, appropriate investigations should be performed. These include standard, orbital, plain film radiographs to detect radioopaque foreign bodies. Computed tomography (CT) with axial and coronal cuts is helpful in the evaluation of both intraocular and periocular structures as well as the presence or degree of periocular damage. It may also show whether a patient has sustained an intracranial injury, such as subdural haemorrhage. Ultrasound is useful to localize nonmetallic intraocular foreign bodies and detect choroidal haemorrhage, posterior scleral rupture, retinal detachment and subretinal haemorrhage.

Details regarding the setting of the injury are important and give an idea of what to look for and exclude in the physical examination.

The equipment required to perform an initial eye examination includes: vision card, penlight, topical anaesthetic eye drops, direct ophthalmoscope, sterile fluorescein strips, gauze, eye pads, eye shields, Q-tips and irrigating solution.

Topical anaesthetic may be needed to control the pain and discomfort before physical examination can begin. However, if an open injury of the globe is evident or suspected, it is important not to instill such medications in order to prevent toxicity to the intraocular structures. In badly traumatized eyes, only a cursory examination may be possible in the clinic and detailed evaluation may have to be performed in the operation theatre under general anaesthesia – often prior to surgical repair.

It is important to assess the visual acuity as soon as possible. This is not only an important factor in the initial assessment and a parameter for monitoring progress, but is also necessary for medicolegal reasons. If a Snellen acuity chart is not available, newspaper or magazine print can be used to provide a rough idea of the impairment in visual function.

The initial evaluation should include inspection of the brow and lids for lacerations, bruising and haematoma. The presence of air in the periorbital tissues will be detected by the presence of crepitus on palpation and is an important sign denoting damage to the sinuses adjacent to the eye. A penlight is used to obtain oblique illumination of the eye, which may reveal damage to the conjunctiva, cornea, anterior chamber, pupil, iris and lens:

1. The conjunctiva should be inspected for haemorrhage, laceration and foreign bodies. The presence of a bloody bag of conjunctiva – termed chemosis, is often an indicator of underlying globe rupture. This is due to damage to the vascular choroid which leads to the extravasation of blood which collects under the loosely adherent conjunctival tissue. If foreign bodies are suspected, then the upper eyelids should be everted as foreign bodies are often present on the surface of the tarsal conjunctiva and these can usually be removed easily with a Q-tip.
2. The cornea is then examined for any foreign body, abrasions or lacerations. Abrasions can be outlined easily by fluorescein dye. The patient is asked to look up while the examiner pulls down the lower lid and applies the sterile fluorescein strip into the pool of tears in the lower fornix. The fluorescein strip may also be wetted with sterile eye drops before being applied to the conjunctival sac.
3. The clarity and depth of the anterior chamber should be assessed and compared with the other eye. The presence of hyphaema (collection of blood with a level in the anterior chamber) can be identified even with a penlight.
4. The shape, size and symmetry of pupils must be noted. A peaked pupil with low intraocular pressure usually signifies a ruptured globe. The pupillary reactions to light, both direct and consensual, must also be tested. A positive relative afferent pupillary defect usually implies significant afferent pathway damage; for example, massive retinal detachment or optic nerve damage.
5. The examination of ocular motility and periorbital deformities is essential for assessing the possibility of orbital wall defects and extraocular muscle problems. The red fundal reflex can be produced easily with a direct ophthalmoscope. Abnormal fundal reflex may signify medial opacity, such as lens cloudiness (traumatic cataract), vitreous haemorrhage or retinal detachment.

Patients should be referred promptly to an ophthalmologist if the following conditions are suspected:
- fractured orbit;
- lid laceration involving the lid margin or canalicular system;
- ruptured eyeball (including corneal or scleral laceration);
- hyphaema;
- traumatic cataract;
- lens subluxation or dislocation;
- vitreous haemorrhage;
- retinal detachment;
- choroidal rupture;
- optic nerve damage.

In the event of chemical or thermal injury – in addition to performing the detailed evaluation described above, it is important to thoroughly irrigate the eye with clean, cold saline to minimize contact of the deleterious agent with the ocular structures. The irrigation can be performed by having the patient lie down on a couch and after instilling topical anaesthetic drops, a speculum is inserted to keep the eyelids separated. An intravenous line is connected to the bottle of saline on a stand, and the fluid is run into the patient's eye – in the case of chemical injury, the use of a litmus paper will allow determination of the endpoint of irrigation – it is performed till there is no colour change in the litmus paper.

OCULAR INFECTION

Common symptoms of ocular infection include eye redness, pain, discharge, foreign body sensation, photophobia, eyelid crusting and swelling. The type of discharge, characteristics of conjunctival reaction and distribution of eye redness are essential features to note during the examination. Visual acuity, pupillary light reflex and extraocular movements should also be noted. Apart from clinical findings, microbiological investigations also play an important role in the diagnosis and management of the disease. Specimens from simple eye swab, corneal scrapings, anterior chamber and vitreous tap may be needed.

Among the symptoms of ocular infection, red eye is by far the commonest. Although conjunctivitis is the commonest cause of red eye, there are more sinister causes. For example, when the redness is located at the perilimbal area (ciliary injection), acute closed-angle glaucoma, anterior uveitis or corneal diseases are the more likely diagnoses. Prompt ophthalmological referral is indicated for these conditions. Also, when there is an associated drop in visual acuity, photophobia, restricted eye movements, severe eye pain or abnormal pupil reflex, the condition could be serious and early referral is needed.

As for all infections, prompt diagnosis, identification of the causative pathogen(s), and early and appropriate treatment are the keys to successful management.

Eyelid

Blepharitis

This is the commonest external eye disease encountered in clinical practice and is associated with staphylococcal infection and seborrhoea. Itching, burning, foreign body sensation, crusts around the eyelids with prominent blood vessels and inspissated oil glands at the lid margins are the usual clinical presentations. Lid hygiene, topical antibiotics, such as erythromycin or bacitracin ointments, and/or systemic tetracycline are useful treatments. Crucial in the treatment is the patient's compliance with the proper lid hygiene instructions.

External hordeolum (stye)

This is a small abscess caused mainly by acute staphylococcal infection of a lash follicle or its associated glands. Examination shows a tender, inflamed swelling in the lid margin, at the base of an eyelash. This condition is common in patients with blepharitis. Most styes resolve spontaneously with or without discharge of their contents. Hot compresses and antibiotic ointments may aid resolution. If there is acute pain and a pointing abscess, removal of the infected eyelash allows drainage of the pus, and quick resolution of pain. Surgical incision and drainage (I&D) is only required in the rare instance of a large abscess formation.

Orbit

Preseptal cellulitis

This infection involves tissues anterior to the orbital septum and is sometimes preceded by trauma or sinusitis. *Staphylococcus aureus*, streptococci and *Haemophilus influenzae* are the common pathogens. Examination reveals eyelid erythema, swelling, warmth and tenderness, but there is neither proptosis nor restriction in ocular motility. Radiographs or CT scans may show signs of sinusitis or evidence of trauma. Systemic ampicillin combined with penicillinase-resistant antibiotics is the treatment of choice. Surgical treatment is indicated in unresponsive cases or for the treatment of associated sinusitis. While this condition in adults is relatively simple to treat, in infants and young children, this can constitute an emergency. The definition of the orbital septum in these cases is poor and it is not difficult for the infection to track through the septum into the tissues of the orbit. Since the orbit contains many vital structures, infection in this region can cause serious visual loss and thus, these children must be hospitalized and treated with intravenous antibiotics – preferably a fourth-generation cephalosporin.

Orbital cellulitis

Although uncommon, this is a sight-threatening condition and hospitalization is required. Apart from eyelid swelling, proptosis and restricted ocular motility with pain on attempted eye movement, the patient may also complain of reduced vision. Systemic symptoms may include malaise and fever. The warning signs of orbital cellulitis are a dilated pupil, marked ophthalmoplegia, loss of vision, afferent pupillary defect, papilledema, perivasculitis and violaceous lids. Systemic sepsis work-up, including CT scan of sinuses, orbits and brain, blood culture or even lumbar puncture, is needed if meningeal or cerebral signs develop. Urgent ear, nose and throat (ENT) consultation should be arranged and systemic intravenous broad-spectrum antibiotics, covering Gram-positive, Gram-negative and anaerobic organisms are indicated. Surgical drainage may be needed in selected cases.

Conjunctiva

Bacterial conjunctivitis

This is a common condition, often caused by *Staphylococcus epidermidis*, *S. aureus*, *Haemophilus* and *Streptococcus* spp. There is usually conjunctival hyperaemia, which is maximal in the fornices, mild papillary reaction, purulent or mucopurulent discharge and mild lid crusting. Although topical antibiotics are often prescribed, the infection usually resolves in about 2 weeks, even without treatment.

Viral conjunctivitis

The commonest pathogen is adenovirus. The contagious nature of the disease makes thorough hand washing important after examination. Examination shows follicular reaction and periauricular lymphadenopathy is often present. Topical antibiotics to prevent secondary infection are usually prescribed. Additional antihistamine eye drops are sometimes used to decrease the eye congestion and symptoms. Topical steroids are reserved for severe cases. Conjunctivitis can rarely be followed by keratitis and such patients may become steroid dependent.

In both conditions, it is important to inform the patient about the need to maintain basic personal hygiene to avoid transmitting the condition to others.

Cornea

Bacterial keratitis

In general, corneal infections are assumed to be bacterial until proven otherwise. Predisposing factors for bacterial keratitis includes chronic infections of the ocular adnexa, underlying corneal disease, dry eye, contact lens wear, neurotrophic or exposure keratopathy and use of steroids. This is a condition that requires prompt referral and treatment. Urgent identification of the pathogen by corneal scraping and eradication of organisms by hourly fortified broad-spectrum antibiotics (tobramycin or gentamycin with cefazolin or vancomycin) should be commenced as early as possible.

Viral keratitis

Herpes simplex virus is a relatively common causative agent, although some cases are subclinical. Antiviral ointments, such as acyclovir eye ointment, should be applied to the eye 5 times per day. Secondary infections can occur and should be watched for.

Fungal keratitis

This is a rare infection and the patient usually presents with a history of trauma – often by vegetable matter. *Fusarium*, *Aspergillus* and *Candida* are the usual causative organisms. Topical antifungal agents such as natamycin, amphotericin B and miconazole are used. A systemic antifungal agent is indicated in severe cases.

Acanthamoebic keratitis

Improper contact lens wear and care are the most important risk factors. The condition is easily confused with herpes keratitis and if not properly diagnosed and treated, blindness is a common outcome. Patients usually present with severe eye pain and photophobia. The classical finding is a ring infiltrate in the cornea and the symptoms are usually much greater than the signs. Since *Acanthamoeba* is a neurotrophic organism, the presence of enlarged and prominent corneal nerves is an important clue to this condition. Treatment is difficult and requires prolonged use of relatively toxic medications like neosporin, dibromopropamidine, propamidine, polyhexamethylene biguanide and chlorhexidine.

INFLAMMATORY DISORDERS OF THE EAR, NOSE, SINUSES AND THROAT

The ear

Preauricular sinus

Preauricular sinus is a common congenital condition particularly in the Orientals. There is no need for any treatment unless it becomes infected (Fig. 20.1). It may then present with pain, swelling and discharge. If seen at an early stage,

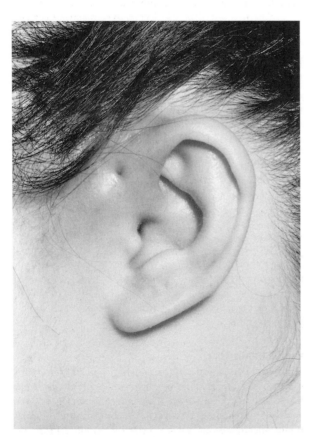

Figure 20.1. An infected preauricular sinus.

infected preauricular sinus may be controlled with antibiotic. If a patient presents with a preauricular abscess, I&D together with antibiotic become necessary. The site of incision should be through the sinus opening so as to minimize branching of the sinus tract. This is particularly important with recurrent preauricular abscess. Abscess formation or recurrent infections are indications that the sinus tract should be excised. It is important that all sinus tracts should be excised to prevent recurrence. If in doubt, any soft tissue adherent to the tract should be excised as deep as the temporalis fascia. The supra-aural approach is a suitable choice with good results.

Auricular haematoma

The pinna, because of its exposed and protruding position, is frequently traumatized. Blunt injury may lead to formation of an auricular haematoma. The haematoma typically form in the subperichondrial plane. If treatment is delayed, the haematoma may dissect along the subperichondrial plane and result in unsightly deformity. Thus auricular haematoma need to be evacuated promptly and pressure dressing applied to conform with the shape of the pinna by means of through and through stitches. A prophylactic course of antibiotics is indicated to minimize secondary infection.

Auricular perichondritis

Perichondritis may complicate any external ear trauma. It is a serious condition and need to be treated with full respect. Once developed, perichondritis rapidly spread to involve the whole pinna sparing only the ear lobule (as the lobule has no cartilage). The patient will have severe pain and itchiness in the affected ear. Prompt treatment with antibiotics that cover both Gram-positive and Gram-negative organisms (especially pseudomonas) should be started without delay. Less severe cases may be treated as outpatient with a course of quinolones (e.g. ciprofloxacin). More severe cases should be admitted to hospital and treated with intravenous antibiotics. Again, quinolones or combination of a second-generation cephalosporin and an aminoglycoside is a good alternative. Further antibiotic treatment should be guided by the result of culture and sensitivity tests. Antibiotics should be given till all signs of infections have subsided. If abscess develops during therapy, this should be incised and drained immediately. The cavity irrigated with aminoglycoside solution to treat or prevent pseudomonas infection. Once becomes clean, the cavity should be closed by pressure dressing applied to conform with the contour of the pinna. Some deformity is often inevitable, however, with prompt and proper treatment a cauliflower ear should be avoidable.

Otitis externa

Otitis externa is a very common ear condition. It usually occurs following minor trauma, often self-inflicted, to the external auditory canal (EAC). Treatment is usually straightforward with local toilet and topical medications. In severe cases, the external canal should be packed with an otowick or ribbon gauze impregnated with a steroid-containing antibiotic cream. The dressing should be changed daily or as required by the condition. When the condition becomes recurrent or is resistant to treatment, an underlying cause should be excluded. Conditions like diabetes mellitus and a chronic dermatosis may need to be treated simultaneously. Otomycosis may sometimes complicate chronic otitis externa especially when prolonged or recurrent courses of topical antibiotics had been used. Rigorous aural toilet and topical antifungal eardrops should be used. Repeated local toilets and antifungal therapy are often needed as the fungal spores are very resistant to treatment. Occasionally, stenosis of the EAC may be the cause and need to be treated surgically.

Necrotizing otitis externa

Necrotizing otitis externa is also known as 'malignant otitis externa'. It is not that the condition may become malignant, but because of the occasional fatal outcome. This typically occurs in elderly patient who is diabetic or is immunocompromised for other reasons. There is usually a long history of ear discharge and otalgia is frequently present and pronounced. The causative organism is *Pseudomonas pyocyanea*. The clinical features of 'necrotizing otitis externa' are often misleading and deceptive in the early phase of the disease. However, the response to standard treatment is poor and the condition may suddenly deteriorate. Ear examination often shows exuberant granulation tissue. A biopsy should be taken for microbiological work-up and for histological examination to exclude malignancy. Infection and the necrotizing process may spread to involved the temporal bone causing osteomyelitis. The first indication is often facial nerve palsy. In advanced disease, the jugular foramen may also be affected by osteomyelitis resulting in ninth, tenth and eleventh cranial nerves palsies. Thrombosis of the internal jugular vein and retrograde cavernous sinus thrombosis may also occur.

If the condition is suspected, the patient should be treated vigorously with intravenous antibiotics. A combination of a second-generation cephalosporin, an aminoglycoside and metronidazole should be used. These together will have coverage for Gram-positive, Gram-negative (including pseudomonas) and anaerobes. CT scanning of the temporal bone should be performed to delineate the extent of the disease. In diabetic patients, the control of blood sugar level plays an important role. Hyperbaric oxygen therapy has been used in patients with severe disease with good result. Surgical treatment of this condition is purely secondary. The traditional mastoidectomy is rarely useful as the disease does not spread through the mastoid air cells. However, aggressive debridement of surrounding necrotic soft tissues and drainage of secondary local abscesses are important.

Acute otitis media

Acute otitis media most commonly occurs in young paediatric patients less than 6–7-year old. It typically occurs, following an upper respiratory tract infection (URTI), as ascending infection through the Eustachian tube. The natural course of acute otitis media is best described in four stages: hyperaemic, inflammatory, suppurative and resolution phases. In the hyperaemic phase, the patient has otalgia without hearing loss and otoscopy reveals a hyperaemic eardrum. The inflammatory phase that follows is characterized by increasing otalgia and hearing loss. Fever is usually present at this phase. Otoscopy reveals a hyperaemic eardrum and middle ear effusion. The disease reaches a climax at the suppurative phase. The patient often becomes irritable because of intense otalgia and hyperpyrexia is frequently present. Otoscopy reveals pus collecting behind a bulging and intensely hyperaemic eardrum. The eardrum is now under severe tension and may rupture spontaneously. Once the eardrum ruptures, the condition enters the resolution phase. All the symptoms especially otalgia resolves rapidly.

The natural course of acute otitis media may be altered by therapy. The underlying URTI will need to be treated. Nasal decongestant is useful to reduce the oedema of the Eustachian tube. A second-generation cephalosporin is a logical choice for initial antibiotic therapy. Acute otitis media usually settles quickly with medical therapy. If the facial nerve canal is dehiscent, facial nerve palsy may very rarely complicate the condition. If this occurs, myringotomy is indicated to hasten resolution of the suppurative phase and recovery of the facial nerve function.

Otitis media with effusion

Otitis media with effusion (OME) is a condition with complex etiologies including anatomical variations, allergy, infections and inflammation. The interplay of these factors lead finally to structural and/or functional abnormality of the Eustachian tube resulting in OME. The more horizontal lie of the Eustachian tube and frequent attacks of URTI contribute to the high prevalence of OME in infants and young children of any race. The reported cumulative incidence of first episode of OME reaches almost 100% by the age of 3 years. The incidence drops sharply after the age of 7 so much so that the condition is uncommon amongst teenagers and rare in adults. However, in places where nasopharyngeal carcinoma (NPC) is endemic, deafness associated with OME is a common presenting symptom of the disease. In these areas, NPC should be excluded in any adult with unilateral OME.

Clinical diagnosis is straightforward when otological examination shows a fluid level (Fig. 20.2) or bubbles behind the eardrum. In more subtle cases, tympanometric studies may be required. The finding of a flat (type b) tympanogram is diagnostic. Initial treatment of OME should be conservative. Coexisting allergic rhinitis, URTI should be adequately treated. The use of antibiotics is controversial. However if there is any evidence of acute otitis media, a course of antibiotics is advisable. Persistent OME is more effectively treated with myringotomy and insertion of a grommet (Fig. 20.3). In infants and young children, adenoidectomy

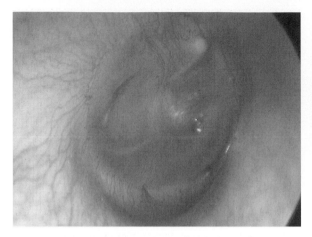

Figure 20.2. Otitis media with effusion. (*Note*: The presence of a fluid level behind the eardrum.)

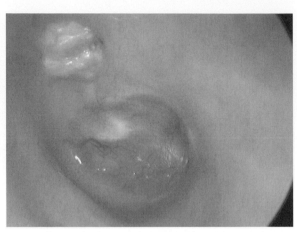

Figure 20.4. A CSOM with cholesteatoma. (*Note*: The attic defect above the eardrum.)

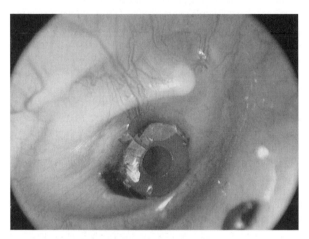

Figure 20.3. An OME treated by myringotomy and grommet insertion. (*Note*: The grommet in place across the eardrum.)

will reduce the risk of recurrent OME. OME associated with NPC should be treated more conservatively as there is a higher incidence of otorrhoea and otalgia in these patients also receiving radiotherapy.

Chronic suppurative otitis media

Chronic suppurative otitis media (CSOM) is the commonest form of chronic otitis media. Clinically it is characterized by otorrhoea and conduction hearing loss of variable severity. Otoscopy reveals a perforated eardrum. The condition is classified into the safe (tubotympanic) and unsafe (atticoantral) variety depending on the likelihood of coexisting cholesteatoma.

The safe variety is CSOM without cholesteatoma. It can be further classified into active or inactive depending on whether there is infection or not. Safe inactive CSOM can be managed either conservatively or surgically. Safe active CSOM should be treated initially conservatively to control the infection. A tympanoplasty procedure should then be performed to prevent recurrent infection.

The unsafe variety is CSOM with cholesteatoma (Fig. 20.4). The presence of cholesteatoma is usually obvious on otoscopy. Occasionally, cholesteatoma may be more difficult to diagnose. If otoscopy reveals granulation tissue, aural polyps or middle ear infection that is resistant to conservative treatment, cholesteatoma should be excluded. Traditionally, in the presence of a marginal perforation or a deep retraction pocket, CSOM is considered potentially unsafe. However with modern endoscopic equipment and CT, assessment of the middle ear becomes much more accurate than before. Diagnostic uncertainty occurs only rarely. The treatment of unsafe simple chronic otitis media (SCOM) is surgical as cholesteatoma can cause serious complications that may be fatal. The type of surgical procedure to employ is controversial. The classical radical mastoidectomy, modified radical mastoidectomy or the 'combined approach tympanoplasty' may be chosen depending on the extent of cholesteatoma and more importantly on the experience of the surgeon. Whatever the procedure chosen, the aim of the surgery is to remove all the disease and to give the patient a safe, dry and functioning ear.

The nose and sinuses

Rhinitis

'Rhinitis' which literally means inflammation of the nasal mucosa is a non-specific term. The multifactorial aetiology and overlapping symptomatology makes 'rhinitis' extremely difficult to classify. Up to date, the classification proposed by the '*International Rhinitis Management Working Group*' in 1994 is the most comprehensive one although is still far from being universally accepted. The commonest cause being allergy. For a long time, allergic rhinitis is classified as seasonal or perennial. More recently, it is being reclassified as intermittent or persistent depending on the total duration of the symptomatic period. Management of rhinitis is dependent on the underlying cause. Superimposed infection is not uncommon and should be treated accordingly.

Sinusitis

Sinusitis is a better defined clinical condition. The pathogenesis of sinusitis is better understood nowadays after the importance of mucous transportation is realized. Sinusitis is usually unilaterally its symptoms are better appreciated in four levels:

1. Primary (Level 1) symptoms of sinusitis are unusual as the sinuses have no specific function. However if the involved sinus becomes totally blocked, local pain and tenderness may occur as tension develops within the sinus.
2. Secondary (Level 2) symptoms develop as entrapped and frequently infected secretion overflows from the involved sinus. The patient may then present with mucopurulent rhinorrhoea.
3. Tertiary (Level 3) symptoms develop as the mucopus collects around the Eustachian tube causing middle ear dysfunction.
4. Quaternary (Level 4) symptoms develop if a totally obstructed sinus also becomes infected or develops into a mucocele. Under these situations, progressive tension will develop and may decompress itself along line of weakness. Patients may then present with orbital or intracranial complications.

Acute sinusitis

This commonly follows an URTI and presents acutely with fever local pain and tenderness over the involved sinus. Nasal symptoms may not be prominent. Nasal endoscopy reveals local congestion and pus may be seen streaming down from the diseased sinus. A pus swab should be taken for microbiological work-up and meanwhile the patient should be treated symptomatically with an analgesic and antipyretic. A 2-week course antibiotic with coverage for Gram-positive and Gram-negative organisms should be started immediately. The regime may need to be revised if clinical progress is slow or as determined by culture and sensitivity results. Most acute sinusitis resolves with conservative treatment.

Chronic sinusitis

This usually present with chronic nasal congestion and recurrent mucopurulent rhinorrhoea (Level 2 symptoms). There is usually an underlying cause such as nasal polyposis, a septal deviation, an abnormal middle turbinate, etc. The presence of any condition which obstructs mucous transportation out of the sinus will lead to recurrent infection and sinusitis becomes chronic. Therefore, surgery is frequently required as a definitive procedure. Functional endoscopic sinus surgery (FESS) which aims at re-establishing normal

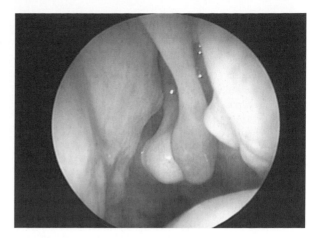

Figure 20.5. Nasendoscopic picture of the nose showing a solitary nasal polyp coming out of the middle meatus.

mucous transportation is now a well-established operation for this condition. When considering any patient for FESS, coronal CT scanning of the sinuses must be done so that the full extent of disease and any variation in sinus anatomy are known to the surgeon.

Nasal polyposis

Nasal polyposis is a common condition of obscure aetiology. The true incidence in the general public is unknown but it is one of the few common causes for visits to the ENT clinics around the world. Whatever the cause may be, the final common pathophysiological pathway is believed to be inflammatory. The condition is highly associated with aspirin intolerance, adult onset asthma and cystic fibrosis. The polyps are typically arising from the lateral nasal wall especially around the narrow middle meati (Fig. 20.5). Diagnosis is based on clinical examination. If the diagnosis is in doubt, for example when the polyp is unilateral and with a rough surface, a biopsy to exclude a tumour is necessary.

Treatment is either medical or surgical. Medical treatment with topical steroid is indicated for patients with small polyps. Patients with larger or diffuse polyposis are more effective treated with endoscopic nasal polypectomy. For polyps that affect the paranasal sinuses, full FESS may be needed. Overall, nasal polyposis has a high chance of recurrence with any treatment in the region of 25–30%. Those with diffuse sinonasal polyposis have the worse results while those with solitary nasal polyp have a high chance of cure with surgery. For recurrent nasal polyposis, sometime a short course of systemic steroid may prove very useful.

The throat

Tonsillitis

Acute tonsillitis is a very common condition in children. Clinically it is characterized by acute sore throat and fever.

It is usually part of an URTI and mostly viral in origin. On examination, the tonsils are usually enlarged and erythematous. Treatment is mainly symptomatic. Isolated follicular tonsillitis is less common and is frequently due to streptococcal infection. On examination, the tonsils are usually slightly enlarged with a rough surface. The roughness is due to the presence of numerous follicles. Treatment should include an antibiotic. Exudative tonsillitis is much less common and usually means a more severe infection. A blood sample must be taken from the patient for haematological evaluation to exclude infectious mononucleosis. If an antibiotic is needed as in patients with hyperpyrexia, ampicillin should be avoided. Membranous tonsillitis is extremely rare but potentially serious. In a developing country, one must think of diphtheria. In a developed country, a haematological malignancy should be excluded. It is not uncommon for patients who have had 'tonsillectomy' to present with sore throat, in these instances, lingual tonsillitis should be excluded by a mirror examination.

Quinsy

Acute tonsillitis may sometimes be complicated by abscess formation. Quinsy, which is peritonsillar abscess, commonly follows inadequately treated acute tonsillitis. Patients with quinsy typically present with fever and progressive sore throat that becomes localized to one side. Some degree of trismus will be present due to irritation of the pterigoid muscles by the abscess. Examination will reveal a unilateral tonsillar swelling with red-hot mucosa. The diagnosis is confirmed when pus is obtained by fine needle aspiration (FNA). The pus should be sent for microbiological work-up. The treatment should consist of high-dose intravenous penicillin and I&D of the abscess. It is important that the site of the abscess is well localized by FNA, as the carotid artery may be pushed forward by the abscess and be injured by during I&D of the abscess. The response to treatment is usually prompt. If progress is slow, the cause has to be determined. Additional anaerobic cover should be added or the antibiotic regime modified according to culture and sensitivity results. Sometimes the incision site may need to be open again with a pair of sinus forceps to ensure no recollection of pus. Hot tonsillectomy may, very rarely, be indicated for prevention of sepsis extending to the deep neck spaces. After the acute episode, patients with quinsy should have an interval tonsillectomy if there is previous history of quinsy or recurrent tonsillitis. An isolated attack of quinsy is considered only as a relative indication for interval tonsillectomy.

Acute supraglottitis

'Acute epiglottitis' is a misnomer and 'acute supraglottitis' (Fig. 20.6) should be used instead. Anatomically, there is no boundary to separate the epiglottis from the rest of the supraglottis. Therefore, the whole supraglottis will inevitably be involved by an inflammatory or infective process. In the past, the condition is typically caused by *H. influenzae* type b

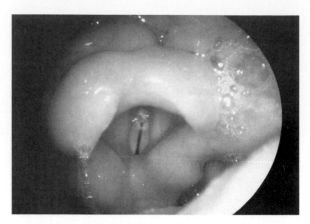

Figure 20.6. Acute supraglottitis. (*Note*: The whole supraglottitis is swollen sparing only the vocal cord.)

(Hib) and affect almost exclusively paediatric patients. However with universal vaccination against Hib in developed countries, supraglottitis-affecting adults have increasingly been reported in the recent literature. In children, the condition usually presents with airway obstruction. Adult patients usually present with sudden severe sore throat. Respiratory distress may occasionally be the presenting symptoms. Children suspected to have the condition should be taken to the operation theatre immediately for direct laryngoscopy under general anaesthesia. Both the anaesthetist and the surgeon should be experienced to deal with the paediatric airway. If the diagnosis is confirmed, endotracheal intubation should be performed and the patient be observed in the intensive care unit. In adult patients without respiratory distress, the diagnosis should be confirmed by mirror examination or flexible laryngoscopy. Carefully performed, these examinations will not precipitate airway obstruction. It is safer to have a correct diagnosis by a gentle examination. In adult patients with respiratory distress, they should be treated as in the case of children. Adult patients with supraglottitis and stable airway should be observed in intensive care unit where facilities and expertise for endotracheal intubation is readily available. Tracheostomy is not needed in most cases as prolonged intubation is unlikely. The pathogens associated with the condition are more variable nowadays including various streptococcal species, anaerobes as well as Hib. The choice of antibiotics should be guided by the prevalence of pathogens and varies from place to place. In general, a second-generation cephalosporin is recommended as the initial treatment.

FOREIGN BODIES IN THE ENT

Aural foreign bodies

Foreign body in the ear typically entraps in the EAC. Diagnosis is usually straightforward. Foreign bodies may be classified as living insects, vegetable and inorganic materials. Living insect

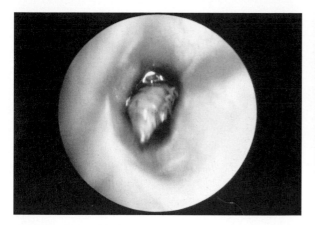

Figure 20.7. Cockroach in the EAC.

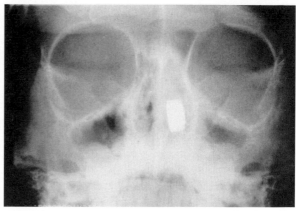

Figure 20.8. Plain X-ray of the nose showing a button battery in the left nasal fossa.

in the EAC (Fig. 20.7) is most disturbing. It should first be killed with a non-irritant eardrop such as olive oil, paraffin oil or cooking oil. The insect should then be removed by suction or by fine forceps. Vegetable foreign bodies are best removed by curettage and suction. Syringing is contraindicated as the foreign body may swell and subsequent removal is more difficult. Inorganic foreign bodies if diagnosed early may be removed with forceps, suction, syringing or curettage depending on their shape. Inorganic foreign bodies, being inert, can be left in the external canal for a long time without much symptoms. Foreign bodies left in the EAC can sometimes become very adherent to the canal skin and may require general anaesthesia for their removal. For young children or the mentally deranged individuals in general, whenever a foreign body is found in one ear, the other ear and perhaps the nostrils should also be checked. Simultaneous multiple foreign bodies may rarely be present. Multiple attempts at removing any foreign body in an uncooperative patient is inadvisable as tympanic membrane perforation and ossicular chain injury may occur. Under this circumstance, general anaesthesia may be warranted.

Nasal foreign bodies

Nasal foreign body occurs almost exclusively in young children and mentally deranged individuals. Live insects are extremely rare to enter the nose probably because of the nasal airflow, high humidity and the heat inside the nose. Thus common nasal foreign bodies are either vegetable or inorganic matters. Most foreign bodies present as such and diagnosis is simple. Vegetable foreign bodies are irritant to the nose and induce a strong local reaction. In the absence of a definite history, they usually present with unilateral obstruction and foul smelling nasal discharge for weeks or months that respond poorly to conservative treatment. Inorganic nasal foreign bodies, being inert, may present as rhinoliths with non-specific nasal symptoms for years. Whenever the diagnosis is in doubt,

nasendoscopy should be performed. Nasal foreign bodies should always be removed with a blunt hook. The hook should be lubricated with K-Y jelly and be passed upside the foreign body. The movement of the hook should always be towards the floor and the front of the nose in order to avoid pushing the foreign body further backward. Multiple attempts should be avoided especially in struggling patients otherwise the foreign body may be dislodged and inhaled. General anaesthesia should be used instead.

Button battery nasal foreign body (Fig. 20.8) deserves special mention because significant damage may occur if it is left for any length of time. As a result of the contour of the nose, the poles of button battery will fit tightly between the septum and the inferior turbinate. Four types of injury may occur resulting in serious morbidity:

1. Mechanical injury may occur due to the tight mucosal contact.
2. Electrical injury may arise as the battery is short circuited by contact with the moist nasal mucosa.
3. Electrochemical injury may occur as electric current passes through the mucosa causing electrolysis.
4. Chemical injury may occur due to leakage of chemical from the battery.

It is the author's observation that the maximum damage done to the nose always corresponds to the side in contact with the negative pole and this happens with both new and old battery. We believe the most significant damage occur as a result of chemical injury. In order to avoid serious injury (such as septal perforation, alar collapse), this type of foreign body should be removed without any delay. A course of antibiotic should always be used afterwards. Although there are no scientific proof, a short course of systemic steroid may also be helpful.

Ingested foreign bodies

As a result of the eating habit, ingested foreign bodies are extremely common amongst the Chinese. The presentation

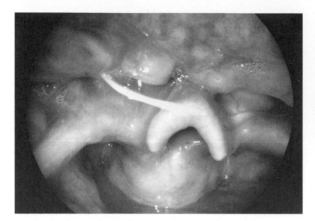

Figure 20.9. Fish bone in the tongue base.

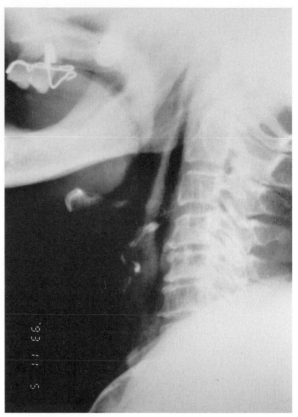

Figure 20.10. Plain X-ray of the neck showing free gas in the retro-pharyngeal space due to perforation of the oesophagus after oesophagoscopy.

varies depending on whether the patients can make a clear complaint. Thus in the prelingual children and in the mentally retarded patients, the presentations may be refusal of feed, vomiting or they may present with complication such as a neck abscess. Otherwise patients always present with foreign body sensation immediately following the episode of foreign body ingestion. The commonest foreign body ingested is fish bone (Fig. 20.9). Others include pig's bone, chicken bone, skeleton of shrimps and lobsters, etc. The commonest metallic foreign body is coin.

A careful history is very useful both in making a diagnosis and localization of the foreign body. Symptoms that lateralize to one side and localize at a site at or higher than the cricoid are usually very accurate. Symptom that migrates downward is pathonomonic of an ingested foreign body.

There will be hardly any physical signs in the uncomplicated cases. Therefore, the purpose of physical examination is to confirm or exclude the presence of any foreign body. Larger and more blunt foreign bodies, for example coins, chicken or pig's bone tend to be trapped by the narrowest part of the upper aerodigestive tract at the cricopharyngeus. Smaller and sharp foreign bodies such as fish bone may be impacted anywhere from the tonsils, tongue base to anywhere down the oesophagus. Most of the impacted foreign bodies will be found on clinical examination with a tongue depressor or a laryngeal mirror. When no foreign body is found, a direct flexible pharyngolaryngoscopy should be performed. This gives a better and dynamic view of the hypopharynx as the patients are instructed to phonate and swallow. Most ingested foreign bodies can be removed by simple means with a pair of Tilly's forceps or with flexible laryngoscopy. Oesophagoscopy may occasionally be required to remove foreign bodies. Rigid oesophagoscopy gives a better view of the cervical oesophagus while flexible oesophagoscopy is preferred below the thoracic inlet.

The usefulness of a plain lateral X-ray of the neck depends on the type of foreign body and the site of impaction. Thick bones like chicken bone, pig's bone, pigeon's bone, etc. are radio-opaque and will readily be picked up by a plain X-ray. Similarly, metallic foreign bodies such as coins will be clearly shown on plain X-rays. Most fish bones are radiolucent and therefore can easily be missed by plain X-rays. When foreign bodies are impacted above the cricopharyngeus, radiological investigations will not be as accurate as clinical examination. Foreign bodies impacted below the thoracic inlet is difficult to be shown on plain X-rays as the view will inevitably be overlapped by the vertebrae and the thoracic skeleton. The cervical oesophagus is the only segment of the upper digestive tract that plain X-rays are reliable enough to be clinically useful.

Complications of 'ingested foreign bodies' may arise as a result of the impaction or passage of the foreign bodies. They can also be iatrogenic from attempts to remove the foreign bodies. These include perforation of the pharynx or oesophagus (Fig. 20.10), retropharyngeal or mediastinal abscesses. Coexisting fever and leucocytosis should be taken as warning signs of a potential serious complication. Surgical emphysema either clinical or radiological is diagnostic of a perforation in the pharynx or oesophagus.

EPISTAXIS

Epistaxis is an extremely common complaint, it is estimated that up to 60% of people will experience one episode in their lifetime with 6% requiring medical attention. The underlying cause should be sought whenever possible in order to apply treatment logically. In the majority of the cases, however, the bleeding is idiopathic. When a cause can be identified, epistaxis is usually secondary to nasal trauma, a local nasal pathology, a blood vessel abnormality or a blood dyscrasia.

Isolated mild epistaxis probably requires no specific treatment. However, if this happens in an adult patient, a careful examination of the nose and nasopharynx should be performed, so that a tumour will not be missed. For patients with recurrent epistaxis, the primary cause, if identified, should be treated. Systemic causes should be treated medically and local causes controlled with local measures. The commonest local cause is due to self-inflicted injury to some engorged vessels in the Little's area. Chemical cautery of the vessels in the Little's area under topical anaesthesia is a useful measure. Sometimes if the bleeding is more profuse, electrocautery should be used instead.

For patients with severe epistaxis, the initial management aims to control the bleeding. Attempts should be made to stop anterior nasal bleeding with an anterior nasal pack while for posterior bleeding, balloon tamponade is more effective. When balloon tamponade is used, the pressure should be adjusted to the minimum required to arrest the bleeding. When nasal packs are used for more than 48 h, it is advisable to give prophylactic antibiotics. It is only in the most unusual situation will surgery may require to stop bleeding or to prevent recurrent epistaxis.

Surgical treatment for epistaxis is controversial with many options being available. The controversy relates more to the timing and what type of surgical intervention than how to perform a particular operation. In general surgical intervention is indicated when there is bleeding of any of the following type:
- continuous bleeding despite adequate conservative management;
- re-bleeding immediately after nasal packs are removed;
- frequent and significant re-bleeding.

Surgical intervention can be logically considered in three steps: identification of the bleeding source; surgery for local control of bleeding and arterial ligation.

Identification of the bleeding source

Although the cause of epistaxis may not be found, the site of bleeding should not be difficult to identify. Nowadays with modern endoscopes and the necessary accessories the nose can be adequately examined even in the presence of active bleeding. When the source of bleeding is found, a more logical approach to management can be planned.

Surgery for local control of bleeding

This part in the management of epistaxis has largely been neglected. In fact, there is a lot to be done for local control if the source of bleeding can be localized. Most of the bleeding vessels inside the nose are within 1 mm and should easily be controlled with diathermy. Occasionally, a septal spur may need to be removed before the bleeding point will become accessible. If the bleeding point is in the nasopharynx or at the back of the nasal septum, the combined approach to the nasopharynx may be employed.

Arterial ligation

Arterial ligation, although not cause specific, is an effective means of epistaxis control and should be considered when: rapid control of epistaxis is critical; other methods to control the bleeding have failed or there is recurrent severe epistaxis. The aim of arterial ligation for the control of epistaxis is to lower the perfusion pressure so that bleeding will stop or may be stopped more easily by local measures.

In general, the more distal the site of ligation the more effective the procedure as the development of anastomotic channels will be less likely. The decision to ligate an individual artery or a combination of arteries will depend on whether the site of bleeding is identified or not. A clear understanding of the principle of arterial ligation and the blood supply of the nose is necessary. When the bleeding is from the roof of the nose, the ethmoidal arteries should be dealt with first. On the other hand, when the bleeding is from the lower part of the nasal fossa or the lateral nasal wall, the maxillary or the external carotid artery should be ligated. When the bleeding is profuse and the source is poorly localized a combination of arteries from both systems may need to be ligated.

The external carotid artery can be ligated in the neck close to its origin. This approach has the advantage of being a simple procedure. The external carotid is identified by demonstrating at least two of its branches. It is then doubly ligated in continuity with O silk distal to its lingual branch. Although complications are rare, however, blindness may occur if the ophthalmic artery originates from the middle meningeal branch of the external carotid artery.

The tributaries of the maxillary artery to the nose begin in the pterygopalatine fossa. This can be approached transantrally and is the ideal site to ligate the maxillary artery and its branches to the nose. As the main trunk of the maxillary artery comes from a deeper aspect than its branches, it can occasionally be missed. The infra-orbital branch may be mistaken for the main trunk of the maxillary artery. Complications are uncommon, although isolated cases of total ophthalmoplegia have been reported in the literature.

The internal carotid system contributes much less to the nasal blood supply than the external carotid. The anterior and posterior ethmoidal arteries, both being derived from the ophthalmic artery, are conveniently reached in the orbit.

The anterior ethmoidal artery is the larger of the two and contributes more to the blood supply of the nose. In many instances, only the anterior ethmoidal artery requires ligation. The ethmoidal vessels perforate the medial orbital wall into the anterior and posterior ethmoidal canal, respectively, at or close to the fronto-ethmoidal suture. The anterior ethmoidal artery will be encountered at a distance about 1.5–2 cm from the lacrimal fossa. The posterior ethmoidal artery will be encountered about 0.5–1 cm further back. The anterior ethmoidal artery can be absent in as high as 14% of cadaver dissections unilaterally and 2.5% bilaterally. This is especially important to bear in mind if both the anterior and posterior ethmoidal arteries are to be clipped. The optic nerve may then be mistaken as the posterior ethmoidal artery and clipped resulting in blindness.

Transnasal endoscopic ligation

Endoscopic endonasal surgery is gaining popularity nowadays. Transnasal endoscopic ligation of the sphenopalatine artery has been reported with good result for epistaxis control. This is particularly useful for the prevention of recurrent epistaxis. In patients with active profuse bleeding, any endoscopic surgery will be extremely difficult if not impossible. The technique itself is simple. The middle meatus is cleared by performing an uncinectomy, the ethmoidal bulla is removed if prominent. The natural maxillary ostium is identified and enlarged if necessary so as to allow visualization of the posterior antral wall. A convenient vertical mucosal incision is made just in front of the imaginary medial projection of the posterior antral wall. The sphenopalatine artery should then be easily identified and clipped as it passes medially from the sphenopalatine foramen.

Hereditary haemorrhagic telangiectasia

Epistaxis requiring surgery in most patients arises from arterial bleeding. However, in the case of hereditary haemorrhagic telangiectasia epistaxis is due to both arterial and capillary bleeding. Results of any form of therapy, including arterial ligation are poor. These patients usually require a combination of arterial ligation (or embolization) together with local control. It is important to cause as little mucosal damage as possible as there is always need for repeated local therapy. A proactive approach is advisable, it is much more effective to treat and cauterize potential bleeding points regularly than to tackle major epistaxis once in a while. Both the carbon dioxide (CO_2) and potassium titanyl phosphate (KTP) lasers have proved useful in the management of this condition.

ENDOSCOPY OF THE ENT

Modern endoscopes are equipped with excellent optics and designed for ease of handling. There is a choice between the flexible fibrescope or the rigid rod endoscope. The fibrescope, being flexible, can overcome long curvy passage and always give you an undistorted end-on view. The rigid rod endoscopes, on the other hand, give a better picture and can be controlled with one hand. Coupled with camera and recording system, they can be used for diagnosis, treatment, monitoring and documentation of disease. With suitable instrument, the ENT are all accessible to direct endoscopy.

Otoscopy

A 4-mm wide-angled rigid rod endoscope is preferred. Earwax may need to be removed if it is in the way; otherwise, there is no need for any local preparation. The tip of the endoscope should be treated with anti-fog solution before use. The EAC should be straightened by pulling the pinna outward, backward and upward while the otoscope is being introduced under vision. There is no need to go deep in the EAC as long as the whole eardrum can be visualized. It is important to set the light intensity low, otherwise the heat generated at the tip of the endoscope may induce a caloric effect and the patient may complain of vertigo.

Nasendoscopy

Both the nasal cavity and nasopharynx are accessible to direct endoscopy. In any case, the procedure should be performed under topical anaesthesia both for patient's comfort and to enable a biopsy to be taken if necessary. Adequate surface anaesthesia and vasoconstriction can be achieved by applying cotton pledgets soaked in 5% cocaine solution or a mixture made up of 4% xylocaine with 1 in 10 000 adrenaline.

A narrow end-viewing flexible fibrescope is most versatile and suited for this examination. It gives an undistorted view and provides the flexibility required to inspect the area in detail. Alternatively a rigid 4 mm 0° wide-angled (viewing angle greater than 110°) rod endoscopes are also suitable for direct inspection of the nose and nasopharynx. When the depth of the nasal meati or the spheno-ethmoidal recess need to be examined in details, a 30° wide-angled nasendoscope should be used. Most pathologies of the nose and nasopharynx can easily be picked up this way. However, as the view of the nasopharynx obtained with this antegrade approach is from front to back, the depths of the fossae of Rosenmüller will be hidden by the inwardly projecting Eustachian cushions. A simple manoeuvre, by asking the patient to say 'ah' (mouth sound), 'ng' (nasal sound) and then to swallow (opening and closing the Eustachian tube) will expose and obviate any small lesion in the fossae of Rosenmüller for inspection.

The nasopharynx can also be examined by transoral retrograde nasopharyngoscopy with either a 70° or 90° endoscope. This technique is technically more demanding but it provides a paramount wide-angled view of the entire nasopharynx with superb clarity of detail. As the view obtained is centred from below and behind, the fossae of Rosenmüller on both sides are wide open for evaluation.

Pharyngolaryngoscopy

The larynx and the pharynx are intimately related both anatomically and functionally. They are normally evaluated together. Transnasal flexible endoscopy with the fibrescope is ideal for this purpose. The endoscope should be well lubricated with K-Y jelly for ease of passage through the nose. In sensitive patients, the nasal mucosa may be similarly prepared as for nasendoscopy. Gag reflex is usually not a problem, should it happen, the oropharynx and hypopharynx may be treated with a few puffs of 10% xylocaine spray. The examination is usually straightforward and pathologies easily picked up. However, some cul-de-sac areas need some simple manoeuvers to be examined in details. The valecullae for example can only be clearly visualize when the patient protrudes the tongue forward. Similarly, the pyriform fossae open up fully only when the patient is phonating a high-pitch sound. When the procedure is performed for therapeutic purpose such as removal of an impacted foreign body, an instrument with a working channel and an assistant is necessary.

HEAD AND NECK TUMOURS

Successful management of head and neck tumours requires early detection, correct histological diagnosis and a thorough understanding of the biological behaviour of the tumour. For malignant lesions, a multidisciplinary approach provides the best care. A head and neck tumour conference involving the head and neck surgeon, otolaryngologist, plastic surgeon, neurosurgeon, oncologist, radiotherapist, radiologist and pathologist offers the best environment for interdisciplinary review and interaction.

Skin

The skin is the largest organ of the body. The head and neck region, being largely exposed and susceptible to the carcinogenic effect of sunlight (ultraviolet light A and B), is the site of most skin cancers.

Seborrhoeic keratoses

These are benign superficial, brown-black hyperkeratotic lesions that are commonly present on the sun-exposed face as multiple raised, thickened plaques of variable sizes that may mimic a mole or a melanoma. Treatment is by electrosurgery and curettage. Occasionally, excisional biopsy is warranted to exclude melanoma.

Actinic keratoses (solar keratoses)

These are small, erythematous, scaly papules commonly found on the sun-exposed face. Biopsy shows hyperkeratoses and parakeratoses with dysplasia in the epidermis. About 5% progress to squamous cell carcinoma. Treatment is preferably by cryosurgery or excision.

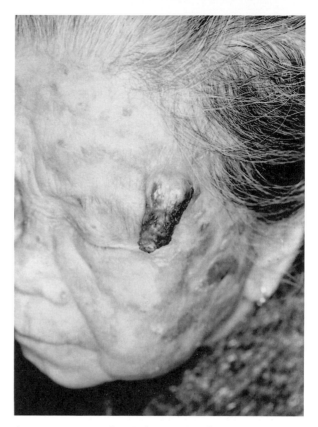

Figure 20.11. Cutaneous horn with squamous cell carcinoma in the base.

Cutaneous horn

The clinical term 'cutaneous horn' is a hard, horn-like growth that may develop from the base of an actinic keratoses, seborrhoeic keratoses (benign superficial, brown-black hyperkeratotic lesions) or squamous cell carcinoma. Therefore, nodular growth in the base of cutaneous horn usually represents squamous cell carcinoma (Fig. 20.11). Treatment is by surgical excision.

Bowen's disease

Bowen's disease is squamous cell carcinoma *in situ* (cytological atypia confined to epidermis). This commonly presents as a circumscribed scaling erythematous patch. About 10% develop into invasive squamous cell carcinoma and therefore should be surgical excised.

Lentigo maligna melanoma (Hutchinson's freckle)

This is melanoma *in situ* (Clark's Level I). The treatment is surgical excision with clear margin.

Keratoacanthoma

This is a common, rapidly enlarging nodular skin growth with central keratinous crater that occurs mainly on sun-exposed areas in the elderly. Excisional biopsy is required to distinguish it from squamous cell carcinoma.

Naevus sebaceous of Jodassohn

A warty epidermal naevus typically occurring in or near the scalp region. It can give rise to appendiceal tumours, basal cell carcinoma and, occasionally, squamous cell carcinoma in adulthood. Full-thickness surgical excision is usually required. For selected thin lesions, CO_2/erbium laser resurfacing can be attempted.

Basal cell carcinoma

Basal cell carcinoma is the commonest skin cancer. It can present as an ulcer (rodent ulcer), a nodule, a black-pigmented lesion or an erythematous patch (sclerosing or morpheaform). For basal cell carcinoma of the face, treatment is preferably by surgical excision with frozen section evaluation of the excised margins or Moh's surgery (microscopically controlled excision with radial and vertical fresh tissue sections for clearance of tumour margin). A microscopic surgical margin of 1 mm is acceptable. A cure rate of 98% or more is expected when surgical margins are clear. Cryosurgery is only suitable for small superficial basal cell carcinoma.

Squamous cell carcinoma

Squamous cell carcinoma of skin is more directly related to ultraviolet radiation than basal cell carcinoma. Other predisposing factors or conditions include radiation, chemical exposure (arsenic and organic hydrocarbons), burn scars and non-healing venous ulcers. *Verrucous carcinoma* is a low-grade or well-differentiated squamous cell carcinoma of skin or mucus membrane that presents as an exophytic verrucous, keratotic mass that grows slowly. It may involve the skin as well as the mucus membrane of the oral cavity (Fig. 20.12). Superficial biopsy typically shows hyperkeratoses and histological evidence of malignancy can only be diagnosed from the entire excised mass. Therefore, treatment by surgical excision should be undertaken based on clinical correlation. Squamous cell carcinoma should be treated by excision with at least 1 cm margins and clinically detected regional metastasis should be treated by radical or modified radical neck dissection.

Melanoma

Melanoma peaks at age 20–45 years, typically in fair-skinned persons with a history of severe sunburn. Other risk factors are past history of melanoma and family histories of melanoma and dysplastic naevi. Clinical types are superficial spreading melanoma, nodular melanoma and acral lentiginous melanoma (occurring in palm, sole, nail bed and mucus membrane). If possible, total excisional biopsy is preferred.

The extent of treatment, risk of regional metastasis, risk of recurrence and overall prognosis is dependent on tumour thickness which is best determined by Breslow scale on

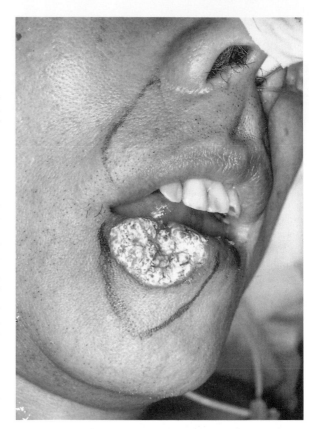

Figure 20.12. Verrucous carcinoma of the lower lip.

the biopsy specimen:
- minimum risk <0.76 mm;
- low risk 0.76–1.50 mm;
- intermediate risk 1.51–4.0 mm;
- high risk >4.0 mm.

Historically, Clarks levels of histological invasion also predict prognosis:
- *Level I*: *In situ*, above papillary dermis.
- *Level II*: Penetrates papillary dermis.
- *Level III*: Involves papillary dermis.
- *Level IV*: Enters reticular dermis.
- *Level V*: Enters subcutaneous fat.

Treatment is by surgical excision of skin and subcutaneous tissue with 1.5–3 cm of margin depending on the site and thickness of the melanoma. The best data available show no difference in outcome between removing the underlying fascia and not. Elective regional lymph node dissection is optional for tumour thickness over 1.5 mm. For lesions arising in the temporal or upper cheek area, total parotidectomy as well as neck dissection may be required to treat adequately regional nodal metastases. In recent years, sentinel node biopsy is increasingly accepted for melanoma over 1.5 mm in thickness.

Merkel cell carcinoma

This is an uncommon neuroendocrine tumour occurring in the face and neck of elderly patients. It is an aggressive dermal nerve cell tumour that has a propensity for regional and distant metastasis. Treatment is wide surgical excision with consideration for regional lymph node dissection or sentinel node biopsy. Post-operative radiotherapy can also be considered.

Sentinel lymph node biopsy

In recent years, sentinel lymph node (SLN) mapping and biopsy have been well established for intermediate to thick melanoma and clinically node-negative breast cancer. In a study of 114 patients (from Emory University School of Medicine) with thick melanoma (≥4 mm), 32.5% had a positive SLN biopsy, half of which had a single-positive lymph node after dissection. The overall 3-year survival for SLN-negative patients was 82% versus 57% for node-positive patients.

Typical SLN mapping technique involves peri-tumour injections of 10–40 mbq (99 m) Technetium labelled albumin colloid. Lymphoscintigraphy with dynamic and static imaging followed in the antero-posterior and lateral projections. Vital blue dye may also be added during surgery. Typically 1–2 ml of 2.5% patent blue dye or isosulfan blue dye was injected around the tumour. Hand held gamma probe was used to identify and remove blue-stained lymph nodes with small incisions. The SLN may be identified by dye alone, gamma probe alone or a combination of both. If SLN is not successfully identified (vary from 1 to 5 in number), traditional regional lymph node dissection may be considered. SLN biopsy is a minimally invasive procedure for patients at risk of harbouring subclinical regional metastasis. Frozen section may be used to provide prompt evaluation of the disease status of excised lymph nodes.

Currently, the role of positron emission tomography (PET) using (18)F-flusoo-deoxy-glucose (FDG) and sentinel node imaging and biopsy in the preoperative staging of the clinically node-negative neck in patients with oral squamous cell carcinoma are under active investigation. Early results suggested that sentinel node imaging and biopsy with probe and patent blue dye-guided harvest may be more useful than (18)F-FDG PET scan in identifying true disease status of the regional lymphatics.

Scalp

The scalp has six anatomical layers: skin, subcutaneous layer, galea (aponeurosis), subgaleal layer and periosteum. All of the above tumours can occur in the scalp especially, if the scalp has long-standing sun exposure as a result of alopecia. In addition, carcinoma of skin appendages may arise from the scalp. *Carcinoma of sebaceous gland* can occur in the scalp as well as the eyelids. It usually presents as an ulcerated nodular mass. The scalp of the elderly is also a common site for *angiosarcoma* which typically presents as multifocal, superficial spreading purple patches and plaques that blanch on pressure.

The principle of surgical treatment of malignant scalp lesion is by excision of the entire full-thickness of involved scalp, including the periosteum. Extension of tumour into the bony calvarium calls for resection of the involved bone as well. Reconstruction is by split-thickness skin graft (the intact vascularized bone will allow a skin graft to take) or by rotation scalp flap.

Oral cavity and oropharynx

Anatomy

The oral cavity extends from the lips to the junction of the hard and soft palate above and to the circumvallate papillae of the tongue below and consists of six anatomical sites: lip, buccal mucosa, gum, floor of the mouth, hard palate and anterior two-thirds of the tongue (oral tongue). The oropharynx consists of the faucial arch (Waldeyer's ring), which includes the soft palate, uvula, tonsillar pillar, tonsillar fossa and tonsil, base of tongue and posterior pharyngeal wall (Fig. 20.13).

History

Strong predisposing factors for squamous cell carcinoma of the oral cavity and the upper aerodigestive tract include smoking and drinking of alcoholic beverages and the carcinogenic effects of these are additive. Other observed pre-disposing factors to oral cavity cancer include continuous trauma by ill-fitting dentures or sharp teeth, chewing of betel nuts or tobacco and regular use of alcohol-containing mouth washes.

Physical examination

The entire oral cavity should be thoroughly inspected with a good light and a tongue depressor paying attention to mucosal abnormalities arising from the various anatomical

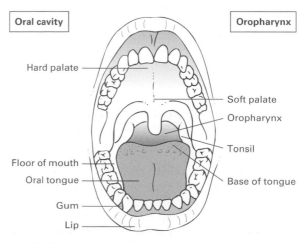

Figure 20.13. Anatomical sites of the oral cavity and oropharynx.

sites. The tonsils should be inspected. The oral tongue and base of the tongue should be palpated and bimanual examination should be done for the floor of the mouth and submandibular glands. The neck should be palpated systematically to look for enlarged lymph nodes, bearing in mind that oral cavity and oropharyngeal tumours tend to metastasize to submental, submandibular and upper jugular or jugulodigastric lymph nodes before spreading to lower level lymph nodes (mid- and lower jugular lymph nodes).

Diagnostic tests and procedures

Ultrasound examination of the neck is performed to detect nodal metastases. For a complex mucosal tumour or neck mass, CT or magnetic resonance imaging (MRI) will be more useful for clinical staging and treatment planning. High-resolution CT scanning with three-dimensional view is useful in delineating the local extent of the tumour in relationship to adjacent vascular and other important structures. Incisional or punch biopsy of mucosal lesions is usually required for diagnosis. Excisional biopsy is done for small lesions. FNA for cytology is routinely done for palpable neck nodes. This is usually carried out with a 21- or 23-G needle with the aspirated contents placed on a glass slide to make a smear or injected directly into 50% alcohol for examination by a cytopathologist. Excisional biopsy of a suspected malignant cervical node should be avoided unless lymphoma is suspected or when the primary remains unknown after a diligent search that includes panendoscopy (nasopharyngolaryngoscopy, esophagoscopy and bronchoscopy), CT or MRI and examination under general anaesthesia. A PET scan is very useful in detecting distant metastasis, recurrent cancer and in the search of an unknown primary with metastatic cervical lymph nodes.

Erythroplakia

Erythroplakia is defined as a red, erythematous, granular mucosal plaque or lesion that bleeds easily and is likely to represent the earliest sign of asymptomatic cancer. On biopsy, approximately 60% of erythroplakia contain *in situ* or invasive squamous cell carcinoma.

Leukoplakia

This is a clinical term which refers to any white plaque or patch of oral mucosa. Histology may reveal a wide variety of lesions ranging from inflammation, lichen planus dysplasia and micro invasive cancer. Those with dysplasia can be considered to be premalignant. Leukoplakia should be biopsied and those showing dysplasia excised with a cold knife or CO_2 laser.

Squamous cell carcinoma

Squamous cell carcinoma is the commonest (90%) malignancy of the upper aerodigestive tract (others are lymphoma,

adenocarcinoma arising from minor salivary glands and sarcoma). It presents typically as a painful ulcerative lesion or mass and has a propensity to metastasize to cervical lymph nodes as tumour volume increases.

The tumour, node, metastases (TNM) staging of oral cavity and oropharyngeal tumours is by size of primary tumour:
- T1 tumour <2 cm;
- T2 tumour <4 cm;
- T3 tumour >4 cm;
- T4 tumour >4 cm and with deep invasion to involve antrum, pterygoid muscles, root of tongue or skin of neck and extent of cervical nodal involvement:
- N0: no clinically positive node;
- N1: single-positive node >3 cm;
- N2: positive node >3 cm but <6 cm, or multiple-positive nodes, or bilateral/contralateral nodes;
- N3: positive node >6 cm.

Treatment

Treatment of early disease (T1 and early T2) by either surgery or radiation gives equivalent survival rates. However, most lesions are conveniently treated by surgery which is generally preferred by patients. Advanced disease (late T2, T3, T4 or clinically positive neck node) is best treated by surgery followed by post-operative radiotherapy.

The aim of surgical treatment is excision of the primary tumour with a 1–2 cm margin, with tumour clearance confirmed by frozen section. For access to posteriorly located tumours, lower cheek flap or mandibular swing (median mandibulotomy) may be required. Reconstruction of the surgical defect after resection of a large tumour may require a latissimus dorsi myocutaneous flap, pectoralis major myocutaneous flap or a free forearm flap with microvascular anatomosis of the radial artery and forearm vein to the recipient neck vessels (Figs 20.14 and 20.15). Surgical treatment of clinically positive neck nodes requires comprehensive neck dissection in the form of radical neck dissection or modified radical neck dissection. *Radical neck dissection* is *en bloc* removal of lymph node-bearing tissues in the submental, submandibular, upper jugular, mid-jugular, lower jugular and posterior triangle region along with the submandibular gland, internal jugular vein stern-ocleidomastoid muscle and the spinal accessory nerve.

Modified radical neck dissection differs from radical neck dissection in that the spinal accessory nerve is preserved to maximize shoulder function. The use of selective neck dissection in the form of *supraomohyoid neck dissection* (*en bloc* removal of submental, submandibular, upper- and mid-jugular node-bearing tissues) is limited to the management of a clinically negative neck, and confirmation of microscopic disease on frozen section generally requires conversion to a comprehensive neck dissection. The complication rate of radical neck dissection, even in the previously irradiated neck, is low and may include wound haematoma, wound infection, flap necrosis and, rarely, carotid artery

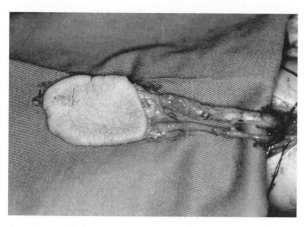

Figure 20.14. Free forearm flap based on the radial artery.

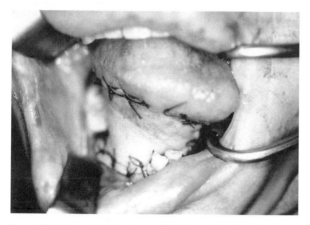

Figure 20.15. Reconstruction of a surgical defect of the floor of the mouth by free forearm flap.

rupture. When a myocutaneous or free flap is used for the reconstruction of oral cavity defect, orocutaneous fistula and partial or complete flap necrosis may occur.

Induction chemotherapy with 5-fluorouracil and cis-platinum may make surgical resection of a locally advanced tumour possible; concurrent chemotherapy and radiotherapy may also be of benefit to locally advanced tumour.

Typical 5-year survival rates for early disease (Stages I and II) is 60–80% and advanced disease (Stages III and IV) is 20–40%.

Minor salivary gland tumours

These tumours arise from the mucosal minor salivary glands distributed throughout the upper aerodigestive tracts. The majority of these minor salivary gland tumours are malignant and occur predominantly in the oral cavity. Adenoid cystic carcinomas make up over one-third of the minor salivary carcinomas. Other carcinomas include adenocarcinoma and mucoepidermoid carcinoma. These tumours have a low rate of cervical lymph node involvement but a high rate of distant metastasis. Their 5-year cure rates following surgical resection are typically lower than for a squamous carcinoma of the same site.

Nasopharynx

Anatomy

The nasopharynx serves as a conduit for air, nasal and paranasal sinus secretion, and is lined by squamous, respiratory and transitional epithelium. It lies above the level of the soft palate and posterior to the choanae (Fig. 20.16). The lateral wall consists of the Eustachian tube opening, the lateral

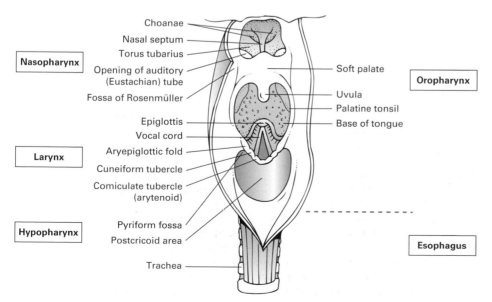

Figure 20.16. Anatomical sites of the nasopharynx, oropharynx, hypopharynx and larynx.

pharyngeal recess (fossa of Rosenmüller) and the cartilaginous medial end of the Eustachian tube (torus tubarius). The fossa of Rosenmüller is a cleft-like pouch lined by the pharyngobasilar fascia and it extends to the parapharyngeal space within which runs the internal carotid artery, internal jugular vein, cranial nerves IX–XII and the sympathetic nerve (Fig. 20.17).

Nasopharyngeal cancer

The first sign of NPC is often an enlarged metastatic cervical node in the posterior triangle. Common local signs and symptoms include nasal (blood-stained discharge, obstruction), aural (serous otitis media, tinnitus, conductive hearing loss) and neurological symptoms (diplopia due to abducen nerve paralysis). Diagnosis is by flexible fibreoptic nasopharyngoscopy and biopsy. Elevated blood levels of antibodies to Epstein–Barr virus capsid antigen (IgA-VCA) and early antigen (IgA-EA) are often seen. CT and MRI are useful in staging the disease and in detection of recurrence. Radiation is the first-line treatment for NPC of all stages because of the radiosensitivity of undifferentiated carcinoma. For recurrent disease after radiotherapy, surgical resection of the nasopharynx by the transoropalatal approach, mandibular swing or maxilla swing approach are recently established surgical salvage procedures that are preferred over re-irradiation which is associated with complications including radiation myelitis, encephalopathy, cranial nerve palsy, otitis media, hearing loss, trismus, cataract formation and osteoradionecrosis of the maxilla and mandible. For recurrent disease limited to the neck, radical neck dissection provides excellent control of the neck disease.

Juvenile nasopharyngeal angiofibroma

This is a benign but locally destructive vascular tumour of the nasopharynx occurring exclusively in boys. Surgical resection is facilitated by maxilla or mandibular swing.

Larynx and hypopharynx

Anatomy

The larynx consists of three single cartilages (epiglottis, thyroid cartilage and cricoid cartilage) and three smaller paired cartilages (cuneiform, corniculate and arytenoid cartilages). The larynx can be divided into three sub-sites: the supraglottic larynx consists of the epiglottis, aryepiglottic folds, arytenoids and ventricular bands (false cords); the glottic larynx consists of true vocal cords; and the subglottic larynx is the region below the glottis bounded by the cricoid cartilage (Fig. 20.17).

The recurrent laryngeal nerve innervates the vocal cord muscle and dysfunction results in hoarseness. The internal branch of the superior laryngeal nerve provides laryngeal and hypopharyngeal mucosal sensation and dysfunction may cause aspiration. The external branch of the superior laryngeal nerve innervates the cricothyroid muscle which is the tensor of the vocal cord and injury leads to a weak voice.

The hypopharynx extends from the level of the hyoid bone to the level of the cricoid cartilage. It emcompasses the pyriform sinus, the postcricoid area (posterior surface of the larynx) and the lower posterior pharyngeal wall. The cervical oesophagus is below the hypopharynx (Fig. 20.17).

Clinical evaluation

Vocal cord polyps and tumours may cause hoarseness. Large laryngeal tumours and infraglottic tumours cause airway obstruction. Hypopharyngeal tumours frequently cause dysphagia or pain on swallowing. Following examination of the neck and oral cavity, the larynx and upper portion of the hypopharynx is best examined by mirror examination (indirect laryngoscopy) and direct laryngoscopy by flexible fibreoptic nasopharyngolaryngoscopy which is done as an outpatient procedure. For more complete examination of the hypopharynx, direct laryngoscopy with rigid laryngoscope under general anaesthesia is required.

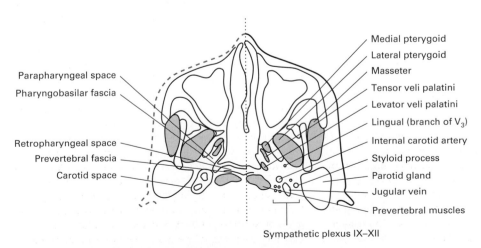

Figure 20.17. Parapharyngeal space at the level of the nasopharynx.

Panendoscopy

The term 'panendoscopy' means examination of the entire upper aerodigestive tract including the pharynx, larynx, oesophagus, trachea and bronchus with a combination of flexible and rigid laryngoscope, bronchoscope and oesophagoscope. Panendoscopy is essential in delineating the extent of deep-seated tumours, in the detection of a synchronous second primary and in searching for an unknown primary, causing cervical nodal metastasis.

Second primary

The risk of multiple primary tumours in the head and neck area is higher than elsewhere because of the field cancerization theory related to susceptibility of head and neck mucosa to common carcinogens (smoking and alcohol). Of 573 patients with squamous cell carcinoma of head and neck (lung cancer excluded) observed over a 4½ year period, 2.4% had multiple second primary carcinoma (69% with synchronous primary tumours) and 63% of all second primary tumours occurred in the oesophagus (Fig. 20.18).

Laryngeal papilloma

The *juvenile form* is believed to be acquired during birth from maternal vaginal warts. The condition does not manifest, however, until months or years later when significant papillomata develop. In general, those who present early usually present with airway obstruction, while older children usually present with progressive hoarseness. Treatment is extremely difficult and frequent recurrence is a rule rather than exception. At laryngoscopy, there is usually extensive involvement of the whole larynx; simultaneous tracheal and pharyngeal involvement by the papillomata is not uncommon. Repeated CO_2 laser therapy offers the best control of the disease. In severe cases, antiviral therapy including interferon therapy may be tried. Although the effectiveness of treatment is unpredictable, spontaneous regression of the papilloma may occur at any age.

The *adult form* typically presents with progressive hoarseness and laryngoscopy, and reveals either a solitary papilloma or multiple but discrete papillomata. These usually affect the true cord. Histologically, they are squamous papilloma and should be considered a premalignant lesion. The papilloma should be removed for histological evaluation and the base of the lesion treated with a CO_2 laser. The patient should refrain from smoking and be closely followed up for recurrence.

Laryngeal and hypopharyngeal cancer

Over 90% of these malignancies are squamous cell carcinoma. The remaining malignancies arise from minor salivary gland or from supporting tissue such as fibrosarcoma, chondrosarcoma and rhabdomyosarcoma. Early stage squamous cell carcinoma of the larynx is usually treated by external radiation. Early or intermediate stage supraglottic laryngeal carcinoma can be treated by conservation surgery (supraglottic subtotal laryngectomy) and localized glottic carcinoma can be treated by hemilaryngectomy. When there

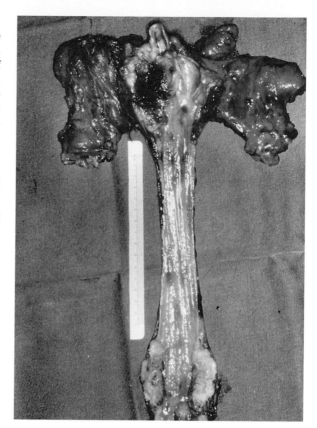

Figure 20.18. Patient with obstructing pyriform fossa squamous cell carcinoma requiring pharyngolaryngoesophagectomy and bilateral neck dissections. Surgical specimen revealed a synchronous oesophageal second primary.

is cord fixation or extension of disease into the hypopharynx or when hypopharynx cancer causes fixation of the hemilarynx, total laryngectomy is usually required. Hypopharyngeal cancer requires partial or total pharyngectomy in addition to laryngectomy. Reconstruction of the pharyngeal defect is by regional myocutaneous flap (based on the latissimus dorsi or the pectoralis major muscle), free forearm flap (Fig. 20.14), free jejunal segment or gastric pull up. Extrathoracic gastric pull up or colon interposition is required to reconstruct the oesophagus when total oesophagectomy is carried out for upper cervical oesophageal disease (Fig. 20.18). Voice rehabilitation is by learning oesophageal speech, use of an electrolarynx or by creation of a tracheo-oesophageal fistula for insertion of a Blom–Singer prosthesis. Advanced stage laryngeal/hypopharyngeal cancer often requires concomitant neck dissection for a clinically positive neck followed by postoperative radiotherapy. Induction chemotherapy with 5-fluorouracil and cis-platinum in selected patients may allow preservation of the larynx since complete response to chemotherapy may allow the patient to proceed to radiotherapy without undergoing surgery.

Tracheostomy

Tracheostomy is indicated for airway control after major oropharyngeal surgery, especially when the mandible continuity is disrupted, and in severe maxillofacial trauma to prevent aspiration of blood. A transverse skin incision is preferred. With retraction of the thyroid isthmus upward, the pretracheal fascia is incised in order for a transverse incision to be made between the second and third tracheal rings. Initial tracheostomy care includes humidification and frequent suctioning. The tracheostomy tube is usually changed after the first 5 days when the track in the subcutaneous tissue is established.

Cricothyroidotomy

In an urgent situation, a cricothyroidotomy allows quick access to the airway by insertion of a small size tracheostomy tube through the cricothyroid membrane into the trachea. To avoid subglottic stenosis, a formal tracheostomy should be performed within 24 h.

Paranasal sinuses

Of paranasal sinus tumours, 80% occur in the maxillary sinus with the rest arising from the ethmoid, frontal and sphenoid sinuses. The maxillary sinuses are lined by ciliated columnar epithelium and the majority of the malignant epithelial neoplasms are squamous cell carcinoma. Oral signs and symptoms appear early while nasal obstruction and bloody nasal discharge are late symptoms. Invasion of the orbit is associated with ocular signs, including unilateral proptopsis and diplopia. Anterior extension leads to facial asymmetry and deformity. Extension of tumour posteriorly leads to destruction of the pterygoid plates and invasion of the infratemporal fossa. There may be unilateral deafness and facial palsy. Both axial and coronal CT scans are required to define the extent of the paranasal tumour since extension of tumour to adjacent sinuses and structures are common due to delay in presentation and in diagnosis.

Localized tumour can be successfully treated by subtotal maxillectomy, including the orbital floor, hard palate and lower pterygoid plates. Rehabilitation with dental prosthesis is required. For cancer extending to or arising from the ethmoid sinus, a craniofacial resection is required safely to resect the roof of the ethmoid sinus (i.e. the cribriform plate). For extensive malignant tumours not amenable to curative surgical resection, palliation by combined chemotherapy and external radiotherapy may give useful control of the disease. Regional metastasis is uncommon at presentation and distant metastasis is rare.

Esthesioneuroblastoma

This is a neurogenic tumour of the olfactory region. It may involve the nasal turbinate, paranasal sinuses or cribriform plate. It can extend intracranially and metastasize to cervical nodes or to distant sites. Surgical resection by craniofacial resection offers the best chance of cure.

Neck masses

History

Age group is important. Congenital lesions are more likely to occur in children, whereas in the adult, persistent cervical lymphadenopathy represents malignancy until proven otherwise. Inflammatory lesions may have a history of recent onset, rapid increase in size and pain. Tuberculosis (TB) is associated with fever and night sweats. Whereas, upper aerodigestive malignancy is usually associated with chronic intake of alcoholic products and smoking, and there may be symptoms of hoarseness, haemoptysis, dysphagia and weight loss.

Physical examination

A complete head and neck examination and a general examination should be carried out. The emphasis of the latter is the detection of peripheral lymphadenopathy, hepatosplenomegaly and abdominal mass. Initial head and neck examination includes examination of the oral cavity and oropharynx by direct inspection. The neck is palpated to note the location, size, consistency, mobility, surface topography and tenderness of the mass. Associated lymphadenopathy or thyromegaly is noted.

Investigations

If an inflammatory cause is considered, a complete blood count and sedimentation rate are obtained. In patients who are at risk of developing NPC, blood levels of IgA-VCA and IgA-EA are determined. When the neck mass is consistent with lymphadenopathy, flexible fibreoptic nasopharyngolaryngoscopy is carried out to look for a possible head and neck primary. Any suspicious mucosal lesions should be biopsied. FNA can be carried out on all neck masses, including salivary gland tumours. Exceptions are pulsatile masses with bruit which may represent high-flow carotid body tumour, arteriovenous malformation and haemangioma. The aspirate is sent for cytology and, for suspected inflammatory lesions, is also sent for Gram and Ziehl Nissen stain for acid–fast bacilli. Plain X-ray is not used in the routine evaluation of a neck mass. The neck mass is best studied by an ultrasound examination which can confirm the anatomical location of the mass, its composition (cystic or solid) and relationship to adjacent structures as well as associated lymphadenopathy in the neck. More sophisticated imaging such as CT scan, MRI and digital angiography are indicated in the evaluation of a complex mass or a suspected vascular lesion. The diagnosis of a haemangioma can also be established by red blood cell (RBC) scintigraphy, using sodium pertechnetate radioisotope.

The long list of differential diagnosis for neck mass can be simplified by considering four major categories:
1. congenital;
2. inflammatory (viral, bacterial, fungal, granulomatous);
3. neoplastic (benign, malignant);
4. miscellaneous (Zenker's diverticulum).

Congenital masses

Common congenital neck masses include thyroglossal duct cyst, branchial cyst, cystic hygroma, teratoma (mostly in infants) and haemangioma.

Thyroglossal duct cyst

The thyroglossal duct cyst originates from the epithelial remnants of the thyroglossal tract and therefore is typically located in the midline between the isthmus of the thyroid gland and the foramen caecum of the tongue base. It can be at, below or above, the level of the hyoid bone. The typical thyroglossal duct cyst moves with swallowing and protrusion of the tongue because of its adherence to the hyoid bone and adjacent strap muscles. It may or may not have a ductal connection to the tongue base. Ultrasound examination is useful in ruling out ectopic thyroid and in confirming the presence of a normal thyroid gland in the lower neck. Treatment is by Sistrunk's operation (excision of entire cyst with a small central segment of hyoid bone and any ductal connection to the tongue base). Small thyroglossal duct cysts with no history of infection can be observed as the risk of malignant change is well under 1%.

Branchial cyst

During the fifth embryonic week, the branchial apparatus, which is phylogenetically related to the primitive fill slits, develops into five paired mesodermic arches separated by four pairs of invaginations of ectoderm and endoderm known, respectively, as branchial clefts and pouches. Each branchial arch develops into cartilage, artery, nerve and muscles. Branchial anomalies in the form of a cyst, sinus (communicates to the viscera or skin) or fistula (communicates to both skin and viscera) can form from vestigial remnants of branchial pouches and clefts. Branchial anomalies are lined by squamous epithelium or respiratory epithelium or both. First branchial anomalies are rare and are of two types. A type I lesion is usually postauricular in location (commonly mistaken as postauricular sebaceous cyst) and represents a duplication of both membranous and cartilaginous portions of the EAC. A type II lesion typically presents as a cyst or sinus in the preauricular or upper neck with the fistula tract intimately related to the parotid gland and the facial nerve. Second branchial anomalies commonly present as a cyst in mid-neck (Fig. 20.19). It may course between the external and internal carotid artery and may reach the tonsillar fossa. Third branchial lesions are uncommon. They present lower in the neck and may track posterior to the internal carotid artery to exit near the pyriform fossa. In children, an inflamed third branchial cyst may present clinically as acute thyroiditis. Differential diagnosis of a branchial cyst includes nodal metastasis of papillary carcinoma of thyroid or squamous carcinoma with cystic change and other inflammatory mass. Ultrasound examination and CT scan are useful to help differentiate branchial cyst anomalies from other conditions. Treatment of branchial anomalies is surgical excision. Surgical treatment of type II first branchial anomalies requires facial nerve dissection.

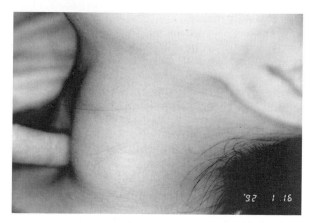

Figure 20.19. Large second branchial cyst.

Cystic hygroma

These are congenital malformations of lymphatic channels (lymphangioma) commonly occurring in the posterior neck. They are usually present at birth. They may be cystic or cavernous and the cavernous form tends to infiltrate diffusely adjacent tissues and structures. Surgical resection should be considered in childhood.

Teratomas and dermoid cysts

These are developmental cysts composed of trigeminal components foreign to the site of origin. In the head and neck region, true teratomas tend to arise from embryonic tissue near the primitive streak and notochord. According to Batsakis, teratomas include dermoid cyst and related cystic lesions (epidermoid or epidermal cyst, teratoid cyst and teratoma of the neck). *Epidermoid cyst* is lined by simple squamous epithelium, dermoid cyst is an epithelial-lined cavity with skin appendages, and *teratoid cyst* may contain squamous epithelium or ciliated respiratory epithelium. Dermoid cyst of the floor of the mouth may present in the midline submental area. Teratomas of the neck are commonly present at birth and the mass effect may be associated with respiratory distress and dysphagia. Therefore, surgical excision is always indicated. Malignant teratoma of the neck is rare.

Haemangioma

In the head and neck area, haemangioma typically present as diffuse, soft, subcutaneous masses that may gradually increase in size over many years. Unless localized, haemangioma is best treated conservatively once the diagnosis has been confirmed by ultrasound, CT scan or RBC scan. Haemangioma of skin (port-wine stain) can be treated by pulsed dye laser. Nodular or deep haemangioma can be treated by pulsed dye laser (585–590 nm) and/or long pulsed Nd : YAG laser (1064 nm) in multiple treatment sessions. Radiation should not be used for the treatment of haemangioma.

Inflammatory masses

Inflammatory neck masses include lymphadenitis of viral, bacterial, fungal and granulomatous aetiology as well as bacterial abscesses of the neck:

- In *viral lymphadenitis*, pharyngitis or tonsilitis have associated cervical nodal enlargement that is usually self-limiting, <1.5 cm in size and resolves in 2 weeks.
- *Infectious mononucleosis*, due to Epstein–Barr virus usually cause pharyngitis and cervical lymphadenopathy in older children and young adults. Monospot (heterophile agglutination) test is positive.
- *Bacterial lymphadenitis*, in children, streptococcal tonsillitis is commonly associated with cervical lymphadenitis. Peritonsillar abscess, odontogenic infections or bacterial lymphadenitis can lead to neck abscesses.
- *Ludwig's angina* is gangrenous cellulitis and abscess of the submandibular region that can progress to mediastinitis, empyema and death. Common causes are mandibular molar infection, floor of mouth perforation and extension of a peritonsillar abscess. Treatment is antibiotics and emergency surgical drainage.

Granulomatous lymphadenitis

In areas such as Asia where TB is largely still endemic, patients with *scrofula or cervicofacial myobacterial infections* commonly present with multiple tender, matted, posterior or supraclavicular lymph nodes that may progress to form 'cold abscesses'. Less than 10% of patients with scrofula have associated extranodal TB. When FNA of involved cervical node fails to yield acid–fast bacilli on Ziehl Nissen stain, incisional or excisional biopsy is required for diagnosis. A longer course of drug treatment than for pulmonary disease is usually required. *Actinomycosis* may cause persistent facial–cervical abscess and draining sinuses. It is caused by a bacterium with microaerophilic and anaerobic growth requirement. Typical sulphur granules (branching filaments with calcium phosphate) may be microscopically demonstrated. *Cat-scratch disease* is due to a cat scratch or bite. The cervical lymphadenitis is associated with a small rod-shaped bacillus. No specific treatment is required.

Neoplasms

Neoplasms can be benign or malignant. Malignant lesions can be primary or metastatic.

Benign neoplasms

These include thyroid tumours, salivary gland tumours and soft-tissue tumours (e.g. lipoma). Madelung's disease (multiple symmetrical lipomatosis) is a rare disease of unknown aetiology. Rarer benign tumours include paraganglioma, carotid body tumour, schwannoma (solitary-encapsulated nerve tumour) and neurofibroma (non-encapsulated, usually multiple).

Von Recklinghausen's disease is an inherited autosomal dominant trait. Affected patients have cafe-au-lait spots neurofibroma of the skin (multiple neurofibromatosis) and Lisch nodules (pigmented iris hamartomas). Acoustic neuroma and other tumours of the central nervous system can occur. *Carotid body tumours* arise from the paraganglion cells of the carotid body located at the bifurcation of the carotid artery. They are usually benign, firm, slow-growing masses that may occur bilaterally. The tumour may involve adjacent cranial nerves. Surgical excision by an experienced surgeon is recommended.

Angiolymphoid hyperplasia with eosinophilia (Kinura's disease)

This is an unusual soft-tissue tumour arising frequently in the parotid or submandibular area causing gradual nodular enlargement. In some patients, there is peripheral eosinophilia. Surgical excision is required to confirm the diagnosis and to rule out malignancy.

Fibromatosis

This is a group of aggressive fibroblastic proliferative lesions that is benign but locally infiltrative. The term fibromatosis is generally preferred over extra-abdominal desmoid.

Malignant neoplasms

Malignant causes of lymph node enlargement may be due to primary involvement by lymphoma or secondary involvement by head and neck primary (upper aerodigestive squamous cell carcinoma, salivary gland carcinoma and thyroid gland carcinoma) as well as by infraclavicular primary (breast, lung, stomach, colon, kidney and ovary). Ultrasound is useful in differentiating lymphoma and cervical metastatic lymph node.

Rarely, malignancy may arise from extranodal soft tissues of the neck (e.g. sarcoma and dermatofibrosarcoma protruberans).

Miscellaneous

Miscellaneous neck masses that may be palpable include *Zenker's diverticulum*, which is a herniation of pharyngeal mucosa through a weakness between the inferior constrictor muscle and the cricopharyngeous muscle. Symptoms include regurgitation of undigested food, dysphagia. Treatment is by surgical repair.

Kikuchi's disease

This is a self-limiting necrotizing lymphadenitis, possibly of autoimmune basis. Patient presents typically with non-tender, persistent cervical lymphadenopathy. Excision biopsy of the enlarged lymph node is required for diagnosis. Some patients may have associated lupus erythematosis; therefore, serology for anti-nuclear antibody and rheumatoid factor should be obtained.

Salivary gland disease

Salivary gland inflammation

Acute parotitis causing diffuse enlargement of the parotid gland may be due to viral infection (e.g. mumps) or bacterial infection. Submandibular sialadenitis is usually associated with obstruction of the Wharton's duct by calculus. *S. aureus* and *Streptococcus viridans* are the main pathogens. Intravenous antibiotic is required for the treatment of acute bacterial parotitis. Mycobacterial infection may also involve the parotid gland causing nodular enlargement. Chronic recurrent enlargement of bilateral parotid gland is seen in Sjögren's syndrome which is usually associated with keratoconjunctivitis sicca, xerostomia (dry mouth) and rheumatoid arthritis. Benign lymphoepithelial lesions and lymphoma may arise in a parotid gland affected by longstanding Sjögren's syndrome.

Salivary gland tumours

Benign and malignant salivary gland tumours can arise from the parotid gland, submandibular gland and rarely the sublingual gland. They typically present as a parotid or submandibular mass. Approximately 10% of parotid and 50% of submandibular gland tumours are malignant. Both ultrasound and FNA are useful in delineating the nature of the salivary gland lesions. A CT scan may be required to evaluate a complex mass such as deep lobe tumours and invasive tumours. Common benign tumours are *pleomorphic adenoma* and *Warthin's tumour (papillary cystadenoma lymphomatosum)*. Pleomorphic adenoma is usually rubbery firm in consistency and may recur if not excised with an adequate margin. Warthin's tumour may be bilateral and tends to occur in the elderly. *Malignant salivary gland tumours* include mucoepidermoid carcinoma, adenoid cystic carcinoma, acinic cell carcinoma, adenocarcinoma, undifferentiated carcinoma, squamous cell cacinoma and lymphoma. Metastases to the parotid gland can originate from the scalp, cheek, nasopharynx and oral cavity. Superficial parotidectomy via a preauricular incision is the recommended minimal surgical procedure. Open incisional biopsy should be avoided due to the concern for facial nerve damage and unsightly scarring. When malignancy is confirmed by intraoperative frozen section, total parotidectomy and sampling of the jugulodigastric lymph node are recommended. The facial nerve is preserved unless directly involved by the tumour. When the facial nerve or its major branches are scarified, a nerve graft is desirable. Radical neck dissection is necessary in the presence of clinically evident cervical nodal metastasis. Prognosis is dependent on the size and grade of the malignant tumour. For high-grade tumours, postoperative radiotherapy is recommended.

Parapharyngeal space tumours

The parapharyngeal space (lateral pharyngeal space) is a pyramid-shaped loose fascial plane around the pharynx

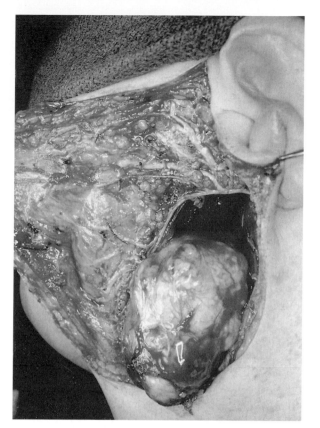

Figure 20.20. Pleomorphic adenoma of the deep lobe of the parotid gland being dissected out of the parapharyngeal space.

between the skull base and the hyoid bone (Figs 20.17 and 20.20). Tumours of the parapharyngeal space can present as an upper neck mass or submucosal oropharyngeal mass. They may be salivary gland tumours, neurogenic tumours, carotid body tumours, vascular tumours, lymphomas and miscellaneous soft-tissue tumours (e.g. lipoma). Treatment is surgical excision by transcervical or parotidectomy approach.

FURTHER READING

Choy ATK, Van Hasselt CA, Chisholm EM, Williams SR, King WWK, Li AKC. Multiple primary cancers in Hong Kong Chinese patients with squamous cell cancer of the head and neck. *Cancer* 1992; **20**: 815–820

Hughes GB (ed.). *Textbook of Clinical Otology.* New York: Georg Thieme Verlag, 1985

International Rhinitis Management Working Group. International Consensus Report on the Diagnosis and Management of Rhinitis. *Eur J Allergy Clin Immunol* 1994; **49**(Suppl.)

Kanski JJ. *Clinical Ophthalmology,* 3rd edn. London: Butterworth-Heinemann, 1994, pp. 1–150

King WWK. Head and neck cancer. *J HK Coll Radiol* 1998; **1**(Suppl. 2): 88–93

King WWK, Li AKC. Nasopharyngeal cancer. In: Morris PJ, Wood WC (eds), *Oxford Textbook of Surgery*, Vol. 3, 2nd edn. New York: Oxford University Press, 2000, pp. 2925–2937

King WWK, Teo PML, Li AKC. Patterns of failure after radical neck dissection for recurrent nasopharyngeal carcinoma. *Am J Surg* 1992; **164**: 599–602

King WWK, Ku PKM, Mok CO, Teo PML. Nasopharyngectomy in the treatment of recurrent nasopharyngeal carcinoma: a twelve year experience. *Head Neck* 2000; **5**: 215–222

Maran AGD (ed.). *Logan Turner's Diseases of the Nose Throat and Ear*. Rome and London: Butler & Tanner Ltd., 1988

McGuirt WF. Neck mass: patient examination and differential diagnosis. In: Cummings CW, Fredrickson JM, Harker LA, Krause CJ, Schiller DE (eds), *Otolaryngology – Head and Neck Surgery*, Vol. 2. CV Mosby: St. Louis, 1986

Mygind N, Lildholdt T (ed.). *Nasal Polyposis – An Inflammatory Disease and Its Treatment*. Munksgaard: Copenhagen, 1997

Rosenfeld RM, Bluestone CD (ed.). *Evidence-Based Otitis Media*. Hamilton London Saint Louis: B.C. Decker, 1999

Soo KC, Spiro RH, King W, Harvey W, Strong EW. Squamous carcinoma of gums. *Am J Surg* 1988; **156**: 281–285

Stammberger H (ed.). *Functional Endoscopic Sinus Surgery*. Philadelphia: B.C. Decker, 1991

Walters DAK, Ahuja AT, Evans RM, Chick W, King WWK, Metrewel C, Li AKC. Role of ultrasound in the management of thyroid nodules. *Am J Surg* 1992; **164**: 654–657

21

The Central Nervous System

James Palmer

Department of Neurological Surgery, Derriford Hospital, Plymouth, UK

CONTENTS

Anatomy	**415**
Brain	415
Cranial nerves	418
Cerebral arteries	420
Cerebral veins	421
Pituitary gland	422
Autonomic nervous system	422
Spinal cord	422
Neurophysiology	**423**
Cerebrospinal fluid	423
Cerebral circulation	423
Investigations	**424**
Imaging	424
Neurophysiological investigations	425
Further reading	**439**

ANATOMY

Brain

The *scalp* is extremely vascular with blood supply coming from the external carotid arteries; anteriorly from the superficial temporal arteries which are branches of the maxillary arteries and posteriorly the occipital arteries. Since these vessels enter the scalp from the base upwards towards the vertex and since the supply is very good, provided the location of these supplying vessels is borne in mind, scalp incisions can be made almost anywhere with impunity without devascularizing the scalp. The layers of the scalp can be remembered by a mnemonic:

S *s*kin
C sub*c*utaneous tissue
A the *a*poneurosis (galea)
L *l*oose areola tissue (the scalp is reflected back by dissecting this layer)
P *p*ericranium (periosteum)

When suturing a scalp wound absorbable sutures are used to close the galea and then clips or sutures in the skin. As all the significant vessels lie within the subcutaneous tissue this two layer closures tamponades the vessels and can control all scalp edge bleeding.

The *skull* is a complex series of connected bones. In the neonate the vault bones are only loosely attached at sutures and these join with cartilagenous fusion at 18 months. The skull reaches 90% of its adult size at approximately 7 years, and maximum size at puberty; the suture lines can be seen on skull radiographs throughout life but tend gradually to obliterate with advancing age. The skull varies in thickness in differing areas, being thickest in the parieto-occipital area and thinnest in the temporal area just above the mandibular articulation. It is divided into three fossae – anterior, middle and posterior (Fig. 21.1).

There are a number of foramina though which pass specific structures (Table 21.1).

Structure and function

The brain is composed of neurons, neuroglia, and blood vessels. Each neuron is composed of a cell body, dendrites, which are short non-myelinated processes, and one or more axons whose length varies from a few millimetres to over 1 m. Neurons may be unipolar, bipolar or multipolar; the first two are primarily afferent and convey sensory information from receptor endings to the central nervous system (CNS). The majority of neurons in the CNS are of the multipolar type. In the peripheral nervous system (PNS), axons are ensheathed by neurilemmal cells which form myelin in myelinated axons, although unmyelinated axons have a sheath but no myelin. The myelinated axon has regular gaps in the myelin called nodes of Ranvier. In the CNS, axons may be myelinated or unmyelinated, and some neurons, such as those in the anterior horn cell of the spinal cord, have very long axons.

In both the CNS and autonomic nervous system, axons make contact with a neuron, a dendrite or another axon through a synapse. At most synapses a nervous impulse is chemically mediated and is due to the release of a specific transmitting substance stored in the axonal ending and thus transmission is unidirectional. Synapses may be excitatory

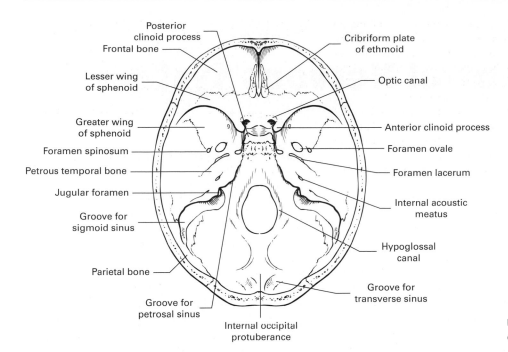

Figure 21.1. Internal surface of the skull base.

Table 21.1. **Foramina of the skull.**

Foramen	Structures passing through
Optic	Optic nerve, ophthalmic artery
Superior orbital fissure	Occulomotor nerve, trochlear nerve, abducens nerve, trigeminal nerve (ophthalmic division V1)
Foramen rotundum	Trigeminal nerve (maxillary division, V2)
Foramen ovale	Trigeminal nerve (mandibular division, V2), lesser petrosal nerve
Foramen spinosum	Middle meningeal artery, meningeal branch of mandibular nerve
Foramen lacerum	Carotid artery enters into side above closed inferior portion
Carotid canal	Carotid artery, sympathetic plexus
Stylomastoid	Facial nerve (exit)
Internal acoustic meatus	Facial nerve, cochlear nerve, superior and inferior vestibular nerves, labyrinthine artery and vein
Jugular foramen	Glossopharyngeal nerves, vagus nerve, accessory nerve, sigmoid sinus, inferior petrosal sinus
Foramen magnum	Spinal cord, hypoglossal nerve, vertebral arteries, spinal arteries, cervical accessory nerve

or inhibitory. There are many synaptic substances within the brain (central transmitters), the best known being dopamine, noradrenaline, adrenaline, serotonin, acetylcholine, and gamma amino-butyric acid (GABA). Excitation of a neuron gives rise to a propagated action potential which travels along the axon by a wave of depolarization at constant speed. In myelinated fibres, conduction is faster since depolarization jumps from one node of Ranvier to the next (saltatory conduction). All this depends on the permeability of the cell membrane to sodium and potassium, and the sodium–potassium pump.

Neuroglia are cells which neither form synapses nor conduct impulses. Oligodendrocytes predominate in the white matter and play the same role as the neurilemmal cells in the PNS. Astrocytes are larger and stellate in form and though extremely numerous much remains to be learnt regarding their influence on neuronal activity. Microglia are derived from mononuclear cells which migrate from blood vessels and can become macrophagic in response to brain injury or disease. Ependymal cells are ciliated and line the ventricles and the central canal of the spinal cord. The neurilemma are described above.

Aggregations of neurons are called nuclei and collections or bundles of axons, fibre tracts.

General morphology
The brain comprises two hemispheres. At the base of these runs the brain stem containing fibre tracts running to and from the brain to the rest of the body as well as the nuclei of the cranial nerves (III–XII inclusive); the cerebellum is attached to posterior aspect of the brain stem.

The cerebral hemispheres are separated in the midline by the fold of dura called the falx at the bottom of which lies the major hemispheric connection the corpus callosum. For descriptive reasons the brain is divided into four lobes which must not be thought of as discrete or isolated from one another. The surface of the brain is convoluted with the hollows called sulci and the ridges, gyri. Two main sulci and two small ones help divide the brain into these four lobes; the Rolandic (central) sulcus lies approximately half way between the anterior and posterior poles of the hemisphere and on the lateral aspect of the hemisphere runs obliquely forward to meet the Sylvian fissure; one of the small ones is the pre-occipital notch about 5 cm in front of the occipital pole laterally and the other is the parietopital sulcus which lies mainly medially. The four lobes are thus:

- frontal lobe: area above the Sylvian fissure and anterior to the Rolandic sulcus;
- temporal lobe: area below the fissure and anterior to a line joining the occipital notch and the parieto-occipital sulcus;
- parietal lobe: area posterior to the Rolandic gyrus above the Sylvian fissure;
- occipital lobe: posterior part of the brain.

The cerebrum consists essentially of cortex, which is grey matter containing neurons, and deep to this is the white matter consisting mainly of fibre tracts. Deeper still is further grey matter of the thalamus and hypothalamus and beside the thalamus there are the basal ganglia. The cortex consists of differing types of neurons and is organized differently in differing areas. The white matter consists of commissural fibres connecting the two hemispheres (corpus callosum being the greatest), association fibres between gyri and projection fibres, the largest of the latter being the corona radiata lying close to the lateral ventricle which lower down becomes the internal capsule through which run fibres going to and away from the cortex.

There is some localization of function within the cerebrum with some areas having a predominant function:

- precentral gyrus – voluntary movement;
- post central gyrus – somatic sensation;
- prefrontal cortex – control of intellect and personality;
- inferior and medial frontal cortex – visceral and emotional activity;
- medial temporal cortex – memory and smell;
- inferior frontal gyrus, superior temporal gyrus and part of the parietal lobe – speech functions (in a right-handed person these are on the left of the brain and in left-handed people, dominance can be either right or left, and thus approximately 95% of people are left hemisphere dominant for speech);
- occipital lobe, in particular the cingulate gyrusvision;
- thalamus – animal behaviour;
- hypothalamus – control of autonomic nervous system and anterior pituitary gland and also makes antidiuretic hormone (ADH) which passes down to the posterior pituitary gland.

Examination

Conscious Level

The examination of the conscious level is integral to any surgical assessment. Many vague terms can be used to describe

Table 21.2. The AVPU Scale.

A	alert
V	responds to verbal stimuli
P	responds to painful stimuli
U	unresponsive

Table 21.3. The Glasgow Coma Scale.

Eye opening	
E4	Spontaneous
E3	To speech
E2	To pain
E1	None
Verbal response	
V5	Orientated
V4	Confused
V3	Words
V2	Sounds
V1	None
Motor response	
M6	Obeys commands
M5	Localizes to a painful stimulus
M4	Normal flexion to pain
M3	Abnormal flexion to pain
M2	Extending to pain
M1	None

the state of consciousness which is very difficult to define and communicate to other clinicians. A coma scale is therefore used to describe the conscious level. The surgeon should use in modern practice one of two commonly used scales. The alert voice pain unresponsive (AVPU) Scale is found described in the advanced trauma life (ATLS) System (Table 21.2). The author recommends that the surgeon should not use the AVPU system but use the Glasgow Coma Scale (GCS, Table 21.3) as the same stimuli need to be utilized for both assessments. The examination starts with asking the patient to open their eyes (if not spontaneously open) and to lift up their arms. Asking the patient where there are and what day it is establishes all of the verbal response criteria. If the patient failed to obey commands then a painful stimulus is applied to determine the eye opening and motor response. The site of the painful response in the initial assessment is preferred to be pressure on the supraorbital nerve. Upward thumb pressure in the supraorbital groove consistently produces pain. The neural pathway is through the Trigeminal Nerve and to the brain and not via spinal nerves and the spinal cord.

It has become common practice to summate the scores of the GCS into a score out of 15 with a GCS of 8 or less indicating a severe head injury. For clinical practice this should not be done, it is more meaningful to indicate the separate parts of the scale such as E1V2M5. Reserve the summated score for research studies. Continuous regular recording of the GCS is essential to monitor progress or decline.

Two abnormal postures of the patient can be seen in the patient with brain injury. The first is where the upper limbs are flexed due to damage of fibres in the subcortical cerebral white matter and basal grey matter the 'decorticate posture'. The second is where the upper limbs are extended where there is a preponderance of damage to the afferent fibres of the upper brain stem the 'decerebrate posture'. The painful stimulus can demonstrate these postures early after injury. The postures usually do not become spontaneous until some hours after injury.

Higher cerebral function

If the patient can talk then an assessment of higher functions is undertaken. The patient may not be able to obey commands because of a receptive dysphasia, there may be difficulty constructing a sentence because of expressive dysphasia. Disorders of naming of objects (nominal dysphasia), recognizing objects (agnosia), reading (dyslexia), writing (dysgraphia), serial 7s (dyscalculia) are all malfunctions of the dominant hemisphere that can be easily assessed. Disorders of drawing two intersecting pentagons (constructional apraxia), dressing (dressing apraxia) are malfunctions of the non-dominant hemisphere.

Memory disturbance

The surgeon will frequently meet a patient with a mild or moderate head injury. It has been shown that post-traumatic amnesia (PTA) can indicate the severity of the brain injury. Assessing this amnesia is quite difficult. Asking the patient for the first event that followed the injury, such as getting into the ambulance, assesses antegrade amnesia. The memory for the last event before the injury is retrograde amnesia. To determine PTA the examiner needs to establish whether the patient has continuous short-term memory, by asking a series of verifiable questions of the day's activities such as 'what did you eat for breakfast and lunch, who came to see you today, what have you been watching on TV?' PTA is therefore quite difficult to assess in the A&E department. The Galveston Orientation and Amnesia Test (GOAT) can be used in structured way to assess PTA.

Cranial nerves

I (olfactory) nerve

The fibres originate from the olfactory cells lying in the upper nasal mucus membrane. These are collected together and pass through the cribiform plate of the ethmoidal bone and end in the olfactory bulb. They are the organs of smell and recognition of finer tastes. They can be tested by presenting a variety of smells, one at a time, to the patient and closing the other nostril. Lack of smell (anosmia) can occur after head injury as the movement of the frontal lobe

of the brain can disrupt the fine nerve fibres passing through the cribiform plate.

II (optic) nerve

The fibres of the II nerve originate in the ganglion layer of the retina which converge on the optic disc and then pierce the retina, choroid and sclera to form the optic nerves. The nerve is pierced by the central retinal artery and vein 12 mm from the sclera. It runs through the muscle cone and then through the optic foramen. Once inside the skull, the nerve runs obliquely and medially to join its fellow nerve from the opposite side to form the optic chiasm lying just under the hypothalamus. In the chiasm, fibres from the nasal half of the retina, including the nasal half of the macula, cross the midline and join with the temporal fibres from the opposite retina and macula to form the optic tract which runs through the brain to the occipital cortex. Visual acuity can be grossly checked using newspaper print or the Jaeger book of different text sizes. Ideally acuity should be tested with the Snellen chart at 6 m from the patient. Visual fields are tested in each eye sequentially and then both eyes together. Lesions of the optic pathway lead to different impairments of the visual fields: optic nerve unilateral blindness (trauma); optic chiasm bitemporal heminopia (pituitary tumour, craniopharyngioma); optic tract homonymous hemianopia (tumour). Bilateral damage to the visual cortex and lead to reduced vision uniformly distributed in the visual field with preserved pupil reflex (cortical blindness).

Opthalmoscopy in a surgical examination is essentially looking for the presence or absence of papilloedema. The optic disc is swollen and elevated with a blurred margin and streaks radiating from the disc. Veins are enlarged due to stasis and small haemorrhages may appear along the disc margin. It normally takes about 24 h for raised intracranial pressure (ICP) to develop papilloedema. Open subarachnoid spaces must be present for papilloedema to be present. A classical surgical eye examination is optic atrophy in one eye (from direct compression) and papilloedema in the other eye (from raised ICP) can be seen with large slowly growing tumours in the anterior fossa.

III (occulomotor), IV (trochlear) and VI (abducens) nerves

In a patient with a low GCS pen-torch assessment of pupils is a vital early part of the surgical examination, an abnormality could indicate a level of urgency that curtails further detailed examination. A dilated pupil can indicate pressure on the III nerve along its course. Arising from the nucleus in the floor of the aqueduct of Sylvius in the midbrain the III nerve runs between the superior cerebellar and posterior cerebral arteries and then forwards alongside the free edge of the tentorium to run in the lateral wall of the cavernous sinus. In brain herniation such as following head injury the medial part of the temporal lobe (the uncus) squeezes into the gap between the medulla and the free edge of the tentorium compressing the nerve. A complete paralysis of the III nerve leads to ptosis, external strabismus due to the unopposed action of the lateral rectus and superior oblique dilatation of the pupil and loss of accommodation and reaction to light. The route of the papillary reflex is via optic nerve, optic chiasm, optic tract, Edinger Westphal nucleus in the brainstem, oculomotor nerve making a synapse in the ciliary ganglion. A Horner's Syndrome (unilateral miosis, ptosis, decreased sweat production and conjunctival vasodilatation) is a result of decreased sympathetic innervation such as infarction of medulla oblongata, apical lung tumour.

The VI nerve nucleus is in the pons, the fibres emerge at the junction of the pons and the medulla. It has a long extracerebral course up the clivus and enters the lateral wall of the cavernous sinus. The IV nerve (trochlear) nucleus lies in the midbrain at the level of the caudate colliculus, fibres cross the midline and the nerve leaves the posterior side of the brainstem and continues around it to the front where it enters the cavernous sinus innervating the superior oblique muscle. Examination of occular movements is achieved by asking the patient to follow the finger which is moved in the shape of an H. Loss of lateral movement of the eye indicates a VI nerve palsy and induces a diplopia. A VI nerve palsy can be what is termed a 'false localizing sign' as raised intracranial pressure without direct nerve compression can cause impairment of nerve function. A IV nerve defect requires careful observation of the adducted eye when looking down, for example if you ask the patient to look to the left and downward the left eye looks downward innervated by the III nerve the right eye does not look downward if there is a IV nerve palsy.

V (trigeminal) nerve

The fibres of the sensory root arise from cells of the trigeminal ganglion which lies near the apex of the petrous temporal bone. The central fibres pass to the pons and the peripheral fibres are divided into three main nerves – ophthalmic and maxillary (which are wholly sensory) and mandibular (which is a mixed motor and sensory nerve). V1 (ophthalmic) runs in the lateral wall of the cavernous sinus and divides into three branches which all run through the superior orbital fissure. It supplies sensation to the eyeball, conjunctiva, part of the mucus membranes of the nose and skin of the nose, eyelids, and scalp from the frontal region as far posteriorly as the lambdoid suture. V2 (maxillary) runs through the lateral wall of the cavernous sinus, leaves the skull through the foramen rotundum, and then passes through the pterygopalatine fossa and enters the orbit through the inferior orbital fissure (as the infraorbital nerve). It supplies sensation to the lower side of the nose, lower eyelid, skin, and mucus membrane of the cheek, and upper lip as well as the inside of the upper mouth and upper teeth. V3 (mandibular) leaves the skull through the foramen ovale. The motor root supplies the muscles of mastication as well as the tensor palati and tensor tympani. The sensory root supplies the teeth and gums of the mandible, lower lip, anterior two-thirds of the tongue, and floor of the mouth. The chorda tympani nerve of the 7th nerve hitches a lift in the lingual branch of the mandibular nerve to supply taste to the anterior two-thirds of the tongue. Examination of facial sensation should include the cornea and usually just requires light touch only. Facial sensation is a function of the V Nerve (trigeminal) through three subdivisions: V1 forehead; V2 cheek, V3 mandible. The masseter is innervated through motor fibres within the nerve. Deficits of trigeminal nerve function can be due to tumours in the region of the petrous apex such as meningioma or schwannoma of the nerve itself.

VII (facial) nerve

This nerve possesses a motor and sensory root. The sensory root is the chorda tympani mentioned above. The motor root supplies the muscles of the face (facial expression), the scalp, buccinator, stapedius, stylohyoid, posterior belly of the digastric and the platysma. The motor nucleus lies in the pons and the sensory nucleus in the medulla. The two roots join and emerge from the pons and run through the cerebellopontine angle close to the 8th nerve and into the internal auditory meatus. The nerve then runs a tortuous course through the petrous bone and is close to the tympanic antrum before leaving the skull through the stylomastoid foramen. Thereafter, the nerve runs through the parotid gland and divides into branches to supply the muscles listed above.

Paralysis may occur from central or peripheral lesions. In central cerebral lesions the lower part of the face is particularly affected and the upper part of the forehead may be relatively spared. Peripheral paralysis affects the whole face. The nerve is very vulnerable to a variety of pathological processes due to its long tortuous course through the cerebellopontine angle, petrous bone and skull base, and the parotid gland. It behoves any surgeon operating in this area to study and learn the detailed anatomy in order to attempt the preservation of facial expression.

VIII (auditory) nerve

The VIII nerve is a sensory nerve comprising two sets of fibres: one forms the vestibular nerve which relays information on the position of the head with respect to gravity from the semicircular canals in the petrous bone; and the other the cochlear nerve which relays hearing from the cochlear. Both nuclei lie within the pons.

Vestibular function is part of the overall function of balance and it is not surprising that there are many complicated relays between the vestibular nucleus, cerebellum, 3rd, 4th and 6th nerve nuclei, and the spinal cord. If total damage occurs to one nerve or the semicircular canals, the opposite side can function quite well, but problems occur when there is partial damage and then imbalance between the two sides resulting in vertigo and ataxia.

Auditory function is complex and has two main components – the transmission of sound across the middle ear (tympanic cavity) to the tympanic membrane and the conversion of these transmissions by the cochlear into nerve impulses; thus two main types of deafness or partial hearing loss may occur – conduction (mechanical) or sensorineural. Using a tuning fork, a clinical assessment can be carried to establish which is better heard by the patient – air or bone conduction – remembering that the norm is for air to be better than bone conduction. Detailed assessment of hearing is carried out by audiometry.

Disease processes in the middle ear can lead to hearing loss as well 7th nerve damage. Disease processes in the petrous bone such as infections, neoplasms, and fractures from head injuries can cause hearing deficit as can lesions in the intracranial cerebellopontine angle such as acoustic neuromas.

IX (glossopharyngeal) nerve

This is a mixed motor and sensory nerve. The sensory part supplies fibres to the pharynx and tonsil and both sensation and taste to the posterior one-third of the tongue. The motor fibres supply the stylopharyngeus muscle and the secretomotor fibres to the parotid gland. The nuclei are in the medulla and the nerve leaves this to exit the skull through the anterior part of the jugular foramen.

X (vagus) nerve

This is a mixed motor and sensory nerve and has probably the most extensive distribution of any nerve in the body. The nuclei are within the medulla and the nerve leaves this to exit the skull through the jugular foramen. It then runs down the neck within the carotid sheath lying between the internal jugular vein and internal carotid artery proximally and the internal jugular vein and common carotid artery distally. Thereafter the course is different for each side. On the right, the nerve crosses the subclavian artery and thence into the superior mediastinum; then it passes behind the right main bronchus and behind the oesophagus and picks up some fibres from the left vagus and runs through the diaphragm as the posterior vagal trunk. On the left, the nerve enters the mediastinum between the left common carotid and subclavian arteries. It crosses the root of the left lung and forms the anterior vagal trunk with some fibres from the right vagus and enters the abdomen as the anterior vagal nerve on the front of the oesophagus.

Both nerves give branches off during their course; in the neck they supply the muscles of the soft palate (except the tensor palati) and the pharynx. They also supply sensation to the mucus membrane of the larynx. The recurrent laryngeal nerve has a different course on each side on the right going round the subclavian artery and on the left around the arch of the aorta; it supplies the muscles of the larynx except the cricothyroid, in particular those muscles moving the vocal cords and paralysis leads to dysphonia. It is particularly at risk in neck surgery of the thyroid and parathyroid glands as well as anterior vertebral column surgery.

The vagus supplies the heart, stomach, first part of the duodenum, liver, and kidneys. Due to its wide distribution, detailed knowledge of its anatomy is necessary for neurosurgeons, eye nose throat (ENT) surgeons, faciomaxillary surgeons, cardiothoracic, and abdominal surgeons.

XI (accessory) nerve

The XI nerve is unusual in having a small cranial root and a much larger spinal root. The latter is formed from anterior horn cells as far down as the 5th cervical nerve. The fibres coalesce and run upwards through the foramen magnum and then leave the skull again through the jugular foramen. It supplies the sternomastoid and trapezius muscles.

XII (hypoglossal) nerve

This is the motor nerve of the tongue. The nucleus lies in the floor of the 4th ventricle and the fibres emerge as rootlets and pass through the anterior condylar foramen. It passes behind the internal carotid artery, then in front of the vagus nerve and enters the tongue on top of the hyoglossus muscle. Due to its course, it is particularly vulnerable to pathology and more particularly surgery in this region. Paralysis leads to failure to protrude the tongue on that side and the tongue deviates to that side as a result of unopposed action of the contralateral muscles.

The term bulbar palsy is used to describe malfunction of the lower cranial nerves from the IX to XII and is of lower neuron type; it may be bilateral or unilateral. Pseudobulbar palsy used to describe malfunction of these nerves when the lesion is higher and is of the upper motor neuron type.

Cerebral arteries

Arterial blood is delivered to the brain through four main arteries: the two internal carotid arteries and the two vertebral arteries. The internal carotid artery enters the skull through the carotid canal in the petrous temporal bone and then passes through the cavernous sinus to emerge through the dura close to the anterior clinoid process and as it does so it gives off the ophthalmic artery which supplies the structures off the orbit, including the central retinal artery. Thereafter the internal carotid artery forms part of the circle of Willis.

The two vertebral arteries arise from the subclavian arteries. On each side the artery ascends to run through the foramina transversaria of the upper six cervical vertebrae, runs across the lateral mass of the atlas into the vertebral canal and through the foramen magnum. The anterior and posterior spinal arteries are given off as is the posterior inferior cerebellar artery before the two vertebral arteries join to form the basilar artery.

The circle of Willis is a ring of arteries at the base of the brain formed in the front by the internal carotid arteries bifurcating to give the middle cerebral arteries, and the anterior cerebral arteries which are joined by a channel,

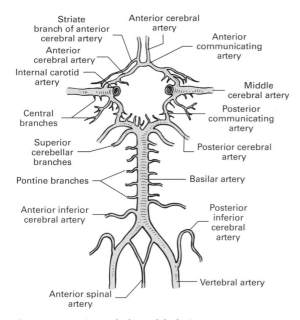

Figure 21.2. Arteries on the base of the brain.

the anterior communicating artery, which has very variable configurations (Fig. 21.2). The internal carotid arteries before their bifurcation give off the posterior communicating artery which runs backwards to join the posterior cerebral artery which is formed by the bifurcation of the basilar artery.

The middle cerebral artery through its branches supplies the lateral hemisphere above and below the Sylvian fissure (Fig. 21.3). The anterior cerebral artery supplies the medial aspect of the hemisphere as far back as the occipital lobe which is supplied by the posterior cerebral artery as is the medial aspect of the temporal lobe. Deep structures are supplied by perforating arteries from the circle of Willis. Although the arteries anastomose on the surface of the brain, once they enter the brain substance they become terminal (end arteries).

Cerebral veins

The vast majority of venous drainage of the brain is through the sagittal sinuses (Figs 21.4 and 21.5: the superior, and the straight which is the continuation of the inferior) which

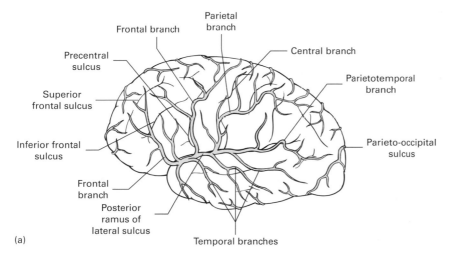

(a)

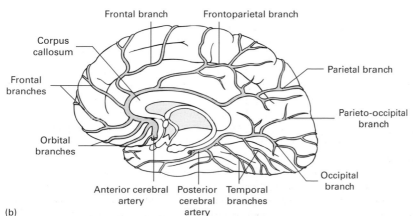

(b)

Figure 21.3. (a) Arteries of the superolateral surface of the left cerebral hemisphere and (b) of the medial and tentorial surfaces.

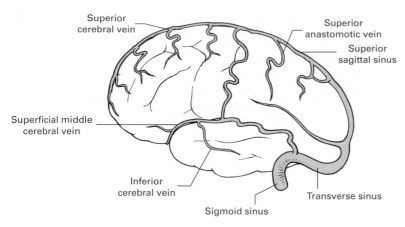

Figure 21.4. Veins of the superolateral surface of the hemisphere.

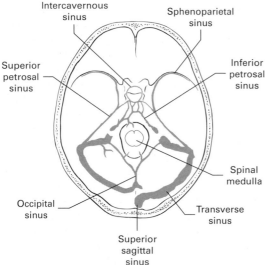

Figure 21.5. Floor of the cranial cavity, illustrating the main venous sinuses.

join together at the confluence of sinuses inside the inion. There the lateral sinuses are formed which run around the posterior fossa to become the sigmoid sinuses which become the internal jugular veins to leave the skull and run through the neck in the carotid sheath. There are no valves in the sinuses.

There is no lymphatic drainage of the brain, although the scalp and face do have lymphatic drainage initially to superficial lymph glands (parotid, mastoid, submental, and occipital) and thence into the deep cervical glands.

Pituitary gland

The normal pituitary gland is situated at the base of the brain and connected to it by the pituitary stalk which runs from the hypothalamus. It measures $12 \times 9 \times 6$ mm and lies within the sella turcica of the skull base. It is surrounded by pituitary capsule which is similar to dura mater and the superior surface (diaphragma sellae) has an opening through which the stalk

runs; in approximately 20% of people the diaphragma sellae is deficient and only arachnoid covers the gland at this point.

Autonomic nervous system

As elsewhere in the body, the autonomic nervous system is composed of two parts which often have opposing action – the sympathetic and parasympathetic systems. The outflow for the sympathetic system to the head is from the upper (usually T1 and T2) spinal cord segments and the nerves relay in the superior cervical ganglion and thereafter the nerve fibres hitch a lift in or around several structures, the most important of which is around the internal carotid artery.

In the eye, the pupillary and ciliary muscles are controlled by the sympathetic system which produces pupillary dilatation and accommodation for distant vision, and by the parasympathetic which produces pupillary constriction and accommodation for near vision; the origin of the parasympathetic fibres is from the Edinger–Westphal nucleus in the midbrain. The lacrimal gland produces tears under the control of the parasympathetic from the facial nucleus in the pons. The salivary glands are controlled by the sympathetic and the parasympathetic from salivary nuclei of the facial and glossopharyngeal nuclei in the pons and medulla.

Spinal cord

The spinal cord begins at the foramen magnum as the continuation of the medulla oblongata and runs down the vertebral canal to finish opposite the 1st lumbar vertebra in the adult. As it finishes it tapers as the conus medullaris and then a fibrous cord, the filum terminale, runs down further to the lower sacral canal. Since the spinal cord is shorter than the vertebral column, the neural segments do not correspond to the bony segments.

The grey matter is central and H-shaped and is larger in the cervical and lumbar areas. This is surrounded by columns of myelinated nerve fibres – anterior, lateral and posterior. The main columns are laterally the corticospinal dealing with voluntary movement and superficial to these are the lateral spinothalamic, which deal with pain; posteriorly the dorsal columns dealing with sensation. The anterior grey matter (anterior horns) is almost exclusively efferent whilst the posterior horns are afferent and have a number of connections and relays with the incoming afferent fibres. The spinal nerve roots are posterior (afferent), entering the spinal cord close to the posterior horns, and anterior (efferent), emerging from the spinal cord close to the anterior horns. The cell bodies of the posterior root fibres are in the dorsal root ganglion outside the spinal cord and those of the anterior root mainly arise in the anterior horn. The two roots join mechanically together to form the spinal nerve, one to each side, which emerge from the vertebral column through the intervertebral foramina. The spinal nerve then immediately divides into the posterior ramus which supplies the skin and muscles of the back and the anterior ramus which supplies the anterior body wall, limbs, and other appendages.

The segmental arrangement of the spinal cord and spinal nerves is preserved in the thoracic regions, although for the limbs there is complicated crossing over and linking in plexi, for the arm the brachial plexus and for the buttocks and legs the lumbosacral plexus. A myotome is the muscle tissue supplied by a single spinal motor root and the dermatome is the area of skin which sends sensory information inwards through a single spinal sensory root.

NEUROPHYSIOLOGY

Cerebrospinal fluid

Each day 500 ml of Cerebrospinal fluid (CSF) is secreted mostly by the choroids plexus within the lateral and with the 3rd and 4th ventricles. Very little appears to change the production rate of CSF other than quite markedly raised intracranial pressure which reduces it. The CSF flows from the lateral ventricles through the foramina of Munro into the 3rd ventricle and thence down the aqueduct of Sylvius situated in the midbrain and upper pons. Once in the 4th ventricle, a very small amount passes down the central canal of the spinal cord but the vast majority flows out through the lateral foramina of Luschka and the central foramen of Magendie. Thereafter the CSF can flow down the subarachnoid space in the spine or pass upwards; eventually all CSF passes upward in the subarachnoid spaces around the midbrain and thence over the cerebral hemispheres and particularly to the parasagittal areas. It is reabsorbed into the blood stream through the arachnoid villi which protrude into the great venous sinuses, the superior sagittal sinus in particular.

Hydrocephalus

Hydrocephalus is an increase in CSF volume usually resulting from impaired absorption. Excess CSF production occurs only from a rare neoplasm, choroid plexus papilloma. Obstruction to the passage of CSF within the brain or within the subarachnoid spaces leads to an obstructive hydrocephalus; causes of this are a mass lesion, or meningitis from bacteria or blood. Failure of absorption of CSF leads to a communicating hydrocephalus; causes include infection, subarachnoid haemorrhage or carcinomatous meningitis. As hydrocephalus develops the ventricles dilate and CSF permeates into the periventricular white matter leading to raised intracranial pressure. In young children the head size increases and the anterior fontanelle is tense, there can be impaired upward gaze leading to the 'setting sun' appearance of the eyes. In the neonate and young child, the skull may expand if the sutures between the skull bones give way (suture diastasis) and for this reason, the monitoring process for children includes plotting of measurements of skull circumference on appropriate percentile charts. Acutely developing hydrocephalus can lead to impaired consciousness and vomiting, gradual onset leads to dementia, gait ataxia and incontinence.

Two main patterns are seen on computerized tomography (CT) or magnetic resonance (MR) imaging: one is where all the ventricles are dilated which suggests a communicating hydrocephalus; the second is where the 4th ventricle remains a normal size with dilatation of the lateral and 3rd ventricle which suggests obstructive hydrocephalus most commonly at the level of the aqueduct of sylvius, aqueduct stenosis.

Specimens of CSF can be obtained by lumbar puncture, or by a burrhole and tapping the lateral ventricle with a brain cannula. If there is any suspicion of a mass lesion, a brain scan should be performed first, since a lumbar puncture in the presence of a mass lesion and/or raised intracranial pressure is dangerous and may lead to sudden brain displacements; a burr hole is much safer since CSF is drained above any mass lesion and displacements are much less likely to occur.

Any causative mass lesion should be excised if possible. If such resection does not settle the hydrocephalus or if there is no causative mass lesion surgical CSF diversion is required. This diversion can be temporary by placing a ventricular drain through a frontal burr hole and CSF is collected into a measuring chamber. For aqueduct stenosis the treatment of choice is an endoscopic 3rd ventriculostomy where the floor of the 3rd ventricle is directly visualized and punctured. Most patients will require a permanent CSF shunt which is implanted subcutaneously between one of the lateral ventricles and the peritoneal cavity. These shunt systems use a valve to regulate the flow of CSF to prevent over-drainage, many of these valves have components that prevent siphoning of the CSF and can be programmable by utilizing a magnet over the valve rested on the scalp.

Cerebral circulation

The brain accounts for only 2% of the total body weight yet its blood flow represents 15% of the resting cardiac output and it uses 20% of the oxygen used by the whole body at rest. Cerebral blood flow (CBF) has been studied by the passage of biochemically inert gases (e.g. nitrous oxide, krypton and xenon) through the brain. The value for a normal conscious human at rest is 50–60 ml of blood/100 g brain tissue/min. Each day the brain requires about 1000 litres of blood in order to obtain 71 litres of oxygen. Cessation of blood flow causes unconsciousness within 5–10 s.

The brain can regulate the blood flow in accordance to its metabolic need. The cerebral vasculature can adjust to changes in arterial blood pressure keeping the flow constant within certain limits, this is called cerebrovascular autoregulation. The CBF is autoregulated within certain parameters:

- CBF is maintained at systemic mean arterial pressures between 60 and 150 mmHg. Below systemic blood pressures of 60 mmHg, CBF lessens such that if the pressure falls rapidly to 20 mmHg, CBF virtually ceases. Slower falls under controlled conditions, such as hypotensive anaesthesia, can be tolerated to 40 mmHg before CBF starts to lessen. When the systemic arterial pressure is raised, CBF remains constant until 150 mmHg when an increase occurs, often described as breakthrough of autoregulation. In chronically hypertensive patients, this limit may be higher at around 170 mmHg.
- Arterial blood gases have a major influence on CBF. CBF and cerebral blood volume increases when the arterial $PaCO_2$ is raised due to dilatation of pial arterioles. When the arterial PaO_2 falls, CBF starts to rise.

When CBF falls to 25–30 ml/100 g/min, neurological dysfunction occurs leading to cellular chemical events culminating in neuronal death. Some areas are particularly sensitive including not only the deep nuclei but also the boundary areas of the cortex where the distal branches of the major vessels of the circle of Willis meet and as a consequence the circulation and perfusion is less resistant to falling CBF (these areas may infarct giving rise to the so-called boundary zone lesions/infarcts). These changes have major implications not only for intracranial pathological processes such as stroke, head injury and neoplasia, but also for systemic processes such as shock and severe respiratory dysfunction. Therefore, it is imperative to attempt to normalize blood pressure and arterial blood gases and reduce raised intracranial pressure (ICP) when it occurs.

The difference between the arterial pressure and the intracranial pressure is the cerebral perfusion pressure (CPP). In patients where autoregulation is impaired such as after head injury falls in the CPP will lead to cerebral ischaemia and infarction. It is currently recommended to keep the CPP above 70 mmHg following severe head injury. Often the intracranial pressure after head injury can be in the region of 30 mmHg, it therefore follows that the mean arterial blood pressure (MABP) should be maintained at around 100 mmHg until the intracranial pressure can be directly measured.

INVESTIGATIONS

At the outset it must be stated that the clinical history and clinical examination are the most important clues to the underlying pathology of any patient with suspected disease of the nervous system. A tentative clinical diagnosis can frequently be made and then, if necessary, taken further by special investigations.

Imaging

Radiographs

Plain radiographs of the skull, face and vertebral column can yield important data. Their use is becoming more limited as multi-slice CT scanners become more widely available. Today skull radiographs can be important in the emergency department in patients with a head injury looking for skull fractures. Radiographs of the facial skeleton can also be useful, although CT scanning probably yields more information. Skull radiographs are not used in the assessment of suspected intracranial mass lesions since CT and MR scanning are so much more useful. Radiographs of the vertebral column can be useful in suspected spinal injuries, spondylosis, metastatic and primary neoplasms and spinal infection. Chest radiographs are mandatory for any suspected intracranial mass lesion, in particular looking for possible bronchogenic carcinoma.

CT scanning

CT scanning uses ionizing radiation; scintillation detectors measure and a computer localizes the absorption characteristics at all points within a planar cross-section (the thickness of each varying from 1 to 10 mm). Absorption is expressed on the Hounsfield scale between 1000 (bone), 0 (water) and 1000 (air), but in practice the images are viewed on a grey scale of about 15 shades between black and white. CT is good at detecting mass lesions, particularly if these are enhanced by giving the patient an intravenous injection of iodinated contrast medium before a second scan. An unenhanced scan is good at detecting blood, bone anatomy and pathology. The main disadvantage of CT is the relatively high dose of ionizing radiation needed and if possible repetitive scans should be kept to a minimum.

MRI imaging

MRI imaging has become rapidly the primary tool for investigation of the CNS. MRI is based on the fact that a nucleus can have one of two magnetic spins with differing energy levels. The nucleus will preferentially hold the lower energy state but can be changed to the higher state through a radiofrequency pulse which once withdrawn allows the nucleus to relax and give up off the absorbed energy. It is the relaxation time of giving up this energy is the basis of MRI. The unit of magnetic field strength is the Tesla, the MR scanning magnets into which the patient is inserted are 0.5–2.0 Tesla.

MR contrast is due to how water in different tissues responds to magnetic disturbance. There are two main types of sequence T1 and T2 that are used in imaging and gadolinium is used as a contrast media. Water is seen as black on T1 and white on T2 images. Intrinsic brain tumours can be seen on the T1 scan as areas with lower density than surrounding brain, gadolinium enhancement in these tumours suggests malignancy. T2 images can show the extent of brain oedema around the tumour. The various pathologies in the CNS have differing characteristics on the images.

MRI can also determine the chemical content of the tissue through a technique of nuclear magnetic resonance (NMR) Spectroscopy, by determining areas of higher glucose metabolism functional MR can define areas of the brain such as the speech centres which can help in surgical planning.

Myelography

Myelography today is only used when there is no access to an MR scanner or if the patient suffers from claustrophobia and is unable to enter the scanner. A non-ionic iodine-containing substance is injected into the subarachnoid space, usually by lumbar puncture, and the patient lies on a tilting table which is used to run the dye up and down the spine. On its own, a myelogram can only demonstrate a lesion as a filling defect in the column of dye or show a swollen spinal cord, although the information can be considerably enhanced by CT scanning of the level of the lesion with the dye *in situ*.

Angiography

This technique is used to demonstrate the blood vessels, in particular the arteries. In adults it is performed under local anaesthesia. A non-ionic iodine-containing medium is injected into the arteries. It is usual to catheterize the femoral artery and advance the catheter retrogradely up the aorta, placing its tip in the carotid and vertebral arteries in the neck, at the skull base or even within the branches of the circle of Willis. The images are computer enhanced which reduces the amount of iodine required and produces better images (digital subtraction angiography (DSA)) unobscured by overlying bone. Angiography is used to determine the cause of intracerebral haemorrhage and to assess the blood supply of mass lesions. For examination of the carotid and vertebral arteries in the neck for suspected atheroma, it is now considered safer to use the non-invasive technique of Doppler Duplex ultrasound.

The interventional neuroradiologist now has technology of microcatheters that can be manipulated up the carotid or vertebral arteries to most locations in the brain. Detachable coils can be fed up the catheters into aneurysms, packing them internally, stents can be passed that expand and hold open narrowed vessels, substances that harden (e.g. Onyx) can be injected in liquid form. These techniques are rapidly changing the therapies available to CNS vascular pathology. In tandem with these developments diagnostic angiography obtained by MRI or CT is now able to produce images very close to conventional angiography.

Neurophysiological investigations

The two commonest techniques are the electroencephalogram (EEG) and nerve conduction studies. EEG is used in the investigation of epilepsy and suspected brain damage after hypoxia and drug poisoning. Nerve conduction is used to confirm and localize disease of peripheral nerve and, in particular, is used in suspected compression neuropathies before attempting surgical release.

Head injury
Pathology
Head injury leads to about 5000 hospital deaths per year. Head injuries can occur in isolation or with multiple trauma. They result either from deceleration of the head, for example in road traffic accidents, or acceleration, for example in assaults with blows to the head or face. The head may come into contact with an object, resulting in damage to the scalp and/or skull, or the body may decelerate/accelerate without direct contact to the head. Since the brain is soft and jelly-like, there is an inertia between it and the skull and it oscillates and is often forced against the skull several times along the line of force; damage is caused in this way, particularly in high-speed road traffic accidents. Penetrating missile injuries are unusual in the UK but common in some countries and in war zones; they cause impact damage, as above, but also focal damage along the missile tract within the brain.

Lesions are classified as primary if they occur at the time of injury and secondary if as a result of complications. Primary lesions may be:

- *intracerebral haemorrhages.* These may be single or multiple and vary in size from large to petechiae;
- *localized areas of contusion.* These (like a bruise elsewhere on the body) are softened swollen brain with haemorrhages and occur maximally in the temporal, frontal and occipital lobes. The term contre-coup contusion is used to describe the oscillation of the brain whereby it is contused at the opposite pole from the impact;
- *laceration and diffuse axonal injury.* Lacerations occur either from an open direct penetration or within a closed injury and can occur anywhere on the cerebral cortical surface or even in the corpus callosum. In diffuse axonal injury (DAI) there is widespread damage to the white matter of the cerebral hemispheres and fibre tracts within the brain stem.

Secondary lesions include:

- *oedema.* Oedema around contusions and lacerations adds to the local mass effect and there is an increase in brain tissue water and increased permeability of blood vessels. There may be diffuse brain swelling which is thought to be most likely due to vascular engorgement, although if the brain becomes hypoxic there may be cytotoxic oedema as well;
- *displacement of brain and internal herniations.* The brain may be herniated under the falx or the undersurface of the temporal lobe forced into the tentorial opening leading to compression of the midbrain;
- *surface haematomas.* These may be subdural or extradural. The former arise from tearing of surface veins or the cerebral cortical substance and tend to spread over the

cerebral hemisphere. Extradural haematomas result from either tearing of one of the meningeal vessels or from a fracture site; in either event the dura is stripped from the overlying bone for some surrounding distance and the haematoma develops in the potential space. Most frequently, extradural haematomas occur in the middle fossa, but can occur in the anterior or posterior fossae. Both subdural and extradural haematomas lead to secondary displacement and compression of the underlying brain.

The compounding effects of poor pulmonary gaseous exchange and falling systemic blood pressure upon an already damaged and deranged brain can never be overestimated (see above).

Clinical features

Neurological deficits

Focal or generalized neurological deficits can occur either from the primary or secondary injuries. Their nature varies depending on the site and severity of brain damage. These may include limb disturbance with weakness, dyspraxia and sensory loss. Eye movement disorders may occur from damage to the III, IV and VI nerves or to the midbrain. I nerve damage can occur and is irrecoverable if total and bilateral. Ataxia of the trunk with balance and gait disturbance is common after severe injuries.

Some of the most serious deficits are cognitive and speech disorders. Speech disorders may include dysphasia and dysarthria. Cognitive disorders can be severe and distressing, yet are often not appreciated in the early phases after a head injury. They include reduction of short-term memory, learning and ability to retrieve new information and logical thought. Personality changes can also occur and often best recognized by relatives and friends.

Management

The acute management of head-injured patients can be divided temporally and logistically into three phases:
• scene of the incident;
• emergency department;
• (if required) inpatient admission and care.

The scene of the incident is attended by the Ambulance Service whose paramedics are trained in resuscitation. Any unconscious patient requires immobilization of the neck in a firm collar during retrieval back to the emergency department. The airway needs protection if the patient is still unconscious.

At the emergency department, patients can be triaged into major, moderate and mild injuries. The key element of managing a patient with a head injury is the routine ABC of trauma care to ensure airway patency, adequate breathing and circulation. Following that attention is given to the exclusion of intracranial mass lesions that cause the secondary injuries as described above. Patients who have a decreased conscious level after head trauma have a high risk of an intracranial mass lesion and most of these patients will require a CT scan to exclude. The presence of a skull fracture also greatly

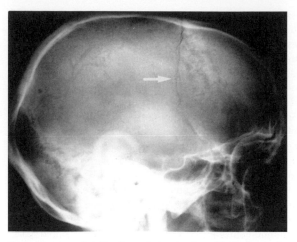

Figure 21.6. Lateral skull radiograph showing linear fracture (arrow) of 45-year-old man with blow to the head.

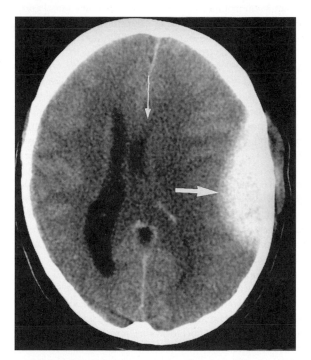

Figure 21.7. CT scan of the same patient as in Fig. 21.6 showing extradural haematoma (large arrow). Note also severe shift of the brain (thin arrow).

increases the risk of an intracranial mass lesion and if an X-ray demonstrates a fracture then a CT must follow in most cases (Figs 21.6 and 21.7).

Small children, in particular, are vulnerable and a full GCS assessment is often difficult to achieve, and the vast majority of these should be admitted. If alcohol is detected, care must be taken in assessing the patient and any confusion or reduction of GCS must not be exclusively attributed to the alcohol, irritating though this may be to the medical and nursing staff. Patients with medical conditions that might have a bearing upon their response to a head injury should also be admitted, for example diabetes mellitus, epilepsy, respiratory and cardiac conditions and also patients who are taking anticoagulants or corticosteroids.

Observations, including the GCS, should be performed half-hourly and any decline in the GCS and the development of neurological deficits or both should alert the clinician to a complication and a cause should be immediately sought. Investigations including an urgent CT scan should be performed.

Patients who are present in coma after head injury present major problems and immediate attention must be given to the establishment and maintenance of their airway and the maintenance of normal cardiovascular status. The upper airway must be protected, if necessary by an airway or endotracheal intubation. Adequate gaseous exchange must be checked by arterial blood gas analysis, and if abnormal, reasons sought and the necessity for artificial ventilatory support considered. The cardiovascular status must be checked by measuring blood pressure, pulse volume and heart rate. The patient must be checked for other injuries by using the log-roll procedure and full frontal and posterior examination carried out. After resuscitation, a GCS score is derived and note taken of any injuries about the head, face and neck. Any suspected areas about the body must be radiographed and a lateral radiograph of the cervical spine taken before the collar is removed. CT scanning is necessary for all patients with a GCS of eight or less. Following this, the nearest neurosurgical department should be contacted; if no CT scanner is available, the neurosurgical department should be contacted as soon as possible.

If transfer to a distant neurosurgical department is deemed necessary, the patient should be stabilized with respect to his pulmonary and cardiovascular status as quickly as possible before being transported by ambulance and accompanied by an anaesthetist and surgeon.

The control of pain from injuries outwith the brain can be difficult, since opiates depress the level of consciousness and lead to pupillary constriction. Codeine, as a milder opiate, can be given but if there is severe pain, morphine may be required and its use agreed between surgeons and anaesthetists.

Epilepsy can occur early after head injury. Whilst it is important to prevent further seizures, it must be appreciated that intravenous anticonvulsants (e.g. phenytoin and diazepam) may not only make neurological assessment more difficult, but can induce apnoea as well as cardiac dysrhythmias and an anaesthetist with full resuscitation equipment must be present when the drug is administered. Epilepsy requires treatment but there is no need for routine prophylactic anticonvulsants simply because the patient has suffered a head injury.

CSF fistulae may occur through the nose or ear. In these cases prophylactic antibiotics are not currently recommended but vigilant observation and investigation of all potential pyrexia are essential. CSF rhinorrhoea requires investigation and possibly repair by a neurosurgeon, as does persisting CSF otorrhoea.

Surgery

Scalp lacerations   The scalp is very vascular and patients can lose quite large volumes of blood from extensive lacerations. In an emergency situation, a pressure dressing can be applied. After assessment and/or resuscitation and skull radiographs, a scalp laceration requires exploration and any rough irregular edges with possible skin damage require debridement. The wound is then sutured, preferably in two layers with absorbable sutures to the galea and sutures to the skin; if done properly, haemostasis will be achieved. Skin sutures can be removed after 5 days. If there is loss of scalp, this requires urgent surgery by a neurosurgeon or a plastic surgeon.

Burr holes   It must be realized that only liquid haematomas can effectively be removed though burr holes, and therefore this form of surgery is only suitable for a fluid chronic subdural haematoma. However, burr holes are the starting point for a craniectomy or craniotomy (see below). A burr hole is performed by making a linear 4 cm long incision down to the pericranium, which is then scraped to each side. A Hudson brace with a perforator is then used to drill as far as the dura. The perforator is changed for a conical or spherical burr which enlarges the hole to about 15 mm. The exposed dura is then incised in a cruciate fashion to expose the brain.

Craniectomy and craniotomy   Ideally, it is better to perform a craniotomy, although for the less experienced surgeon, a craniectomy can be life-saving for the patient. For a craniotomy, four burr holes are drilled at the corners of a square with sides at least 6–8 cm in length. Three of the four burr holes are connected with a saw and the 4th side is broken to keep the pericranium and/or temporalis muscle intact, thereby rendering the bone flap osteoplastic such that the bone will survive.

A craniectomy is performed by drilling a burr hole and then, with a bone rongeur, nibbling bone away to give sufficient exposure (the minimum being at least 5 cm in diameter); adequate exposure is vital and bone defects can always be repaired at a later date. An extradural haematoma is immediately encountered if the burr hole is in the right place; this will be solid and requires suction removal. The dura should be opened if a subdural haematoma is also suspected. The cause of the haematoma needs to be sought; if it is from the skull fracture this requires smearing with bone wax, but if it is from a tear of a branch of the middle meningeal artery, diathermy is required. The exposed dura must then be hitched, by interrupted sutures, over the bone edge to the pericranium to prevent further stripping of the dura and further extradural haematoma formation. A suction drain must be inserted and left for at least 24 h postoperatively.

Depressed skull fracture Compound depressed skull fractures require a CT scan and need to be fully explored by a neurosurgeon, since bone fragments or other solid objects may be driven into the brain and lead to subsequent brain abscess. Simple depressed fractures require elevation only if they are significant and in a cosmetically important area. In the child under 3 years of age, considerable remodelling of the skull is possible and only severe depressions require elevation.

Missile injuries Penetrating missile injuries demand particular expertise in their management, ideally by a neurosurgeon.

Rehabilitation

Any patient who suffers a head injury requires rehabilitation, although in the case of minor injuries the patient may require advice rather than major rehabilitation. A head injury with a PTA of <1 h may take 1–2 months, but often less, for full recovery. Whilst it is important to get the patient back to his former life style, it is also important to ensure he is fully recovered before so doing. Headaches are a frequent problem and are variable in intensity and duration but usually subside after a few months; if they continue, a CT scan is required to check for chronic lesions such as a subdural haematoma or hydrocephalus.

Patients with longer PTAs and those with neurological deficits need longer to recover and may have continuing cognitive problems that require assessment by a clinical neuropsychologist. Those with severe problems require the services of a fully trained rehabilitation team, which will include a neurosurgeon, rehabilitation expert, physiotherapist, occupational therapist, speech therapist and neuropsychologist or, in the case of children of school age, an educational psychologist. The CNS is slow to repair and reorganize and 2 years is usual time span for maximal recovery to take place. Relatives are particularly important since they often have to bear the heavy burden of a difficult patient in the home environment and they need support; they can also often make useful contributions in rehabilitation.

Post-traumatic epilepsy requires treatment. Patients at greatest risk for this complication have penetrating brain injuries with the dura being breached, long PTAs, intracranial haematomas, and early post-traumatic epilepsy. In the UK, such patients should not drive a motor vehicle until they have reported themselves to the Chief Medical Officer and to the Driving and Vehicle Licensing Authority (DVLA), who may suspend them from driving for between 6 and 12 months, or longer if they have epilepsy or neurological deficits.

Brain death

As a result of resuscitation and intensive care, patients who are deeply comatose and unresponsive may be maintained on artificial ventilation. In these circumstances if brain death is diagnosed it is appropriate to withdraw ventilatory support.

For a diagnosis of brain death to be made, all of the following must coexist:
- Patient is deeply comatose and there is no suspicion that this is due to narcotics, hypnotics or neuroleptic drugs. There should be no hypothermia and the core body temperature must be 35°C or above. There should be no major metabolic or endocrine disturbance and the serum glucose and electrolytes should be normal or nearly normal;
- Patient is maintained on a ventilator because spontaneous respiration had become inadequate or ceased. Neuromuscular blocking drugs should not be present, or if they have been used they should have been stopped at least 24 h previously;
- There should be no doubt that the patient's condition is due to irremediable brain damage and the reason for this has been fully established.

Tests to confirm brain death must be performed as a set closely together in time as follows:
- *Brain stem reflexes* are absent:
  - pupils are fixed and dilated and do not respond to light;
  - no corneal reflex;
  - no eye movements when 20 ml of ice cold water is slowly perfused through each external auditory meatus.
- No *motor response* can be elicited in any area of the body by painful stimuli.
- No *gag reflex* in response to bronchial stimulation by passing a catheter down the trachea.
- No *respiratory movements* occur on stopping the ventilator for 10 min. Samples can be checked both pre- and post ventilatory arrest to confirm that the CO_2 has risen to levels which would drive respiration.

The tests should be carried out by two doctors who have both been registered for at least 5 years.

Transplantation/organ donation

Homologous cadaveric organ donation features heavily in any organ transplant programme, particularly with respect to kidneys, heart, liver and pancreas and currently potential recipients exceed potential donors. It is incumbent on the treating doctors to raise this issue with the relatives and it also possible that the patient may carry a donor card or have expressed premorbid wishes. If consent is possible, the transplant team should be informed and will make the necessary arrangements; it must be made absolutely clear to relatives that the treating team and transplant team are completely separate.

Spinal injuries

In the UK, the great majority of spinal injuries are closed and occur from the indirect effect of violence applied to the vertebral column. In military practice open and compound from penetration by missiles of various sorts are found. The distributions of spinal injuries are as follows: 10% occur in the cervical region, 10% in the upper thoracic, 50% in the lower thoracic and 30% in the lumbar. Approximately 50%

are the result of road traffic incidents, 30% from industrial incidents and most of the remainder from sport or falls. Approximately 75% occur in patients under 40 years and 80% are males.

The effects can most easily be described by considering spinal cord and vertebral column injury separately, although clearly these are intertwined.

Spinal cord injury

Spinal concussion is the transient loss of neurological function which may recover quickly and fully, and is similar to minor concussion of the brain. Spinal contusion involves swelling and haemorrhages in the spinal cord and very quickly there may be a central necrosis. The myelin sheaths are broken up, the axons are ruptured and neurons degenerate. Eventually the swelling subsides; some neural tissues may recover but those that have died are replaced by gliosis. An occasional late complication is the development of a syrinx (cyst) within the cord.

If injury is severe, there is an immediate and total loss of function at the level of the contusion and in the distal cord. Paralysis is complete and flaccid and there is total sensory loss. The bladder ceases to function. It is generally agreed that if there is no return of function within the first 48 h after injury, then the lesion is a complete functional transection and there will be no subsequent return of functions running up and down the spinal cord. If the lesion is partial and if there is some distal function remaining or returning, the neurological deficits are variable from one case to the next, as is the extent of recovery.

Spinal shock is the term used to describe the early phase lasting several weeks after injury; muscles are flaccid and there is also paralysis of the bladder and intestinal tract. As spinal shock wears off, distal spinal cord function returns but is shut off from the brain. Spinal cord reflexes return, the major one being the mass reflex, that is limbs reflexively withdraw on stimulation, the rectum and bladder evacuate and there is profuse sweating.

Cervical spinal cord injuries bring particular problems dependent on the level of injury. The lower the lesion in the cervical spinal cord, the more arm function is preserved, remembering that the main neurological supply to the arm is between C5 and T1. The higher the lesion, the greater the problems with respiration, since if the injury is at C4 or above not only are the intercostal muscles paralyzed but so are the diaphragm muscles due to loss of the phrenic nerve innervation and the patient can only survive by artificial ventilation or by electrical pulsed stimulation of the phrenic nerves.

Vertebral column injury

The types of vertebral column injury are many and only a brief account is given here. One important concept to grasp is the difference between a stable injury which will not displace further and an unstable injury which may displace further and cause further neurological damage.

The upper two cervical vertebrae are more complex and different from those lower down the neck. Three main types of fracture occur:

- Jefferson fracture involves the ring of the atlas and is usually a stable fracture;
- Hangman's fracture involves both sides of the neural arch of the axis, thus separating the arch from the body;
- The dens (odontoid) may fracture at variable distances from the body of the axis, which is unstable and may lead to avascular necrosis of the dens above the fracture line.

In the cervical spine, fracture dislocations may occur as well as compression (burst) fractures. Dislocations can also occur when the facet joints dislocate unilaterally or bilaterally. All these injuries should be regarded as unstable and require some form of fixation. In any suspected injury, the whole cervical spine needs to be viewed on radiographically with the neck in a neutral position and this may involve pulling down the shoulders during the examination so that the whole cervical spine, including C7, is visualized.

It must also be appreciated that patients with pre-existing cervical spondylosis are less tolerant of acute flexion or hyperextension and the osteophytes may contuse the spinal cord without there necessarily being a vertebral column injury.

Thoracolumbar injuries are usually due to violent hyperextension or vertical compression when a heavy object falls on the shoulders. If the posterior ligaments remain intact, there may only be a crush (compression) fracture of the vertebral body.

Management

At the scene of the incident, great care must be taken to avoid causing further damage, particularly to the spinal cord. In the case of suspected cervical spinal injuries, ideally a hard collar should be applied but if none is available, one person should hold the neck in a neutral position and apply gentle traction by holding the patient around the mandibular angles and pulling gently backwards. The patient must be kept flat and moved in a straight position onto a stretcher, which requires four people.

On arrival in hospital, the same precautions must continue. Plain radiography is performed or in many institutions now multi-slice CT scanning can cover the whole of the spine rapidly. Any suspected unstable cervical spinal injury requires skull traction and this is best done using the Gardner–Wells, which can be applied to the skull above the ears in under 60 s, and thereafter a pull of at least 3–5 kg weight. A full neurological examination is required. In the past decade there has been a thrust to give large doses of methylprednisolone early in an attempt to diminish some of the spinal cord damage; the evidence for the efficacy of this is limited.

Inpatient care involves the following:

- The patient must be given details of his injury and any prognosis; maintaining his morale is of paramount importance;

- Skin care is critical particularly in those patients with sensory loss. The prevention of bedsores is a real challenge to the nursing staff who may be helped by turning beds, such as the Stryker frame, or motorized beds that constantly change position;
- Respiratory care is essential though the intensity depends on the level of the lesion. Upper cervical lesions will require ventilatory support, though all patients require regular chest physiotherapy;
- The bladder requires drainage to prevent back-flow, urinary damage and infection. In the long term for lesions above the conus medullaris, reflex bladder action may return stimulated by manual compression or by implanted electrodes. If there is no reflex bladder action, the bladder can be drained by an indwelling catheter or by teaching the patient self-catheterization. Renal function must be carefully and regularly monitored;
- Joints rapidly deteriorate if not moved passively and gently and the prevention of contractures is vital;
- Blood pressure must be watched since patients with severe high lesions develop orthostatic hypotension. G-suits can be used when attempting to elevate the patient beyond the horizontal;
- Deep venous thrombosis must be carefully looked for since not only is the muscle pump inefficient or non-existent but pain is also diminished or lost and as a result the patient may not complain of calf or thigh pain;
- The gastrointestinal tract may not function normally in the early phases and there may even be a paralytic ileus and thus parenteral nutrition is necessary. Thereafter, nutritional requirements must be carefully assessed;
- Further displacement may occur at the fracture/dislocation site and further plain radiology is essential to monitor this area;
- Sexual and reproductive function may be possible even in patients with quite severe neurological deficits, although details of treatment are for specialists in spinal injuries.

Surgery
The role of surgery is relatively limited and the indications few; some of the techniques are quite complex. The indications for possible surgery are:
- Further deterioration in an incomplete lesion requires urgent radiography in the form of CT or MR scanning. If there is evidence of cord compression from the impingement of bone or disc fragments or an extradural haematoma, then urgent decompression by the appropriate route is indicated;
- Unstable injuries require fixation after they have been reduced. This is mostly by internal fixation, but in some cases of cervical injury, a skull halo and body fixation may be used. The vertebral column is slow to heal and any external fixation may be required for 3–6 months.

Although all the above management can be carried out in any good general hospital, in the UK it is usual to transfer the patient to a regional spinal injuries unit where there are facilities for acute care, rehabilitation and long-term follow-up.

Spinal cord compression
The spinal cord lies within the vertebral canal from the foramen magnum to approximately the first lumbar vertebra, and thereafter continues as the nerve roots of the cauda equina. It is surrounded by the three meningeal layers of dura, arachnoid and pia. There is very little spare room within the vertebral canal and space-occupying pathological processes soon lead to spinal cord compression. To some extent the symptomatology depends on the vertebral level, the layer of meninges containing the pathological process and the speed of onset of compression – the faster the onset, the poorer the prognosis for recovery even with expeditious treatment, and the converse applies for slowly compressing lesions.

In the cervical region, compression expresses itself as sensory and motor symptoms and signs of numbness and weakness in the upper limbs, which may be flaccid or spastic depending on the level, and weakness of the trunk and lower limbs, which will have increased tone or even spasticity. If vertebrae are involved in the pathological process, there is often neck pain (or referred interscapular pain), but intradural lesions are often painless.

In the thoracic region if the bone is involved, there is often pain in the spine and girdle pain around the chest wall in the distribution of the appropriate intercostal nerve, unilaterally or bilaterally. The arms are unaffected but the legs develop weakness and increased tone, and there is usually a sensory level in the trunk and lower limbs distal to the affected level. Bladder function is often compromised.

In the lumbar region there is a motor and sensory paraparesis with bladder dysfunction, depending on the level of cord or cauda equina compression.

Neurological dysfunction of the bladder (the neurogenic bladder) is particularly important to recognize. In the early phases, there is failure fully to empty the bladder such that the bladder enlarges, eventually building up back pressure on the ureters and kidneys. Finally, the patient goes into urinary retention which is often painless due the involvement of the sensory pathways. In the male, neurogenic bladder is accompanied by failure of penile erection and ejaculation.

Causes
Vertebral column
Malignancy may be secondary or primary. Metastases occur most commonly in the thoracic spine and may weaken the bone leading to collapse. Malignant tissue may also spread into the extradural space as well as into the paraspinal tissues. The single commonest primary site is bronchogenic carcinoma but other sites are carcinomas of breast, prostate and kidney. Less commonly, other primary malignancies may metastasize to the spine. Malignancies from the reticuloendothelial system

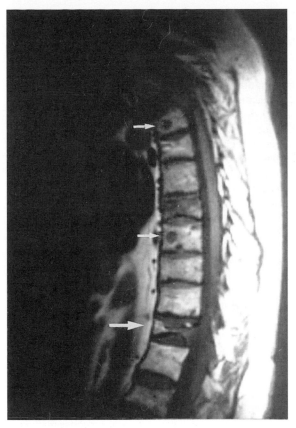

Figure 21.8. Magnetic resonance scan of the thoracic spine in 60-year-old man with a pathological collapse fracture of vertebra (large arrow) and multiple vertebral body lesions (small arrow). The diagnosis was found by needle biopsy to be multiple myeloma.

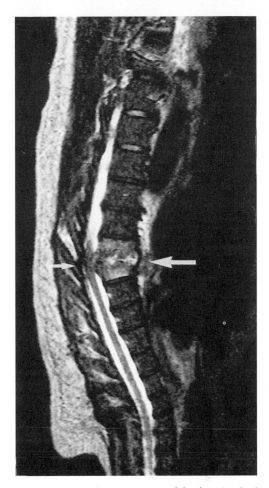

Figure 21.9. Magnetic resonance scan of the thoracic spine in 40-year-old man showing collapse with abnormal signals of two contiguous vertebrae in mid-thoracic region (large arrow). Note some preservation of intervertebral disc. Note also spinal cord compression (small arrow).

and blood-forming tissues also occur, either as part of widespread disease or starting primarily in the spine; these include myeloma (Fig. 21.8), Hodgkin's and non-Hodgkin's lymphoma and reticulosarcoma (see Ch. 11).

Primary neoplasms occur in the spine and are similar to those occurring in bones elsewhere in the body such as osteogenic sarcoma, osteoclastoma, chondroma and chrondrosarcoma. In children, Ewing's sarcoma may occur in the vertebrae and neuroblastoma within the extradural space. In patients with osteoporosis, particularly in post-menopausal women, collapse fractures can occur spontaneously or with minimal trauma (pathological fractures). Such fractures may be single or multiple. Osteomalacia can also lead to pathological fractures (see Chapter 20).

The spine can be infected by tuberculosis or pyogenic bacteria such as staphylococci. As the infection takes hold, the bone is weakened although the intervertebral disc is more resistant (Figs 21.9 and 21.10). Pus may be formed and the abscess spreads both inwards into the extradural space and outwards into the paraspinal tissues.

A small proportion of defective intervertebral discs may protrude centrally and cause spinal cord or cauda equina compression often fairly acutely, although more chronic compression may develop from osteophytes in spondylosis of the spine.

Intradural lesions

Intradural lesions may be either in the subdural space but extrinsic to the spinal cord, or intrinsic within the spinal cord. The commonest subdural extrinsic neoplasms are meningiomas and neurofibromas; the latter may also grow through an intervertebral canal and enlarge outside the spine (dumbbell tumour). The commonest intrinsic neoplasms are ependymomas and astrocytomas and both can compress and destroy the spinal cord from within outwards. Rarely, subdural pyogenic abscesses may form in the subdural space and can spread for quite long distances within the vertebral canal.

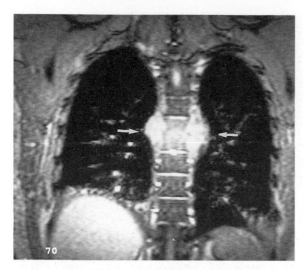

Figure 21.10. Same case as Fig. 21.8 with coronal images. Note paravertebral mass (arrows). The patient was explored and an abscess found with osteomyelitis due to *Staphylococcus aureus*.

Investigations

Recognition of acute spinal cord compression demands real urgency. Often patients have been previously well but primary malignancies elsewhere should be suspected. However, even if there is an antecedent proven malignancy elsewhere in the body, it is unwise to assume that cord compression is due to metastasis since there may be an alternative unrelated process in the spine.

Radiological tests play a key part in the investigation. Plain radiographs of the spine should be performed looking for destruction of bone and paraspinal masses. At the same time, a chest radiograph is mandatory to look for bronchogenic carcinoma. The spine must be imaged by MRI of the whole spine, or if this is not available then by myelography and CT of any areas of myelographic block or indentation.

Management

Emergency referral to a neurosurgeon is essential for consideration of decompression of the cord compression, usually by laminectomy and excision or drainage of the pathological process. The patient should have an indwelling urinary catheter inserted for free drainage of urine. In the case of metastasis, partial excision is all that can be effected, although this does have the additional merit of yielding a histological tissue diagnosis. If the cord compression is incomplete, needle biopsy of the spine can be performed under radiological guidance. Instability of the spine is treated by instrumented fixation with products now specifically designed for all parts of the spine. The treatment thereafter of a metastasis is usually radiotherapy of the affected portions of the spine and treatment of the primary malignancy. Abscesses require drainage and in the case of the thoracic spine, this is usually performed through a thoracotomy and an anterolateral approach to the spine.

The general care of patients with neurological deficits is as for patients with spinal injuries (see above), although special treatments may be necessary and obviously the prognosis will depend on various factors outlined above.

Intracranial neoplasms

Cerebral neoplasms may be primary or secondary (metastasis). In the latter case, they may occur in patients already diagnosed as suffering from malignancy elsewhere in the body or may be the first manifestation of malignancy from an initially occult primary neoplasm. Primary neoplasms may be classified as benign or malignant: benign intracranial neoplasms have some of the same histological hallmarks as benign neoplasms elsewhere in the body, although their mass effect may kill the patient; malignant primary intracranial neoplasms invade and spread into the brain locally and may metastasize through the CSF pathways but only extremely rarely do they metastasize outwith the CNS. Another description that is used is extrinsic, that is within the skull but not part of the CNS, or intrinsic, that is within the skull and deriving from the CNS. Knowledge of the amazing variety of primary neoplasms is only essential to the neurosurgeon, although a few common types are mentioned below.

In the young child without fusion of the sutures, gradually expanding lesions, with or without accompanying hydrocephalus, may lead to enlargement of the head, but the skull of the older child and adult cannot expand.

In discussing pathophysiology it is simplest to subdivide neoplasms into those that occur above and those that occur below the tentorium in the posterior fossa.

Supratentorial neoplasms

The supratentorial site is the most common location for adult brain tumours. Tumours occur in about six persons per 100 000 per year. Epilepsy can be the first presenting feature in about 30% of patients. The effects of an expanding space-occupying lesion may lead to raised intracranial pressure or cerebral or cranial nerve dysfunction. Most neoplasms, whether benign or malignant, are surrounded by local swelling of the brain which is seen on CT scan as a pale area with a high water content; this has the effect of compounding the mass volume effect of the lesion, often by 2–3 times. Focal neurological defects can occur and usually steadily deteriorate; the type of defect depends on its site. As the lesion enlarges, the brain may be pushed aside and displaced and other more remote areas of the brain may be compressed against the skull and/or dural partitions such as the falx or tentorium. Eventually, raised ICP occurs since the compensating mechanisms, such as squeezing CSF outside the skull, often fail quite quickly. In the chronic phase, the patient complains of headache which is often worse in the morning; fundoscopy may reveal papilloedema and in severe cases retinal haemorrhages. With higher levels of ICP, CBF is reduced, the midbrain and thalamus are compressed and there is a steadily decreasing level of consciousness.

Infratentorial neoplasms

The infratentorial site is the most common location for childhood brain tumours. Hydrocephalus is very common and is usually of the obstructive type since the passage of CSF through the Sylvian aqueduct or exit from the 4th ventricle or both is held up. If the process is slow, the ventricles can enlarge and cause cognitive defects without necessarily leading to raised ICP; if there is more rapid expansion, raised ICP with papilloedema may ensue. Focal neurological defects may occur depending on the site of the lesion and there is often concomitant truncal ataxia with disorders of balance and gait.

Investigations

A careful clinical history and examination of the patient may suggest a mass lesion and give a clue to its site. A brain scan is then performed with contrast enhancement – iodine for CT and gadolinium for MRI. MRI is a little more sensitive and can show small multiple metastases better and has become the investigation of choice. Thallium single photon emission computed tomography (SPECT) scanning can show increased metabolism in malignant tumours, positron emission tomography (PET) scanning will become more widely available. A CT of the chest and abdomen are indicated to determine the primary source of disease when a Metastatic tumour is suspected.

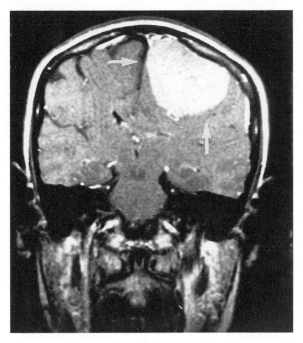

Figure 21.11. Coronal magnetic resonance scan of a 45-year-old woman showing large meningioma (arrows). Note the distortion of the brain in particular the midline.

Management

The two main goals are to remove the lesion and to preserve neurological function; sometimes these are incompatible and the neurosurgeon has to settle for the latter as the prime goal even if this means only partially excising lesions. Dexamethasone is used to treat the associated brain swelling which reduces ICP and can reverse deficits of neurological function. If there is hydrocephalus, this can be controlled either by excising the lesion or draining the ventricles by a temporary external ventricular drain through a frontal burr hole or permanently with a ventriculoperitoneal shunt.

Benign primary neoplasms

Other than pituitary adenomas (see below), the commonest benign neoplasm is a meningioma which is a neoplasm of arachnoid cells arising from the inner surface of the dura mater or the arachnoid granulations. The commonest sites are parafalcine, over the convexity of the cerebral hemispheres (Fig. 21.11), the tentorium and skull base. Treatment is by surgical excision which should be total but may be subtotal particularly in the case of meningiomata involving the skull base. Residual tumour following surgery may remain sessile but stereotactic radiosurgery has become the treatment of choice when the tumour show signs of enlargement.

Acoustic neuromas, or more accurately vestibular schwannomas, arise on the vestibular portion of the VIII nerve and expand in the cerebellopontine angle (Fig. 21.12). They have a variable growth potential and may be of variable size. They can

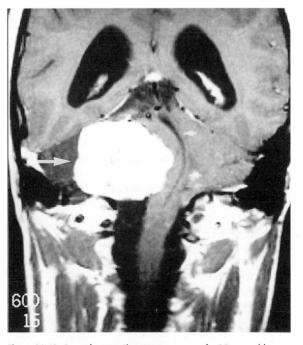

Figure 21.12. Coronal magnetic resonance scan of a 25-year-old man showing large acoustic neuroma (large arrow). Note also the distortion of the brainstem and fourth ventricle (small arrows).

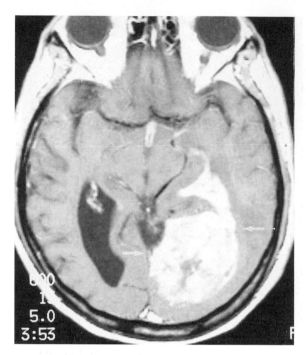

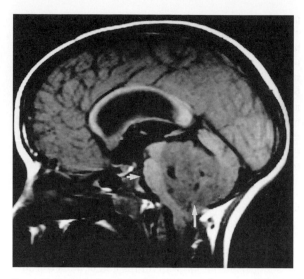

Figure 21.14. Magnetic resonance sagittal scan of a 9-year-old boy with large medulloblastoma of the vermis cerebelli (large arrow). Note also the compression of the brainstem (small arrow).

Figure 21.13. Magnetic resonance basal scan of a 60-year-old man with large parieto-occipital glioma (arrows). Note combination of mass effect and brain replacement.

occur in association with Type 2 neurofibromatosis where they may be bilateral. When small, they may be detected by sensorineuronal nerve deafness on audiometry. Treatment is by surgical excision either through the posterior fossa or through the labyrinth or by stereotactic radiosurgery. Even with large lesions, preservation of the facial nerve is now possible in most patients.

Malignant primary neoplasms

Gliomas are neoplasms that arise from the glial cells of the brain. The commonest are the astrocytomas which may occur at any site (Fig. 21.13). They show variable degrees of malignancy and are graded into four types. The grade I and II tumours are called low grade. Grade III tumours are called anaplastic astrocytoma and the most malignant of all is the glioblastoma multiforme (grade IV) which has tumour necrosis. Low grade neoplasms undergo surgery and no radiotherapy if they have symptoms and surgery can be completed with low risk of deficit. Maximally resective surgery and radiotherapy are used for high grade tumours unless resection would cause too greater a risk of deficit when a needle biopsy is used. Surgery is commonly guided by image guidance and biopsies by stereotactic techniques. Adjuvant chemotherapy, can also be used but affects on survival are small, local wafers of carmustine are now used intraoperatively for some indications. The results for the more malignant grades are

poor with few cures. In children, a subset called juvenile astrocytoma which occurs principally in the cerebellum is virtually benign and although total excision is preferable, subtotal excisions can often preserve good quality of life for up to 30 years.

The main other type of glioma is an oligodendroglioma, which has a propensity to haemorrhage. In immunosuppressed patients (e.g. transplanted patients on immunosuppressive therapy) or immunocompromised patients (e.g. human immunodeficiency virus (HIV)-positive patients) lymphomas can occur; these are usually non-Hodgkin lymphomas which can be B cell, T cell or mixed and are usually highly malignant.

Primitive neurectodermal tumours (PNET) occur principally in childhood. The commonest were previously called medulloblastomas (Fig. 21.14), but since they contain elements from both ependymomas and medulloblastomas, though in variable proportions, they have been renamed. They are thought to be embryonic tumours. They can be highly malignant and can seed through the CSF pathways. Treatment is by as radical excision as possible followed by radiotherapy to the whole neuraxis, including the spinal cord, in an attempt to sterilize the CSF pathways. They are radiosensitive and chemotherapy is also used. The 5-year survival rate is approximately 50% and the cure rate is 25%. Ependymomas occur close to the lining ependyma of the CSF pathways and within the spinal cord and conus medullaris and treatment is by surgical excision, followed by radiotherapy.

Secondary neoplasms (metastasis)

Almost any primary malignant neoplasm outwith the CNS may metastasize to the brain; however the commonest primary sites are the breast and lung which are of course common malignancies. Other sites which metastasize to the brain are renal, melanoma, prostate, stomach and ovary. The metastases may be solitary or multiple or can be widespread within the CSF pathways leading to carcinomatous meningitis and hydrocephalus. A single metastasis can be excised giving symptomatic relief and thereafter the treatment is as for the primary site and metastases elsewhere. Not infrequently, a cerebral metastasis appears without any obvious primary malignancy being found elsewhere in the body for some time. Multiple metastases are considered inoperable. Dexamethasone has a beneficial effect in dealing with pressure effects. Stereotactic radiosurgery is a developing treatment for metastases.

Pituitary gland

This is an endocrine gland in two parts: the adenohypophysis and neurohypophysis. The anterior pituitary secretes six hormones:

- Growth hormone (GH) is essential for skeletal growth in the pre-pubertal child and in the adult for regeneration of tissues and its release is controlled by the opposing hypothalamic hormones of somatostatin (inhibition) and growth hormone releasing hormone (GRH);
- Prolactin (PRL) is necessary for lactation but it is also released in the normal male and its action here is uncertain; production and release is controlled by a variety of factors and inhibition is under the control of dopamine;
- Adrenocorticotrophic hormone (ACTH) controls the release of corticosteroids from the adrenal gland;
- Thyroid stimulating hormone (TSH) has an effect on the thyroid gland and is controlled by thyrotrophic releasing hormone (TRH);
- The gonadotrophins – luteinizing (LH) and follicular stimulating (FSH) – have an effect on the gonads to control sexual characteristics, ovulation and spermatogenesis.

The posterior pituitary releases antidiuretic hormone (ADH) which is involved in the control of osmoregulation through an effect on the kidneys.

Adenomas

Pituitary neoplasms are virtually all benign adenomas. They arise from cells producing one or more of the anterior hormones, from cells producing partially formed hormones or from inactive cells. They cause symptoms through endocrinological effects, pressure mass effects on the optic nerves and chiasm which lie above the pituitary or in the case of very large adenomas on the cerebral structures such as the hypothalamus (Fig. 21.15).

Excess GH leads to acromegaly in the adult and gigantism in the pre-pubertal child. Acromegaly is characterized by overgrowth of hands, feet and the facial skeleton and distortion of other parts of the skeleton leading to progressive osteoarthritis. Internally, it leads particularly to visceromegaly and insulin-resistant diabetes mellitus.

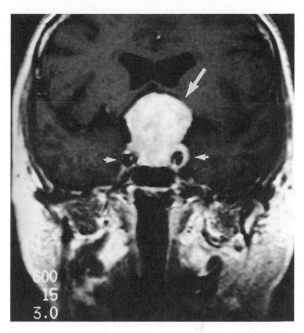

Figure 21.15. Magnetic resonance coronal scan of a 65-year-old woman with a large pituitary adenoma (large arrow). Note also the compression of the brainstem (small arrow).

Prolactinomas in pre-menopausal women lead to amenorrhoea, infertility and galactorrhoea and in men to impotence and loss of secondary male sexual characteristics.

ACTH adenomas lead to Cushing's disease. Cushing's syndrome involves loss of elastic tissue in the body with easy bruising of the skin, increased deposition of fat, myopathy and systemic hypertension. The syndrome can be due to one of three causes: a pituitary adenoma (Cushing's disease), an adenoma or carcinoma of the adrenal cortex, or oat-cell carcinoma of the bronchus leading to ectopic ACTH production.

Gonadotrophinomas lead to similar problems as prolactinomas without galactorrhoea. Thyrotrophinomas lead to secondary hyperthryroidism.

It is important to realize that a hypersecretory adenoma may compress the pituitary gland, leading to anterior hypopituitarism of other hormones. Anterior hypopituitarism leads eventually to deficiencies in all the pituitary hormones and the attendant effects on the target endocrine glands such that there is hypothyroidism, amenorrhoea or early menopause, infertility or loss of secondary sexual characteristics and loss of the cortisol response to physical stress. The onset may be insidious and may not be easily recognized.

Investigations Investigation of patients with suspected adenomas is by a full endocrinological biochemical assessment, testing the visual acuity and fields and an MR scan.

Management The two main aims of treatment are to normalize endocrine function and remove pressure mass effects. These can be effected by surgical excision, radiotherapy or hormone/antihormone therapy or by combinations of these. When surgical excision is employed, this is performed in over 90% of patients by the trans-sphenoidal route; basically, this involves going behind the nose, through the vomer and into the sphenoid air sinus and then cutting a bone window in the sellar floor and thence into the sella and excising the adenoma and leaving the pituitary gland behind. Occasionally, for very large adenomas, a frontal craniotomy is performed and the adenoma approached from above within the cranial cavity. Radiotherapy can be given to the sella, particularly in the case of inadequately excised adenomas, and over a number of years will usually eliminate the adenoma but at the expense of also killing most of the normal gland as well.

Antihormones are also used – for acromegaly, this is with somatostatin given by injection or occasionally a dopamine-agonist, bromocriptine. The latter, given by tablet or capsule, is much more effective in reducing excess PRL, has no obvious teratogenic effect and can be maintained through pregnancy. More recent analogues, for example cabergoline, only need to be taken every 3 days. In the case of Cushing's disease, the preferred option is surgery since this is a fatal disease and the antagonist metyrapone is effective for a limited period only.

Replacement hormones are given, except for PRL deficiency:

- GH is replaced in children by injection until they have grown sufficiently and recent trials suggest adults may also benefit;
- TSH deficiency is replaced using thyroxine;
- ACTH deficiency is replaced by hydrocortisone which is required twice daily for ordinary life, but if the patient has an intercurrent illness or undergoes surgery for lesions elsewhere in the body, it is absolutely essential that the dose is at least doubled whilst the physical stress lasts, and if the patient cannot take or absorb oral fluids then hydrocortisone must be given parenterally; the patient must also carry a blue steroid card with him at all times;
- ADH deficiency is replaced with the synthetic drug 1-deamino-8D-arginine vasopressin (DDAVP) which can be given orally, by nasal inhalation or by injection.

Intracranial vascular disease

Stroke and transient ischaemic attacks

The management of these conditions consumes about 5% of health service hospital costs within the UK. Stroke is not a diagnosis as such but is merely a description of a symptom complex ending in a cerebral infarct or haemorrhage as a result of a variety of vascular diseases.

A transient ischaemic attack (TIA) is an sudden onset episode of focal neurological deficit due to inadequate blood supply to the brain which resolves within 24 h and leaves no residual deficit. The majority occur in the internal carotid artery territory, although they can occur in the vertebrobasilar territory as well. Following TIA 5–10% of patients will have a stroke in each year after the event, the risk is highest in the first few days and weeks. Most TIAs are embolic and due to disease in the carotid arteries or heart. Such patients require urgent investigation of the heart by electrocardiogram and, possibly echocardiography of the carotid arteries by Doppler/duplex ultrasound and of the brain by CT scanning. If there is a carotid stenosis of >70%, then consideration needs to be given to carotid endarterectomy.

Of strokes, 85% are due to thromboembolic disease and 15% to haemorrhage (5% secondary to subarachnoid haemorrhage and 10% to intracerebral haemorrhage); the clinical distinction between occlusive and haemorrhagic stroke is often extremely difficult and CT scanning is required. The vast majority of strokes are treated medically but intracranial aneurysms, arteriovenous malformations and a small number of intracranial haemorrhages without obvious structural abnormality are treated surgically.

The risk factors for stroke include increasing systemic hypertension, cardiac disease, diabetes mellitus, and smoking. Hypertension is the most important risk factor and lowering blood pressures to the norm corrected for the patient's age is essential; in the non-urgent surgical case, referral should be made to a physician and surgery delayed until the blood pressure is controlled; in the emergency case it is essential to discuss the problem with the anaesthetist who will try and stabilize the situation during induction and maintenance of anaesthesia, although it must also be appreciated that sudden lowering of blood pressure can be dangerous.

Intracranial haemorrhage

Spontaneous intracranial haemorrhage may occur within the brain substance or subarachnoid space, and less commonly in the subdural space. The commonest cause is rupture of an intracranial aneurysm; rarer causes are rupture of a cerebral arteriovenous malformation, haemorrhage from a neoplasm or a bleeding diathesis (most commonly iatrogenically induced by the anticoagulant warfarin, Fig. 21.16).

The patient complains of a sudden very severe headache the like of which they have never experienced before. They may then lose consciousness (coma-producing haemorrhage) or remain unwell without going into coma (non-coma producing); approximately 20% die immediately or very soon after the haemorrhage. The survivors develop meningism due to the blood passing into the spinal subarachnoid space; meningism causes painful stiffness of the neck and lumbar region, which worsens with movement, and must not be confused with spinal pathology (see Chapter 20). Patients may develop neurological deficit either from the site of the aneurysm (e.g. a 3rd nerve palsy from an aneurysm of the internal carotid artery) or from ischaemia resulting from spasm of the major vessels and/or narrowing or occlusion of more distal vessels within the cerebral substance.

The diagnosis of a subarachnoid haemorrhage (SAH) is confirmed by the finding of blood on CT brain scan provided the scan is completed within 48 h of the ictus. If the scan is negative then a lumbar puncture is indicated but this is best left to

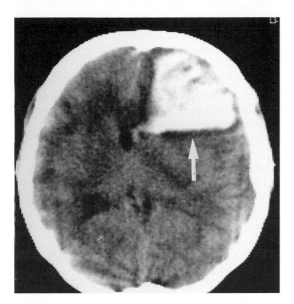

Figure 21.16. CT scan of a 30-year-old woman on uncontrolled warfarin. Note the large frontal spontaneous intra-cerebral haematoma (arrow).

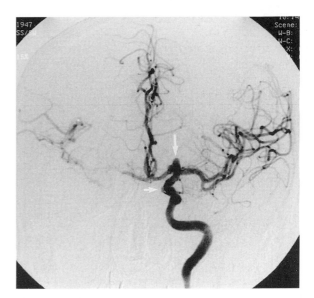

Figure 21.17. Digital subtraction angiogram anterior projection in 40-year-old woman with subarachnoid haemorrhage showing an aneurysm of bifurcation of internal carotid artery (large arrow) and posterior communicating aneurysm (small arrow).

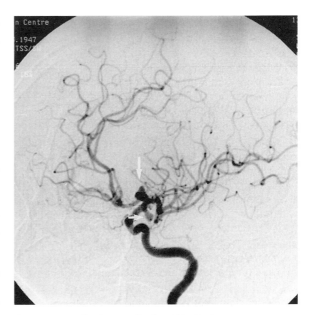

Figure 21.18. As for Fig. 21.17 but lateral projection.

longer than 6 h after the ictus if the patient's condition allows, SAH is confirmed by the finding of uniformal blood staining or xanthochromia. Thereafter, referral should be made to a neurosurgeon who will then obtain cerebral angiography of all four major vessels (both internal carotid and both vertebral arteries) to ascertain the cause of the haemorrhage.

Aneurysms are true aneurysms. They are nearly always situated at junctions of the major vessels of the circle of Willis, most commonly the anterior communicating complex, the internal carotid close to the junction with the posterior communicating artery and the trifurcation of the middle cerebral artery (Figs 21.17 and 21.18). If they occur in the young, they are thought to be congenital and they may also be familial. The majority occur from 40 years onwards and in these are thought to arise from a slight pre-existing weakness of the arterial wall which is then further weakened by atheroma and/or systemic hypertension. Once rupture has occurred, there is a propensity for further rupture and treatment is directed towards early obliteration of the aneurysm by inserting coils inside the aneurysmal sac and inducing clotting by interventional radiology or if this is not possible by craniotomy and placing of a spring clip across the neck thus excluding the aneurysm from the circulation.

Arteriovenous malformations (AVM) can occur anywhere in the cerebral substance. The majority are mainly capillary in structure and they all have arteriovenous shunts leading in some to increasing demands for blood and as a result further enlargement (Fig. 21.19). They cause problems in three main ways: haemorrhage, epilepsy and cerebral steal whereby blood is diverted from normal areas of brain to feed the AVM and thus causes neurological deficits. There is

usually no normal neural tissue within an AVM and treatment is by surgical excision, embolization by interventional radiology and/or stereotactic radiosurgery.

Occasionally, intracranial haematomas without an obvious structural aetiology require evacuation; this particularly applies to haematomas of the cerebellum. The patient on warfarin presents particular problems and haemorrhage

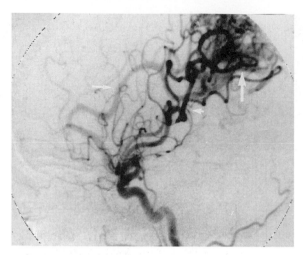

Figure 21.19. Lateral digital subtraction angiogram of a 38-year-old woman with subarachnoid and intra-cerebral haemorrhage showing arteriovenous malformation (large arrow). Note the enlarged feeding artery (smallest arrow) and cerebral steal with filling of contralateral artery (middle sized arrow).

usually occurs as a result of an elevated international normalized ratio (INR). If evacuation of the haematoma is thought necessary, warfarin must be temporarily stopped and in an emergency situation actually reversed. Thrombolysis for myocardial infarct or stroke can lead to intracerebral haemorrhage, emergency surgery is preceded by the administration of aprotinin to reverse the thrombolytic state.

CNS infections

The CNS is particularly sensitive to infection and the infective agents can be bacterial, viral and fungal or agents such as prions (small-chain deoxyribose nucleic acid (DNA) fragments) which are the suspected causative agents in Creutzfeldt–Jakob disease. Bacteria and fungi cause meningitis or brain abscess, viruses lead to encephalitis and prions to spongiform encephalopathies.

Meningitis

Acute bacterial meningitis

An acute infection of the subarachnoid space which invokes an inflammatory reaction from the meninges. Bacteria gain access to the CSF pathways through a variety of routes such as through the sinuses, if the dura has been breached such as through a CSF fistula, or most commonly indirectly through the bloodstream. The common infecting organisms vary at different stages of life. In neonates gram negative bacilli such as *E. coli*, in children haemophilus influenzae, in adults pneumococcus or meningococcus. In immuno-compromised patients, for example those on immune suppressing therapy and those with HIV infection, the bacteria may be opportunistic, that is usually commensal elsewhere in the body of a healthy patient and thus harmless, but in these patients somehow gain access

to the CSF and grow. In this context, it should be realized that one of the commonest causes of death in a patient with HIV infection is intracranial infection with the commonest bacterium being Listeria monocytogenes.

A purulent exudates forms in the basal cisterns and the brain becomes oedematous and ischaemic. The process of acute inflammation in the subarachnoid space can lead to an external obstructive hydrocephalus. Infarction of the brain can occur as the inflammation leads to an arteritis or venous thrombophlebitis.

Clinically, meningitis manifests as fever, headache, neck stiffness, photophobia and a deteriorating level of consciousness. A transient petechial skin rash can occur in meningococcal meningitis. Seizures, cranial nerve signs including deafness can develop. Focal neurological deficits can occur usually from focal ischaemia or the development of an abscess.

Diagnosis is suspected clinically and confirmation is by examination of the CSF by lumbar puncture. If there is focal neurological deficit, decreased conscious level or papilloedema, it is essential to perform a CT brain scan first to look for any space-occupying lesion. The CSF must be taken immediately to microbiology where a white cell count will be performed together with a Gram-stained film (gram +ve cocci – pneumococcus, gram −ve bacilli – haemophilus, gram −ve intra and extracellular cocci – meningococcus). A raised white cell count in the CSF is diagnostic (100–10 000 cells/mm^3); the glucose is reduced; the causative organisms can only be correctly identified by culture. Further investigations are then needed to determine the source of the infection for example chest X-ray, sinus X-ray, skull X-ray.

The main mode of treatment is with antibiotics which should be started immediately after diagnosis. Antibiotics must penetrate the blood brain barrier, be in appropriate doses, and the causal organism must be sensitive. Benzylpenecillin, cefotaxime, and Gentamicin are the most commonly used drugs. Treatment is continued until the patient is asymptomatic and a follow-up lumbar puncture shows resolution of the white cell count; the minimum period should be at least 10 days.

Tuberculous meningitis

Tuberculosis involves the CNS in 10% of infected patients. Following a bacteraemia foci of infection can lodge in the meninges, cerebral or spinal tissue, or choroids plexus. The basal meninges are most severely affected and hydrocephalus is common. The illness is progressive over months with a dementia. In the CSF a lymphocyte pleocytosis is present, the CSF protein is elevated, the CSF glucose is usually significantly lowered compared to the blood glucose. Microscopy using a Ziehl Neelsen stain can reveal the acid fast bacilli, CSF culture confirms the diagnosis but takes many weeks, most laboratories have polymerase chain reaction (PCR) tests available to detect the bacterial DNA. Treatment is with antibiotics usually including Isoniazid, Rifampicin and Pyrzinamide, steroids may be used if the conscious level is deteriorating and hydrocephalus may need CSF drainage.

Viral meningitis

CNS involvement in viral infection can occur through massive viraemia or along peripheral nerves. The infection not only can lead to meningitis but also cause encephalitis, cerebritis or myelitis. Infection of the motor neurons and spinal nerves is poliomyelitis and of the dorsal root ganglia radiculitis. The commonest causal organisms are enteroviruses, mumps virus, or herpes simplex. The meningeal phase of infection with headache photophobia and drowsiness usually lasts about 7–10 days. CSF cell count is elevated and if obtained early can contain the virus. Treatment is for the symptoms apart from severe herpes simplex meningitis where acyclovir is used.

Abscess

Intracerebral abscess can occur either as a result of haematogenous emboli of bacteria with for example congenital heart disease, bronchiectasis or by direct spread from the nose and paranasal sinuses or from the middle ear and mastoid cavities (Fig. 21.20), through compound depressed fractures, infected dental caries. In either event the bacteria grow and initially lead to an area of septic encephalitis. Thereafter, the centre liquefies and the surrounding brain reacts by forming a gliotic capsule and thus a true abscess develops. In direct spread from sinusitis or mastoiditis, the bacteria either spread intracranially through a hole in the dura or by retrograde spread along a draining emissary vein and the commonest sites are in the frontal or temporal lobes. Also direct spread can lead to extradural or subdural abscess formation; occasionally the bone is involved and develops osteomyelitis (see Chapter 20).

Clinically, an abscess is suspected in a patient with symptoms and signs of raised intracranial pressure, focal neurological deficit and only occasionally fevers. Systemic signs of infection can be often absent. An infectious source may or may not be apparent. Diagnosis is by CT scanning although MRI is able to show multiple lesions not seen on CT and lumbar puncture is contraindicated. Emergency referral should be made to a neurosurgeon who in the majority of cases will perform a burr hole and aspirate the pus for microbiological analysis. Treatment is by appropriate antibiotics, abscess drainage. The infectious source must be found and dealt with early to prevent further abscesses forming. Persistent abscesses may require excision by craniotomy particularly those in the cerebellum as do subdural and extradural abscesses. Intracerebral and subdural empyema are accompanied by a very high incidence of epilepsy and anticonvulsants are usually necessary. The patient must be informed that he should report himself to the Driving Licensing Authority before recommencing driving.

Creutzfeldt–Jakob disease

One of the prion diseases characterized by the accumulation of a modified cell membrane protein within the central nervous system. The infective agent is resistant to heat and

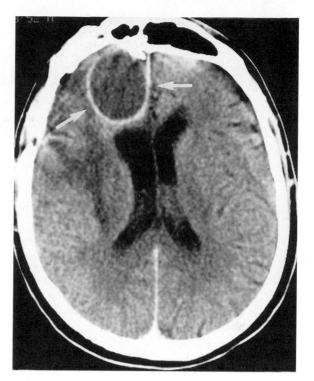

Figure 21.20. CT scan of a 40-year-old-man who 8 years previously had a head injury with fracture of the frontal bone. Note the frontal intra-cerebral abscess (arrows).

radiation therefore is potentially transmissible through contaminated surgical instruments. Creutzfeldt–Jakob disease (CJD) has an incidence of 1 in 1 million and presents with rapidly progressive myoclonus, ataxia, and dementia. The new variant form vCJD presents in younger patients with a slower time course and has been linked to bovine spongiform encephalopathy (BSE). Other prion diseases include Gestmann Straussler syndrome similar to CJD and Kuru spread by cannibalism in Papua New Guinea.

FURTHER READING

Apuzzo MLJ (ed). *Brain Surgery: Complications, Avoidance and Management*. New York: Churchill Livingstone, 1993

Crockard A, Hayward R, Hoff JT (eds). *Neurosurgery: The Scientific Basis of Clincal Practice*. Oxford: Blackwell Scientific Publications, 1992

Findlay G, Owen R (eds). *Surgery of the Spine*. Oxford: Blackwell Scientific Publications, 1992

Lindsay KW, Bone I (eds). *Neurology and Neurosurgery Illustrated*. Churchill Livingstone, 1997

Palmer JD (ed). *Manual of Neurosurgery*. New York: Churchill Livingstone, 1996

Russell DS, Rubinstein LJ. *Pathology of Tumours of the Nervous System*. London: Edward Arnold, 1989

Schmidek HH, Sweet WH (eds). *Operative Neurosurgical Techniques: Indications, Methods and Results*. Philadelphia: WB Saunders, 1995

22

Musculoskeletal System

Simon P Frostick and Vishal Sahni

Department of Orthopaedics, Royal Liverpool University Hospital, University of Liverpool, Liverpool, UK

CONTENTS

Fractures	**440**
Fracture healing	441
Clinical assessment	442
Investigations	443
Management	443
Specific fractures	445
Complications of fractures	447
Compartment syndromes	449
Joints	**450**
Clinical assessment	450
Arthritis	451
Joint injuries	452
Joint replacement	455
Amputations and prosthetics	**458**
Amputations	458
Prosthetics	460
Tendon injuries	**461**
Diagnosis	461
Management	461
Hand injuries	**462**
Clinical assessment	462
Palmar compartments and spaces	462
Bone trauma (including 'crush injuries')	462
Fractures (open and closed) and fracture dislocations	463
Hand infections	464
Disorders of the foot	**464**
Clinical assessment	464
Investigation	465
Ankle disorders	465
Hindfoot disorders	466
Forefoot disorders	467
Bone and joint infections	**469**
Acute osteomyelitis	469
Chronic osteomyelitis	470
Brodie's abscess	471
Septic arthritis	471

Bone and joint pain	**473**
Cervical spine pain	473
Shoulder pain	474
Clinical assessment	475
Back pain	476
Sciatica	479
Clinical features	479
Metabolic bone disease	**480**
Osteoporosis	480
Rickets	481
Osteomalacia	483
Malignant disease of bone and soft tissue	**483**
Clinical assessment	483
Investigations	485
Management	488
Common disorders of infancy and childhood	**489**
Congenital dislocation and developmental dysplasia of hip	489
Congenital talipes equinovarus (club foot)	489
Intoeing gait	490
Perthes' disease	490
Transient synovitis of the hip	491
Slipped upper femoral epiphysis	491
Further reading	**492**

This chapter describes common orthopaedic conditions with heavy emphasis on the relevant clinical details that should be elucidated on history and examination. With a firm grasp of the principles of clinical orthopaedic assessment, a differential diagnosis can be formulated and appropriate investigations performed subsequently.

FRACTURES

Fractures can be divided into the following types:
- *Green stick fractures*: These occur in children. One cortex is splinted and the other is intact.

- *Closed fractures*: There is no communication between the fracture haematoma and the environment outside the integument. The skin and soft-tissue envelope remain intact.
- *Open ('compound') fractures*: There is breach of the integument and soft-tissue envelope surrounding the fracture such that the fracture haematoma communicates with the outside environment. These fractures are associated with an open wound and there is increased risk of deep infection, which may have catastrophic consequences for the healing of bone and soft tissues and subsequent usage of the affected part. Therefore, such fractures invariably require surgical treatment and constitute an orthopaedic emergency. Compound fractures may also be associated with delayed union.
- *Pathological fractures*: These occur in bone weakened by a pre-existing disease, for example metastatic deposits or a generalized bone disease such as osteoporosis. Therefore, the resultant force required to fracture the bone is less than that required to fracture normal bone.
- *Stress fractures*: These usually occur in otherwise normal bone, typically the shaft of the second metatarsal in military recruits, that is subjected to repeated stresses that it is unaccustomed to and over a long period of time.

The commonest fractures presenting in adults are:
- distal radial fractures;
- fractured necks of femur;
- fractures involving the medial and lateral malleoli of the ankle;
- phalangeal/metacarpal fractures;
- long-bone fractures of the upper and lower limbs, particularly from contact sports and road traffic accidents;
- fractures and dislocations involving joints (e.g. glenohumeral joint).

The equivalent list in children is:
- epiphyseal fracture of the distal radius;
- complete or incomplete fractures of the radius/ulna;
- fractures of the long bones of the lower limbs;
- displaced fractures of the distal humerus.

Fracture healing

There are two types of fracture healing: primary and secondary.

Primary healing of a fracture is a direct attempt by the cortex to re-establish itself thereby restoring mechanical continuity. This occurs when rigid fixation has been achieved and is most commonly seen after dynamic compression plating (DCP) of fractures. The bone resorbing cells on one side of the fracture form a tunnel and re-establish new haversian systems by providing pathways for the penetration of blood vessels. Osteoclasts form cutting cones that advance across the fracture line forming a resorptive cavity.

Secondary healing can be categorized into three broad phases:

1. *Inflammatory phase* (haematoma and granulation tissue formation): When a bone fractures, the periosteal and endosteal vessels are torn and bleed. A blood clot forms between the fracture ends. Osteocytes in their lacuna at the fracture ends loose their nutrition supply and undergo necrosis. The clotting of blood to form a haematoma takes approximately 48 h. There is an acute inflammatory response with local vasodilatation and infiltration with white cells. The blood clot is invaded by macrophages and osteoclasts which remove any dead bone. The haematoma is invaded by newly formed capillaries from the endosteum–periosteum and other connective tissue cells, and over the ensuing 2 weeks it changes to granulation tissue. The granulation tissue osteoblasts proliferate and have the capacity to produce new bone. Clinically this stage is associated with pain, swelling and heat.

2. *Reparative phase* (fibrocartilaginous callus and bony callus formation): Over the next 2–6 weeks, the granulation tissue matures into a mass of callus which stabilizes the fracture fragment by bridging the gap between the fracture ends. (The exception is in the healing of cancellous bone, where little callus is formed.) The callus consists of osteoid tissue. Essentially, subperiosteal and endosteal callus formation surrounds the fracture ends and within this mass ossification begins to form mature bone. The early woven bone, although stable, has some mobility at the fracture ends. As ossification continues between 6 and 12 weeks, the woven bone changes to dense lamella bone. At this stage the fracture is clinically stable and when the callus is fully mature, usually between 12 and 26 weeks, the fracture is considered to have united. Clinically this stage corresponds to early clinical union by fibrous and cartilaginous tissue.

3. *Remodelling phase*: Over the ensuing months, the newly formed bone adapts to the stresses applied within it (e.g. weight bearing in a lower limb bone). The capacity for remodelling is greater in children and any deformity following the fracture may be partially corrected. The remodelling process can continue for 1–2 years.

Fracture healing is affected by local and general factors. The former include:
- blood supply to the fracture area;
- type of bone involved and location of fracture within a particular bone;
- interposition of soft tissue between fracture ends;
- whether the fracture is open or closed and presence of infection within the fracture site;
- gap between the fracture ends.

General factors influencing fracture healing are:
- patient's age,
- patient's nutritional status,
- various metabolic factors.

Delayed union

This is when a fracture takes longer than normal to unite. Factors contributing to delayed union include poor local blood supply and displacement of fracture fragments leading to a significant gap between fracture ends, with or without associated soft-tissue interposition in between. Inadequate initial treatment of the fracture may also contribute to delayed union. This may take the form of inappropriate or inadequate immobilization of the fracture allowing excessive movement which prevents the appropriate soft-tissue response between the fracture ends that is essential for mature bone formation. Operative treatment may also interfere with fracture healing as it may predispose the fracture site to infection and surgical exposure can further disrupt what may already be an attenuated blood supply and in addition drains the fracture haematoma which has an immense healing potential by virtue of its cellular elements.

Non-union

This is when a fracture fails to unite (Fig. 22.1) unless external intervention is undertaken. The healing process fails completely and the fracture ends remain separate. They may be bridged by scar tissue. There may be a surrounding capsule of fibrous tissue with a fluid-filled cavity between the fracture ends (pseudoarthrosis).

There are two types of non-union: atrophic and hypertrophic. *Atrophic non-union* is usually associated with a poor local blood supply and minimal or no callus formation. The fracture ends undergo necrosis and atrophy. In such cases the biological environment is responsible for non-healing of

the fracture and without bone grafting, the fracture will not unite. This usually involves surgical exposure of the fracture ends and removal of any pseudoarthrosis and false capsule together with associated scar tissue. Osteogenic activity is promoted by means of the bone graft (see below). Then the fracture is immobilized either by internal or external fixation. *Hypertrophic union* is characterized by massive callus formation which can become ossified but there is incomplete bridging between the fracture ends and the fracture remains mobile. In such cases the biomechanics of the fracture are at fault and the usual cause is inadequate immobilization of the fracture. This type of non-union is best addressed by stable fixation.

Malunion

When a fracture unites but in a non-anatomical position, this is referred to as malunion (Fig. 22.2). Malunion can be translational, angulational and rotational.

Clinical assessment

There is usually an history of acute trauma to the injured part and this is important to determine whether a fracture is pathological or not. It should also be determined if there is a history of prior problems with the affected part which preceded the acute trauma. If there are any conditions, either local or general which may predispose to the development of fractures, this may also affect patients' recovering rehabilitation.

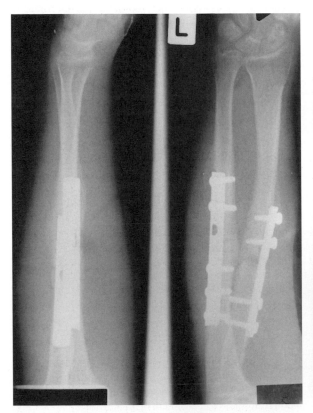

Figure 22.1. Radial non-union. Plated radius (left) and ulna (right).

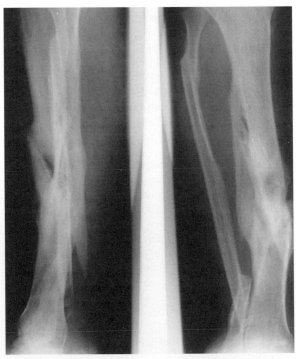

Figure 22.2. Malunion of a fractured tibia (left) and fibula (right).

Clinical features are usually:

- *Pain* is usually of sudden onset and localized to the region of the fracture; however, it may radiate to an area remote from the fracture (e.g. fractured neck of femur). In pathological fractures, there may have been pre-existent mild bone symptoms prior to the sudden onset of severe pain.
- Due to the associated bleeding into the soft tissues secondary to the fracture, *swelling* can be marked around the fracture site. The soft tissues are distended and in a limb fracture this may present as a fusiform swelling of the affected part of the limb. Bleeding into the subcutaneous region also leads to *bruising*.
- The fracture area is exquisitely *tender* and on palpation, abnormal movement and/or crepitus may be detected at the fracture site due to mobility between the fracture ends.
- If the fracture is displaced or angulated, the affected bone and therefore the affected body part will lose their normal anatomical contour. The *deformity* must be assessed not only in the coronal and sagittal planes, but also by looking for rotational deformity as this must be corrected as the capacity for rotational remodelling is limited.
- Due to the above, there is acute *loss of function* of the affected part. However, a patient may also present with deformity and swelling but no pain or tenderness because of damage to the peripheral nerves. Under these circumstances, the patient may tolerate the disturbed function and their presentation may be delayed.

Investigations

The diagnosis of the vast majority of fractures is confirmed by plain radiographs. Radiological evaluation of the fracture configuration should include a radiograph in at least two planes at 90° to one another as a single radiograph in one plane may not be sufficient to detect all fractures. The joint above and below the fracture of a long bone should also be visualized to exclude associated but remote fractures of adjacent bones or the involvement of the joint surface. Depending on the area for investigation, more specialized radiographs can be performed to detect particular sorts of fractures. If the clinical suspicion is high but plain radiographs do not confirm the presence or absence of a fracture, then more sophisticated imaging techniques, namely radioisotope, magnetic resonance imaging (MRI) or computed axial tomography (CAT) scanning, can be performed.

A fracture needs to be described according to the following features:

- simple – isolated fracture separating the bone into two fragments, or comminuted – multiple fragments are identifiable;
- region of the bone in which it occurs – diaphysial, metaphyseal or epiphysial;
- extra- or intra-articular involving an adjacent joint surface;
- displaced (in coronal, sagittal or rotational) or undisplaced.

The neurovascular supply to the affected part with associated soft-tissue or visceral injuries must also be assessed, including for compartment syndromes (see below) and acute vascular disruption rendering the limb ischaemic.

Management

Pain relief

Adequate temporary immobilization of the fracture, be it with plaster of Paris backslabs or casts, various splints or special frames which allow traction of the affected limb, usually results in prompt relief of acute pain. This is usually supplemented with adequate analgesia if there is no specific contraindication and also regional nerve blocks, but only after the patient has been assessed for associated nerve injury. Discomfort from swelling may be relieved by elevating the affected limb.

Early reduction

If there is a substantial initial displacement of the fracture in the surrounding soft tissues and neurovascular supply to the distal part of the limb, then the fracture should be reduced to an acceptable position and appropriately immobilized. Displaced fractures can compromise the local blood supply to soft tissues, particularly the skin and if not treated urgently, can result in localized necrosis which may render a closed fracture into an open one and increase the risk of subsequent sepsis and problems with union. This is particularly common with fracture dislocations. Once the fracture has been temporarily reduced and immobilized, radiographs should be taken to assess the adequacy of the reduction.

Definitive fracture treatment

To reduce the risk of infection, patients with open fractures must be taken to theatre as early as possible and undergo appropriate and adequate debridement of the soft tissues and the fractured ends of the bones under the cover of appropriate antibiotic prophylaxis (see below) and copious lavage with at least 3 l of saline. This can be combined with appropriate internal or external fixation of the fracture.

If the fracture is closed and there is no associated neurovascular deficit, the decision to use either conservative or operative treatment will depend on general and local factors. Both forms of treatment have their disadvantage and advantages. General factors include the patient's:

- age;
- general fitness;
- employment;
- involvement in sporting activities and hobbies;
- social and domestic situation;
- ongoing medical conditions that may be debilitating;
- functional demands;
- psychological makeup, which has a dramatic influence on the patient's ability to cope with a particular fracture treatment and the required postfracture rehabilitation.

Local factors include:
- site of fracture;
- degree of comminution of the fracture (influences stability of fracture);
- whether the fracture involves an articular surface (also influences stability of fracture);
- quality of the bone stock;
- quality of surrounding tissues, particularly the overlying skin;
- most importantly, the tissue environment for the healing of the fracture.

Conservative treatment

Closed reduction can be achieved by skilful manipulation of the fracture, often under image intensifier control with the patient adequately anaesthetized. The fracture, and possibly the joints above and below it, then need to be immobilized using bandaging, plaster of Paris casts (Fig. 22.3) or specialized splints (e.g. Thomas splint). Check radiographs are usually performed after application of a cast or splint to assess the alignment of the fracture.

The advantage of conservative treatment is that there is no formal operation under anaesthesia and the patient is not left with a scar. As the skin integument is not breached, risk of developing a deep infection at the fracture site should be precluded and as the soft tissue is not disrupted, the local environment for the healing of the fractures should not be adversely influenced. Also, conservative treatment precludes the necessity of a second operation which may be required to remove any metallic hardware.

The disadvantage is the necessity of external immobilization, usually of the joint above and below the fracture site, for a prolonged period of time, which results in stiffness of the joints with bone and soft-tissue atrophy, which is called as 'the fracture disease'. Exact anatomical alignment is often not achieved with closed means of treatment and there may therefore be residual deformity.

Operative treatment

This usually involves internal or external fixation of the fracture. External fixation involves the use of specialized frames to maintain the fracture alignment. Internal fixation can involve the use of percutaneous pins or the formal open reduction of the fracture site and then stabilizing the fracture fragments with a combination of screws, plates and pins which are left *in situ* (Fig. 22.4). Depending on the bone involved and the site of the fracture, intramedullary nails or special internal fixation devices designed for specific fracture configurations can also be used. When the fracture is deemed unfit for fixation or for instance when an elderly patient sustains an intracapsular femoral fracture, a replacement prosthesis is an excellent option.

The advantage of open surgical treatment is that the exact anatomical alignment is often obtained. With good internal

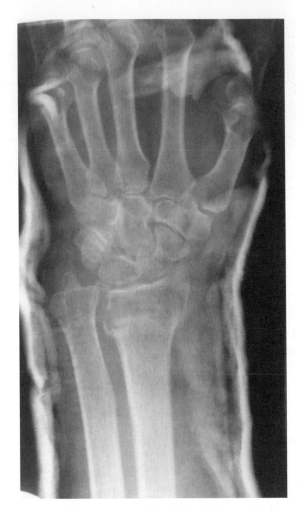

Figure 22.3. Colles fracture treated in a plaster of Paris cast.

fixation, no external fixation is required to augment stability of the fracture. This allows early active mobilization of the joints above and below the fracture, which prevents the development of postfracture stiffness and tissue atrophy, and aids in the rehabilitation of the affected parts. It also allows the patient to get back to work in a shorter time.

The main disadvantage is that the patient requires an anaesthetic. An open procedure is involved and this predisposes to the development of infections. There is a risk of damage to vital structures such as nerves and vessels, and also the local tissue environment of the healing fracture may be affected if there is disruption of the blood supply to the fracture fragments. The combination of loss of fracture haematoma which has factors essential for fracture healing and devascularization of the bone by surgical handling can lead to delayed union or non-union. The patient is left with a postoperative scar that may be cosmetically important to some individuals. Depending on the site and duration of operation, the patient may also require a blood transfusion.

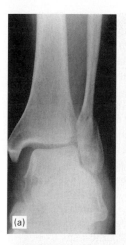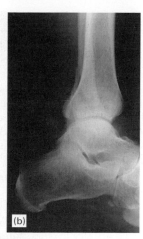

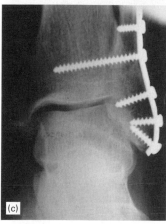

Figure 22.4. Fractured lateral malleolus with talar shift (a & b) and following open reduction and internal fixation (c).

Thromboembolic phenomena, particularly with lower limb fractures, can occur with either conservative or operative treatment. If the patient remains confined to bed for prolonged periods, particularly in skeletal traction where an affected limb is immobilized, antithromboembolic prophylaxis is required. If surgical fracture fixation is satisfactory, then early mobilization may reduce the risk of deep venous thrombosis (DVT); however, if the patient cannot be mobilized early, operative treatment may actually increase the risk of thromboembolic phenomena. The important risk factors in development of a thromboembolic phenomena are past history of DVT, currently taking an oral contraceptive pill, patients with malignancy, prolonged and major surgery on the lower limb and inherited or acquired hypercoagulability.

Bone grafting

Four types of bone grafts are usually recognized:

- *Autografts*: Donor bone is transferred from one site on the patient to another site. The donor site is typically the iliac crest of the pelvis and grafts are cancellous chips or corticocancellous strips which are laid between and over the exposed fracture ends to encourage union at a fracture site or to achieve fusion across a joint.
- *Isografts*: Grafts transferred between identical twins.
- *Allografts*: Grafts transferred between individuals of the same species but with a different genetic makeup. Typically this involves the use of cadaveric bone transferred to a living individual as a structural graft.
- *Xenografts*: Transfer of a graft from a member of one species to a different species.

Autografts are commonly used in the treatment of delayed unions and non-unions to enhance fracture healing, act as a structural support and, as fresh bone grafts contain cells which can theoretically form new bone, possibly to replace lost bone. By using vascularized bone grafts, most commonly fibular grafts, the blood supply to a fracture area can be enhanced and therefore one of the conditions necessary for fracture healing improved.

Early rehabilitation

The fragment must be adequately healed and clinically stable before a plaster cast or splint is removed and movement of the affected part is allowed. The effects of prolonged immobilization – disuse osteopaenia of the bones, contracture of soft tissues and stiffness of associated joints, which may take a prolonged period to overcome – must be weighed against too early removal of the splintage before the fracture is solid with subsequent loss of fracture alignment necessitating remanipulation.

With internal fixation, the associated joints are encumbered by external splintage and therefore rehabilitation may begin early but only if the internal fixation is of a satisfactory standard to avoid the problem of loss of fixation.

Regardless of the method of fracture stabilization, once fractures are clinically solid, ancillary treatment (physiotherapy and hydrotherapy) must endeavour to return the affected part to its pre-injury function as early as possible.

Specific fractures

Hand fractures are dealt with under the later section on the hand.

Distal radial fractures

These are the commonest fractures in adults, particularly the elderly. Distal radial fractures may be extra- or intra-articular, displaced or undisplaced and comminuted (Fig. 22.5). Grossly unstable fractures with significant dorsal angulation and displacement of the distal radial fragments usually involves a high degree of comminution with radial shortening and are often associated with a fracture of the ulnar styloid (Fig. 22.6). The commonest way of immobilizing relatively uncomplicated fractures of the distal radius is closed reduction with

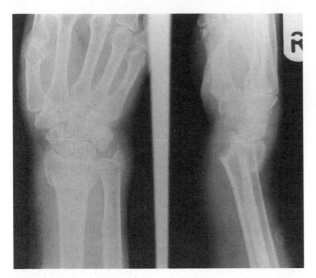

Figure 22.5. Colles fracture.

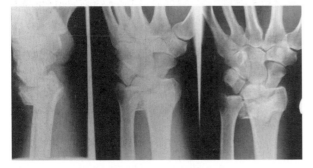

Figure 22.6. Comminuted displaced intra-articular fracture of the distul radius.

local, regional or general anaesthesia and immobilization for 4–6 weeks in a well-moulded below-elbow cast. Complicated fractures may require either the application of an external fixator or open reduction and internal fixation with metallic plate, screws and pins. A significant bony defect remains once acceptable reduction has been achieved and fixation may need to be augmented with an autogenous bone graft, synthetic bone substitutes or bone cement.

Ankle fractures

Fractures involving the ankle joint commonly involve the lateral malleolus with or without involvement of the medial and posterior malleolus. Lateral malleolar fractures in isolation may be associated with medial ligamentous disruptions. Ankle fractures that also involve external rotation abduction can also result in proximal spiral fractures of the fibula with associated medial soft-tissue damage. These may often go

unrecognized but are important because they involve significant instability of the ankles. As these fractures are generally intra-articular, they require accurate reduction to maintain normal alignment of the joint surfaces (Fig. 22.7). The decision to operate is mainly based on the talar shift, age of the patient and co-morbidities if present. Talar shift is the gap between the talus and the medial malleolus and indicates malalignment of the ankle joint. The ankle joint is very sensitive to even very little malalignment and 1 mm of talar shift can cause almost 13% malalignment of the joint.

If the fractures are undisplaced or minimally displaced, and if there is no talar shift they may be treated conservatively with plaster immobilization in a below-knee cast. Whether the patient can weight bear through the cast is a clinical decision depending on radiographical assessment of the alignment of the fracture. Immobilization for 6 weeks in a below-knee cast is usually adequate after which mobilization with crutches, and partial weight bearing increasing to full weight bearing is instituted.

However, the vast majority of ankle fractures are usually displaced on presentation. They may be associated with dislocation of the tibiotalar joint with resultant ischaemic changes in the overlying skin. This requires prompt reduction. The ankle should then be immobilized in a below-knee plaster slab and the leg elevated whilst awaiting definitive surgical treatment. Surgical treatment usually involves open reduction and internal fixation of the medial and lateral malleolar fragments with metallic screws and plates. Radiographs are obtained on the operating table to ensure good anatomical reduction of the articular surface, the fracture site and also appropriate placement of the implant. If the internal fixation is satisfactory, then there is no need for external plaster immobilization and the joint can be mobilized early with range of movement exercises. However, the implants are not strong enough to tolerate body weight and therefore the patient is mobilized, non-weight bearing on the affected leg, with crutches. This regimen is continued for 6 weeks and then the patient is allowed to weight bear.

Fractured neck of femur

Fractured necks of femur may be classified as intra- or extracapsular. The former are either displaced (Fig. 22.8) or undisplaced. Undisplaced intracapsular fractures are generally treated by pinning them *in situ* with cannulated screws in the operating theatre under X-ray control. The blood supply to the femoral head is somewhat precarious in displaced intracapsular fractures and the risk of avascular necrosis of the femoral head is high. Therefore, these fractures are generally treated with prosthetic replacement of the femoral head in the older age group, which precludes the development of avascular necrosis and allows early relief of pain and early mobilization with full weight bearing from the outset. The other main complication of displaced intracapsular fractures is non-union. The incidence of non-union in these

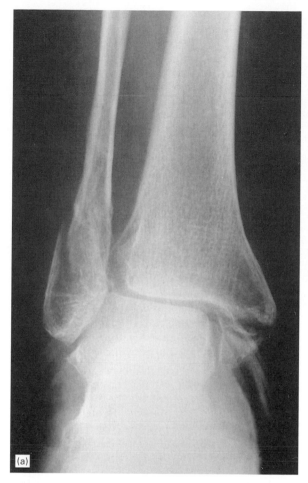

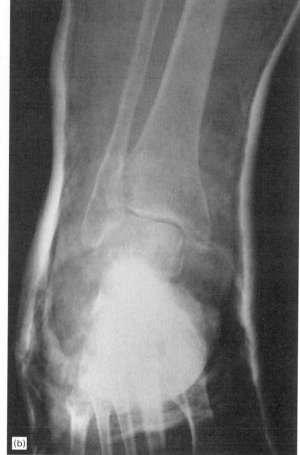

Figure 22.7. Bimalleolar fracture treated with a plaster of Paris cast.

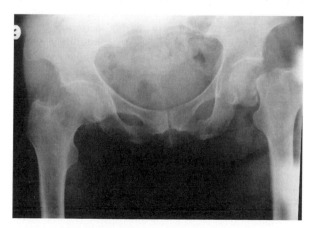

Figure 22.8. Displaced intracapsular fracture of the left neck of femur.

fractures is higher than other fractures because of the biomechanical disadvantage whereby shearing forces act on the fracture and also due to the fact that synovial fluid has angiogenic inhibiting factors.

Extracapsular fractures usually involve the pertrochanteric, intertrochanteric or subtrochanteric regions of the proximal femur and may be displaced or undisplaced, simple or comminuted. They are usually unstable but because of the risk to the elderly of prolonged immobilization in bed, the accepted form of treatment is usually screw and plate implants, which are designed to allow collapse of the fracture into a stable configuration. The most commonly used implant is a dynamic hip screw (DHS). A proximal femoral nail (PFN) is another option for these fractures. Elderly patients are often unable to co-operate with a non- or partial-weight-bearing regimen postoperatively but the implant allows full weight bearing from the start.

Complications of fractures

Immediate complications

Associated vascular injuries resulting in ischaemia to parts distal to the fracture must be treated as an emergency or necrosis of tissues distal to the fracture site can result with the possibility of developing gangrene, necessitating amputation. Other local complications include neural injury from laceration of a nerve or secondary to external compression, for example neurovascular complications in supracondylar fractures of the humerus in children. It is also important to recognize the development of compartment syndrome (see below).

Other immediate problems can be shock, associated injuries to the neurovascular structures, injuries to joints, intra-articular fractures and fracture dislocations, and also disruption of the integument resulting in a compound fracture.

Delayed complications
Infection
Compound fractures that are not treated as a surgical emergency with aggressive debridement of soft tissue and fracture ends, can result in subsequent infection of the soft tissues and of the fracture haematoma. If not appropriately treated, infection can delay union or result in non-union and chronic osteomyelitis. Early and judicious appropriate intravenous antibiotics should be given as prophylaxis and swabs and soft-tissue specimens sent to microbiology to identify any early organisms that may contaminate the wound.

Volkman's ischaemic contracture
This is usually a result of an unrecognized compartment syndrome where there is alternate necrosis of the muscles within a compressed myofascial compartment. Once the muscle tissue is necrotic, it is replaced by scar tissue. As the scar tissue matures it contracts, resulting in joint contractures and deformity across which the muscles act. This is most commonly seen in children after distal humeral fractures wherein the forearm muscles are commonly affected resulting in clawing of the hand, though it may also affect myofascial compartments in the leg, foot and very rarely in the thigh.

Treatment in chronic cases is very difficult. It often requires prolonged physiotherapy with serial splintage to try and correct some of the residual deformity. However, in the established case, surgical release of the scarred muscles popularly known as the muscle slide procedures, with or without tenotomies, and joint contractures may be appropriate. To restore active function in the joints, tendon transfers may be appropriate.

Fat embolism
The exact aetiology of this condition remains somewhat obscure. It is thought to be a generalized metabolic derangement secondary to release of fat particles from the marrow within the medullary cavity into the general circulation. Its main effect appears to be at the gas-exchange interface within the lungs. An inflammatory response within the alveoli causes an interstitial exudate to form between the alveolar membrane and the capillary lining. There is also necrosis of specific cells within the alveoli that are important in the production of surfactant, resulting in alveolar collapse. This causes a

thickening of the interface at the gas–blood membrane which interferes with gas exchange between alveolar air and capillary blood, resulting in hypoxaemia which manifests clinically as disturbed mental function. A clinical diagnosis is made on the basis of tachycardia, tachypnea, fever, hypoxaemia and a petechial rash that appears on the upper anterior body areas like chest, neck, axilla and upper arm, and is considered a pathognomonic sign of fat embolism syndrome. As the condition becomes established, the patient's general condition deteriorates and treatment in intensive care with artificial ventilation is required. There is a definite mortality associated with this syndrome, although, with early aggressive therapy, namely oxygen and intermittent positive pressure ventilation, treatment of any associated multiorgan failure, mortality and morbidity can be reduced.

Myositis ossificans
This is a post-traumatic event that usually involves ossification of the soft tissues and the haematoma surrounding a fracture, typically in the anterior aspect of the elbow. It results in progressive stiffness of the joint and if untreated can result in a totally rigid joint. The patient may notice an increased degree of warmth around the elbow associated with increasing stiffness and occasionally pain. At a later stage, a palpable lump in the region of the fracture may be detected. The initial treatment usually involves resting the injured part. However, the entire process may take years to resolve and once the ossification mass is mature it may warrant surgical excision.

Late complications
These usually involve abnormalities of fracture union, namely malunion, non-union and delayed union. Even later sequelae are degenerative osteoarthrosis of the associated joints and tardy nerve palsy. Malunion can involve shortening of the affected limb or a residual deformity. In the younger age group, deformity may be reduced by remodelling an overgrowth of the bone; however, in adults, particularly with respect to rotational deformity, remodelling is extremely limited in its ability to correct residual deformity.

Epiphyseal plate injuries
These occur in the paediatric age group and may result in ongoing deformity if there has been disruption of the growth plate.

Avascular necrosis
This commonly affects fractures where the blood supply to the bone is tenuous (e.g. fractures of the femoral neck, scaphoid and talus). As a result of the fracture, the blood supply to a segment of bone is disrupted and will not be reinstituted even with accurate reduction and appropriate immobilization; over a period of time the bone undergoes necrosis and ultimately collapses often leading to arthritis of the joint.

Sudeck's atrophy

A not uncommon sequelae of fractures and their associated treatment is reflex sympathetic dystrophy or Sudeck's atrophy. Many names have been attributed to this condition and the most recent name in vogue is complex regional pain syndrome type II. This most commonly occurs following hand or wrist fractures, though it can occur in the lower limbs. The exact aetiology is unknown but it is thought to be related to autonomic nervous system dysfunction, particularly involving the sympathetic branch. It is difficult to predict which patients will be predisposed to developing this condition. The joints distal to the fracture are usually stiff and the affected part is usually swollen with shiny, smooth, mottled skin which may be excessively sweaty or cold to palpation depending on the stage of the condition. Skin creases are usually lost and the nails and hair become atrophic. Any attempted movements of the joints results in severe pain despite fracture union. Radiographically, there is marked osteopaenia of the involved bones. The patient is extremely reluctant to move the affected part because of the pain this induces and this triggers a vicious cycle of further lack of movement resulting in further pain, stiffness and swelling. Treatment usually revolves around braking this cycle by first relieving the patient's discomfort using guanethidine or regional sensory nerve blocks and then aggressive physiotherapy to mobilize the affected joints. If this proves unsuccessful, sympathectomy may be deemed necessary.

Compartment syndromes

Compartment syndromes have multiple aetiologies, the commonest of which is raised intracompartmental pressure secondary to trauma. The application of tight dressings which goes unrecognized may also exacerbate this condition. The commonest areas where compartment syndromes occur are the volar compartment of the forearm and the anterolateral and lateral compartments of the leg. However, potentially, any closed fascial compartment is prone to the development of a compartment syndrome.

Increased tissue pressure within a closed bony and fascial compartment compromises the microcirculation. With raising intracompartmental pressure, the venous outflow is obstructed. There is continued extravasation of blood from damaged capillaries into the extracellular space resulting in increased swelling of the tissues, a raised extravascular pressure with compression of the arterial circulation and therefore closure of the microcirculation within the compartment which restricts local tissue perfusion. This results in ischaemia of the tissues, particularly the muscles within the compartment, and if not recognized and treated, eventually results in necrosis with irreversible tissue changes.

Symptoms and signs

- *Pain*: A compartment syndrome secondary to trauma, particularly when associated with fractures, results in pain which is unremitting and is not controlled by immobilization of the fracture or standard analgesics. The patient remains restless and agitated. The compartment itself feels extremely tense to palpation and is characterized by exquisite tenderness. Passive stretching of the involved muscles markedly exacerbates the symptoms. With established tissue ischaemia, active contraction of the involved muscles is restricted due to the severity of the pain. Severe, persistent, poorly localized pain out of proportion to the injury and requiring regular doses of strong analgesic is the most reliable sign of a compartment syndrome.
- *Pallor*: Discolouration of the affected limb distal to the compromised fascial compartment is not an altogether reliable sign. The distal extremity may show signs of pallor or cyanosis but adequate perfusion does not exclude a compartment syndrome.
- *Paraesthesia*: Ischaemia of the sensory fibres of a peripheral nerve transversing an affected compartment may result in paraesthesia over the cutaneous distribution of that particular nerve. This may or may not be an early sign of compartment syndrome and its absence does not discount an imminent or established compartment syndrome. Hyperaesthesia and/or anaesthesia may be late signs of compartment syndrome.
- *Paralysis*: Loss of muscle function due to irreversible muscle necrosis, as early as 6 h from the onset of ischaemia, results in paralysis but this is a very late sign and signifies irreversible changes within the fascial compartment. The patient may demonstrate 'pseudoparalysis' with an inability to perform muscle contraction because of the severity of pain; this does not signify irreversible changes and requires careful monitoring to detect it. If true paralysis of the involved musculature is detected, the pathological process is well advanced.
- *Pulselessness*: This is also an unreliable sign. The enclosed fascial compartment, particularly the anterolateral compartment of the leg and volar compartment of the forearm, may be completely ischaemic in the presence of normal distal pulses. However, if distal pulses are absent, secondary to soft-tissue swelling, then the process is well advanced and signifies minimal chance of recovery even with surgical treatment.

Diagnosis

Early diagnosis relies on a high index of suspicion for the development of a compartment syndrome. Close and careful monitoring of the patient's progress is required with regular assessment of the patient's degree of pain and neurovascular status of the affected limb by testing sensation, muscle power, peripheral pulses and passive movement of affected muscle groups to see if this markedly exacerbates the patient's discomfort. It is also important to assess the capillary return of the affected limb and the temperature of the skin in comparison with the unaffected side.

Various systems have been devised for monitoring, generally by manometric assessment, intracompartmental pressures in comparison with the unaffected limb. They rely on a standardized technique for accuracy and the clinician must be familiar with the particular technique to achieve reliable results. A fine needle is inserted into the affected compartment and then connected via tubing to a mercury manometer air-filled syringe. Various studies have shown that the intracompartmental pressure should be 0 mmHg: if it rises to within 10–30 mmHg of the patient's diastolic blood pressure, there is tissue ischaemia, and if it equals the patient's diastolic blood pressure, there is no effective tissue perfusion.

Treatment

The first principle in the management of compartment syndromes is early recognition. If the diagnosis is confirmed or suspected, the relevant compartment must be decompressed urgently. Constrictive dressings must be released, particularly circumferential plaster casts. A plaster cast must be completely split, including the woollen padding beneath the plaster. Once split, it should preferentially be spread or more appropriately bivalved to allow part of the cast to be removed while the limb remains in the remainder to support the injured part.

If this does not result in significant improvement of symptoms, or a fall in intracompartmental pressure measurements, then surgical treatment is warranted. This involves splitting the fascial membrane which encloses the compartment in the operating theatre. A tourniquet is *not* used. It is important to divide the fascia along the length of the entire compartment, so as to achieve adequate decompression. The viability of the tissues within the compartment, particularly the muscle bellies, can then be assessed. Viable muscle should bleed and contract on mechanical stimulation. Any necrotic muscle should be debrided as it only serves as a potential culture medium for infection. The skin wound is closed over a deep drain if feasible. The deep fascia is *not* sutured. If there is any doubt as to the tension within the compartment with skin closure, the wound should be left open and resutured later. Different surgical approaches are used for the different compartments within the upper and lower limbs.

JOINTS

Clinical assessment

Many patients present with joint symptoms involving one or multiple joints, symmetrically or asymmetrically. These symptoms include:
- pain,
- swelling,
- stiffness,
- deformity,
- loss of function.

History

On questioning the patient, the clinician must determine:
- Exact symptoms, particularly the nature of any pain, their duration and particular precipitating, aggravating and alleviating events.
- If a single or multiple joints are involved.
- Exact site of injury and side dominance of a patient (right or left handed).
- If the symptoms occur at rest or are purely mechanical in nature, such as pain on weight bearing, history of giving way or locking (Fig. 22.9).
- If there are any system symptoms, particularly those involving the genitourinary and gastrointestinal symptoms, and also pertaining to the eyes and skin, namely rashes and conjunctivitis. A history of urethral diseases may be significant.
- If there is a history of recent infections, either viral or bacterial, or recent overseas travel, particularly to third world countries. Of particular relevance, is whether the patient may have been exposed to tuberculosis.
- If there is a recent or more distant past history of trauma to the joint and whether this was a single event or recurrent trauma (see below).
- If there is any family history of diseases involving the joints, particularly at a young age.

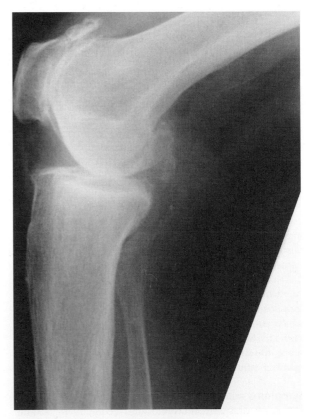

Figure 22.9. Patellofemoral osteoarthritis.

- The nature of any treatment, conservative or operative, instituted in the past: standard pain killers, anti-inflammatory agents, steroids, immunosuppressive agents or antibiotics; bracing of the joint for stability or pain relief, physiotherapy, walking aid, surgical procedure, etc.
- If past treatment has been successful and if there has been a recurrence of symptoms.
- Most importantly, the degree to which the symptoms have interfered with the patient's quality of life and his ability to remain in gainful employment. Have they just prevented the patient from taking part in sporting activities or hobbies or are symptoms of such a severe nature that the patient has difficulty with personal hygiene, dressing or feeding, thereby resulting in loss of independence?

Clinical examination

An accurate and thorough clinical examination of the patient in general and also the particular joint or joints involved is essential to determine the cause of an arthropathy. Clinical examination involves assessing the alignment and stability of the joint and associated soft-tissue swellings, including any effusion within the joint. Scars or sinuses suggesting surgery and infections must be noted. It is important to palpate for local temperature (warm in case of inflammatory pathologies and hot in acute infections) any bony areas for tenderness and to assess the range of both active and passive movements. General examination must assess other joints involved as well as the musculoskeletal system, looking for signs that may confirm an inflammatory or infective arthropathy. The format most popular in *orthopaedics* is *look*, *feel*, *move* (*in*spection, *p*alpation, *m*ovements) followed by *special tests* for specific pathologies suspected, neurological assessment, vascular assessment, assessment of other joints and Gait.

Arthritis

A simple pathological classification of arthritis is:
- *inflammatory*: rheumatoid arthritis (Fig. 22.10), ankylosing spondylitis;
- *degenerative*: osteoarthritis;
- *infective*: tuberculosis, postseptic arthritis (Fig. 22.11);
- *post-traumatic*: an arthropathy may be secondary to trauma causing premature degenerative changes within the joint because of loss of bone stock, soft-tissue support or alignment;
- *idiopathic*: avascular necrosis (Fig. 22.12);
- *metabolic*: gout and pseudo-gout secondary to inflammation resulting from crystal deposits in the synovium (crystalline arthropathies);
- *haematological*: haemophilia (Fig. 22.13).

The pathological changes within the joint will vary depending on the aetiology; however, the final common pathway generally involves destruction of the articular cartilage to the

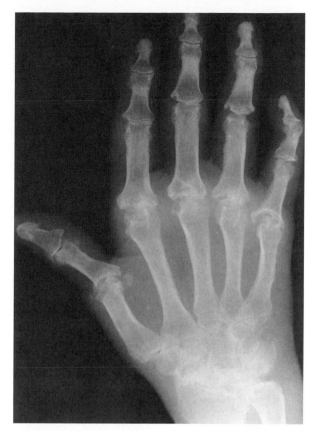

Figure 22.10. Rheumatoid arthritis of the hand.

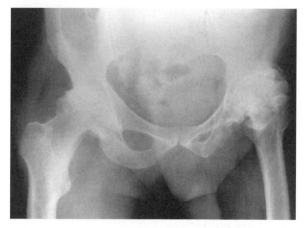

Figure 22.11. Degenerative changes involving the left hip secondary to previous septic arthritis.

subchondral bone, loss of the normal elasticity of the capsular tissues and acute or chronic inflammation of the synovium. Capsular contractures result in stiffness and deformity of the joint, together with restriction of the range of movement. Erosion of the articular cartilage together with destruction of the subchondral bone due to abnormal load through the

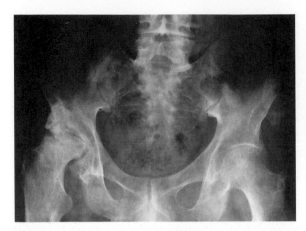

Figure 22.12. Avascular necrosis of the right hip.

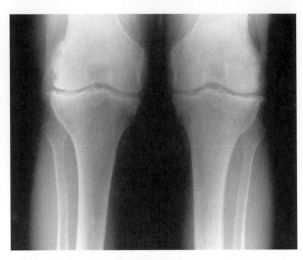

Figure 22.14. Osteoarthritis of the knee.

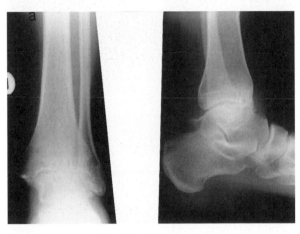

Figure 22.13. Haemophilic ankle with degenerative changes.

Inflammatory arthropathies include rheumatoid arthritis (Fig. 22.10), arthropathy associated with inflammatory bowel disease and the spondyloarthropathies, particularly ankylosing spondylitis. Appropriate serological investigations include latex glutination tests, HLAB 27 serology and antinuclear antibody screens.

Diagnosis of a purely idiopathic degenerative condition essentially relies on clinical assessment with the assistance of plain films (Fig. 22.15). Arthropathies secondary to metabolic conditions or coagulopathies, in particular haemophilia, rely on the appropriate biochemical assays, haematological screening for clotting factor deficiencies radiological assessment of changes specific to these conditions (Fig. 22.13).

If all the above investigations fail to confirm an exact diagnosis, then it may be appropriate to obtain a specimen of joint fluid by aspirating the synovial effusions. This must be performed under strict aseptic conditions so as not to cause an iatrogenic infective arthritis. This specimen is sent to the laboratory for appropriate investigation, particularly cytological assessment, polarizing microscopy to look for crystals and routine culture of anaerobic or aerobic organisms and tuberculosis. The latter is necessary even if skin testing for tuberculosis has been performed.

Joint injuries

Common injuries can be classified as:
- subluxation,
- dislocation,
- fracture/dislocation.

Joints commonly injured are:
- shoulder,
- interphalangeal (IP) joints,
- metacarpophalangeal (MCP) joint of thumb,
- elbow,
- hip,

joint or chronic inflammation also results in loss of alignment (deformity) and normal smooth gliding of the articular surfaces over one another (pain and stiffness) (Fig. 22.14).

Acute or chronic inflammation involving the synovium produces either haemorrhagic or seropurulent effusions within the joint that result in distension, together with loss of mobility and associated pain and stiffness. The secondary effects of the pathological process involving the joint result in loss of use with subsequent atrophy of the muscles involved in movement of the joint. Osteopaenia from a degree of disuse further aggravates loss of function, not only within the joint itself but also in the involved limb.

Appropriate investigations of an arthropathy include plain X-rays of the joint and long films of the entire limb to assess alignment. Routine blood investigations, particularly looking at the white cell count and various acute phase reactants (erythrocyte sedimentation rate (ESR) and C-reactive protein (CRP)) are performed, as well as appropriate serological tests if a postviral arthropathy is suspected.

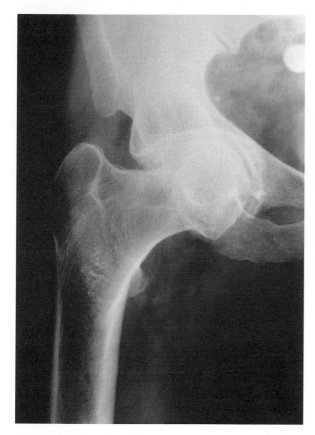

Figure 22.15. Osteoarthritis of the hip.

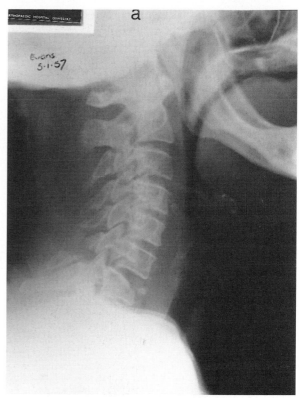

Figure 22.16. Fracture-dislocation of the cervical spine (C6/C7).

- ankle,
- subtalar joint,
- spinal facet joint (cervical) (Fig. 22.16).

The history should elicit:

- mechanism of injury;
- degree of violence;
- associated injuries;
- previous injury to affected joint and duration since;
- history of generalized joint and other joint laxity;
- family history of joint instability;
- previous treatment regimens, including hospitalization;
- effect on occupation, domestic and social activities.

The examination should include early and adequate evaluation of:

- the joint involved;
- remainder of the affected limb;
- neurovascular status;
- overlying skin/soft tissues;
- associated injuries, for example if hip joint dislocation, check posterior cruciate ligament (PCL) of ipsilateral knee.

One should also:

- Document any neurovascular deficits prior to attempted reduction as the procedure for reduction may result in neurovascular injury.

- Document any associated injuries/fracture prior to reduction as manipulation can result in fracture of involved bones, for example fracture of surgical neck of humerus with reduction of shoulder dislocation.

Investigations

Radiographs in at least two planes are needed to assess adequately for dislocation/subluxation and to exclude associated fractures. This can prove technically difficult, for example axillary lateral in shoulder dislocation. Further information as regards associated fracture configuration can be gained from specialist views, for example Judet views of acetabulum, swimmers view for lower cervical spine or CT scan of joint to assess for intra-articular fragments following fracture dislocation and tomograms of spine to assess facet joint fracture dislocations.

Associated neurological and vascular injuries can be investigated by:

- Electromyogram (EMG) nerve conduction studies,
- MRI,
- angiography.

However, performance of investigations must not delay prompt reduction of the joint. If satisfied that the dislocation is straightforward, for example recurrent glenohumeral joint dislocation/ankle joint dislocation (especially if there is overlying ischaemia of skin or neurovascular deficit), then reduction may be performed without further investigations. However, performance of post-reduction imaging is mandatory to:

- assess adequate reduction of the joint,
- document that the joint has been reduced,
- assess for any associated fractures (Fig. 22.17).

Management

This involves:

- Early/rapid reduction of joint to: relieve/prevent ischaemic damage to overlying soft tissues (e.g. skin); avoid traction/ischaemic damage to nerves; prevent/relieve external pressure effects on vascular structures; limit damage to articular cartilage.
- Technique of reduction/manipulation depends on the joint involved and can be either closed manipulation or open reduction with or without soft tissue/skeletal stabilization. Associated fractures should be treated simultaneously or in a delayed procedure.
- Post-reduction the joint should be adequately immobilized or stabilized for long enough to allow soft tissues to heal.
- Early and appropriate joint and soft-tissue rehabilitation should be performed to: protect joint surfaces; minimize risk of recurrence; prevent post-traumatic stiffness; regain range of movement and power; regain function of affected joint or limb.
- Patient education as regards: risks of recurrence/instability; prognosis for long-term degenerative changes in joint; timing of return to employment and sporting activities.
- Adequate follow-up, especially in high-risk patients for recurrence or joint degeneration.

Specific joints

Shoulder

This is one of the commonest joints affected by dislocation of which the vast majority are anterior dislocations (Fig. 22.18). Posterior dislocations are associated with electrocution and epileptic seizures. Anterior dislocation is particularly associated with violent contact sports injuries (e.g. rugby). It is not uncommon to sustain injuries to the axillary nerve or brachial plexus, although the former may spontaneously recover. In the older age group, glenohumeral joint dislocations are associated with rotator cuff tears and fractures of the greater tuberosity. The pathological lesion in younger age groups is the Bankart lesion and predisposes the shoulder to recurrent dislocation. It is an avulsion or tear of the anterior labrum off the glenoid articular margin with capsular striping off the anterior neck of the glenoid. It may be associated with a small fracture off the anterior rim of the glenoid ('bony Bankart lesion'). Dislocation is associated with early degenerative changes in the joint.

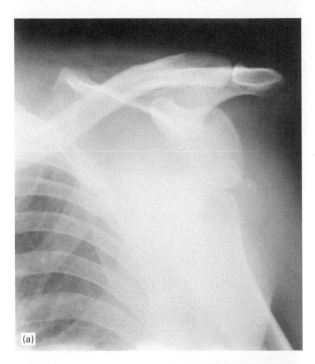

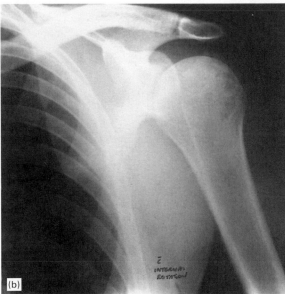

Figure 22.17. Anterior fracture-dislocation of the glenohumeral joint pre (top) and post (bottom) reduction.

Anteroposterior and axillary lateral (especially in the case of possible posterior dislocation) plain radiographs are required as well as specialized views (e.g. Wallace view) if it is impossible to obtain an axillary lateral view due to pain. Associated bony lesions should be looked for and assessed, for example impression fracture of posterior humeral head

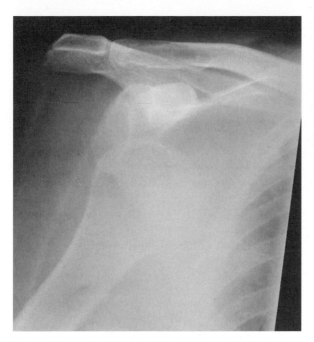

Figure 22.18. Anterior dislocation of the glenohumeral joint.

(Hill Sachs lesion) and fracture of anterior glenoid (bony Bankart lesion). Recurrent dislocation should be investigated with MRI and arthroscopic evaluation of the joint.

The patient should be given analgesia, sedation and muscle relaxant (but beware of hypoventilation) and closed reduction attempted with the Hippocrates or Kocher techniques or traction/countertraction. Prompt reduction reduces the risk of neurovascular damage. If unsuccessful, the dislocation should be manipulated under general anaesthesia; open reduction is rarely required unless it is associated with fracture of the surgical neck of humerus. Treatment of recurrent dislocation is by arthroscopic or open anterior soft-tissue stabilization (i.e. repair of Bankart lesion).

Following reduction, the shoulder should be immobilized with a sling and swathe. The duration of immobilization is controversial for anterior (ranging from 0 to 6 weeks), with some arguing that immobilization makes no difference to the recurrence rate.

Hip

Dislocation can be anterior (Fig. 22.19), posterior or central, where it is associated with fracture of the acetabular floor. Major trauma is usually involved and care should be taken to note associated injuries to pelvis, vasculature, sciatic nerve and ipsilateral knee. Urgent reduction is required, generally under general anaesthesia (Fig. 22.20). As hip dislocation is often associated with fractures of acetabular wall, prolonged skeletal traction may be required post-reduction or simultaneous open internal fixation to stabilize the joint. This

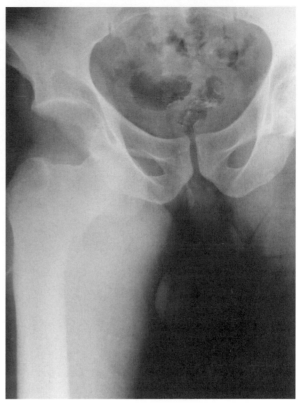

Figure 22.19. Anterior dislocation of the hip.

allows early mobilization. There is a significant risk of long-term degenerative changes within the joint.

Elbow

This is a relatively uncommon dislocation and is usually posterior. It can be associated with minor trauma. There is the possibility of neural injury: median, ulna and radial. Elbow dislocation requires prompt reduction, which can be performed under sedation. Post-reduction radiographs should be checked for associated fractures of the radial head, capitellum and trochlea with resultant intra-articular base bodies. These may predispose to locking of the joint. Early mobilization of the joint is essential to avoid post-traumatic stiffness and a hinged cast brace to prevent full flexion or extension should be used. Loss of extension is very common following elbow injuries and myositis ossificans (see above) is a not uncommon sequelae.

Joint replacement

The aims of joint replacement are to reduce pain and improve mobility and quality of life. Joint replacements allow patients to maintain their independence, may reduce

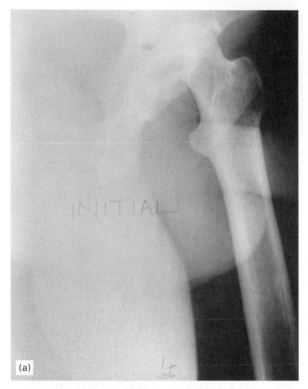

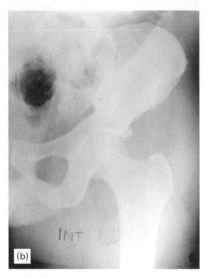

Figure 22.20. Posterior fracture-dislocation of the hip pre (a) and post (b) reduction.

their reliance on walking aids and may even allow the housebound patients to re-enter the community.

Indications for joint replacement include severe pain interfering with the patient's activities of daily living and quality of life, increasing severity of deformity and joint stiffness, and loss of independence. The requirement of large doses of analgesics to control symptoms, interruption to sleep pattern due to persistent pain and failure of conservative means of treatment such as the use of walking aids, physiotherapy and possibly bracing are also relevant.

The disease process may be an isolated phenomenon affecting a particular joint or be part of a generalized arthropathy (e.g. rheumatoid arthritis) where multiple limbs may be affected either symetrically or asymetrically. As such the patient may require multiple joint arthroplasty involving both upper and lower limbs, and if this is the case, the sequence and timing of joint replacement are important considerations. Bilateral joint replacements can also be performed sequentially or at the same operation (e.g. bilateral total hip replacements).

The decision to perform joint replacement or arthroplasty, whether it involves the upper or lower limb, depends on both local and general factors. The latter relate mainly to an assessment of whether the patient requires a joint replacement, his general fitness and suitability for major surgery and extensive rehabilitation. The patient's loss of independence through an inability to perform daily activities of living and its impact on him must be enquired about. Age is not generally a contraindication to joint replacement. In generalized disease processes such as diabetes or patients who are immunocompromised, for example renal transplant patients on immunosuppressive agents, there is an increased risk of complications of joint arthroplasty, particularly infection.

The local factors which need to be assessed prior to joint replacement surgery include an assessment of the quality of soft tissues and bone, the neurovascular status of the limb, particularly where the surgery involves the lower limb and the alignment of the limb together with associated deformity of the joint. If there are any concerns regarding the vascular status of the limb, then a preoperative vascular opinion should be sought.

Evaluation, especially in the context of patients who have had previous surgery to the affected joint, involves:

- *Skin*: previous surgical scars, especially if there have been multiple operations around the joint, may affect the surgical approach to the joint. The surgeon needs to be aware of the presence of chronic skin conditions, especially chronic ulcers, around the joint that may be in close proximity to the surgical incision as this can predispose to infection.

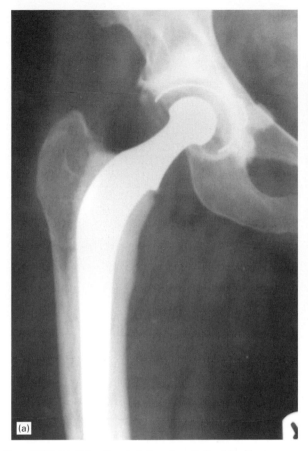
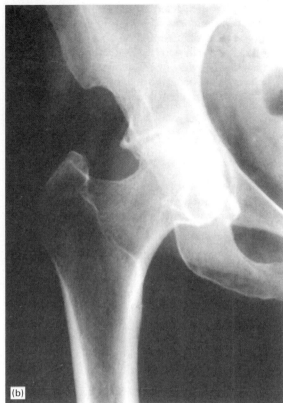

Figure 22.21. Total hip arthroplasty for osteoarthritis of the hip.

- The quality of the *subcutaneous tissues and muscles* is important as adequate coverage of the prosthesis is needed. This is usually a problem in the knee and elbow or small joints of the hand. Ligamentous stability also needs to be assessed as this may affect which type of prosthesis is used.
- The amount and quality of *bone* is carefully assessed radiographically as this is the main supporting tissue for any prosthetic implant (Fig. 22.21). Patients with poor bone stock or quality due to generalized bone disorders (e.g. osteoporosis) may require a specialized prosthesis or a different surgical technique compared with those who have good bone quality without major loss of the bone stock.
- Alignment of the joint or loss thereof due to *deformity* secondary to loss of bone stock and soft-tissue contracture is important in the weight-bearing joints of the lower limbs. Alignment is assessed both clinically and radiologically and influences the surgical technique as well as choice of prothetic implant. In the case of the knee joint, only one compartment may be involved in degenerative disease.

Unicompartmental prostheses are available to allow the most affected compartment to be addressed while preserving bone stock.

Following clinical assessment, appropriate radiographs of the involved joint, and if necessary the contralateral joint, are taken for comparison. In some cases, full-length films of the limb may be required, particularly with regards to total knee arthroplasty.

Once the decision has been made to proceed with joint replacement surgery, on the basis of clinical and radiological findings, a lengthy discussion needs to be undertaken with the patient to inform him of the details of the procedure to be undertaken, the expected outcome and the complications involved. Only under these circumstances, can a patient give informed consent to undergo a major surgical procedure. The patient also needs to be informed of the usual postoperative course, any rehabilitation that will be required, the expected life of any prosthetic implant and the consequences of having to undergo revision surgery. The patient should be advised that implants can dislocate and loosen (Fig. 22.22) or fail (Fig. 22.23). The patient should

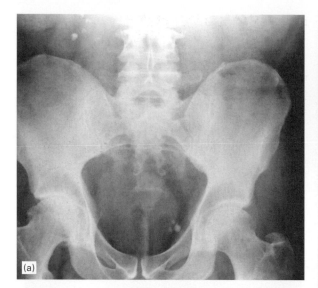

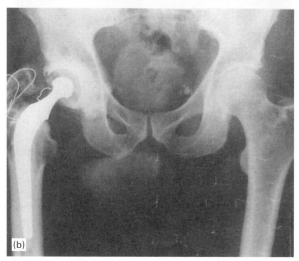

Figure 22.22. Total hip arthroplasty for osteoarthritis of the hip-arthroplasty now painful and possibly loose.

either be reviewed on a regular basis long term or advised as to what symptoms to expect in the event of problems with the implant.

AMPUTATIONS AND PROSTHETICS

Amputations

There are two types of amputations: disarticulations in which the amputation is carried out through a joint surface; and amputations directly through bone and soft tissues at a particular level depending on the disease process. Amputations are recorded in the earliest medical literature and have subsequently been refined, not only from the perspective of the

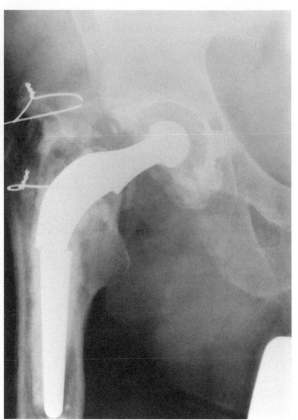

Figure 22.23. Total hip replacement – implant failure with a broken femoral stem.

disease process but also the functional and prosthetic requirements that are required following amputation to enhance the rehabilitation of the patient. Amputations have come a long way from being regarded as the last step of failed management to being the first stride in successful rehabilitation of a patient!

The indications for amputations can be broadly classified as:

* *Peripheral vascular disease*: The vast majority are patients with atherosclerotic disease or vessel disease secondary to diabetes mellitus. In diabetics with small vessel disease developing trophic ulcers with subsequent infection and osteomyelitis, the level of amputation is determined by the patient's age, his functional requirements and mobility and the extent of the disease process. This latter requires a careful assessment of the vascular supply of the limb. The requirements of proximal resection so as to ensure good stump healing must be balanced against those of maintaining adequate stump length for prosthetic fitting so as to encourage the patient to become independent again.
* *Post-traumatic*: In young adults, particularly men, road traffic and industrial accidents account for the majority of amputations performed in this age group. Most involve the

lower limb and the injuries usually have acute vascular and/or neural damage to the limb with associated massive bone and soft-tissue injury. Under some circumstances the damage is irreparable and primary amputation may be the best course of action. In other situations, attempts may be made to debride the damaged soft tissues, stabilize the bony skeleton and repair the neural and vascular supplies in an attempt to maintain the viability of the distal part of the limbs. This approach may restore some functional anatomy but often a prolonged course with multiple surgical procedures is required. The decision between salvage or amputation of a severely injured limb is one of the most difficult decisions an orthopaedic surgeon has to make. Several scoring systems have been devised to predict the results of limb saving surgery. The common ones are MESS (Mangled Extremity Severity Scale), PSI (Predictive Salvage Index) and NISSA (Nerve injury, Ischaemia, Soft-tissue and skeletal injury, Shock, Age of patient). They attempt to quantify the severity of trauma and provide guidelines to decide between amputation and salvage. However it cannot be overemphasized that the final decision must rest on the surgeon's assessment and clinical acumen rather than any scoring system. In those cases where attempted repair proves unsuccessful, a delayed amputation may be deemed necessary. In patients with severe burns, it may be best to delay any consideration of amputation until an accurate demarcation between the viable and non-viable tissues can be delineated.

- *Tumours*: The commonest indication for amputation in this category of patients is malignant tumours without evidence of metastatic spread where curative resection is the aim. This requires accurate clinical and radiological evaluation to determine the extent of spread of the tumour within the affected limb. Amputation may also be undertaken in patients in whom metastatic spread may have occurred but where the tumour is ulcerating, necrotic and gangrenous and its removal will improve quality of life if not the duration. It is uncommon for benign tumours to require amputation; however, some may interfere with the function of surrounding soft tissues and neurovascular structure to such an extent that amputation and prosthetic replacement may restore a greater degree of functional independence to the patient than local resection. The majority of amputations performed in the paediatric age group are either for malignancy or congenital anomalies (Fig. 22.24). In the last few years advances in chemotherapy, radiotherapy, surgery and the availability of custom made implants and prostheses have considerably improved prognosis and quality of life in these patients.

- *Neural deficits*: Patients with isolated neural injuries, either post-traumatic or -surgical, and left essentially with a flail limb may also benefit from amputation and prosthetic replacement using the remaining functional muscles to manipulate the prosthesis. Common examples are brachial plexus lesion with a subsequent flail upper limb and

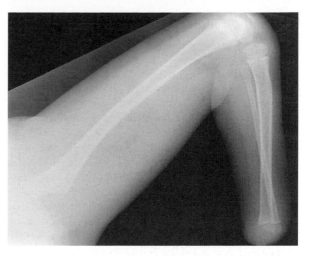

Figure 22.24. Congenital amputation of the foot at ankle joint level.

gunshot or traumatic injuries involving the sciatic nerve and leaving the lower limb flail below the knee. Attempts are being made to repair such neural injuries acutely; however, the recovery period can be prolonged and somewhat unpredictable.

- *Infection*: Acute infections such as gas gangrene rapidly spreading throughout the soft tissues with associated generalized septicaemia may precipitate the need for amputation to save the patient's life. The level of amputation depends on the degree of septic involvement of the limbs. Other causes of less virulent infection, such as chronic osteomyelitis that fails to resolve following other forms of surgical management, chronic tuberculous involvement of part of a limb or secondary neoplastic involvement of chronic discharging sinuses may also warrant amputation.

Surgical considerations

There are many different types of amputations at different levels through the upper and lower limbs, often associated with eponymous names. Depending on the patient's age, his fitness for surgery must be assessed. In the older age group with diabetes mellitus and generalized atherosclerosis, the cardiorespiratory, renal and peripheral vascular status of the patient must be assessed. The postoperative functional requirements and general mobility of the patient must also be taken into account; that is, the postoperative considerations for a patient who is wheelchair bound preoperatively will differ from those for a patient who is ambulant with or without walking aids.

The biological amputation level is the distal-most functional amputation level with a high probability of supporting wound healing. To determine the optimal amputation level, biological amputation level is combined with the rehabilitation potential that provides maximum function.

Once the exact level of the amputation has been defined, the local surgical considerations involve meticulous care of the soft tissues, appropriate fashioning of the bony stump to accommodate the prosthesis and adequate fashioning of skin flaps to achieve good soft-tissue coverage and maximum potential for stump healing.

Limb amputations are generally carried out with a tourniquet; however, prior to stump closure, the tourniquet must be released to make sure that all bleeding vessels have been carefully ligated. Nerves must be carefully divided proximally so that they can retract into the soft tissues and will not be irritated by the scar at the tip of the stump; thus neuromatous pain is avoided. In the closed amputation technique, which is used particularly in diabetics, skin flaps must be repaired without undue tension so as to avoid the possibility of postoperative sepsis and dehiscence of the stump.

In the open amputation technique, following removal of the affected part of the limb, the stump is left open. This is a common technique in cases of massive sepsis where repeat debridements may be necessary. Once adequate haemostasis has been achieved and the soft tissues have been adequately repaired to cover the tip of the stump, a careful stump dressing is applied. This is necessary to support the soft tissues at the end of the stump and to help reduce the risk of marked soft-tissue swelling that can occur following such surgery. Sequential stump dressings are applied over the days following surgery. Once the wound has healed satisfactorily, consideration may be given to the application of interim prostheses to allow the patient to begin the rehabilitation programme as early as possible.

Apart from the general and local medical considerations, the psychological effect of such surgery on the patient must not be overlooked. This needs to be carefully assessed and treated by both pre-, peri- and post-operative counselling and also aggressive rehabilitation.

Complications

Haematoma formation

This is generally due to inadequate haemostasis or inadequate postoperative drainage. It is very important to release the tourniquet after the amputation has been performed to ensure that all bleeding vessels are cortorized or ligated. If there is persistent ooze from remaining soft tissues, deep drains may be appropriate. It can also be difficult to achieve adequate haemostasis from the cut ends of a long bone. The formation of a postoperative haematoma can delay wound healing, predisposes to infection and also delays the rehabilitation programme due to the fact that it is difficult to fit an interim prosthesis. If the haematoma is massive and is likely to take a long time to resolve, it may be appropriate to return the patient to theatre, drain the haematoma surgically, pay meticulous attention to haemostasis and repair the stump soft tissues over deep drain tubes. Small haematomas usually resolve given time.

Postoperative infection

This is particularly common in diabetics. However, it may occur in any amputation where adequate attention is not given to management of soft tissues and wound tension during repair. It is encouraged by haematoma formation and necrosis of skin edges or soft tissues which can occur if the stump flaps are sutured under excessive tension over the bone. A careful surgical technique with perioperative antibiotic prophylaxis reduces this risk. Small superficial areas of cellulitis in the wound may be treated appropriately with a course of antibiotics. However, deep persistent infection may require the patient to be returned to theatre for further debridement with complete excision of all infected tissue. It is important to try and avoid the sequelae of stump osteomyelitis involving the resected bone ends. It may be necessary to shorten the bone to allow the skin and soft-tissue flaps to be closed without undue tension. Multiple swabs and soft-tissue specimens should be sent for laboratory assessment to try and identify any growing organisms and appropriate antibiotic therapy instituted until the stump as healed.

Stump necrosis

Skin necrosis may be minor at the wound edges through to full-thickness necrosis of the soft-tissue flaps requiring extensive refashioning of the stump.

Neuroma formation

This can commonly occur at the cut ends of nerves, particularly if they are entrapped in scar tissue at the tip of the stump and irritated by traction. It is important to divide nerves as proximally as possible to allow them to retract into the proximal soft tissues away from the scar tissue at the tip of the stump. If a neuroma proves to be particularly troublesome, the prosthesis can be adjusted to take some of the pressure away from the neuromatous area and the neuroma injected with local anaesthetic temporarily to relieve the symptoms. Alternatively, surgical exploration allows the scared tip of the cut nerve to be excised and the nerve formally buried in soft tissues away from the tip of the stump.

Joint contracture

This is usually secondary to contracture of the soft tissues surrounding the joint just proximal to the amputation. It is usually secondary to disuse of the joint following the amputation surgery and can be best avoided by aggressive mobilization and physiotherapy to the joint so as to maintain suppleness and flexibility in the surrounding soft tissues. It is imperative to avoid joint contractures just above the stump as these will hinder prosthetic use and functional rehabilitation.

Prosthetics

There are two main groups of prostheses.

- *Passive prostheses*: These may provide a minor degree of function but their main aim is to attempt to restore normal anatomical appearance.

- *Functional prostheses*: These may be body powered or externally powered prostheses. The former are controlled by the remaining normally functioning muscle groups; the latter have an external power supply. Upper limb body-powered prostheses can be cable motivated. Externally powered prostheses can be gas or electrically operated and their control is usually initiated by normal joint function proximal to the amputation level or by feedback from elec-tromyographical signals. Contraction of muscle can be detected transcutaneously by appropriately placed elec-trodes. Some prostheses, particularly those which attempt to restore upper limb function, may be a combination of these types (carrier tool prostheses).

The requirements of a prosthetic device are usually that it is robust, not too heavy as to be cumbersome and provides a reasonable cosmetic appearance. Prostheses may be articu-lated or non-articulated.

TENDON INJURIES

Diagnosis

Diagnosis of tendon injury relies on careful clinical assess-ment, particularly if *flexor or extensor tendon injuries* of the hand are not to be missed. Each individual tendon should be tested in isolation with awareness that partial division of tendons may weaken the tendon function but does not result in complete loss of function. The same applies to div-ision of one of the slips of flexor digitorum superficialis to the digits.

Achilles tendon rupture is another tendon injury that is commonly missed. It is usually degenerative in nature and is not normally secondary to penetrating injuries. The patient notices difficulty standing on the toes of the affected side. The patient can often continue walking but with some diffi-culty and may present several days to weeks after the initial injury. The patient usually presents with sudden onset of pain in the hindfoot and often describes a sensation of being kicked in the posterior aspect of the ankle. Severe pain in the calf is often misdiagnosed as a muscle sprain. Again, the diagnosis will not be missed if the patient is carefully exam-ined lying prone on the examining couch.

Swelling over the Achilles tendon and loss of the normal contour of the lower part of the calf and hindfoot will be apparent due to soft-tissue swelling. A palpable defect may be found within the substance of the Achilles tendon and this if often very tender. The most important test to perform is the calf squeeze test. The patient lies prone on the exam-ining couch and flexes both knees to 90°. This allows the pos-ture of both feet to be observed under the influence of gravity. The affected limb will show less plantar flexion at the ankle joint than the non-affected side and is relatively dorsi-flexed. The calf of the non-affected limb is squeezed and passive plantar flexion of the foot observed. When this is repeated on the affected side, pain will be elicited but more importantly no passive plantar flexion at the foot will be observed. This test is called the Simmons–Thompson test and is the most reliable test of assessing integrity of the Achilles tendon. It must be performed on any patient who presents with the above history.

Management

Treatment of a ruptured Achilles tendon can be either con-servative or operative. In the acute situation, the patient can be treated in an equinus plaster for 6–8 weeks, followed by a heel raiser for a further 4 weeks. In the older age groups, par-ticularly if the diagnosis is delayed, the benefits of surgery may be outweighed by the possible complications and the loss of plantar flexion may have to be accepted.

The patient must be informed of the pro and cons as well as the complications involved. Operative treatment carries the risk of deep infection (1%), fistula (3%), skin necrosis (2%) and re-rupture (2%). However, with conservative treat-ment the re-rupture rate can be up to 30%. Ruptures treated after 1 week have greater incidences of re-rupture and less plantar flexion strength. Once the decision has been made to repair a lacerated tendon surgically, it is important that the tendon ends are carefully exposed. In the hand, this requires appropriate skin incision and dissection through the subcuta-neous tissue. The more proximal of the divided tendon ends may have retracted proximally within the finger or into the palm. This may require a separate incision to retrieve the tendon through the fibrous flexor sheath. Once both ends have been retrieved, the divided tendon ends are accurately apposed, ensuring there is no displacement of the tendon edges or malrotation of the tendon ends. Displacement makes the repair bulkier and therefore limits free gliding of the tendon within the fibrous flexor sheath and particularly past the pulleys.

Many different techniques have been described for sutur-ing together the divided tendon ends. The important aspects of the repair are that the suture knots used to appose the ten-don ends are buried within the substance of the tendon and that the tendon ends are not crimped together tightly as this makes the repair bulkier. When exposing the tendon ends, it is particularly important to preserve the vinculae and there-fore the blood supply to the tendons. The dissection should be limited to the area of the divided tendon rather than on extensive exposure. All these procedures are designed to minimize the degree of scarring within the fibrous flexor sheath so as not to limit tendon function.

The pulley mechanism of the flexor aspect of the digits is very important for normal tendon function. Integrity of the tendon pulleys avoids the problems of bow stringing and thus loss of range of motion of the tendon within the sheath. Any such loss of motion will ultimately affect the degree of movement of the IP and MCP joints. It is therefore important at the time of surgical repair to try and maintain the integrity of the tendon pulleys. If this is not possible, then they should be accurately repaired once the tendon reconstruction is complete.

Once complete, the integrity of the repair must be assessed by passively flexing and extending the finger and wrist joints while observing the passive posture of the affected finger. Affected digits should be slightly flexed and in line with the other non-affected digits. On flexion and extension of the IP, MCP and wrist joints, the tendon should glide freely within the fibrous flexor sheath, particularly past the pulleys, without any catching that may cause triggering. On full extension of the joints, there should be no separation of the tendon ends if the repair is satisfactory. Assessment can be done on the operating table with the patient anaesthetized.

Splintage is then applied to protect the repair. There are several postoperative mobilization regimens, for example the Kleinert or Belfast regimens, which rely on passive flexion of the affected digit with limited active extension. This is achieved either with an extension block splint or elastic bands attached to the volar aspect of the fingers so as to restrict extension. This form of splintage protects the tendon repair while allowing early movement so as to minimize the degree of scarring and adhesions within the fibrous sheath which may restrict tendon motion and therefore reduce the range of movement of the affected finger. Such regimens are generally continued for approximately 6 weeks postoperatively when the scarring has matured and the tendon repair is thought to be solid.

The patient is followed regularly in the outpatient clinic to ensure that flexion contractures of the digit are not forming and also that with combined active and passive movement, the tendon repair remains intact. At 6 weeks, when the protective splintage is removed to allow full range of motion exercises, a static nocturnal splint may be used for a limited period until full function has been regained.

HAND INJURIES

Hand injuries, particularly those involving the dominant hand, can be a seriously debilitating long-term problem if appropriate early treatment is not instituted. A working knowledge of the anatomy of the hand is needed for accurate diagnosis of acute injuries.

Injuries to the hand can be broadly classified as bony, soft tissue or combined. Bony injuries include fractures of the phalanges and metacarpal bones and also fracture dislocations involving the IP, MCP and carpometacarpal joints. Soft-tissue injuries commonly include lacerations which may or may not involve tendon and/or digital nerve injuries. Some penetrating wounds may result in superficial or deep infections involving either the palmar spaces or the tendon sheaths.

Clinical assessment

When examining the hand after an acute injury, function of the individual components of the hand must be accurately assessed, particularly the long flexor and extensor tendons to the digits, and also the function of the digital nerves. This is vital so as not to miss any damage to deep structures that may cause long-term problems after the skin wound has healed. As regards flexor tendons, it is important to assess the function of the superficialis and profundus tendons in isolation for each digit and also the function of extensor tendons to all digits as well as flexor and extensor pollicis longus (see above). Assessment of digital nerve function involves testing sensation to light touch and a pinprick over each digit individually and comparing response with the normal uninjured hand.

Flexor and extensor pollicis longus are assessed by testing the power of contraction of the IP joint of the thumb when flexed and extended, respectively. The flexor digitorum profundus to the digits can be assessed in isolation by testing the power of flexion of the distal IP joint to each digit, while maintaining the MCP and proximal IP joint in the extended position so as to avoid superimposed action of the superficialis tendon which may mask damage to the profundus tendon.

Assessment of the superficialis tendons to each digit involves extending the IP and MCP joints to all other digits passively and allowing only the digit being examined to attempt flexion. This isolates the superficialis tendon to that particular digit and avoids the effect of mass action of the superficialis tendons masking an injury to one superficialis tendon to a single digit. The extensor tendons are also assessed in isolation by testing extension at individual MCP joints. This must be differentiated from extensor action at the IP joints by the intrinsic muscles of the hand by assessing bone extensor function with MCP joints internal extension not flexion.

Palmar compartments and spaces

Broadly speaking, the palm is divided into three main deep fascial compartments: thenar space, hyperthenar space, and mid-palmar space. The main fascial compartments involving the digits are the tendon sheaths. Deep infections within these closed fascial compartments can damage the structures within, particularly the flexor tendons. Infections can also transgress the intermetacarpal spaces and involve the dorsum of the hand.

Bone trauma (including 'crush injuries')

The problem with bone injuries to the hand, including crush injuries, with or without associated fractures is soft-tissue swelling and oedema. Due to the fact that the soft-tissue compartments in the palm and digits are enclosed by tight fascial membranes, the function of structures in these compartments can be compromised by severe soft-tissue swelling. If adequate treatment is not instituted early, adhesions develop within the fascial compartments restricting free movement, particularly within the tendon sheaths, and resulting in stiffness of the small joints of the hand with subsequent limitation of function. The majority of such injuries are industrial accidents and they occur in manual workers, often involving the dominant hand. As such, it is essential that early and correct management is followed by aggressive rehabilitation if there is to be any hope that the patient will return to his former employment with a normally functioning hand.

Early management of soft-tissue injury swelling and oedema comprises the RICE regime which stands for rest, ice, compression and elevation. Rest prevents further injury and promotes the body's own healing process. Ice decreases bleeding by vasoconstriction. Compression limits the swelling and elevation allows gravity to drain fluid thereby reducing swelling. The patient's pain must be controlled with adequate analgesia to the extent that he can begin early mobilization of the hand under the supervision of a physiotherapist. The hand must be temporarily splinted in a functional position with the wrist joint either in neutral or slightly dorsiflexed, the MCP joints flexed 60–90° and the IP joints maintained in the extended position. Early on, the patient must be encouraged to remove the splint and begin early mobilization exercises.

Burst lacerations of the skin must be appropriately debrided and irrigated, preferably in the operating theatre. Where these occur in the digits, it is important that lacerations are left open as with the ensuing swelling over the next 24 h, sutures only predispose to soft-tissue necrosis and subsequently infection. Compound fractures must be formerly debrided in the operating theatre together with appropriate prophylactic antibiotics. Any underlying fractures secondary to crush injuries with associated bursting lacerations of the skin, must be treated as compound. It is important to remember that crush injuries involving the finger tip with associated nail avulsion and nail-bed laceration associated with an underlying fracture must also be treated as a compound fracture. Individual fractures can be treated with appropriate internal fixation if treatment is early, which avoids the problems of prolonged splintage and allows early mobilization.

The postoperative regimen includes elevation, regular analgesia, appropriate splintage and early physiotherapy to expedite range of movement exercises of the small joints and therefore hasten return of function of the affected hand.

Fractures (open and closed) and fracture dislocations

Common fractures and fracture dislocations of the hand involve the metacarpals, the phalanges and the IP joint.

Closed fractures

Treatment of fractures involving the metacarpals and phalanges is governed by the resultant deformity of the hand, the instability of the fracture and the reliability of the patient to adhere to a rehabilitation programme. It is important to assess the alignment of the digits not only in the coronal and

sagittal planes but also whether there is any rotational malalignment of the fingers. This can be assessed by looking at the fingers and assessing the alignment of the finger nails with all fingers fully extended. All digits should remain aligned and comparison can be easily made with the normal unaffected hand. Ask the patient to flex all MCP and IP joints together. Check the direction the fingertips are pointing in. It is important that all digits point toward the tubercle of the scaphoid to reveal rotational malalignment that may not be apparent on initial inspection. Where metacarpal fractures are involved, it is essential to assess the degree of extensor lag of the MCP joint.

Clinically, fractures present with pain, swelling, loss of function, point tenderness and deformity. Fracture stability is generally assessed clinically and radiographically. As a general rule, stable fractures may be treated with minimal splintage and early mobilization to avoid the problems of small joint stiffness. Unstable fractures, particularly those with significant deformity, may best be treated by open reduction and internal fixation. This avoids the necessity of cumbersome external splints which may not give adequate stability or correction of deformity. If internal fixation is adequate, early mobilization may be instituted. With intra-articular fractures, it is vital to reconstitute the joint surface, which can often only be achieved with internal fixation. However, if the degree of comminution is so severe that it is not possible to fix the fragments internally, the position may have to be accepted and early mobilization relied upon to achieve the best functional results.

Dislocations and fracture dislocations

These most commonly involve the IP joints and often occur during sporting activities. The diagnosis is usually relatively straightforward as there is marked clinically deformity and this is confirmed by appropriate radiographs. IP joint dislocations or fracture dislocations may be reduced by the patient at the time of injury. This often dramatically relieves the pain and corrects the deformity, but the joint may remain unstable, particularly if there is an associated intra-articular fracture. Careful radiographical assessment is then warranted.

Simple closed dislocations of the IP joints, if stable, may be treated with early mobilization. Those involving intra-articular fractures or volar plate injuries remain unstable even after adequate reduction. Under these circumstances, extension block splintage may be necessary as this prevents redislocation while allowing some movement to occur early, so as to reduce the inevitable problem of joint stiffness.

Open fractures

Open fractures of the small bones of the hand must be treated aggressively. The principles of treatment are early and adequate surgical debridement, which is repeated at regular intervals as necessary; appropriate stabilization of the fracture by external or internal fixation; adequate prophylactic antibiotics; postoperative elevation; and early mobilization to avoid post injury oedema and stiffness. An appropriate physiotherapy regimen should be begun early to enhance the chances of good functional recovery. As mentioned above, crush injuries of the finger tip with avulsion of the nail from the bed and associated with an underlying fracture of the distal phalanx must be treated as compound fractures and referred urgently to an orthopaedic specialist.

As with all hand injuries, open fractures often require an intensive rehabilitation programme. It is important to impress upon the patient the necessity of regular follow-up and close monitoring of progress is vital if there is to be any chance of good functional recovery. Patients who are lost to follow-up may represent after a prolonged period with marked stiffness of the small joints of the hand and adhesions within the soft tissues, particularly the tendons, which may prove refractory to all forms of treatment.

Hand infections

Deep-seated hand infections are generally due to penetrating injuries. Lacerations resulting from objects as varied as human teeth, sharp industrial implements and sports kit, can lead to a variety of organisms infecting hand tissue.

Diagnosis

It is important to remember that the actual size of the skin wound may not reveal the degree of damaged tissues within the confined space beneath the skin. With all hand injuries, it is very important to assess not only the bony structures and joints for stability but also the neurovascular and tendinous structures for impaired function.

Management

Early and adequate irrigation and debridement is especially important for injuries that are grossly contaminated with soil or other foreign material (e.g. injection paint-gun injuries). Patients should be taken to theatre as early as possible. The skin wound should be opened by an extensile approach to display all the contaminated tissue. Neurovascular structures and tendons should be inspected at the time of surgical debridement. Wherever possible, it is essential to preserve and these structures intact and repair them.

For those patients who present late with a chronic deep infection secondary to trauma or where the diagnosis has been missed, surgical debridement is again necessary. The affected part is laid open to allow drainage of all pus and adequate debridement of all necrotic tissue. At the time of surgery, swabs are taken and tissue specimens are sent for microbiological evaluation to try and identify any infecting organism.

Appropriate antibiotic prophylaxis should be given in adequate dosage and for an appropriate duration. Swabs should initially be taken in either the emergency department or at the time of surgery, together with tissue specimens if appropriate, for culture. While awaiting definitive microbiological evaluation, a broad-spectrum antibiotic should be given. The choice of antibiotic can be changed depending on any organisms identified together with their specific antibiotic sensitivity. The initial 24–48 h of antibiotic therapy may be administered intravenously depending on the severity of contamination and this can be followed up by an appropriate oral course of antibiotics.

The wound should be inspected 24 h after debridement for further evidence of purulent discharge of necrotic tissue. If necessary, the patient should return to theatre for repeat debridements until all contamination or affected tissue has been removed. Following surgical debridement, the hand is splinted in the position of function. A plaster of Paris split may be used initially followed later by a removable thermoplastic splint. The hand is also elevated to try and reduce the development of soft-tissue oedema.

Mobilization of hand injuries should not be delayed until all soft tissues have healed, which may take several weeks. Instead, under the supervision of a physiotherapist, early active and passive mobilization should be performed depending on the individual injury. The patient should be instructed to perform his own physiotherapy so that this can be continued following discharge from hospital.

Regular follow-up is important with vigilance for the development of chronic infections. These are usually secondary to inadequate initial treatment, misdiagnosis or a late presentation. If chronic infection occurs, the principles of treatment are essentially the same as above.

DISORDERS OF THE FOOT

Clinical assessment

History

History must elucidate the following:

- Presenting symptoms, which are usually pain, stiffness, swelling, deformity, problems with footwear and loss of function.
- Exact nature of the pain and whether it is purely related to weight bearing or also occurs at rest. The exact distribution of the pain may localize the pathology.
- Duration of symptoms is important and whether they are improving or deteriorating with time.
- Whether the patient has received any treatment, including surgical procedures, in the past and whether this has been effective.
- Whether there is any family history of foot disorders. Did the patient have trouble with his feet as a child or is there any history of spinal anomalies since birth?

Examination

For the clinical examination, the patient's entire lower limbs need to be exposed. The patient's gait needs to be assessed and his footwear checked for signs of abnormal wear. It is helpful to see if the patient can heel walk and toe walk as this may exacerbate pain and also allows some assessment of motor power around the ankle and foot. Careful inspection of the feet, including the soles, for abnormal pressure patterns is important. Any deformity of the toes, midfoot or hindfoot should be noted. In particular, look for previous surgical scars, atrophic skin changes and ulceration over bony prominences.

The vascularity of the foot must be carefully assessed, not only testing the pulses in the lower limbs but also the capillary return. A careful neurological assessment is also important, particularly assessing sensation over the foot. The active and passive movement must be assessed of the ankle, subtalar, midtarsal, tarsometatarsal, metatarsophalangeal (MTP) and IP joints. Depending on the history, the joints should be tested individually. It is also important to assess motor power of individual tendons on the plantar and dorsal aspects of the foot and ankle. Assessment of the plantar arches usually involves standing behind the patient and asking him to stand on his toes. In the patient with flat feet, this test gives an idea as to whether the fallen arches are dynamic or structural. If the latter is the cause of collapsed arches, the arch will not be reconstituted when the patient stands on his toes. All bony prominences should be palpated for tenderness depending on the localization of the pain. It is important also carefully to examine the patient's spine, looking for surface anomalies that may suggest an underlying spinal dysraphysm.

Investigation

Investigations usually involve plain radiographs in the first instance, followed by more specialized investigations, namely a computed tomography (CT) scan and MRI to help further elucidate the diagnosis.

Ankle disorders

Recurrent lateral ligament instability

This condition commonly occurs in sportsmen. It is usually secondary to recurrent inversion injuries to the ankle, which result in complete tears usually of the anterior talofibular and lateral calcaneofibular ligaments. There is often a history of an initial traumatic injury treated conservatively. Alternatively, there may be a history of recurrent minor strains associated with less trauma. The patient complains of a feeling of instability of the ankle, particularly on walking on uneven ground. There is usually a positive anterior drawer sign of the ankle suggesting incompetence of the anterior talofibular ligament. There may be excessive inversion of the affected hindfoot compared with the contralateral side. Stress inversion radiographs performed on both ankles show excessive talar tilt on the affected side.

Treatment may be conservative or operative. The former usually consists of physiotherapy with muscle strengthening and proprioceptive exercises. If these prove unsuccessful, then surgical reconstruction of the lateral ankle ligaments may be necessary. This usually involves use of one of the peroneal tendons to act as a substitute for the damaged anterior talofibular and calcaneofibular ligaments. The Christman and Snook procedure is one such popular procedure which involves the reconstruction of the anterior talofibular and calcaneofibular ligaments. In this, the peroneus brevis tendon attaches the fibula to the base of the fifth metatarsal in substitution of the anterior talofibular ligament, and to the calcaneus to substitute the calcaneofibular ligament.

Osteoarthritis of the ankle joint

This may rarely occur as a primary disorder; however, degenerative arthritis of the ankle joint is more commonly secondary to recurrent episodes of trauma from lateral ligament instability or from the sequelae of intra-articular fractures involving the ankle joint. It may also occur as a secondary phenomenon to avascular necrosis of the talar dome secondary to talar neck fractures. The long-term outcome of septic arthritis of the ankle joint which damages the articular cartilage may be degenerative osteoarthrosis.

The presenting symptoms and signs are usually pain, swelling and stiffness of the joint. The pain is markedly exacerbated by weight bearing. Restriction of movement usually affects dorsiflexion.

Initial treatment usually revolves around conservative measures (i.e. walking aids, supportive footwear, analgesics, anti-inflammatory agents and physiotherapy). If these fail, injection of intra-articular anaesthetic and steroid may be considered to give temporary symptomatic relief and operative treatment may be necessary. This usually takes the form of an ankle joint arthrodesis which relieves pain effectively but permanently stiffens the joint.

Osteochondritis dissecans of the talus

This is one of the osteochondritides, as is Freiberg's (Fig. 22.25) and Kohler's disease (Fig. 22.26). The exact aetiology is unknown but may be related to trauma. It usually occurs in younger age groups and may present as pain and swelling around the ankle joint, with or without episodes of mechanical locking secondary to loose body formation, depending on the stage of the disease. Early in the disease process a small fragment of the dome of the talus, usually in the anteromedial corner, separates from the body of the talus and may eventually form a loose body within the ankle joint. The radiographical appearance can vary from a small fragment of bone separate but still attached to the dome of the talus, to a defect in the dome of the talus, with or without an obvious radio-opaque loose body visible within the joint.

Treatment depends on the stage of the disease. If the fragment is still attached, internal fixation may be attempted in the hope that it will heal. However, if the bony fragment is loose, then its surgical removal from the joint is required.

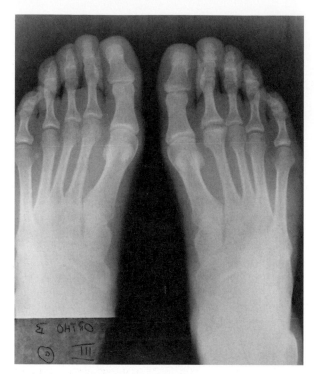

Figure 22.25. Frieberg's disease of second metatarsal head (right).

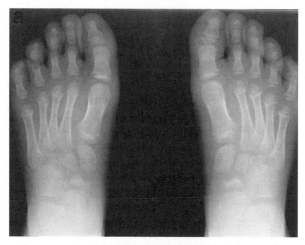

Figure 22.26. Kohler's disease of the tarsal navicular (right).

Avascular necrosis of the talus

This is usually secondary to displaced talar neck fractures where the blood supply to the talar dome is disrupted. As with the femoral neck and the scaphoid, the dome of the talus has a tenuous blood supply which runs either subperiosteally across the neck of the talus or enters the dome via the sinus tarsi. Displaced fractures of the talar neck are often associated with disruption of the subtalar joint and therefore the sinus tarsi. In these circumstances, the periosteal and endosteal blood supplies to the talar dome are disrupted as well as the vessels entering via the sinus tarsi. Even accurate surgical reduction does not guarantee that the talar dome will be revascularized. If it remains avascular, it eventually undergoes necrosis and will collapse under the load of weight bearing. This results in deformity of the ankle joint and secondary degenerative changes.

The usual treatment in delayed cases where conservative treatment has failed is ankle arthrodesis to relieve the pain from secondary degenerative changes within the ankle joint.

Hindfoot disorders

Rheumatoid arthritis

This generalized systemic disease can affect the ankle joint as well as the hindfoot, namely subtalar joint. The erosive arthropathy destroys the joint surfaces, resulting in loss of bone stock, osteopaenia, collapse of bony architecture and resulting hindfoot deformity. This is usually a valgus hindfoot and is secondary not only to destruction of the joint surfaces but also damage to the associated ligaments and soft tissues. This affects both the ankle and subtalar joint and the deformity is generally rigid if the disease process is well established.

Clinically, an abnormal wear pattern is found in the patient's shoes. On standing behind the patient, there may be marked valgus of the hindfoot which does not correct when the patient stands on his toes. The ankle and subtalar joints may be stiff and irritable to movement. There may also be hindfoot swelling, tenderness to palpation and tenosynovitis of the peroneal or posterior tibial tendons and tendon rupture may occur.

Conservative treatment consists of modifying footwear to try and relieve weight on pressure points and give some added support to the hindfoot. If the hindfoot deformity is still mobile, as it may be early in the disease, then bracing with special orthoses may be appropriate to try and maintain the hindfoot in normal alignment. Due to the relentless nature of the disease, conservative measures often prove fruitless and therefore surgical intervention is necessary. There are three main categories:

• *Osteotomy*: usually involves realigning the os calcis beneath the tibia to correct hindfoot valgus. This does not affect the joint surfaces and the deformity can recur.
• *Arthroplasty*: involves resurfacing the joint; however, due to the stresses placed through the joint, this often fails and the prosthesis can loosen.
• *Arthrodesis*: involves bony fusion across the ankle, hindfoot or midfoot joints. 'Double arthrodesis' may be preferred in younger, more active patients. It involves arthrodesis of calcaneocuboid and talonavicular joints. 'Triple arthrodesis' is a popular procedure which involves

arthrodesis of subtalar, calcaneocuboid, and talonavicular joints. It has a high union rate in rheumatoid arthritis and can improve ambulatory status in more than 80% patients and can provide pain relief in up to 90% patients. 'Pantalar' arthrodesis is the term used for fusion of the ankle, subtalar, talonavicular and calcaneocuboid joints. This is often used to permanently stabilize the hindfoot.

Osteoarthritis of the subtalar joint

This is most commonly secondary to displaced intra-articular fractures of the os calcis and results in disruption of the articular surfaces and the normal complex alignment of the subtalar joint. Subsequent degenerative changes occur resulting in pain and stiffness of the hindfoot. The patient has particular difficulty walking on uneven ground and clinically there is marked restriction of inversion and eversion and the patient finds these movements quite painful. Conservative treatment usually consists of appropriate footwear to try and support the hindfoot, but if this fails, a subtalar joint arthrodesis can be undertaken which again permanently stiffens the joint but may relieve the patient's discomfort.

Sever's disease

This is a traction apophysis at the insertion of the Achilles tendon into the os calcis. The condition is commonest in pubertal boys and the only treatment required is a heel raiser. It is usually a self-limiting condition.

Ruptured Achilles tendon

This is discussed under the section Tendon injuries, above.

Plantar fasciitis

This is an uncommon cause of hindfoot pain. It emanates from the plantar aspect of the heel where the plantar muscles and fascia arise from the os calcis. It presents as a sharp stabbing pain, particularly on weight bearing and can cause considerable discomfort. Clinically, there is an area of localized tenderness on the plantar aspect of the heel. Radiographically, there may be a plantar calcaneal spur, however this may be a coincidental finding. Underlying treatment usually involves neoprene heel inserts for the footwear, injections of local anaesthetic and steroid into the tender area and if these measures fail, surgical release of the plantar fascia of the os calcis.

Hallux rigidus

This is osteoarthritis of the first MTP joint. The exact aetiology is unknown. The patient usually presents with pain and stiffness of the great toe. The patient may complain of throbbing or aching at rest, but usually the symptoms are most pronounced on weight bearing, particularly the take-off phase of the gait. It is often an isolated phenomenon and other joints in the foot are not affected. The patient is generally middle aged. Clinically, there is swelling in the joint with restricted range of movement, particularly dorsiflexion at the MTP joint. There may be an associated osteophyte on the dorsum of the joint.

Radiographs of the affected joint generally reveal marked degenerative changes with loss of joint space, osteophyte formation and subchondral sclerosis.

Conservative treatment usually involves the application of a metatarsal bar to the sole of the shoe, the rigidity of which helps to release some of the stress across the MTP joint. If this proves unsuccessful, surgical treatment can be undertaken. The surgical options are:

- *Cheilectomy*: involves excision of the prominent dorsal osteophyte of the first metatarsal head.
- *Excision arthroplasty*: involves removal of the arthritic joint by excising the base of the proximal phalanx and trimming the osteophytes off the metatarsal heads. This defunctions the great toe leaving it floppy and may affect the patient's gait, particularly the push off component.
- *Arthrodesis*: involves permanent stiffening of the MTP joint by achieving bony fusion with screw fixation.

Forefoot disorders

Hallux valgus

This is a deformity of the forefoot involving the great toe. The great toe deviates laterally crowding the lesser toes. It may be unilateral or bilateral. It is often associated with a bunion or painful callosity over the medial aspect of the first MTP joint. This is generally due to a large osteophyte at the base of the proximal phalanx or head of the first metatarsal.

The aetiology is unknown but may be familial. Poor footwear is often blamed as the cause, but this usually aggravates the symptoms rather than initiating the problem.

Clinical examination reveals a valgus deformity of the great toe. If this is severe, there can be resultant deformity of the second toe with it eventually overriding the great toe. There may be a large prominence over the medial aspect of the first metatarsal head with associated callosities. It is often irritated by footwear and there may be an underlying bursa. There may be mild irritability of the first MTP joint.

Plain X-rays may reveal an increased intermetatarsal angle between the first and second metatarsal. There is also a valgus malalignment of the great toe relative to the axis of the forefoot (Fig. 22.27). There may be mild degenerative changes within the first MTP joint and the possibility of an exostosis over the medial aspect of the first metatarsal heads.

Various splints and braces have been tried to passively hold the great toe in alignment if it is passively correctable. Patients often find them cumbersome and a hindrance. The most appropriate management, having initially enquired about the patient's footwear, is recommendation of the use of flat shoes that have a broad toe box. This particularly applies to women who tend to wear high-healed shoes with a narrow toe box. Most patients find that this alleviates the symptoms but they must be warned that this will not correct the deformity.

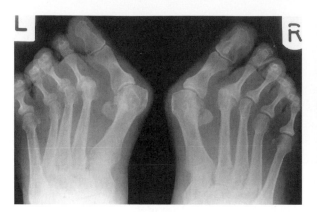

Figure 22.27. Bilateral hallux valgus.

There are five main methods of surgical treatment:

- *Soft-tissue procedures like the McBride operation*: involves release of adductor hallucis, transverse metatarsal ligament and lateral capsule combined with excision of medial eminence and plication of the capsule medially.
- *Excision arthroplasty* (Keller's arthroplasty; Fig. 22.28): involves excising the proximal third of the proximal phalanx of the great toe and forming a medial exostosectomy of the prominence of the first metatarsal head. Due to the bowstring effect of the extensor hallucis longus tendon, this is lengthened by Z-plasty so as to allow correction of the valgus deformity. However this procedure must be reserved for the elderly population with very limited demands as the results of this procedure in high-demand patients are not good.
- *Arthrodesis*: is more commonly performed in patients with hallux rigidus (Fig. 22.29), but is also more appropriate than excision arthroplasty if there are significant degenerative changes within the first MTP joint or the patient falls into the younger age group. The first MTP joint is usually transfixed with a single screw. It is important when performing this procedure that the valgus malalignment of the great toe is not overcorrected, which can result in an extremely disabling hallux varus deformity. It is also important to determine the nature of the shoes the patient will be wearing on a regular basis, so that the great toe may be fused in an appropriate degree of dorsiflexion.
- *Metatarsal osteotomy*: involves the first metatarsal shaft and can either be proximally or distally based. The advantage is that there is no disruption to the MTP joint. This option is often reserved for patients who have a markedly increased angle between the first and second metatarsals. In younger patients basal osteotomies are favoured where the aim is to lateralize the distal segment of the first metatarsal so as to achieve secondary correction of the obstacle near the great toe. Many different procedures have been described and they are often combined with

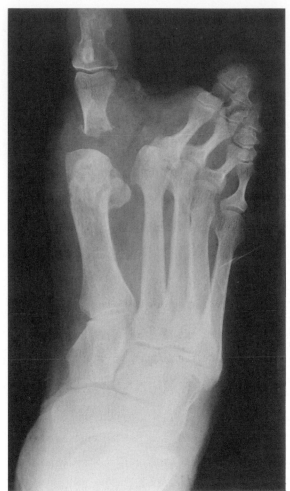

Figure 22.28. Keller's arthroplasty.

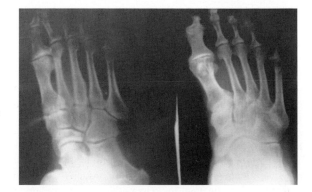

Figure 22.29. Hallux rigidus.

soft-tissue procedures, particularly around the first MTP joint.

- *MTP joint Arthroplasty*: involves patients who undergo metatarsal osteotomies or arthrodesis need to be immobilized in a plaster boot for up to 6 weeks. It is important that the patient is observed carefully so as to avoid any pressure sores developing from the plaster boot. The patient should be able to fully weight bear if the plaster boot is comfortable. Patients who undergo an excisional arthroplasty do not require such immobilization other than appropriate strapping of the foot until the wound is healed. These patients must be warned preoperatively that the great toe will remain floppy after the procedure.

Morton's metatarsalgia

This is due to neuroma formation at the intersection of the plantar digital nerve. It commonly involves the junction of the medial lateral plantar nerve in the third intermetatarsal space, but can also occur in other intermetatarsal spaces. It is thought to be due to irritation of the nerve.

The patient typically complains of forefoot pain with a sharp burning sensation radiating up adjacent sides of the affected toes, commonly the third and fourth, if the neuroma involves the third metatarsal space. There is usually point tenderness in the affected intermetatarsal space on palpating from the plantar aspect of the forefoot. Symptoms may be reproduced by squeezing the forefoot manually (Nelson's sign). It is uncommon to find altered sensation along the adjacent borders of the affected toes.

If diagnosis is still in doubt from the clinical findings, an ultrasound of the forefoot is sometimes helpful. MRI has been used, usually to rule out more serious pathology.

Conservative treatment involves adjustment of footwear to give appropriate support to the metatarsal head with an insole metatarsal arch support. If conservative treatment fails, the neuroma can be excised. This is often performed through a plantar approach with a longitudinal incision, but it is vital to confirm with the patient preoperatively exactly which intermetatarsal space is involved by noting the exact location of the tender area.

Freiberg's disease

This is essentially an osteochondritis of either the second or third metatarsal head. It usually affects young adolescents and the aetiology is unknown. A segment of the metatarsal head becomes avascular and over a period of time there is collapse of the metatarsal head with some disruption of the MTP joint. The patient generally complains of forefoot pain, particularly on weight bearing, and there may be associated swelling and tenderness around the affected metatarsal head. There is also irritability of the relevant MTP joint.

The diagnosis is usually confirmed by plain X-rays (Fig. 22.25). These show deformity of the affected metatarsal head, usually the second or third with collapse. In the early stages, the articular surface may be preserved but later there is disruption of the joint and there may be degenerative changes if the condition is long-standing nature.

The condition is often self-limiting but some cases may be refractory. Adjustments to footwear with metatarsal arch supports may give symptomatic relief but will not alter the course of the disease. Occasionally, symptoms persist and are incapacitating. Many different surgical procedures have been tried and all have met with varying degrees of success:

- osteotomy through the neck of the metatarsal,
- excision of the metatarsal head,
- open bone grafting of the metatarsal head.

BONE AND JOINT INFECTIONS

The specific case of hand infections is dealt with under the section above on Hand injuries.

Acute osteomyelitis

This can be classified as acute, acute on chronic or chronic and most commonly affects children. The organisms commonly involved are *Staphylococcus aureus*, *Streptococci*, *Brucella* spp. In sickle cell anaemia, *Salmonella* spp. are important causes. Causes of infection are haematologous spread from remote source, for example skin infection, dental abscess, genital infection, direct penetration from sharp trauma and blunt trauma resulting in subperiosteal haematoma.

The epiphyseal end of a long bone becomes seeded with organisms spread by the blood stream which lodge in fine capillaries. Pus forms within the canals and, due to the confined space, causes a necrosis of bone. As pus extends into the subperiosteal region, the periosteal blood supply is disrupted, and direct pressure and thrombosis of small vessels cause further bone necrosis. Islands of dead bone are formed within the porous cavity. Pus may burst through the periosteum discharging into a body cavity or skin forming a sinus. Further periosteal stripping occurs with further necrosis of bone. The body's response, apart from the acute inflammatory response, is new bone formation. This surrounds the dead bone forming a porotic cavity containing an involucrum which may extend the entire length of a long bone.

Clinical features

General symptoms include fever, sweats, malaise, anorexia, weight loss and apathy. Tachycardia and elevated temperature are consistent with a patient who is toxaemic. Local features are pain relieved by rest, swelling of the affected limb, immobility of associated joints, paralysis in the chronic situation and tenderness in the region of the epiphyseal region of the long bones.

There is a spectrum of presentation depending on the stage of the disease. In the early stages, symptoms may be absent, whereas in the delayed situation, the patient may be septicaemic and any palpation of the affected part may cause excruciating pain. Presentation may also be complicated if the patient has already received a course of oral antibiotics as this may suppress but not cure the infection and therefore mask the signs so that the diagnosis is missed.

The differential diagnosis is:

- septic arthritis,
- transient arthritis,
- subperiosteal haemotoma secondary to trauma,
- inflammatory arthropathy (e.g. rheumatoid arthritis),
- fracture,
- chronic subcutaneous infection.

Investigations

Haematological tests may find a raised white cell count with neutrophilia. There may also be a raised ESR and CRP. Blood cultures may help to identify the causative organism.

In the early stages, plain radiographs may be normal. In later stages, when there has been periosteal stripping with new bone formation and bone necrosis, evidence of subperiosteal new bone formation, bone necrosis with sequestral formation, cavitation with the metaphyseal region and areas of lacunae may be seen. It usually takes approximately 10 days for radiological changes to become apparent and the first change is usually rarefaction of the bone.

Management

This depends on the stage of the disease. In acute osteomyelitis it consists of:

- Analgesia.
- Resting the affected part.
- High-dose intravenous antibiotics, initially given intravenously until symptoms settle and blood parameters, CRP and ESR begin to return to normal. This may take up to 2 weeks and then the patient is transferred to an appropriate oral regimen of antibiotics to complete a total course of 6 weeks.
- Excision and drainage of periosteal collections may allow decompression of the metaphyseal region of the bone and also allows acquisition of specimens to help isolate an organism and therefore improve antibiotic choice.

Complications

- Chronicity (chronic osteomyelitis, see below).
- Infections (infection can spread into adjacent joints resulting in septic osteoarthritis).
- Limb length discrepancy due to damage to adjacent epiphyseal growth plate.
- Septicaemia if condition is untreated.

Chronic osteomyelitis

Chronic osteomyelitis is usually the sequelae of unsuccessful or partially treated acute osteomyelitis. The infection was never eradicated from the affected bone due to the inability of antibiotics to penetrate an abscess cavity. The pus continues to spread with further subperiosteal stripping, bone necrosis and new bone formation with extension of the involucrum and further sequestrum formation. This is often accompanied by multiple sinus formation.

The patient usually has a history of treatment for an acute episode of osteomyelitis which may have occurred many years previously. Infection was never completely eradicated and the patient is left with intermittent flare-ups of the condition which are associated with pain, swelling and tenderness, but settle with further courses of antibiotics. Alternatively the patient may present with a persistent or intermittently discharging sinus.

Clinical features

These include:

- chronic discharging sinus;
- pathological fracture;
- deformity (possibly associated with limb length discrepancy);
- current acute episodes of swelling of the femur, associated with toxaemia (acute on chronic osteomyelitis).

Investigations

If the patient is experiencing an acute flare-up of the condition, there may be an elevated white cell count with moderately elevated acute phase reaction such as ESR and CRP. Blood cultures are generally negative. Swabs taken from any discharging sinuses will often just grow skin flora and there is extreme difficulty in isolating an organism in these individuals as they have often had multiple courses of antibiotics.

Plain radiographs may show a complete alteration of the architecture of a long bone with an abnormal shape, marked new bone formation surrounding a cavity that contains sclerotic bone or sequestra or an involucrum extending along the length of the diaphysis, depending on the extent of the disease. There may be destruction of associated growth plates with resultant shortening of the bone. If there has been antigen spread into an adjacent joint with resultant septic arthritis, there may be complete destruction or degenerative changes within the adjacent joints.

Management

The patient may remain on a long-term antibiotic selected according to any organisms previously isolated. Alternatively, the patient may only receive antibiotics during flare-ups, when the patient becomes temporarily toxaemic, with increased tenderness, swelling or associated discharge from the affected site. Some patients may find that their function is reasonable even in the presence of chronic infection and they can cope with having a short course of antibiotics during acute flare-ups to control symptoms. However, these patients must be warned of the long-term sequelae of chronic infection, particularly amyloidosis with resultant renal failure and the possibility of neoplastic transformation at the margins of discharging sinuses.

Decompression, antibiotic suppression and curettage of the abscess cavities are also unlikely to eradicate infection. Cure is achieved with more extensive treatment:

- Massive open debridement of all affected tissue, both bone and soft tissue, with excision of involucrum and excision of cavity. This may leave a large defect in the bone which requires bridging either with bone transport or bone grafting. Multiple surgical procedures are involved with prolonged hospital stay. Eradication of the infection is not guaranteed and there are sequelae for the function of the limb.
- A more radical option is amputation of the affected part, particularly a distal part of a limb which is suitable for prosthetic replacement. This may be a more viable option if the patient wishes to return to normal activity as soon as possible and avoid prolonged hospital treatment. On the other hand, amputation is not acceptable to many patients.

Brodie's abscess

This is a chronic walled-off abscess generally containing sterile fluid and necrotic debris with inflammatory granulation tissue. It was originally described only in the tibia but can occur in other long bones. The lesion can be present for many years. Symptoms usually include intermittent pain and swelling of the affected part.

Plain X-rays reveal a well circumscribed radiolucent area with a sclerotic well-defined margin. Lesions usually occur in the metaphyseal region of long bones. Aspiration often reveals a sterile fluid but may contain bacteria (staphylococci). The treatment is surgical evacuation by drilling or open drainage under antibiotic cover with curettage of the wall of the cavity.

Septic arthritis

This generally refers to bacterial arthritis although it may be tuberculous. Pus is extremely chondrolytic and leads to rapid destruction of cartilage in septic arthritis. Untreated the condition can cause rapid destruction of the joint and therefore septic arthritis requires rapid decompression of the joint to preserve the articular cartilage followed by a prolonged course of antibiotics.

The organisms involved are: *Staphylococcus aureus* and *S. epidermidis*, *Streptococcus*, *Pseudomonas*, *Gonococcus*. In patients less than 3 years of age *H. influenzae* is the commonest organism whereas in all patients older than 3 years of age, *Staphylococcus aureus* is the commonest. Hence empirical treatment initially starts with broad-spectrum antibiotics to cover these commonest organisms. In immunosuppressed individuals fungi and mycobacteria are important causative organisms, as well as coliforms and tuberculous (Fig. 22.30). Their mode of spread is haematogenous (from cardiac valves, skin, oral cavity, genitourinary or respiratory tract), direct

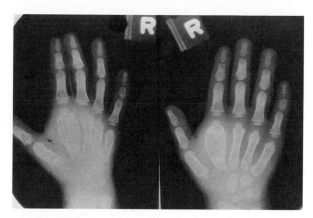

Figure 22.30. Tuberculous dactylitis.

penetration of the joint from the exterior usually due to trauma/surgery, and contiguous spread from an adjacent focus of osteomyelitis (Figs 22.31 and 22.32).

Predisposing factors are:

- rheumatoid arthritis,
- immunosuppressive agents,
- steroids,
- lymphoproliferative disorders,
- leukaemias,
- human immunodeficiency virus (HIV) infection,
- alcoholism,
- diabetes,
- age.

The offending organism bulges in the synovium of the joint causing inflammation. This results in a purulent synovitis with purulent exudate forming within the joint cavity. Enzymes within the exudate rapidly destroy the articular cartilage matrix, especially when under pressure within the confined joint space. This results in early destruction of the joint with fibrosis and/or ankylosis leading to early degenerative changes.

Clinical features

- severe unremitting pain;
- immobility of the affected joint (any movement causes severe pain);
- swelling of the joint secondary to effusion;
- muscle wasting if chronic which accentuates the relative swelling of the joint;
- erythema of the surrounding soft tissues, especially if there is an associated cellulitis;
- children tend to hold the limb immobile and refuse to weight bear if a lower limb joint is involved;
- an associated systemic upset;
- fever, sweats, rigors;
- anorexia;
- toxaemia.

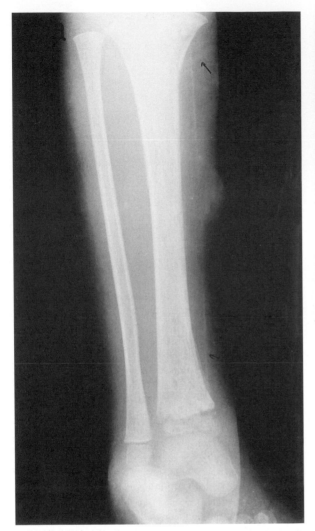

Figure 22.31. Osteomyelitis of the distal tibia.

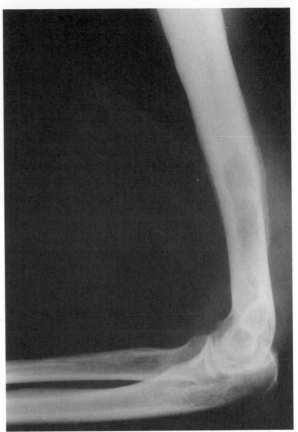

Figure 22.32. Osteomyelitis of the distal humerus.

Investigations

- *Haematological*: leucocytosis/neutrophilia if bacterial; raised ESR and CRP; positive blood cultures.
- *Microbiological*: sputum and urine culture.
- *Plain radiograph*: may be normal early in the disease process but later distension of the joint, effusion, loss of the joint space, sclerosis and joint destruction may be seen.
- *Ultrasound*: effusion may be detected compared with the normal joint and is especially useful in assessing hips in neonates. It is quick and non-invasive. However, ultrasound cannot confirm that an effusion is infected or secondary to a reactive synovitis.
- *Aspiration*: Obtaining joint fluid for culture is the definitive test. Fluid should be sent for urgent Gram stain, culture and sensitivity. Local antibiotics should be given

when cultures are obtained, unless the patient is toxaemic when antibiotics should be commenced on a 'best guess' basis. Aspiration under strict aseptic conditions is mandatory if a diagnosis of septic arthritis is suspected.

Beware partially treated septic arthritis. This usually involves a case where a course of oral antibiotics has been prescribed which masks the symptoms but does not resolve the condition. If an aspiration is performed in this situation, an organism may not be isolated from the joint fluid. There may be pus cells only and this can sometimes be confused with crystalline arthroplasty in adults.

Management

Urgent decompression of the joint, usually via an arthrotomy, and copious lavage with saline to ensure the breakdown of all loculi within the joint in chronic cases is performed. In some joints the procedure can be performed arthroscopically. This is followed by a prolonged course of antibiotics, usually given parenterally in the first instance. At the time of surgery, multiple specimens should be sent for microbiological analysis, especially the synovial fluid and synovium itself.

Antibiotic must be administered in high doses to achieve a therapeutic level and be appropriately chosen according to bacterial sensitivities on culture. Serum antibiotic levels should be monitored together with white cell count, ESR and CRP, as well as the clinical condition of the patient to ensure the sepsis is resolving.

If the Gram stain of the aspirate is negative, then the patient can be carefully observed and haematological and biochemical parameters measured while and definitive culture results are awaited. If the Gram stain is positive, arthrotomy drainage should be instituted immediately. Negative joint aspirations, that is no fluid is obtained, may occur if the pus is too thick to withdraw, but if clinical suspicion is high, arthrotomy should also be the next step in such a case. 'Best guess' antibiotics should be commenced as soon as all specimens have been obtained and then adjusted as soon as culture results are available. Specimens should also be routinely sent for tuberculous culture. Identification of the causative organism is imperative if the appropriate antibiotic is to be given for the appropriate duration.

Early rehabilitation of the joint once the acute symptoms subside is necessary to regain range of movement, power and therefore function. In the early stages, rest in a splint and analgesics should be prescribed to relieve the severe pain.

Complications
- Sinus formation.
- Chronicity: fibrosis/ankylosis.
- Destruction of the joint surfaces.
- Early degenerative arthritis.
- Metatastic infection.

BONE AND JOINT PAIN

Cervical spine pain

Pain emanating from the cervical spine may be localized to the back of the neck radiating into the intercapsular region or be diffusely referred to the shoulder girdle. Radiculopathy implies damage to the nerve root exiting from the spinal cord. It may be secondary to compression or inflammation. Myelopathy implies damage to the spinal cord itself and one can use symptoms and signs to localize the level of myelopathy. Radicular pain follows a typical nerve root distribution and is easy to discern by careful history taking. Very commonly, rather diffuse pain is difficult to isolate to any one particular structure in the cervical spine, be it a disc, facet joint or ligament. To assess these patients accurately, a good working knowledge of the anatomy of the cervical spine is needed as well as of the myotomal and dermatomal distribution of the cervical nerve roots to the upper limbs. There may be confusion as to whether the pain emanates from structures within the cervical spine or shoulder joints. However, careful clinical assessment should help to elucidate this.

A simple pathological classification of diseases involving the cervical spine is:
- *Congenital spinal dysraphysm*:
  - spinal dysraphysm
- *Klippel Feil syndrome.*
- *Developmental.*
- *Acquired*:
  - *Degenerative*: cervical spondylosis (Fig. 22.33), prolapsed cervical intervertebral disc, facet joint arthropathy, foraminal stenosis.
  - *Neoplastic*: primary bone tumours, metastatic tumour, primary intradural/extradural tumour.
  - *Inflammatory*: rheumatoid arthritis, HLAB 27 spondyloarthropathy.
  - *Infective*: bacterial vertebral osteomyelitis, infective discitis + epidural abscess.
  - *Post-traumatic*: traumatic cervical disc prolapse, cervical instability.
  - *Psychogenic.*
  - *Miscellaneous*: diffuse idiopathic skeletal hyperostosis, anterior longitudinal ligament calcification.

Clinical assessment

History must determine:
- The nature of the symptoms – have they been experienced before or do they represent an exacerbation of recurrent symptoms? Does the pain wake the patient at night? Are there any associated systemic symptoms or neurological deficits involving the limbs?
- If there has been recent or past trauma to the cervical spine, particularly from road traffic accidents.
- If the patient has experienced weight loss, development of swellings in the neck, tumours involving other body systems.
- If the patient smokes.

The neck should be inspected for any deformity, swelling, scars, etc. This is followed by palpation, both anteriorly and posteriorly, looking for tender areas or masses. These may be inflammatory masses arising from the prevertebral region or cervical nodes. The supraclavicular fossae should be examined bilaterally, looking for masses which may be swollen lymp nodes or a cervical rib.

Examination should involve assessing the range of movement of the cervical spine in six directions: flexion, extension, lateral rotation to the left and right, and lateral flexion to the left and right. It should be determined if any or all such movements are restricted and to what extent and whether they exacerbate the patient's pain. If the pain is diffusely referred to the shoulder girdle, movement of the shoulder should be assessed to see if this is restricted or reproduces the pain.

An accurate neurological examination of the upper and lower limbs should include a detailed motor and sensory examination and including superficial and deep tendon reflexes. Examination for long-track signs suggestive of cervical myelopathy is also vital together with an assessment of sphincter function.

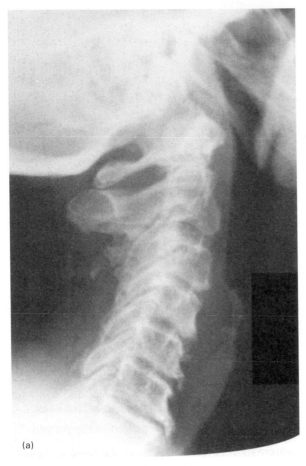

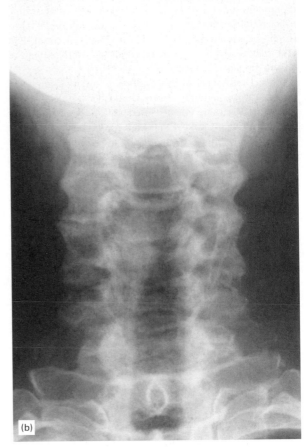

(a)

(b)

Figure 22.33. Cervical spondylosis.

Investigations

Depending on the differential diagnosis, investigations generally include serological tests, haematological evaluations and radiographical assessment of the cervical spine. If the diagnosis is still in doubt, more advanced techniques such as CT, myelography, MRI, neuroelectrophysiological studies and tissue biopsy can help to confirm a diagnosis.

Management

Treatment is determined by the diagnosis. The commonest course of diffuse cervical pain is generalized degenerative disease involving the cervical spine (Fig. 22.34), but a more sinister condition must not be overlooked. Treatment for degenerative cervical spine, with or without radiculopathy, is either conservative or operative. The former usually involves analgesics, anti-inflammatory agents, cervical supports, namely soft and hard collars, and physiotherapy. The patient may have to adjust his employment or social activities until the acute symptoms subside. If conservative treatment fails, symptoms are incapacitating or there is a deteriorating neurological deficit, surgical options can be considered.

Operative treatment for degenerative disc disease usually involves cervical fusion. If there is an associated radiculopathy, this requires nerve root decompression and this may be performed either posteriorly, with laminotomy or foraminotomy, or anteriorly, when it is combined with disc excision and intervertebral body fusion.

The results of treatment are variable. On occasions, the patient's symptoms may remain refractory despite multiple forms of treatment.

Shoulder pain

Shoulder pain may be referred from the cervical spine or be localized to a particular structure within the shoulder girdle. The pain may arise from the acromioclavicular joint, rotator cuff, long head of biceps or the glenohumeral joint. The diagnosis as always relies on careful clinical examination.

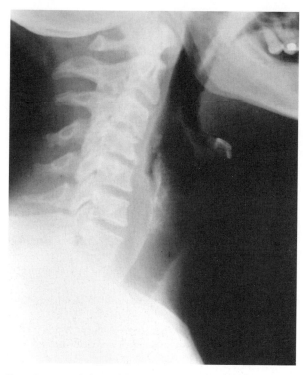

Figure 22.34. Cervical spondylosis and C2/C4 subluxation.

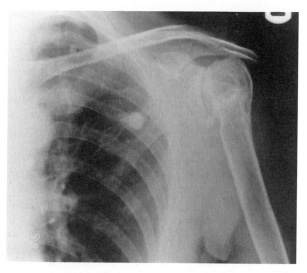

Figure 22.35. Cuff tear arthropathy of the shoulder.

Diagnosis varies according to the patient's age. In the younger age group, patients will generally present with symptoms of instability. This may be unidirectional and post-traumatic, or multidirectional and atraumatic. The symptoms are often recurrent in nature. The middle age group usually presents with symptoms of subacromial impingement, rotator cuff degeneration and frozen shoulder. The older age group presents with symptoms consistent with acromioclavicular joint osteoarthritis, subacromial impingement, rotator cuff tears or glenohumeral joint degeneration. This degeneration may be secondary to inflammatory arthritis (rheumatoid arthritis), post-traumatic arthritis, primary osteoarthritis or a massive rotator cuff tear (cuff tear arthropathy, Fig. 22.35).

Clinical assessment

Patients generally complain of pain, stiffness, swelling and loss of function. It is important to elicit a history of:

- Previous trauma to the shoulder, particularly that of dislocation of the glenohumeral joint, the circumstances under which this occurred and what the original treatment was.
- Past treatment, including surgery and injections around the shoulder joint, and whether this has been successful.
- Any sudden marked loss of movement in the shoulder girdle, especially following minor trauma.
- Difficulty performing activities above the head.
- Pain interfering with the patient's sleep pattern.

Examination of the shoulder girdle involves looking for scars from previous surgery, at its contour, and for any evidence of muscle wasting or deformity of the clavicle or proximal humerus. It is important also to look in the axilla for any scars or sinuses. The first hint of a rotator cuff tear, a common disorder in patients over 50 years of age, is obvious wasting of the supraspinatus and infraspinatus. The scapulothoracic rhythm and winging of the scapula must be noted.

Palpation involves not only assessing the cervical spine and supraclavicular fossae for tenderness but feeling all the bony landmarks around the shoulder girdle (i.e. the lateral end of the clavicle, acromioclavicular joint, acromion and proximal humerus). It is also possible to palpate the region of the long head of biceps in the bicipital groove. The tip of the coracoid process can also be palpated at the proximal end of the deltopectoral groove.

Assessing movement involves evaluating both the active and passive components. The patient's active range of shoulder movement should be examined in flexion, extension, abduction, adduction, internal and external rotation, comparing both sides simultaneously. This assessment is then repeated for passive movement. Active movement may be limited by a mechanical block or by pain. On assessing passive movement, an increased range may be found if the limitation is purely due to pain, but it is important not to cause the patient undue discomfort. The patient's face must be observed at all times to see if the examination elicits a painful response.

It is important to see if the patient can get the hand of his affected side behind his head or how far into the small of the back he can place his hand. This should be compared with the non-affected side.

Ancillary tests are then performed to diagnose common disorders like subacromial impingement, acromioclavicular joint arthritis, biceps tendon lesions, rotator cuff tears, instability of shoulder (unidirectional or multidirectional) and glenohumeral arthritis. For example the function of the rotator cuff is determined by assessing its individual components, that is:

- subscapularis by testing internal rotation against resistance and comparing this with the normal side;
- supraspinatus by testing the power of resisted abduction at approximately 30° of abduction;
- infraspinatus and teres minor by testing the power of external rotation against resistance.

Internal and external rotation are normally assessed with patient with his elbows tucked into his sides and flexed 90°. The patient is asked to rotate internally and externally while the examiner opposes such movements from behind. This allows a quick assessment and ready comparison of both sides.

Apprehension tests can also be performed to assess the stability of the joint. The commonest is the anterior apprehension test which is performed by standing behind the patient with the affected shoulder abducted to 90° and externally rotated with the elbow flexed to 90°. The examiner then applies an external rotation force to the shoulder whilst simultaneously applying an anteriorly directed force to the back of the humeral head. If there is any anterior instability such as an anterior labral tear, this will elicit apprehension in the patient.

Management

Treatment depends on the specific diagnosis. For instability problems in the shoulder, physiotherapy is used to strengthen the shoulder stabilizers, especially the rotator cuff muscles. With unidirectional instability secondary to trauma, surgical stabilization is required. Subacromial impingement with or without acromioclavicular joint arthritis requires conservative treatment initially. This involves physiotherapy combined with a series of subacromial injections of local anaesthetic and steroids. If the patient's symptoms fail to respond to this regimen, then surgical decompression of the subacromial space via an anterior acromioplasty and excision of the acromioclavicular joint may be warranted.

Rotator cuff tears are treated keeping in mind the patients symptoms, co-morbidities, functional loss, size and extent of tear and quality and retraction of the edges of the torn tendon. Massive un-repairable rotator cuff tears may require formal debridement performed arthroscopically or as an open procedure. Small- to medium-sized repairable tears are best managed by arthroscopic repair provided skills are available. Otherwise a mini open rotator cuff repair involving a 5–6-cm long incision may be indicated. Degenerative or inflammatory diseases involving the glenohumeral joint can be treated with total shoulder arthroplasty.

Frozen shoulder affects the middle or older age groups and its aetiology is entirely unknown. It may run a refractory course, particularly in diabetics where it may also be bilateral. The mainstays of treatment are adequate analgesia and anti-inflammatory agents together with prolonged aggressive physiotherapy to try and regain shoulder movement. In situations where conservative treatment fails, manipulation under anaesthesia may be of benefit.

Back pain

Due to almost epidemic proportions of patients presenting to general practitioners, general orthopaedic clinics, and accident and emergency departments, a working knowledge of the assessment of the patient presenting with back pain, as well as an idea of the possible causes and their treatment is essential. The vast majority of patients presenting with back pain of a musculoskeletal origin will have symptoms secondary to degenerative spinal disease. Other conditions can occur such as trauma, infections and inflammatory spondyloarthropathies. Visceral causes can also represent with very symptoms that mimic back pain.

A simple pathological classification of spinal disorders includes:

- *Congenital lesions* (e.g. spina bifida, sacral agenesis, diastematomyelia).
- *Developmental anomalies* (e.g. scoliosis (Fig. 22.36), Schuermann's kyphosis, isthmic or dysplastic spondylolisthesis, spondylolysis (Fig. 22.37)).
- *Acquired conditions*:
  - *Degenerative* (e.g. degenerative lumbar disc disease, spondylolisthesis, facet joint arthropathy).
  - *Traumatic* (e.g. burst fractures to the vertebral body, fracture dislocations thoracolumbar junction resulting in a post-traumatic kyphosis).
  - *Infective* (e.g. tuberculosis of the spine, bacterial vertebral osteomyelitis, discitis).
  - *Inflammatory* (e.g. HLAB 27-positive spondyloarthropathy, seronegative spondyloarthropathies).
  - *Neoplastic* (e.g. primary bone or soft-tissue tumours, metastases mainly from the kidney, thyroid, prostate, lung, breast, bowel).
  - *Iatrogenic* (postsurgical) (e.g. postlaminectomy syndrome).
  - *Psychogenic*.
  - *Metabolic*.
  - *Miscellaneous* (e.g. 'visceral' abdominal aortic aneurysm, pancreatitis, renal/ureteric calculi, soleus abscess, peptic ulceration).
  - *Idiopathic*.

Clinical assessment

An accurate history must be obtained including:

- Duration of symptoms, whether acute onset or deterioration of a chronic problem, any associated precipitating events such as a traumatic incident and factors that exacerbate or relieve the pain.
- Precise location of pain and whether there is any referred pain to the lower limbs.

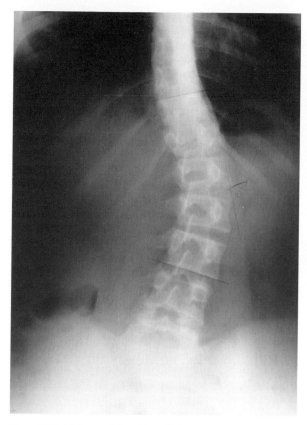

Figure 22.36. Adolescent idiopathic scoliosis.

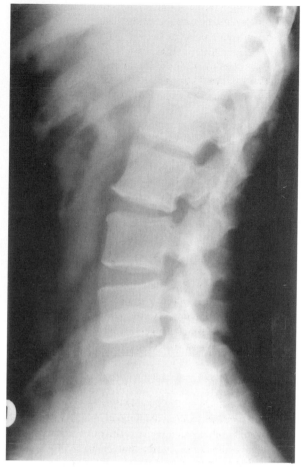

Figure 22.37. Spondylyosis at L2/L3.

- Accurate systems review, particularly with regard to weight loss, fevers, sweats and a nocturnal component to the pain; genitourinary or gastrointestinal pathology or associated ocular symptoms.
- Sphincter disturbance and any neurological deficits in the lower limbs associated with back pain.
- Extent to which symptoms interfere with the patient's lifestyle, namely domestic and social duties, employment, sports and hobbies.
- Nature of any past treatment, be it conservative or operative, and how effective it has been. Has the patient's requirement for analgesics and anti-inflammatory agents increased recently?
- Whether the patient is a smoker.
- Family history of back problems or history of spinal deformity diagnosed in childhood and any treatment undertaken for this.

Although the vast majority of patients presenting to the orthopaedic clinic with symptoms of back pain generally have degenerative lumbosacral spine disease, vigilance is required to ensure symptoms representative of tumours or infections of the spine are not overlooked. These are comparatively uncommon but if the diagnosis is missed the consequences are catastrophic. The clinician should be wary of patients who present with back pain that falls in the following categories:

- Elderly patients who present with recent onset of back pain that has never been experienced before, especially when associated with systemic symptoms such as weight loss.
- Patients who are troubled by persistent severe nocturnal back pain.
- Patients with interscapula/midthoracic pain.
- Any patient with associated neurological deficit.
- Patients presenting with back pain with bilateral radicular pain referred to the lower limbs.
- Any patient with perianal sensory disturbance or loss of sphincter control.
- Any patient with a previous diagnosis of malignant disease involving other organ systems.

A thorough clinical examination is imperative and involves:

- Identification of the exact source of the pain if possible and also any referred pain pattern into the limbs. In those with diffuse thoracic and lumbar spinal pain, assessment of respiratory excursion is also important.

- Any limitation in the range of movement of the spine and paravertebral muscle spasm.
- Tender areas must be accurately identified, whether they be over the spinous process or interspinous ligaments. Any palpable defect or step in the spinous processes should also be recognized by careful palpation.
- Spinal deformity should be noted in both the coronal and sagittal planes.
- Accurate lower limb neurological examination, including assessment of perianal sensation and anal tone. Any neurological defects need to be elucidated, including performing a rectal examination.
- Careful abdominal examination to exclude any intra-abdominal masses such as aortic aneurysms, pancreatic pseudocysts, retroperitoneal lymphadenopathy, bladder distension, secondary to neurogenic sphincter disturbance.
- General assessment for signs of generalized arthropathy and ocular, integumentary and cardiac manifestations that may accompany an inflammatory spondyloarthropathy.

Investigations

The investigations performed depend on the differential diagnosis. They normally include a series of plain radiographs of the whole or part of the spine, depending on the pathological process and the area localized by symptoms. Routine serological and haematological parameters are assessed, particularly if there an inflammatory or infective aetiology is being considered. Specialized investigations may be requested if the diagnosis is in doubt, that is radionuclide scanning to assess for increased tracer uptake in both the soft tissues and the bony skeleton; CT scanning to give a better appreciation of the bony anatomy, particularly in the horizontal plane (useful in trauma and post-traumatic situations); MRI scanning, especially if there is an associated neurological deficit, to visualize not only the intervertebral discs but also the intrathecal contents and nerve roots.

If the diagnosis is still in doubt, particularly if there is a mass lesion involving the spine, then a biopsy may need to be performed with either a fine needle under radiographical control or formal open surgical biopsy. Tissue specimens are routinely sent for histological and microbiological evaluation, including assessment for anaerobic and aerobic bacteria and tuberculosis.

Management

Once a formal diagnosis has been made, treatment depends on factors such as:
- Patient's age and general medical fitness, especially if the disease process involving the spine is part of a widespread systemic illness.
- Actual or perceived incapacity of the patient, particularly with regards to employment, loss of quality of life.
- Severity and duration of the symptoms.
- Failure of previous treatment, either conservative or operative.

- Presence of associated neurological deficit, for example cauda equina lesion or isolated radiculopathy resulting in deferred pain with or without motor or sensory loss.
- Psychological makeup of the patient, particularly as regards depressive illness which may be secondary to the severity of the symptoms or a premorbid condition which results in the development of psychogenic symptoms involving the back.

In general, conservative treatment of patients with degenerative back pain without neurological sequelae consists of analgesics, anti-inflammatory agents, walking aids if appropriate, spinal supports and braces, and physiotherapy. Alteration of lifestyle, change of employment, cessation of particular sporting activities or hobbies that may aggravate symptoms also need to be considered. Symptoms may persist despite aggressive conservative treatment. If symptoms are refractory and incapacitating, then surgical management, either spinal fusion or neural decompression, can be considered and again will depend on the exact diagnosis.

Any compressive lesion of the spinal cord is an emergency and must be treated aggressively. Spinal cord, cauda equina or nerve root compromise is most commonly secondary to extrathecal compressive lesions due to metastatic tumours arising from the vertebral body, retropulsed bony fragment into the spinal canal (associated with spinal fractures) or large prolapsed intervertebral discs (which may effect an isolated or multiple nerve roots resulting in cauda equina lesions). Tumours may be treated conservatively by either radiotherapy or chemotherapy or surgical decompression. Disc prolapse requires surgical decompression. Cauda equina lesions also require urgent decompression by surgical means to relieve pressure on the nerve roots and cornus so as to maintain neurological function. The most important consideration here is loss of sphincter control which necessitates urgent treatment.

For isolated nerve root lesions resulting in radicular pain in the lower limb, it needs to be determined if the nerve root irritation results in referred pain alone or if there is an associated neurological deficit. If the latter, is it static or deteriorating with time? This most commonly occurs secondary to compressive lesions from a degenerative lumbar spine, be it disc prolapse or compression of the nerve root secondary to foraminal stenosis as it exits the spinal canal. As to whether these conditions are treated conservatively or operatively depends on the timescale of the neurological deficit and whether there is associated pain. If the neural defect is of a long-standing nature with no ongoing deterioration, it may be treated conservatively with appropriate analgesics, bracing and physiotherapy, and progress monitored carefully.

If the neurological deficit is of acute onset and appears to be rapidly deteriorating, surgical decompression may be the chosen treatment to:
- prevent further deterioration,
- possibly improve the chances of recovery of the neural deficit.

Despite all forms of treatment, the patient may still fail to improve. Under these circumstances, appropriate backup from other medical disciplines such as pain control clinics and physiotherapists do help patients cope with the secondary effects of their debilitating symptoms.

Sciatica

Lumbar spinal anatomy

The lumbar spine consists of individual motion segments which comprise the vertebral body, intervertebral disc and facet joints. The spinal canal is made up of a bony-ligamentous ring which consists of the posterior aspect of the vertebral body and intervertebral disc anteriorly, pedicles and intervertebral foramina laterally together with the laminae and ligamentum flavum posteriorly. The articular processes of the facet joints are posterolaterally. The facet joints are enclosed within the facet joint capsules. Along the posterior aspect of the vertebral bodies, extending down the posterior fibres of the annulus fibrosis, is the posterior longitudinal ligament.

This bony-ligamentous ring of each motion segment completes the spinal canal posterior to the vertebral body. Contained within the canal are the thecal contents. The spinal cord ends at the lower border of the L1 vertebral body. Below this the cauda equina trails down from the conus medullaris, the individual nerve roots exiting through the intervertebral foramina at their appropriate levels and extending of the dural sleeve of the intervertebral foramen.

The anatomy of the intervertebral foramina, through which the individual nerve roots exit, consists of the pedicle of the corresponding body superiorly, posterolateral aspect of the vertebral body and intervertebral disc anteriorly, adjacent superior and inferior articular processes of the corresponding facet joint posteriorly and pedicle of the vertebral body below inferiorly.

As the nerve root exits through the foramen, it can be subjected to compression from a disc herniation medially, facet joint capsule hypertrophy and osteophytes on the facet joints laterally and also from the stenosis of the exit foramen due to collapse of the intervertebral disc with resultant loss of height of the intervertebral disc space, thus narrowing the exit foramen. A combination of all three pathological processes may occur simultaneously also resulting in circumferential stenosis of the exit foramen. All these processes can impinge extradurally on the exiting nerve root resulting in a radiculopathy. The symptoms and signs of this are generally referred to as sciatica but the overall clinical picture is determined by which individual nerve roots are compromised, their myotomal and dermatomal distribution.

Clinical features

The patient with sciatica usually presents with referred pain to the lower limb emanating from nerve root irritation in the lumbar spine. The exact site and distribution of the referred lower limb pain depends on which nerve root is being irritated. The leg pain may or may not be associated with mechanical back pain. The compromise in the function of the nerve root, be it motor, sensory or combined is referred to as radiculopathy.

As a general rule, the pain resulting from nerve root irritation follows the dermatomal distribution of that particular nerve root, for example irritation of the L1 root may result in groin pain and may be confused with local pathology in the hips; fifth lumbar nerve root irritation can result in pain extending down the posterior aspect of the thigh, lateral aspect of the leg and dorsum of the foot; first sacral nerve root irritation can result in posterior thigh and calf pain extending into the sole of the foot. However, this may not always be the case. Referred pain to the lower limb may emanate from facet joint arthropathy or disc degeneration without specific nerve root impingement and may mimic sciatica although it is not typical radicular pain. To help differentiate radicular pain from diffuse pain referred into the lower limb, clinical examination as well as a careful history must be relied upon.

Physical signs

Irritation of the nerve root resulting in radicular pain in the lower limb can be identified by eliciting the nerve root tension signs. This essentially involves stretching the nerve root with specific movements of the lower limb which will exacerbate (positive nerve root tension sign) the pain in a distribution typical of the compromised root. All the tests below are designed to elucidate radicular pain referred to the lower limb secondary to nerve root irritation.

- *Well straight leg test*: With the patient lying flat on his back on the examining couch, the non-affected limb is passively raised off the couch by the examiner with the knee in an extended position. The angle of the elevated straight leg with the couch which reproduces the patient's contralateral leg pain should be recorded. The reproduction of pain in the contralateral limb is described as a positive well leg raising test and is an unequivocal sign of contralateral nerve root irritation.

- *Straight leg raising test*: The patient lies supine on the examining couch. Instead of the non-affected limb being raised in the extended position, the affected leg is passively elevated, with the knee extended, by the examining physician. The elevation continues passively until the patient's limb pain is reproduced and the angle at which this occurs is recorded. A positive test is classified as one which reproduces the patient's lower limb pain in the same distribution. It is not positive if it only reproduces low back pain. Discomfort from hamstring tightness must be differentiated from exacerbation of the patient's lower limb pain and again does not constitute a positive test. Reproduction of buttock pain only is also not a positive test.

- *Bowstring test*: The patient lies supine on the examining couch. The hip and knee of the affected limb are flexed to

90°. The examiner's thumb is placed in the patient's popliteal fossa on the lateral hamstring tendons, adjacent to the common peroneal nerve. With the hip and knee flexed to 90°, pressure is applied over the common peroneal nerve with the examiner's thumb. Holding this pressure with the hip maintained at 90° flexion, the knee is passively extended by the examiner to see if this reproduces or exacerbates the patient's lower limb pain.

- *Laseque's test*: This test is similar to the bowstring test but pressure over the common peroneal nerve and the popliteal fossa is not applied. Instead, with the hip maintained at 90° flexion, the knee is passively extended by the examiner and a positive sign is noted if this reproduces or exacerbates the patient's leg pain.

- *Straight leg raising test with augmentation*: This test is performed in a similar fashion to the straight leg raising test with the patient lying supine on the examining couch. The affected limb is passively elevated by the examiner, maintaining the knee in an extended position. When the patient's pain is reproduced, the angle at which this occurs is noted. With the straight leg maintained in this position, the ankle joint is passively dorsiflexed, theoretically stretching the sciatic nerve if this exacerbates the patient's lower limb pain.

- *Femoral nerve stretch test*: The patient lies prone on the examining couch with the knee of the affected limb flexed to 90°. The examiner then passively extends the hip joint applying a stretch across the anterior aspect of the hip. If this reproduces the patient's typical anterior thigh pain, then it is classified as a positive test. Reproduction of back pain is not a positive test. Alternatively, the test can be performed with the patient lying on his side with the affected limb uppermost. The examiner stands behind the patient and places one hand on the pelvis to stabilize the hips. The knee of the affected limb is flexed to 90° and the ipsilateral hip is maintained in the extended position. With the examiner standing behind the patient, the hip joint is passively extended by pulling the leg posteriorly. The test is positive if this reproduces and/or exacerbates the patient's anterior thigh pain.

Lower limb neurological assessment of the myotomal and dermatomal distribution of the individual nerve roots will help identify any neurological deficits. This relies on accurate assessment of sensation and power in individual muscle groups supplied by particular nerve roots.

In patients who have radicular symptoms, particularly those with bilateral radicular pain, that sphincter function must be assessed. This involves testing perianal sensation by light touch and pinprick and performing a rectal examination to evaluate anal tone and sensation.

Investigations

Investigations to confirm a diagnosis of nerve root compression include plain X-rays of the lumbosacral spine, looking for evidence of degenerative change such as osteophytic lipping at the edges of the vertebral bodies and collapse of disc height with degenerative changes within the facet joints, particularly involving the level corresponding to the clinical assessment. Very occasionally, radicular pain may result from neoplastic or infective lesions irritating the nerve root, but the commonest causes are a prolapsed intervertebral disc impinging on the nerve root (Fig. 22.38) and stenosis due to degenerative changes (Fig. 22.39).

Other more specific investigations include CT myelography, where a contrast media is injected into the thecal sac to outline the nerve roots, but this has essentially been superceded by MRI which gives excellent images of the intrathecal contents and surrounding soft tissues and bony anatomy.

Management

Treatment is directed by the specific diagnosis. If sciatica is secondary to nerve root impingement from a disc prolapse, treatment can be conservative or operative. The former usually consists of analgesics, anti-inflammatory agents and rest in best for short periods where appropriate followed by a physiotherapy regimen. If these measures fail, consideration may be given either to epidural injection or operative intervention. The usual indications for operative treatment include:

- severe intractable radicular pain that fails to respond to conservative treatment;
- progressive neurological deficit;
- cauda equina symptoms with loss of sphincter control;
- recurrent incapacitating episodes of sciatica that interfere with employment or daily life.

Operative treatment usually involves decompressing the nerve root either by discectomy for a prolapsed disc or spinal canal decompression (e.g. laminectomy for spinal canal stenosis).

METABOLIC BONE DISEASE

This can be classified into diseases due to:

- reduction in the skeletal bone mass (osteoporosis);
- inadequate osteoid synthesis;
- inadequate osteoid mineralization (rickets/osteomalacia).

Osteoporosis

The World Health Organization (WHO) has established criteria for making the diagnosis of osteoporosis, as well as determining levels which predict higher chances of fractures. These criteria are based on comparing bone mineral density (BMD) in a particular patient with those of a 25-year-old female. BMD values which fall well below the average for the 25-year-old female (stated statistically as 2.5 standard deviations below the average) are diagnosed as 'osteoporotic'. If a patient has a BMD value less than the normal 25-year-old female, but not 2.5 standard deviations below the average, the bone is said to be 'osteopaenic' (means decreased BMD, but not as severe as osteoporosis).

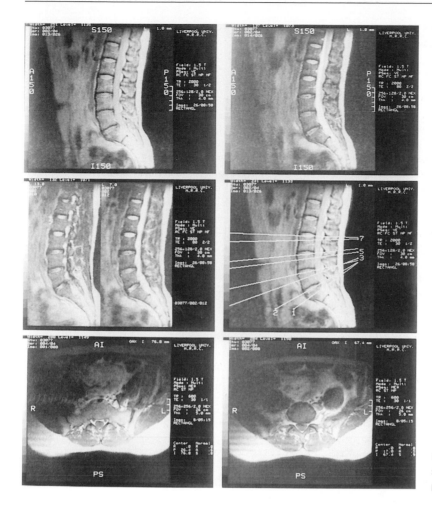

Figure 22.38. MRI scan of lumbosacral spine: sagittal and axial views showing L5/S1 prolapsed intervertebral disc.

This disease is secondary to a decrease in the actual skeletal bone mass and is commonest in postmenopausal women, especially those over the age of 65 years. The pathogenesis is thought to be related to oestrogen deficiency but many factors ultimately play a role.

The usual presenting symptoms are back pain, generalized bone and joint pain, fractures secondary to relatively minor trauma and increasing kyphosis of the dorsal spine due to vertebral body collapse. Fractures most commonly involve the distal radius and neck of femur.

Radiological changes include cortical and trabeculae thinning, and vertebral body collapse. The skeleton in general becomes more radiolucent.

Treatment once the condition is established is difficult. Prevention involves encouraging a healthy diet and regular exercise to maintain the normal body bone mass as long as possible. Hormone replacement therapy may maintain skeletal mass if instituted around the time of or within 5 years of the menopause. Other treatments include: diphosphonates, calcium supplements, fluoride supplements and vitamin D metabolites. In general, no treatment is absolutely satisfactory and the complications of the disease tend to be treated as they arise (i.e. bone pain and pathological fractures).

Rickets

Although rarely seen in the UK, rickets is still a problem in many parts of the world. It is currently ranked among the top five childhood diseases in developing countries. Inadequate vitamin D, from dietary sources or sunlight, has long been thought to be the cause of rickets.

Rickets is the inadequate osteoid mineralization in the growing skeleton as in osteomalacia, osteoid production is normal. It is due to a deficiency of calcium, phosphorus, or both. The deficiency may be secondary to:

• inadequate intake in the diet;
• problems with absorption from the gut – diseases of the bowel or pancreas which restrict absorption of fat-soluble vitamins;

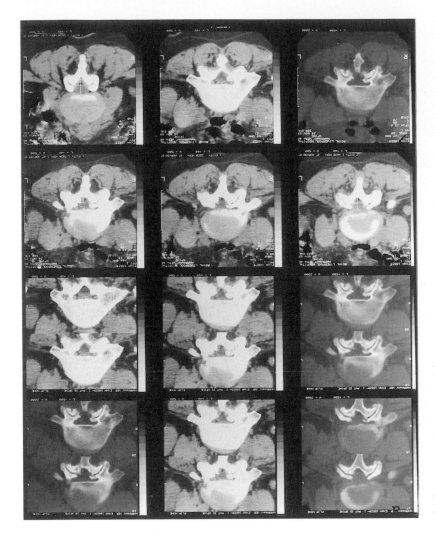

Figure 22.39. CT scan of lumbar spine: axial views showing spinal canal stenosis.

- diseases of the kidney with failure of conservation of calcium and phosphorus or enzymatic disturbances involving the vitamin D pathway.

Rickets is characterized by softening of the skeleton resulting in characteristic deformities.

Rickets is rare nowadays and is most obvious in the first 3 years of life. The clinical features are:

- frontal bossing;
- thinning of the skull;
- kyphoscoliosis of the spine;
- acetabular protrusion;
- bowing of lower limbs, especially the tibiae;
- shortness of stature due to stunted growth;
- rachitic rosary due to enlargement of the costochondral junctions;
- 'Harrison's groove' due to the traction from the diaphragm and softening of the thoracic margins.

Biochemically, the serum calcium is normal due to maintenance from the skeleton. Parathyroid hormones release calcium from the bone to keep this serum calcium normal and this may result in hyperplasia of the parathyroid glands (see Chapter 15). There is excessive loss of phosphate from the kidney and therefore the serum phosphate level is low.

Radiographical changes include:

- widening of the epiphyseal growth plates;
- cupping of the end of long bones;
- widening of cranial sutures;
- green stick fractures;
- bowing, especially of long bone of lower limbs.

Treatment is directed at the cause of the condition: that is dietary supplementation, correction of malabsorption or renal disease, or bypassing the defective step in the metabolic pathway with supplements of the required metabolite for the next step.

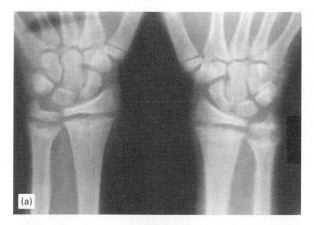

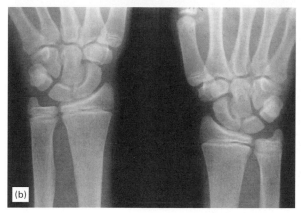

Figure 22.40. Renal rickets before (a) and after (b) treatment.

Renal rickets

This is also known as renal osteodystrophy and is due to disease of the kidneys with inability to convert vitamin D3 to 1, 25-dihydroxycholecalciferol which is essential for absorption of calcium from the gut (see Chapter 15). Serum calcium is low and due to this the osteoid matrix is not mineralized and the bones remain soft which has skeletal manifestations (Fig. 22.40). In an effort to elevate the chronically low serum calcium, the parathyroid glands undergo secondary hyperplasia so as to mobilize calcium salts from the skeleton.

The clinical features include those of other forms of rickets together with manifestations of chronic renal disease. Treatment is directed primarily at the kidney disease but calcium and vitamin D supplements are required to overcome the chronic deficiencies.

Osteomalacia

This is lack of osteoid mineralization in the adult and can be caused by dietary deficiency, malabsorption syndromes or renal disease. The condition is not uncommon even in the West.

Clinical features include:
- deformity or bending of weight-bearing bones of the lower limbs,
- flattening or splaying of the pelvis,
- degenerative changes in joints,
- complaints of generalized bone pain,
- poor general condition with malnutrition.

Radiographical changes include:
- Psuedofractures which are focal areas of demineralization, most commonly at the medial border of the scapula and inferior ramus of the pubis.
- Looser's zones which are regions of deossification which cause radiolucent lines on radiographs. They occur on the concave side of long bones, pubic bones, medially on the neck of the femur, on the axillary border of the scapula, radius and ulna.

Alkaline phosphatase is elevated and depending on the cause, the serum calcium may be normal or low. If the condition is due to renal disease with loss of phosphate in the urine, serum phosphate will be low.

Osteomalacia can be difficult to diagnose either clinically or radiologically and the patient may ultimately require a bone biopsy (usually from the iliac crest) to confirm the diagnosis. Treatment is determined by the exact cause of the condition. Dietary deficiencies are corrected by the appropriate supplements and improving the nutritional status of the patient. Vitamin D, calcium and phosphate are given in high doses depending on the patient's biochemical profile.

MALIGNANT DISEASE OF BONE AND SOFT TISSUE

A simple classification of bone tumours is:
- benign;
- malignant: primary, secondary, metastatic.

Primary bone tumours occur *de novo* and are rare. Secondary bone tumours occur in bone with a pre-existing condition (e.g. Paget's disease). Metastatic involvement of bone occurs more commonly with increasing age and is the commonest cause of neoplastic involvement of the bony skeleton in the elderly.

Clinical assessment

The following factors should be elicited in the history:
- age of the patient (Fig. 22.41);
- family history of bone diseases;
- genetic predisposition to conditions that may be associated with bone tumours (e.g. diaphyseal aclasis (Fig. 22.42));
- previous medical history (e.g. Paget's disease (Fig. 22.43));
- previous history of cancer;
- smoking;
- industrial exposure to carcinogens (i.e. employment history/occupation);

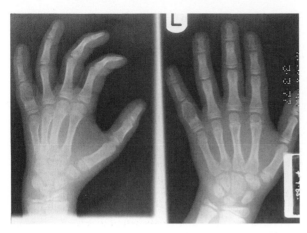

Figure 22.41. Echondroma of the proximal phalanx of the little finger.

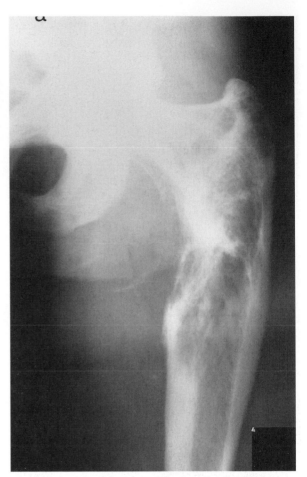

Figure 22.43. Malignant change in Paget's disease of the upper femur.

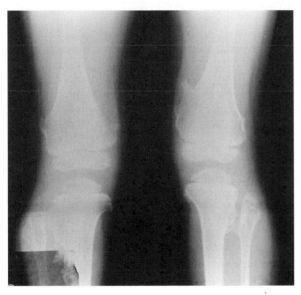

Figure 22.42. Diaphyseal aclasis.

- *Neural/vascular impairment.*
- *Associated systemic symptoms*: loss of weight, anorexia, apathy, loss of interest, disturbed mental function, cachexia, night sweats, icterus.
- *Associated features*: pathological fracture (Fig. 22.46).
- *Impairment of surrounding structures*: nerves, vessels, tendons, joints, ligaments, for example solitary exostosis impairing function of hamstring tendons (Fig. 22.47).
- *Limp/abnormal gait.*
- *Spinal involvement* either primarily or secondarily: cord/cauda equina/radicular involvement from extradural compression (Fig. 22.48).
- *Cerebral involvement* (from metastases): disturbed mental capacity/function.
- *Biochemical upset*: hypercalcaemia, hyponatraemia, hypoalbuminaemia.

In the case of metastases to the bony skeleton, consideration must be given to the site of the primary. This may not always be clinically obvious. The commonest organ tumours to

- environmental factors;
- geographical factors (e.g. UV light exposure);
- other predisposing factors such as previous DXRT for benign/malignant conditions or HIV infection.

Clinical features to be described are:

- *Pain*: site, characteristics, nocturnal component, aggravating/relieving factors, distribution, intensity/severity, duration, associated swellings/lumps/nodes.
- *Swelling*: site, size, shape, tenderness, etc. (Fig. 22.44), regional/distant nodal involvement, associated visceromegaly (liver, spleen).
- *Deformity* (Fig. 22.45).
- *Loss of function* of affected part.

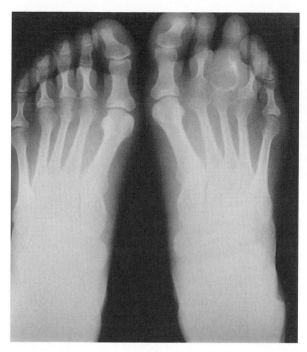

Figure 22.44. Giant cell tumour of the proximal phalanx of the third toe.

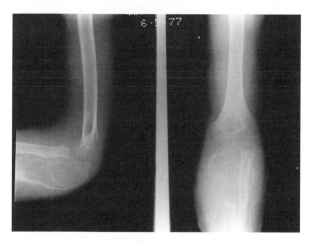

Figure 22.45. Aneurysmal bone cyst of the proximal ulna.

metastasize to bone are breast (Fig. 22.48), lung (Fig. 22.49), thyroid, kidney and prostate. Therefore, it is essential to identify a general examination of a patient presenting with malignant disease involving the skeleton to locate a primary tumour at a remote site. Assess for:

- neck lumps/swelling;
- respiratory symptoms (chest pain, productive cough, haemoptysis);
- breast lumps, previous mastectomy/lumpectomy scars;
- urinary symptoms/haematuria;
- rectal examination for rectal masses and assess the prostate.

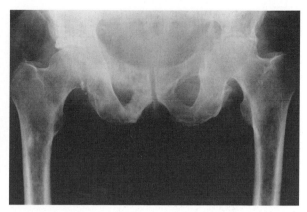

Figure 22.46. Carcinoma of the prostate with pelvic metastases: pathological fracture of the left acetabulum.

Investigations

A differential diagnosis is best formulated with the help of plain radiographs. The radiographical features of a lesion indicate if the tumour is benign or malignant, and the latter, whether it is a primary tumour of bone, a malignant change in a pre-existing condition or a metastasis (Fig. 22.50). It is important to perform radiographs in at least two planes so as to demonstrate all the radiological features (Fig. 22.51).

Further investigations suggested by the differential diagnosis are:

- *Haematological*: full blood count, ESR/CRP, renal function tests, liver function tests including serum calcium, thyroid function tests, acid phosphatase/prostatic specific antigen.
- *Cytological*: sputum cytology, urine analysis.
- *Nuclear medicine*: bone scan to look for other areas of bony involvement and to determine if the lesion is 'hot' (Fig. 22.52). However, note that some tumours can show cold spots on bone scan or be negative.
- *Further plain X-rays*: skeletal survey depending on results of bone scan, radiographs of other hot sports on the scan, chest X-ray to assess for pulmonary metastases.
- *CT scan*: to assess the bony architecture of the lesion in an axial plane, extent of the tumour and presence or absence of cortical penetration. CT scan of the chest for metastases, especially for soft-tissue tumours.
- *MRI*: to assess for extracompartmental spread of tumours and degree of soft-tissue involvement. Also important in preoperative planning for clearance biopsies, extent of marrow involvement, measurement of resection margins and planning surgical approach for prosthetic implantation.

If curative resection is to be attempted, then it is important to stage malignant tumours, especially those involving the soft tissues and the above investigations should be helpful in aiding staging and should preferably be undertaken prior to a biopsy, as open–open biopsies in particular can disrupt the

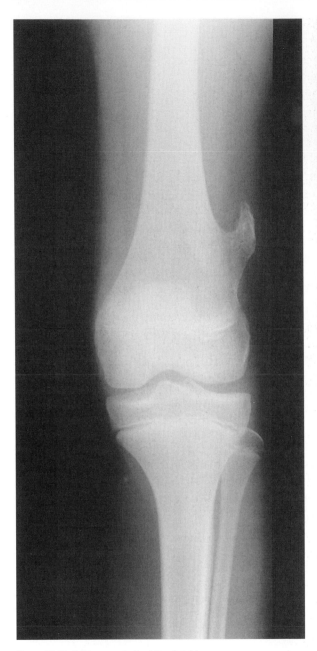

Figure 22.47. Solitary exostosis of the distal femur.

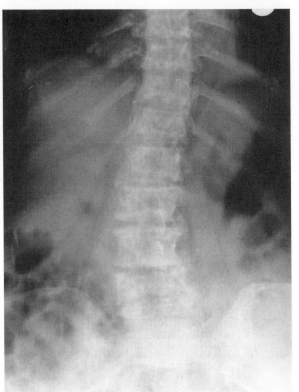

Figure 22.48. Carcinoma of the breast with spinal secondary deposits.

soft-tissue planes and therefore interfere with interpretation of the radiological and MRI characteristics of tumours.

Biopsy

Biopsies can be taken by:
• fine needle aspiration (FNA)
• Trucut needle biopsy
• open biopsy.

The choice of biopsy technique is guided by discussion with the radiologist as to the differential diagnosis. FNA is less invasive then an open biopsy but there is a greater possibility of not obtaining adequate or diagnostic tissue. The site of entry needs to be carefully planned, especially with open biopsies, so that the surgical biopsy tract can be excised adequately at the time of the definitive resection. Open biopsies should ideally be performed by the surgeon who will ultimately undertake the definitive operation. The incision for open biopsy is usually longitudinal and the pathology department must be informed well in advance of the biopsy being sent for examination. The radiographs and clinical findings should be discussed with the pathologist. Strict haemostasis must be achieved while taking open biopsy and if a drain is required it must exit the wound or close to the wound, in such a manner to allow excision of the drain tract during definitive surgery to prevent potential seeding.

Pathological fractures biopsy specimens can be taken at the time of internal fixation if the treatment is palliative rather than an attempt at curative resection. At the time of open biopsy in theatre, multiple specimens should be obtained especially from the margin of the lesion to improve the chances of making the correct diagnosis. Biopsy of the centre may only show necrotic tissue. It cannot be over-emphasized that the clinical features of the lesion should be relayed to the histopathologist as this will make formulating a diagnosis easier.

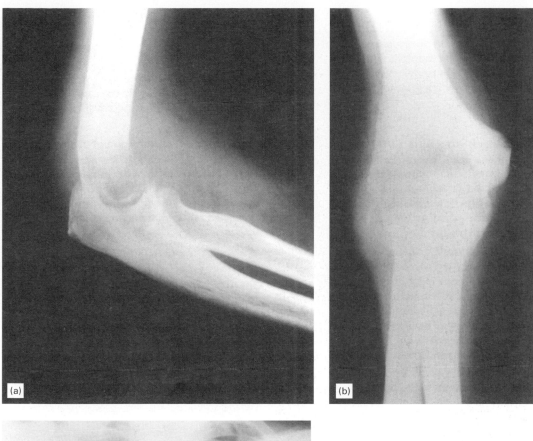

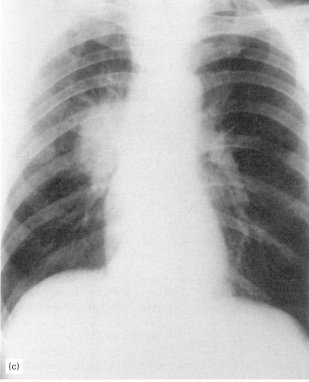

Figure 22.49. Carcinoma of the bronchus with metastasis to the distal humerus.

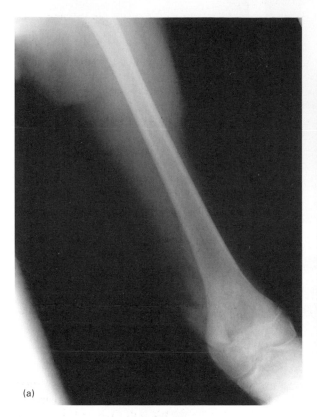

(a) (b)

Figure 22.50. Osteosarcoma of the distal femur.

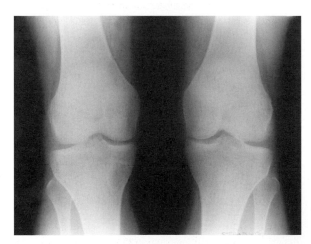

Figure 22.51. Fibrous cortical defects of the proximal right fibia.

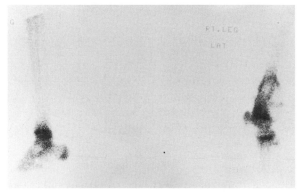

Figure 22.52. Isotope bone scan of osteosarcoma of the distal femur.

tumours but are not generally absolutely diagnostic. It is difficult to perform frozen sections on bone biopsies as they need to be decalcified first which may take a week.

Management

The definitive treatment of a lesion is determined by the diagnosis. This may be conservative treatment (e.g. chemotherapy

The mode of transport of the specimen to the laboratory should be discussed with the histopathologist. Some specimens can be transported fresh to the laboratory and others placed in formalin which acts as a preservative and fixing agent. Frozen sections may be performed on soft-tissue or radiotherapy). Surgical treatment can be curative (complete resection of the lesion) depending on the staging of the tumour; or it can be palliative if the disease is widespread and the aim is to relieve the patient's pain and improve his quality of life.

COMMON DISORDERS OF INFANCY AND CHILDHOOD

Congenital dislocation and developmental dysplasia of hip

Previously this condition was known as congenital dislocation of the hip (CDH). However the correct term is developmental dysplasia of hip (DDH) because in many cases the condition is not present at birth but rather develops after birth. Secondly in a majority of cases there is no frank dislocation but a dysplasia (poorly developed acetabulum) leading to instability of the hip joint.

This process covers a spectrum of conditions from acetabular dysplasia through to complete dislocation of the hip joint. Incidence has not declined (in the UK approximately 1.5 in 1000 live births); however, misdiagnoses have reduced with routine screening of infants using Barlow's and Ortolani's tests. CDH is thought to have a genetic predisposition, some geographical variation and joint laxity may be an aetiological factor. Girls are more commonly affected than boys and left side is more commonly affected than the right.

Clinical features

In infants CDH may manifest as asymmetry of the hips, a clicking hip or difficulty abducting a hip to wash the baby's perineum or apply nappies. The toddler may have an abnormal gait or a leg-length discrepancy.

Diagnosis depends on routine examination of the hips of all neonates. This usually involves Barlow's and also Ortolani's test. The former is click or clunk on dislocation of the hip, and the latter, a cluck on reduction of the hip. Examination also notes that when the hip is flexed 90° there may be reduced abduction compared with the normal side.

Investigations

Plain radiographs may be used but these may be difficult to interpret in the neonate due to the lack of appearance of the upper femoral epiphysis. In CDH, development of the upper femoral epiphysis tends to be delayed. There may be some pelvic asymmetry and various angles (acetabular) and lines (Perkin's) can be drawn in the absence of visualization of the upper femoral epiphysis to assess for acetabular dysplasia and congenital subluxation or dislocation.

Ultrasound with or without arthrography may also be helpful in assessing acetabular dysplasia with CDH and determining whether there is an inverted limbus or an hourglass constriction of the hip joint capitals.

Management

When the condition is diagnosed early, appropriate splinting using either a pelvic harness or immobilizing splint for up to 12 weeks may alleviate the condition. The splints tend to hold the hips in a reduced and stable position, with the hips flexed and slightly abducted. Careful follow-up is required to monitor acetabular and femoral head development.

When a late diagnosis is made, patients may require a closed reduction with initial traction followed by manipulation under anaesthetic with application of a plaster of Paris splint with the hips in abduction and internal rotation. If this is unsuccessful, surgery may be required with open reduction after removal of the inverted limbus and resection of the hourglass constriction of the capsular structure. A plaster of Paris splint is then applied with the hips in abduction and internal rotation.

Very late diagnosis, when the femoral head and acetabulum have already undergone maldevelopment, may require bony procedures to achieve reduction of the femoral head into the acetabulum, for example procedures on the femoral neck, such as rotational osteotomies, or acetabular or pelvic osteotomies such as the Salter, Kiari or acetabular rotational osteotomy.

Congenital talipes equinovarus (club foot)

This can be classified as either flexible or rigid. In the former condition, the deformity is fully correctable and will generally resolve spontaneously with time. In the rigid type, the deformity requires treatment.

The aetiology of this condition is unknown. Both genetic and environmental factors are probably important in its pathogenesis, which may be related to atrophy or contracture of the muscles of the calf and foot. It may also be related to associated bony anomalies or deformities within the foot. The incidence of the condition in the UK is 1.2 in 1000 live births and it is commoner in males.

Clinical features

The appearance of the foot is one of plantar flexion equina foot varus, inversion and supination. The hindfoot is held in varus and is plantar flexed. The forefoot is adducted and supinated. In true club foot, the deformity is rigid and uncorrectable. There is obvious calf wasting compared with the normal side.

Investigations

Plain radiographs in the neonate are often unhelpful. Epiphyseal centres may not have appeared or may be very immature and therefore interpretation of plain radiographs is difficult.

Management

In the neonatal period, this takes the form of serial casts or splints. These casts or splints are changed weekly for the first 6 weeks and then fortnightly up to the age of approximately

3 months. The deformity of the foot should be corrected slowly so as not to damage the cartilaginous anlage of the bone of the foot which in the neonate are much weaker than the soft tissues. The order of correction is:

1. reduce forefoot supination,
2. correct forefoot adduction,
3. correct hindfoot varus,
4. reduce plantar flexion.

If between 8 and 12 weeks, the surgeon feels that adequate correction has not been achieved, then surgical treatment must be considered. This involves both bony and soft-tissue procedures. Soft-tissue releases can be performed up to the age of 5 years and usually entail surgical release of tight structures posteriorly, posteromedially and on the plantar aspect of the foot. Bony procedures are generally performed after the age of 5 years and take the form of:

- *Osteotomies*: calcaneal osteotomy (Dwyer).
- *Procedures involving the joints*: laterally-based wedge excision of the calcaneocuboid joint (Evans).
- *Triple arthrodesis*: fusion of the calcaneocuboid, talonavicular and subtalar joints with appropriate resection of bone so that the final fused position maintains the foot in a plantar grade position.

Intoeing gait

There are three causes.

Anteversion of the femoral gait

This allows an excessive range of internal rotation which is clinically manifest by the ability internally to rotate the hips almost 90°. This condition usually spontaneously corrects itself and no treatment is necessary.

Metatarsus adductus

In this condition, the forefoot is adducted but there is a normal hindfoot. Again this condition usually spontaneously corrects itself. However, if by the age of 3 the condition has not corrected or is rigid, it requires treatment with serial plaster casts carefully and gently moulded to reduce the forefoot adduction deformity. If serial casts are unsuccessful, surgical procedures can be undertaken; these can involve either soft-tissue release (division of the adductors along the medial border of the foot) or bony carpentry. A new procedure involves multiple metatarsal osteotomies.

Before the age of 3, some authors feel that regular passive stretching of the medial aspect of the forefoot may be beneficial, although this is debatable.

Flat foot

Flat foot may be classified as flexible (mobile) or rigid. In the flexible flat foot, this condition may be apparent due to the plantar flat pad in children. There may be some increased laxity in the soft tissues of the foot. The child also has poor control of the intrinsic muscles of the foot and this may have

some effect on flexible flat foot in children. However, this condition spontaneously corrects and does not generally require any treatment.

Rigid or spastic flat foot can be associated with talocalcaneal or calcaneonavicular bars which form a synostosis either between the talus and calcaneus, or the calcaneus and the navicular. These have been termed tarsal coalitions and are often associated with spasm in the peroneal muscles. This anatomical anomaly is commoner in males. The foot is everted and pronated and this is not passively correctable. Any attempt to correct the deformity causes painful spasm within the peroneal muscles.

Investigation can take the form of plain radiographs which may reveal a bony bar between the tarsal bones. Further elucidation can be obtained with a CT scan.

Treatment can be either conservative or operative. Conservative treatment consists of serial below-knee casts to try and alleviate the symptoms. However, it will not spontaneously correct the deformity. Surgical treatment is usually required in the form of excision of the bar or synostosis. In severe refractory cases, a triple arthrodesis may be necessary.

Perthes' disease

This is a cause of limp in childhood and the aetiology is unknown. It is caused by a disruption of the blood supply to the upper femoral epiphysis. The usual age range for the condition is 4–8 years. It is commoner in boys and can be bilateral. The condition is characterized by softening of the upper femoral epiphysis, resulting in distortion of the shape and collapse of the femoral head with consequent disruption of the hip joint biomechanics.

Clinical features

The child generally has a limp which may be painless. There is restriction of motion of the hip joint, particularly internal rotation and extension. There may be some shortening of the affected leg but this often presents late in the condition. The natural history of the disease may last for as long as 2 years. The resultant outcome depends on the degree of femoral head involvement and the degree of collapse of the upper femoral epiphysis.

Investigations

In the early stages, plain radiographs may only show a widening of the joint spaces and increased density of the upper femoral epiphysis. In the later stages, there is fragmentation of the head with collapse of the femoral epiphysis. Catterall devised a classification of Perthes' disease depending on the severity of the condition and the amount of involvement of the upper femoral epiphysis. Increasing severity of the process is associated with a higher grade in the classification. With worsening collapse and fragmentation of the upper femoral epiphysis, there is associated widening of the metaphysis with extrusion of the softened femoral head from the acetabulum. There may be some cystic formation within the femoral head and the metaphyseal region of the neck. There may also be a V-shaped sequestrum within the medial aspect of the femoral head (Gage's sign).

Management

In the acute stages, if the condition is painful, treatment is generally rest. However, the condition is often not associated with anything other than a painless limp. The general approach to treatment is to contain the femoral head within the acetabulum until the revascularization process of the upper femoral epiphysis is completed. As stated above, this may take up to 2 years. During this phase the aim must be to relieve weight bearing through the softened upper femoral epiphysis so as to prevent collapse of the head and therefore deformity. Non-surgical treatment consists of splintage of the hips in an abducted position and use of weight-relieving callipers. Surgical treatment takes the form of various osteotomies around the femoral neck to contain the femoral head within the acetabulum.

The prognosis is poor in those categories where there is greater femoral head involvement as this may lead to early degenerative changes within the hip joint.

Transient synovitis of the hip

This is the commonest cause of irritable hip in the paediatric age group. It is characterized by hip pain and refusal to weight bear in a child who may be otherwise systematically well. The haematological and biochemical parameters are generally normal. Plain X-rays may reveal widening of the joint space due to an effusion or they may be normal. The child is generally apyrexial, although there may have been recent history of a concomitant viral infection.

The important differential diagnosis is septic arthritis. The clinician needs to be sure that it is transient synovitis of the hip that is being treated rather than septic arthritis as the latter condition can rapidly destroy the hip joint if not treated aggressively. Investigations must be performed to exclude septic arthritis and if there is any doubt as to the exact diagnosis, a specimen of hip-joint fluid must be obtained for culture to exclude septic arthritis.

Treatment in the acute phase consists of rest, with or without the use of traction, until the symptoms subside. The patient is then mobilized as pain allows. The symptoms often resolve spontaneously.

Slipped upper femoral epiphysis

This condition occurs in the rapid growth phase of early adolescence (age range is 10–14 years). It is thought to be due to failure of the upper femoral epiphyseal growth plate. It is commoner in boys and can often be bilateral. Therefore, the clinician needs to be aware that there may be an asymptomatic

hip on the contralateral side. The aetiology is unknown but various theories have been advanced but remain unproven, such as a sex hormone imbalance, thyroid disturbance, trauma to the upper femoral epiphyseal growth plate and also an association with obesity.

Clinical features

The presentation may be acute or chronic. In the acute condition, there may be a sudden onset of severe pain in the affected hip. This has the presentation of an acute fracture involving the upper femoral epiphyseal plate. The patient is unable to weight bear on the affected limb and the leg rolls into the external rotation. There is extreme irritability of the hip and resistance to any movement. In acute and chronic situations, onset is more gradual. The patient may only present with a painless limp in the chronic condition. Clinically, a restriction of internal rotation is found. There may be only minor irritability of the hip or none at all. In the case of a gradual slip, the symptoms may be very mild.

Loder et al., classified a slip as unstable if the child had such severe pain that walking was not possible even with crutches, regardless of the duration of the symptoms. They classified a slip as stable if walking and weight bearing wherever still possible, with or without crutches. In unstable slips the position of the slip may be improved by gentle skin traction but not in the stable slips (and also should not be attempted). In their study 96% of patients in the stable group had a good prognosis whereas only 47% of patients in the unstable group had a good prognosis.

Investigations

Plain radiographs of the hip, including an anteroposterior view of the pelvis and lateral view of the affected hip, are vital. Note must be taken of the relationship between the femoral epiphysis and the midline of the neck in both the anteroposterior and lateral films. It is essential to check both hips radiographically as the condition can be bilateral or one hip may be asymptomatic. The radiographical signs include Capener's and Trethowran's sign. New bone formation may be seen along the medial corner of the metaphysis of the femoral necks. The degree of slip is judged by the percentage displacement of the upper femoral epiphysis on the femoral neck, which is best assessed on lateral radiographs.

Management

This is generally surgical as any further deterioration in the slip must be prevented if the slip is only mild. On the other hand, if there is a significant degree of slipping of the upper femoral epiphysis on the femoral neck, which will result in significant deformity of the hip, reduction of the slip must be attempted and the upper femoral epiphysis stabilized in the reduced position. Both procedures are not without the risk of complications.

In an acute slip which is <30°, the surgeon may opt to pin the upper femoral epiphysis *in situ*. This can be performed with cannulated screws which are placed up the femoral neck into the femoral epiphysis so as to encourage premature fusion of the upper femoral epiphyseal growth plate and therefore prevent any further slip. The operation is performed under general anaesthetic and image intensifier control. The procedure can often be performed percutaneously. Postoperatively, the patient is mobilized on crutches with protected weight bearing until there is evidence of fusion of the upper femoral epiphysis.

In an acute slip of >30°, reduction of the degree of slip can be attempted before undertaking surgical stabilization. Closed reduction can be attempted either using of traction where the reduction is gradual or by manipulation under anaesthetic in theatre just prior to surgical stabilization. If the reduction is satisfactory, the upper femoral epiphysis can be pinned in the reduced position.

In the acute and chronic situation where there is a significant degree of slip, an open reduction followed by internal fixation may be opted for.

In a chronic slip which is apparent radiographically with new bone formation along the medial corner of the femoral neck metaphysis, reduction of the slip is not possible. Various geometrically designed femoral neck osteotomies are used to realign the femoral head on the femoral neck.

Complications

Avascular necrosis of the upper femoral epiphysis can occur secondary to disruption of the blood supply to the epiphysis caused by reduction of the slip. The risk of a vascular necrosis is greater with open reduction but even with closed reduction there is still a significant incidence of this complication.

Chondrolysis can occur following surgical stabilization. This is often associated with penetration of pins or screws through the cortex of the upper femoral epiphysis into the hip joint at the time of internal fixation. Clinically, increasing pain and stiffness within the joint is noted. Radiographically, there is progressive loss of the joint space. This is quite a debilitating complication as it leads to early degenerative changes within the hip joints. As stated previously, care must be taken that asymptomatic contralateral slip does not go unnoticed and both hips must be monitored carefully with regular follow-ups.

The main long-term sequelae of slipped upper femoral epiphysis is early degenerative changes within the hip joint and this may be a complication of the slip itself or of the treatment.

FURTHER READING

Dandy DJ. *Essential Orthopaedics and Trauma*, 2nd edn. Edinburgh: Churchill Livingstone, 1993

Rose GK. Principles of splints and orthotics. In: Owen R, Goodfellow J, Bullough P (eds), *Orthopaedics and Traumatology*. London: Heinmann, 1980

Mark Miller. *Review of Orthopaedics*, 4th edition. W.B. Saunders Company, 2004

Canale, S. Terry. *Campbell's Operative Orthopaedics*, 10th edn. Mosby Publications, 2002

McRae, Ronald. *Clinical Orthopaedic Examination*, 5th edn. Churchill Livingstone

ONLINE READING

1. http://www.worldortho.com/database/etext/
An electronic textbook, edited by Eugene Sherry, for medical students and orthopaedic residents/registrars.

2. http://www.orthoteers.co.uk/
This site was originally developed for postgraduate orthopaedic trainees preparing for the FRCS (Trauma and Orthopaedics) examination in the UK.

3. http://www.wheelessonline.com/
This textbook was derived from a variety of sources, including journal articles, national meetings, lectures, and other textbooks. Nina Lightdale MD and Justin Field MD are the resident editors.

4. http://www.eatonhand.com/index.htm
The electronic textbook of hand surgery.

23

Paediatric Surgery

Paul KH Tam

Chair of Paediatric Surgery, Department of Surgery, Queen Mary Hospital, University of Hong Kong, China

CONTENTS

Surgical physiology	**494**
Temperature	494
Fluid and electrolytes	494
Nutrition	495
Respiration	495
Sepsis	495
Endocrine and metabolic response to surgery	495
Transfer of surgical patients	**495**
Surgical techniques	**495**
Head and neck	**496**
Congenital cysts and sinuses	496
Haemangioma	496
Cleft lip and palate	497
Chest	**497**
Oesophageal atresia and/or tracheo-oesophageal fistula	497
Congenital diaphragmatic hernia	499
Cystic lesions of the lung	499
Mediastinal masses	500
Chest wall deformity	500
Gastrointestinal tract	**500**
Gastro-oesophageal reflux	500
Abdomen	**501**
Neonatal gastric perforation	501
Gastric volvulus	501
Pyloric atresia	501
Swallowed foreign bodies	501
Peptic ulcer	501
Neonatal intestinal obstruction	501
Duodenal atresia and annular pancreas	501
Malrotation	502
Jejunal and ileal atresia	503
Gastrointestinal duplications	503
Meconium ileus	504
Meconium peritonitis	504
Anorectal anomaly	504
Hirschsprung's disease	505
Meconium plug syndrome	506
Necrotizing enterocolitis	506

Hypertrophic pyloric stenosis	507
Intussusception	508
Abdominal pain	509
Acute appendicitis	510
Acute non-specific abdominal pain	510
Abdominal masses	510
Abdominal wall	510
Umbilical granuloma	512
Umbilical and midline abdominal hernias	512
Acquired anorectal disorders	512
Hepatobiliary disorders	**513**
Biliary atresia	513
Choledochal cyst	513
Groin and scrotum	**514**
Inguinal hernia and hydrocele	514
Inguinal hernia	514
Hydroceles	515
Inguino-scrotal emergencies	515
Testicular torsion	515
Torsion of testicular appendages	516
Epididymo-orchitis	516
Acute idiopathic scrotal oedema	516
Undescended testes	517
Varicocele	517
Paediatric urology	**518**
Multicystic dysplastic kidney	518
Pelviureteric junction obstruction	518
Duplex system	518
Vesicoureteric reflux	518
Vesicoureteric junction obstruction	519
Ureterocele	519
Posterior urethral valve	519
Wetting	519
Hypospadias	520
Phimosis	520
Paediatric solid tumours	**521**
Wilms' tumour	521
Neuroblastoma	521
Soft tissue sarcoma	522
Other tumours	522
Further reading	**523**

The specialty of paediatric surgery has developed in recognition of the facts that infants and children differ from adults in their anatomy, physiology and psychology as well as in the diseases they encounter. It is a broad specialty and is defined by age rather than by organ systems. There are two levels of specialization: specialist paediatric surgery and general paediatric surgery.

Specialist paediatric surgery consists of:

- *Neonatal surgery* from birth to postconceptional age of 44 weeks;
- Surgery of *major or complex conditions* in infants and older children, including neoplasms, hepatobiliary diseases, specialized gastrointestinal conditions, thoracic anomalies, major trauma, etc.;
- *Paediatric urology.*

General paediatric surgery encompasses relatively common and less demanding disorders, including elective conditions such as inguinal hernia and emergency conditions such as appendicitis in older children.

The outcome of infants and children requiring surgery has improved enormously in recent years as a result of a better understanding of physiology of children, improvement of surgical techniques, advances in paediatric anaesthesia and intensive care and the adoption of a multidisciplinary approach. Attention to the psychological needs of children, involvement of the family in the management process and more effective postoperative pain relief further enhance the quality of care for these children.

SURGICAL PHYSIOLOGY

Children are not 'small adults'. The differences between children and adults are greatest immediately after birth as the infant adapts to extrauterine life: these are further accentuated in preterm babies.

Temperature

The infant is vulnerable to hypothermia because of the high surface area: body weight ratio and the small amount of subcutaneous fat. This is aggravated in the operating theatre when the viscera are exposed to a low ambient temperature. Increased heat production is needed to maintain body temperature resulting in increased oxygen consumption and metabolic acidosis. Meticulous care to preserve body heat must therefore be undertaken before, during and after operation to prevent the development of hypothermia.

Fluid and electrolytes

The total amount of fluid and electrolytes required by a child daily is determined by the maintenance requirements and replacement needs of abnormal losses. The maintenance fluid requirement is age- and weight-dependent (Table 23.1). It can also be conveniently summarized in the 4–2–1 rule for infants and children after the first week of life: 4 ml/kg/hr

Table 23.1. Maintenance fluid requirements (ml/kg/day).

Day 1	40
Day 2	60
Day 3	80
Day 4	100
Day 5	120
Day 10	150
Infants	100
Pre-school	80
Adolescent	60

Table 23.2. **Normal values.**

Age	Pulse rate (min)	Blood pressure (mmHg)	Urine output (ml/kg/day)
Infant	160	80	100
Pre-school	120	90	60
Adolescent	100	100	30

for the first 10 kg of body weight, 2 ml/kg/h for the second 10 kg of body weight and 1 ml/kg/h thereafter. The maintenance requirements of sodium, potassium and chloride are 2–4 mmol/kg/day. Infants and small children become dehydrated easily because of a high surface area: body weight ratio and immature regulating mechanisms. Surgical conditions often incur abnormal losses, for example water loss from exposed bowel in gastroschisis and loss of gastric contents (fluid and electrolytes) in intestinal obstruction, etc. An intravenous line and nasogastric tube are the best first steps in the management of a child with a surgical problem. Infants become hypoglycaemic easily, hence the need for dextrose in the intravenous fluid for any significant period of fasting. A useful solution is 0.18% saline in 10% dextrose (neonates) or 5% dextrose (children). Potassium is added as required.

Severe electrolyte disturbances can lead to acid–base imbalance, as can poor tissue perfusion, respiratory distress, etc. In addition to acid–base correction, the cause of the imbalance needs to be identified and treated.

Changes in circulatory volume are reflected in the vital signs and urine output (Table 23.2). Tachycardia, cool extremities, hypotension and oliguria (<1 ml/kg/h) indicate shock and demand vigorous fluid resuscitation. The blood volume of infants and young children is approximately 80 ml/kg, that of older children approaches the adult value of 70 ml/kg. The low body weights of small infants means that blood loss which would be considered inconsequential in adults represents a substantial proportion of the infant's circulating blood volume, for example 20 ml represents 20% of the blood volume of a preterm infant. Paediatric surgeons must take meticulous care to minimize intraoperative blood loss, using diathermy.

Nutrition

Infants and young children have relatively higher metabolic rate and energy requirements than adults. In addition to maintenance needs, the child requires nutrition for growth. Enteral feeding is the preferred method of providing fluid, calories (carbohydrate, protein and fat), minerals and vitamins but may not be possible in critically ill or postoperative patients having paralytic ileus. Refinements in parenteral nutrition have undoubtedly been a major factor in the improved outcome of major surgery for infants and children. As a rule, parenteral nutrition should be considered in neonates when there is a delay of >4 days before adequate enteral feeding can be established. Long-term parenteral nutrition in infants carries the same risks as in adults (metabolic complications, sepsis, venous access problems, etc.) but infants appear to be particularly prone to develop cholestasis which can lead to liver failure.

Respiration

The respiratory rate in children is 40 breaths/min in infants, 30 min in pre-school children and 20 min in adolescents.

The mechanisms controlling respiration are inadequately developed in infants. Preterm infants are particularly at risk of developing apnoea and need close monitoring for at least 24 h after even relatively minor surgical procedures such as inguinal hernia repair. The presence of hyaline membrane disease in low birth weight babies demands expert neonatal care. Abdominal distension, shock and sepsis can compromise the fragile respiratory status of a neonate, and trigger the need for mechanical ventilation.

Sepsis

Infants are predisposed to septic complications because of their immature defense system. Neonatal sepsis may not always be accompanied by fever or leukocytosis and may present with non-specific features, for example lethargy, intolerance of feeds. Neonatal sepsis needs to be treated empirically and rapidly once cultures have been taken and before results are available. Once septicaemia becomes established, shock, disseminated intravascular coagulation, and multiple system organ failure may follow.

Endocrine and metabolic response to surgery

Surgery represents a major stress, the metabolic effects of which are more pronounced in infants than adults. In response to surgery, there is an increase in plasma concentrations of adrenaline, noradrenaline, insulin, glucagon, glucose, lactate, pyruvate and alanine. The response is directly proportional to the severity of surgical stress. Cortisol and prolactin levels are also increased postoperatively. Cytokines which mediate the host response to injury, are also implicated. Plasma levels of interleukin-6 and interleukin-8 are increased postoperatively and the increase is exaggerated when postoperative complications arise.

The metabolic complications induced by operative stress may be sufficient to upset the delicate metabolic balance in a sick surgical infant with limited body reserves and immature defence mechanisms. As a result, for similar surgical procedures, infants have a higher morbidity and mortality than adults. To minimize the metabolic consequences in children undergoing surgery, much emphasis is now placed on the need for correction of metabolic abnormalities preoperatively.

TRANSFER OF SURGICAL PATIENTS

The principle of safe transfer of sick infants and young children to centres with adequate facilities and expertise is well established. There are few conditions under which a sick infant will benefit from being 'rushed to theatre' in a hospital without proper paediatric anaesthetic, intensive care and surgical support. Upon recognition of a paediatric surgical condition requiring specialist attention, the principles of surgical physiology outlined above should be observed and arrangements made for transfer of the patient. The child should be resuscitated, kept in a warm, humidified environment and well hydrated. Measures to prevent respiratory complications should be undertaken including orogastric drainage to minimize the risk of aspiration. Good communication with the referring centre is essential. For very sick patients, a doctor should accompany the patient during transfer. Results of simple investigations such as complete blood picture, serum biochemistry, blood grouping and plain radiographs, when available should be transferred with the patient.

Increasingly congenital anomalies are diagnosed by antenatal ultrasound examination. This allows parental counselling, and referral to specialist centres for delivery and planned surgical treatment. Fetal surgery is seldom indicated, and should only be performed in highly specialized centres for a few carefully selected life-threatening conditions.

SURGICAL TECHNIQUES

Most incisions should be placed along the skin crease to improve healing. The 'squareness' of the abdomen of infants and young children means that laparotomy can usually be accomplished with a transverse incision. For thoracotomy, ribs should be spared and not removed. Haemostasis must be meticulous because children have a small blood volume, hence diathermy is used liberally. Instead of non-absorbable sutures, the fascia is repaired with slowly absorbable synthetic sutures. Skin is approximated with absorbable subcuticular sutures or adhesive tapes. Intestinal anastomosis is often accomplished with a single layer of interrupted, mucosa-inverting (or extramucosal), absorbable sutures.

In addition to routine analgesics, postoperative pain relief measures should include local wound infiltration of 0.25% bupivacaine intraoperatively, regional anaesthesia, spinal anaesthesia, epidural anaesthesia or patient/parent/nurse-controlled analgesia with intravenous morphine infusion (see Chapter 3).

Minimally invasive techniques are increasingly adopted in paediatric surgery. With advances in the miniaturization of instruments and improved endosurgical experiences, most procedures that previously required open surgery can now be performed with laparoscopic or thoracoscopic approach. Operations that range from appendicectomy, pyloromyotomy and herniotomy to fundoplication, splenectomy, pyeloplasty and even repair of oesophageal atresia can be achieved endoscopically using ports of 2–5 mm in diameter. Short-segment Hirschsprung's disease can be treated by one-stage transanal pullthrough with or without laparoscopy assistance, without a laparotomy incision or colostomy. The potential advantages of the minimally invasive approach are improved cosmesis, reduced postoperative pain, decreased adhesion formation, and shorter hospital stay.

HEAD AND NECK

Congenital cysts and sinuses

External angular dermoid

This is typically a pea-sized subcutaneous swelling above the lateral end of the eyebrow. Excision is curative.

Dermoid cysts

A dermoid cyst in the scalp is not uncommon. Communication with the dura has been recorded rarely and where present is usually associated with midline lesions. Treatment is with excision.

Preauricular sinus

Preauricular sinus is an ectodermal inclusion related to aberrant development of the auditory tubercles. It is prone to infection and may be bilateral. The tract with a pin-sized external opening anterior to the helix leading to the auricular cartilage has to be completely excised during the quiescent phase to prevent recurrence.

Ranula

A ranula is a cyst of the floor of the mouth. Small lesions are excised and large ones marsupialized.

Tongue tie

A tight frenulum which impedes speech development or causes feeding problem should be divided.

Thyroglossal cyst

A thyroglossal cyst is a midline neck lesion with a tract originating from the foramen caecum and therefore moves upwards on protrusion of the tongue. The cyst can be situated above, at or below the hyoid level, but the tract is invariably embedded in the inner surface of the central part of the hyoid bone. A 1 cm segment of hyoid must be excised together with the cyst and the tract followed to the foramen caecum to prevent recurrence (Sistrunk's operation).

Branchial sinus and branchial cyst

A branchial sinus is usually a remnant of the second branchial cleft with an external opening anterior to the sternomastoid muscle in the lower neck. The condition may be familial and may be complicated by infection. The tract which courses upward along the carotid sheath between the external and internal carotid arteries and ends in the tonsillar fossa needs to be completely excised, sometimes requiring two incisions. The treatment for a branchial cyst which is situated laterally at the upper neck is similar.

Cervical lymphadenopathy

Hyperplastic lympadenopathy associated with viral illnesses usually resolve on observation. Acute suppurative lympadenitis is treated with antibiotics; progression to pyogenic abscess requires aspiration or drainage. Chronic lymphadenopathy caused by atypical mycobacteria is managed by surgical excision. Lymphoma, leukaemia, and metastatic neoplasms can present with enlarged cervical lymph nodes which should be biopsied for diagnosis.

Torticollis

Torticollis, which is the result of a shortened fibrosed sternomastoid, is often associated with a 'sternomastoid tumour' or haematoma. It results in rotation and tilting of the head. The condition is benign and the majority respond to physiotherapy. Very rarely, surgical division of the muscle contracture is required.

Cystic hygroma

Cystic hygroma is a multiloculated lymphangioma most commonly occurring in the neck (75%), sometimes in the axilla (20%) and other parts of the body (5%). Enlargement, which may be precipitated by infection, bleeding or trauma, can result in airway obstruction or dysphagia. Excision is the preferred treatment but may be challenging because of the multicystic nature and possible extension to the mediastinum, oral cavity, etc. Sclerotherapy (e.g. OK-432, bleomycin) has been reported to be of use but the results are inconsistent.

Haemangioma

There are many forms of *haemangiomas* but the commonest is juvenile or strawberry capillary haemangioma (with or without cavernous components). The lesion, usually undetected in the first few days or weeks of life, appears as a red spot which grows in size at an alarming rate in the next few months. The majority resolve spontaneously between 1–4 years of age. First there is the arrest of growth and subsequently the appearance of pale areas. Intervention is only rarely indicated in the presence of complications, for example platelet trapping, haemodynamic disturbance or interference with important functions such as acquisition of visual-cortical circuitry in the case of a haemangioma blocking the eye. Short-course high-dose steroid therapy is sometimes effective. Alpha interferon therapy may be attempted for steroid-resistant cases, but is associated with significant side-effects and costs. Lesions persisting into adolescence may require excision. Vascular malformations do not involute and should be distinguished from haemangiomas.

Cleft lip and palate

Cleft lip and palate affects 1 in 5000 births, singly or in combination. The defect may be unilateral or bilateral. A complete cleft lip and palate is a severe anomaly affecting appearance, speech, feeding, breathing, hearing, etc. Management is long-term and multidisciplinary involving the surgeon, orthodontist, speech therapist and supporting staff. Cleft lip is generally repaired at the age of 3 months and cleft palate at 9 months. Secondary procedures may be necessary in later life.

CHEST

Respiratory distress of the newborn may be caused by abnormalities of the chest or other parts of the body (Fig. 23.1).

Oesophageal atresia and/or tracheo-oesophageal fistula

This is one of the most challenging conditions in neonatal surgery. It affects 1 in 4000 live births. The anatomical variations in

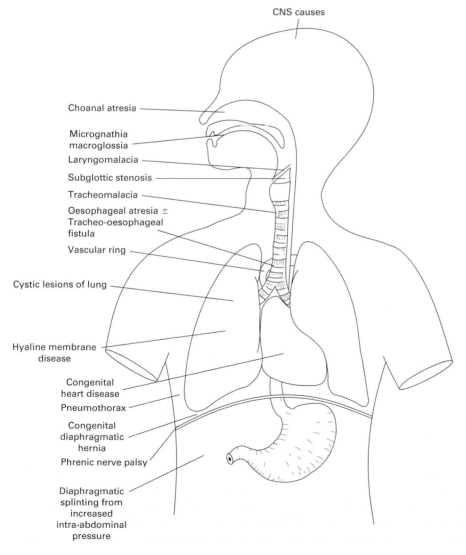

Figure 23.1. Major causes of respiratory distress in the newborn.

order of frequency are following:
- proximal oesophageal atresia with distal tracheo-oesophageal fistula (85%);
- pure oesophageal atresia without a fistula (10%);
- H-type tracheo-oesophageal fistula without atresia (4%);
- oesophageal atresia with proximal tracheo-oesophageal fistula (0.5%);
- oesophageal atresia with proximal and distal tracheo-oesophageal fistulae (0.5%) (Fig. 23.2).

There is a high incidence of associated anomalies (50%), the best known of which is the vertebral anal cardiac tracheal eesophageal renal limb (VACTERL) association:
- *v*ertebral anomaly (e.g. hemivertebra, 13th rib);
- *a*norectal anomaly;
- *c*ardiac anomaly;
- *t*racheo-oesophageal fistula and o*e*sophageal atresia
- *r*enal and *l*imb anomalies (e.g. radial aplasia).

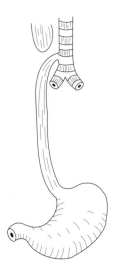

Proximal oesophageal atresia, distal tracheo-oesophageal fistula

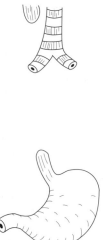

Pure oesophageal atresia

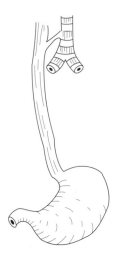

H-type tracheo-oesophageal fistula

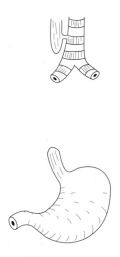

Oesophageal atresia, proximal tracheo-oesophageal fistula

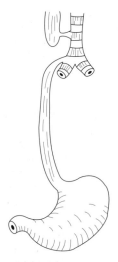

Oesophageal atresia, double tracheo-oesophageal fistula

Figure 23.2. Anatomical types of oesophageal atresia and tracheo-oesophageal fistula.

The CHARGE syndrome describes:

- *c*oloboma (cleft eyelid);
- *h*eart anomaly;
- choanal *a*tresia;
- *r*etarded growth and development;
- *g*enital hypoplasia;
- *e*ar anomaly with deafness.

The survival rate of this once fatal condition is now much improved but mortality remains substantial in infants with major congenital cardiac anomalies and low birth weight.

Diagnosis

There is often maternal polyhydramnios. Pure oesophageal atresia may be diagnosed antenatally – the stomach is small due to a lack of swallowed amniotic fluid. A newborn infant with oesophageal atresia has frothy salivation and develops cyansosis and choking if feeds are given. An orogastric tube cannot be passed >10 cm from the gum margin – this can be confirmed by plain radiography. Aspiration pneumonia should be prevented by constant oropharyngeal suction – the use of a Replogle tube (sump mechanism) minimizes tissue trauma.

Management

In the common form of oesophageal atresia with a distal tracheo-oesophageal fistula, the major risk is reflux of gastric acid via the fistula into the tracheo-bronchial tree. Surgical treatment should be undertaken in a specialist centre. The aim is to divide and ligate the tracheo-oesophageal fistula (via right thoracotomy, 4th interocostal space, extrapleural approach; thoracoscopic repair has also been reported) within 24 h of birth. Primary anastomosis of the oesophageal segments is attempted. In the presence of a long gap, this may be facilitated by mobilization of the upper pouch and techniques such as circular myotomy, and postoperative mechanical ventilation with paralysis for several days. Pure oesophageal atresia is characterized by a long gap between the proximal and distal oesophagus. It is recognized by the absence of gas in the stomach radiologically and can be managed initially with a gastrostomy and oropharyngeal suction. Delayed primary anastomosis can be undertaken a few weeks to a few months later to allow time for the oesophagus to grow. Where anastomosis is not possible, a cervical oesophagostomy is performed and the oesophagus is later substituted by an intestinal segment (most often the colon or stomach).

Complications include:

- anastomotic leak;
- anastomotic stricture;
- recurrent tracheo-oesophageal fistula;
- tracheomalacia, gastro-oesophageal reflux;
- incoordination of swallowing, etc.

As a result, the child may develop repeated chest infection and failure to thrive. Long-term follow-up is necessary to anticipate and avert these problems.

Congenital diaphragmatic hernia

This occurs in 1 in 4000 live births or 1 in 2000 births if still-births are included. The defect is usually left-sided (85–90%) and affects the foramen of Bochdalek which is situated in the posterolateral aspect of the diaphragm. The parasternal foramen of Morgagni is rarely affected. The size of the defect varies from a small opening with a good muscle rim to a near-complete absence of diaphragm (diaphragmatic agenesis). A left-sided hernia usually contains small bowel, stomach, spleen, colon and occasionally the left lobe of the liver. In right-sided hernias, the right lobe of the liver and intestines are the usual contents. Herniation of the intestine results in its non-rotation. Associated anomalies, especially cardiac anomalies, are present in 20–40% of cases and affect the outcome adversely. Gastro-oesophageal reflux is also common.

The most important pathophysiological consequences of diaphragmatic herniation during fetal development are pulmonary hypoplasia and pulmonary hypertension. Development of the ipsilateral lung is most affected but the contralateral lung can also be involved as a result of the mediastinal shift and compression. The abnormal pulmonary arterioles have hypertrophied muscular walls which constrict in response to hypoxaemia. As a result, a vicious circle of hypoxaemia and pulmonary hypertension is established. This mechanism is thought to be responsible for the deterioration of the infant's respiratory status following a 'honeymoon' period.

The survival rate for infants who are symptomatic within the first few hours of life has remained at about 60% despite the introduction of new treatment measures. This is a result of improved diagnosis and transfer of severely affected infants who previously would have failed to reach the referral centres.

Diagnosis

Increasingly, the condition is discovered during antenatal ultrasound examination. Diagnosis before 24 weeks' gestation, liver herniation into the chest and low lung-to-head ratio are associated with severe pulmonary hypoplasia and a high mortality. The typical presentation of a left-sided diaphragmatic hernia is respiratory distress (cyanosis, dyspnoea) within the first few hours of life, apparent dextrocardia and a scaphoid abdomen. In the ipsilateral chest, air entry is reduced and bowel sounds may be present. Infants who remain asymptomatic for >12 h after birth have good pulmonary reserve and a good prognosis. Plain radiography is usually diagnostic.

Management

An orogastric tube should be inserted for gastrointestinal decompression. Face mask resuscitation is contraindicated as gas pushed into the gastrointestinal tract in the chest aggravates compression of the lungs. Instead, the infant should have endotracheal intubation. Mechanical ventilation is usually necessary and care must be taken to avoid barotrauma from excessive pressures. Vital signs, oxygen saturation and arterial blood gases are closely monitored.

In the past, emergency surgery was thought to be necessary. In fact, incarceration of the contents of a diaphragmatic hernia is very rare. Attention has shifted to the physiological needs of the infant and operative repair is only undertaken after a period of stabilization. The systemic circulation is maintained by appropriate fluid and inotropic therapy. Adequate arterial oxygenation should be achieved with low-pressure ventilation (conventional or high frequency oscillatory ventilation) and moderate permissive hypercapnia. Pulmonary hypertension is treated with inhaled nitric oxide. Infants who are resistant to conventional therapies may benefit from support of extracorporeal membrane oxygenation (ECMO). The effectiveness of new therapies such as surfactant replacement, liquid (perfluorocarbon) ventilation has yet to be proven. Fetoscopic tracheal occlusion has been attempted to encourage the severely hypoplastic lung to grow in utero, but clinical trials have so far not shown survival benefit for fetal surgery for severe congenital diaphragmatic hernia.

Surgical repair of diaphragmatic hernia is carried out transabdominally, usually via a left subcostal incision. The visceral contents are reduced and the defect is closed primarily. For very large defects, muscle flaps or synthetic patches (e.g. Gortex) may be necessary. The chest is not routinely drained.

Cystic lesions of the lung

Cystic lesions can be congenital or acquired, the latter often occurring as a complication of staphylococcal pneumonia. Congenital causes include simple lung cyst, congenital cystic adenomatoid malformation, pulmonary sequestration and lobar emphysema. The condition may be asymptomatic but is more often associated with chest infection or respiratory distress. While acquired lesions may respond to expectant treatment, congenital cystic lesions require excision.

Mediastinal masses

Mediastinal masses can be either cystic or solid (Table 23.3). A teratoma normally has both cystic and solid components and can be benign or malignant. A lymphangioma may be either entirely in the chest or more often an extension from a cystic hygroma in the neck. Neural tumours may be benign (neurofibroma, ganglioneuroma) or malignant (neuroblastoma). A mediastinal mass is often discovered incidentally but may also be associated with:
- chest infection;
- airway obstruction;
- swallowing difficulties;
- superior vena caval syndrome;

Table 23.3. Mediastinal masses.

	Cystic	Solid
Anterior mediastinum	Teratoma	Teratoma
	Lymphangioma	Lymphoma
	Thymic cyst	Thymoma
	Pericardiac cyst	Thyroid goitre
Middle mediastinum	Bronchogenic cyst	Lymphoma
Posterior mediastinum	Bronchogenic cyst	Pulmonary sequestration
	Oesophageal duplication	Neural tumours

- neurological symptoms such as spinal cord compression, Horner's syndrome, etc., depending on the location and nature of the lesion.

Surgical excision is often needed for diagnosis and treatment.

Chest wall deformity

The commonest chest wall deformity is pectus excavatum, or funnel chest, which is characterized by a sharp posterior curvature of the sternal body. Most children are asymptomatic. Some authors have described limitation of cardiopulmonary functions on extensive testing but many surgeons believe the deformity (especially the mild-to-moderate lesions) is more a cosmetic than a physiological problem. For surgical treatment, the minimally invasive Nuss procedure that involves elevation of the sternum by a bar without resection or division of costal cartilages is becoming increasingly popular.

GASTROINTESTINAL TRACT

Gastro-oesophageal reflux

Gastro-oesophageal reflux is common in infants. In the majority, it resolves with simple measures. In a minority, however, reflux is persistent and potentially harmful. Gastric acid (and sometimes bile) refluxes into the oesophagus when one or more of the protective mechanisms becomes defective. The protective mechanisms are as follows:
- a high pressure zone in the lower oesophagus;
- an intra-abdominal segment of the oesophagus;
- the acuteness of the gastro-oesophageal angle (angle of His);
- mucosal folds at the gastro-oesophageal junction.

The commonest complication is reflux oesophagitis which causes upper gastrointestinal bleeding and may develop into a stricture. Barrett's oesophagus (columnar metaplasia) predisposes to malignancy. Acid reflux into the tracheobronchial tree results in respiratory complications.

Diagnosis

Non-bilious vomiting is the commonest symptom. Other oesophageal symptoms include feeding problems, pain, bleeding and dysphagia. Respiratory symptoms include aspiration pneumonia, apnoea, bronchospasm, near-miss sudden infant death syndromes, etc. Rarely, there may be seizure-like events and dystonic posturing (Sandifer syndrome).

The gold standard for diagnosis is 24h oesophageal pH monitoring. Upper gastrointestinal endoscopy allows evaluation of oesophagitis and Barrett's oesophagus. Contrast studies have a low sensitivity but are occasionally performed to identify anatomical abnormalities such as hiatus hernia, oesophageal stricture, malrotation or delayed gastric emptying. The latter is often better assessed by radioisotope scintigraphy ('milk scan').

Management

Uncomplicated gastro-oesophageal reflux is usually managed by a combination of upright posturing, small frequent feeds, milk thickeners, antacids (e.g. alginates), H_2-receptor antagonists/proton pump inhibitors and prokinetic agents (e.g. metaclopramide). Surgery is indicated for failure of medical treatment (persistence of failure to thrive) and for severe complications (near-miss sudden infant death syndrome, oesophageal stricture and unresponsive oesophagitis). Patients with underlying pathological conditions, for example neurological deficits, oesophageal atresia, etc. may respond poorly to medical treatment.

The commonest form of antireflux surgery is Nissen's fundoplication. The procedure is effective but may be associated with dumping, retching, gas-bloat and recurrences. Alternative procedures with partial wraps, for example Thal procedure, cause less gas-bloat but may be less effective. Surgery can be accomplished by a laparotomy but increasingly it is performed laparoscopically. Concommitant gastrostomy may be performed for children with neurological deficit who have feeding problems. Oesophageal strictures need to be dilated, preferably by balloon dilators. Persistent strictures may require resection.

ABDOMEN

Neonatal gastric perforation

This is a rare condition, possibly due to mechanical disruption but may also be related to stressful clinical settings resembling necrotising enterocolitis (see below). There is an acute onset of abdominal distension which may be accompanied by respiratory distress and vomiting. Pneumoperitoneum is evident. At laparotomy, the defect, often in the greater curvature, is excised and repaired.

Gastric volvulus

This is also rare: the stomach may rotate around the axis connecting the cardia and pylorus (organo-axial), or less commonly the axis connecting the midpoints of the curvatures (mesenterico-axial). Typically there is acute epigastric distension and pain, unproductive attempts at vomiting and failure of passage of a nasogastric tube. Emergency laparotomy is necessary for derotation and fixation of the stomach.

Pyloric atresia

Atresia, web or membrane can affect the pylorus, resulting in non-bilious vomiting. Pyloric atresia may be associated with epidermolysis bullosa or may occur as part of a familial multiple intestinal atresia. A single enlarged gastric bubble without distal bowel gas is evident on plain radiograph. Gastroduodenostomy is curative.

Swallowed foreign bodies

Foreign bodies that are impacted in the oesophagus, for example bones, coins need to be removed endoscopically. Blunt objects that have passed into the stomach can usually be observed. Bezoars, or collections of hair (trichbezoar) or vegetable matter (phytobezoar) are typically found in stomach of children with psychiatric illnesses and require surgical removal.

Peptic ulcer

Children with peptic ulcer can present with pain, bleeding, perforation, or obstruction. Primary peptic ulcer is usually associated with helicobacter pylori, and its eradication is curative. Secondary peptic ulcer usually occurs in children with severe stress and injuries and initial treatment is acid reduction.

Neonatal intestinal obstruction

Features of neonatal intestinal obstruction are:
- bilious vomiting in a newborn is abnormal and has to be considered as indicative of intestinal obstruction until it is proved otherwise (Table 23.4);
- abdominal distension (the degree of which depends on the level of obstruction);
- constipation/failure to pass meconium.

Plain abdominal radiography is a useful investigation of intestinal obstruction in neonates for whom air is an excellent contrast. It is, however, difficult to distinguish between large and small bowel in neonates on plain radiographs because of the lack of haustra in infant colon. In addition the sigmoid colon can be very redundant in infants and young children and may not be restricted only to the left lower quadrant. All infants with intestinal obstruction will require initial resuscitation with intravenous fluid therapy and gastric decompression. These general points will not be repeated and only specific points of treatment for individual conditions are presented.

Duodenal atresia and annular pancreas

Duodenal atresia occurs in about 1 in 10 000 live births. Obstruction may be complete (atresia), or incomplete

Table 23.4. **Causes of neonatal intestinal obstruction.**

	Intraluminal	Intramural	Extramural
Organic obstruction			
Duodenum		Duodenal atresia	Annular pancreas
			Ladd's band
			(Malrotation)
Small intestine	Meconium ileus	Jejunal and ileal atresia	Midgut volvulus
		Duplications	complicating malrotation
			Meconium peritonitis
			Hernia
Large intestine	Meconium plug	Colonic atresia	
		Anorectal anomaly	
Functional obstruction			
Hischsprung's disease (intestinal aganglionosis)			
Necrotising enterocolitis			
Medial causes: sepsis, prematurity, hypothyroidism, hypoglycaemia			

(stenosis, diaphragm, 'windsock' web) and may occur at any level of the duodenum but most commonly near the ampulla of Vater. The pathogenesis is thought to be due to a failure of recanalization following a solid core phase during early embryonic development. The most important association is Down's syndrome, which is present in a third of duodenal atresias. Other associated anomalies include cardiac anomalies, oesophageal atresia and malrotation.

Annular pancreas is believed to arise from the failure of rotation of the ventral anlage to fuse with the larger dorsal anlage. There is often an associated duodenal atresia.

The presentation of congenital duodenal obstruction is vomiting, which is bilious in postampullary lesions. Classically, there is a 'double-bubble' on the plain abdominal radiograph showing the distended stomach and the first part of the duodenum. Distal gas is absent in duodenal atresia but present in stenosis. Treatment is by duodeno-duodenostomy. Postoperative feeding may be delayed because of dysmotility of the excessively dilated proximal duodenal segment. Tapering of megaduodenum is sometimes recommended but its value is unproven. Transanastomotic tube feeding or preferably parenteral nutrition may have to be implemented until full oral feeding is established. Results of treatment are highly satisfactory.

Malrotation

This is an extremely important condition to recognize as its complication, midgut volvulus, carries devastating consequences. The exact incidence is difficult to estimate as the majority is asymptomatic: an incidence of 1 in 500 autopsies has been recorded.

During the 4th–10th weeks of normal embryological development, the midgut, which grows at a faster rate than the coelomic cavity, takes up temporary residence in a physiological hernia in the umbilical cord and rotates 90° anticlockwise. As the midgut returns to the abdomen in the next 2 weeks, it undergoes a further 180° anticlockwise turn. The 270° rotation results in the passage of the duodenojejunal loop from above the superior mesenteric artery to the left of it and the caecocolic loop from below the superior mesenteric artery to the right of it. Fixation of the duodenum and ascending colon to the posterior peritoneum results in a wide root of mesentery running from the duodenojejunal flexure in the left upper quadrant to the ileocaecal junction in the right lower quadrant. Failure of this normal process results in malrotation. In conditions such as exomphalos and diaphragmatic hernia, non-rotation invariably exists.

Malrotation results in a narrow pedicle of mesentery, predisposing to midgut volvulus. Ladd's bands which arise from the posterior parietal peritoneum to the abnormally situated ascending colon may compress the duodenum leading to obstruction.

Diagnosis

The commonest presenting symptom is vomiting. When midgut volvulus supervenes, there may be rectal passage of blood, acute abdominal distension, peritonitis, shock and metabolic acidosis. Sometimes the symptoms are milder and intermittent, suggesting twisting and untwisting episodes. Occasionally, chronic duodenal obstruction is the only feature.

To diagnose midgut volvulus, a high level of clinical awareness is necessary. Plain abdominal radiographs may show a dilated stomach and duodenum. An upper gastrointestinal contrast study is the most useful investigation, revealing an abnormal position of the duodenojejunal junction to the right of the midline. The duodenum may be dilated and have a corkscrew appearance. A barium enema may demonstrate an abnormal position of the caecum but this test is less reliable than a barium meal. Ultrasonography may be helpful in showing an abnormal relationship of the superior mesenteric artery and vein.

Management

Malrotation should be treated surgically before midgut volvulus sets in. If the latter is present, the bowel is untwisted and its viability assessed. All abnormal adhesions are divided. The duodenum is 'straightened'. The intestines are replaced with the duodenum and small intestines on the right and the caecum and colon on the left of the abdomen. If the appendix is not removed, the family should be made aware of its abnormal position to avoid diagnostic difficulties in case appendicitis develops in the future. Massive bowel gangrene and resection results in short gut syndrome. The lack of sufficient absorptive area to satisfy nutritional and fluid and electrolyte needs for maintenance and growth poses a devastating long-term problem, most often managed by parenteral nutrition. Some adaptation takes place, particularly if the ileocaecal valve is intact. Patients with intractable intestinal failure who cannot tolerate parenteral nutrition (e.g. due to cholestasis) may ultimately require small bowel transplantation. This is associated with severe immune reaction and very significant morbidity and mortality.

Jejunal and ileal atresia

Unlike duodenal atresia, jejunoileal atresia is believed to be a result of an intrauterine mesenteric vascular accident leading to localized intestinal ischaemia, infarction and resorption. This theory of pathogenesis was supported by the result of Louw and Barnard's classical experimental study in puppies in 1955. Clinical evidence of vascular events such as complications of malrotation, volvulus, gastroschisis, meconium ileus, etc. was present in 40% of neonates in one series. Extra-abdominal associated anomalies are uncommon. Morphologically, atresias are classified into following:
- stenosis;
- Type I atresia (membrane/web);
- Type II atresia (blind ends joined by a fibrous cord);
- Type III A atresia (disconnected blind ends);
- Type III B atresia (apple-peel or Christmas tree deformity in which the distal bowel coils round a solitary supplying vessel which arises from the ileocolic or right colic vessel);
- Type IV atresia (multiple atresias); some cases of multiple atresias are familial and probably have a non-vascular pathogenesis.

Diagnosis

Proximal small bowel atresia may be suspected from antenatal ultrasonography (dilated bowel segments). The neonate presents with bilious vomiting. There may be abdominal distension depending on the level of obstruction. Failure of passage of meconium may be a feature but this is not invariable as the causative intrauterine mesenteric ischaemia may occur after intestinal contents have passed into the distal bowel. Plain abdominal radiographs are usually diagnostic showing dilated loops of proximal bowel with fluid levels and absent distal bowel gas. *Distal ileal atresia* may be difficult to differentiate from, and in some instances may coexist with, other causes of low intestinal obstruction, for example meconium ileus. A contrast enema in such circumstances is helpful. In both cases, there is microcolon due to disuse atrophy but reflux of contrast into the terminal ileum will reveal the typical findings of impacted meconium in meconium ileus. Total colonic aganglionosis may also cause confusion.

Management

Surgical treatment involves resection of atretic bowel and primary anastomosis. It is essential to check for patency of distal bowel by intraluminal saline infusion as multiple atresias may exist. The outcome of treatment of isolated intestinal atresia is highly satisfactory.

Gastrointestinal duplications

Duplications are rare congenital anomalies which may occur anywhere along the alimentary tract; 80% are located within the abdomen, most commonly at the ileocaecal region. Most duplications are cystic and are non-communicating; some are tubular and may or may not communicate with the adjacent bowel. Typically, duplications are situated on the mesenteric aspect of the bowel as opposed to the antimesenteric location of Meckel's diverticulum. All duplications have a muscle wall and are intimately attached to at least one point of the alimentary tract with which they share a common blood supply. The inside of duplications are lined with gastrointestinal epithelium, occasionally ectopic gastric mucosa. The pathogenesis is unknown. For those associated with vertebral anomalies, the most popular explanation is an abnormal splitting of the notochord.

Diagnosis

The majority of duplications present in early childhood. Presentations include:
- asymptomatic masses;
- space-occupying effect;
- haemorrhage;
- infection;
- perforation;
- intussusception.

Diagnosis may be made by imaging studies, for example ultrasonography, computerized tomography (CT), etc. Especially for foregut lesions, exclusion of associated vertebral anomalies is advisable.

Management

The preferred treatment is complete surgical excision. Rarely, this may not be possible because of the location, extent and size of the duplication and alternative approaches such as mucosal stripping or internal drainage into normal bowel may have to be adopted.

Meconium ileus

Meconium ileus is the commonest intraluminal cause of neonatal intestinal obstruction in Caucasians and is nearly always associated with cystic fibrosis (95–100%). Cystic fibrosis is transmitted as an autosomal recessive trait and represents the commonest inherited disease in Caucasians (carrier rate 5%, incidence 1 in 2000 births). Meconium ileus occurs in 10% of neonates with cystic fibrosis. Abnormal exocrine secretions result in thickened meconium obstructing the terminal ileum. The distal ileum is inspissated with pellets of hard meconium, proximal to which the meconium is putty-like. There is microcolon because of disuse.

Diagnosis

Half of the neonates present with uncomplicated intestinal obstruction while the remainder present with complications associated with volvulus (twisting of dilated bowel segment) and its sequelae, including perforations, meconium peritonitis and atresia. Neonates with simple meconium ileus develop bilious vomiting, abdominal distension and failure to pass meconium in the first 48 h. The presentation, in complicated cases, is more acute and more severe. Bowel loops distended with meconium or giant cystic collections may be palpable.

Abdominal radiographs reveal dilated loops of bowel. There are no fluid levels as meconium is viscid, giving a soap bubble or 'ground glass' appearance instead in the right lower quadrant. If meconium ileus has been complicated by intrauterine perforation, calcification may be apparent.

Management

For *uncomplicated* meconium ileus, a contrast enema may be both diagnostic and therapeutic. Gastrografin is the most commonly used medium for non-operative treatment. Reflux of the hyperosmolar gastrografin (1800 mosm/l) into the terminal ileum results in shifting of fluid into the intraluminal compartment, disimpacting the meconium. A wetting agent (Tween 80) may be added. To avoid drastic fluid depletion, a 1 : 3 dilution of gastrografin is more commonly used and attention to intravenous fluid therapy must be meticulous. A 50% success rate is recorded for uncomplicated cases.

For *complicated* meconium ileus, and failed non-operative treatment of simple cases, there are a number of surgical options. Non-viable bowel needs to be resected – the ends can be exteriorized or anastomosed primarily. As a variation, one end may be exteriorized, with the other end joined to its side (Bishop–Koop anastomosis), thus giving external access to irrigate and disimpact thick meconium. If the bowel is viable and distension is not severe, enterotomy, irrigation and primary closure can be performed. A variation involves insertion of a T tube for subsequent irrigation.

The diagnosis of cystic fibrosis should be confirmed by a sweat test. Genetic screening of ΔF508, which accounts for 70% of mutations, is advisable. Comprehensive management of cystic fibrosis, including respiratory care, should be implemented.

Meconium peritonitis

Meconium peritonitis results from gut perforation in the last 6 months of the intrauterine period after meconium has formed. The peritoneal reaction gives rise to adhesions and radiologically is characterized by intra-abdominal calcifications. The gut perforation is usually secondary to an underlying pathology, for example intestinal atresia, meconium ileus, etc. but occasionally a primary cause cannot be found. At birth, the perforations may or may not have been sealed off. Surgical treatment consists of laparotomy, identification of possible gut perforation and treatment of underlying pathology.

Anorectal anomaly

Anorectal anomaly, or imperforate anus, occurs in 1 in 4000 births. Boys are slightly more affected than girls. There is a wide spectrum of anomalies and these are classified according to the relationship of the terminal bowel to the puborectalis muscle and presence/absence of a fistula to the urinary tract/vagina (Table 23.5). In low imperforate anus, bowel terminates below the puborectalis (usually within 1 cm of skin level), without an internal fistula. These lesions are suitable for perineal procedures without colostomy. Intermediate, high and rare malformations as well as cloaca are complex anomalies requiring colostomy and total surgical reconstruction.

Boys tend to have more high than low lesions, the commonest defect being rectourethral fistula. In girls, the commonest anomaly is vestibular fistula which may be anal (low) or rectal (intermediate), requiring different treatments.

Associated anomalies are common, especially with high lesions. VACTERL association is discussed above. The commonest associated anomaly is urological: 60% in high and 20% in low lesions. Sacral agenesis involving two or more vertebrae is associated with poor bowel control; some may also develop neurogenic bladder.

Diagnosis

Careful inspection of the perineum should be an integral part of neonatal examination. Occasionally the diagnosis of anorectal anomaly may be delayed because of adequate bowel decompression through a perineal/vestibular fistulous opening and failure to recognize the correct position of the anus. Rarely, in rectal atresia, there is a normal anal opening and the diagnosis is suspected on failure of attempts to pass a rectal thermometer. An abnormal skin tag (the so-called 'bucket handle' deformity) or a 'covered' anus with bulging meconium underneath may provide sufficient information for a diagnosis of low imperforate anus to be made. In boys, meconium-stained urine denotes intermediate/high anomaly. In girls, the relationship of the three pelvic structures – urethra, vagina and rectum – must be carefully defined.

An invertogram is a plain radiograph aimed at showing the most distal extent of the rectal gas shadow which rises when the baby is held upside down. It is done after the first 24 h of

Table 23.5. Simplified 'Wingspread classification' of anorectal anomalies.

Male	Female
Low	*Low*
Anocutaneous fistula	Anocutaneous/anovestibular fistula
Anal stenosis	Anal stenosis
Intermediate	*Intermediate*
Rectourethral fistula	Rectovestibular fistula
Anal agenesis without fistula	Anal agenesis without fistula
High	*High*
Anorectal agenesis with or without	Anorectal agenesis with or without
rectoprostatic fistula	rectovaginal fistula
Rectal atresia	Rectal atresia
Rare malformation	*Rare malformation*
	Cloaca

life (to allow adequate passage of swallowed gas to distal bowel) and may be helpful in differentiating high and low lesions. A lateral radiograph with the baby prone and buttocks elevated serves the same purpose. More sophisticated investigations to define the level of involvement may include ultrasonography, fistulogram, CT and magnetic resonance imaging (MRI). Pelvic musculature can also be assessed by MRI.

Management

For low imperforate anus, anoplasty is satisfactory. For all other lesions, a colostomy is recommended. Subsequent definitive surgery is often undertaken via a posterior sagittal midline approach. After isolation and repair of the fistula to the urethra/vestibula/vagina, the rectum is brought to the perineum through the sphincter complex, after which the sphincter complex is reconstructed posteriorly. More recently laparoscopic anorectoplasty has been described. Some patients may have persistent faecal incontinence despite reconstructive surgery because of deficient pelvic musculature and require treatment with the antegrade continence enema (ACE) procedure using the appendix as a conduit.

Hirschsprung's disease

Hirschsprung's disease is characterized by an absence of intrinsic nerve cells in the rectum (congenital rectal aganglionosis). The aganglionosis can extend proximally for varying lengths. The majority (70%) have rectal/rectosigmoid involvement (short segment Hirschsprung's disease); the remainder (30%) have so-called 'long segment' involvement. About 10% of patients have total colonic aganglionosis. Rarely, innervation is absent from most or all of the small bowel as well.

The distal aganglionic bowel segment fails to relax and results in functional intestinal obstruction. The proximal normoganglionic bowel becomes secondarily dilated and hypertrophied, giving a paradoxical abnormal appearance (congenital megacolon). The intervening hypoganglionic bowel tapers into a transitional zone.

During normal embryonic development, neural crest cells migrate via the vagi into the oesophagus and colonize the entire alimentary tract in a craniocaudal direction. Hirschsprung's disease results from interference with the migration, proliferation, differentiation or survival of the enteric neuroblasts. The molecular and cellular mechanisms involved have not been completely worked out but the recent discovery of genes associated with Hirschsprung's disease (RET, endothelin B receptor and SOX10 genes) provide an important clue to the pathogenesis of this anomaly.

Hirschsprung's disease affects 1 in 5000 births. There is a 4–8% incidence of familial involvement, especially with long segment cases. A male preponderance exists in short segment cases. There is a known association with chromosome anomalies such as Down's syndrome, deletions of chromosome 10 and 13 and malformation syndromes such as Waardenburg syndrome (pigmentary disorder), Ondine's curse (central hypoventilation), etc.

The most dreaded complication of Hirschsprung's disease is enterocolitis which occurs in 20–58% of cases and can be rapidly fatal. Another serious complication is bowel perforation which may be a result of enterocolitis or obstruction. Early diagnosis and treatment of Hirschsprung's disease is therefore important.

Diagnosis

Functional intestinal obstruction in Hirschsprung's disease can be acute, recurrent or chronic. Although the majority of cases nowadays are recognized in the neonatal period, some are still diagnosed at older ages. Nevertheless, even for such cases, symptoms can usually be traced to early infancy. Typically, the infant presents with bilious vomiting, delayed passage of meconium (>24 h) and abdominal distension.

Examination reveals a tight anus and an empty rectum – this is in sharp contrast to the finding of a dilated rectum which is impacted with faeces down to the anal verge in acquired megacolon or idiopathic chronic constipation. In Hirschsprung's disease, withdrawal of the finger or instrument (e.g. thermometer) from the rectum is often accompanied by an explosive passage of flatus or meconium.

Diagnosis of Hirschsprung's disease is established by the histological finding of aganglionosis in a rectal biopsy specimen. Suction rectal biopsy is often adequate in infants; open biopsy is only occasionally necessary. Acetylcholinesterase staining is helpful in demonstrating abnormal proliferation of nerve fibres in lamina propria and hypertrophy of nerve trunks which accompany the aganglionosis. Ancillary investigations include contrast enema (demonstration of a transitional zone) and anorectal manometry (failure of anal sphincter relaxation in response to rectal distension) – these are helpful but not essential for the diagnosis of Hirschsprung's disease.

Management

The conventional treatment of Hirschsprung's disease is initial colostomy (ileostomy for total colonic aganglionosis). This reduces the risk of enterocolitis substantially. At an older age, for example 6 months, resection of aganglionic bowel and pullthrough of histologically proven normoganglionic bowel is undertaken. There are different approaches of pullthrough – rectorectal (Duhamel), endorectal (Soave) and abdominoperineal (Swenson, State-Rehbein). For short-segment Hirschsprung's disease, many surgeons now prefer a primary transanal endorectal pullthrough procedure which avoids the need of an initial colostomy and an abdominal incision. Frozen section examination of biopsy samples obtained intraoperatively is essential to ensure that normoganglionic colon is used for anastomosis.

Hirschsprung-like disease

Some patients have bowel dysmotility despite the presence of ganglion cells on rectal biopsy. The best described condition is intestinal neuronal dysplasia which is characterized by hyperplasia of the submucous and myenteric plexuses and giant ganglia and treatment is in the first instance conservative. Other conditions include hypoganglionosis, immature ganglia, internal anal sphincter achalasia, smooth muscle disorders, and the generally fatal megacystis-microcolon-intestinal hypoperistalsis syndrome.

Meconium plug syndrome

Occasionally, a meconium plug in the rectum may cause intraluminal intestinal obstruction. This readily resolves after an enema with the passage of a tenacious strip of meconium. Hirschsprung's disease and cystic fibrosis have to be excluded before such a diagnosis is established.

Necrotizing enterocolitis

In the past 30 years, necrotizing enterocolitis (NEC) has emerged as the commonest and most lethal neonatal abdominal condition requiring emergency surgery. Unlike most other causes of acute abdomen in the newborn, NEC is an acquired condition which classically affects sick, low birth weight infants. The most distinctive feature of early NEC is pneumatosis intestinalis. The terminal ileum is the most frequently affected site, followed by the colon and other segments of the small bowel. In 10–20%, there is extensive involvement of the intestine, resulting in high mortality.

The most important causative components of NEC are intestinal ischaemia and bacterial proliferation. Enteral feeding facilitates the progression of NEC. Risk factors of NEC include low birth weight and persistent stress events such as hypoxia, polycythaemia, exchange transfusion, umbilical catheterization, etc. A popular hypothesis of the pathogenesis of NEC suggests that perinatal events, such as hypoxia in a premature infant, cause a redistribution of blood flow to vital organs (heart and brain) resulting in relative splanchnic ischaemia – the so-called 'dive reflex'. The ensuing mucosal injury allows translocation of bacteria. Intramural proliferation of bacteria is aided by nutrient from enteral feeds. An alternative hypothesis emphasizes the role of the immature gut barrier to permit bacterial invasion.

The incidence of NEC varies between 1% and 6% of admissions to a neonatal unit and increases with decreasing birth weights. There is often clustering of cases.

Diagnosis

The early clinical picture consists of systemic symptoms (lethargy, apnoea, etc.), poor feeding, vomiting, abdominal distension and blood in stool. On progression to the definite stage of NEC, these clinical features deteriorate and pneumatosis intestinalis becomes radiologically apparent. Occasionally gas can be detected in the portal vein and a worse outcome is predicted. Advanced NEC is associated with septicaemic shock and disseminated intravascular coagulopathy (thrombocytopenia, metabolic acidosis, etc.), peritonitis and pneumoperitoneum.

Management

The cornerstones of management of NEC are as follows:
- early diagnosis;
- correction of predisposing factors;
- cessation of feeding;
- orogastric decompression;
- intravenous fluid and electrolyte therapy;
- intravenous antibiotics;
- close clinical, biochemical and radiological monitoring.

About 30% of cases fail to respond to such measures and require surgery. The main indications for surgery are bowel perforation and gangrene. The timing of surgery is critical. Operating too early will fail to select out potential responders to conservative treatment and will not allow sufficient demarcation of necrotic and viable bowel segments in those requiring resection. Operating too late may result in irreversible septicaemia and multiorgan failure.

At laparotomy, non-viable bowel is resected and the bowel ends are exteriorized. In well-selected cases, primary anastomosis can be undertaken. Very sick, premature infants with bowel perforation may benefit from initial peritoneal drainage: laparotomy is undertaken when haemodynamic and respiratory stability is restored. Pan-intestinal NEC can result in massive bowel loss and short gut syndrome. Intestinal strictures can complicate successful medical or surgical treatment and require contrast studies for diagnosis and bowel resection for treatment.

Hypertrophic pyloric stenosis

Infantile hypertrophic pyloric stenosis is the commonest surgical cause of non-bilious vomiting in Caucasian infants outside the newborn period. Hypertrophy of the pyloric muscle (mainly the circular muscle layer) narrows the pyloric lumen and results in gastric outlet obstruction. The pathogenesis remains unknown. Myenteric ganglia are present in the affected pylorus but defective innervation involving fibres which contain neuropeptides and nitric oxide synthase has been documented. There are also disturbances of gastrointestinal hormones such as hypergastrinaemia. However, it is unclear as to whether these changes are the cause or result of pyloric stenosis.

Pyloric stenosis occurs in 3 in 1000 Caucasian births; it is uncommon in Asians and Blacks. The male : female ratio is about 4 : 1. First borns are more often affected (40–60% of all cases). With an affected father, there is a 5% risk for the son and 2.5% risk for the daughter developing pyloric stenosis. With an affected mother, the risks rise to 20% and 7%, respectively. Overall there is an 18-fold increase in incidence in first-degree relatives compared to the general population. These data suggest a sex-modified, polygenic inheritance. The neuronal nitric oxide (nNOS) gene has been implicated as a susceptibility locus for pyloric stenosis. Associated anomalies may be present. Association with Smith–Lemli–Opitz syndrome, chromosomal disorders, joint hypermobility, and early exposure to macrolide (e.g. erythromycin) has been described.

Diagnosis

Typically, a previously well baby develops non-bilious, projectile vomiting at the age of 3–4 weeks. Occasionally symptoms occur as early as the newborn period and as late as several months of age. Delayed recognition, rare nowadays, can result in dehydration and starvation changes – constipation, 'starvation diarrhoea', passage of greenish 'hungry stool', failure to thrive, weight loss and lethargy. Occasionally haematemesis occurs as a result of oesophagitis/gastritis. Jaundice due to hepatic glucuronyl transferase deficiency

occurs in 2% of cases and resolves after surgery. The hydration and nutritional status of the infant should be assessed on examination. There is often a 'worried' facies. Gastric peristalsis is often visible. The definitive sign of pyloric stenosis is a palpable olive-shaped mass, the so-called 'tumour', in the right upper quadrant. Detection is facilitated by a small feed with dextrose water and improves with the examiner's experience.

When a pyloric 'tumour' is felt, further studies for diagnosis are not required. For equivocal cases, provided the expertise is available, ultrasonography is the investigation of choice. The usual criteria for diagnosis are:
- a pyloric muscle thickness of 4 mm or more;
- an anteroposterior diameter of 15 mm or more;
- an elongated pyloric canal of 19 mm or more.

Alternatively, a contrast study may be used to confirm the diagnosis or to evaluate possible alternative causes of vomiting such as malrotation and gastro-oesophageal reflux.

The characteristic biochemical change is hypochloraemic alkalosis (serum bicarbonate >26 mmol/l, chloride <106 mmol/l) as a result of loss of gastric juice. Sodium and potassium are also depleted. 'Paradoxical aciduria' occurs in severe alkalosis.

Management

Surgical management of pyloric stenosis begins with rehydration and correction of biochemical abnormalities. There is no place for 'emergency operation'. The infant is fasted and an orogastric tube is inserted for gastric decompression and estimation of gastric fluid loss. Mild curds and mucus are removed from the stomach by irrigation. Fluids and electrolytes, usually a combination of dextrose, saline and potassium supplements, are administered intravenously in accordance with the patient's clinical and biochemical status which is regularly reassessed. With sufficient hydration and repletion of chloride and sodium deficits, alkalosis will be reversed.

Ramstedt's pyloromyotomy is the standard operation for pyloric stenosis. An umbilical or right upper quadrant transverse incision is made. The pyloric 'olive' is delivered out of the wound and is held between the thumb (duodenal end) and finger (antral end). An incision is made along the length of the mass anterosuperiorly and the hypertrophied muscle is split either by using a pyloric spreader or by twisting the blunt end of a scalpel holder (the author's preferred method) until the submucosa bulges out. Special care is taken at the duodenal end where there is a projection of duodenal mucosal folds into the pylorus. This is the commonest site of perforation during myotomy. Laparoscopic pyloromyotomy is increasingly popular in specialized centres. Results of surgery are excellent and most patients can be discharged from hospital within 2 postoperative days. Complications, including duodenal perforation, incomplete myotomy, bleeding, wound dehiscence, wound infection and incisional hernia, are mostly avoidable.

Intussusception

Intussusception, the invagination of a segment of bowel (intussusceptum) into the distal bowel (intussucipiens), is a common and important cause of intestinal obstruction in infants and young children. Although intussusception can occur at any age, the peak incidence is at 5–9 months and over 80% occur before the age of 2 years. Males are more often affected (60–70%).

The majority of cases (90%) are idiopathic. The commonest (>90%) site of involvement is the ileocaecal region: ileocolic intussusception usually begins several centimeters proximal to the ileocaecal valve and advances into varying lengths of the colon, occasionally presenting at the rectum. Ileo-ileal and jejuno-jejunal intussusception may be secondary to a pathological lead point or previous surgery. In Africa, there is an increased incidence of colo-colic intussusception which tends to affect older children. The risk of intussusception lies in delayed diagnosis and treatment, which can result in bowel strangulation and perforation.

In primary idiopathic intussusception, lymphoid hyperplasia in the terminal ileum is thought to provide a lead point. A preceding viral illness, often related to adenovirus and rotavirus, is aetiologically implicated in 30–50% of cases. A weaning diet, loss of maternal immunity and differences in diameters of an infant's ileum and caecum has also been speculated to have contributory roles in its pathogenesis.

Secondary intussusception (2–12%) should be suspected in those with atypical presentations, older children, ileo-ileal intussusception and recurrent intussusception. The commonest pathological lead point is Meckel's diverticulum; other known causes include polyp, neoplasm especially lymphoma, duplication, appendiceal stump, intramucosal haematoma (e.g. Henoch–Schönlein purpura), intraluminal lesions (e.g. inspissated stool in cystic fibrosis, ascaris), etc.

Postoperative intussusception occurs rarely; most often following certain intra-abdominal or retroperitoneal procedures. The small bowel is most commonly involved and diagnosis is seldom made before operative treatment because of atypical presentation.

Most intussusceptions are acute. Occasionally, chronic intussusception occurs in the older child and may be associated with pathological lead points.

Diagnosis

The classical presentation of intussusception is abdominal pain (85%), vomiting (85%) and rectal bleeding (50%): the complete triad is only found in 30% of cases. Typically, a previously healthy baby develops screaming episodes of abdominal colic, each of which lasts for a few minutes. The colic is often accompanied by circumoral pallor and drawing up of the legs. The child is initially well in between attacks but becomes restless as the frequency of attacks increases. Food is refused and this is followed by bilious vomiting. Rectal passage of blood and mucus (from venous congestion of intussusception)

results in 'red currant jelly' stool. If the condition remains unrecognized, dehydration and septicaemia set in. The child becomes lethargic and paradoxically quiet. Coma and convulsions may be mistaken for meningitis.

On examination, a sausage-shaped mass is palpable in 60% of cases, most often in the right hypochondrium. There may be a sense of emptiness in the right iliac fossa (Dance's sign). Rectal examination confirms the presence of blood and rarely reveals the apex in an intussusception. Shock, abdominal distension, peritonitis and hyperpyrexia are signs of advanced disease.

For diagnosis, a high index of suspicion is necessary. A plain abdominal radiograph may reveal absence of gas in the colon and a soft tissue mass in the right iliac fossa/ hypochondrium. Ultrasonography has emerged as a highly sensitive and specific investigation for intussusception which gives rise to a 'target' sign in the transverse section (Fig. 23.3a) and a 'pseudokidney' sign in longitudinal section (Fig. 23.3b). Rarely, a pathological lead point, such as duplication, lymphoma, Meckel's diverticulum, etc., may be identified. Barium enema typically demonstrates a mass and the 'coiled spring' sign (Fig. 23.3c).

Management

Intussusception is potentially lethal. It has been estimated that up to 60% of deaths in intussusception are preventable. The key points for successful management in intussusception are as follows:

- early diagnosis;
- adequate resuscitation;
- effective reduction.

Adequate resuscitation begins with intravenous fluid therapy. Administration of antibiotics and nasogastric aspirations are essential for advanced cases. Reduction of intussusception may be non-operative or operative, depending on the clinical condition. Irrespective of the choice of method of reduction, preparation for surgery is essential as non-operative reduction may fail or result in perforation. Blood is cross-matched. The operating theatre is made available and the aneasthetist is informed. The surgeon is the primary clinician for intussusception and should initiate treatment, decide on the method of reduction and should be present at (non-operative) or carry out (operative) the reduction.

Non-operative reduction should generally be attempted for most cases of acute intussusception. The contraindications are perforation, peritonitis indicating bowel necrosis and profound shock. Non-operative reduction is usually unsuccessful if a pathological lead point is present and the primary pathology usually requires operative treatment. A long history (>48 h), radiological evidence of small bowel obstruction and extremes of age are associated with lower success rates but are not absolute contraindications to non-operative reduction.

Non-operative reduction can be hydrostatic or pneumatic. The child is sedated with morphia, diazepam or,

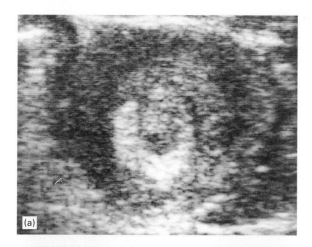

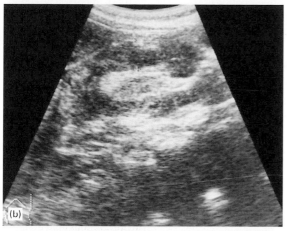

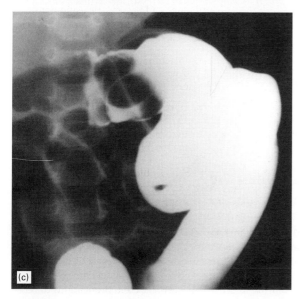

Figure 23.3. Intussusception. (a) Ultrasonography: target sign; (b) Ultrasonography: pseudokidney sign; (c) Barium enema: coiled-spring sign.

rarely, general anaesthesia. Traditionally, hydrostatic reduction is achieved with a barium enema. Barium is introduced via a rectal balloon catheter with the buttocks strapped. The hydrostatic pressure should not exceed the equivalence of 1 mH$_2$O for a maximum of 10 min. The procedure is monitored fluoroscopically. Reduction is indicated by a free flow of barium into the terminal ileum, expulsion of faeces and gas with the barium and resolution of symptoms and signs. Alternatively, hydrostatic reduction can be carried out using Hartmann's solution or saline under ultrasonographic guidance, which avoids the risk of irradiation. Successful reduction rates vary between 50% and 90%. Pneumatic reduction is performed with manometric and fluoroscopic control. If perforation occurs, leakage of air, Hartmann's solution or saline is less damaging than leakage of barium (peritoneal reaction) or the hyperosmolar gastrografin although it should not be forgotten that entry of intestinal contents and bacteria into the peritoneal cavity will cause peritonitis, and this will require emergency surgery.

Surgery is undertaken when non-operative reduction is contraindicated or has failed. A right supra- or sub-umbilical transverse incision is made. The intussusception is milked back proximally by progressive compression of bowel just distal to the intussusception. If viability of the reduced bowel is doubtful, warm packs are applied. Bowel resection is carried out for irreducible intussusception, gangrenous bowel and pathological lead points.

With proper management, the mortality rate of intussusception should nowadays be <1%. Recurrent intussusception occurs in about 10% of cases after non-operative reduction and 1–4% of cases after operative reduction, usually within 1–36 months of reduction, peaking at about 8 months. First recurrences can be treated by non-operative reduction. Second recurrences should be managed operatively. Multiple recurrences suggest the presence of pathological lead points. Adhesive intestinal obstruction is a late complication (3–6%) of operative reduction.

Abdominal pain

Causes of acute abdominal pain in childhood are:
- *Surgical conditions*:
  appendicitis;
  intussusception;
  mesenteric adenitis;
  peptic ulceration/gastritis;
  constipation;
  Meckel's diverticulum;
  malrotation/volvulus;
  adhesive intestinal obstruction;
  ovarian cyst;
  rare miscellaneous conditions (primary peritonitis, pancreatitis, cholangitis/choledochal cyst, inflammatory bowel disease, mesenteric/duplication cyst, etc.).

- *Medical conditions*:
  pneumonia;
  urinary tract infection;
  gastroenteritis;
  parasitic infestation;
  rare miscellaneous conditions (Yersinia infection, Henoch–Schönlein purpura, haemolytic uraemic syndrome, blood dyscrasias, for example leukaemia, sickle cell crisis, diabetes mellitus, meconium ileus equivalent, etc.).
- *Acute non-specific abdominal pain*:
  Acute appendicitis and acute non-specific abdominal pain each account for about one-third of hospital admissions for this complaint.

Acute appendicitis

Acute appendicitis affects all ages and is discussed in detail in Chapter 12. The specific points relevant to the paediatric age group are presented here. Older children are more often affected; pre-school children account for just 5% of children with acute appendicitis. Neonatal appendicitis is rare, and underlying conditions such as Hirschsprung's disease and necrotizing enterocolitis should be excluded.

Diagnosis

The commonest triad of symptoms is vomiting, abdominal pain and fever but a normal temperature does not exclude appendicitis and may be present in 80% of affected pre-school children. The diagnosis is particularly difficult in the young child because of inability to communicate, atypical presentation and other associated illness – diarrhoea, upper respiratory tract infection, otitis media, etc. may coexist with or precede appendicitis. Physical examination reveals right lower quadrant tenderness, muscle spasm and involuntary guarding. Rovsing's sign is positive when palpation of the left lower abdomen elicits pain at McBurney's point. Pain is elicited by extension of the right thigh (psoas sign), or passive internal rotation of the flexed right thigh (obturator sign).

Investigations are needed only when the clinical picture is atypical. Leukocytosis is present in 80% of cases. Abdominal radiograph may show a faecolith, sentinel bowel loops (due to localized ileus), and lordosis away from the right side. Ultrasonography may reveal an enlarged, non-compressible appendix, and exclude tubo-ovarian pathology in adolescent girls. Computed tomography is not recommended as a routine in children.

Management

There is often a delay in seeking a surgical opinion both from parents and general practitioners. The delay in diagnosis, and possibly the thin-walled paediatric appendix, results in a greater risk of perforation (30–45%). Perforation is associated with a greater morbidity. Successful management begins with early diagnosis, achieved by a detailed history, careful examination and repeated reassessment. The importance of fluid resuscitation and safe anaesthesia cannot be overemphasized. Antibiotic prophylaxis is valuable in all cases and should be continued postoperatively in perforated cases. Appendicectomy can be performed via a grid-iron incision or laparoscopically. The commonest postoperative complications are wound infection, intra-abdominal abscess, and small bowel obstruction.

Acute non-specific abdominal pain

This is not a label given on hospital admission but is a diagnosis made only after a period of 'active observation'. It must be emphasized that for the diagnosis of acute non-specific abdominal pain (ANSAP), repeated reassessments and re-examination, preferably by the same surgeon, are essential to exclude a known surgical cause of abdominal pain. During a period of several hours to 48 h, there will be gradual improvement in symptoms and signs, allowing safe discharge of the patient.

Abdominal masses

Abdominal masses may be a presenting or associated clinical feature of a variety of conditions, most of which are discussed in other sections:

- *Gastrointestinal system*: faecal impaction, duplication cyst, appendix mass, intussusception, hypertrophic pyloric stenosis, Crohn's disease, etc.;
- *Urinary system*: distended bladder, hydronephrosis (pelviureteric junction obstruction, advanced vesicoureteric reflux, posterior urethral valve, etc.), polycystic/multicystic kidney, Wilms' tumour;
- *Genital system*: ovarian mass (cyst), uterus (haematocolpos);
- *Liver, spleen, pancreas*: hepatosplenomegaly (blood dyscrasias, neoplasms), choledochal cyst, pancreatic pseudocyst;
- *Solid tumours*: neuroblastoma, rhabdomyosarcoma, teratoma, lymphoma, etc.;
- *Other cysts*: mesenteric cyst, omental cyst.

It is important to determine the age, sex, presence of associated symptoms, duration of symptoms, rate of growth, size, location, solid or cystic nature and other signs so that appropriate investigations are carried out for diagnosis.

Abdominal wall

Gastroschisis and exomphalos (omphalocoele)

Gastroschisis (Fig. 23.4a) and exomphalos (or omphalocele) (Fig. 23.4b) are two distinct types of major congenital abdominal wall defects (Table 23.6), each accounting for about 1 in 5000 births. In recent years the incidence of gastroschisis appears to be increasing.

Gastroschisis is a small full thickness defect of the anterior abdominal wall just to the right of the umbilicus. The aetiology is unknown but is believed to be either an *in utero* rupture of a small exomphalos or a localized infarction related

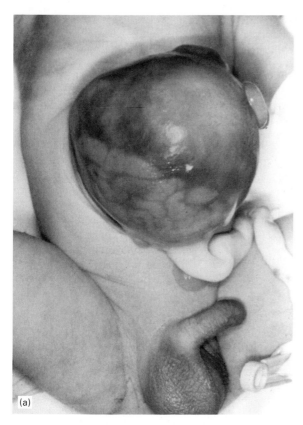

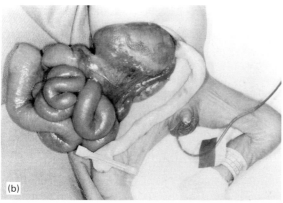

Figure 23.4. (a) Exomphalos; (b) Gastroschisis.

Table 23.6. **Abdominal wall defects.**

	Exomphalos (omphalocele)	Gastroschisis
Location	Umbilical ring	Right side of umbilical cord
Defect size	Large	Small
Sac	Present	Absent
Contents	Liver, bowel, etc.	Bowel
Bowel		
Appearance	Normal	Matted; inflamed, thickened wall
Non-rotation	Present	Present
Atresia	No additional risk	Additional risk
Function	Normal	Prolonged ileus
Abdominal cavity	Small	Small
Associated anomalies	Common (30–70%)	Uncommon (except bowel atresia 10–15%)
Syndromes	Common: Beckwith–Wiedemann, Trisomy 13–16, 16–18, 21, Lower midline syndrome, Pentalogy of Cantrell	None
		None

Exomphalos is a central defect involving the umbilical ring and its neighbouring abdominal wall. It is likely to be a persistence of the anatomical arrangement in the early embryological period (3rd–12th weeks) during which the rapidly elongating midgut resides in the extracoelomic yolk sac. The size of the defect varies. Small defects (2–4 cm) are sometimes called hernia of the umbilical cord and contain only portions of small bowel (sometimes related to Meckel's remnants). Associated anomalies are uncommon and prognosis is excellent. These small defects can be considered as a separate entity from exomphalos. Large exomphalos has a poorer prognosis. The umbilical cord inserts onto a peritoneal sac which often contains nearly the entire gastrointestinal tract as well as the liver, spleen, etc. The sac is intact in 90% of cases and therefore, unlike in gastroschisis, the bowel is relatively unaffected. Associated anomalies are common (30–70%), involving the cardiovascular (most frequent), gastrointestinal, genitourinary, musculoskeletal, central nervous and respiratory systems. There is association with a number of chromosomal abnormalities (trisomy 13–15, trisomy 16–18, trisomy 21) and syndromes (Beckwith–Wiedemann syndrome characterized by exomphalos, gigantism, macroglossia, visceromegaly and hypoglycaemia due to islet cell hyperplasia). Extension of the defect in the upper midline is classically known as pentalogy of Cantrell (abdominal wall, sternal, anterior diaphragmatic, pericardial and cardiac effects). In the lower midline, exomphalos may coexist with bladder or cloacal extrophy.

to abnormal involution of the right umbilical vein. Unlike exomphalos, there is no peritoneal sac in gastroschisis and the eviscerated bowel is exposed to the damaging effects of amniotic fluid in the intrauterine period. The bowel becomes matted and foreshortened and its walls are inflamed, thickened and covered with fibrin. Prolonged ileus can be expected. There is invariable non-rotation and frequently bowel atresia (10–15%) as a result of intrauterine mesenteric occlusion at the tight hernia ring. Other viscera are seldom involved and extra-abdominal associated anomalies are rare.

Diagnosis

Increasingly, gastroschisis and exomphalos are recognized antenatally by ultrasonography. An elevated maternal serum a-fetoprotein is also seen in gastroschisis and ruptured exomphalos. Amniocentesis for chromosomal analysis may be considered for large exomphalos.

Management

Delivery at a regional centre with specialist paediatric surgical expertise is advisable. With few exceptions a diagnosis of exomphalos or gastroschisis does not in itself constitute an indication for caesarian section. Infants with exomphalos and gastroschisis are often born premature. At birth, a warm aseptic environment is provided for the baby. A transparent plastic cover, for example clingfilm, helps to prevent excessive heat and water loss. An orogastric tube is inserted to prevent aspiration and distension of the gastrointestinal tract due to air swallowing. Intravenous fluid and antibiotics are given.

Nowadays, most major abdominal wall defects can be repaired surgically. Surgery is carried out as soon as possible. The ideal treatment is primary fascial repair which is achieved with good paralysis, decompression of the gastrointestinal tract and, if necessary, manual stretching of the abdominal wall at operation to enlarge the small abdominal cavity. Excessively tight closure, however, may result in diaphragmatic splinting and caval compression, compromising respiration and circulation, respectively. If the fascia cannot be approximated comfortably, one option is to achieve skin cover only, leaving the ventral hernia to be managed at an older age. Alternatively, a prosthetic sheet may be used for the fascial defect.

Recently, minimal intervention management for gastroschisis has been described. This consists of elective delayed midgut reduction and umbilical port capping using the umbilical cord in the neonatal surgical unit under no anaesthesia.

Defects which cannot be repaired primarily are most often managed by staged repair. A strong prosthetic (e.g. silastic) sheet is sutured to the edge of the abdominal wall defect in the form of a chimney or 'silo' to provide temporary cover for the viscera. Pre-made silastic silo with a wire-ring covered base is commercially available as an alternative option. The top of the silo is hung from the ceiling of the incubator to encourage gradual return of viscera into the abdominal cavity. Over a period of 7–10 days, the size of the silo is gradually reduced by rolling in or suturing the top of the silo. At the second stage operation, the silo is removed and closure of fascia and skin is achieved.

A period of postoperative ventilation and paralysis is often necessary. For gastroschisis, there is often a delay in return of normal gastrointestinal function, requiring total parenteral nutrition for support.

Rarely, for massive exomphalos with an intact sac or infants with life-threatening medical conditions, non-operative management may be adopted. Epithelialization is encouraged by daily topical application of escharizing agents such as silver sulfadiazine.

Umbilical granuloma

Umbilical granuloma often results from low-grade infection of the stump of umbilical cord after delivery and usually clears up on regular dressing. Healing may be expedited by topical application of silver nitrate. Rarely, a persistent granuloma may need local excision.

Occasionally umbilical discharge becomes persistent. The presence of mucosa in the umbilicus and gastrointestinal or urinary contents in the discharge may point to an underlying pathology: a patent vitello-intestinal duct or urachal remnant, for which exploration and excision is indicated.

Umbilical and midline abdominal hernias

Umbilical hernia is common in the newborn period and results from a delay in the closure of the umbilical ring. The intestinal contents are easily reducible and complications are extremely rare. The majority will resolve spontaneously. Surgery (repair of fascial defect with a periumbilical incision) is indicated only in the minority of cases which persist after the age of 4 years. Hernias with a diameter greater than 1.5 cm are unlikely to close spontaneously. Umbilical hernia related to increased intra-abdominal pressure, for example ascites, is a separate clinical entity and management is directed at the underlying cause.

Hernias in the midline of the abdominal wall excluding the umbilicus represent abnormal defects in the fascia and are most commonly located near the umbilicus: *paraumbilical hernia, supraumbilical hernia*. They may also be located anywhere along the midline between the xiphisternum and the umbilicus: *epigastric hernia*. Usually, an extraperitoneal pad of fat (or occasionally the omentum) protrudes through a small defect, presenting as a pea-sized swelling which is best felt by rolling the fingers along the midline of the abdominal wall. There may be a history of abdominal pain. Surgical repair is indicated. It is essential that the site of hernia is marked preoperatively as the hernia may be difficult to locate when the child is anaesthetized and in a reclined position.

Divarication of recti occurs commonly in infants and requires no treatment.

Acquired anorectal disorders

Anal fissure is the most common cause of minor rectal bleeding in infants and toddlers, and is associated with constipation and painful defaecation. The tear in the anal mucosa is typically located in the posterior midline. Chronic fissure is sometimes associated with a sentinel skin tag at 12 o'clock position. Treatment consists of stool softener, sitz bath and local anaesthetic gel application. Occasionally a chronic fissure requires topical nitroglycerin therapy or lateral sphincterotomy. Rarely, Crohn's disease and immunodeficiency can present with laterally located anal fissures.

Rectal polyp causes painless rectal bleeding in school aged children. The juvenile polyp is a harmatoma and sometimes autoamputate. A rectal polyp which persists can be removed endoscopically with a diathermy snare. More than one polyp may be found in up to 25 % of patients upon colonoscopic examination. The condition is benign and should be distinguished from diffuse adenomatous polyposis in Peutz–Jeghers syndrome and familial polyposis coli.

Perianal abscess occurs commonly in infants and is treated by incision and drainage. Approximately one third of abscesses develop into a *fistula-in-ano*. Fistulas which persist after infancy are treated by fistulectomy. Crohn's disease should be considered in older children with multiple fistulas.

Rectal prolapse usually occurs in the toilet training age group and is often associated with constipation. The prolapse usually involves the mucosa only and responds to conservative treatment. Persistent prolapse may require hypertonic saline injection or Thiersch procedure using a strong nylon suture. The possibility of cystic fibrosis should be considered.

HEPATOBILIARY DISORDERS

Biliary atresia

Neonatal jaundice is most frequently physiological and is associated with unconjugated hyperbilirubinaemia:
- physiological jaundice of newborn;
- Rh, ABO incompatibility;
- breast feeding;
- haemolytic disease.

Persistent conjugated hyperbilirubinaemia is, however, abnormal and requires investigations. Causes are:
- Anatomical disorders:
  - extrahepatic: biliary atresia, choledochal cyst, spontaneous bile duct perforation, inspissated bile syndrome;
  - intrahepatic: bile duct hypoplasia;
- Infection:
  - neonatal hepatitis: idiopathic giant-cell hepatitis; B, A or non-A, non-B hepatitis;
  - systemic: septicaemia, cytomegalovirus, rubella, toxoplasmosis, syphilis, etc.
- Metabolic:
  - α1-antitrypsin deficiency, galactosaemia, cystic fibrosis, etc.
- Endocrine:
  - hypothyroidism, hypopituitarism, etc.;
  - iatrogenic;
  - parenteral nutrition-induced cholestasis.

Biliary atresia is an important surgical cause of conjugated hyperbilirubinaemia. It is characterized by an obliteration of the extrahepatic bile ducts which represents the end-result of an inflammatory destructive process. Unrelieved, progressive intrahepatic damage will occur, leading to the histological findings of cholestasis, portal tract proliferation and inflammation with giant-cell infiltration. Cirrhosis and liver failure are the eventual outcome.

Biliary atresia affects 1 in 10 000 births. Associated anomalies occur in 10–20%, most commonly polysplenia, situs inversus, preduodenal vein, etc. Biliary atresia is classified into:
- Type 1: atresia of common bile duct (10%);
- Type 2: atresia of common hepatic duct (2%);
- Type 3: atresia of most or the entire extrahepatic ducts including porta hepatitis (88%).

Type 1 biliary atresia has been termed correctable type and a biliary-enteric anastomosis for drainage is possible. The majority of cases of biliary atresia had been termed uncorrectable until Kasai demonstrated that in the early course of the disease, the fibrous remnant at the porta hepatitis contains patent bile ductules and adequate bile drainage may be obtained by portoenterostomy.

Diagnosis

As the best results of surgery are achieved before 6–8 weeks of age, early investigation and referral to a specialist centre is advisable. Deepening jaundice, darkening urine and clay-coloured stool are observed. Serial liver function tests reveal persistent or increasing levels of conjugated bilirubin as well as enzyme derangement. Other known causes of jaundice, for example αa1-antitrypsin deficiency, must be excluded. Ultrasonography may identify choledochal cyst (see below). A radioisotope (HIDA) scan typically shows absence of excretion into the gastrointestinal tract. Duodenal intubation shows absence of bile. Endoscopic retrograde cholangiography has been attempted in selected centres. Liver biopsy is helpful. Despite all investigations, distinction between neonatal hepatitis and biliary atresia can still be difficult and certain diagnosis is only achieved by laparotomy, exploration and operative cholangiogram.

Management

On confirmation of the diagnosis of biliary atresia, the fibrous remnant is excised up to the level of the porta hepatis (proximal to the posterior surface of the bifurcation of portal vein) and portoenterostomy is performed with a Roux-en-Y jejunal loop. Better results are achieved with early surgery and in patients with large bile ductules in the fibrous remnant.

Under ideal circumstances, clearance of jaundice can be accomplished in 70–80% of infants treated with portoenterostomy. There are ongoing risks of cholangitis, portal hypertension and liver failure – it is estimated that 50–60% of patients will require liver transplantation in the long-term.

Choledochal cyst

Choledochal cyst is a rare congenital cystic dilatation of the biliary tree affecting 1 in 100 000 births. The aetiology is believed to relate either to reflux of pancreatic enzymes associated with anomalous junction of the pancreatic and common bile ducts (long common channel), or distal common bile duct stenosis. It is classified into:

- Type I: cystic or fusiform dilatation of common bile duct (commonest type);
- Type II: diverticulum of bile duct;
- Type III: choledochocele;
- Type IV: intrahepatic and extrahepatic cysts;
- Type V: intrahepatic cysts only (Caroli's disease).

Diagnosis

Most cases present in childhood but diagnosis may also be made antenatally and in adulthood. Jaundice, pain and mass are the commonest clinical features but presentation with the complete triad is infrequent. Occasionally, patients may present with vomiting, failure to thrive and complications including cyst perforation, cholangitis, gallstones, pancreatitis, portal hypertension, cirrhosis and malignancy.

In addition to abnormal liver function tests, the plasma amylase level may be elevated. Ultrasonography is frequently diagnostic. CT, MRI and endoscopic retrograde cholangio-pancreatography (ERCP) may be used selectively for better anatomical delineation.

Management

Treatment consists of excision of the cyst and hepatico-enterostomy with a Roux-en-Y loop. Simple drainage procedures are no longer considered to be satisfactory because of long-term risk of malignancy and anastomotic stricture.

GROIN AND SCROTUM

Inguinal hernia and hydrocele

Inguinal hernia (Fig. 23.5) and hydrocele are common groin and scrotal conditions in infancy and childhood. Repair of inguinal hernia represents one of the most frequently performed operations in childhood. Inguinal hernia and hydrocele in childhood are different from the same conditions in adulthood both in their aetiology and treatment.

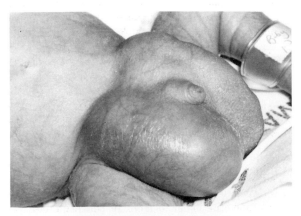

Figure 23.5. Bilateral inguinal hernia in a preterm infant.

Childhood inguinal hernia and hydrocele are congenital anomalies resulting from a persistence of processus vaginalis. As the testis descends from its retroperitoneal position to beyond the internal ring, it carries with it an anteromedial diverticulum of peritoneum (the processus vaginalis). The process of obliteration of the processus vaginalis begins at 32 weeks gestation and may continue for the first 2 years of life. A widely patent processus vaginalis which allows the passage of visceral contents results in an indirect inguinal hernia. A narrowly patent processus vaginalis which allows the passage of peritoneal fluid results in a communicating hydrocoele. An inguinal hernia does not regress whereas most infantile hydroceles will resolve spontaneously upon completion of the process of obliteration of the processus vaginalis. Occasionally, the fluid collection may persist after closure of the processus vaginalis resulting in a hydrocele of cord (hydrocele of canal of Nuck in females) or a non-communicating hydrocele.

Inguinal hernia

The incidence of inguinal hernia in term neonates has been estimated to be 1–5%. Preterm infants have an even higher incidence (10%). Boys are more commonly affected – male : female ratio is 8 : 1. Right-sided hernias are commoner than left-sided hernias. Bilateral occurrence is common: 10% in children and 40% in infants with hernia.

Cryptorchidism is a common associated condition. In addition to prematurity, other conditions which relate to a higher incidence of inguinal hernia include various causes of raised intra-abdominal pressure, connective tissue disorder (Marfan syndrome, Ehlers–Danlos syndrome), testicular feminization, etc.

Diagnosis

The commonest presentation of an inguinal hernia is a swelling in the groin, with or without extension into the scrotum (labia majora in females). The swelling appears on straining and is reducible. In some children, the swelling is not obvious on examination and a thickening of the cord or the 'silk-glove' sign is looked for instead. The usual contents of a hernia are intestine (giving rise to a gurgling sensation on reduction), or ovaries and fallopian tubes in females.

There is a high risk of incarceration (10% in children, 30% in infants). Incarceration is diagnosed when the hernia becomes irreducible and tender and can result in intestinal obstruction and strangulation as well as gonadal ischaemia (compression of testicular vessels in the inguinal canal in males, incarceration of ovaries in females). To avoid incarceration, early elective surgery should be arranged once the diagnosis of inguinal hernia is made.

Management

The surgical procedure for a childhood inguinal hernia is herniotomy. Unlike the case in adults, there is no need to repair the posterior wall of the inguinal hernia. A groin crease incision is made. In infants, the inguinal canal is short and need not be opened for herniotomy; in older children, the external oblique aponeurosis is incised. After careful dissection to avoid damage of the vas and testicular vessels, the sac is removed at its neck and transfixed. At the end of the procedure, the testes must be retracted back into the scrotum to avoid the complication of iatrogenic high testes.

Urgent reduction is necessary for an incarcerated hernia to avoid complications. Upon sedation, the hernia either spontaneously reduces or is manually reduced. To avoid recurrent incarceration, elective surgery is undertaken 24 h after reduction when the oedema of the hernia sac has settled. A hernia which is persistently irreducible or shows signs of strangulation requires emergency exploration after resuscitation.

A preterm infant with an inguinal hernia presents a special problem. There is a higher risk of anaesthesia and postoperative apnoea. Surgical repair is undertaken at a specialist centre when the infant is medically fit for discharge from the special care baby unit. Monitoring for apnoeic attacks is undertaken for 24 h after herniotomy.

Herniotomy in a preterm infant can be a very difficult procedure. The difficulty increases when herniotomy is performed on an emergency basis for incarcerated hernia and a higher complication rate can be expected. Complications of herniotomy include recurrence, scrotal haematoma, testicular atrophy, high testes and wound infection. There is controversy as to whether contralateral groin exploration should be undertaken because of the relatively high incidence of bilateral hernia. The conventional approach is not to explore because not all patent processus vaginalis (30% contralateral patency) will become symptomatic inguinal hernias (10% contralateral hernia). It is now possible to visualize the contralateral processus vaginalis with a mini-laparoscope inserted via the hernia sac during open herniotomy. Alternatively, hernia repair, whether unilateral or bilateral, can be achieved by laparoscopic suture obliteration of internal inguinal opening/s via three miniports (2 mm in diameter) in the abdomen.

Hydroceles

Although a hydrocele may fluctuate in size due to gravitation of peritoneal fluid during the day, the swelling does not disappear completely like a reducible hernia. Rarely an acute tense hydrocele may present – however, unlike an incarcerated hernia, a hydrocele is not tender. A hydrocele transilluminates brilliantly but sometimes a hernia in an infant also transilluminates because of the thin bowel wall.

Most infantile hydroceles will resolve and can be safely observed until the age of 1 year. High ligation of processus vaginalis, similar to herniotomy, is performed for persistent hydrocele.

Direct inguinal hernia and *femoral hernia* are rare in childhood and the diagnosis is often missed pre- and intra-operatively.

Inguino-scrotal emergencies

Causes of an acute scrotum in childhood are:
- testicular torsion;
- torsion of testicular appendage;
- epididymo-orchitis;
- idiopathic scrotal oedema;
- incarcerated inguinal hernia;
- acute tense hydrocele;
- Henoch–Schönlein purpura;
- acute leukaemia;
- testicular tumour;
- testicular trauma.

Testicular torsion

Testicular torsion is one of the commonest and most important causes of acute scrotum and there are two types:
- extravaginal (neonatal) (Fig. 23.6a);
- intravaginal (adolescent) (Fig. 23.6b).

Extravaginal testicular torsion occurs in the perinatal period and is characterized by a twist of the whole spermatic cord above the testis and tunica vaginalis. Intravaginal testicular torsion occurs from infancy to young adulthood, peaking in adolescence and is characterized by a twist of the testis inside the tunica. Normally, the tunica envelopes only the anterior two-thirds of the testis, leaving the posterior surface of the testis fixed to the posterior scrotal wall. Abnormal complete enclosure of the testis by the tunica results in the testis being freely suspended within the space ('bell-clapper' deformity). Contraction of the cremaster muscle may initiate intravaginal torsion of the spermatic cord. Alternatively, intravaginal torsion of the mesorchium of the testis may occur. The testis is often in a transverse lie.

Diagnosis

Neonatal testicular torsion may be relatively painless and presents as a firm discoloured scrotal swelling which does not transilluminate. Intravaginal testicular torsion causes acute scrotal pain which may be associated with lower abdominal pain, nausea and vomiting. The left testis is twice as commonly involved as the right. There may be a history of similar, milder complaint, suggesting previous twisting and untwisting of the testis. The testis is tender, swollen and often elevated. The contralateral testis may have a transverse lie.

Testicular torsion is an emergency as delay in diagnosis and treatment will result in testicular infarction: necrosis occurs within 6 h of the onset of symptoms and few testes will survive >24 h of torsion. The commonest differential diagnoses are torsion of testicular appendages and epididymo-orchitis (see above). Doppler ultrasound and radioisotope scan demonstrating reduced testicular blood flow in testicular torsion have been advocated for use in doubtful cases but these should only be attempted if the expertise is available and the tests can be performed without delay. Prompt scrotal

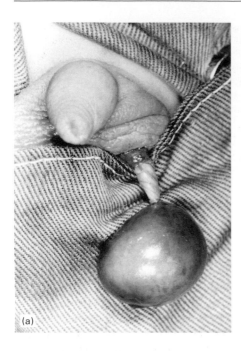

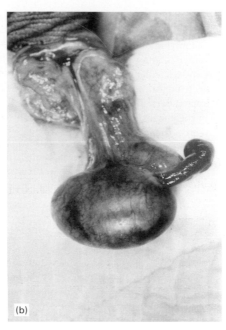

Figure 23.6. Testicular torsion:
(a) Extravaginal (neonatal);
(b) Intravaginal (adolescent).

exploration is the safest approach for any child with the slightest doubt in testicular torsion.

Management

The treatment of testicular torsion is to untwist the testis. Bilateral fixation of the testes with non-absorbable sutures is performed since the contralateral testis may have the same anatomic abnormality which predisposes to torsion. Viability of the testis may be assessed by the colour and bleeding on incision of the tunica albuginea. The testis in neonatal torsion is seldom viable. Retention of a non-viable testis may result in persistent symptoms and possible abscess formation and subsequently subfertility through an autoimmune reaction. After removal of a necrotic testis, prosthetic insertion may be considered for psychological reasons.

Torsion of testicular appendages

Torsion of the appendix testis or appendix epididymis (remnants of Mullerian and mesonephric ducts, or hydatids of Morgagni) gives rise to acute scrotal pain which is usually less severe compared to testicular torsion. The peak incidence is at the age of 10 years. In the early stage, there may be a 'blue-dot' sign – discolouration at the upper pole of the testis where a tender pea-sized swelling can be felt separate from a normal testis. Later on, oedema spreads to obscure these localized findings. Treatment may be conservative (analgesics) if the diagnosis is certain but more often exploration and excision of testicular appendage is performed, leading to speedy recovery.

Epididymo-orchitis

Most commonly epididymo-orchitis occurs in young adults and is related to sexually-transmitted infection. In pre-school children, epididymo-orchitis (infective or chemical) is often related to urinary tract pathology. Viral orchitis, for example mumps and epididymo-orchitis secondary to blood-borne infection are rare.

The presentation is gradual scrotal pain. The scrotal swelling and tenderness may be bilateral and mainly involves the epididymis. The testis is usually normal. Urine microscopy may be helpful. As emphasized, exploration is required for doubtful cases to exclude testicular torsion. Antibiotic treatment is usually effective. Ultrasonography of the urinary tract and micturating cystourethrogram should be performed in children with epididymo-orchitis unrelated to sexually-transmitted infection to exclude urinary tract abnormalities.

Acute idiopathic scrotal oedema

Acute idiopathic scrotal oedema can present with sudden painless oedema of the scrotal skin (unilateral or bilateral) with or without extension to the neighbouring skin, for example perineum, lower abdomen. The child is otherwise healthy and asymptomatic. An allergic or infective cause has been postulated but not proven. There is no tenderness and the testis is normal on palpation. Treatment is reassurance as the oedema resolves spontaneously within 2–3 days.

Undescended testes

Undescended testes, or cryptorchidism (which literally means hidden testes), is a common male anomaly, affecting 1–2% of boys. Intra-abdominal descent of the testis from the posterior abdominal wall occurs in the first 28 weeks of gestation. Further descent along the inguinal canal into the scrotum occurs in the last 12 weeks of gestation and may continue for another 3 months postnatally. Cryptorchidism may result from an arrest of descent along the normal pathway or rarely an aberrant descent into an ectopic position, for example perineal or femoral. The commonest location of an undescended testis is the superficial inguinal pouch (just above and lateral to the external inguinal ring), which is not considered as ectopic. Other positions of arrested descent are 'canalicular' or less commonly, intra-abdominal.

Undescended testes must be differentiated from retractile testes. Retractile testis results from an overactive cremasteric reflex and can be coaxed into the scrotum. Most retractile testes will descend spontaneously and do not require treatment. There is some recent evidence to suggest that a small group of high retractile testes may actually ascend (the ascending testes) rather than descend, requiring follow-up and intervention if necessary.

Management

Surgery is recommended for children with undescended testes for three main reasons:

1. *Subfertility*: Evidence of impaired germ-cell development (reduction of spermatogonia, abnormalities of seminiferous tubules) is present in the undescended testes after the age of 1 year. This is believed to be related to the higher temperature associated with the undescended position (35–37°C) than the normal scrotal position (33°C). Hormonal function is not affected.

2. *Risk of malignancy*: Approximately 10% of testicular tumours arise in undescended testes. The risk of malignancy in an undescended testis is estimated to be 10–40 times higher than normal; the risk is increased further by 6-fold in intra-abdominal testes. Placement of an undescended testis in the scrotal position allows early detection of malignant changes in later life. There is no proof, but some suggestion, that early orchidopexy may lower the risk of malignancy.

3. *Psycho-cosmetic reasons*: An empty scrotum may be detrimental to the psycho-social development of a child or young adult.

Ancillary reasons for treating undescended testes include the need to treat concomitant hernia and increased risks of torsion and trauma.

Orchidopexy is now recommended between 6 months and 1 year of age if the expertise is available. For the inexperienced surgeon, the advantage of early orchidopexy has to be balanced against the risk of testicular vessel damage in a young infant. Orchidopexy is carried out via a groin incision. The gubernaculum is divided. The patent processus vaginalis, which is often present, is isolated, divided and ligated. The testicular pedicle is mobilized sufficiently to allow tension-free transfer of the testis to the scrotum. The testis is fixed in the dartos pouch.

Of undescended testes, 20% are *impalpable* and these constitute a special management problem. Impalpable testes can represent absence of testes, intra-abdominal testes or canalicular testes. Testicular absence accounts for 20–40% of impalpable testes. Most cases of testicular absence result from degeneration following intrauterine torsion (vanishing testes) rather than agenesis. Unilateral congenital testicular absence or mono-orchidism is commoner (1 in 25 cases of undescended testes) than bilateral absence of anorchidism (1 in 20 000). For bilateral impalpable testes, XY karyotyping and human chorionic gonadotrophin (HCG) stimulation test to demonstrate the presence of testosterone-secreting tissue should be performed. Appropriate endocrine therapy is implemented for anorchidism.

Although orchidopexy is usually a satisfactory operation for lower undescended testes, surgery for high undescended testes, and in particular intra-abdominal testes, remains a major challenge. Pre- or peri-operative localization is indicated as some procedures for high undescended testes depend on an intact collateral blood supply to the testes which may be disturbed by unplanned exploration. Imaging studies, including ultrasonography, CT, arteriography and venography, have limited accuracies or are invasive and are not widely practised. MRI with contrast enhancement is more useful. At present, laparoscopy is the most accurate method for the localization of testes. For high undescended testes which cannot be brought to an intra-scrotal position by standard orchidopexy, the following surgical options are available:

- *Staged orchidopexy*: at the initial operation, the testis is fixed to the pubis, and together with the cord, is encased in a silastic sheet. A second operation is undertaken 8–16 months later.
- *Testicular vessel division* (Fowler–Stephen's procedure): a high undescended testis is often associated with a long-loop vas which provides collateral circulation to the testis, allowing the testicular vessel to be divided high above the testis in one- or two-stage orchidopexy. This is the most popular procedure and can be done laparoscopically.
- *Microvascular orchidopexy*: with the available expertise, transfer of testes to the scrotum can be achieved by anastomosis of the testicular and inferior epigastric vessels.
- *Orchidectomy*: for post-pubertal man with a unilateral intra-abdominal testis and a normal contralateral testis, orchidectomy and prosthesis insertion may be considered.

Varicocele

Varicocele represents a dilatation of the testicular veins in the pampiniform plexus and occurs predominantly in the left hemiscrotum, probably related to the drainage of the left spermatic vein into the left renal vein at a 90° angle. It usually presents in an adolescent as a 'bag of worms', which decreases as he lies supine. There is a risk of subfertility. Surgical treatment consists of high ligation/clipping of spermatic vein via a groin incision or preferably laparoscopically. For a young child with a varicocele, the possibility of an underlying neoplasm such as Wilms' tumour should be considered.

PAEDIATRIC UROLOGY

Urinary tract infection in infants and children is most often caused by urinary stasis which can result from vesicoureteric reflux, obstructive uropathy, neuropathy/dysfunction of urinary tract, or rarely stones; ascending infection can occur in girls after bubble-bath because of the short urethra. A urine culture is obtained and antibiotics given. All young children should be investigated after the first documented episode of urinary sepsis with ultrasonography and micturating cystourethrogram.

Hydronephrosis can be caused by severe reflux nephropathy or urinary obstruction due to pelviureteric junction (PUJ) obstruction, primary obstructive megaureter or posterior urethral valve. Unilateral PUJ obstruction results in unilateral hydronephrosis, unilateral vesicureteric obstruction or reflux manifests as unilateral hydronephrosis and hydroureter, whereas posterior urethral valve causes bilateral hydronephrosis, hydroureters, thickened bladder and dilated proximal urethra.

Multicystic dysplastic kidney

This condition is distinguished from polycystic kidney disease which is a rare genetic disorder. Multicystic dysplasia is usually unilateral and may be detected by ultrasonography both ante- and post-natally. The cysts are unconnected and there is no functioning renal parenchyma. Many multicystic dysplastic kidneys will atrophy with age and may not require treatment. Nephrectomy is carried out for persistent and symptomatic (urinary infection) lesions. The risk of late malignancy is considered very unlikely.

Pelviureteric junction obstruction

PUJ obstruction is a common congenital anomaly which results in hydronephrosis without hydroureter. There is typically a narrow segment at the pelviureteric junction with disorganized musculature and fibrosis and often an aberrant artery crossing it anteriorly. Rarely it can be caused by a kink, band, valve or polyp. It is commoner in boys and on the left side; 5% is bilateral.

Diagnosis

The condition is increasingly detected antenatally by ultrasonography (1 : 100 pregnancies, although only 1 in 1000 have persistent uropathy). An abdominal mass in infants is often renal in origin (50%), and 40% can be attributed to hydronephrosis secondary to PUJ obstruction. Loin pain (known as Dietl's crisis when intermittent and associated with vomiting, followed by diuresis and resolution of symptoms) and urinary infection are common symptoms. Occasionally haematuria, hypertension or stone occurs. In addition to anatomic diagnosis by ultrasonography, renal function and degree of obstruction should be assessed by intravenous urography, or preferably a radioisotope renal scan: mercaptoacetyltriglycine (MAG3) or diethylenetriaminepentaacetate (DTPA).

Management

Mild hydronephrosis due to incomplete pelviureteric junction obstruction, which is diagnosed by antenatal ultrasonography but remains asymptomatic, may be observed. Antenatal pelvic dilatation ≤12 mm (anteroposterior diameter) is considered minimal, and ≥20 mm severe. An infant with significant antenatal hydronephrosis should be given antibiotic prophylaxis until a micturating cystourethrogram is performed as 30% has vesicoureteric reflux.

Surgery is indicated when the hydronephrosis is symptomatic, complicated or shows deteriorating renal function on periodic isotope renography (≤35% differential renal function). The standard procedure is dismembered pyeloplasty (Anderson–Hynes) which can be performed by the open or laparoscopic approach. Endopyelotomy is less effective. For kidneys with <10% of overall renal function, nephrectomy is performed instead.

Duplex system

There are varying degrees of duplication of the urinary tract, some of which are inconsequential, for example partial bifid ureter. In accordance to embryology, the lower pole ureter generally inserts more lateral and cephalad into the bladder than the upper pole ureter which has a more medial and caudal orifice that is sometimes ectopic. As a consequence, the lower pole ureter is more prone to reflux, whereas the upper pole ureter is more often obstructed (Weigert–Meyer law). The commonest entity requiring treatment consists of a poorly functioning upper kidney moiety drained by an ectopic ureter. The ureter may open into a ureterocele in the bladder, or rarely outside the bladder in which case the child typically wets in between normal voids. Urinary infection is more commonly the presenting symptom. Treatment consists of upper pole nephroureterectomy. Associated anomalies, for example ureterocele, may require additional procedures.

Vesicoureteric reflux

Vesicoureteric reflux is found in 1% of children, and is a common cause of urinary infection (20–50%). There is a female preponderance (85%) and a familial tendency (30% incidence in siblings of affected patients, suggesting an autosomal dominant inheritance with variable penetrance). The oblique course of an intravesical, submucosal ureteral segment normally functions as a valve, failure of which (e.g. a short ureteral tunnel) results in reflux. Vesicoureteric reflux is only harmful when complicated by infection. Repeated urinary infection is associated with renal scarring, loss of renal function and eventually hypertension and renal failure.

Diagnosis

Vesicoureteric reflux is diagnosed by micturating cystourethrography and the severity is graded as follows:
- Grade I: partial filling of an undilated ureter;
- Grade II: total filling of an undilated upper tract;
- Grade III: dilated calyces;
- Grade IV: blunted fornices;
- Grade V: massive hydronephrosis and tortuous ureter.

A radioisotope (DMSA) renogram delineates the degree of renal scarring and loss of function.

Management

Treatment of vesicoureteric reflux may be medical or surgical. Especially for mild grades of reflux, prophylactic antibiotics are often adequate in preventing urinary infection and allow spontaneous resolution of reflux which usually completes by the age of 4 years (Grade I: 90%, Grade II: 75%, Grade III: 50%, Grade IV: 25%, Grade V: 0–5%). Surgery is considered for children with severe reflux or failure of medical treatment, for example breakthrough urinary infections, progressive renal scarring, drug intolerance or non-compliance, and associated anomalies. Conventional antireflux surgery consists of ureteric reimplantation, the most popular method being submucosal, transtrigonal reimplantation (Cohen). More recently, subureteric transurethral injection of teflon or its biodegradable equivalent, Deflux STING has become popular. The paste injected into the lamina propria behind the submucosal ureter in the trigone excites a fibrous reaction which prevents reflux. Proponents of STING claim high success rates with this procedure, especially for mild–moderate degrees of reflux, although there are doubts about the long-term outcome of foreign particle implantation in children.

Vesicoureteric junction obstruction

Occasionally, the lower end of the ureter is stenosed, resulting in urinary infection and megaureter. This should be excised and the ureter (which may need tapering) implanted.

Ureterocele

Ureterocele is a cyst-like dilatation at the lower end of a ureter. Occasionally, it is small and orthotopic, originating from a single ureter. More commonly, it is associated with an ectopic ureter which usually drains an upper kidney moiety of a duplex system. Apart from obstruction to the ureter, reflux may coexist. Urinary infection is the commonest presentation. Occasionally, a large ureterocele may cause bladder outlet obstruction or even prolapse outside. Treatment of ureterocele varies individually. In sick young infants with severe urinary sepsis, endoscopic incision of ureterocele can be life-saving. The most radical procedure is excision of ureterocele, reimplantation of orthotopic ureter and removal of ectopic ureter and ectopic kidney moiety.

Posterior urethral valve

Posterior urethral valve is the most common life-threatening urological anomaly in the newborn. The common form of posterior urethral valve originates from the inferior margin of the verumontanum that extends anteriorly and distally as two leaflets; rarely it presents as a perforated diaphragm. There are varying degrees of bladder outlet obstruction on micturition. Antenatal ultrasound could reveal oligohydramnios, bilateral hydronephrosis, megaureters and a distended thick-walled bladder. Severe oligohydramnios can lead to pulmonary hypoplasia. The newborn boy may develop urosepsis, renal failure and rarely urinary ascites – the sick baby should be stabilized initially with appropriate fluid and electrolyte management, antibiotics and bladder catheterization with a fine feeding tube. Older children can present with voiding dysfunction such as wetting, poor stream, acute urinary retention, etc. A micturating cystourethrogram typically shows a dilated posterior urethra with abrupt distal narrowing. Ablation of the valve can usually be achieved endoscopically but the sequelae of obstructive uropathy may give rise to long-term bladder dysfunction (valve bladder).

Wetting

Wetting in children can be caused by anatomic incontinence (ectopic ureter, bladder obstruction, extrophy), neurogenic incontinence (spinal dysraphism, trauma, tumours), functional incontinence (urge syndrome, fractional voiding), enuresis (nocturnal, diurnal), and other conditions (urinary infection, polyuria). Incontinence is characterized by failure of voluntary bladder control and incomplete emptying whereas in enuresis emptying is complete and the child is often unaware when wetting occurs.

Neurogenic bladder can result from a variety of causes which interfere with the innervation of the bladder, the commonest congenital anomaly being a neural tube defect (myelomeningocele or spina bifida). Urinary incontinence and infection are the main problem. Evaluation is achieved by urodynamic studies. Intermittent self-catheterization is the most important ingredient in its treatment. Bladder augmentation, urinary diversion and artificial urinary sphincters are procedures which may be applicable in individual instances.

A child with urge syndrome has frequent voiding and a small bladder. A child with fractional voiding has infrequent, incomplete voiding and a large bladder. These are treated with retraining and anticholinergics.

Primary nocturnal enuresis (defined as wetting ≥2 times per week for ≥3 months in a child ≥5 years) affects 15–20% of 5 year old children. The natural course is spontaneous resolution, at a rate of 15% of patients per year. Even though enuresis causes no physical harm, adverse psychological consequences may be sustained. The diagnosis of primary nocturnal enuresis is achieved by exclusion, starting with a good history including psychological evaluation, and proper physical examination. The child has never been dry in primary enuresis whereas in secondary enuresis the child has been dry for ≥6months. Primary enuresis is essentially monosymptomatic; workup for other causes of wetting is necessary when enuresis is polysymptomatic. The parents are reassured by counselling on the epidemiology and natural history of enuresis. Behavioural therapy is enhanced with star chart and alarms, and a success rate of 60–80% has been reported. Medical treatment may be necessary in resistant/recurrent cases. Imipramine (a tricyclic antidepressant) has anticholinergic and central effects, and gives 10–50% response. Desmopressin (DDAVP), an antidiuretic hormone analogue increases the urine-concentrating ability, and is deemed more effective.

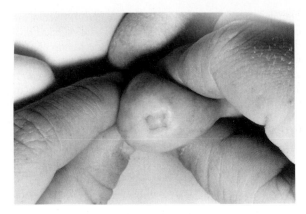

Figure 23.7. Phimosis resulting from BXO.

Hypospadias

Hypospadias is characterized by a proximal location of the urethral meatus ventrally. There is a spectrum of severity: glandular, coronal, subcoronal, mid-shaft, penoscrotal and perineal. Except for very mild hypospadias, there is often an associated chordee, a ventral curvature of the penis, which is exacerbated on erection. The foreskin has an abnormal appearance of a dorsal hood. Some degree of torsion of the axis of the penis often exists.

Hypospadias affects 1 in 300 boys. There is a familial tendency: 8% of fathers and 14% of brothers of patients are affected. Associated anomalies include undescended testes (9%), hernia-hydrocele (9%), and upper urinary tract anomalies (2–3%).

Management

It is important to recognize the condition as circumcision is absolutely contraindicated: the dorsal hood of foreskin is a valuable piece of tissue for reconstruction. Uncorrected, the penile curvature and abnormal urination and semen delivery could lead to major psychological and sexual sequelae and infertility. The goal of surgery is to straighten the penis, provide a urethra which opens at its tip and achieve a normal appearance. A variety of techniques have been employed. Most are repaired at around the age of 1 year. A single stage operation is performed except for very severe hypospadias. If chordee is present, this is excised completely. For proper placement of the new urethral opening, a short distance may be covered by meatal advancement and glanuloplasty. In moderate and severe hypospadias, a neourethra has to be fashioned, usually from penile skin which commonly is meatal-based or pedicled from the dorsal hood, or by tubularizing the urethral plate. Complications include meatal stenosis, urethrocutaneous fistula, stricture, diverticulum, etc. Bladder or buccal mucosa grafts may be needed for secondary procedures.

Phimosis

True phimosis affects only 1% of boys and is usually the result of a chronic inflammatory process, balanitis xerotica obliterans (BXO) (Fig. 23.7). BXO is probably a form of lichen sclerosis, which leads to a scarred and non-retractile foreskin. Circumcision is indicated for true phimosis.

Non-retractility of foreskin in early life is, however, normal (physiological phimosis) as the epithelial layers of the glans and foreskin are fused at birth. This probably protects the infant from ammoniacal excoriation and hence neonatal circumcision has no medical grounds. This procedure is commonly performed in United States (US) for reasons of 'hygiene', 'perhaps lowering the risk of urinary infection', 'social habit', etc. The other major non-medical reason for circumcision is religion, notably for Jews and Muslims. Natural separation of foreskin usually occurs so that by the age of 4 years, the foreskin becomes retractile in 90% of boys. Prior to this, sometimes anxious parents may discover pea-sized swellings underneath the foreskin. These are collections of smegma, are harmless and will resolve when foreskin separation is complete.

Balano-prostitis may also be a concern and repeated attacks after the age of 4 years constitute a relative indication for intervention.

Rarely, a foreskin with a narrow preputial ring which has been retracted cannot be pulled forward, resulting in acute, painful swelling, that is *paraphimosis*. This needs to be reduced manually with sedation. A dorsal slit under anaesthesia is sometimes required. When the inflammation has settled, elective circumcision is arranged.

Circumcision is usually performed as a day-case procedure under general anaesthesia. Complications include bleeding, infection, meatal stenosis, fistula formation, excessive/inadequate skin removal, etc. It is important that penile abnormalities, for example hypospadias, buried penis, webbed penis, etc. are excluded before circumcision.

Alternatives to circumcision include preputioplasty and separation of preputial adhesion under general or local anaesthesia.

PAEDIATRIC SOLID TUMOURS

Management of malignant neoplasms is one of the great success stories of paediatric surgery, witnessing an improvement of survival rates from <20% in the 1950s to >60% currently. The most important factors responsible for this phenomenon are effective chemotherapy ± radiotherapy and formation of large multicentre cancer study groups with pooling of patient materials to allow scientific and evidence-based evaluation of new treatment protocols and identification of risk factors.

Wilms' tumour

Wilms' tumour and neuroblastoma (see below) are the commonest abdominal malignant tumours in children, affecting 8–10 per million population. Wilms' tumour, or nephroblastoma, is a large and heterogeneous renal embryonoma which is usually confined within a pseudocapsule but can invade neighbouring tissues, especially the renal vein. Histologically, there is a mixture of primitive blastemal, stromal and epithelial cells. There may be associated anomalies, for example congenital aniridia, hemihypertrophy, genitourinary anomalies, mental retardation, chromosomal abnormalities, Beckwith–Wiedemann syndrome, etc. Loss of heterozygosity of WT1 gene on chromosome 11p13 is found in half of patients with Wilms' tumour. The WT2 gene located on chromosome 11p15 is associated with Beckwith–Wiedemann syndrome. Chromosomes 16q and 1p are also associated with Wilms' tumour.

Diagnosis

The majority presents before the age of 5 years, usually as an asymptomatic abdominal mass. There may be non-specific constitutional symptoms such as abdominal pain, malaise, weight loss, anaemia, hypertension, and occasionally haematuria. Rarely, a left variocele arises from tumour occlusion of the left renal vein. Investigations should include ultrasonography, chest and abdominal X-rays and CT scan with intravenous contrast.

Management

Treatment is multimodal and depends on staging and histology. Anaplasia or sarcomatous changes (rhabdoid or clear cell) are unfavourable indicators. Rhabdoid tumours frequently metastasise to the brain, and clear cell tumours to the bone. The National Wilms' Tumour Study Staging System (NWTS-3) is:

- Stage I: tumour limited to kidney, completely excised;
- Stage II: tumour extends beyond kidney, completely excised;
- Stage III: residual tumour with abdomen;
- Stage IV: haematogenous metastasis;
- Stage V: bilateral renal tumour.

Treatment for stages I and II is surgery and chemotherapy and for stages III, IV and unfavourable histology (any stage) radiotherapy is added. Treatment of stage V is individualized. The duration and intensity of chemotherapy increase with advancing stages. The most commonly used chemotherapeutic agents are vincristine and actinomycin D. Advanced stage, unfavourable histology and age >2 years are poor prognostic indicators. The overall survival rate of Wilms' tumour now approaches 90%.

Congenital mesoblastic nephroma was initially regarded as a variant of Wilms' tumour, but now has been identified as a separate entity. It is the most common renal neoplasm detected in the antenatal and neonatal periods. The tumour is benign in nature and surgical resection results in virtually 100% survival.

Neuroblastoma

Neuroblastoma arises from the neural crest, most commonly in the adrenal medulla, but can be found anywhere along the sympathetic ganglion chain in the neck, thorax, abdomen and pelvis. The tumour is vascular, nodular and locally invasive. The typical histological features are small round blue cells with scanty cytoplasm arranged in rosettes with fine nerve fibres in the centres. There are varying degrees of differentiation with the most mature form being the benign ganglioneuroma. Very rarely, spontaneous maturation of neuroblastoma to ganglioneuroma occurs, resulting in 'cure'. Associated anomalies include Hirschsprung's disease (neurocristopathy), Klippel–Feil syndrome, Beckwith–Wiedemann syndrome, di George syndrome, Ondine's curse (congenital central hypoventilation) and trisomy 18.

Diagnosis

The commonest presentation of abdominal neuroblastoma is a mass;

- thoracic lesions may give rise to respiratory symptoms;
- cervical tumours may cause Horner's syndrome;
- pelvic tumours are associated with urinary and bowel dysfunctioning;
- paraspinal tumours often have dumb-bell extensions into the spinal canal resulting in neurological symptoms.

Rarely, excessive catecholamine or vasoactive intestinal peptide production leads to hypertension or diarrhoea respectively. Systemic symptoms are often prominent and are sometimes related to metastasis. Over 90% of neuroblastomas show an elevated urinary level of vanillylmandelic acid, a metabolite of catecholamines. A plain radiograph may show calcification. Ultrasonography, CT and MRI provide useful anatomical information. Metastasis is evaluated by bone marrow aspiration, skeletal survey and more recently ^{131}I scan using MIBG (m-iodobenzylguanidine), which is taken up by neuroectodermal tumours.

Shimada pathologic classification divides neuroblastomas into stroma-rich and stroma-poor categories, with prognostic values. Stroma-rich tumours have a favourable pronosis, unless a nodular pattern is present. The prognosis of stroma-poor tumours depends on age at presentation, differentiation, and the mitosis–karyorrhexis index(MKI);older age, undifferentiation and MKI < 100/5000 cells are unfavourable.

Staging

- Stage I: localized tumour;
- Stage II: tumour extends beyond organ but not across midline;
- Stage III: tumour extends beyond midline;
- Stage IV: distant metastasis;
- Stage IVs: small primary lesion with metastasis confined to liver, skin or bone marrow without cortex involvement in infants <1 year of age.

Management

Stage I and II tumours are excised and chemotherapy is given for stage II. For stage III tumours, resection is undertaken if possible followed by chemotherapy and radiotherapy. For unresectable tumours, chemotherapy + radiotherapy is given to reduce the size of the tumour which is then resected. Stage IV disease is treated with chemotherapy (cisplantin, VP-16, adrimycin, melphalan). Stage IVs is treated by surgery; occasionally respiratory distress may develop from a rapidly enlarging liver, requiring low dose irradiation or insertin of a temporary 'silo' as in the treatment of gastroschisis/exomphalos.

The prognosis of neuroblastoma is worse than Wilms' tumour with overall survival rates of only 30–50%. Advanced stage, age >2 years, unfavourable histology, multiple copies of N-*myc* oncogene, diploidy, etc. are poor prognostic factors. Stage IVs unlike stage IV disease is associated with a good prognosis.

Neonatal screening programmes based on urinary catecholamine studies for early detection of neuroblastoma have failed to provide survival benefits.

New strategies for treatment of advanced diseases include high-dose chemotherapy with total body radiation and allogeneic or autologous bone marrow transplantation, immunotherapy, target therapy with monoclonal antibody antiganglioside GD2, retinoids to induce differentiation, and gene therapy.

Soft tissue sarcoma

Rhabdomyosarcoma is the commonest soft tissue tumour in childhood and can occur in any part of the body except the brain and bone arising from embryonic tissue capable of muscular differentiation. It is slightly less common than Wilms' tumour and neuroblastoma. Rhabdomyosarcoma is a small round cell tumour, characterized by positive staining with antibodies against actin and myosin. There are five histologic subtypes: embryonal (60%), botryoid (6%), alveolar (20%), undifferentiated (20%) and pleomorphic (1%). There are two peak age incidences, before 5 years and at 12–18 years. Familial tendency, and association with neurofibromatosis, Li Fraumeni syndrome and p53 mutation have been described. Clinical features relate to the location of the tumour which can occur anywhere in the body, but commonly at the head and neck, distal urogenital tract (young children), trunk and paratesticular site (adolescents). Lung and bone are common metastatic sites. Diagnosis is made by biopsy after imaging studies (ultrasound, CT, MRI) and workup for metastasis. Treatment is multimodal (surgery, chemotherapy, radiotherapy) and depends on staging (stage I: localized disease, completely resected, no lymph node involvement; stage II: localized or regional disease with grossly total resection but with microscopic residues; stage III: incomplete resection; stage IV: distant metastasis). Overall survival (65%) is better than for neuroblastoma but worse than for Wilms' tumour. Prognosis is dependent on stage, pathology (embryonal type is favourable, alveolar and undifferentiated are unfavourable), and location (orbit, and genital organs have a favourable prognosis).

Other tumours

Germ-cell tumours may occur in any part of the reproductive system or ectopically as a result of abnormal migration of primitive germ cells. Histologically, these may be teratoma, seminoma, dysgerminoma, yolk sac tumour or choriocarcinoma. The presentation is often a mass or pain. Dysgerminoma secretes hormones resulting in precocious puberty. Serum markers such as α-fetoprotein and human chorionic gonadotrophin are helpful for diagnosis and follow-up monitoring. Benign teratoma (a common cause of ovarian mass) is simply excised. Malignant tumours require multimodal treatment (surgery, chemotherapy, radiotherapy). Testicular tumours should always be excised via a groin incision, *not* a scrotal incision. Sacrococcygeal teratoma most commonly presents in the newborn period and the majority are benign, responding to excision which should always include the coccyx.

Lymphoma is a common malignancy in childhood but the majority are treated by chemotherapy and radiotherapy. Gastrointestinal lymphoma can be treated by surgery.

Malignant *liver tumours* are relatively rare. There are two histological types:
- hepatoblastoma;
- hepatocellular carcinoma.

Hepatoblastoma affects infants and young children and is associated with a good prognosis. Hepatocellular carcinoma occurs in older children, often complicating underlying liver disease. Serum α-fetoprotein is elevated and in some hepatoblastomas, human chorionic gonadotrophin level is also raised. Hepatic resection is the main form of treatment. Children are noted for their excellent capacity for hepatic regeneration, allowing resection of up to 80% of the liver. Hepatoblastoma is chemosensitive. Inoperable hepatocellular carcinoma may be palliated by transarterial oily chemo-embolization (TOCE). Overall survival for hepatoblastoma is 70% and for hepatocellular carcinoma 13%. Liver transplantation may be attempted in selected patients.

FURTHER READING

Glick PL, Pearl RH, Irish MS, Caty MG (eds). *Pediatric Surgery Secrets*, Philadelphia: Hanley & Belfus, Inc, 2001

Majid AA, Kingsnorth AN (eds). *Advanced Surgical Practice*, London: Greenwich Medical Media, 2003

O'Neill Jr JA, Grosfeld JL, Fonkalsrud EW, Coran AG, Caldamone AA (eds). *Principles of Pediatric Surgery*, 2nd ed. St. Louis: Mosby, 2003

Spitz L, Coran AG (ed). *Rob & Smith's Operative Surgery: Paediatric Surgery*, 5th ed. London: Chapman and Hall Medical, 1995

Tam PKH. *Laparoscopic surgery in children.* Archives of Disease in Childhood 2000; **82**: 240–243

Index

A

ABCs 91, 97, 121, 426
Abdominal hernias 276, 512
Abdominal injuries 98–101, 361
  computed tomography 99
  laparoscopy 99
  laparotomy 99–100
  management 100–1
  peritoneal lavage 99
  ultrasound 99
Abdominal mass
  gastrointestinal system 510
  genital system 510
  imaging, laparoscopy 242
  liver, spleen, pancreas 510
  solid tumours 510
  urinary system 510
  see also Cysts
Abdominal pain
  acute conditions 510
  ectopic pregnancy 390
  endometriosis 390
  infants and children
    acute non-specific 510
    medical conditions 509–10
    surgical conditions 509
  ovarian cysts 390
Abdominal wall
  conjoint tendon 270
  defects, infants 510–11
  external anatomy, surface markings 267–8
  external oblique aponeurosis 269–70
  fascia transversalis, the space of Bogros 270
  peritoneum 270–1
  subcutaneous layer 268
  superficial nerves 268–9
Abdominal wounds
  closure 76
  dehiscence 83–4
Abortion, ethics 185, 186
Abscesses
  anorectal 253–4, 260
  breast 330
  Brodie's 471
  drainage 86–7
  intracerebral 439
  lung 363
  peritonsillar 398, 412
  subdural, epilepsy association 439

Acanthamoebic keratitis 394
  contact lens wear 394
Achalasia 234, 237, 367
  oesophagus 367
Achilles tendon rupture 461
Acidemia 131
Acinic cell carcinoma 413
Acoustic neuroma 412, 433
Acquired immune deficiency syndrome 220–2
Acromegaly, growth hormone (GH) 435, 436
ACTH and cortisol 107–8
Actinic keratoses 403
Actinomycosis 412
Activated partial thromboplastin time 210
Acute abdomen 390, 509–10
Acute lung injury and ARDS 139–41
Acute lung injury (ALI) 139, 140
Addisonian crisis, adrenal suppression 9, 11
Adenocarcinoma 309, 364
  Barrett's mucosa 368
  bladder 385
  kidney 381
  prostate gland 387
  skeletal radionuclide and CT scans 365
Adenoid cystic carcinoma 407, 413
Adenoids 205
Adenoma
  ACTH 435
  hypersecretory, pituitary gland compression 436
Adenovirus, viral conjunctivitis 393
Adhesion molecules 62, 110, 162, 341
Adhesive strips 76
Adjuvant therapy 246–7, 258
Adnexa oculi, bacterial keratitis 393
Adrenal glands
  disorders 315–17
Adrenal glands, anatomy and physiology 313–14
Adrenal hyperplasia, congenital 317
Adrenal masses 317
  cysts 317
Adrenal suppression, steroid-induced 11
Adrenaline, action 314–15
Adrenocorticotrophic hormone (ACTH) 107, 313, 314, 435, 436
  congenital adrenal hyperplasia 317
  pituitary gland 320

  secretion in trauma 107
Adult respiratory distress syndrome (ARDS) 139–41
Advanced Trauma Life Support (ATLS) system 90–1
  diagnostic peritoneal lavage 99
Aetiology
  exertion and herniation 272
Age, preoperative assessment 2–3
Age of dissection 265
Agglutination reaction 213
AIDS *see* HIV infection and AIDS
Airway
  artificial *see* Intubation
  laryngeal mask 24, 133
  oropharyngeal aperture, classification 20
  preanaesthesia assessment 17–18
  trauma care 90–1
  see also Ventilation
Airway obstruction
  early hypoxaemia 30–1
  following thoracic surgery 354, 361
Alcohol, alcoholism
  anaesthesia risks 10
  carcinogenesis 155
Aldosterone, secretion 314
Alfentanil, characteristics 23, 27, 35
Algorithms
  asystole 122
  nutritional support 50
  pulseless ventricular tachycardia 122
  ventricular fibrillation 122
Allen test 116
Alpha-adrenergic blocking agents 386
Alveolar hypoventilation, early hypoxaemia 30
Amine precursor uptake decarboxylase (APUD) cells 319, 320
Amino acids, metabolism after trauma 108
Aminoglutethimide 315
Aminoglycosides, treatment of sepsis 68
Amnesia
  post-traumatic (PTA) 418, 428
  retrograde 418
Amputation 291–2, 458–60
  chronic osteomyelitis 471
  classification 458–9
  complications 460
  congenital anomalies 459
  haematoma formation 460

Amputation (*Contd*)
  indications 458–9
  joint contracture 460
  neural deficits 459
  neuroma formation 460
  peripheral vascular disease 458
  post-traumatic 458–9
  postoperative infection 460
  psychological assessment 460
  stump necrosis 460
  stump osteomyelitis 460
  surgical considerations 459–60
  tumours 405
Amrinone 119
Amylase, serum, abdominal injuries
    100, 101
Anaemia
  aplastic anaemia 214
  autoimmune haemolytic 222
  implications for surgery 214
  preoperative assessment 9
Anaesthesia 16
  ASA classification of illness 1, 14, 20
  assessment 17–21
    examination 19–20
    risk stratification 20
  awareness 17
  complications 16–18
  definitions 16
  emergencies
    cardiac arrest 34
    cardiorespiratory collapse 34
    failure to intubate 33–4
    rapid sequence induction 33
  induction 23–4
    inhalational/intravenous 23
  local agents 34–5
    toxicity 34–5
  local anaesthesia technique 275–6
  maintenance, inhalational/intravenous
    24–5
  monitoring 29–30
  premedication 21–2
  preoperative assessment 1–3
    concurrent drugs 11–13
    lifestyle risks 10–11
  previous, history 17–18
  prophylaxis of thromboembolic
    disease 13–14
  recovery 30–3
  stages 16–17
  tourniquets 37
  ventilation 37–8
  see also Local; Regional anaesthesia
Anaesthesia
  emergency 33–4
Anaesthetic agents
  inhalational agents 25–6
  interactions with concurrent drugs
    18–19
  intravenous anaesthetic agents 26–7
  local agents 34–5, 44
  neuromuscular blocking drugs 27–8
  pharmacology 25–8
  regional agents 35–7
Anal and perianal disorders
  anorectal abscesses 254

anorectal anomaly 504–5
anorectal manometry 250
fissure 260–1
injury 101
Anal cancer 260
Analgesia 16, 25, 27
Anaphylaxis, anaesthetic agents 17
Anastomosis
  gastrointestinal 84, 88
  leaks 84
  principles 87–8
  vascular 84, 88
Anatomy of
  biliary system 231
  duodenum 231
  hepatic system 231
  oesophagus 230–1
  pancreas 231
  portal venous system 231
    stomach 230
Anderson–Hynes dismembered
    pyeloplasty 384
Androgens, secretion 313–14
Aneuploidy 172
Aneurysms 279, 287, 296
  anastomotic 298
  degenerative 287, 295
  intracranial 436, 437
Angina
  grading 3
  Ludwig's 412
  preoperative assessment 3
Angiography 425
  central nervous system investigations
    415
  digital subtraction (DSA) 425, 437, 438
  magnetic resonance (MRA) 289
  see also Endoscopic retrograde
    cholangio-pancreatography
    (ERCP)
Angiolymphoid hyperplasia with
    eosinophilia 412
Angioplasty 290, 291, 293
Angiosarcoma 405–6
Angiotensin converting-enzyme
    inhibitors
  action 114
  interactions with anaesthetic agents 19
Animal models, ethics 187
Ankle and brachial pressure index (ABPI)
    288
Ankle disorders 465–6
  avascular necrosis of the talus 448
  osteoarthritis 466
  osteochondritis dissecans of the talus
    465
  recurrent lateral ligament instability 465
Ankle fractures 446
Ankylosing spondylitis 451, 452
Anorectal *see* Anal and perianal disorders
Anorectal conditions
  anal fissure 260–1
  fistula-in-ano 260
  haemorrhoids 261
  prolapse 261
Anorectal disorder 262–3
  anal incontinence 262–3

constipation 262
Anorectal manometry 506
Antibiotics
  ICU 144
  prophylactic 64–5
  treatment of sepsis 67
Antibodies
  classes 212–13
  cold 222
  molecular structure 212
  receptors 212
  warm 222
Anticholinergics, characteristics 24
Anticoagulants
  interactions with anaesthetic agents
    19
  prophylaxis of thromboembolic
    disease 12
Antidiuretic hormone (ADH) 417, 435
Antigen matching 228
Antigens 212
  prostate-specific antigen 172, 376
Antihypertensives, kidney disease 374
Antiinflammatory mediators 59
Antiplatelet agents, prophylaxis of
    thromboembolic disease 13
Antisense oligonucleotides 150, 177
Aorta
  intra-aortic balloon pump 120
  transection 98
Aortic aneurysms 296, 298
Aortic rupture, thoracic trauma 361
Apache II scoring system, ICU 147
Aplastic anaemia 214
Apoptosis 153
Appendicitis, acute
  diagnosis 510
  management 510
Appendix
  acute appendicitis 276
  carcinoid tumours 319–20
Appendix epididymis torsion 516
Aprotinin 438
APUD cells, multiple endocrine neoplasia
    320
Arrhythmias 32, 122, 360
Arterial anastomosis 87–8
Arterial anatomy and physiology 286–7
Arterial blood gases
  normal values 131
  and pH 41, 131
  pulse oximetry 29, 131
Arterial bypass 291, 293
Arterial diameter 288
Arterial disease 286
  abdominal aortic aneurysms 296
  aneurysms 287
  arterial trauma 297
  collateral circulation 286
  degenerative aneurysmal disease 295
  diabetic foot 296–7
  epidemiology, clinical features and
    management 287–8
  intermittent claudication 292
  intracranial 436–8
  investigation 288–9
    angiography 289

ankle/brachial pressure index (ABPI)
    288, 301
B-mode ultrasound 288
computed tomography angiography
    289
Duplex ultrasonography 288, 289
exercise testing 288
magnetic resonance angiography
    (MRA) 289
lower limb 298–9
management
    complications of surgery 297–8
    pathology 287
    surgical techniques 289–92
mesenteric 294
pathophysiology 298–9
surgery 286
Arterial endarterectomy 291, 293, 295
Arterial grafts 290–1
Arterial injuries 103, 297
Arterial pathology 287 see also Arterial
    disease
Arterial pressure, mean 40, 424
Arterial thrombosis 219
Arteriovenous malformations (AVM) 252,
    253, 437
Arthritis 451–2
    ankylosing spondylitis 451
    avascular necrosis 452
    classification 451
    degenerative 451
    gout and pseudo-gout 451
    haemophilia 452
    postseptic 451
    post-traumatic 451
    septic 471–3
        clinical features 471
        investigations 472
        management 472–3
    tuberculosis 451
    see also Rheumatoid arthritis
Arthrodesis
    ankle 466–7
    hallux rigidus 467
    hallux valgus 467–9
    rheumatoid arthritis 466–7
Arthropathy
    cuff tear 475
    inflammatory bowel disease
        association 452
Arthroplasty
    hallux rigidus 467
    hallux valgus 467–9
    Keller's 468
    rheumatoid arthritis 466–7
Asbestos exposure, malignant
    mesothelioma 365
Aspergillus sp., fungal keratitis 393
Aspiration, prevention 24
Aspirin, interactions with anaesthetic
    agents 19
Asthma
    preoperative assessment 6
    URTIs 6
Astrocytomas
    juvenile 434
    spinal cord 434

Asystole 122
Ataxia–telangiectasia gene 175
Atelectasis, postoperative 48
Atheroma 292
Atherosclerosis, peripheral vascular
    disease 458
Atherosclerosis, occlusion disease 292–5
Atracurium, characteristics 28
Atresia
    biliary atresia 513
    classification 503
    distal ileal 503
    duodenal 502–3
    jejunoileal 503
    oesophageal 367, 497–9
    proximal small bowel 503
    pyloric 501
Atrial fibrillation, postoperative 47
Atropine, characteristics 22
Audit 191–2
Auditory cranial nerve 419–20
Autoantibodies
    Graves' disease 222–3
    idiopathic thrombocytopenic purpura
        222
    myasthenia gravis 223
    systemic lupus erythematosus 223
Auto-immune diseases 222–3
Autonomic nervous system 422
Autonomy 185
Avascular necrosis 446, 448
    complications, 492
    osteoarthritis 465
    talus, 466
Awareness during anaesthesia 17
Axilla, anatomy and physiology 324
Axonotmesis, bone injury 102

B

B cell deficiencies 220
B cells, structure/function 202, 212
Back pain 476–9
    clinical assessment 476–8
    investigations 478
    loss of sphincter control 478
    management 478–9
    pathological classification 476
Bacteria, development of sepsis 60–1
Balanitis 389
Balanitis xerotic obliterans (BXO) 520
Bandaging, graduated compression 303
Bankart lesion, shoulder joint 454
Barium enema 250, 256, 502
Barium imaging 366
Barlow's test, CDH 489
Barrett's mucosa, adenocarcinoma 368
Barrett's oesophagus 500, 501
Basal cell carcinoma 404
Basic fibroblast growth factor 154, 162,
    172
Basophils, structure/function 202
Beckwith–Wiedemann syndrome 511,
    521
Bedsores, prevention 430
Benzodiazepines, characteristics 22
Beta-adrenergic blocking agents

interactions with anaesthetic agents
    19
phaeochromocytoma 316–17
Bicarbonate, Henderson–Hasselbach
    equation 131
Bier's block, regional anaesthesia 36
Bile acids, gallbladder 244
Biliary atresia
    Classification 513
    Diagnosis 513
    Management 513
Biopsy
    bone 486
    breast 328–9
    excisional, video-assisted thorascopic
        surgery (VATS) 357–8
    types 85
Bladder
    developmental anomalies 371
    diverticular disease involvement 390
    functional abnormalities 386
    inflammation 385
    neurogenic 385
    pain 373
    spinal pathology 386
    stones 385
    surgical anatomy 370–1
    trauma 386
    tumour
        adenocarcinoma 385
        superficial 385
        transitional cell carcinoma 385
    ultrasound scan 376
Bladder contractions,
        overactive/underactive, symptoms
        372–3
Bladder injury 101
Bladder neck, continence mechanisms 371
Bladder neck dyssynergia 386
Blebs, distinguished from bullae 363
Bleeding
    lower GI, management 253
    upper GI 253
Bleeding disorders 9, 218–19
Bleeding time 210
Blepharitis 392
Blom–Singer prosthesis 409
Blood group antigens 228
Blood loss, sepsis 60
Blood pressure
    as indication of haemorrhage 91
    intra-arterial 29
    non-invasive 29
    postoperative 40
Blood pressure monitoring
    arterial catheterization 115–16
    central venous catheterization 116
    central venous pressure 116–17
    PA catheterization 117–18
    pulse contour cardiac output 118
Blood products transfusion 215
    administrative errors 215
    autologous donation 215
    haemolytic transfusion reactions 217
    red blood cells 215
    safety 215
Blood salvage 43

Blood tests, genitourinary investigations 375–6
Blood transfusion 42–5
  autologous techniques 43, 215
  blood products 215
  complications 215–217
  sepsis 60
Blood viscosity, factors 286–7
Blunt, penetrating and missile injury 92–3, 103
BMR, calorie requirements, Harris–Benedict equation 105
Boarehaave rupture 363
Bochdalek hernia 353
Body temperature, monitoring 40–1
Bohr equation, physiological dead space 130
Bone
  infections 469–473
  malignant disease
    biopsy 486–8
    classification 483
    investigations 485–8
    management 488–9
  metabolic disease 480–3
Bone and Soft tissue, malignant disease
  clinical assessment 483–5
  Investigation 485–8
  Management 488–9
Bone grafting
  types 445
Bone injury 102–3
  reduction and fixation 102–3
Bone marrow
  anatomy 200
  failure 214–215
  transplantation 227–8
Bone pain 473–80
Bone scan 378
Bony Bankart lesion, shoulder joint 454, 455
Boundary zone lesions/infarcts 424
Bowel, short gut syndrome 503, 507
Bowel anastomosis, leaks 84
Bowel atresia 503
Bowel gases, explosion hazards 79
Bowel injury 100
Bowel obstruction 245, 256
Bowel preparation 250, 251, 253
Bowel, large 250, 260
Bowel, small 46, 253, 319–20, 368, 502
Bowel surgery
  prophylactic antibiotics 64–5
Bowel tumour 260
  Carcinoid tumour 319–20
Bowen's disease 403
Bowstring test 479–480
Brain
  anatomy 415
  computed tomography 424
  morphology 416–17
  MR scanning 424–5
  radiography 424
  structure and function 415–16
  see also Cerebral; Head injury; Intracranial
Brain abscess 438

Brain death, diagnosis 428
Branchial cyst 411
Breast 322
  ageing changes 325
  anatomy and physiology 322–5
  congenital abnormalities 325
  lymphatics 323
  and menstrual cycle 325, 332
  pregnancy and lactation 325, 349
  screening programs 349–350
Breast (benign) disease 336
  cysts 334
  epitheliosis 335
  fat necrosis 335
  fibroadenomas 333–4
  fistula 330
  galactocole 334
  gynaecomastia 336
  infections 329–30
  lactating breast 330
  mammary duct ectasia 330
  mammary dysplasia 334–5
  Mondor's disease 335
  sclerosing adenosis 335
Breast carcinoma 336
  clinical presentation 342
  diagnosis 343
  inheritance 159, 161
  male 349
  mammographic appearance 325–7
  marker genes (BRCA1) 159, 160, 337
  metastases 347
  microcalcification 326
  pathological types 338–9
  pregnancy and lactation 349
  prognostic factors 340–1
  spinal metastases 488–9
  staging 341–2
  treatment 343
    adjuvant therapy 346
    axillary lymph nodes 344–5
    breast reconstruction 345–6
    chemotherapy 346
    hormone therapy 346–7
    LABC 343–4
    myocutaneous flaps 346
    nipple and areola reconstruction 346
    primary tumours 343
    principles 342
Breast disease
  bilateral 348–9
  diagnostic modalities 325–9
    biopsy 329
    fine needle aspiration cytology 327–8
    mammography 325–7
    ultrasound 327
  elderly patients 348
  epidemiology and risk factors 336–8
    alcohol consumption 338
    benign disease vs carcinoma 336
    diet 338
    exercise 338
    genetic factors (BRCA1 and 2) 161, 337
    hormonal factors 337
    incidence, various countries 336
    ionizing radiation 337

    smoking 338
  mastalgia
    cyclical/non-cyclical 332
    pathogenesis 332
  nipple discharge 330–1
  nipple retraction (inversion) 331–2
  phylloides tumour 348
  see also Breast (benign) disease
Breast reconstruction 345–6
Breathing
  controlled ventilation 24
  trauma care 90–1
Breathlessness, pulmonary function loss 356
Breslow scale assessment, melanoma 404
Brodie's abscess 471
Bromocriptine 333
Bronchial anatomy 352–3
Bronchial obstruction 366
Bronchial tree 352
Bronchiectasis 363
Bronchitis see Chronic obstructive airways disease
Bronchopleural fistula, following pleural surgery 358, 359–60
Bronchoscopy 354–5
Bronchospirometry, smokers 356
Bronchus-associated lymphoid tissue (BALT) 204
Brucella spp., acute osteomyelitis 469
Bucket handle deformity 504
Bulbar palsy 133, 420
Bullae, distinguished from blebs 363, 364
Bupivacaine 35, 44, 72
Burkitt's lymphoma, Epstein–Barr virus infection 157, 158
  and nasopharyngeal cancer 157–8
Burns 82–3, 103–6
  assessment 104–5
  electrical 82
  heat loss 104
  infections 104
  management 82–3, 105–6
  metabolic rate 104
  metabolism 104
  pathophysiology 103
  smoke inhalation injury 104
Burr holes 423, 427
Bypass procedures 120, 121, 291

C

C-reactive protein 108, 452
Cafe-au-lait skin lesions 366, 412
Calcitonin 304, 311, 320
Calcium channel blockers
  P-glycoprotein 176
  interactions with anaesthetic agents 19
Calf phlebectomy 301
Calories, Harris–Benedict equation 105
Cancer 149
  advanced 257
  cancer cell, signalling pathways 150–2
  cancer families 159
  early 256–7
  elderly patients 182
  epidemiology 163–6

immune responses 224
invasion and metastases 162–3
malignant change 153
management 149
metastatic 257–8
molecular biology 149
    cancer cell 152–3
    carcinogenesis 155–9
    inheritance 159–61
    metastases 162–3
    molecular genetics 153–5
quality of life 181–2
screening 166–9
staging 169–73
    C-factor, R-category 169–70
    TNM classification 169–70
treatment 173–8
    chemotherapy 175–6
    curability 173
    novel therapies 176–8
    pain relief 178–81
    photodynamic therapy 175
    radiotherapy 174–5
    surgery 173–4
tumour markers 171–3
Candida, fungal keratitis 393
Cantrell, pentalogy 511
Capener's sign, slipped upper femoral
        epiphysis 491
Capnography, CO₂ analysers 23, 34, 130
Carbepenems, treatment of sepsis 68
Carbohydrates
    metabolism after trauma 108
    polysaccharides, non-starch 156
Carcinoembryonic antigen 171–2
Carcinogenesis 155–9
Carcinoid syndrome 319–20
Carcinoid tumours 319–20
Cardiac arrest, during anaesthesia 34
Cardiac arrest and resuscitation 121–2
Cardiac arrhythmias
    following pulmonary surgery 358–60
    post-anaesthesia 32
    postoperative 49
Cardiac catheterization 115–16
Cardiac cycle 113
Cardiac failure, postoperative 40
Cardiac function tests 15
Cardiac muscle 112–13
Cardiac muscle contraction 119
Cardiac output 113–14, 117
    low 30, 32
    radio isotope scan 118
Cardiac postoperative complications
        46–9
Cardiac risk factors 3–4, 21
Cardiac support 118–21
Cardiac tamponade 123–4
    following thoracic surgery 361
Cardiogenic shock 125–6
Cardiopulmonary bypass 120–1
Cardiopulmonary resuscitation 121–2
Cardiorespiratory collapse, during
        anaesthesia 34
Cardiovascular disease, preanaesthesia
        assessment 18
Cardiovascular support

extracorporeal circulation 120–1
inotropes 118–19
intra-aortic balloon pump 120
vasopressors 119
vasoregulatory agent 119
Cardiovascular system 3–5, 111
    anatomy 111–13
    investigations 118
    monitoring 115–18
    pharmacology 118
    physiology 113–15
    see also Cardiac
    preanaesthesia assessment 19–20
    preoperative assessment 3–5
    response to injury 108
Caroli's disease 514
Carotid artery disease 289
Carotid body tumour 410, 412
Carotid subclavian bypass 295
Cat-scratch disease 412
Catecholamines, action 314–15
Catheters
    antegrade uretogram 377
    genitourinary investigations 354–6
    intercostal
        complications 358–60
        management 358
        pneumonectomy 358–60
        three-bottle system 358, 360
    micturating cystourectrogram 377
    retrograde ureterogram 377
    Seldinger technique 289–90
    sepsis 63–4, 138
    urethrogram 377
    vasogram 377
Cauda equina lesions, decompression
        478
Cauliflower ear 394
Cell adhesion 157, 162, 172, 341
Cell cycle 152
    apoptosis 152
    thymidine labelling index 172
Cell signalling pathways 150–2
Cellulitis
    orbital 393
    preseptal 393
Central nerve blocks, regional
        anaesthesia 36–7
Central nervous system 6–7, 415
    anatomy 415–23
    dementia 7
    epilepsy 6–7
    examination 417–18
    imaging 424–5
    infections 438–9
    investigations 424–6
    neurophysiology 423–4
Central venous pressure 41, 116–17
Cephalosporins, treatment of sepsis 68
Cerebral, see also Intracranial
Cerebral arteries 420–1, 436, 437, 438
Cerebral artery disease 295
Cerebral blood flow (CBF) 423–4
    autoregulation 424
Cerebral neoplasms 432
Cerebral perfusion pressure (CPP) 424
Cerebral veins 421–2

Cerebrospinal fluid (CSF) 423
    excess production 423
    fistulae, following head injury 425
Cervical carcinoma, pathophysiology 157
Cervical fusion 474
Cervical ribs 354
Cervical spinal cord injury 133, 429
Cervical spine
    anterior longitudinal ligament
        calcification 473
    compression fractures 429
    congenital spinal dysraphysm 473
    degenerative diseases 474
    diffuse idiopathic skeletal hyperostosis
        473
    fracture dislocations 429
    infective diseases 473
    inflammatory diseases 473
    Klippel–Feil syndrome 473
    neoplastic diseases 473
    nerve root decompression 474
    pain 473–4
    post-traumatic diseases 473
    psychogenic diseases 473
    spondylosis 473, 474, 475
Cervicofacial mycobacterial infections
        413
Chamberlain procedure 355
CHARGE syndrome 499
Cheilectomy, hallux rigidus 467
Chemical carcinogens 155, 374
Chemotherapy 175–6
    resistance 176
Chest injury 97–9
Chest pain, respiratory disease symptom
        354
Chest radiograph 97
    preoperative assessment 14–15
    respiratory disease investigation
        354, 355
    scout film 376
Chest wall deformities 362
    infants and children 500
Children
    chest wall deformity 500
    common disorders 489–92
    endocrine and metabolic response to
        surgery 495
    nutrition 495
    respiration 495
    sepsis 495
    see also Paediatric surgery
Chlorhexidine, skin preparation 64
Cholecystectomy gallbladder 234, 245–6,
        267
Cholecystitis
    acalculous 234–5
    acute 234–5
Choledochal cyst
    classification 513–14
    diagnosis 514
    management 514
Choledocholithiasis 236
Cholesteatoma, unsafe CSOM 396
Chondrolysis 492
Choroid plexus papilloma 423
Chromium EDTA clearance 378

Chronic obstructive airways disease
chest shape 354
lung transplantation 360
preoperative assessment 7
spontaneous pneumothorax 363
therapy 6
Chronic renal failure
diabetes 7
dialysis 382
hyperkalaemia 7
preoperative assessment 7
transplantation 382
Circle of Willis 420–1
Circulatory support
Contraindication 92
haemorrhage control 91–2
Circumcision 389, 520–1
contraindication 520
Cleft lip and palate 497
Clinical audit 191
Clinical research see Research projects
Clinical studies
analytical epidemiology, interventional
vs observational 165
case–control 165
cohort studies 165
meta-analyses 166
Club foot
bony procedures 490
clinical features 489
investigations 489
management 489–90
CO_2 analysers 29
Coagulating agents 78
Coagulation disorders, preoperative
assessment 9–10
Coagulation factors 209–10
deficiencies 219
Cocaine 35
Codeine, use 180
Coeliac plexus block 181
Cognitive disorders, head injury 426
Cohort studies 165, 193
Coiled spring' sign, intussusception 508
Cold abscesses 412
Colectomy, ileostomy 253, 257, 506
Colles fracture 444, 446
Colon see Bowel, large
Colonoscopy 250, 253, 259
Colony-forming units, model of
hemopoiesis 207
Colony-stimulating factors 206, 207
Colorectal cancer 251, 255
aetiology 255–6
management 256–7
non-surgical treatment 258–60
pathology 258
preoperative staging 256
Colorectal carcinoma 243
inheritance 159
metastases 243
obstruction 241
Colorectal emergencies
anorectal sepsis 253
colorectal injury 254
diverticulosis 252
foreign body 254

lower GI haemorrhage 252
obstruction 250–2
Coma, Glasgow Coma Scale (GCS) 95,
147, 417
Common bile duct (CBD) 231, 514
Compartment syndromes 292, 294, 298
intracompartmental pressure 449–50
pseudoparalysis 449
symptoms and signs 449
Compensatory anti-inflammatory
response syndrome (CARS), vs
SIRS 62
Complaints 190
Complement cascade 206
Compound fractures
infection 441
Compression sclerotherapy 300
Computed tomography scanning 233
head injury 93
Concussion and contrecoup injury 93
Conditions, upper GI
gallstones 245–6
gastro oesophageal reflux disease
247–8
jaundice 244–5
peptic ulcer 246–7
portal hypertension 246
Confidential Enquiry into Perioperative
Deaths (CEPOD) 20
Confidentiality, legal considerations 188,
189
Congenital dislocation of the hip (CDH)
489
clinical features 489
investigations 489
management 489
screening of infants 489
Congestive cardiac failure, preoperative
assessment 4
Conjunctiva, ocular injury 391
Conjunctivitis, bacterial and viral 393
Conn's syndrome 315–16
Consciousness, level of 432, 438
Consensus guidelines 197
Consent, legal considerations 188
Consent, preoperative assessment 1
Contact lens wear
acanthamoebic keratitis 394
bacterial keratitis 393
Contre-coup contusion 425
Cooper's ligament 269–70
Cornea, ocular injury 393
Corneal disease 392, 393
Coronary arteries
anatomy 112
blood flow 112
Coroner's court 191
Corticotrophin-releasing factor (CSF) 314
Cost-benefit analysis 272
Cost-effectiveness analysis 272
Cost-minimization analysis 272
Cost-utility analysis 272
Cough, respiratory disease symptom 354
Courvoisier's law 241, 244
Cranial nerves
I (olfactory) nerve 418
II (optic) nerve 418

III (occulomotor), IV (trochlear) and VI
(abducens) nerves 418–19
V (trigeminal) nerve 419
VII (facial) nerve 419
VIII (auditory) nerve 419–20
IX (glossopharyngeal) nerve 420
X (vagus) nerve 420
XI (accessory) nerve 420
XII (hypoglossal) nerve 420
Craniectomy and craniotomy 427
Creatinine measurement, 24-hour urine
collection 375
Creutzfeldt–Jakob disease 438, 439
Cricopharyngeal spasm 367
pharyngeal pouch, Killian's dehiscence
367
Cricothyroid membrane 351, 359
Cricothyroidotomy 97, 133, 410
Crush injuries, hand 462–3, 464
Cryoprecipitate 43
Cryptorchidism 514, 517
Crystalloids
contents 28
contraindications 92
replacement and maintenance, burns
105
Cushing's disease 315, 318, 435
management 315
Cushing's reflex 94
Cutaneous horn 403
Cystic fibrosis
association with meconium ileus 504
lung transplantation 360
Cystic hygroma 411, 496
Cystic lesions of the lung 497, 500
Cystitis 373, 385
Cystoureterogram, micturating 377, 380
Cystometrogram
videourodynamics 379
Cystoscopy, haematuria investigations
379
Cystourethroscopy 379
Cysts
abdominal mass 510
branchial 411, 496
choledochal 509, 510, 513
congenital 500, 513–14
video-assisted thoracoscopic
approach 355
dermoid 411, 496
duplication 362, 367, 503
epidermoid 411
excision 82, 84
lung, congenital 361
mesenteric 510
omental 510
ovarian cysts 390
paraoesophageal developmental 367
ranula 500
and sinuses, congenital 496
teratoid 411
teratoma 500
thyroglossal 310, 411, 496
Cytokines
Anti-cytokine therapy 68
mediators of inflammatory response
61–2, 205

neuroendocrine response to injury 107–10
overexpression 176
signal transduction 205, 206
Cytological sampling 85–6
Cytoplasmic oncogenes 154

D

Damage-control surgery 100
Danazol 333
Dance's sign, intussusception 508
Death certification 163
Decision making, ethical 186
Declaration
    of Geneva 185
    of Helsinki 185, 187
    of Oslo 185
    of Tokyo 185
Deep vein thrombosis see Venous thrombosis
Delerium, postoperative, causes 48
Dendritic cells, structure/function 203
Denonvilliers fascia 371
Dens fracture, vertebral column injury 429
Dermatome, defined 420
Dermoid cysts 84, 411, 496
Desflurane, characteristics 26
Detrusor instability 372
Detrusor
    overactivity 372
    underactivity (DUA) 373, 386
    failure 386
    symptoms 373
Dextrose–saline, composition 45
Diabetes mellitus
    amputation 458–60
    preoperative assessment 8
Diagnosis of lymphadenopathy 225
Diagnostic peritoneal lavage 99, 225
Dialysis
    haemodialysis 382
    peritoneal 382
    renal failure 382
Diaphragm
    agenesis 499
    anatomy 353–4
    eventration 353
    rupture 361
Diaphragmatic hernia
    congenital 499–500
        diagnosis 499
        management 499–500
        pulmonary hypertension 499
        pulmonary hypoplasia 499
    neonatal emergency 353
Diathermy
    capacitance coupling 79
    incisions 73
    monopolar/bipolar machines 79
    principle 78–9
Diazepam, characteristics 22
Dicyclomine 181
Diet
    cancer-protective substances 155–7
    carcinogenetic substances 155–7
    micronutrients 155

Dietary fibre 156, 262
Diffuse axonal injury (DAI) 93–4, 425
Diffuse idiopathic skeletal hyperostosis 473
DiGeorge syndrome 220
Digital nerve blocks 72–3
Digital subtraction angiography (DSA) 289, 425
Digoxin 119
Dimercaptosuccinic acid (DMSA), renogram 378, 500
Diphtheria 398
Dipstick testing 373, 375
    haematuria 373
Dislocation, shoulder joint 453, 454–5
Disseminated intravascular coagulation 143, 219–20
Disseminated intravascular coagulopathy 10, 43, 506
Distributive shock 127
Diuretics
    interactions with anaesthetic agents 19
    kidney disease 374
Dive reflex 506
Diverticular disease, bladder involvement 390
Diverticulitis 144, 252, 276
Diverticulum 367
DMSA see Dimercaptosuccinic acid
DNA, genetic code 149–50
DNA probes 161
DNA viruses 154, 157
    carcinogenesis 154
Dopamine 119, 142
Doppler ultrasound, cardiac output 118
Down's syndrome, Hirschsprung's disease association 505
Dressings 77–8, 82
Driving, cessation 424
Drug treatment
    preoperative 11
Drugs, non-prescription, and preoperative assessment 11
Dukes' stage
    classification 258
Dumb-bell tumour 521
Duodenal ulcer
    Zollinger–Ellison syndrome 319
Duodenum
    anatomy 231
    atresia 501–2
    injury 101
Duplex scanning, arterial disease 290
Duplex system 518
Dupuytren's contracture 83
Dysphagia 234, 239, 368
    defined 367

E

Ear
    foreign bodies 398–9
    inflammatory disorders 394–8
ECG
    monitoring 47, 92, 147
    perioperative assessment 15, 32
    preoperative assessment 4
    stress 4

Echocardiography 118
    applications 4
Echondroma 484
Economics
    hernia repair 272–3, 275
    laparoscopic surgery 281–2
    normal activity and work, return 273
Ectopia vesicae 371
Ectopic pregnancy, abdominal pain 390
Effectiveness, assessment 191–8
Effusion, exudate vs transudate 354, 355, 356
Ehlers–Danlos syndrome 514
Elbow joint
    injuries 455
    myositis ossificans 448
Electroencephalogram (EEG) 425
Electrolytes 45–6, 142, 375–6
    monitoring 57
    paediatric surgery 494
Elloesser procedure 362
Embolectomy 138, 293–4
EMLA cream, characteristics 22
Emphysema see Chronic obstructive airways disease
Empyema 245, 362, 439
Encephalitis 438, 439
Endarterectomy 291, 293, 295
Endocrine preoperative assessment 8
Endocrine surgery 304
Endocrine system 8–9
    adrenal insufficiency 9
    diabetes 8
    hypothyroidism 8
    hyperthyroidism 8–9
    phaeochromocytoma 9
Endometriosis, abdominal pain 390
Endoscopic retrograde cholangio-pancreatography (ERCP)
    biliary atresia 513
    choledochal cyst 513
    duodenal perforation 231
    upper GI 233
Endoscopy
    ENT 402
    upper gastrointestine 233
Endothelial cell mediators, platelets 208–9
Endothelial cells, structure/function 208–9
Endothelin 110, 209
Endotoxins 60, 61, 62
Endotracheal intubation see Intubation
Energy, nutritional requirements 52–3
Enflurane, characteristics 26
Enoximone 119
Enteral nutrition 52, 53–5
    complications 54–5
    disease-specific diets 64–5
    polymeric diets 53
    response, post injury 110
Enterocolitis, necrotizing 506–7
Eosinophilia, angiolymphoid hyperplasia 412
Eosinophils, structure/function 202
Ependymomas, spinal cord 431, 434

Epidemiology
analytical 165–6
arterial disease 287
cancer 163–4
descriptive 163–5
Epidermal growth factor 154
Epidermoid cyst 411
Epididymis, appendix epididymis torsion
516
Epididymo-orchitis 374, 516
Epidural block 36, 37, 45
Epigastric hernia 512
Epilepsy
driving 439
intracerebral and subdural abscess 439
post-traumatic 428
supratentorial neoplasms 432
Epiphyseal plate injuries 448
Episodic desaturation 31
Epistaxis 402–3
arterial ligation 401–2
bleeding source 402
external carotid artery ligation 401
hereditary haemorrhagic telangiectasia
402
internal carotid system 401
maxillary artery ligation 401
posterior ethmoidal artery caution
402
surgical intervention 401
transnasal endoscopic ligation 402
Epstein–Barr virus infection 412
Burkitt's lymphoma 157–8
Error, research projects 192
Erythroplakia 406
Erythropoietin
recombinant human 207
Escherichia coli, CSF fistula 438
Esthesioneuroblastoma 410
ESWL *see* Extracorporeal shockwave
lithotripsy
Ethical committees 186–7
Ethical decision-making 186
double effect 186
lesser of two evils 186
slippery slope 186
Ethics 184–8
Etomidate, characteristics 27
Ewing's sarcoma 431
Exercise testing 288
Exomphalos 510–12
Experimental studies 194–5
Explosion and fire hazards, operating
theatres 79
Extracorporeal shockwave lithotripsy
(ESWL) 246, 380
Exudate effusion, vs transudate 354

F

Facial cranial nerve 419
Faecal DNA analysis, colorectal cancer
260
Faecal occult blood testing, colorectal
cancer 259
Fasciotomy 102, 291
Fat, and carcinogenesis 156

Fat embolism 102, 448
Fatty acids, essential (EFA), and mastalgia
332
Fatty acids, non-essential (NEFA)
metabolism post injury 108
neuroendocrine response to injury 107
Femoral epiphysis
avascular necrosis 448
Perthes' disease 490–1
slipped 491–2
Femoral exostosis 486
Femoral gait, intoeing 490
Femoral hernia
three open approaches 282
open prosthetic repair 282
laparoscopic repair 282–3
Femoral metastases 484–5
Femoral nerve stretch test 480
Femur, osteosarcoma 488
Femur neck fractures 446–7
Fentanyl, characteristics 23, 27, 35
Fertility 389
α-Fetoprotein 171, 243
Fever, postoperative causes 48
Fibre, dietary 155
Fibrinolysis 210, 220
Fibroblast growth factor 154, 162, 172
Fibroblasts
structure/function 203
wound healing 81, 82
Fibromatosis 412
Finger clubbing, respiratory disease
symptom 354
Fistula-in-ano 260, 513
FK506, immunosuppressant 229
Flail chest 91
following thoracic surgery 361
Flat foot 490
Flexible sigmoidoscopy, colorectal cancer
250, 259–60
Fludrocortisone 316
Fluids
crystalloids, composition 28
and electrolytes, paediatric surgery 494
overload, cardiac failure 47
replacement and maintenance 46
resuscitation 66
Follicular stimulating hormone (FSH),
pituitary gland 318, 435
Foot disorders
clinical assessment 464–5
examination 464–5
Freiberg's disease 469
hallux rigidus 467
hallux valgus 467–9
history 464
investigation 465
Morton's metatarsalgia 469
osteoarthritis of the subtalar joint 467
plantar fasciitis 467
rheumatoid arthritis 466–7
Sever's disease 467
see also Ankle disorders
Foreign bodies
aural 398–9
ENT 398–400
ingestion 399–400

nasal 399
Fournier's gangrene 254, 388
Fowler–Stephen's procedure 517
Fractures 440
ankle 446
avascular necrosis 448
bimalleolar 446, 447
bone grafting 445
clinical assessment 442–3
closed fractures 441
colles fracture 444, 446
compartment syndromes
diagnosis 449–50
intracompartmental pressure 449, 450
pseudoparalysis 449
symptoms and signs 449
treatment 450
complications 447–9
delayed 448
immediate 447–8
late 448–9
compound 441, 448, 463, 464
infection 441, 448
definitive treatment 443–5
conservative 444
operative 444–5
delayed union 441–2
descriptions for imaging 443
distal radial 445–6
early reduction 443
early rehabilitation 445
epiphyseal plate injuries 448
fat embolism 448
femur neck 446–7
green stick 440
hand injuries 462–4
healing 441–2
inflammatory phase 441
non-union, atrophic/hypertrophic
442
pseudoarthrosis 442
remodelling phase 441
reparative phase 441
infection 448
investigations 443
malunion/non-union 442
management 443–5
myositis ossificans 448
open ('compound') fractures 441
pain assessment and relief 443, 449
pallor 449
paraesthesia 449
paralysis 449
pathological 441
osteoporosis 431
plaster of Paris casts 444
pulselessness 449
specific 445–7
stress 441
Sudeck's atrophy 449
thromboembolic phenomena 445
Volkmann's ischaemic contracture 448
Frank–Starling mechanism 114
Freiberg's disease 469
Fresh frozen plasma 43, 217
Frozen shoulder 476
Fusarium sp., fungal keratitis 393

G

Gait
anteversion of the femoral gait 490
flat foot 490
metatarsus adductus 490
Gallbladder
ultrasound 234
Gallstone ileus 245
Gallstones 245–6
Gangrene, Fournier's gangrene 254, 388
Gas exchange 129
Gastrectomy, Zollinger–Ellison syndrome 319
Gastric, *see also* Stomach
Gastric Carcinoma 240–1
Gastric perforation, neonatal 501
Gastric ulcers 238, 247
Gastric volvulus, neonatal 501
Gastrin, assay 319
Gastrinoma 319
Gastro-oesophageal reflux
diagnosis 500–1
disease (GORD) 234, 239, 247–8
infants 500
management 501
Nissen's fundoplication 501
pH monitoring 234
treatment 247–8
Gastrograffin swallow, rupture site identification 363
Gastrointestinal, *see also* Abdominal
Gastrointestinal atresia 503
Gastrointestinal duplications
diagnosis 503
management 503
Gastrointestinal malrotation 502
Gastrointestinal motility, irritable bowel syndrome 256
Gastrointestinal secretions
composition 45
gastric acid 247, 319
Gastrointestinal surgery
abdominal mass 510
anatomy and physiology 230–2
bleeding 237–8, 253
complications, postoperative 49
and malignant disease 256
manometry 234
oesophageal function test 233
paediatric surgery 500–1
pH monitoring 235
preexisting disease assessment 18
selective digestive decontamination (SDD) 63
surgical techniques 272–6
Gastrointestinal system
abdominal mass 510
paediatric surgery 500–1
Gastrointestinal tumours 318–20
Gastroschisis and exomphalos 510–11
Gastrostomy, enteral nutrition 53–5
Gaussian distribution 195
Gelofusine, composition 125
Gene testing 160
Gene therapy 177
Genetic code 149–50

Genetics
linkage analysis 160
segregation analysis 159–60
two-hit hypothesis 154
Genital anomalies 280
Genitourinary system 369
abdominal mass 510
anatomy and developmental anomalies 369–72
diseases and treatment 380
investigations 375–80
functional tests 377–9
pain 373–4
urological conditions 379–80
Germ-cell tumours 522
Giant cell tumour 485
Gillick case, consent 189
Glasgow Coma Scale (GCS) 95, 417
Glaucoma 392
Glioblastoma multiforme 434
Gliomas
grading systems 434
Glomerulonephritis 380
haematuria 373
Glossopharyngeal cranial nerve 420
Glucagon, action 321
Glucagonoma 319
Glucocorticoids, secretion and action 314
Glutathione 176
Glycogenolysis, neuroendocrine response to injury 108
P-Glycoprotein, *mdr*-gene 176
Glycoprotein hormones, erythropoietin 207
Glycoproteins, imunogenicity 212
Glycopyronium, characteristics 22
Gonadotrophinomas 435
Gonadotrophins, pituitary gland 435
Gonococcus, septic arthritis 471
Goserelin 333
Gout and pseudo-gout
arthritis 451
Grafts
arterial 290–1
autologous vein 290
bone, allo, auto, iso, and xenografts 445
bypass 293
donor, and recipient 227
infection 298
rejection 228–9
renal 313
Granulation tissue 80
Granulomas, spontaneous pneumothorax 363–4
Granulomatous disease, chronic 220
Graves' disease 222–3
Groin and scrotum, paediatric surgery 514–18
Groin hernias, children
diagnosis 277–8
incarceration and strangulation 277–8
operation 278
Growth hormone (GH)
acromegaly 435
pituitary gland 435
Growth hormone releasing hormone (GRH), pituitary gland 435

Gunshot injury 93
Gut decontamination, selective (SDD) 63–4
Gut-associated lymphoid tissue (GALT) 204
Gynaecology, urological problems 390
Gynaecomastia 336

H

Haem, structure 207–8
Haemaccel, composition 46
Haemangioma 411
juvenile 496–7
strawberry capillary 496–7
Haematocrit, postoperative 46
Haematology, preoperative assessment 9–10, 14
Haematoma
auricular 394
intracranial 94, 95, 437–8
subdural 94, 95, 425–6
wound 47
Haematuria 373
dipstick testing of urine 373
investigations 379
pain associated 373
schistosomiasis 374
vaginal bleeding 390
Haemodialysis 382
Haemoglobin
blood transfusion 42–4
chronic renal failure 7
correction in anaemia 9
measurement 131, 207–8
oxygen dissociation curve 129, 208
structure 207
Haemophilia A and B 219
arthritis 451, 452
Haemophilus influenzae
acute supraglottitis 398
preseptal cellulitis 393
Haemophilus spp., bacterial conjunctivitis 393
Haemopneumothorax, spontaneous 364
Haemopoiesis 207
Haemopoietic and lymphoreticular systems
anatomy 200–5
pathology 214
physiology 205
Haemopoietic organs, cellularity changes 200
Haemopoietic system
anatomy and physiology 200–14
pathological states 214–29
Haemoptysis, respiratory disease symptom 354
Haemorrhage
bone injuries 102–3
coma-producing 436
control 91–2
gastrointestinal 252
intracranial 436–7
postoperative complications 46
sepsis 98
subarachnoid 436–7
vascular surgery 298

Haemorrhage control, circulatory
     support 91–92
Haemorrhagic telangiectasia, hereditary
     10, 402
Haemorrhoids 261
Haemostasis 78–9, 208–10
   preoperative assessment 9–10
   wounds 78
Haemothorax 98
   following thoracic surgery 361
Hallux rigidus 467, 468
   arthrodesis 467
   arthroplasty 467
   cheilectomy 467
Hallux valgus 467–9
   arthrodesis 468
   excision arthroplasty 468
   metatarsal osteotomy 468
Hallux varus deformity 468
Halothane
   characteristics 25
   toxicity 25–6, 32
Hamartomas 362
Hand hygiene 64
Hand infections
   diagnosis 464
   management 464
Hand injuries 462–4
   bone trauma 462–3
   clinical assessment 462
   closed fractures 463
   crush injuries 462–3
   dislocations and fracture dislocations
     463
   open fractures 463–4
   palmar compartments and spaces 462
   tendons 461–2
Hangman's fracture, vertebral column
     injury 429
Harris–Benedict equation, calories 105
Harrison's groove 482
Hartmann's fluid, composition 28, 45
Hartmann's procedure, acute
     diverticulitis 252, 257
Hashimoto's thyroiditis 223, 308, 309
Head injury 93–5
   brain death 428
   brain displacement and internal
     herniations 425
   cerebrospinal fluid fistulae 427
   clinical features 426
   epilepsy 427
   headaches 428
   intracerebral haemorrhages 425
   laceration and diffuse axonal injury 425
   localized areas of contusion 425
   management 426–7
   missile injuries 428
   neurological deficits 426
   oedema 425
   pathology 425–6
   pathophysiology 94
   rehabilitation 428
   surface haematomas 425–6
   surgery 427–8
Head and neck
   paediatric surgery 496–7

treatment 406–7
tumours 403–13
   see also Neck masses
Headaches, head injury 428
Health Service Commissioner,
     Ombudsman 190
Heart see Cardiovascular system
Heart rate 40
   as indication of haemorrhage 91–2
Heart valves
   anatomy 111
   preoperative assessment 4–5
   prostheses, preoperative assessment
     10
Helicobacter pylori, peptic ulcer 236–7,
     501
Heller's myotomy 367
Hemofiltration 142–3
   in ARF 142
   renal replacement therapy 142
Henderson–Hasselbach equation,
     bicarbonate 131
Henoch–Schönlein purpura 508, 510, 515
Heparin
   dosages 289
   half-life 289
   management of surgery 289–92
   prophylaxis of thromboembolic
     disease 13
Hepatic encephalopathy 143–4
Hepatitis B, and sepsis, surgical 69
Hepatitis C, and sepsis, surgical 69
Hepatobiliary disorders, paediatric
     surgery 513–14
Hepatoblastoma, infants and young
     children 522
Hepatocellular carcinoma (HCC)
   older children 522
   pathophysiology 157, 243
Hepatosplenomegaly 410, 510
Hereditary haemorrhagic telangiectasia
     9–10, 402
Hereditary non-polposis colorectal
     cancer (HNPCC) syndrome 159
Hernia 264
   Bochdalek 353
   diaphragmatic 353–4
     neonatal emergency 353
   epigastric 512
   femoral 279, 282–3
   groin 277–8
   incisional 284–5
   inguinal 281, 514–15
   Littre' 277
   Morgagni 353
   paraumbilical 512
   Richter's 277
   sites 353
   sliding 353
   supraumbilical 512
   umbilical 283, 512
Hernia general complications
   incarceration, obstruction,
     strangulation 276–7
   Littre's hernia, Meckel's diverticulum
     277
   Richter's hernia 277

Hernia management 264
   abdominal wall anatomy 267–71
   aetiology 271–2
   anaesthesia 275–6
   economics 272–4
   femoral hernia 279–80, 282–3
   general complications 276–7
   groin hernias, children 277–8
   incisional hernia 284–5
   inguinal hernia, adults 280–1
   laparoscopic groin hernia repair 281–2
   laparoscopic repair, inguinal hernia 267
   lump diagnosis, adult 278–80
   principles, hernia surgery 274
   prosthetic biomaterials 274–5
   tension-free hernia repair 267
   umbilical hernia, adults 283
Hernia surgery, principles 274
Heroin 180
Herpes simplex, viral keratitis 393
Hexachlorophene, skin preparation 64
Hiatus hernia 231–2, 247
High-dependency unit (HDU) 66, 90, 146
Hill Sachs lesion, shoulder joint injury
     454–5
Hip joint
   dislocation, congenital (CDH) 489
   injuries 455
   replacement surgery 456, 457
   transient synovitis 491
Hippocratic Oath 184, 185
Hirschsprung's disease 505–6
   Down's syndrome association 505
   Ondine's curse association 505, 521
   Waardenburg syndrome association
     505
Histamine, wound healing 80
HIV infection and AIDS 221, 222
   HIV natural history 158
   intracranial infection 438
   retroviruses 154, 157
   spontaneous pneumothorax 363–4
   surgical sepsis 69
Hordeolum, external 393
Hormone replacement therapy 255, 481
Horseshoe kidney 370
Human chorionic gonadotrophin,
     tumour marker 171, 376, 522
Human papilloma viruses (HPV) 157, 260
Hutchinson's freckle 403
Hydatid of Morgagni 388, 516
Hydralazine 114
Hydrocele 515
   see also Inguinal hernia
Hydrocephalus 423, 432, 433
   infratentorial neoplasms 433
Hydronephrosis 383–4, 518
5-Hydroxy-indole-acetic acid (5-HIAA) 320
Hyoscine, characteristics 22
Hyperaldosteronism 315–16
Hyperbilirubinaemia 244, 513
Hypercalcaemia, and parathormone 311,
     312
Hypercarbia, hypoventilation 31, 32
Hyperkalemia
   cardiac resuscitation 121
   side-effects of suxamethonium 28

Hyperparathyroidism 312–13, 320, 376
Hypersplenism 226, 244
Hypertension
    diabetes mellitus 8
    preoperative assessment 4
    vasodilatation 32
Hyperthyroidism (Graves' disease) 222–3
    preoperative assessment 8–9
    secondary 435
Hypocalcaemia
    and parathormone 311
    post-operative 313
Hypoglossal nerve 420
Hypoparathyroidism 312, 313
Hypopharyngeal cancer 409
Hypopharynx see Larynx and
        hypopharynx
Hypospadias 371–2, 520
Hypotension
    causes 32
    differential diagnosis 46
Hypothalamic–pituitary–adrenal axis,
        neuroendocrine response to injury
        107
Hypothalamus
    anatomy and physiology 317–18
    hormones 318
    Pituitary tumour 318
Hypothermia, infant 494
Hypothyroidism, preoperative
        assessment 8
Hypoventilation, hypercarbia 31
Hypovolaemia, on recovery from
        anaesthesia 30
Hypovolaemic shock 126
Hypoxaemia
    early
        airway obstruction 30
        alveolar hypoventilation 30
    late
        episodic desaturation 31
        respiratory dysfunction 31
    primary, causes during anaesthesia
        34
    recovery from anaesthesia 30
Hypoxia, diffusion 30
Hysterectomy, ureter damage 390

I

131I-MIBG scanning,
        phaeochromocytoma 316
Ileal conduit urine diversion 385–6
Ileostomy 253, 257, 506
Ileus
    differential diagnosis 49
    meconium 504
    paralytic 59, 430, 495
Iliac artery stenosis 290
Immune responses, cancer 224
Immunity
    acquired 211–14
    innate 210–11
Immunodeficiency, and cancer 224
Immunodeficiency disorders 220–2
Immunodiagnosis 224
Immunofluorescence 214

Immunoglobulins
    classes 212–13
    serology 213–14
Immunosuppressants 11, 218
    FK506 229
Immunosuppression, leukaemias 221
Immunotherapy 224
Impotence 389
Incisional hernias 48, 284
    aetiological factors 284
    incidence 284
    principles, open repair 284–5
Incisions 73, 87
    closure 74–6
    cutting diathermy 73
    muscle-sparing 357
Incontinence 386–7
    bladder neck 387
    investigations 380–1
    and prostate gland 387
    stress 373, 379, 387
    urge 372
Infants see Children; Paediatrics
Infections
    burns 103–5
    intensive care unit (ICU) 144–5
    local and systemic response 59
    postoperative causes 48
    postsplenectomy 226
    surgical wound complications 47–8
    see also Sepsis, surgical
Infectious mononucleosis 412
Infiltrative myelopathies 214
Inflammatory bowel disease 252, 254,
        256, 453
    arthropathy association 452
    Crohn's disease (CD) 255, 256–7
    ulcerative colitis (UC) 254–5, 256
Inflammatory reaction 59
Inflammatory response 61–2, 210–11
Infratentorial neoplasms, hydrocephalus
        434
Inguinal hernia 278–9, 514
    anterior open repair 280
    diagnosis 280, 514
    double-breasting technique 280
    and hydrocele 514
    Lichtenstein technique 280–1
    management 514–15
    postoperative care 281
    'silk-glove' sign 514
    strangulated hernia 281
Inguino-scrotal emergencies 515
Inhalational agents, pharmacology 25–6
Injury see Trauma; Wounds
Inotropes 118–19
Insulinoma 318–19
    provocation tests, contraindications
        318
Integrins 162, 201, 209
Intensive care unit 145
    Apache II scoring system 147, 235
    criteria for admission 94–5, 146–7
    discharge 146–7
    equipment 115–16
    admission 146–7
    infections 144–5

nosocomial pneumonia 144–5
    organization 145–6
    principles 145
    scoring 147–8
    staffing 145–6
Intercellular communication 205–7
Intercostal catheters 358
Intercostobrachial nerve 324–5
Interferon 206, 381, 497
Interleukins 108, 206
    mediators of inflammatory response 62
Intermittent claudication 292
International Rhinitis Management
        Working Group, rhinitis
        classification 396–7
Intervertebral discs 431
    discectomy 480
Intestinal mucosal barrier, disruption
        59–60
Intra-aortic balloon pump 120
Intra-vascular catheter-related infection
        in ICU 145
Intracerebral abscess 439
Intracranial, see also Brain; Cerebral
Intracranial aneurysm 436
Intracranial haematomas 94, 438
    warfarin 438
Intracranial haemorrhage 436–8
Intracranial infection, HIV infection 438
Intracranial neoplasms 432–6
    investigations 433
    management 433
    metastatic 433
Intracranial vascular disease 436–8
Intradural lesions
    spinal cord compression 431
Intrathoracic pressure, intercostals
        catheter 358
Intravenous regional anaesthesia 36, 73
    anaesthetic agents 25, 26–7
Intravenous urogram (IVU) 376, 377
    disadvantages 377
    uses 377
Intubation 23
    advantages/disadvantages 24
    failure 33–4
    oesophageal 29
    endotracheal 132–3
Intubation, difficult 17, 33
    predictors 20
Intussusception 508
    'coiled spring' sign 508
    Dance's sign 508
    diagnosis 508
    Henoch–Schönlein purpura 508, 509
    management 508–9
    Meckel's diverticulum 508
    'pseudokidney' sign 508
    'red currant jelly' stool 508
Invasion and metastases
    development 162–3
Invasive colorectal surgery 263
Iodo-cholesterol scanning 316
Ionizing radiation
    carcinogenesis 155
    energy 174
    risk factor for breast disease 337

Iron metabolism 208
Irritable bowel syndrome 256
Ischaemia
    management 294
    Raynaud's phenomenon 223, 294
Ischaemic heart disease, preoperative
        assessment 3–4
Ischemia–reperfusion injury 60
Isoflurane, characteristics 26
Isosorbide dinitrate 114
Isotopic scanning, ventricular ejection
        fraction 4
Ivor Lewis resection, carcinoma in lower
        oesophagus 368

J

Jaundice 244–5
    liver failure, acute 143–4
    neonatal 513
    postoperative 48
Jefferson fracture, vertebral column
        injury 429
Jejunoileal atresia 503
Jejunostomy, enteral nutrition 54
Joints
    clinical assessment 450
    clinical history 450–1
    infections 469–73
    injuries 452–5
        classification 452–3
        examination 453
        history 453
        investigations 453–4
        management 454
        specific joints 454–5
    pain 473–80
    replacement 455–8
        clinical assessment 456–7
        implant failure 458
Jugular venous bulb, oxygen assessment
        94
Juvenile haemangioma 496–7

K

Keller's arthroplasty 468
Keratitis
    acanthamoebic 394
    bacterial 393
    fungal 393
    viral 393
Keratoacanthoma 403–4
Keratoconjunctivitis sicca, bilateral
        parotid gland enlargement 413
Kidney 312
    anatomy 369–70
    embryological development 370
    horseshoe 370
    surgical anatomy 369–70
    trauma 381
    ultrasound scan 376
    see also Renal
Kikuchi's disease 412
Killian's dehiscence, pharyngeal pouch
        367
Kinura's disease 412

Klippel–Feil syndrome 473, 521
Klippel–Trenaunay syndrome 303
Knee joint
    osteoarthritis 452
    replacement surgery 457
Kohler's disease 465
Kupffer cells, structure/function 203

L

Lactation, breast changes 325
Langerhans cells 203
Laparoscopic groin hernia repair 281
    disadvantages 282
Laparoscopic repair, hernia 267, 282–3
Laparoscopy 99, 239, 242, 278
Laparotomy 99–100
    avoiding 100
Laplace's law 252
Large intestine see Bowel, large
Laryngeal mask airway 24, 122, 133
Larynx and hypopharynx
    anatomy 408
    clinical evaluation 408
    tumours 408
        second primary 409
Laseque's test, sciatica 480
Lasers
    types 79
    uses 79
Legal considerations 188–91
Lentigo maligna melanoma 403
Leukaemias
    immunosuppression 218
    pharmacological sanctuaries 175
Leukocytes, wound healing 80
Leukoplakia 406
Leukotrienes 204
Li–Fraumeni syndrome 159, 337, 522
    mutation site 155
Life style influences
    herbal products 11
Ligatures 76, 78
Lignocaine 35, 44, 72
Limb see Lower limb
Linkage analysis 160
α-Linoleic acid 156
γ-Linolenic acid 333
Lipid mediators 206
Lisch nodules 413
Listeria monocytogenes, HIV infection
        438
Liver 7
    abdominal mass 510
    anatomy and access 231
    failure 8
    portal venous system 231–2
Liver cancer 156, 157, 244
Liver disease, preanaesthesia assessment
        18
Liver failure, acute 143–4
    clinical presentation 143–4
    etiology 143
Liver function tests 242–3, 244, 245
Liver injury 100–1
Liver metastases, carcinoid tumours 322
Liver tumours 522–3

Lobar collapse
    muscle-sparing incision 357
    radiographic appearance 356
Lobectomy, cancer in elderly patients 360
Local anaesthesia 34–5, 44–5, 72–3, 275–6
    infiltration 44, 72
Local invasion, colorectal cancer 256
Loin incision 369
Loin pain 380, 518
Looser's zones, osteomalacia 483
Lorazepam, characteristics 22
Lower gastrointestine (GI)
    anal cancer 260
    anorectal cancer 260–2
    anorectal disorders 262–3
    colorectal cancer 255–8
    colorectal cancer, non-surgical
        treatment 258–60
    colorectal emergencies 250–4
    colorectal investigations 250
    inflammatory bowel disease 254–5
    invasive colorectal surgery 263
    surgical anatomy 249
Lower limb 298–303
    anatomy 298
    pathophysiology 289–9
Ludwig's angina 412
Lumbar puncture 423, 425
    intracerebral abscess 439
    meningitis 438
Lumbar spinal anatomy 479
Lumbosacral spine
    MRI 481
    nerve root compression 480
    stenosis 482
Lung, lymphatic drainage 352
Lung abscess 363
Lung cancer 364–6
    bone metastases 485, 487
    lobectomy for elderly patients 360
    MRI 365
    non-small cell 364–5
    pleural-based tumours 365–6
    secondary tumours 365
    small cell 364
    TNM staging system 365
    WHO histologic classification 364
Lung surgery see Pulmonary surgery
Lung transplantation 360
Lung volume reduction 360–1
Lung volumes, spirometry 5, 129
Lungs, pulmonary perfusion 130–1
Luteinizing hormone (LH), pituitary
        gland 318, 435
Luteinizing hormone releasing hormone
        (LHRH)
    analogue 333
    prostate cancer 388
Lymph glands, structure/function 204–5
Lymph node surgery, malignant disease
        224
Lymphadenitis
    bacterial 412
    granulomatous 412
    viral 412
Lymphadenopathy
    periauricular 393

Lymphangio-leiomyomatosis,
    spontaneous pneumothorax 363
Lymphatic channels and nodes
    breast 324
    and cancer 174
    drainage, lung 352
    post-surgical leak 298
Lymphocytes
    structure/function 202, 204–5, 212
    see also B and T cells
Lymphoma 522–3
    salivary gland 413
Lymphoreticular system
    anatomy and physiology 199–214
    pathological states 214
Lymphoreticular systems, pathological
    states 214–29
Lynch syndrome 337–8

M

Macrophages
    MODS 138
    structure/function 203
Madelung's disease 412
Magnetic resonance
    angiography (MRA) 289, 425
    cholangio-pancreatography (MRCP) 233
    imaging 233, 250
    mammography 327
Major histocompatibility (MHC) antigens
    212, 227–8
Malignant hyperpyrexia, anaesthetic
    agents 17
Malignant melanoma 260, 403, 404
Malignant mesothelioma, asbestos
    exposure 365
Malignant pleural effusion 366
Malnutrition 50–1, 60
    and sepsis 67
Malrotation 502
    diagnosis 502
    management 503
Mamillary body 317
Mammography 325–7
Manometry
    oesophageal 234
Marfan's syndrome 514
    spontaneous pneumothorax 363
Mast cells 203–4
mdr-gene, P-glycoprotein 172, 176, 177
Mean arterial pressure (MAP) 40
Meckel's diverticulum 277, 508, 509
Meckel's remnants 511
Meconium ileus
    cystic fibrosis association 504
    diagnosis and management 504
Meconium peritonitis 504
Meconium plug syndrome 506
Mediastinitis 363
Mediastinoscope 355
Mediastinotomy 357
Mediastinum
    anatomy 353
    divisions 353
    glands, positron emission tomography
        (PET) 354

masses 500
    tumours 353
Mediators 224
    effector response 207
Mediators of inflammatory response
    antiinflammatory mediators 62
    proinflammatory mediators 62
Medulloblastomas 434
Melanoma, Breslow scale assessment 404
Meningiomas
    sites 433
    spinal cord 431
Meningism 436
Meningitis
    clinical manifestation 438
    lumbar puncture 438
    tuberculous 438
Menstrual cycle, breast changes 325
Mercaptoacetyltriglycine (MAG 3)
    renogram 377–8
Merkel cell carcinoma 405
Mesenteric arterial disease 287
Mesenteric cyst 510
Mesothelioma, malignant 365–6
Meta-analyses, clinical studies 166
Metabolic bone disease 480–3
Metabolic rate, burns 104, 108
Metabolism and utilization, energy
    substrates, 108
Metanephrines 314, 316
Metastatic disease, colorectal cancer 258,
    259
Metatarsal osteotomy, hallux valgus 468
Metatarsalgia 469
Metatarsus adductus 490
Methotrexate, action 175, 176
Methylprednisolone, spinal cord damage
    429–30
Metronidazole, treatment of sepsis 65, 68
Metyrapone 315, 436
Microglial cells 203
Micrometastases 173, 346, 389
Micronutrients 57, 155, 156–7
Microorganisms, development of sepsis
    60–1
Midazolam, characteristics 22
Midgut volvulus
    diagnosis 502
Milligan–Morgan technique 261
Milk scan 501
Milrinone 119
Minitracheostomy, Seldinger technique
    134, 351, 359
Minor histocompatability (MHC)
    antigens 228
Minoxidil 114
Mixed venous saturation 115, 116, 117
Mondor's disease 335
Monoamine oxidase inhibitors
    anaesthetic risks 12
    interactions with anaesthetic agents 19
    pre-surgery 12
Monoclonal antibodies 214, 228, 382, 522
    therapy 178
Monocytes, structure/function 201–2
Mononucleosis, infectious 412
Morgagni hernia 353

Morphine 27, 44
    characteristics 23
    complications 180–1
    use 181
Morton's metatarsalgia 469
Mucoepidermoid carcinoma 407, 413
Mucosa-associated lymphoid tissue
    (MALT) 204, 205, 213
Mucositis 181
Multi-organ dysfunction syndrome
    (MODS)
    acute liver failure 143–4
    acute lung injury, ARDS 139–41
    acute renal failure 141–3
    definition 138
    infections in ICU 144–6
    pathophysiology 138–9
    prevention and therapy 139
    SIRS in 138
    treatment 139
Multicystic dysplastic kidney 518
Multiple endocrine neoplasia
    APUD cells 320
    hyperparathyroidism 312–13
    MEN I and II 309, 316, 320
Multiple sclerosis, bladder function 374,
    386
Murphy's sign, acute cholecystitis 234
Muscle-sparing incision, lobar collapse
    357
Musculoskeletal system 440–92
Myasthenia gravis 223
Mycobacterial infections 413
Myelodysplastic syndrome 214
Myelography, central nervous system
    investigations 425
Myelopathies, infiltrative 214
Myocardial contusion, following thoracic
    surgery 98, 121–2, 361
Myocardial infarction
    confusion with spontaneous
        pneumothorax 363
    postoperative 45
    preoperative assessment 3
    reinfarction risk 21, 297
Myocardial ischaemia, perioperative 32
Myocardial protection, cardiopulmonary
    bypass 120–1
Myofibroblasts, structure/function 203
Myositis ossificans 448
    following elbow injury 455
Myotome, defined 423

N

Naevus sebaceous of Jodassohn 404
Naftidrofuryl 292
Naloxone 41, 181
Nasal obstruction, button batteries 399
Nasopharyngeal carcinoma, Epstein–Barr
    virus infection 157, 408, 412
Nasopharynx
    anatomy 407–8
    angiofibroma, juvenile 408
    cancer 408
National Institute for Clinical Excellence
    (NICE) 272, 274

National Wilms' Tumour Study Staging System (NWTS-3) 521
Natural killer cells, structure/function 202
Nausea and vomiting 55
  cancer 181
  postoperative 33, 49
Neck, *see also* Cervical spine
Neck dissection
  radical 406, 408, 413
  supraomohyoid 406
Neck injuries 97
Neck masses
  congenital 411
  history 410
  imaging 410
  inflammatory 412
  investigations 410
  physical examination 410
  ultrasound examination 411
Necrotizing enterocolitis (NEC)
  diagnosis 506
  management 506–7
Needle biopsy 85, 328
Needle catheter jejunostomy 54
Needles, types 77
Negligence 190–1
Nelson's syndrome 315
Neoadjuvant therapy 258–9
Neonates
  diaphragmatic hernias 353–4
  gastric conditions 501
  intestinal obstruction 501
    annular pancreas 501–2
    causes 502
    duodenal atresia 501–2
    gastrointestinal duplications 503
    jejunal and ileal atresia 503
    malrotation 502–3
    meconium ileus 504
  oesophageal atresia 367
  sepsis 495
  surgery 494
Neoplasia 252–3
Nephroblastoma *see* Wilms' tumour
Nephrolithotomy 380
Nephroureterectomy 381, 384, 518
Nerve blocks
  digital 72
  field 73
  regional anaesthesia 35
Nerve conduction 425
Neuroblastoma
  diagnosis 521–2
  management 522
  staging 522
Neuroendocrine
  Hypothalamo-pituitary-adrenal axis 107–8
Neuroendocrine response to injury 106–7
Neurofibroma 366, 412, 500
  posterior mediastinum 353
  spinal cord 431
Neurofibromatosis, mutation 155
Neurogenic bladder 430, 504, 519
Neurogenic shock 128
Neurological assessment 92
Neuromuscular paralysis 24, 25

Neurophysiological investigations 425–6
Neurotmesis, bone injury 102
Neutrophils
  mediators of inflammatory response 61–2
  structure/function 201
  transfusion 215
Nifedipine 294
Nissen's fundoplication, gastro-oesophageal reflux 247, 501
Nitrates, interactions with anaesthetic agents 19
Nitric oxide 110, 209
Nitrogen, nutritional requirements 52–3
Nitroglycerin 114, 512
Nitroprusside 114, 317
Nitrous oxide
  characteristics 26
  diffusion hypoxia 26, 30
Nonsteroidal anti-inflammatory drugs
  analgesia 25
  cancer pain 178–81
  postoperative pain 32–3, 44–5
Noradrenaline, action 314
Normal distribution 195, 196
Nose, foreign bodies 399
Nose and sinuses, inflammatory disorders 396–7
Nosocomial pneumonia 144–5
Nuclear isotope renography
  bone scan 378
  chromium EDTA clearance 378
  dimercaptosuccinic acid 378
  MAG3 renogram 377–8
Nuclear oncogenes 154
Nutrition, *see also* Diet
Nutritional support
  enteral nutrition 52, 53–5
  energy, nitrogen requirements 52–3
  indications 50–1
  planning algorithm 51
  routes of administration 53–4
  total parenteral nutrition 52, 55–7

O

Obesity
  and breast carcinoma 338
  morbid
    anaesthesia risks 10
    perioperative problems 10
Observational studies 193–4
Obstructive shock 126–7
Obstructive sleep apnoea 6
Obturator hernia 276–7, 277, 280
Occlusion, tests 288–9
Ocular infection 392–4
  conjunctiva 393
  cornea 393–4
  eyelid 392–3
  orbit 393
Ocular injury 391–2
Odontoid fracture, vertebral column injury 429
Odonyphagia, defined 367
Oedema
  increased permeability 140

Oesophageal atresia 367
  anatomical variations 497–8
  anomalies 498–9
  CHARGE syndrome 499
  complications 499
  diagnosis 499
  management 499
  maternal polyhydramnios 499
  VACTERL association 498, 504
Oesophageal diseases 366–8
Oesophageal function tests
  manometry 234
  pH monitoring 234
Oesophageal speech 409
Oesophagectomy
  oesophageal carcinoma 368
  transhiatal 368
Oesophago-gastro-duodenoscopy (OGD) 233, 253
Oesophagoscope 366, 409
Oesophagus
  achalasia 367
  anatomy 353
  atresia 367, 497–9
  Barrett's 239, 248
  carcinoma 239–40
    oesophagectomy 368
    radiotherapy 368
  cervical, repair using small bowel graft 368
  diseases 366–8
    motility problems 367
  manometry 234
  pH measurement 235, 367
  pressure measurement 367
  rupture, following thoracic surgery 361
  strictures 233, 267–8, 501
Oestrogen receptor 156, 341
  assay 172
Oestrogens, and cancer 158–9
Olfactory cranial nerve 418
Oligodendroglioma 434
Oligonucleotides, antisense 177
Ombudsman, Health Service Commissioner 190
Omental cyst 510
Omphalocoele 510–11
Oncogenes 154
Ondine's curse, Hirschsprung's disease association 505
Operating theatres, explosion and fire hazards 79
Operations
  classification 20
  high-risk surgical patients 21
Opioids 22, 27
  characteristics 23
  combination preparations 180
  episodic desaturation 31
  postoperative 36, 44
  routes of administration 36
  strong 180–1
  weak 180
Optic cranial nerve 418
Oral cavity
  anatomy 405
  diagnostic tests and procedures 406

history 405
physical examination 405–6
tumours 406–7
Oral contraceptives
anaesthetic risks 13
and breast disease 337
Orbital cellulitis 393
Orchidectomy 159, 388, 389, 517
Orchidopexy 374, 517
Orchitis 388, 516
Organ donation 428
Organ transplantation
graft rejection 227, 228–9
histocompatibility antigens 227–8
Oropharynx
tumours 405–7
Ortolani's test, CDH 489
Osteoarthritis
ankle joint 465
hip 453, 457, 458
knee 452
patellofemoral 450
subtalar joint 467
Osteoarthropathy, hypertrophic,
symptom of respiratory disease
354
Osteochondritis, Freiberg's 469
Osteochondritis dissecans of the talus
465–6
Osteomalacia 431
clinical features 483
dietary deficiencies 483
radiographic changes 483
Osteomyelitis 395, 439
acute
clinical features 469–70
complications 470
differential diagnosis 471
investigations 470
management 470
chronic
amputation 471
amyloidosis 470
clinical features 470
investigations 470
management 470–1
Osteopaenia 449, 452
Osteoporosis 480–1
vertebral column 431
Osteosarcoma 158
isotope bone scan 488
Osteotomy
metatarsal, hallux valgus 468
rheumatoid arthritis 466
Otitis externa 394–5
malignant 395
necrotizing 395
Otitis media
acute 395
chronic suppurative 396
classification 396
effusion 395–6
Otorrhoea, following head injury 396, 427
Ovarian ablation 347
Ovarian cancer, BRCA1 gene 159
Ovarian cysts, abdominal pain 390
Oxpentifylline 292

Oxygen
and metabolic rate 121
pulse oximetry 29, 41, 131, 208
saturation 208
transcutaneous monitoring 131
Oxygen assessment, jugular venous bulb
94
Oxygen consumption, physiology of
cardiovascular system 115
Oxygen delivery, physiology of
cardiovascular system 114–15
Oxygen dissociation curve 129
Oxygen extraction ratio, physiology of
cardiovascular system 115
Oxygen therapy
cardiopulmonary resuscitation 121–2
delivery and utilization 114–15, 131, 208
face masks, fixed vs variable
performance 31–2
hyperbaric oxygen therapy, necrotizing
otitis externa 395
postoperative 31–2
in sepsis 67–8

P

p53 products 172, 341
Paediatric surgery 493–523
abdomen 501
chest 497–500
circulatory volume 494
clinical categories 510
endocrine and metabolic response to
surgery 495
fluid requirements 494
gastrointestinal tract 500–1
groin and scrotum 514–18
head and neck 496–7
hepatobiliary disorders 513–14
nutrition 495
physiology
fluid and electrolytes 494
temperature 494
respiration 495
safe transfer of patients 495
sepsis 495
solid tumours 521–3
surgical techniques 495–6
urology 494, 518–21
Paget's disease 483
femur 484
nipple 339, 348
Pain
abdominal 509–10
acute non-specific abdominal pain
(ANSAP) 510
analgesic ladder 179–81
arterial disease 288–9
bladder and prostate gland 373
bone and joint pain 473–80
cancer 178–81
claudication 292, 294
complications 36–7, 45
fractures 449, 463, 491
genitourinary system 373–4
kidney and ureter 373
loin 373, 380, 518

management, principles 178–81
mastalgia 332–3
opioid-resistant 181
palliative care 178
pathways and mechanism 44
post-surgery 32, 44–5
renal colic 373, 374, 380
rest pain 292, 293
scrotum and penis 373–4
shoulder pain, clinical assessment 474–6
TENS 181
see also Abdominal pain; Back pain
Palliative therapy, colorectal cancer, 259
Pancreas
abdominal mass 510
annular 501–2
carcinoma 241–3
function, intubation tests 242–3
glucagonoma 319
injury 101
insulinoma 318
vipoma 319
Pancreatitis
acute 236–7
Pancuronium, characteristics 28
Panendoscopy 409
Papaveretum 27, 180
Papillary cystadenoma lymphomatosum
413
Papilloedema, supratentorial neoplasms
432
Papilloma
laryngeal
adult form 409
juvenile form 409
Paracetamol
with opioids, compound preparations
180
postoperative 33
Paraganglioma 412
Paranasal sinuses, tumours 410
Parapharyngeal space 408
tumours 413
Paraphimosis 389, 520
Parasympathetic nervous system 422
Parathormone 311
Parathyroid glands
anatomy and physiology 310–11
disorders 312–13
embryology 310
hyperplasia in renal osteodystrophy
(rickets) 482, 483
Parathyroidectomy 310, 312
post renal graft 313
Parenteral nutrition 52, 55–7, 495
Parkinson's disease, bladder function 374
Parotid gland
enlargement 413
metastases 413
Parotitis 413
Patellofemoral osteoarthritis 450
Patients' Charter 188
Pectus carinatum 362
Pectus excavatum 362
Pelvic floor dysfunction weakness
symptom 373
Pelvic fractures 101–2

Pelviureteric junction obstruction 384
  diagnosis 518
  differential diagnosis 379
  management 518
Penicillins, treatment of sepsis 67–8
Penis
  developmental anomalies 371–2
  erectile dysfunction 389–90
  inflammation 389
  pain 373–4
  squamous carcinoma 389
  stricture 389
  surgical anatomy 371
  trauma 389
  tumour 389
Pentagastrin test 320
Peptic ulcers 236–7, 246–7, 501
  Zollinger–Ellison syndrome 319
Percussion, assessment of respiratory
      disease 5, 354
Perforated viscus
  oesophagus 237
  peptic ulcer 236–7
Perforator surgery 302
Pericardial tamponade 123–4
Perichondritis, auricular 394
Perioperative deaths (CEPOD) 20
Periorbital deformities, ocular injury 392
Peripheral vascular disease, amputation
      458
Peritoneal dialysis 382
  in ARF 142
Peritoneal lavage 99, 225
Peritoneal macrophages 203
Peritoneum-associated lymphoid tissue
      (PALT) 204
Peritonitis
  causes 236
  leak in bowel anastomosis 84
  treatment 236
Perkin's lines, CDH 490
Personality changes, head injury 426
Perthes' disease
  Catterall classification 490–1
  clinical features 490
  investigations 490–1
  management 491
Pethidine, characteristics 23, 44
Peyer's patches 204, 205
Peyronie's disease 374
pH, and arterial blood gases 41, 131
pH monitoring, gastro-oesophageal
      reflux 234
Phaeochromocytoma 9, 316–17, 320
Pharyngeal pouch, Killian's dehiscence 367
Pharynx see Hypopharynx; Throat
Phenothiazines, characteristics 32
Phenoxybenzamine 318
Phentolamine 316
Phimosis 520–1
Phlebitis, postoperative complication 48
Phosphodiesterase inhibitors 6, 118,
      389–90
Phospholipase, signal transduction 206
Photodynamic therapy, treatment of
      cancer 175
Phrenic nerve, anatomy 353

Phylloides tumour of breast 348
Physiological dead space, Bohr equation
      130
Phytoestrogens 156
Pituitary ablation 181
Pituitary gland 422, 435
  adenomas 318, 435
    antihormones 436
    investigations 435
    management 435
    replacement hormones 436
    trans-sphenoidal procedure 436
  anatomy and physiology 317–18
  hormones 318
Placebos 194
Plantar fasciitis, hindfoot 467
Plasma, transfusion 42, 43
Plasma membrane, receptors 206
Plasminogen activator 209, 210
Platelet disorders 218–19
  preoperative assessment 9
Platelet-activating factor, lyso 206
Platelet-derived growth factor 154, 206
Platelet count, haemostasis 210
Platelets
  concentrates 43, 215
  endothelial cell mediators 209
  structure/function 202, 209
  transfusion 43, 215
Pleomorphic adenoma 174, 413
Pleural biopsies, video-assisted
      thorascopic surgery (VATS) 355,
      357–8
Pleural effusion 365, 366
Pleural space, anatomy 352–3
Pleural-based lesions, video-assisted
      thorascopic surgery (VATS) 358
Pleural-based tumours, lung cancer 365–6
PNET see Primitive neurectodermal
      tumours
Pneumocystis carinii, spontaneous
      pneumothorax 363
Pneumonectomy
  catheters 358
  ventilation-perfusion scan 360
Pneumonia
  nosocomial 144–5
  postoperative 49
  causes 60
Pneumothorax
  open, following thoracic surgery 361
  simple 98
  spontaneous 363
    video-assisted thorascopic surgery
        (VATS) 357–8
  tension 91, 127
    following thoracic surgery 361
Poland's anomaly 362
Poland's syndrome 325
Polyhydramnios, oesophageal atresia 499
Polyposis coli, mutation site 155
Polysaccharides, non-starch 156
Porphyria, anaesthetic agents 17
Port-wine stain 411
Portal hypertension, treatment 246
Portal venous system, anatomy and
      access 231–2

Positron emission tomography (PET),
      mediastinal glands 344, 354
POSSUM score 192
Post-traumatic amnesia (PTA) 418
Postoperative management 39–49
  blood transfusion 42–4
  complications 46–9
  critical care 41–2
  fast-track surgery 49
  fluid and electrolytes 45–6
  monitoring 40–1
  pain 44–5
Potassium
  dangers of infusion 46
  preoperative, in CRF 7
Potter's syndrome 370
Preadmission clinics 14
Preauricular sinus 394, 496
Pregnancy
  breast changes 325
  and lactation, breast carcinoma 338, 349
Preoperative assessment 1
Preoperative management 1
  anaesthesia 3–11
  preadmission clinics 14
  routine investigations 14–15
  skin preparation 64, 71–2
Priapism 390
Prilocaine 35, 72
Primitive neurectodermal tumours
      (PNET) 434
Probability and significance 196
Prochlorperazine 180
Prokinetics, characteristics 22
Prolactin (PRL), pituitary gland 435
Prolactinomas 435
Proliferation, markers 172
Propofol, characteristics 25, 26–7
Prostacyclin 209, 294
Prostaglandins 209, 320
Prostate gland 387
  adenocarcinoma 387
  and bladder pain 373
  cancer 387–8
    LHRH 388
    pelvic metastases 485
    PSA levels 376
  continence mechanisms 371
  inflammation 387
  pain 373
  surgical anatomy 371
  transurethral resection (TURP) 371, 387
  ultrasound scan 376
Prostate-specific antigen (PSA) 172, 376,
      387
Prostatitis 387
Prostheses
  passive/functional 460–1
  replacement joints 455–8
Prosthetic biomaterials 274–5
Protein kinase C 151, 152
Protein metabolism, response to injury
      108
Protein synthesis 150
Protein–energy malnutrition 50
Proteus mirabilis, staghorn renal calculus
      380

Prothrombin time 210
Proto-oncogenes 154
Pseudo-obstruction 251–2
Pseudoarthrosis 442
Pseudobulbar palsy 420
'Pseudokidney' sign, intussusception 508, 509
Pseudomonas, septic arthritis 471
Pulmonary artery, catheterization 42, 117–18, 126
Pulmonary collapse 356
Pulmonary compliance 130
Pulmonary contusion 98, 361
Pulmonary embolism 29, 137–8
    postoperative 48
Pulmonary fibrosis, lung transplantation 360
Pulmonary function 356
    test 129–30
Pulmonary hypertension, diaphragmatic hernia, congenital 499
Pulmonary hypoplasia, diaphragmatic hernia, congenital 499
Pulmonary macrophages 203
Pulmonary oedema 139, 141
    postoperative 31
Pulmonary perfusion 131–2
Pulmonary sequestration 362, 500
Pulmonary surgery 360–1
    complications 358–60
    contusion following 98, 361
Pulse oximetry 29, 41, 131
Pulseless ventricular tachycardia
    algorithm 123
    sinus 122–3
Pulsus paradoxus 124
Pupils, ocular injury 392
Pyelonephritis 380
Pyloric atresia 501
Pyloric stenosis
    diagnosis 507
    management 507
Pyloric 'tumour' 507

Q

Quality of life (QALYs) 181–2
    EORTC 170, 181
    screening for cancer effectiveness 166–9
Quinolones, treatment of sepsis 68
Quinsy 398

R

Radial fractures 445–6
Radiation effects
    carcinogenesis 155–9
    resistance of tissues 176
Radiculopathy 473, 474, 479
Radioimmunoassay 213–14
Radioisotope scans 118
Radiotherapy
    brachytherapy and teletherapy 174
    treatment of cancer 173–8
Ramstedt's pyloromyotomy 507
Randomization 169

Ranula 497
Rarities 280
Rathke's pouch 317
γ-rays, radiotherapy 174
Re-anastomosis 384, 389
Receptors 206
Recombinant genes 160
Rectal, *see also* Anal; Bowel; Colorectal carcinoma
Rectal aganglionosis, congenital 505
Rectal injury 101
Rectourethral fistula 504, 505
Red blood cells
    function, 207–8
    salvage 43
    structure 200–1
    transfusion 215–17
'Red currant jelly' stool, intussusception 508
Reflex sympathetic (Sudeck's) atrophy 449
Regional anaesthesia
    advantages/disadvantages 36
    Bier's block 36, 73
    central nerve blocks 35, 36–7
    indications/contraindications 36
    intravenous 36, 73
    intravenous drugs 26–7
    techniques 36–7
Regression to mean 193
    multiple 196
Renal, *see also* Kidney
Renal disease
    adenocarcinoma 381
    antihypertensives 374
    colic 373, 374
    developmental anomalies 369–72
    diuretics 374
    hydronephrosis 383–4
    inflammation 380
    multicystic dysplastic 518
    pain 373–4
    preanaesthesia assessment 17–18
    transplantation 382
    tumour 381
Renal failure, acute 141–3, 382
    causes 141, 382
    diagnosis 141–2
    treatment 142–3
    prognosis 143
Renal failure, chronic 382
    dialysis 382
    transplantation 382
Renal injury 101
Renal osteodystrophy (rickets) 483
Renal pelvis, Transitional cell carcinoma (TCC)
    bladder 381, 385
    ureter 384
Renal replacement therapy 142–3
Renal stones 369, 376, 380–1
    Proteus mirabilis 380
Renal transplantation, parathyroidectomy 313
Renography
    nuclear isotope 377–8
        bone scan 378

chromium EDTA clearance 378
    DMSA 378
    MAG 3 377–8
Renoscopy 379
Reproductive factors in cancer 158–9
Research projects
    cohort studies 193–4
    Declaration of Helsinki 185, 187
    error 192
    ethical committees 186–7
    experimental studies 192, 194–5
    observational studies 192, 193
    regression to mean 193
    sensitivity and specificity 192–3
    statistical considerations 195–7
Resource allocation, ethics 187–8
Respiratory center 128
Respiratory disease
    ARDS 139–41
    symptoms 354
Respiratory failure
    hypercapnic 132
    hypoxemic 132
    risk indicators 5
Respiratory function
    investigations 129–31
    physiology 128–9
    previous anaesthesia assessment 17
    preoperative assessment 5
    risk factors 5
    test in asthma 6
    see also Ventilation
Respiratory system
    artificial airways 132–4
    failure 131–2
    investigations 129–31
    mechanical ventilation 134–7
    obstructive sleep apnoea 6
    physiology 128–9
    pulmonary embolism 137–8
Restriction fragment length polymorphisms 160, 161
Resuscitation, in sepsis 66–7
Reticular cells, structure/function 203
Retinal haemorrhage, supratentorial neoplasms 432
Retinoblastoma, genetics 154, 155
Retroviruses 154, 157, 220
Rhabdomyosarcoma, diagnosis and management 522
Rheumatoid arthritis 223, 466–7
    arthrodesis 466–7
    arthroplasty 466
    bilateral parotid gland enlargement 413
    hand 451
    hindfoot 466–7
    osteotomy 466
Rhinitis 396–7
Rhinorrhoea
    following head injury 427
    mucopurulent 397
Rib fractures 97–8
Rickets
    clinical features 482
    dietary deficiencies 481
    Harrison's groove 482

Rickets (*Contd*)
  radiographical changes 482
  renal rickets 483
Risk assessment
  analytical epidemiology 165–6
  ASA classification 1, 20
  high-risk surgical patients 21
RNA viruses 154
Road traffic accidents *see* Trauma
Rodent ulcer 404
Ropivicaine 35

S

Salivary gland
  inflammation 57, 413
  tumours 407, 413
Salmonella spp., sickle cell anaemia 469
Sandifer syndrome 501
Saphenous vein
  graft 290
  ligation 300
  stripping 300
Sarcoma, soft tissue 522
Scalene gland biopsy 355
Scalp lacerations 427
Scalp tumours 405
Scars 83
Schistosomiasis 374, 376, 383
Schwannoma 366, 412, 433
Sciatica
  bowstring test 479–80
  clinical features 479–80
  discectomy 480
  femoral nerve stretch test 480
  Laseque's test 480
  lumbar spinal anatomy 479
  management 480
  nerve root tension signs 479
  physical signs 479–80
  sphincter function assessment 480
  spinal canal decompression 480
  straight leg raising test with
    augmentation 480
Sclerotherapy, lower limb 300
Scoliosis, adolescent idiopathic 476, 477
Scoring systems, ICU 147–8, 235
Scout film 376
Screening and surveillance, colorectal
    cancer 259
Screening programme 168–9
  breast cancer 349–50
  test, sensitivity vs specificity 166–8
Scrofula 412
Scrotum
  acute idiopathic oedema 516
  fertility 389
  inflammation 388
  pain 389
  trauma 389
  tumours 388–9
Sebaceous gland, carcinoma 405
Secondary tumours, groin swelling
    279–80
Sedation 16, 35
Segregation analysis 159–60
Seldinger technique, catheters 289–90

Selective digestive decontamination
    (SDD) 63
Seminoma 389
Sensitivity and specificity
  research projects 196
  screening test 166–9
Sepsis, neonatal 495
Sepsis, surgical 58
  environmental factors 66
  HIV and viral hepatitis 69
  management 66–9
  mediators 61–2
  pathophysiology 58–60
  prevention 63–6
Septic arthritis 471–3
Seroma, wound 47
Serotonin
  carcinoid tumours 319–20
  wound healing 80
Sever's disease 467
Severe combined immunodeficiency
    disorders 220
Sevoflurane, characteristics 26
Shaving 63, 64
Shock 124–8
  cardiogenic 125–6
  definitions 128
  distributive 127–8
  hypovolaemic 126
  neurogenic 128
  obstructive 126–7
  resuscitation 125
  types 124
  see also Sepsis
Short gut syndrome 503, 507
Shoulder joint
  Bankart lesion 454–5
  cuff tear arthropathy 475
  Hill Sachs lesion 455
  injuries 454
  pain 474–5
  Wallace view 454
Sickle cell anaemia, *Salmonella* spp.
    469
Sickle cell disorders
  preanaesthesia assessment
    17–18
  traits, approach to surgery 18
Signal transduction 206–7
Sinus bradycardia 128
Sinus tachycardia 122
Sinuses and nose
  functional endoscopic sinus surgery
    (FESS) 397
  inflammatory disorders 396–7
  sinusitis 397
Sistrunk's operation 411, 496
  thyroglossal cyst 411, 496
Sjögren's syndrome, bilateral parotid
    gland enlargement 413
Skin, café-au-lait lesions 366, 412
Skin cysts, excision 84–5
Skin preparation 71–2, 80
  explosion hazards 79
Skin tumours 403–5
Skull base, internal surface 416
Skull fracture, depressed 428

Slipped upper femoral epiphysis
  Capener's sign 491
  clinical features 491
  complications 492
  management 491–2
  Trethowran's sign 491
Small intestine *see* Bowel, small
Smoke inhalation injury 104, 105, 106
Smoking
  and breast carcinoma 338
  carcinogenesis 155–9
  perioperative problems 10
  preoperative assessment 10–11
  and pulmonary function 354
Soft tissue
  injury 102
  malignant disease 483–9
    clinical assessment 483–5
Solar keratoses 403
Southern blot 161
Speech disorders, head injury 426
Sphenopalatine artery, transnasal
    endoscopic ligation 402
Spina bifida, bladder function 386
Spinal block 36–7
Spinal cord 422–3
Spinal cord compression 430–2
  bladder, neurological dysfunction 430
  cervical region 430
  intradural lesions 431
  investigations 432
  lumbar region 430
  management 432
  thoracic region 430
  vertebral column causes 430–1
Spinal cord injury
  cervical 429
  management 429–30
  methylprednisolone 429
  surgery 430
  syrinx 429
  see also Vertebral column injury
Spinal cord tumours
  astrocytomas 431
  ependymomas 431
  meningiomas 431
  neurofibromas 431
Spinal disc prolapse, surgical
    decompression 478
Spinal dysraphysm, congenital 473
Spinal injury 95–6
Spinal shock 429
Spinal trauma, bladder function 386
Spine *see* Vertebral column
Spirometry 129, 356
Spironolactone 316, 336
Spleen
  abdominal mass 510
  disorders 225–7
  structure/function 204
  trauma 225–6
Splenectomy 101, 226
  complications 226–7
  indications 226–7
Spondylitis 158, 451
Spondylosis 473, 474, 475
Spongiform encephalopathy 438

Spontaneous pneumothorax 363–4
Sputum production, respiratory disease symptom 354, 360
Sputum retention, following pleural surgery 359
Squamous cell carcinoma 364, 368
  bladder 385
  oral cavity and oropharynx 406
  penis 389–90
  salivary gland 413
  skin 404
  upper aerodigestive tract, TNM staging 406
Staghorn renal calculus, *Proteus mirabilis* 380
Stamm gastrostomy 54
Standard deviation and standard error 196
Staphylococcus aureus
  acute osteomyelitis 469
  bacterial conjunctivitis 393
  preseptal cellulitis 393
  salivary gland inflammation 413
  septic arthritis 471
Staphylococcus epidermidis
  bacterial conjunctivitis 393
  septic arthritis 471
Stapled haemorrhoidectomy 261
Staples 75–6
Statistical considerations
  correlation 196
Statistics
  appropriate tests 197
  research projects 195–8
Stem cells
  model of hemopoiesis 207
  physiology 207
  structure/function 202
  transfusion 202
Sternomastoid tumour, torticollis association 496
Sternum fractures, following thoracic surgery 361
Steroid-induced adrenal suppression 11
Stitches 74–5
  subcuticular 75
Stomach
  anatomy 230
  carcinoma 239–44
  colorectal injuries 255–8
  gastric ulcers 238, 247
  see also Gastric
Stomatitis 181
Stone metabolites, 24-hour urine collection 375
Storage/filling symptom, genitourinary system 372–3
Straight leg raising test 479, 480
Strawberry capillary haemangioma 496–7
Streptococcal tonsillitis 412
Streptococcus spp., bacterial conjunctivitis 393
Streptococcus spp
  acute osteomyelitis 469
  septic arthritis 470
Streptococcus viridans 413
Streptokinase 210, 219
Stress incontinence 373, 375, 379, 387

Stroke, transient ischaemic attacks 436
Stye 393
Sudden infant death syndrome 501
Sudeck's atrophy 449
Supraglottitis, acute 398
Supratentorial neoplasms 432
  epilepsy 433
  papilloedema 432
  retinal haemorrhage 432
Surgery, response, normal patients 214–15
Surgical emphysema 366
Surgical haemorrhoidectomy 261
Surgical implications, lymphoreticular systems 214–15
Surgical instruments, sterilization 65–6
Suture diastasis 423
Sutures 77, 78, 84
  material sizes 76
  materials 290
Suxamethonium
  characteristics 27–8
  side-effects 28
    apnoea 17
    hyperkalaemia 7
    muscle pain 28
Swallowing, oesophageal carcinoma 366–7
Sympathectomy 294
  Sudeck's atrophy 449
Sympathetic nervous system 314
  neuroendocrine response to injury 107
Sympatho-adrenal axis 108
Synchronous lesions, colorectal cancer 256
Synovitis, hip 491
Syrinx, spinal cord injury 429
Systemic inflammatory response syndrome (SIRS) 62
  characteristics 58, 138
Systemic lupus erythematous 223

T

T cell deficiencies 204, 220
T cells
  structure/function 202, 204
  thymus 204
Talipes equinovarus *see* Club foot
Talus
  avascular necrosis 448, 466
  osteochondritis dissecans 465
Tamoxifen 333
  side-effects 346–7
^{99}Tc^m-dimercaptosuccinic acid (DMSA), nuclear isotope renography 377–8
^{99}Tc^m-MAG 3 renography 377–8
Telomeres, construction 152–3
Temazepam, characteristics 22
Tension-free hernia repair 280–1
Tendon injuries 461–2
  diagnosis 461
  hand 462
  management 464
  surgical intervention 461–2
Teratoid cyst 411
Test, sensitivity vs specificity 166–8
Testicular feminization 514

Testicular torsion 515–6
  appendage torsion 516
  'bell-clapper' deformity 515
  'blue-dot' sign 516
  diagnosis 515–16
  extravaginal (neonatal) 515, 516
  intravaginal (adolescent) 515, 516
  management 516
Testis
  cryptorchidism 514, 517
  developmental anomalies 371–2
  fertility 389
  inflammation 388
  surgical anatomy 371
  swellings 388
  torsion *see* Testicular torsion
  trauma 389
  tumours 388–9
  ultrasound scan 376
  undescended 375, 517
    malignancy risk 517
    management 517
    microvascular orchidopexy 517
    orchidectomy plus prosthesis 517
    orchidopexy 517
    psycho-social development 517
    subfertility 517
    surgical options 517
    testicular vessel division 517
    urological history and examination 374–5
Tetanus status 81
Thermodilution, cardiac output 117, 118
Thermoregulation
  and metabolic rate 108
  response to injury 108–9
Thiopentone, characteristics 26
Thoracic diseases and treatment 361–6
Thoracic nerve 324, 345, 357
Thoracic surgery 351
  anatomy 351–2
Thoracic trauma 361
Thoracocentesis, pleural space depth 355–6
Thoracodorsal nerve 324
Thoracotomy 357–60
  anterior 357
  axillary 357
  posterolateral 357
  techniques 357–8
Throat
  foreign bodies 399–400
  inflammatory disorders 397–8
Thrombin time 210
Thrombocytopaenic purpura, idiopathic 222
Thromboembolic disease, and anaesthesia 13–14
Thromboembolic phenomena, fractures 445
Thrombolytic therapy 138
Thrombotic disorders 219–20
Thymidine labelling index, cell cycle 172
Thymomas, anterior mediastinum 353
Thymus 204
Thyroglossal cyst 304, 310, 496
  Sistrunk's operation 496

Thyroglossal tract 304, 310, 411
Thyroid cysts 308
Thyroid gland 304–10
  anatomy 304–5
  blood supply 305–6
  clinical examination 306
  disorders 307–10
  embryology 304
  goitre 304
    diffuse 306, 307
    nodular 308–10
    retrosternal 310
  histology 306
  investigations 306
  physiology 306
  solitary thyroid adenoma 308–10
  solitary thyroid nodule 308
  thyroglossal cyst 310
Thyroid lymphoma 309
Thyroid stimulating hormone (TSH),
      pituitary gland 318
Thyroid storm 8
Thyrotoxicosis, primary 307
Thyrotrophic releasing hormone (TRH),
      pituitary gland 318
Thyrotrophinomas 435
TIA see Transient ischaemic attacks
Tietz's syndrome 332
Tissue injury 214
Tissue markers 172
Tissue plasminogen activator 209
Tissue typing 228
TNM staging 169–71, 239, 240, 241, 365
Tonsillectomy, quinsy 398
Tonsillitis 397–8
  follicular 397–8
  membranous 398
  streptococcal 398, 412
Torticollis, sternomastoid tumour
      association 496
Total parenteral nutrition (TPN) 52, 55–7,
      236
Totally extraperitoneal (TEP),
      laparoscopy 271, 282–3
Tourniquets 37
Tracheo-oesophageal fistula
  Blom–Singer prosthesis 409
  see also Oesophageal atresia
Tracheobronchial rupture, following
      thoracic surgery 361
Tracheobronchial tree 351–2, 366
Tracheostomy 410
  cryco-thyroid puncture 34
  indications 133–4
  and insertion 133–4
  and minitracheostomy 351
  Seldinger technique 359
Transferrin receptor 208
Transfusion-related acute lung injury 218
Transient ischaemic attacks (TIA) 295,
      436
Transient synovitis of the hip, differential
      diagnosis 491
Transitional cell carcinoma 371
Translation 150, 151
Transplantation
  donor 429

kidney 383
lung 360
Trans-sphenoidal procedure, pituitary
      adenomas 436–7
Transudate effusion, vs exudate 355
Transuretero-ureterostomy 385
Trans-abdominal preperitoneal (TAPP),
      laparoscopy 273, 284–5
Transurethral resection of the prostate
      (TURP) 372, 386, 387, 388
Trauma 89
  ATLS system 90–1, 106
  blunt, penetrating and missile 93, 103
  definitive care 93, 106
  'golden hour' 90–3
  history 92
  immediate hospital management 90–3
  normal patients' response to surgery
      214
  pathophysiology 106–10
    acute phase 109
  pre-hospital management 90
  prevention 90
Trendelenberg tourniquet test 299–300
Trethowran's sign, slipped upper femoral
      epiphysis 491
Tricyclic antidepressants, interactions
      with anaesthetic agents 12, 19
Trigeminal cranial nerve 419
Triple therapy, peptic ulcer 247
Tuberculosis (TB) 438, 476, 478
  spinal 431
Tuberculous dactylitis 471
Tumor necrosis factor α and β 206
Tumour markers 171–3
Tumour necrosis factor, mediator of
      sepsis 61–2
Tumour suppressor genes 153, 154–5, 337
  mutations, rare tumours 155
Tumours, immune responses 224
TURP see Transurethral resection of the
      prostate
Tympanoplasty, combined approach,
      unsafe CSOM 396

U

Ulcer, venous 301
Ultraviolet radiation, carcinogenesis 158
Umbilical granuloma 512
Umbilical hernia 512
  adults 283
  Mayo's repair 283
Upper gastrointestine (GI)
  surgery 230
  anatomy 230–2
  investigations 232–4
  emergencies 234–8
    acute cholecystitis 234–5
    acute pancreatitis 235–6
    perforated viscus 236–7
  bleeding 237–8
  malignancy 239–44
  conditions 244–8
Upper GI, malignancy
  cancer, GOJ
    classification 241

gastric carcinoma 240–1
hepatic tumours 243–4
oesophageal carcinoma 239–41
pancreatic carcinoma 241–3
Uretero-sigmoidosctomy 371
Ureterogram, antegrade/retrograde 377
Ureteroscopy 379
Ureters
  damage, hysterectomy 390
  developmental anomalies 370
  duplex 370, 383
  obstruction, sites 383
  pain 373
  surgical anatomy 369–70
  ureterocele 519
  vasicoureteric reflux 518–19
Urethra
  developmental anomalies 371
  erectile dysfunction 389–90
  inflammation 389
  surgical anatomy 371
  tumour 389
Urethral injury 101
Urethral valve, posterior 519
Urethrogram 377
Urethroplasty 389
Urge incontinence 372
Urinary incontinence see Incontinence
Urinary retention 48
  acute 372, 373
  chronic 372, 386
Urinary tract
  injury 101
  stones 380, 384
Urinary tract infections 380, 518
  in ICU 144
Urine diversion 385–6
Urine flow test 378
Urine outflow obstruction 379
  symptoms 372
Urine tests
  24-hour collection 375
  cytology 375
  dipstick testing 375
  genitourinary investigations 375–80
  microscopy and culture 375
Urodynamics 372, 373, 378
Urokinase 210
Urological history 374–5
Urological symptoms 372–4
  paediatric 494
  problems caused by surgery and
      gynaecology 390
Ursodeoxycholic acid 246
Uveitis, anterior 392

V

VACTERL 498, 504
  vestibular fistula association 504
Vagal nerve 353, 420
  anatomy 353
Vaginal bleeding, haematuria 390
Valves see Heart valves
Vancomycin, treatment of sepsis 65
Variance 195–6, 197, 267
Varicocele 517–18

Varicose veins 300
    surgical management 300–1
        complications 300
Vascular anastomosis 88
    leaks 84
Vascular disease
    disseminated intravascular coagulation
        9, 252
    see also Arterial disease; Venous disease
Vascular injuries 103
Vascular purpura 218
Vascular surgery 286
Vasectomy 389
Vasoactive intestinal polypeptide (VIP) 318
Vasodilators 110
Vasogram 377
Vasopressors 119
Vasospastic disorders 287
Vecuronium, characteristics 28
Vegetables, cancer-protective substances
    156
Venous claudication 292
Venous disease
    deep vein thrombosis 226, 302
        intracranial 436–8
        lower limb 298
        ulcer and associated conditions 301
Venous disorders
    classification 299
Venous sinuses, cranial cavity 422
Venous surgery, lower limb venous
    disorders 300
Venous system, hemisphere 422
Venous thrombosis 12, 48–9, 219, 303
Venous ulceration 301–2
    assessment 301
    epidemiology 301
    management 301–2
Ventilation
    airway management 133
    analgesia and sedation 136
    assist control (A/C) 134
    brain death 428
    classes of ventilator 134
    complications 136
    controlled 24
    discontinuation 136
    end-expiratory pressure 38
    independent lung 133
    intermittent mandatory (IMV) 134–5,
        137
    IPPV 38
    levels of support 134
    mechanical
        controlled (CMV) 134
        indications 134
    positive end-expiratory pressure
        (PEEP) 130, 135
    pressure control 134
    pressure support (PSV) 135, 136, 137

    in sepsis 66
    spontaneous 24, 134
    synchronized intermittent mandatory
        (SIMV) 134
    ventilator-induced trauma 136
Ventilation-perfusion scan
    lung volume reduction 360
    pneumonectomy 360
Ventricular dysfunction, diabetes 8
Ventricular ectopics, postoperative 15, 25
Ventricular ejection fraction, isotope
    scanning 4
Ventricular fibrillation, and pulseless
    ventricular tachycardia, algorithms
    121, 122
Vermiculation 370
Verrucous carcinoma 404
Vertebral artery disease 295
Vertebral column
    carcinoma 423
    infections 423
    intervertebral discs 473–4
    osteoporosis 480–1
    pathological fractures 470
    spinal cord compression 430–2
    see also Cervical spine
Vertebral column injury 429
    dens fracture 429
    fracture dislocations 429
    Hangman's fracture 429
    Jefferson fracture 429
    stable/unstable 429
Vesicoureteric junction
    obstruction 519
    reflux 518–19
Vesicoureteric reflux 518–19
    diagnosis 519
    management 519
    STING injection 519
Vestibular fistula 504
    bucket handle deformity 504
    VACTERL association 504
Video-assisted thoracic surgery (VATS)
    357–8
    biopsy 358
    congenital cyst treatment 361–2
Vipoma 319
Viral genes, and cancer 153
Virchow's triad 48
Vital capacity 129
Vitamin D, physiology 311
Vitamins, cancer-protective substances
    155–6
Voice rehabilitation 409
Voiding symptom, genitourinary system
    372
Volkmann's ischaemic contracture 83
Volvulus
    colorectal, 250–2
    gastric, 501

Vomiting see Nausea and vomiting
Von Recklinghausen's disease 412
Von Willebrand factor 43, 209
Von Willebrand's disease 9, 217, 219

W

Waardenburg syndrome, Hirschsprung's
    disease association 505
Wallace view, shoulder joint dislocation
    454
Warfarin, intracranial haematomas 437
Warthin's tumour 413
WDHA syndrome 319
Well straight leg raising test 479, 480
Wheeze, respiratory disease symptom 18,
    354
Whipple's pancreaticoduodenectomy 242
Whipple's triad 318
Wilms' tumour 381, 521
    diagnosis 521
    management 521
    mutation site 155
    staging (NWTS-3) 521
Witzel jejunostomy 54, 56
Wounds
    cavities and raw areas 78
    classification 62, 81
        penetrating and missile 82, 93, 103
    complications 47–8
    contraction and contracture 80, 83
    dehiscence 83–4
    dressings 77–8
    granulation tissue 80, 82
    haemostasis 78
    healing pathophysiology 79–80
    infected 81
        microorganisms causing sepsis 60–1
    management 81–3, 106
        burns 82–3, 103–6
        delayed primary closure 82
    modifying factors 80–1
    postoperative development of sepsis 60
    prevention 63
    scars 83
    see also Trauma

X

Xerostomia, bilateral parotid gland
    enlargement 413

Z

Zenker's diverticulum 412
Ziehl–Neelsen stain 410, 412, 438
Zollinger–Ellison syndrome 246, 319